613.282 BAL
Ballantyne, Sarah

Paleo principles

JAN 25, 2019

DISCARD

JAN 25 2019
956

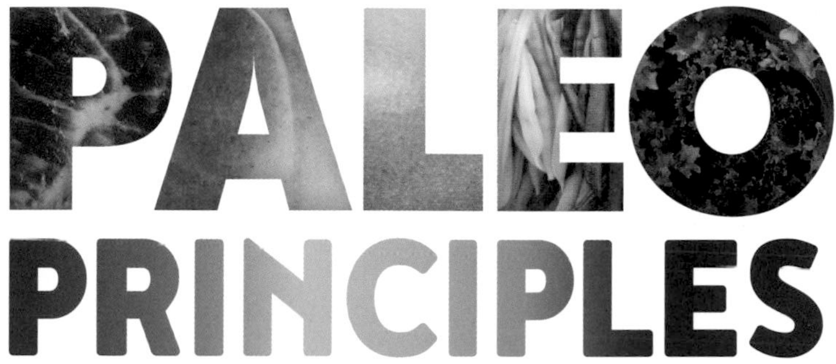

PALEO PRINCIPLES

THE SCIENCE BEHIND THE PALEO TEMPLATE, STEP-BY-STEP GUIDES, MEAL PLANS, AND 200+ HEALTHY & DELICIOUS RECIPES FOR REAL LIFE

by

Sarah Ballantyne, PhD

VICTORY BELT PUBLISHING, INC
Las Vegas

FAIRPORT PUBLIC LIBRARY
1 VILLAGE LANDING
FAIRPORT, NY 14450

For my family.

First Published in 2017 by Victory Belt Publishing Inc.

Copyright © 2017 Sarah Ballantyne

All rights reserved

No part of this publication may be reproduced or distributed in any form or by any means, electronic or mechanical, or stored in a database or retrieval system, without prior written permission from the publisher.

ISBN 13: 978-1-628609-00-4

The information included in this book is for educational purposes only. It is not intended nor implied to be a substitute for professional medical advice. The reader should always consult his or her healthcare provider to determine the appropriateness of the information for their own situation or if they have any questions regarding a medical condition or treatment plan. Reading the information in this book does not create a physician-patient relationship.

Victory Belt ® is a registered trademark of Victory Belt Publishing Inc.

Interior and cover design by Yordan Terziev and Boryana Yordanova

Recipe photography by Kiersten Peterson, NTP, and Sarah Ballantyne, PhD

Printed in Canada

TC0217

TABLE OF CONTENTS

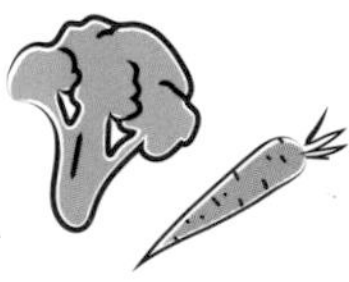

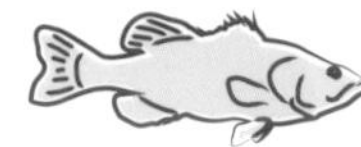

PART 6:
PUTTING PALEO INTO PRACTICE / 379

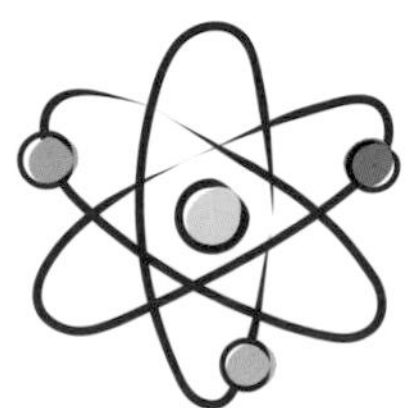

PART 7:
PALEO COOKING BASICS / 443

PART 8:
RECIPES / 479

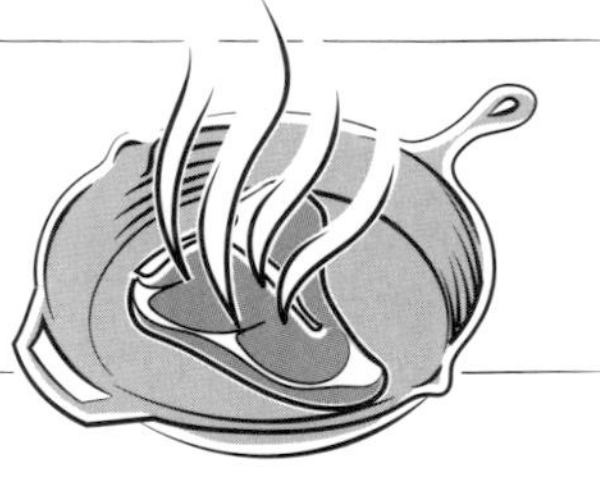

CHAPTER 42:
MAIN DISHES / 534

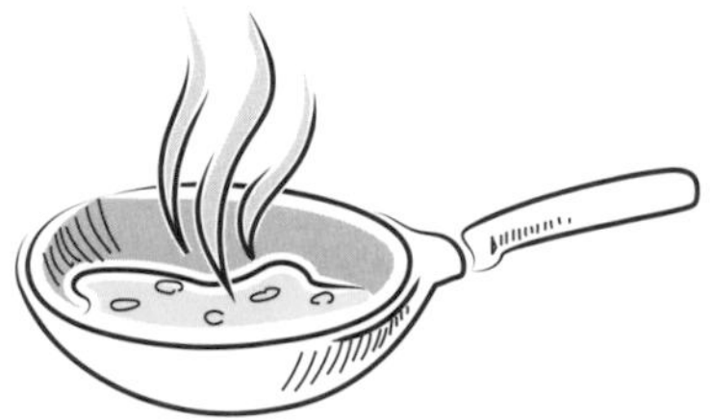

CHAPTER 43:
SIDE DISHES / 548

CHAPTER 44:
BREADS, MUFFINS, AND SNACK FOODS / 562

REFERENCES
The complete list of supporting scientific articles and resources can be viewed or downloaded at:
www.thepaleomom.com/paleo-principles-references

INTRODUCTION

We're sick, we're fat, and we're tired. I wish that statement was hyperbolic, but statistics back it up. More than half of all Americans take two or more prescription drugs, and about one-fifth of us take at least five daily medications prescribed by our doctors. Rates of just about every chronic illness are increasing dramatically. Two-thirds of Americans are overweight, with 40 percent of us being obese or extremely obese. Another 40 percent of Americans report frequently feeling tired during the day, with 10 percent of men and 15 percent of women reporting extreme fatigue or exhaustion most of the time.

This isn't normal. We're not supposed to be so sick that we need multiple medications to get us through each day. We're not supposed to depend on coffee, energy drinks, or an afternoon candy bar boost to perform well at our jobs. We're not supposed to feel so uncomfortable in our bodies that exercise equates to miserably hard work that we avoid in favor of watching TV. Statistically, chronic health problems have become the norm, but they're not normal.

No other animal on Earth is plagued with poor health like humans are. Yet we're at the top of the food chain, dominating every corner of the planet. We didn't get here by luck. It was a combination of ingenuity and adaptability, thanks to our big brains, and resilience, thanks to the inherently good health that we enjoyed for most of human history. Only recently has chronic illness become such a big part of our day-to-day existence that we've forgotten, as a society, not just what it feels like to be healthy, but that healthy is our natural state of being.

Health is sometimes defined as being free of disease. And while mitigating chronic illness is certainly a common path to the Paleo template, those of us in the health and wellness sphere prefer a definition of health that encompasses more than simply the absence of something bad. Health encompasses feeling vibrant, having energy throughout the day, sleeping well and waking up refreshed, having proportional and balanced reactions to life's stresses, feeling motivated at work and school, craving movement and activity, enjoying time spent with friends and family, laughing, feeling happy, having a sense of well-being, and loving life.

The good news is that we can achieve and maintain this broad definition of health through informed day-to-day choices of the foods we eat and the way we live our lives. And all the information you need to guide those choices is in this book!

FOOD AND HEALTH

Let's start with food.

We're fairly used to thinking about how food is related to weight: eat too much of the wrong things and you become overweight; eat the right amounts of the right things and you lose weight. But health is about so much more than whether you could stand to lose a few pounds. And food has a much more profound impact on health than whether you've got a spare tire around your middle.

Food provides all the building blocks used to make every cell, tissue, organ, and structure in our bodies. Food provides all the raw materials for the millions of chemical reactions happening inside our bodies at every moment. And food provides the energy needed to sustain life. When you think about it this way, it's easy to see how eating the right foods is so important for health: without all the building blocks, raw materials, and energy that our bodies need to operate normally (and healthily!), how can we expect them to stay free of disease?

When we make our food choices based on what provides the best raw materials for our bodies, we have what's called a micronutrient dietary focus. Micronutrients are chemicals in foods that are essential for life and health, but are needed in relatively small amounts (see Chapter 1). These include vitamins, minerals, phytochemicals (antioxidants and vitaminlike chemicals found in vegetables and fruits), essential amino acids (the building blocks of proteins), and essential fatty acids (the building blocks of fats, but they're also used to make essential structures in every cell, like the outer cell membrane). In contrast, macronutrients are the constituents of food that provide the energy we need in larger amounts: carbohydrates, protein, and fat (also discussed in detail in Chapter 1). The hallmark of any healthy diet is nutrient sufficiency. That means every day we're getting all the building blocks and raw materials that our bodies need from our food. There's more than one way to accomplish micronutrient sufficiency, and nowhere is this more evident than in hunter-gatherer and traditional cultures.

Depending on where in the world these groups live, their traditional diets vary dramatically, and so do the ratios of protein, fat, and carbohydrate in their diets—in other words, the proportion of animal foods and plant foods. But these cultures are typically extremely healthy, with none of the chronic illnesses that plague first-world countries (like cardiovascular disease, cancer, obesity, and diabetes). For example, the Kitavans, who live on one of the islands of Papua New Guinea and eat a diet rich in starchy tubers, fruit, coconut, and seafood, have virtually no incidence of ischemic heart disease or stroke, despite the fact that nearly 80 percent of them smoke. The Inuit have a vastly different traditional diet—theirs is rich in animal foods and saturated fats—yet they too boast an extraordinarily low prevalence of cardiovascular disease. One of the major contributors to this good health is micronutrient sufficiency. These cultures demonstrate that the human body can thrive on a wide range of macronutrient proportions, so long as we're getting plenty of the full complement of micronutrients.

Modern biological research backs up the necessity of a micronutrient-rich diet as well as metabolic flexibility when it comes to macronutrient ratios. Yet historically, government dietary guidelines have not focused on micronutrients. In fact, current recommendations for a healthy diet fall far short of the mark.

HOW DIETARY GUIDELINES HAVE STEERED US WRONG

Since their beginnings in 1894, various United States Department of Agriculture (USDA) nutrition guidelines have been criticized as not accurately representing scientific information about optimal nutrition and being inappropriately influenced by the agriculture industry. The earliest guidelines justifiably focused on avoiding malnutrition and starvation, problems that were rampant in many areas at that time. The 1916 guidelines introduced food groups, and their recommendation to liberally consume foods from five groups—milk and meat, cereals, vegetables and fruits, fats and fatty foods, and sugars and sugary foods—successfully targeted the issue of gross malnutrition.

In 1943, the USDA updated its guidelines to what was called the "Basic 7," which, flawed as it was, was a noble attempt at creating food groups based on micronutrients. The scientific understanding of essential nutrients was in its infancy in the early 1940s: the roles of many minerals in the human body, as well as the very existence of many of the vitamins that we now know are necessary for survival, had yet to be discovered. However, the Basic 7 guidelines were on the right track with a partial shift away from the previous focus on energy and toward a focus on micronutrients. While some of the earlier food groups remained, vegetables and fruits were divided into three different categories based on the few micronutrients that were known to exist at the time. For example, oranges, tomatoes, grapefruit, salad greens, and cabbage formed one food group based on their high levels of vitamin C. Butter got its own food group thanks to its vitamin A content. While we certainly would come up with different micronutrient-based food groups now, the Basic 7 was a good effort and a move in the right direction.

Unfortunately, the Basic 7 was met with skepticism and confusion by the public. Policymakers decided that, in order to be successful, the dietary guidelines needed to be simplified. And with the newly established Recommended Dietary Allowances providing a target for daily dietary intake of each essential micronutrient, it was simpler to stop basing food groups on nutrients.

The pinnacle of dietary guideline simplicity was achieved in the next update. The "Basic 4" enjoyed the longest reign of all the USDA dietary recommendations, from 1956 until 1992. The rules of how to choose foods could be communicated in 30 seconds or less: two to four servings from the milk group, two or more servings from the meat group, four or more servings from the vegetables and fruit group, and four or more servings from the bread and cereal group, "plus other foods as needed to complete meals and to provide additional food energy and other food values." The problem was that the foods in each group varied widely in terms of nutrients, so choosing foods using that framework in no way ensured adequate nutrition.

When the Basic 4 was finally revamped for subsequent USDA dietary guidelines, including the Food Guide Pyramid, MyPyramid, and MyPlate, vegetables and fruits were divided into their own food groups. Yet the only appreciable differences among all the dietary recommendations of the last sixty years are the number of servings suggested from each food group and the way the information is presented visually.

With the public's rejection of the Basic 7, the idea of basing dietary recommendations on micronutrient content was lost. Instead of dividing foods into groups based on the micronutrients they contain, the guidelines based the food groups on how the foods are produced. As a result, and compounded by the increase in consumption of manufactured and refined foods and other factors discussed in Chapter 1, nutrient deficiencies have become rampant. And nutrient deficiency may be one of the biggest contributors to the rise in chronic illnesses seen in recent decades.

The USDA's 2015-2020 Dietary Guidelines for Americans represent a shift back toward a micronutrient focus, with recommendations to eat a variety of nutrient-dense foods from each of six food groups, a division of vegetables into five subgroups, and an emphasis on avoiding excess caloric intake and added sugar while eschewing refined and manufactured foods. And while many of the advances in this newest revamp are a giant leap in the right direction, another major problem has emerged: hardly anyone is paying attention anymore.

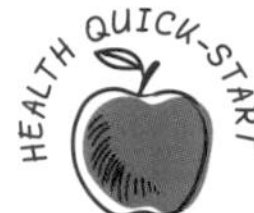

Forget most of the "rules" of healthy eating that you've been taught. Forget about grains being the base of the Food Pyramid, about eggs being full of cholesterol, about saturated fat causing heart disease, about low-fat salad dressing, and about fat-free yogurt. In this book, you'll learn why these foods are mislabeled as healthy choices and which foods form the foundation of a truly healthy diet.

The last sixty years of steadily increasing rates of chronic disease have proven that distilling dietary recommendations to a simple set of rules is not an effective strategy to support public health. Instead, the public has become distrustful of dietary guidelines and the authorities making them, dogmatic in their own approaches to nutrition and more likely to subscribe to fad diets and/or be completely apathetic toward food, feeling like "eating right" isn't worth the effort.

Fewer than 10 percent of Americans choose most of their foods according to the USDA dietary guidelines. This is a strong indicator that it doesn't work to communicate dietary guidelines as a set of rules without explaining why one food is a better choice than another. Humans are instinctively rebellious against arbitrary rules and unmerited authority. If we're expected to follow rules about what we eat, especially when following those rules means avoiding addictive, hyperpalatable junk foods and most convenience foods, those rules had better be well founded, and we need to understand where they come from. Whether dietary guidelines are distilled to recommended servings from four food groups or twenty, what's missing isn't a fancy graphic but the reasoning behind the recommendations.

TAKING BACK OUR HEALTH WITH PALEO PRINCIPLES

Let's turn the tide of public health and rediscover what it feels like to be healthy. Doing so starts with a dietary template that is solidly rooted in physiology and nutritional sciences, uninfluenced by special interests, and communicated with a thorough explanation of the origins of each facet of that template.

Nutritional science has come a long way since the first half of the twentieth century, when its primary focus was identifying micronutrients and establishing their recommended daily intakes. Now, our understanding of how nutrients (both those deemed essential and those currently considered nonessential) and other compounds in food act in the body to promote or undermine health spans many disciplines of science. There are tens of thousands of scientific articles on the topic, each examining one small piece of the puzzle. And while we still don't have all the pieces, when we put together what we do know we find that the average American diet is far from an optimal human diet. And, while the USDA dietary guidelines are finally getting closer to the mark, there's plenty of room for improvement. In this book, we won't be making incremental changes to a flawed dietary guideline system. Instead, we'll be going back to the drawing board and building a template based on current scientific knowledge.

Whether you're looking to lose weight, manage diabetes, reduce risks of cancer and cardiovascular disease, mitigate autoimmune disease, or improve performance or you simply want to experience the best health possible, a diet that is abundant in all the micronutrients and simultaneously omits foods known to be problematic for health is your best bet. What does this diet look like? Its foundation is the most micronutrient-dense foods available, including organ meat, seafood, and both a huge variety and copious quantities of vegetables, with other quality meats, fruit, eggs, nuts, seeds, healthy fats, probiotic and fermented foods, herbs, and spices to round it out. At the same time, it omits foods known to be inflammatory, disrupt hormones, or negatively impact the health of the gut, including all grains, most legumes, conventional dairy products, and all processed and refined foods. Yes, this is the Paleo template.

Over the past decade, Paleo has grown from a relatively underground movement to a diet that dominates news headlines, bestselling books, and even products in the grocery store. But despite its popularity, the scientific rationale for Paleo remains wildly misunderstood and misrepresented. For example, we might know that grains are a no-go, that vegetables are fantastic, and that dietary fat is nothing to be afraid of (despite years of the low-fat push from various health authorities), but why are these guidelines in place? The answer has little to do with reenacting what our early ancestors ate and everything to do with what modern science says is best for our bodies.

In short, Paleo is a nutrient-focused whole-foods diet, with the goal to maximize foods that heal and minimize foods that harm. It improves health by providing balanced and complete nutrition while avoiding most processed and refined foods and empty calories. It's not a way to simply lose pounds quickly (even though it has that effect for many people!), and it's not a fad that dissolves under scientific scrutiny; rather, every Paleo principle is solidly rooted in the latest research and data.

In this book, we'll be exploring the multiple lines of evidence supporting Paleo eating and understanding the science that underlies its tenets. We'll look at why the basic Paleo framework focuses on nutrient density, balanced macronutrients, diverse omnivorism, and biological systems health. We'll look at why specific foods (like seafood, vegetables and fruit, meat, healthy fats, and probiotics) are included, while other foods (like grains, processed vegetable oils, high-fructose corn syrup, and toxic additives) are excluded. And I'll be completely up-front about the foods for which the scientific evidence isn't cut-and-dried. I'll also give you tools to discover your own individual tolerance to suboptimal foods. And of course, I'll provide tons of practical how-tos, including over 200 recipes and 20 meal plans!

HEALTH QUICK-START

You probably already enjoy many meals that are completely Paleo! Scrambled eggs, bacon, and fruit for breakfast; a salad with grilled chicken for lunch; steak with roasted veggies for dinner . . . all great Paleo choices! You can hop on the Paleo train simply by trying to make more of your meals look like these favorites: some kind of meat, veggies, and fruit.

WHAT IS THE PALEO DIET?

Following a Paleo diet is actually pretty simple. There's a huge variety of health-promoting nutrient-dense foods to choose from, including:

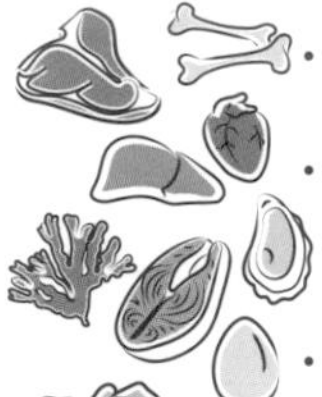
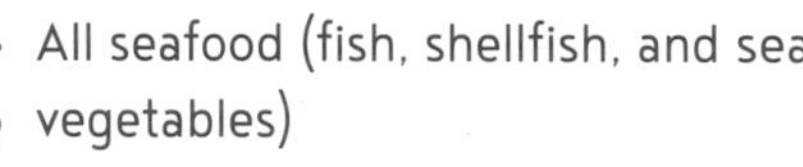
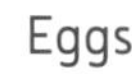
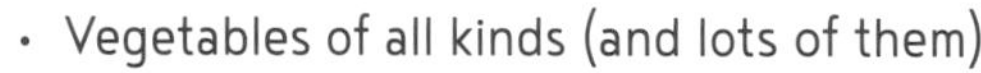
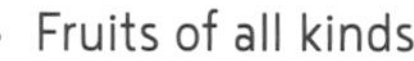
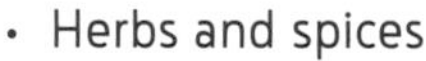

- All meats (and all parts of the animal)
- All seafood (fish, shellfish, and sea vegetables)
- Eggs
- Vegetables of all kinds (and lots of them)
- Fruits of all kinds
- Edible fungi, like mushrooms
- Nuts and seeds
- Herbs and spices
- Healthy unrefined, unprocessed fats from both animals and plants
- Probiotic and fermented foods

At its core, the Paleo diet is a plant-based diet, with two-thirds or more of your plate covered with plant foods and only one-third with animal foods. Of course, meat and seafood consumption is enthusiastically endorsed because it provides vital nutrients that are not obtainable from plant sources. Sourcing the highest-quality food you can buy is encouraged, meaning choosing grass-fed or pasture-raised meat, wild-caught seafood, and local in-season organic fruits and vegetables whenever possible.

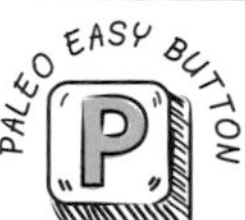

Replace the grains on your plate with vegetables! Swap out pasta for spaghetti squash noodles or zoodles (page 553); swap out rice for cauli-rice (page 555); swap out a dinner roll for a serving of sweet potatoes; swap out sandwich bread for a lettuce wrap. You'll get way more micronutrients and just as much fiber, and you'll avoid the problematic substances in grains (see Chapter 18).

Variety is very important because different foods supply different nutrients. Focusing on as many different whole foods as possible makes it easier to achieve sufficient and synergistic quantities of all the nutrients, potentially including some that haven't been discovered yet. Easy strategies to increase variety include "eating the rainbow," meaning that you choose fruits and vegetables of different colors, and "eating snout to tail," meaning that you eat every part of the animal, including offal (organ meat).

By focusing on the most nutrient-dense foods and eliminating foods that can contribute to hormone dysregulation, inflammation, and gut dysbiosis (where the bacteria in your gut are the wrong kinds, wrong diversity, or wrong numbers and/or are in the wrong part of the gastrointestinal tract), a Paleo diet can improve a vast array of health conditions. Clinical trials demonstrate that a Paleo diet improves cardiovascular disease risk factors, reduces inflammation, improves glucose tolerance, helps with weight loss, and can even improve autoimmune disease. The current status of scientific research on Paleo-style diets is summarized in Chapter 7.

The Paleo diet provides the foundation for a healthy digestive system. It supports healthy growth of a diversity of probiotic bacteria in the gut through its focus on prebiotic and probiotic foods and through its avoidance of foods that contribute to gut dysbiosis. It supports the health of the tissues that form the gut barrier by supplying essential nutrients required for gut barrier integrity and avoiding foods that are inherently difficult to digest, are known to irritate or damage the tissues that form the gut barrier, or are known to stimulate the immune system. And Paleo's focus on eating eight or more servings of vegetables a day is a boon to the microbial community within the gut that relies on quality dietary fiber for sustenance.

The Paleo diet reduces inflammation and supports normal functioning of the immune system. Foods that are inherently inflammatory are avoided, removing this unnecessary stimulus for increased inflammation. Providing the essential nutrients that the immune system requires to regulate itself can modulate an overactive immune system. When supplied with the essential nutrients that it needs to function optimally, a suppressed immune system can recover.

The Paleo diet naturally helps regulate blood sugar through its focus on whole-food sources of slow-burning carbohydrates like starchy roots and tubers and whole fruits. Blood sugar regulation is also a major rationale behind eating full, balanced meals centered on an animal protein and several servings of vegetables, thereby ensuring that we're eating quality carbohydrates, protein, fat, and fiber every time we dine.

The Paleo diet supports detoxification systems by providing the essential nutrients that the liver needs to perform its functions. Hormone regulation is achieved via focusing on foods that contain the nutrients required for hormone balance and avoiding foods known to stimulate or suppress vital hormone systems. Because providing the body with essential nutrients for health forms the basis of the Paleo diet, every system in the body is positively affected by this approach to food.

There are no hard-and-fast rules about when to eat or how much protein versus fat versus carbohydrates to eat (beyond eating some of each with every meal), and there are even some foods (like high-quality dairy and potatoes) that some people choose to include in their diets whereas others do not. This means that there's room to experiment, so you can figure out not just what makes you healthiest but also what makes you happiest and fits best into your schedule and budget.

Best of all, the Paleo diet is not a diet in the sense of being some hard thing that requires a great deal of willpower and self-deprivation until you reach a goal. It's a way of life. Because the focus is long-term health, the Paleo template allows for imperfection but educates you so that you can make the best choices.

Sustainability is an important tenet of the Paleo template, meaning that this is a way of eating and living that you can commit to and maintain for your entire life. You have the flexibility to experiment with your own body to discover what is optimal versus what is tolerable, to find what works best for you and fits into your life for the long term. For some people, flexibility is achieved by following an 80/20 rule (or a 90/10) rule, which means that 80 percent (or 90 percent) of your diet is healthy Paleo foods and the other 20 percent (or 10 percent) is not. Many people find that they are healthiest when their 20 percent (or 10 percent) continues to exclude the most inflammatory foods, such as wheat, soy, peanuts, pasteurized industrially produced dairy, and processed food chemicals.

The foods that are eliminated in a Paleo diet are the ones that provide our bodies with little nutrition (especially for the amount of energy they contain), are difficult to digest (which can cause gut health problems and contribute to gut dysbiosis), and have the ability to stimulate inflammation or mess around with important hormones. Generally, a Paleo diet excludes:

- Grains and pseudograins (such as quinoa)
- Legumes (legumes with edible pods, like green beans, are fine)
- Dairy (especially pasteurized and industrially produced products)
- Refined and processed foods (including refined seed oils like canola oil and safflower oil, refined sugars, and chemical additives and preservatives)

There are additional foods that can be problematic, especially for those with chronic health conditions. These are typically referred to as "middle-ground" foods and are discussed in more detail in Chapter 24.

There are also many foods that might be reintroduced to your diet and tolerated after an elimination phase. Some people enjoy white rice. Others include good-quality (that is, grass-fed) dairy, generally considered a healthful food with the caveat that a large percentage of people are sensitive or intolerant (and might not know it). The best way to know whether these foods work for you is to cut them out completely for a few weeks and then reintroduce them one at a time and see how you feel, which is discussed in more detail in Part 4.

Thoroughly researched and consistent in its overarching principles, a Paleo template is a sustainable way of eating to achieve our best health. Even more, it is a comprehensive approach to health that is steeped in solid science. The Paleo framework looks to evolutionary and contemporary biology to create a solid scientific foundation that informs our day-to-day choices impacting all inputs to our health.

PALEO GOES BEYOND FOOD

Despite being referenced as a diet, Paleo is—on a deeper level—a lifestyle, a framework for making better choices for the rest of our lives. And the principles of the Paleo template go beyond the foods on our plates to incorporate a focus on other inputs to health, including how active we are, how well we manage stress, whether we're getting enough quality sleep, and how connected we are to family, friends, and community.

Yes, health comes from more than just how we eat; it's also about how we live.

While technological advances like the internet, antibiotics, and indoor plumbing have undoubtedly improved our quality of life, our busy modern lives have come at a cost. Never before in human history have we worked as much, spent more of our days indoors, slept less, been more sedentary, or been as relentlessly stressed out as we are now. And this is as big a contributor to chronic illness as diets devoid of vital nutrients and overabundant in refined calories and inflammatory fats.

We can again take clues from hunter-gatherers, whose days are filled with constant gentle movement and positive social interaction while containing little in the way of chronic stressors; instead, these peoples experience the occasional short-lived but intensely stressful event. Hunter-gatherers consistently go to bed within a few hours of sunset, waking up just before dawn, totaling 7 to 8 hours of quality sleep every night. And modern scientific research tells us that each of these aspects of a healthy lifestyle has a direct impact on hormone systems, immune health, and neurological health. Again, no reenactment necessary; every facet of a healthy lifestyle can be integrated into our modern lives thoughtfully and deliberately.

Another reason for focusing on both diet and lifestyle factors is that there's a direct link between them, meaning that making better choices in one arena will help with the other. For example, eating a high-fiber diet and a serving of starchy carbs at dinner can help improve sleep quality. And consuming enough omega-3 fatty acids while limiting caffeine intake is a boon to our stress responses. Conversely, our lifestyle directly affects our food choices—we crave high-sugar and high-fat foods when we're stressed or tired, for example. And people who get at least 7 hours of sleep every night are more likely to choose vegetables and fruits over fast food. In addition, how our bodies respond to diet is influenced by aspects of our lifestyle. For example, studies show that we don't experience the same anti-inflammatory benefits from good food choices when we're stressed. And one night of lost sleep is as detrimental to blood sugar regulation as six months of poor diet.

That's the summary and probably everything you need to know to start following a Paleo template today. But there are a whole lot of pages between here and the recipes! Why?

MORE THAN RULES: USING PALEO PRINCIPLES

Rules don't work: at least 60 percent of people will choose to eat something unhealthy even though they know that they "shouldn't." To truly change the landscape of public health, we need to improve scientific literacy around public health topics. When we have a deep understanding of why a specific choice is unhealthy, we are far more motivated to seek healthier alternatives. Not that we'll be perfect all the time, but the Paleo template isn't about perfection; it's about making a better choice as often as possible while finding enough balance to make eating and living healthfully sustainable for a lifetime.

Rather than handing down from on high a set of new "Paleo rules" for you to learn, this book is about laying down a scientific foundation so that you understand why Paleo choices are better.

The first part of this book explains the scientific rationale behind Paleo, detailing the major principles from which the Paleo template is derived. You'll learn why Paleo is first and foremost a nutrient-focused way of eating, why balanced macronutrient intake supports health, and why choosing a diversity of both plant and animal foods is optimal. You'll also learn about key biological systems and how the health of these systems is impacted by your dietary choices and lifestyle. Finally, I'll discuss avoiding exposure to toxins from food and the environment as a critical factor in regaining and maintaining health.

The second part of this book focuses on the incredible diversity of foods included in the Paleo template, detailing the reason why these foods form the foundation of a health-promoting diet. You'll learn about the importance of eating lots of vegetables and focusing on slow-burning carbohydrates from starchy veggies and fruit. You'll understand the benefits of the most nutrient-dense animal foods, including seafood and organ meat, as well as why sourcing high-quality foods makes such a huge difference nutritionally. I'll also explain what healthy fats are, why probiotic foods are essential, and why herbs are so beneficial. Part 2 is the "what to eat" section of this book, which culminates in some great food lists and quick-start guides in Chapter 16.

It's also important to understand which foods are eliminated on the Paleo diet and why. In Part 3, you'll learn which types of antinutrients, toxins, and carcinogens can be present in food and which foods contain them. You'll understand why we can't cheat sweet, what the problem with refined and manufactured foods is, how grains can undermine health in many ways, and which fats to avoid. Finally, you'll learn how to read nutrition labels to successfully eliminate problematic foods from your diet.

There are boundaries to current human knowledge; Part 4 discusses those foods for which the scientific evidence isn't cut-and-dried. There are both pros and cons to these foods—alcohol, white rice, vegetables of the nightshade family, and others—so whether to incorporate them into your diet is an individual choice. Chapter 24 summarizes these "middle-ground" foods, and Chapter 25 gives you a step-by-step protocol for discovering your individual reactions to them.

Part 5 of this book discusses essential aspects of a healthy lifestyle and how prioritizing sleep, physical activity, and stress management improves health. These recommendations don't go much against the grain of conventional wisdom; however, finding time for beneficial lifestyle choices still tends to take a back seat to just about everything else in our busy lives. The thorough explanations of the scientific rationale behind these inputs to health will motivate you to restructure your priorities to incorporate healthier lifestyle choices, and the practical tips and guides will give you the tools you need to be successful.

Part 6 is where this book switches from scientific foundation to practical day-to-day resources. Chapter 39 summarizes the Paleo principles so that you can get a head start on following the Paleo template while you digest the information in Parts 1 through 5. You'll also learn the best way to transition to the Paleo diet to set yourself up for lifelong compliance. Plus, you'll learn how to modify the Paleo template to address specific health challenges and goals, like losing weight, reducing disease risk, and enhancing performance. Finally, Chapter 42 walks you through various avenues for troubleshooting should the standard Paleo template prove insufficient for your specific needs.

We head to the kitchen in Part 7 for a focus on shopping and cooking basics. You'll find tons of guides on where to shop, what types of foods to keep in stock, and how to manage your time in the kitchen, and you'll get a primer on cooking tools and techniques. You'll also find useful guides like measurement conversions, cooking times and temperatures for common cuts of meat, and ingredient substitutions in the Appendixes at the back of the book.

Part 8 includes more than 200 recipes for delicious everyday Paleo foods that will please the whole family. From healthy re-creations of old favorites, like pancakes, pizza, and pad Thai, to Paleo staples like bunless burgers, kale chips, and roasted sweet potatoes, to treats and transition foods like Paleo bread (page 562) and Molten Lava Chocolate Cake (page 587), this book has you covered! Plus, every recipe is labeled for the top-eight allergenic foods, nightshades, and the Autoimmune Protocol. And Part 9 offers twenty meal plans complete with shopping lists, you'll have everything you need to stay on track and enjoy tasty Paleo meals while you regain your health!

By understanding and embracing the principles of Paleo, we can empower ourselves to be our healthiest selves possible. So let's get started!

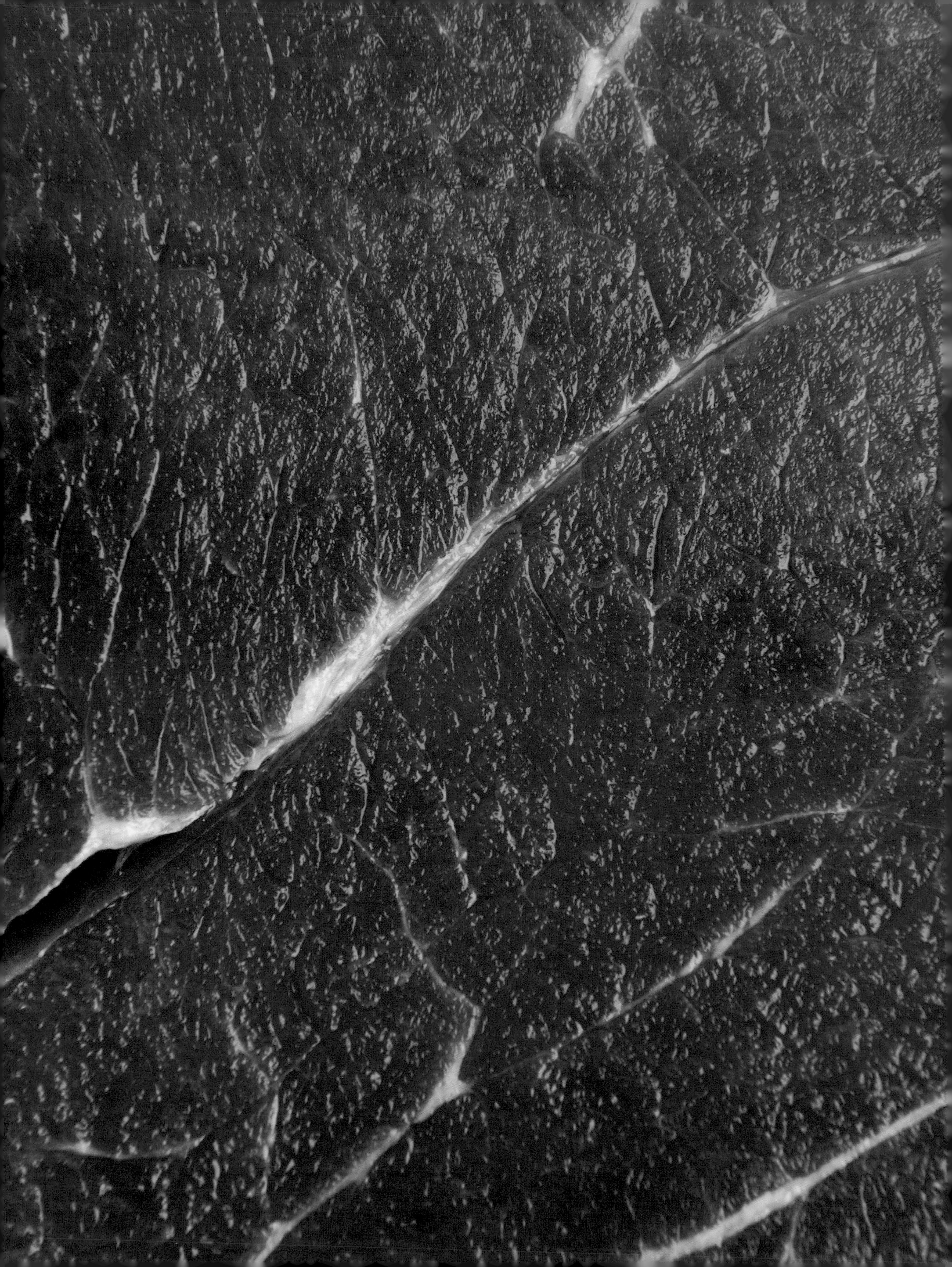

1.

THE RATIONALE: THE SCIENCE BEHIND THE FRAMEWORK

The Paleo template is a framework—rooted in science—for eating and living to support lifelong health.

The dietary component of the Paleo template is a set of nutritional principles compiled using modern scientific health and nutrition research. While the initial insight leading to the Paleo diet was gleaned from studies of Paleolithic man and both modern and historically studied hunter-gatherers, the core support for this way of eating comes from contemporary biology, physiology, and biochemistry. There are thousands of scientific studies that evaluate how components in foods interact with the human body to promote or undermine health. These are the studies used to form the basic tenets of the Paleo diet.

Before we look at the detailed whys behind which specific foods are included (or excluded) on a Paleo diet, let's zoom out to the diet's core principles: *micronutrient density, balanced macronutrients, diverse omnivorism, biological systems health*, and *minimizing toxin exposure*. These fundamental principles form the criteria against which foods are evaluated to determine what role they merit in our diets.

The Paleo template includes an equal emphasis on lifestyle choices because of the huge impact that things like sleep, stress, and activity have on our overall health. While most of us intuitively understand that we should strive for work-life balance and get some exercise, the Paleo lifestyle goes beyond making New Year's resolutions to join a gym and instead integrates a focus on achievable healthy lifestyle choices.

The big-picture principles for both diet and lifestyle discussed in this part are supported by numerous lines of evidence as promoting optimal health. For that reason, they're fundamental components of the Paleo framework.

FAIRPORT PUBLIC LIBRARY
1 VILLAGE LANDING
FAIRPORT, NY 14450
956

Chapter 1:
NUTRIENT DENSITY

First and foremost, the Paleo diet is a nutrient-dense diet. *Nutrient density* refers to the concentration of micronutrients (mainly vitamins and minerals, but also phytochemicals, essential fatty acids, and essential amino acids) per calorie of food. Nutrient-dense foods supply a wide range of micronutrients (or high levels of a specific micronutrient) relative to the calories they contain. Conversely, low-nutrient-density foods supply abundant calories without much in the way of nutrition (what we typically refer to as "junk food").

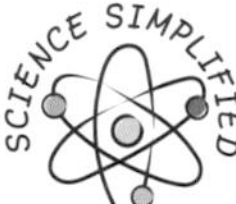

Nutrients are the molecular building blocks of our bodies. Not only are we made up of these raw materials, but our cells also use nutrients when they perform their various functions. This is why we need to continually consume enough nutrients for our cells to stay healthy and keep doing their jobs effectively.

So *why* exactly is nutrient density so important, and why is it central to Paleo?

Micronutrient deficiency is increasingly showing up as a major underlying driver of chronic disease. Many of us think that nutrient deficiencies are mainly a problem in developing nations (whereas in Westernized countries like the United States, our problem is that we have too *much* food!), but this is a misconception. The Standard American Diet is definitely energy-rich, but it's also nutrient-poor: the types of food that many people eat each day are high in added sugars, refined grains, and industrially processed oils, but devoid of the vitamins and minerals (and other health-promoting compounds) found in whole foods. The result is a high prevalence of nutrient deficiency right in our own backyard.

WHERE NUTRIENT DEFICIENCIES COME FROM

Our food system is abundant in calories (the U.S. produces about 6,000 calories' worth of food per person per day), but the Standard American Diet is deficient in most of the essential vitamins and minerals that our bodies need to be healthy. According to one analysis using data from the National Health and Nutritional Examination Survey (looking at food intakes for more than 16,000 Americans over the age of two) and the estimated average requirements (EAR values) for each nutrient:

- 70 percent of the population doesn't consume enough vitamin D.
- 60 percent doesn't consume enough vitamin E.
- 45 percent doesn't consume enough magnesium.
- 38 percent doesn't consume enough calcium.

- 34 percent doesn't consume enough vitamin A.
- 25 percent doesn't consume enough vitamin C.
- 8 percent doesn't consume enough vitamin B6, vitamin B9 (folate), or zinc.
- A smaller percentage (less than 6 percent) doesn't consume enough vitamin B1, vitamin B2, vitamin B3, vitamin B12, phosphorus, iron, copper, or selenium.

Whew! And those numbers include nutrient intakes from regular food, fortified food, *and* supplements combined, so the vitamins and minerals coming from whole-food sources are even lower for most people. For example, 88 percent of the U.S. population would be consuming inadequate vitamin B9 if it weren't for extensive fortification and supplementation.

An analysis of dietary nutrition not including supplements (but including fortified foods) compared to recommended daily allowance from the data collected by the USDA Agricultural Research Service revealed that large percentages of Americans are falling short on thirteen essential vitamins and minerals. In this analysis (see graph above), a whopping 73 percent of Americans over the age of two are not getting enough zinc, 65 percent aren't getting enough calcium, 61 percent are falling short on magnesium, 56 percent aren't getting enough vitamin A, and 53 percent aren't getting enough vitamin B6. And roughly a quarter to a third of us aren't consuming enough B vitamins or vitamin C.

We should keep in mind that these percentages are averages. When we group people based on age, race/ethnicity, and various lifestyle factors, certain groups have higher deficiency rates than others. For example, the CDC's Second Nutrition Report found that menstruating women are more likely to be iron deficient, non-Hispanic blacks are more likely to be deficient in vitamin D, and women ages 20 to 39 are more likely to be iodine deficient. This also doesn't take into account how, for example, different diet and lifestyle factors can increase our nutrient needs and render our intakes insufficient even when we appear to be meeting the Recommended Dietary Allowances. For instance, a high intake of fructose or glucose can increase our requirements for calcium, vitamin C, magnesium, chromium, and vitamin D.

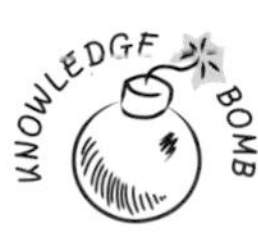

Micronutrient deficiencies are so common that some researchers speculate that nearly all of us are deficient in at least one vital nutrient.

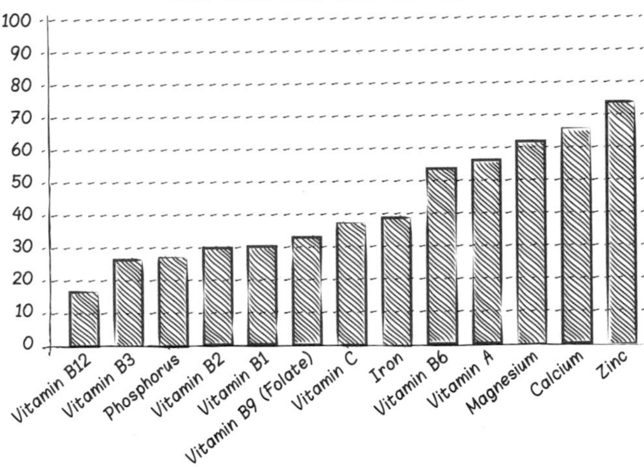

Source: Analysis of USDA Agricultural Research Service data presented in Cordain, L., et al. "Origins and evolution of the Western diet: health implications for the 21st century." *American Journal of Clinical Nutrition* 81, no. 2 (2005): 341-354.

The more processed or refined a food is, the more nutrients are stripped out of it. For example, there is a difference as wide as the Grand Canyon between the superb micronutrient content of beets (which are especially rich in vitamin B9 and manganese but also contain vitamins A, B1, B2, B3, B5, B6, and C, as well as calcium, potassium, magnesium, phosphorus, zinc, copper, and selenium) and the micronutrient content of table sugar, which contains no vitamins or minerals whatsoever, even though many brands are made from sugar beets—in fact, 55 percent of U.S. sugar production comes from sugar beets rather than sugarcane.

	BEETS (100 g or 3/4 cup)	BEET SUGAR (7 g or 2 tsp)
Sugars	7 g	7 g
Vitamin A	2 mcg*	0
Vitamin B1	31 mcg	0
Vitamin B2	40 mcg	1 mcg
Vitamin B3	334 mcg	0
Vitamin B5	200 mcg	0
Vitamin B6	67 mcg	0
Vitamin B9	109 mcg	0
Vitamin C	4.9 mg	0
Calcium	16 mg	0
Potassium	325 mg	0
Magnesium	23 mg	0
Phosphorus	40 mg	0
Zinc	400 mcg	0
Copper	100 mcg	0
Selenium	0.7 mcg	0
Manganese	300 mcg	0
Fiber	2.8 g	0

*A microgram (mcg) is a millionth of a gram (g).

While this example is an extreme one, it's also an effective demonstration of just how detrimental manufactured foods have become in terms of nutrient depletion. The more a food is manipulated to make it shelf-stable, convenient, cheap, and addictively delicious, the fewer valuable nutrients remain in that food. Worse, processing often adds or creates *antinutrients* (substances that hinder the absorption of nutrients from our food; see page 230), not to mention other compounds with dubious health effects (such as preservatives, typically toxic even in moderate quantities; see page 239).

Junk food, white bread, and high-fructose corn syrup aren't the only culprits here. Even eating what many people believe to be a healthy diet can leave our bodies starved for micronutrients. And this falls on the shoulders of dietary guidelines with their long-standing grouping of foods based on how they are produced rather than the nutrients they contain. For example, vegetables, which vary widely in vitamin, mineral, phytochemical, and fiber content, all get lumped together based on both farming practices to grow them and very broad botanical classification. And until the Food Guide Pyramid was introduced in 1992, vegetables were lumped together with fruit, even though fruit typically comes from entirely different kinds of plants and different kinds of fruits vary just as widely in nutrients.

After the guidelines lump all these foods into one or two food groups, they recommend that we "eat the rainbow." The concept of eating a variety of fruits and vegetables of different colors is an excellent one—the pigments that give plants their colors are also micronutrients (phytochemicals and vitamin precursors), so eating many different-colored vegetables and fruits is a great way to make sure that we're getting the full complement of nutrients that plant foods can provide. But what would make far more sense from a public health perspective is to divide fruits and vegetables by color into four groups: blue and purple; green; red, orange, and yellow; and white. Eating two or three servings daily from each group would result in a vastly superior micronutrient intake.

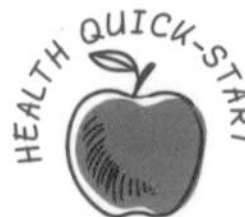

Start thinking about the different color families of vegetables and fruits as their own individual food groups. Aim for two to three servings each day from each color family:

- *Blue and purple*
- *Green*
- *Red, orange, and yellow*
- *White*

And aim for a minimum of eight servings of fruits and vegetables daily. An easy way to do this is to have two servings at breakfast and three servings each at lunch and dinner. For more on what constitutes a serving size, see page 157.

The U.S. dietary guidelines also group together meat, fish, eggs, legumes, nuts, and seeds based on the fact that they all contain protein. While it's great that nutrients are being considered here, this broad classification is misleading. Plant-based proteins are difficult to digest and typically don't contain all the amino acids our bodies need (that's why they're referred to as incomplete proteins; see page 168), yet they get equal billing with meat, fish, and eggs, which are much more useful to our bodies. This nod to vegetarians is respectful from a social perspective, but it implies that kidney beans provide the same sort of nutrition as a steak. They don't. And for those who are not following vegetarian diets for ethical or religious reasons, this is important information. In addition, vegetarians need to make sure that they're eating specific combinations of foods to get all twenty amino acids, and this grouping of foods isn't taken into account. Finally, these foods provide many nutrients other than protein, and they absolutely do not provide them equally. From a micronutrient perspective, it would make far more sense for this food group to be divided into at least four groups:

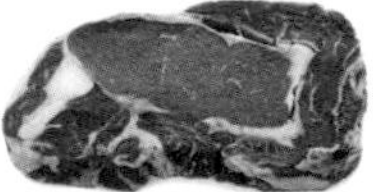
MEAT AND EGGS

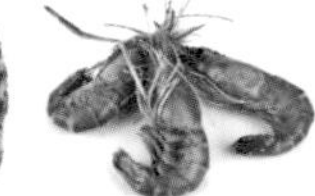
FISH AND SHELLFISH

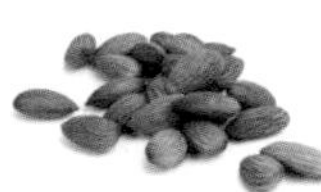
NUTS AND SEEDS

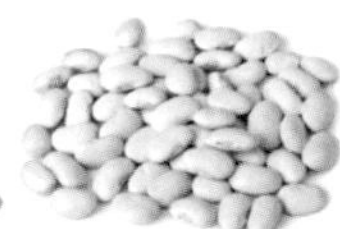
LEGUMES

Organ meat could possibly be celebrated as its own food group—it's one of the most micronutrient-dense foods available in the modern food supply, and it has a very different nutrient profile from other meats.

HEALTH QUICK-START

Fish and shellfish provide the most easily digested complete protein and the healthiest fats, while being extremely rich in vitamins and minerals, including some that are hard to get from other animal foods. Aim for a minimum of three servings a week.

In the dietary guidelines, grains enjoy their own food group despite the fact that even whole grains don't contribute much more than calories to our diets. The fact that whole grains are touted as being the foundation of a healthy diet may be the biggest contributor to the mismatch between the nutrition our bodies need and how much we actually get. Vegetables and fruits contain up to ten times more vitamins and minerals than grains, just as much fiber, and only a fraction of the sugar, plus they have high amounts of health-promoting phytochemicals. There is absolutely no need for grains in a diet that includes vegetables and fruits. Given that so many grain-based products contribute a disproportionately high amount of blood sugar-spiking, too-easily-digested carbohydrate (a contributor to obesity and diabetes) as well as high amounts of the most inflammatory fatty acids, they likely belong in the same grouping of foods as candy, fast food, and other junk.

KNOWLEDGE BOMB

When vegetables take the place of grains in your diet, you win every time.

These graphs show the relative content of vitamins and minerals in grains compared with vegetables, adjusted for caloric content, using eight of the most nutrient-dense whole-grain foods and fifty common vegetables. Values are expressed as the percentage of vitamin and mineral in grains compared with vegetables. For example, grains have about 10 percent of the vitamin E and calcium content that vegetables have.

The only micronutrients for which grains can match vegetables are sodium and manganese. And the only micronutrient in which grains outperform veggies is selenium—but of course, the richest dietary sources of selenium are meats and seafood!

Dairy is the only food group that focuses on a micronutrient: calcium. This group includes all foods made from milk as well as calcium-fortified beverages made from milk alternatives like soy. Of course, there are plenty of amazing sources of calcium that are not included in this food group. Not only do fruits, vegetables, nuts, seeds, and seafood contain substantial amounts of calcium, but there is scientific evidence that we actually absorb more calcium from cruciferous vegetables (like kale) than we do from dairy. In fact, several studies show that fruit and vegetable intake correlates much more strongly with bone health than dairy intake—yes, to prevent osteoporosis and look after your bones, eat your veggies!

PALEO EASY BUTTON

Worried about bone health if you give up dairy? Cruciferous veggies like cabbage, broccoli, and leafy greens; seafood; nuts and seeds; and citrus are all great Paleo sources of calcium! See page 264 for more information.

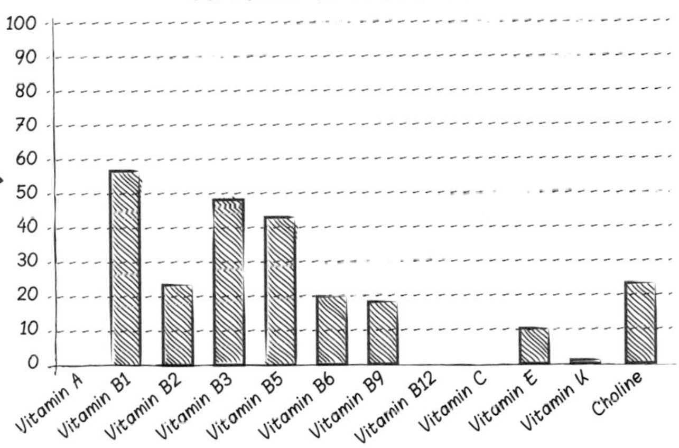

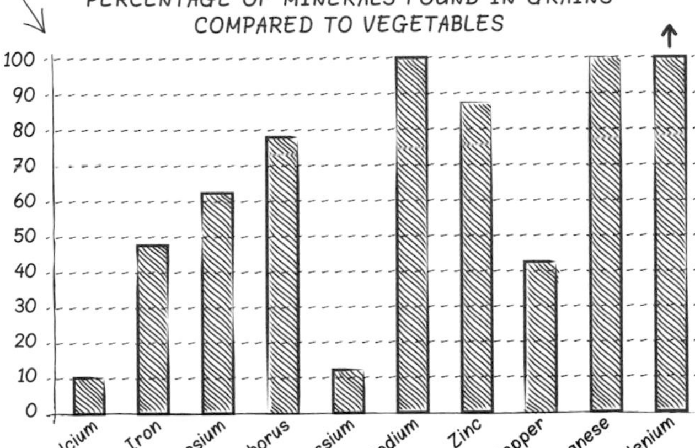

Data obtained from the USDA database.

Of course, even whole vegetables and fruits have less nutrition now than they used to. Between depleted soils, cultivars chosen for long shelf lives and resilience to shipping and handling rather than nutrient density, and nutrient degradation that occurs between the time a fruit or vegetable is picked and when it makes it onto your plate, even these healthy food choices are depleted nutritionally compared to half a century ago, when they were typically grown locally and eaten seasonally.

Vegetables and fruits contain substantially less vitamins than they did in the 1950s.

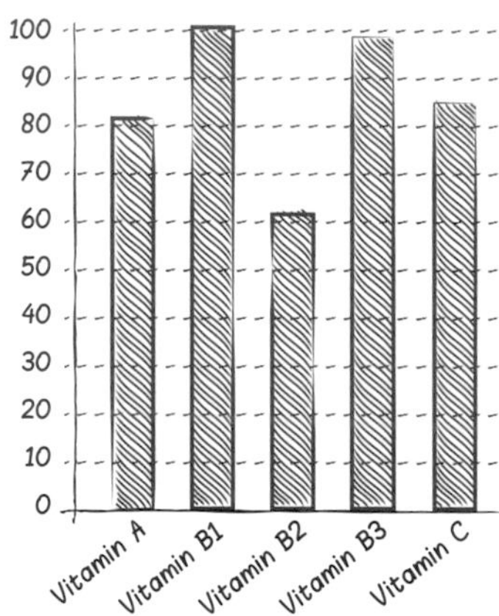

Vegetables and fruits contain substantially less minerals than they did in the 1950s.

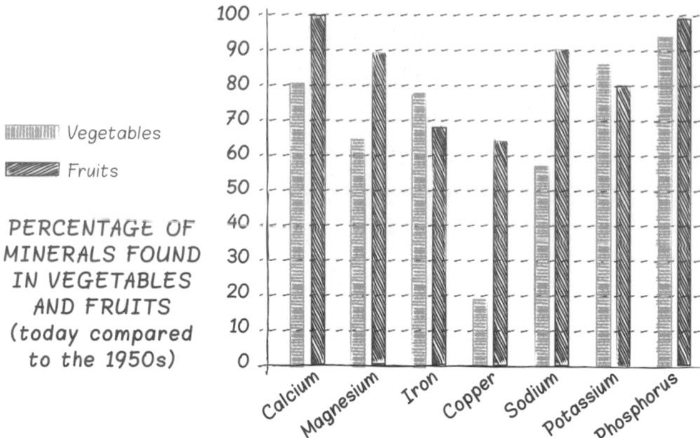

Of course, eating large quantities of vegetables and fruits is essential for human health, so even if our choices aren't quite as good as their equivalents from our grandparents' days, they still need to make it onto our plates! You can also roll back the clock by seeking out locally grown, organic, and in-season produce straight from the farm.

IMPLICATIONS FOR HUMAN HEALTH

So what do micronutrient deficiencies mean for human health? The news isn't good! Specific deficiencies have been linked to a huge spectrum of problems, including:

- Iron deficiency anemia
- Heart disease (vitamin B9 deficiency leads to high homocysteine and impaired endothelial function)
- Greater susceptibility to infection (zinc deficiency leads to impaired immune function)
- Autoimmune disease (detailed in my book *The Paleo Approach)*
- Thyroid disorders (iodine deficiency leads to hypothyroidism and goiters)
- Vision problems (vitamin A deficiency leads to poor retina health)
- Birth defects (vitamin A and vitamin B9 deficiencies lead to neural tube defects and other complications)
- Colorectal cancer and other cancers (vitamin D and selenium deficiencies lead to increased cell proliferation and reduced differentiation and apoptosis)
- Deficiencies of vitamins and minerals involved in glucose metabolism and insulin signaling (which include vitamin D, chromium, biotin, vitamin B1, and vitamin C) have been theorized to underlie diabetes.

What's more, there's evidence that micronutrient deficiencies could even be contributing to our obesity epidemic. The rationale is twofold: first, certain deficiencies are much more common among obese people (for example, vitamin D and vitamin B1 deficiency), and second, vitamin and mineral supplements have been shown to improve appetite regulation and (in some studies) increase body fat loss to a clinically relevant degree. Clearly, focusing on nutrient density is extremely important when establishing a framework for healthy eating—that's why it's a central tenet of Paleo.

In fact, in a real-world setting, the Paleo diet offers far more nutrition than nearly any other diet. And I'm not just talking in comparison to the Standard American Diet. The Atkins Diet, the South Beach Diet, the DASH diet, and other popular eating plans have been evaluated and shown to be nutritionally inadequate when followed as prescribed. (All three of those diets provide inadequate amounts of vitamin E, vitamin B5, biotin, vitamin D, chromium, choline, iodine, potassium, molybdenum, and zinc.) Paleo, on the other hand, has the potential to supply ample amounts of every important micronutrient due to its focus on whole foods, food diversity, food quality, vegetable consumption, and nose-to-tail eating (which I'll discuss in greater depth in Chapter 10).

Even following standard Paleo diet recommendations from the last decade of books and websites is not a guarantee that you're getting all the micronutrients you need to be healthy. And while the foods endorsed by the Paleo diet represent the most nutrient-dense foods in our food supply, reaching micronutrient sufficiency still requires commitment. In fact, analyses of typical Paleo food choices reveal that biotin (abundant in liver and root vegetables), calcium (abundant in its most bioavailable form [meaning that our bodies can easily digest and use it] in dark leafy greens like kale, as well as in whole fish like sardines), and chromium (abundant in dark leafy greens, oysters, and liver) are commonly deficient on the Paleo diet. While the Paleo diet far outstrips other approaches in terms of micronutrient sufficiency, if you just stick to the stereotypical meat, veggies, and coconut oil, you may miss out on important nutrients for optimal health.

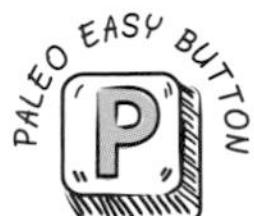

A variety of apps, like MyFitnessPal and CRON-O-Meter, allow you to track essential micronutrients in addition to calories, protein, fat, and carbohydrates. Try recording your food intake for two to three days to see which nutrients you need to focus on getting more of.

A TOUR OF ESSENTIAL AND NONESSENTIAL NUTRIENTS

Nutrient sufficiency is arguably the most important quality of any dietary approach. Every cell, tissue, organ, and system in the human body needs specific amounts of specific nutrients to function efficiently and effectively. Nutrients are used not only to form the components of our bodies but also in the millions of chemical reactions that are occurring in our bodies at every moment. We are made of nutrients, and our bodies need them to do even basic things like breathe. Every tiny detail of every function of every part of the body requires nutrients, and it isn't just the energy supplied by macronutrients—protein, fat, and carbohydrates—that fuel the complex functions of life. Micronutrients—vitamins, minerals, phytochemicals, and other compounds—are necessary resources that get used up, too, and our micronutrient stores must be continuously topped up from the foods we eat. Being even slightly deficient in a single essential nutrient can have negative consequences for our health.

Generally, a nutrients-first approach to eating focuses on micronutrients. When we're getting all the essential amino acids, essential fatty acids, vitamins, minerals, and phytochemicals that our bodies need to thrive, it's nearly impossible not to be consuming sufficient macronutrients.

Micronutrients can be categorized as essential and nonessential. *Essential* means that you'll die without them. *Nonessential* means that you'll go on living without them, though you may not be particularly healthy and indeed, many micronutrients that are considered nonessential are known to improve health. Often, a micronutrient is called nonessential simply because we don't understand exactly what it does to support health—we just know that when we consume more of it, our risk of disease decreases. This is the case for most phytochemicals and many vitaminlike compounds. There are thousands of phytochemicals, and our understanding of their roles in health is so rudimentary that the most we can typically say about them is that they have antioxidant activity (that is, they help prevent damage to molecules in the body from oxidation). Yet we know that the more phytochemicals in our diet, the lower our risk of chronic disease. When you think about it in these terms, it's easy to realize that even nonessential nutrients are pretty darned important.

So let's examine this wondrous world of micronutrients in more detail.

Vitamins and Minerals

We do know the roles that all the known vitamins and many minerals play in the human body. These micronutrients are considered essential, and when we examine how the body uses them, it quickly becomes obvious why we can't enjoy good health without the full complement of essential nutrients.

Vitamins are essential organic molecules needed in small amounts for normal function, growth, and maintenance of body tissues. Our bodies can't synthesize these molecules (in sufficient quantities or at all, depending on which vitamin we're talking about), so we need to get them from food.

The term *vitamin* is derived from the Latin *vita*, meaning "essence of life." Discovered predominantly in the late nineteenth and early twentieth centuries, vitamins were labeled with letters (A, B, C, D, E) as they were discovered, until technological advances permitting the identification of molecular structures changed the nomenclature. Many of the post-E vitamins were later relabeled as vitamins in the B complex, with designations between B2 and B12. For example, vitamin G was renamed vitamin B2 or

VITAMINS AND VITAMINLIKE SUBSTANCES

Vitamin A (retinol): Not to be confused with β-carotene (which is a vitamin A precursor, not vitamin A itself), this vitamin is essential for bone growth, tooth remineralization, skin health, vision, reproduction, and immune function. Retinol is found only in animal foods, including liver, eggs, quality dairy products (see page 288), and seafood (especially shrimp, salmon, sardines, and tuna).

Vitamin B1 (thiamin): Important for energy metabolism, cellular function, and a wide variety of organ functions. Sources include organ meat, pork, seeds, squash, fish (especially trout, mackerel, salmon, and tuna), and legumes.

Vitamin B2 (riboflavin): Aids in the production of two other B vitamins (B3 and B6) and plays an important role in energy metabolism. Riboflavin also acts as an antioxidant. Rich sources include organ meat, mushrooms, leafy green vegetables, eggs, legumes, and squash.

Vitamin B3 (niacin): Helps improve circulation, aids the body in manufacturing stress- and sex-related hormones, and suppresses inflammation. Excellent sources include organ meat, poultry, fish and shellfish, red meat (including beef and lamb), mushrooms, and leafy green vegetables.

Vitamin B5 (pantothenic acid): Along with assisting in energy metabolism (like all B vitamins), vitamin B5 plays a role in manufacturing red blood cells, sex hormones, and stress hormones. It also helps maintain a healthy digestive tract and enables the body to use vitamin B2. Sources include organ meat, mushrooms, oily fish, avocados, red meat (especially beef and lamb), and seeds.

Vitamin B6 (pyridoxine): Important for cell metabolism and the production of hemoglobin, which carries oxygen in the blood. B6 is also vital for producing the key neurotransmitters GABA, dopamine, and serotonin. Sources include a wide variety of plant and animal foods, including leafy and root vegetables, fruits such as bananas, red meat, poultry, and seeds (especially sunflower and pumpkin seeds).

Vitamin B7 (biotin): Involved in many metabolic pathways, especially fat and sugar metabolism. It also helps maintain skin and hair health. Foods high in biotin include eggs, liver, nuts such as almonds and walnuts, root vegetables, and tomatoes.

Vitamin B9 (folate): Plays an important role in methylation (the process of adding a methyl group to different molecules), making it a key player in methylation-dependent processes like detoxification and neuron signaling. Folate is also crucial for cardiovascular health, reproductive function (especially protecting against neural tube defects), and red blood cell production. Rich sources include organ meat, green vegetables (both leafy and non-leafy), legumes, beets, avocados, and fruits such as papayas, strawberries, and pomegranates.

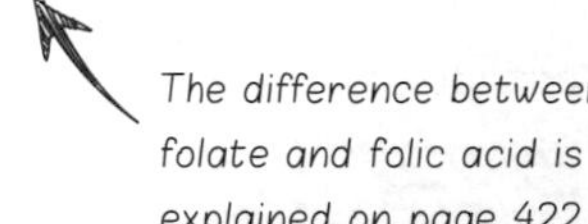
The difference between folate and folic acid is explained on page 422.

riboflavin; vitamin H is now called B7 or biotin; and vitamin M is now called B9 or folate. Other substances originally labeled as vitamins lost their classification once their structure was identified; for example, flavonoids, discussed on page 36, were originally given the name vitamin P. More recently discovered compounds being identified as essential (such as choline, carnitine, inositol, and taurine) may eventually be classified as vitamins but likely will never receive a letter designation.

Vitamins can be broadly divided into two classes:

- **Fat-soluble vitamins,** including vitamins A, D, E, and K, dissolve in fats and oils.
- **Water-soluble vitamins,** including all the B vitamins and vitamin C, dissolve in water.

This property affects the way in which vitamins are absorbed and used in the body. The upshot is that fat-soluble vitamins are generally found in fatty foods (the exception being vitamin K) and water-soluble vitamins tend to come packaged in proteins or carbohydrates. A mineral is a chemical element (that is, a member of

Vitamin B12 (cobalamin): Involved in energy metabolism like the other B vitamins, but also plays a unique role in DNA production. It's vital for maintaining cardiovascular, brain, and nervous system health. Because vitamin B12 is manufactured exclusively by microorganisms, it's found mostly in animal foods that concentrate bacterially produced B12 in their cells, such as fish (especially sardines, salmon, tuna, and cod), shellfish such as shrimp and scallops, organ meat, beef, poultry, and eggs. Some fermented soy products like tempeh also contain vitamin B12.

Choline: Plays an essential role in building cell membranes. It also serves as the backbone for a neurotransmitter called acetylcholine, which is involved in heart health, gut motility (the movement of contents through the digestive tract controlled by the coordinated contraction and relaxation of specialized gut muscle tissue), and muscle movement. Choline is abundant in foods such as fish and shellfish, liver, eggs, poultry, and green vegetables (both leafy and non-leafy).

Vitamin C: A potent antioxidant that's necessary for immune system function and the function of several enzymes (like some that help make collagen, which is why vitamin C deficiency causes scurvy). Foods rich in vitamin C include bell peppers, leafy dark green vegetables, citrus fruits, and other fruits such as papaya, cantaloupe, guava, and berries. Some organ meats are also good sources of vitamin C.

Vitamin D: Assists in calcium absorption, immune system function, bone development, modulation of cell growth, neuromuscular function, and the reduction of inflammation. Although vitamin D can be produced when the sun's UV rays hit the skin and trigger vitamin D synthesis, it also can be obtained from foods, including oily fish (such as salmon, tuna, and mackerel), mushrooms, fish roe, liver, and eggs.

Vitamin E: Actually a group of eight fat-soluble antioxidants, the most well-known of which is α-tocopherol. All forms of vitamin E help protect against free radical damage, reduce the harmful oxidation of LDL ("bad") cholesterol particles in the bloodstream, and boost cardiovascular health. Foods high in vitamin E include nuts, seeds, leafy green vegetables, fatty fish, organ meat, and oily plant foods like avocados and olives.

Vitamin K: Central to maintaining bone health and critical for making important proteins that are involved in blood clotting and metabolism (in fact, the K comes from the German word for blood clotting, *koagulation*). Vitamin K exists in the forms K1, K2, and K3; the K2 form boosts cardiovascular health. The richest sources of vitamin K include cruciferous vegetables (such as broccoli, cauliflower, cabbage, and Brussels sprouts) and leafy dark green vegetables (such as spinach, collard greens, parsley, and Swiss chard), as well as asparagus. Vitamin K2 is found in natto (a fermented soybean product), eggs, butter, and liver.

Ubiquinol: A reduced, more bioavailable form of the vitaminlike compound coenzyme Q10. Ubiquinol is a potent antioxidant and may be helpful in treating or preventing heart and blood vessel conditions, diabetes, gum disease, muscular dystrophy, chronic fatigue syndrome, and breast cancer. Sources include beef, pork, mackerel, yellowtail fish, and chicken; it's also found in smaller amounts in vegetables like broccoli and herbs like parsley.

the Periodic Table of Elements) required as an essential nutrient other than carbon, hydrogen, nitrogen, oxygen, and sulfur (which form the backbone of most organic molecules including amino acids, fatty acids, and vitamins). Dietary minerals may be present in inorganic salts (like table salt, aka sodium chloride) or as part of carbon-containing organic compounds (like magnesium in chlorophyll, the pigment that makes plants green).

Essential minerals can be divided into macrominerals, which we need in excess of 100 milligrams per day to avoid symptoms of deficiency, and trace minerals, which we need in much smaller amounts (1 to 100 milligrams per day). Macrominerals include sodium, chloride, potassium, phosphorus, magnesium, sulfur, and calcium. Trace minerals include copper, chromium, fluoride, iodine, iron, molybdenum, manganese, selenium, and zinc.

ESSENTIAL MINERALS

5 B **Boron:** Supports bone health and is essential for the utilization of vitamin D and calcium in the body. Sources include nuts, avocados, leafy green vegetables, legumes, and a variety of other vegetables and fruits, such as apples, carrots, broccoli, pears, and olives.

20 Ca **Calcium:** In addition to forming bone, calcium is essential to many processes within cells, as well as neurotransmitter release and muscle contraction (including the beating of your heart!). Foods rich in calcium include dark green vegetables, sesame seeds, dairy products, whole sardines (bones included), and squash.

17 Cl **Chlorine:** Required for the production of hydrochloric acid in the stomach and important for electrolyte balance and fluid balance in the body. Foods high in chlorine include seaweed, tomatoes, olives, celery, and lettuce, although most foods contain at least small amounts.

24 Cr **Chromium:** Important for sugar and fat metabolism and particularly critical for blood sugar control. Chromium is found in small amounts in every food group but is most abundant in foods such as oysters, liver, broccoli, green beans, leafy green vegetables, mushrooms, and tomatoes.

29 Cu **Copper:** Involved in the absorption, storage, and metabolism of iron and the formation of red blood cells. Copper is also important for building strong tissue and producing cellular energy. Sources include oysters and other shellfish, legumes, nuts, organ meat, and mushrooms.

53 I **Iodine:** A constituent of thyroid hormones, iodine has diverse roles in the body. It is important for lactation and plays a part in supporting the immune system. Sources include sea vegetables (especially brown varieties such as kelp and wakame), fish, shellfish, eggs, and dairy products.

26 Fe **Iron:** A key component of hemoglobin, the protein in the blood that binds to oxygen and transports it throughout the body. Iron is also important for supporting energy production and proper metabolism in muscles and active organs. You can find iron in foods such as liver, leafy dark green vegetables, red meat, legumes, and olives.

12 Mg **Magnesium:** Necessary for cell life. More than 300 enzymes need magnesium to work, including every enzyme that uses or synthesizes ATP (the basic energy molecule in a cell; see page 267) and enzymes that synthesize DNA and RNA. Magnesium also enhances control of inflammation and maintains nervous system balance. Foods rich in magnesium include green vegetables, nuts and seeds, fish, legumes, and avocados.

25 Mn **Manganese:** Necessary for enzymes that protect the body from and repair damage caused by free radicals. This mineral is important for bone production, skin integrity, and blood sugar control. Foods high in manganese include fish and shellfish, nuts and seeds, legumes, leafy dark green vegetables, and cruciferous vegetables (such as broccoli, cauliflower, cabbage, kale, Brussels sprouts, and turnip greens).

Recommended Dietary Allowance of Essential Vitamins and Minerals

Recommended Dietary Allowances (RDAs) are established by the Food and Nutrition Board of the Institute of Medicine. An RDA is the dietary intake level of a specific nutrient considered sufficient to meet the needs of 97.5 percent of healthy individuals, implying that this intake would be inadequate for just 2.5 percent of the healthy population. RDAs are calculated based on the estimated average requirement for each nutrient, something that some specialists believe is a gross underestimation of our true biological need, since these levels are generally determined based on symptoms of deficiency rather than amounts needed for optimal health.

For some nutrients, no RDA has been established. In those cases, the Institute of Medicine has established a dietary intake level called Adequate Intake (AI), an amount somewhat less firmly believed to be adequate for everyone in the demographic group.

Most of us can target the RDA or AI of each nutrient as a minimum every day. Upper limits have been established for many of these nutrients, although toxicity is typically seen only in the context of

---

42 Mo **Molybdenum:** Necessary for activity of key enzymes that perform detoxification functions in the liver. It also plays an important role in nervous system metabolism. Molybdenum is found in legumes, eggs, tomatoes, lettuce, and a variety of other vegetables, including celery, fennel, and cucumbers.

15 P **Phosphorus:** Plays a role in every metabolic reaction in the body and is important for the metabolism of fats, carbohydrates, and proteins. It also serves a central function in bone support. Phosphorous is abundant in protein-rich foods such as dairy products, fish, shellfish, seeds, and legumes.

19 K **Potassium:** Critical for the function of every cell; it is necessary for nerve function, cardiac function, and muscle contraction. As an electrolyte, it helps conduct electrical charges in the body. Rich sources include leafy dark green vegetables, cruciferous vegetables, some fruits (such as bananas and cantaloupe), legumes, and many orange vegetables (such as carrots, squash, and sweet potatoes).

34 Se **Selenium:** Required for the activity of twenty-five to thirty different enzymes that protect the brain and other tissues from oxidative damage. Selenium also helps support normal thyroid function. Good sources include red meat, poultry, fish and shellfish, Brazil nuts, and mushrooms.

11 Na **Sodium:** Necessary for electrolyte balance; for regulating blood pressure, volume, and pH; for controlling the movement of fluids across cell membranes; and for neuron function. Along with any food doused in table salt or cured in salt, such as olives and some meats, natural sources of sodium include seaweed, celery, turnips, artichokes, and some leafy green vegetables, such as spinach and collard greens. Too much sodium isn't a good thing; it's preferable to get your sodium from whole-food sources and conservative use of unrefined sea salt; see page 198.

14 Si **Silicon:** Required for the formation of connective tissues and bone. It also supports the health of hair, nails, and skin. Sources of silicon include bananas, string beans, legumes, apples, and cabbage.

16 S **Sulfur:** Widely used in biochemical processes, sulfur is a structural component of many proteins and is necessary for the function of many enzymes and antioxidants. It is abundant in cruciferous vegetables, alliums such as onions and garlic, eggs, and other protein-rich animal foods, such as fish, meat, and poultry.

30 Zn **Zinc:** Important for nearly every cellular function, from protein and carbohydrate metabolism to cell division and growth. Zinc also plays a role in skin health and the maintenance of sensory organs (that's why zinc deficiency is associated with a loss of smell and taste) and is a vital nutrient for immune system function. Zinc also plays a vital role in epithelial barrier function by improving tight junction formation (see page 67). The richest source is oysters, but other good sources include red meat, poultry, nuts and seeds, and legumes.

Other trace minerals: We seem to have a biological need for dozens of other minerals, albeit in very small quantities, making them ultra-trace minerals. Vanadium, bromine, titanium, nickel, tin, lithium, aluminum, bismuth, and even gold all have probable essential biological roles, although more research is needed.

supplementation and not via dietary intake of whole foods. It's also worth noting that in many instances, therapeutic doses of essential vitamins and minerals exceed the established upper limits.

	RDA	AI	UPPER LIMIT
Vitamin A	♂3,000 IU ♀2,300 IU		10,000 IU
Vitamin B1	♂1.2 mg ♀1.1 mg		Not established
Vitamin B2	♂1.3 mg ♀1.1 mg		Not established
Vitamin B3	♂16 mg ♀14 mg		35 mg
Vitamin B5		5 mg	Not established
Vitamin B6	♂1.3 mg ♀1.3 mg		100 mg
Vitamin B7		30 mcg	Not established
Vitamin B9	400 mcg		1 g
Vitamin B12	2.4 mcg		Not established
Vitamin C	♂90 mg ♀75 mg		2 g
Vitamin D	600 IU		4,000 IU
Vitamin E	22 IU		1,500 IU
Vitamin K		♂120 mcg ♀90 mcg	Not established
Choline		♂550 mg ♀425 mg	3.5 g
Calcium	1,000 mg		2.5 g
Chromium		♂35 mcg ♀25 mcg	Not established
Copper	900 mcg		10 mg
Fluoride		♂4 mg ♀3 mg	10 mg
Iodine	150 mcg		1.1 mg
Iron	♂8 mg ♀18 mg (18–50 years) ♀8 mg (51+ years)		45 mg
Magnesium	♂400 mg (19–30 years) ♂420 mg (31+ years) ♀310 mg (19–30 years) ♀320 mg (31+ years)		Not established
Manganese		♂2.3 mg ♀1.8 mg	11 mg
Molybdenum	45 mcg		2 mg
Phosphorus	700 mg		4 g
Potassium		4.7 g	Not established
Selenium	55 mcg		400 mcg
Zinc	♂11 mg ♀8 mg		40 mg

**Only RDAs for adults aged 19 to 50 are shown, except where otherwise noted: ♂ are recommendations for adult men and ♀ are recommendations for adult women. See page 425 for RDAs for babies and children. Visit usda.gov for RDAs for other age groups as well as recommendations for pregnant and lactating women.*

Amino Acids

Vitamins and minerals aren't the only essential micronutrients. Amino acids are the basic building blocks of protein, which forms a substantial percentage of our bodies.

Even though we've identified about 500 different amino acids, only twenty are used to build the proteins in our bodies, and only nine of those are considered *nutritionally indispensable,* meaning that we absolutely have to get them from food—our bodies can't make them. These nine essential amino acids are histidine, isoleucine, leucine, lysine, methionine, phenylalanine, threonine, tryptophan, and valine.

Six additional amino acids are considered *conditionally indispensable,* meaning that while other amino acids can be converted into these amino acids, the process is so inefficient that most of the time we still need to get them from food.

The remaining five amino acids are considered *nutritionally dispensable*, meaning that our bodies can make them in sufficient quantities provided that there's enough protein in our diets. While technically we need to get only the nine essential amino acids through diet—our bodies can create the remaining eleven—it is far preferable from a health standpoint to get all of the amino acids from foods. That way, we don't have to rely on often inefficient conversion processes for the amino acids our bodies need to make all the various proteins in our cells and tissues.

Complete proteins provide sufficient quantities of all nine essential amino acids, and for the most part, they come from animals—meat, eggs, seafood, and dairy are all complete proteins. Most plant foods are not complete proteins, and it's not usually easy for our bodies to fully digest and break down plant proteins in order to absorb their amino acids. All proteins from animal foods are easier to digest than proteins from plant foods, and the easiest-to-digest protein is found in fish and shellfish, followed by meat and poultry. While plant foods are extremely important for health, it's misleading to think of them as a good protein source—even legumes, nuts, and seeds, which technically contain way more protein than fruits and vegetables, are not as rich in protein as animal foods (see page 168). Animal foods contain all twenty amino acids and are the only sources of some other key nutrients, including vitamin B12, creatine, taurine, and carnosine (these last three are not considered essential, but they are very important and promote health). Therefore, a micronutrient-sufficient diet must include fish and shellfish at the very least, if not a wide variety of meats.

Recommended Dietary Allowance for Protein

Protein deficiency is detrimental to all of the body's organs and systems, including impacting function of the brain (especially in infants and young children), immune system, gut barrier, and kidneys. Physical signs of protein deficiency include edema (swelling), poor musculature, dull skin, thin and fragile hair, and failure to thrive in infants and children.

Despite understanding the impact of protein deficiency, calculating the daily requirements for the indispensable amino acids as well as establishing a recommended daily allowance for total protein have proven difficult. In fact, these numbers have undergone considerable revision over the last two decades.

The recommended daily allowance of protein is 0.36 gram per pound body weight (0.8 gram per kilogram of body weight). That amounts to 54 grams for a 150-pound person. However, it's important to emphasize that this number is considered a minimum daily allotment, and there is no established upper limit. In fact, many studies have evaluated diets containing three to four times more protein than this minimum and proven benefits to weight management, body composition, hormone regulation, and cardiovascular health.

The following is the World Health Organization recommended daily allowance for the indispensable amino acids (plus tyrosine and cysteine) for adults. Again, these should be considered minimum targets.

AMINO ACID(S)	RDA PER KG OF BODY WEIGHT, FOR ADULTS AGES 19-50*
Cysteine	4.1 mg
Histidine	10 mg
Isoleucine	20 mg
Leucine	39 mg
Lysine	30 mg
Methionine	10.4 mg
Phenylalanine plus tyrosine	25 mg (total)
Threonine	15 mg
Tryptophan	4 mg
Valine	26 mg

** Visit usda.gov for RDAs for other age groups as well as recommendations for pregnant and lactating women.*

Fatty Acids

Fatty acids, the building blocks of fats, are used not only for energy but also for many basic structures in the human body, such as the outer membrane of every single cell. There are many different fatty acids, each with different effects on, and roles in, human health. A fatty acid has two components. The first is called the *hydrocarbon chain,* a bunch of hydrocarbons (a carbon atom bonded with one to three hydrogen atoms, the number of which varies for different fats) bonded together in a string, or chain. The second is the *carboxyl group,* the molecular formula of which is COOH (one carbon atom bound to two oxygen atoms and a hydrogen atom), which is what makes a fatty acid an acid.

Beyond being categorized based on the length of the hydrocarbon chain, fatty acids are broadly categorized as saturated, monounsaturated, and polyunsaturated. These terms reflect the type of molecular bond between the carbons in the hydrocarbon chain (and therefore also the number of hydrogen atoms bound to each carbon atom).

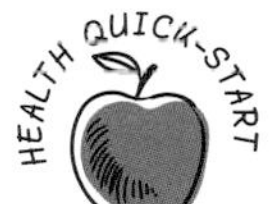

Ditch the low-fat salad dressing! Instead, switch to healthy fats like olive oil, avocado oil, coconut oil, and rendered fats from pasture-raised or grass-fed animals (yep, that includes lard!).

- **Saturated fatty acids.** A saturated fatty acid is one in which all the bonds between carbon atoms in the entire hydrocarbon chain are single bonds (a simple molecular bond in which two adjacent atoms share a single electron). The carbons are then also "saturated" with hydrogen atoms, meaning that each carbon atom in the middle of the chain is bound to two hydrogen atoms. What's special about saturated fatty acids is that they are very stable and not easily oxidized (which means they are not prone to react chemically with oxygen). Beyond making saturated fats highly shelf-stable and excellent for even high-temperature cooking, this means that eating them does not contribute to oxidative stress in the body. They are also the easiest for the body to break apart and use for energy.

THE TWENTY AMINO ACIDS

Alanine: A nutritionally dispensable amino acid involved in sugar and acid metabolism. It can potentially increase exercise capacity, help build lean muscle mass, and improve immunity. Foods high in alanine include animal products (fish, meat, poultry, and dairy), legumes, nuts, and seeds.

Arginine: A conditionally indispensable amino acid that plays a vital role in cell division, wound healing, hormone release, and immune function. Arginine is found in both plant and animal foods, including dairy products, meat, poultry, seafood, nuts, and legumes.

Asparagine: A nutritionally dispensable amino acid involved in cell functions in nerve and brain tissue. It can be synthesized from aspartic acid (see below) but is also found in dietary sources such as plant proteins (legumes, nuts, and seeds), dairy products, beef, poultry, eggs, fish and other seafood, potatoes, and—as you might expect from the similar-sounding name—asparagus.

Aspartic acid: A nutritionally dispensable amino acid that serves as a neurotransmitter and plays an important role in synthesizing other amino acids (asparagine, arginine, lysine, methionine, and isoleucine). It's also involved in the Krebs (see page 267) and urea cycles in the body and plays a role in gluconeogenesis. Foods high in aspartic acid include oysters, wild game, avocado, asparagus, molasses, and seeds.

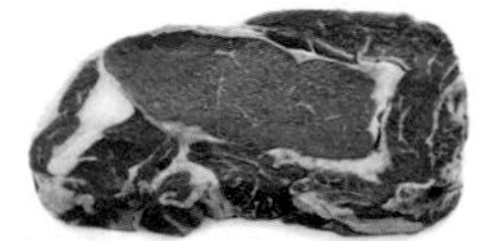

PALEO EASY BUTTON *Aiming for 4 to 8 ounces of meat or seafood with every meal will meet most people's protein needs. Don't forget to round out those meals with plenty of veggies!*

Cysteine: A conditionally indispensable amino acid that helps form the powerful antioxidant glutathione, as well as supports respiratory health and the removal of metal ions and harmful chemicals from the body. Although the body can produce cysteine from another amino acid, methionine (see below), the pathway can be compromised if intake of vitamins B6, B9, and B12 (along with methionine) is inadequate. Dietary sources of cysteine include meat, poultry, eggs, dairy, red peppers, onions, garlic, Brussels sprouts, sprouted lentils, and broccoli.

Glutamic acid: A nutritionally dispensable amino acid that serves as the central nervous system's most abundant excitatory neurotransmitter. It's also a key compound in cellular metabolism and imparts a savory "umami" taste to foods. Sources of glutamic acid include seaweed, meat, poultry, fish, dairy products, and eggs.

Glutamine: A conditionally indispensable amino acid that can help improve intestinal barrier (or gut barrier; see page 67) function and reduce intestinal permeability (which may be associated with many chronic diseases), treat mood disorders, prevent disease-related weight loss, and reduce infection risk. Rich sources include high-protein animal products (fish, meat, poultry, and dairy), legumes, spinach, beets, and parsley.

Glycine: A conditionally indispensable amino acid that plays a number of beneficial roles in the body and may help improve sleep quality, enhance memory, regulate bile acids, and assist in the synthesis of several extremely important proteins. It may also help reverse age-related damage to fibroblasts, a type of cell in connective tissues that produces collagen, and as a result may have antiaging effects. Foods containing glycine include high-protein animal products (fish, meat, poultry, and dairy), spinach, legumes, squash, seaweeds, and cruciferous vegetables.

Histidine: An indispensable amino acid involved in growth, tissue repair, and the manufacture of red blood cells. It helps defend against tissue damage from radiation and heavy metals and plays a role in maintaining the myelin sheaths that protect nerve cells. Histidine is also metabolized into the neurotransmitter histamine, which is involved in immune function, sexual functions, and gastric secretion. Rich dietary sources include high-protein foods like meat, poultry, fish, dairy, beans, and eggs; it is also found in cauliflower, mushrooms, bananas, cantaloupe, rice, bamboo shoots, and citrus fruits.

Isoleucine: An indispensable amino acid that plays an important role in hemoglobin synthesis, blood sugar regulation, and maintenance of energy levels. Foods rich in isoleucine include seaweed, turkey, chicken, fish, lamb, cheese, and eggs.

Leucine: An indispensable amino acid used for a number of metabolic functions, including the formation of sterols in fat and muscle tissue, mTOR activation (which regulates cell metabolism, growth, proliferation, and survival), and direct stimulation of muscle protein synthesis. Leucine is found in hemp seed, beef, fish, almonds, chicken, eggs, beans, lentils, milk, and rice.

Lysine: An indispensable amino acid that is required for growth and tissue repair and that appears to be active against herpes simplex viruses (due to its ability to compete with arginine, an amino acid needed by viruses, for entrance into cells). Dietary sources include red meat, pork, poultry, fish (especially cod and sardines), dairy products, eggs, spirulina, and fenugreek seed.

Methionine: An indispensable amino acid used for angiogenesis (the growth of new blood vessels), the synthesis of cysteine, and the creation of cartilage. It also helps the body produce S-Adenosyl-L-methionine (SAMe), which may benefit psychiatric illnesses and musculoskeletal conditions. Methionine is found in large quantities in eggs, fish, Brazil nuts, sesame seeds, and muscle meats.

Phenylalanine: An indispensable amino acid that supports the structure and function of different proteins and enzymes within the body. It's involved in synthesizing the neurotransmitters dopamine and norepinephrine and can also be converted into the amino acid tyrosine. Phenylalanine is found in most protein-rich foods, including beef, pork, poultry, fish, dairy products, eggs, nuts, and seeds.

Proline: A conditionally indispensable amino acid that's used in collagen production and helps maintain healthy skin, joints, tendons, and cardiac muscle. Foods high in proline include dairy products, meat, poultry, eggs, and seafood, as well as vegetables like broccoli and cabbage.

Serine: A nutritionally dispensable amino acid involved in metabolism, particularly the biosynthesis of purines and pyrimidines. Serine-based molecules are required for the function of many enzymes, fatty acid metabolism, cell membrane structure, muscle growth, and immune function. Rich sources of serine include meat, dairy products, eggs, fish, almonds, asparagus, lentils, pistachios, sesame seeds, cauliflower, fenugreek seed, and beans.

Threonine: An indispensable amino acid that promotes normal growth, supports cardiovascular health, keeps bones and tooth enamel strong, and is involved in liver, central nervous system, and immune system function. Threonine is important for connective tissue and muscle strength and elasticity and may also improve wound healing and recovery from injury. It's found in dairy foods, fish, poultry, meat, lentils, sesame seeds, mushrooms, and leafy vegetables.

Tryptophan: An indispensable amino acid needed for normal growth, nitrogen balance, vitamin B3 synthesis, and making the neurotransmitter serotonin. It's found in most high-protein foods, including eggs, fish, dairy products, turkey, chicken, beef, lamb, sunflower seeds, and sesame seeds.

Tyrosine: A conditionally indispensable amino acid used to produce the neurotransmitters epinephrine, norepinephrine, and dopamine. It also supports adrenal, thyroid, and pituitary gland function and the creation and regulation of hormones. Tyrosine is found in chicken, fish, turkey, almonds, bananas, dairy products, lima beans, pumpkin seeds, sesame seeds, and avocados.

Valine: An indispensable amino acid that works in conjunction with other amino acids (namely isoleucine and leucine) to repair tissues, maintain energy levels, regulate blood sugar, and promote normal growth. Abundant sources of valine include dairy products, nuts, seeds, fish, beans, and mushrooms.

HEALTH-PROMOTING PEPTIDES

Carnosine: Helps slow aging in cells, particularly by protecting against oxidation and DNA damage and slowing the rate of advanced glycation end-product (AGE) formation. It appears to protect against the buildup of atherosclerotic plaque. Foods highest in carnosine include meat, fish, and chicken.

Creatine: Helps supply energy to cells, especially muscle cells. It may help increase muscle strength, boost functional performance, and reduce DNA mutation. Foods high in creatine include animal products like meat, dairy, eggs, poultry, and seafood.

Taurine: Supports neurological development, serves as a major component of bile, and plays a role in water and mineral regulation within the blood (including through membrane stabilization and calcium signaling). It also plays a role in cardiovascular function and the development of skeletal muscle. Taurine is found most abundantly in seafood, dairy products, eggs, seaweed, and certain meats (including beef, lamb, and dark chicken meat).

· **Monounsaturated fatty acids.** A monounsaturated fatty acid is one in which one of the bonds between two carbon atoms in the hydrocarbon chain is a double bond (that is, a molecular bond in which two adjacent atoms share two electrons). This double bond replaces two hydrogen atoms, so the hydrocarbon chain is no longer "saturated" with hydrogen. Monounsaturated fats are less stable than saturated fats and require more enzymes to break apart in order to be used as energy than saturated fats do.

· **Polyunsaturated fatty acids.** A polyunsaturated fatty acid is one in which two or more of the bonds between carbon atoms in the hydrocarbon chain are double bonds (again, replacing hydrogen atoms in the chain). Polyunsaturated fats are easily oxidized, meaning that they are prone to react chemically with oxygen. This reaction typically breaks the fatty acid apart and produces oxidants (free radicals). Consuming oxidized polyunsaturated fats causes oxidative damage to the body.

Polyunsaturated fats are also broadly categorized as omega-3 fatty acids and omega-6 fatty acids. These classifications relate to the location of the first double bond in relation to the end of the hydrocarbon tail. If the first double bond is between the third and fourth carbon atoms, it's an omega-3 fatty acid. If it's between the sixth and seventh, it's an omega-6 fatty acid.

There are only two essential fatty acids. These rather arbitrarily assigned, yet officially deemed essential fatty acids are alpha-linolenic acid (ALA; the smallest omega-3 polyunsaturated fatty acid) and linoleic acid (LA; the smallest omega-6 polyunsaturated fatty acid). The term *essential* is misleading here. The fatty acids with the most profound roles in the human body are arachidonic acid (AA), an omega-6 polyunsaturated fatty acid, and eicosapentaenoic acid (EPA) and docosahexaenoic acid (DHA), both omega-3 polyunsaturated fatty acids. Our bodies can convert any omega-6 polyunsaturated fatty acid to any other omega-6 polyunsaturated fatty acid, and similarly can convert any omega-3 polyunsaturated fatty acid to any other omega-3 polyunsaturated fatty acid—which means that we can make EPA and DHA from ALA and AA from LA. But that conversion can be extremely inefficient, so it's important to get these from food. While ALA and LA are abundant in plant foods, AA, EPA, and DHA are found in seafood, meat, and poultry.

It's also worth noting that the body does best when the ratio of omega-3 fatty acids to omega-6 fatty acids in our diets is somewhere in the range of 1:1 to 1:4. This is one of the exceptions to the "more is always better" approach to micronutrients. Achieving this ideal ratio of omega-3 to omega-6 requires a fair bit of attention to food choices. Omega-6s are abundant in grains, legumes, nuts, seeds, processed "vegetable" oils (like safflower oil or canola oil), poultry (even organic!), and industrially produced meat (the kind that isn't labeled "grass-fed" or "pasture-raised"). On the other hand, the extremely important omega-3s DHA and EPA are found in substantial quantities only in grass-fed meat and seafood (mainly fish and shellfish, but sea vegetables and algae also contain some DHA). Balancing the intake of these fats requires both lowering the amount of omega-6-rich foods in our diets and conscientiously including more seafood.

IMPORTANT HEALTHY FATS

DHA (docosahexaenoic acid): An omega-3 fatty acid that is abundant in the brain and retinas and plays a role in maintaining normal brain function, treating mood disorders, and reducing risk of heart disease (or improving outcomes for people who already have it). The richest sources are fatty fish, such as salmon, mackerel, tuna, herring, and sardines.

EPA (eicosapentaenoic acid): An omega-3 fatty acid that plays a role in anti-inflammatory processes and the health of cell membranes and may help reduce symptoms of depression. Sources include fatty fish (such as salmon, mackerel, tuna, herring, and sardines), purslane, and algae.

CLA (conjugated linoleic acids): A family of naturally occurring *trans* fatty acids that exhibit strong anticancer effects and may improve bone density and increase muscle mass; see page 169. CLAs are found in ruminant meat, such as beef, lamb, and goat, as well as grass-fed dairy.

Monounsaturated fatty acids (MUFA): A type of fat that may help reduce LDL ("bad") cholesterol while potentially increasing HDL ("good") cholesterol and help improve blood sugar control. Foods rich in MUFA include olives, tree nuts like almonds, avocados, and seeds.

Study after study shows that increasing consumption of DHA and EPA, whether via diet or short-term intervention with fish oil supplements, reduces disease severity and symptoms—for instance, it makes the symptoms of rheumatoid arthritis better—and lowers risk of developing certain diseases, such as cardiovascular disease.

No RDA is established for total fat or individual fatty acids; however, the Acceptable Macronutrient Distribution Range (AMDR) is estimated to be between 20 and 35 percent of total calories. This is discussed further in Chapter 2.

Phytochemicals

Phytochemicals are an amazing gift from the plant kingdom. Phytochemicals are compounds in plants that, while not technically considered essential (meaning we must consume them to stay alive), are absolutely vital for optimal health and disease prevention.

Phytochemicals are responsible for giving many fruits and vegetables their rich colors and unique scents, like the deep red hue of tomatoes or the aroma of garlic. They're also a big reason why unprocessed plant foods (fruits and veggies in whole-food form) are found to be disease-protective in study after study. Certain phytochemicals have the ability to slow the growth of cancer cells, help regulate hormones, prevent DNA damage, protect against oxidative stress, reduce inflammation, and induce apoptosis (death) in damaged cells (like a spring cleanup)—just to name a few of their beneficial activities.

Science has only scratched the surface of the 5,000-plus phytochemicals in existence, but we know enough so far to say that many of these compounds are true rock stars! And mounting research suggests that a few classes of phytochemicals in particular play such a major role in human health that their dietary abundance is a necessary feature of any food plan designed to promote health. Another reason why vegetables and fruits feature prominently in the Paleo framework.

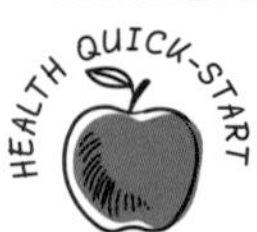

Start eating more veggies! Fresh herbs and high-quality herbal, green, and black teas are also great sources of beneficial phytochemicals.

POLYPHENOLS. Polyphenols are a broad category of phytochemicals that represents the most abundant antioxidants in our diets. In fact, our intake of polyphenols is higher than any other type of phytochemical or vitamin antioxidant. But because of their diversity and complex chemical structures, polyphenols didn't receive much scientific attention until recently (compared to other plant compounds like antioxidant vitamins). As a result, we still have a long way to go before we fully understand how polyphenols exert their health-supportive effects.

For the plants that contain them, polyphenols help protect against sunlight damage (from ultraviolet radiation), deter herbivores, prevent microbial infections, and provide pigmentation (color). And for us humans, polyphenols play a number of important roles as well. Even though polyphenols aren't considered "essential nutrients" (meaning we need them to stay alive), numerous lines of evidence—from epidemiological studies, human trials, animal models, and mechanistic studies—suggest that polyphenols play a huge role in protecting against cancer, heart disease, diabetes, asthma, osteoporosis, neurodegenerative diseases, and other conditions associated with oxidative stress. In fact, a major reason foods like red wine and olive oil (as well as diets rich in both, such as the Mediterranean diet) show up as so beneficial may be due to their high polyphenol content! Along with protecting against chronic diseases, supplementing with polyphenols has been shown to protect against infections and reduce the signs of aging.

So how do polyphenols work? In the body, polyphenols—depending on the specific type—can be absorbed directly in their naturally occurring form, broken down by digestive enzymes, or converted into active metabolites by gut microbes. In any of those cases, once the polyphenols (or their metabolites) finally make it across the small intestine and enter the bloodstream, they can accumulate in tissues all over the body. That's where their health-boosting properties really have a chance to shine!

Polyphenols exert their most potent effects by acting as antioxidants—preventing cellular damage by neutralizing hazardous oxygen radicals and improving cellular health as a result (which, in turn, benefits virtually every system in the body). As a result of their antioxidant properties, polyphenols also boost the immune system and protect against both chronic and acute diseases.

But that's only the beginning of how these powerful molecules work their magic. Polyphenols can also help regulate enzyme function, stimulate cell receptors, modulate the functions of inflammatory cells (including T and B lymphocytes, macrophages, platelets, and natural killer cells; see page 79), alter adhesion molecule expression, affect nerve cells and cardiac muscle cells, and exert antiviral effects. All of these effects translate to polyphenols' amazing disease-protective properties demonstrated over and over in the scientific literature.

Because this class of compounds is so diverse, scientists sometimes divide polyphenols into two subcategories: flavonoids and non-flavonoids (which both encompass even *more* subcategories).

FLAVONOIDS are a diverse group of phytochemicals (including more than 6,000 plant metabolites!) that may help reduce inflammation, exert antibacterial properties, and protect against heart disease and certain cancers. Although flavonoids have a range of different health effects, their benefits seem to be primarily due to helping regulate cell-signaling pathways (rather than by acting as antioxidants, which is a perk many phytochemicals offer). The major flavonoids include:

- **Anthocyanidins and anthocyanins:** These flavonoids give some fruits and vegetables a beautiful blue, purple, or deep red color (think grapes, red cabbage, cherries, eggplant, blueberries, cranberries, raspberries, and blackberries). They appear to have anti-inflammatory and neuroprotective effects and may have pain-relieving properties due to an affinity for certain "pain-sensation" cell membrane receptors in the brain.

- **Flavan-3-ols:** Flavan-3-ols (also called flavanols, not to be confused with flavonols with two o's!) occur in two forms: catechins and proanthocyanidins (also known as condensed tannins). Catechins are found in many types of fruit (apricots are the richest source) as well as red wine and green tea, and proanthocyanidins give certain foods and beverages their astringency—including wine, tea, grapes, peaches, berries, pears, and bitter chocolate. Flavan-3-ols play an important role in vascular health by supporting normal blood flow and maintaining the elasticity of blood vessels, and they may also have anti-microbial, anti-carcinogen, and neuro-protective properties.

- **Flavanones:** Flavanones are a type of phytochemical found abundantly in citrus fruit, and while more research is needed to confirm their effects in humans, studies suggest that they're powerfully cardio-protective. These compounds have been shown to reduce inflammation, reduce hypertension, lower blood lipids, increase insulin sensitivity, and exert antioxidant properties—all of which translate to better protection for the heart.

- **Flavonols:** Flavonols can offer major disease protection by potentially increasing plasma antioxidant capacity, decreasing lymphocyte (a type of white blood cell) DNA damage, increasing activity of an antioxidant enzyme called erythrocyte superoxide dismutase, and decreasing urinary markers of oxidative damage. Flavonols include the cancer- and cardio-protective phytochemicals kaempferol (which can interrupt the growth of a variety of cancers, reduce cardiovascular disease mortality, and protect against diabetes), myricetin (which can protect cells from carcinogenic mutations and protect neurons from oxidative stress while also inhibiting the activity of some viruses), and quercetin (which may suppress inflammation in the brain and promote a healthy gut barrier). Rich sources of flavonols include onions, apples, chives, tomatoes, broccoli, cherries, kale, leeks, and pears.

In addition to flavonoids, non-flavonoid polyphenols play some important roles:

- **Lignans:** Lignans are found abundantly in flax seeds and sesame seeds and in smaller amounts in broccoli, kale, apricots, cabbage, and Brussels sprouts. After we eat lignan precursors, our intestinal bacteria convert them into enterolignans called enterodiol and enterolactone, which can mimic some behaviors of estrogens. Although more research is needed, enterolignans have the potential to protect against hormone-associated cancers (breast cancer, ovarian cancer, prostate cancer, and uterine cancer) by blocking the action of true estrogens. Other studies suggest a role for lignans in reducing inflammation, improving glycemic control, combatting viruses, and protecting against heart disease, but we need more research and better-controlled human trials to clarify whether lignans are responsible versus other components of plant foods.

· **Phenolic acids:** Phenolic acids are powerful antioxidants that can be divided into two categories: derivatives of cinnamic acid (like caffeic acid and ferulic acid) and derivatives of benzoic acid (like gallic acid). The highest sources of phenolic acids are tea (rich in gallic acid), coffee (rich in caffeic acid), and some fruits (including blueberries, kiwis, cherries, plums, and apples). Derivatives of benzoic acid appear to have strong antimicrobial properties, and some studies suggest that cinnamic acid derivatives can protect against heart disease by enhancing cholesterol efflux from macrophages (the key way our bodies protect against atherosclerosis, driven by HDL, where macrophages gobble up cholesterol deposits in blood vessels and return them to the liver for excretion in bile).

· **Tannins:** Tannins are astringent phytochemicals sometimes considered "antinutrients" due to their ability to bind protein and iron. But they actually offer a host of benefits for human health by serving as antioxidants, reducing blood pressure, improving blood lipids, and offering antimicrobial activity. Some tannins can benefit dental health by combating harmful oral bacteria and inhibiting plaque formation. Wine and tea are some of the best-known sources of tannins, but other items include pomegranates, berries, nuts, persimmons, legumes, and certain herbs and spices (cloves, cumin, vanilla, cinnamon, tarragon, and thyme).

· **Stilbenes:** Stilbenes aren't found in very high quantities in most foods, but one particular stilbene—resveratrol—has repeatedly shown up in the scientific literature as having strong anti-cancer properties. Along with its antioxidant effects, resveratrol can thwart all three stages of cancer development (initiation, promotion, and progression) by modulating the pathways involved in cell division, cell growth, cell death, inflammation, angiogenesis (the development of new blood vessels), and metastasis (the spread of tumors). Pretty powerful, huh? Resveratrol is a major reason why red wine (and the grapes it's made from) is strongly disease protective: the richest source is grape skins! Other stilbenes, like rhapontigenin, pinosylvin, and pterostilbene (an analog of resveratrol and the main antioxidant in blueberries), are also being explored for their potential to protect against (or fight existing) cancer, neurological diseases, inflammation, diabetes, heart disease, and stroke. In fact, pterostilbene is emerging as a possible therapy for Alzheimer's disease!

Yep, polyphenols are great! A recent study showed that overall mortality was reduced by 30 percent in participants who ate a diet rich in polyphenols (greater than 650 milligrams/day) as compared with participants who had low polyphenol intakes (less than 500 milligrams/day). For reference, fruits and vegetables typically contain 200 to 300 milligrams per 100-gram serving.

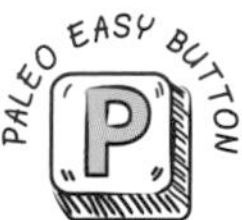

Ever heard that an apple a day keeps the doctor away? Beyond being rich in minerals, vitamins, and fiber, apples are the biggest contributor of polyphenols to the American diet, with about 300 milligrams per apple. When in doubt, an apple is a great addition to a meal or a portable snack!

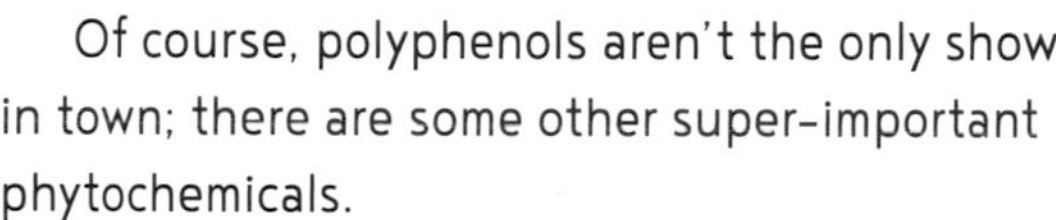

Of course, polyphenols aren't the only show in town; there are some other super-important phytochemicals.

· **Chlorophyll:** Chlorophyll traps light for photosynthesis and is the pigment that gives plants their green color. But this compound plays a beneficial role for humans, too! Chlorophyll is capable of binding to carcinogens (by forming tight molecular complexes) and inhibiting their absorption in the intestines, leading to lower levels reaching body tissues and causing harm. In fact, chlorophyll binds to some of the most widespread foodborne carcinogens, including polycyclic aromatic hydrocarbons (PAHs) and heterocyclic amines (HAs, which can form when cooking meat at high temperatures) and aflatoxin-B1 (which can contaminate peanuts, corn, other cereal grains, pistachios, Brazil nuts, dried spices, and dried fruit—especially when those items were grown and processed in warmer climates).

On top of that, chlorophyll can exert anti-cancer effects through another avenue: inhibiting cytochrome P450 (CYP450) enzymes and increasing the activity of a phase II enzyme called quinone reductase. Enzymes in the CYP450 family are required to turn certain chemicals into active carcinogens, and when their enzymatic activity is reduced, those potential carcinogens don't get converted into truly harmful metabolites. Likewise, phase II enzymes help the body eliminate carcinogens and other harmful substances, so ramping up their activity can also help fight the early phases of cancer.

Where can we find this fantastic phytochemical? Chlorophyll is rich in dark green leafy veggies, especially spinach, parsley, and arugula, as well as green beans and sugar snap peas. Any green veggie will have some, though, and even other colors of vegetables will as well if they're from a part of the plant that grows above ground.

CAROTENOIDS were mentioned briefly earlier, but they're so important that they deserve an even broader discussion. Carotenoids are a group of yellow, orange, and red pigments with potent antioxidant properties. Along with protecting against oxidative stress, carotenoids help facilitate communication between cells by promoting the synthesis of connexin proteins, which create gap junctions in cell membranes that allow small molecules to be exchanged (which is part of how cells "talk" to each other!). This may contribute to carotenoids' cancer-protective properties, since gap junctional communication is reduced in tumors, and increasing it is associated with reduced tumor proliferation. On top of that, carotenoids appear to help protect LDL ("bad") cholesterol from oxidizing.

Most of us are already familiar with β-carotene, but there are actually more than 600 different carotenoids out there. The most extensively studied (and relevant to human health) include lycopene, β-carotene, lutein, and zeaxanthin.

- **Lycopene:** Lycopene is responsible for the red or pink hue seen in tomatoes, pink grapefruit, red peppers, apricots, papaya, peaches, and watermelon. It's best known for supporting prostate health (and potentially reducing the risk of prostate cancer) but can also reduce the risk of other cancers, cardiovascular disease, diabetes, and osteoporosis.

- **β-carotene:** Along with its pro-vitamin A activity (meaning it can be converted into vitamin A by our bodies), β-carotene is a strong immune enhancer that neutralizes free radicals and reduces the risk of some cancers and cardiovascular disease.

- **Lutein and zeaxanthin:** Lutein and zeaxanthin play major roles in maintaining eye health due to their high concentration in the retina and their ability to filter harmful blue-light rays (in turn protecting critical parts of the eye from light-induced oxidative damage). As a result, these two phytochemicals can help prevent and treat age-related macular degeneration, protect against cataracts, and reduce the risk of retinitis pigmentosa. Lutein and zeaxanthin are rich in dark green leafy vegetables, citrus fruit, and broccoli.

By the way, all carotenoids are far more highly absorbed in the presence of fat (even just 3 to 5 grams of fat is enough to do the trick), so be sure to eat carotenoid-rich foods with a little olive oil, butter, ghee, avocado, or other healthy fat (see Chapter 11).

- **Isothiocyanates:** These sulfur-containing phytochemicals are formed by the breakdown of glucosinolates found in cruciferous vegetables (such as broccoli, cabbage, kale, Brussels sprouts, and cauliflower) and are known for their anti-cancer properties (through enhancing tumor suppression and eliminating carcinogens from the body). Some types of isothiocyanates can up-regulate genes involved in protecting against DNA damage, inflammation, and oxidative stress, as well as increase the activity of phase II enzymes (such as quinone reductase and glutamate cysteine ligase) that help remove toxic substances and carcinogens from the body.

- **Organosulfur compounds:** Allium plants (including onions, garlic, chives, shallots, scallions, and leeks) contain a variety of disease-protective phytochemicals called organosulfur compounds, which include dithiolethiones, diallyl sulfide, and sulforaphane. Although these compounds are still being researched, we have strong evidence that they can help protect against stomach and colorectal cancers (due to inhibiting carcinogenesis in various parts of the digestive tract, including the forestomach, esophagus, and colon). Organosulfur compounds exert their effects by modulating important enzymes (the cytochrome P450 family and glutathione S-transferases) that help detoxify carcinogens and prevent DNA adducts from forming. One specific organosulfur compound, diallyl sulfide, also has potent antimicrobial properties and can help fight the stomach bacteria *H. pylori.*

A RAINBOW OF NUTRIENTS

The pigments in different fruits and vegetables are phytochemicals, which is why "eating the rainbow" is important for ensuring that we consume a wide variety of these beneficial compounds. These are the phytochemicals responsible for a fruit or vegetable's color!

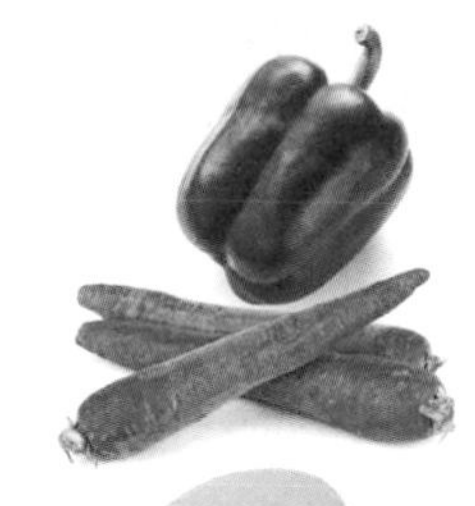

RED: lycopene, anthocyanins

ORANGE: α- and β-carotene, β-cryptoxanthin

YELLOW: β-cryptoxanthin, xanthophylls

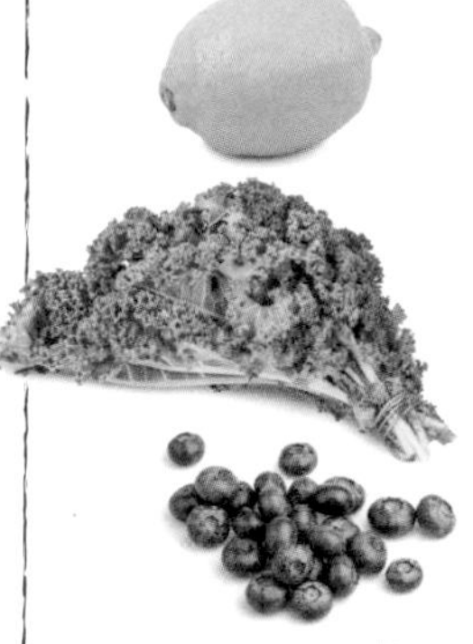

GREEN: chlorophyll, glucosinolates, lutein, zeaxanthin

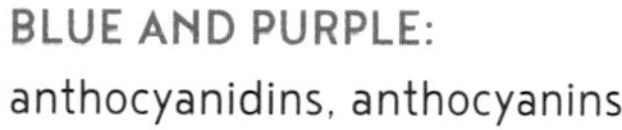

BLUE AND PURPLE: anthocyanidins, anthocyanins

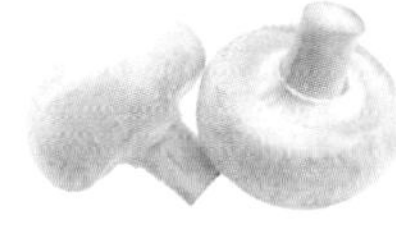

WHITE: anthoxanthins, organosulfur compounds

Of course, there are plenty of other nutrients in fruits and vegetables of different colors, too!

- **Plant sterols and stanols:** Plant sterols and stanols (which are found in nuts, legumes, whole grains, and olive oil, as well as most fruits and vegetables) can help block absorption of cholesterol in the small intestine, due to having a similar chemical structure to animal cholesterol. As a result, these phytochemicals can help reduce high levels of LDL cholesterol in the blood (without impacting HDL levels) and potentially reduce the risk of heart disease.

Whew! That's a pretty impressive array of benefits . . . and remember, it's just a *tiny* sampling of the thousands of helpful phytochemicals that plants contain. These compounds are truly mind-blowing in both their sheer quantity and their value to human health.

Fiber

Plant foods are central to the Paleo framework for a variety of reasons, key among them being fiber. On a basic level, fiber is a type of carbohydrate, meaning that it's simply a long string of sugar molecules (saccharides). Fiber comes from the cell walls of plants. In plant cells, it acts as a skeleton and helps to maintain a plant's shape and structure. There are many, many different types of fiber (different length strings composed of different saccharides, some with branches and some without). The only dietary sources of fiber in Western countries are plant-based foods, including vegetables and fruits (insect and shellfish skeletons contain a type of fiber, but those aren't commonly consumed except in traditional cultures).

HEALTH QUICK-START

Fiber is essential for a healthy gut and endocrine system. Start gradually increasing your fiber intake from whole vegetables and fruits, adding a half serving per day or every other day until you reach a minimum of eight servings of vegetables and fruits per day (see page 156 for more on serving sizes).

What separates fiber from other carbohydrates (starches and sugars) is that the digestive enzymes produced by our bodies that digest carbohydrates by breaking them down into simple sugars (monosaccharides, which are then absorbed across the gut barrier and into the body) are not able to break fiber apart into monosaccharides. Instead, fiber passes through the digestive tract mainly intact.

Some types of fiber (called fermentable fibers) can be digested by the bacteria in our intestines. (These bacteria reside mainly in the large intestine, but there are some in the small intestine, too.) In fact, fiber serves two main functions in the digestive tract: it adds bulk to stool (which makes it easier to pass), and it feeds the probiotic bacteria that live there (which benefits us in many ways). When probiotic bacteria eat fiber, they produce short-chain fatty acids such as acetic acid, propionic acid, and butyric acid. These are extremely beneficial energy sources for the body, including the cells that line the digestive tract, and help to maintain a healthy gut barrier. Short-chain fatty acids are also essential for regulating metabolism and aid in the absorption of minerals, such as calcium, magnesium, copper, zinc, and iron. Healthy gut bacteria have many other important beneficial effects in the body, such as aiding digestion (they release important vitamins and minerals from our food so we can absorb them) and regulating the immune system.

Fiber has other effects, like regulating peristalsis of the intestines (the rhythmic motion of muscles around the intestines that pushes food through the digestive tract), stimulating the release of the hunger-suppressing hormone ghrelin (so we feel more full), and slowing the absorption of simple sugars into the bloodstream to regulate blood sugar levels and avoid the excess production of insulin. Fiber also binds to various substances in the digestive tract (like hormones, bile salts, cholesterol, and toxins) and, depending on the type of fiber, can facilitate either elimination or reabsorption (for the purpose of recycling, which is an important normal function for many substances like bile salts and cholesterol), both of which can be extremely beneficial—if not essential—for human health.

So even though fiber doesn't provide us with energy (like other carbohydrates, fat, and protein) and isn't an essential micronutrient (needed in our diet for survival), it's pretty darned important; in fact, one might argue that its classification as nonessential is erroneous.

Diets rich in fiber also reduce the risk of many cancers (especially colorectal cancer, but also liver, pancreas, and others) and cardiovascular disease, as well as lower inflammation overall. Prospective studies have confirmed that the higher our intake of fiber, the lower our inflammation (as measured by C-reactive protein). In fact, a recent study showed that the *only* dietary factor that correlated with incidence of ischemic cardiovascular disease is low fiber intake (not saturated fat!); the more fiber we eat, the lower our risk. If someone has kidney disease, a high-fiber diet reduces their risk of mortality. If someone has diabetes, a high-fiber diet reduces their risk of mortality. A high fiber intake can even reduce the chances of dying from an infection.

Convinced yet?

So does it matter what types of foods our fiber comes from (and thus what types of fiber we're eating)? Here's why science, once again, supports a high intake of vegetables and fruit. An increasing number of studies support that the health benefits of high-fiber diets really come from a diet high in vegetables (so vegetable fiber) and, to a lesser extent, fruit and nuts (the health benefits are not experienced with a diet high in cereal grains). A high-vegetable diet also reduces cardiovascular disease risk factors and markers of colon cancer risk. How much of this can be attributed directly to the types of fiber in vegetables (mainly insoluble, which I'll expound on next) versus the high vitamin, mineral, and phytonutrient content of vegetables compared to other carbohydrate sources remains unknown. Probably, the benefits come from both.

Now let's look at fiber *types*. Most of us are familiar with soluble and insoluble fiber, at least the terms, if not the details of their definitions. Broadly, soluble fiber dissolves in water, whereas insoluble fiber doesn't. This greatly affects how each type of fiber behaves in the digestive tract.

Soluble fiber forms a gel-like material in the gut and tends to slow the movement of material through the digestive system. Soluble fiber is typically readily fermented by the bacteria in the colon (although not all soluble fiber is fermentable), producing gases and physiologically active by-products (like short-chain fatty acids and vitamins).

Insoluble fiber tends to speed up the movement of material through the digestive system. Fermentable insoluble fiber also produces gases and physiologically active by-products (like short-chain fatty acids and vitamins). Nonfermentable insoluble fiber increases stool bulk, which is believed to be very beneficial in regulating bowel movements and managing constipation.

KNOWLEDGE BOMB *Changing up the type of fiber you consume can make a huge difference to stool quality (assuming you don't have a gut pathology; see page 74). Chronically loose stools? Try eating a more soluble fiber (starchy veggies like sweet potatoes are great sources). Have the opposite problem? Try adding more insoluble fiber (leafy greens are a great source).*

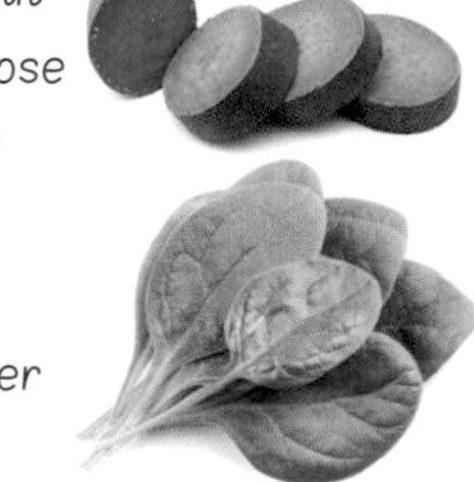

Within these two broad categories, there are many types of fiber, classified based on the types of simple sugars and other components they are made from, the types of bonds between sugars, and the overall structure of the molecule. The major classes of fiber will be discussed in more detail below, but this is how they divide among the soluble versus insoluble categories:

INSOLUBLE	SOLUBLE
Hemicellulose (most)	Hemicellulose (some)
Chitosan (neutral pH)	Chitosan (acidic pH)
β-glucans (some)	β-glucans (most)
Cellulose	Fructan
Lignin	Pectin
Chitin	Gum
Resistant starch	Mucilage

Vegetables and fruits contain a mixture of both soluble and insoluble fiber, but, depending on the specific food in question, might have more of one type than the other.

Classifying a particular fiber as either soluble or insoluble is only one way to describe it. Fiber can also be classified based on whether it is fermentable (if it is, it is considered to be "prebiotic," which just means that it is food for the bacteria that live in our digestive tracts). While soluble fiber has the reputation of being the fermentable fiber, there are plenty of types of insoluble fiber that are fermentable as well, and even some types of soluble fiber that aren't fermentable (or are only weakly fermentable). Fiber can also be classified based on whether it is viscous, meaning how thick it is when it mixes with water and other substances in the digestive tract. (This classification is used to classify soluble fiber because insoluble fiber doesn't dissolve in water.) Many of the health benefits of soluble fiber are specific to high-viscosity fiber. *Functional fiber* is the term for an isolated fiber used as a supplement.

The fibers discussed in more detail below can also be categorized based on whether they are fermentable:

FERMENTABLE	NONFERMENTABLE
Hemicellulose (some)	Hemicellulose (some)
Chitosan	Lignin
β-glucans	Chitin (only weakly)
Fructan	Mucilage (only weakly)
Resistant starch	
Gum	
Pectin	
Cellulose (moderately)	
Mucilage (weakly)	
Chitin (weakly)	

As already mentioned, there are many types of fiber (which are then either lumped into the soluble or insoluble categories or lumped into the fermentable or nonfermentable categories). If we want to understand which types of fiber (or whole-food sources of fiber) are most beneficial to consume, we need to go into far more detail than whether a fiber is soluble or insoluble.

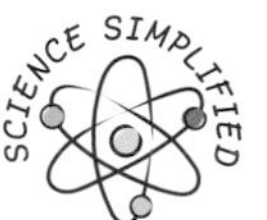

There are many types of fiber, and they all provide slightly different benefits. But if you're getting your fiber from a variety of whole vegetables and fruits, you really don't need to sweat the details!

The main classes of fiber are:

- **Cellulose** is the main component of plant cell walls. Celluloses are identical to starch in the sense that they are long, straight chains of glucose molecules (anywhere from several hundred to more than 10,000 glucose molecules long). However, the links between the glucose molecules are different from those in starch (they are in what is called a β configuration), which make cellulose indigestible to humans. Celluloses are insoluble dietary fibers. The bacteria in our intestinal tracts cannot ferment most cellulose particularly well (although cellulose is partially fermentable). Cellulose is found in all plants, but foods that contain particularly large amounts include bran, legumes, nuts, peas, root vegetables, celery, broccoli, peppers, cabbage and other substantial leafy greens like collards, and apple skins.

- **Hemicellulose** is a common component of the cell walls of plants. In contrast to cellulose, hemicellulose is made of several types of sugar in addition to glucose, especially xylose but also mannose, galactose, rhamnose, and arabinose. Rather than forming long, straight chains like cellulose, hemicellulose may have side chains and branches. Because of these variations, some hemicelluloses are soluble in water and some are insoluble, plus some forms are fermented by bacteria while others are not. Hemicellulose is particularly high in bran, nuts, legumes, and whole grains as well as many green and leafy vegetables.

- **Pectin** is soluble in water and highly fermentable (very little passes through to the colon since it is so readily fermented by bacteria in the small intestine).

Pectins are rich in the sugar galacturonic acid and can be found in several types of configurations (further subdividing this class of fibers by structure). Pectins are found in all fruits and vegetables but are particularly rich in certain fruits, including apples and citrus fruits. They are also found in legumes and nuts.

- **Lignin** is a type of fiber with lots of branches made of chemicals called phenols (rather than sugar molecules). Phenols are currently being studied for a variety of health-related effects, including antioxidant actions (for example, it is the phenolic compounds in olive oil that appear to be responsible for its cardiovascular health benefits). Lignin is unusual because it lacks an overall defining structure. Instead, it consists of various types of substructures that appear to repeat in a haphazard manner. Lignins are insoluble and are not fermentable. Most commonly a component of wood, food sources include root vegetables, vegetable filaments (like the stems of leafy greens and the strings in celery), many green leafy vegetables, and the edible seeds of fruit (such as berry seeds and kiwi seeds).

Hemicellulose, cellulose, and pectin bind together to form a network of cross-linked fibers and together form the walls of most plant cells. Lignin fills the spaces in the cell wall between cellulose, hemicellulose, and pectin components. We get some amount of all four of these whenever we eat any plant-based food.

- **Chitin** is similar to cellulose in the sense that it is made of long chains of glucose (in the case of chitin, it's actually long chains of a particular derivative of glucose called N-acetylglucosamine) and also has amino acids attached. Chitins are insoluble in water and are fermentable, albeit weakly. Chitin is interesting because this fiber is found not only in plants and fungi but also in the exoskeletons of insects and the shells of crustaceans.

- **Chitosan** is similar to chitin in the sense that it is composed of a long chain of N-acetylglucosamine molecules, but it also contains randomly distributed D-glucosamine molecules (like cellulose, linked in a β configuration). Chitosans are naturally found in the cell walls of fungi but are also produced as a functional fiber by treating shrimp and other crustacean shells with sodium hydroxide. Chitosan is a unique fiber. It is soluble in acidic environments, so it starts its journey through the digestive tract as a soluble fiber in the stomach, but when the acidity of the chyme (stomach contents) is neutralized in the small intestine (by pancreatic secretions), it becomes insoluble. It is also fermentable (much more so than chitin).

- **Gums** are a diverse group of fibers that plants secrete when they are damaged. They are complex molecules that contain a variety of types of sugars as well as acids, proteins, and minerals. Gums are soluble and highly viscous fibers and are also fermentable. Isolated (functional fiber) versions are used in food manufacturing as thickening and gelling agents (like guar gum and xanthan gum). Some gums used in food manufacturing increase intestinal permeability through an action on the tight junctions between epithelial cells (one of those cases of the isolated concentrated compound being a problem but the small amount naturally occurring in whole foods being fine); see page 235.

- **β-glucans (more technically β(1,3)-glucans)** are closely related to gums and are also soluble (a minority are insoluble), viscous, and fermentable. They are found in some grains (mainly oats and barley, but also rye and wheat), fungi (yeast and mushrooms, particularly those mushrooms that are used medicinally like shiitake and maitake), and some types of seaweed (mainly algae). β-glucans are the fiber in oats that are mainly responsible for the cholesterol lowering properties of this grain, and, as functional fibers in supplement form, are also known to activate the immune system and may even act as an adjuvant (definitely not good if you have an immune or autoimmune disease).

- **Mucilages** are rich in the simple sugars xylose, arabinose, and rhamnose and have very complex structures. They are soluble and very viscous fibers, forming a thick, gluey substance, and are produced by nearly all plants and some microorganisms. They are particularly concentrated in cacti and other succulents (like aloe), many types of seaweed (like agar agar algae), flax seeds, chia seeds, and psyllium husks. They can also be found in relatively large amounts in a variety of fruits and vegetables, including plantains, bananas, taro root, cassava, and berries. While soluble, mucilages are not particularly fermentable (only partially degraded by bacteria in our digestive tracts). Mucilagenous extracts are often used medicinally, and many of these extracts are known immune modulators or stimulators. For more on mucilage fiber, see Chapter 24.

- **Fructans** are fructose-rich soluble and highly fermentable fibers with simple structures (long chains, some with branches—like the fructose equivalent of cellulose). Shorter chain fructans are called fructooligosaccharides, whereas longer chain fructans are called inulins. Inulin fiber is one of the most heavily studied functional fibers. They are naturally occurring in a variety of plants, including chicory, onions, and Jerusalem artichoke (see "FODMAPs" in Chapter 34).

- **Resistant starch** is really starch (also sometimes called oligosaccharides) and doesn't fit the original technical definition of fiber, which is limited to plant cell wall constituents. Resistant starch is considered to be a fiber because amylase, the enzyme that breaks starch into individual glucose units, doesn't work on this type of starch. Resistant starch is insoluble yet highly fermentable. Green bananas, green plantains, potatoes, and legumes are all sources of resistant starch (particularly when eaten raw). We'll be looking much more closely at resistant starch in our discussion of Paleo starches on page 155.

Whew. And these are only the *major* classes of fiber! Most of these types of fiber can be further divided into sub-subclasses of fiber. They are almost all found to some degree in almost all plants, so when we eat whole vegetables, fruits, nuts, and seeds, we're getting a mix of many of them. We're also getting different forms: the cellulose in an apple peel is different from the cellulose in cabbage, and this may have a slightly different effect in the digestive tract (like so many things in biology/physiology/nutrition, the details have yet to be worked out).

Health Benefits of Soluble versus Insoluble Fiber

So, back to soluble versus insoluble fiber for a moment. Which one is better for us? Many health authorities claim that the answer is soluble. In fact, most of the proposed beneficial effects of fiber consumption are attributed to the viscous and fermentable properties of soluble fiber. In contrast, most studies that evaluate the benefits of soluble versus insoluble fiber show that insoluble is better.

To date, the vast majority of studies evaluating the health benefits of fiber are either correlative studies or studies using fiber supplements. Correlative studies look at a particular group of people, get them to fill out surveys about what foods they eat, and then monitor them for health problems. Then the researchers look to see if there are patterns (like people who ate a particularly high amount of X or Y tended to get Z disease). Fiber supplement studies almost always supplement with soluble, fermentable fibers, most typically inulin or β-glucans. Most of these studies don't (or can't) separate out soluble versus insoluble (and good luck getting more detailed than that!). So mostly what these studies tell us is that our chances of a variety of diseases are lower if we eat a fiber-rich diet (but they can't tell us why or whether the fiber itself is the part that's making the difference). The good news is that there are some studies that are starting to tease out the differences between soluble and insoluble fiber when it comes to health, and these are proving to be very interesting.

Results from prospective cohort studies fairly consistently show that insoluble fiber intake is strongly linked to reduced risk of diabetes. And, while total fiber correlates with decreased risk of cardiovascular disease, this association is much stronger for insoluble fiber compared to soluble. Of course, as is typical in medical research, consensus is hard-won, and there are certainly studies that show the opposite. For example, a study evaluating diet and mortality in type 1 diabetics showed that soluble fiber correlated more strongly than insoluble with reduced risk of complications including death (although both soluble and insoluble fiber reduced risk). Another study in women showed that high soluble fiber intake correlated with reduced risk of developing insulin resistance (but insoluble did not).

Nevertheless, there seems to be a stronger case for health benefits for insoluble fiber compared to soluble, although explanations are still lacking. One possible explanation is the anti-inflammatory effects of insoluble fiber. One prospective study showed that the higher the dietary fiber intake, the lower a person's C-reactive protein (a blood-borne marker of inflammation). The correlation between high fiber and low C-reactive protein levels was even stronger for insoluble fiber than soluble fiber (although both were good).

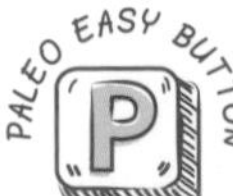

Leafy greens are a great source of insoluble fiber, not to mention vitamins, minerals, and phytochemicals. Aim for a minimum of two to three servings of leafy greens per day.

One team of researchers evaluated the long-term effect of two variations of a diet in mice that would normally cause them to become obese. Two groups of mice were fed high-fat diets identical in every respect (and calorie matched), except one diet contained soluble gum-type fiber and the other contained insoluble cellulose-type fiber. Over the course of the yearlong experiment, the mice fed the soluble-fiber diet became obese, but the mice fed the diet containing insoluble fiber didn't (again, the calories were matched and the two diets were identical other than the type of fiber). The insoluble-fiber group had lower blood sugar levels, too. The researchers made some headway in explaining why. The soluble-fiber group showed markers of happy gut bacteria, like higher breath hydrogen levels and indicators of higher short-chain fatty acid production (which we would expect, since gums are highly fermentable but celluloses are only partially fermentable). But the insoluble-fiber group had lower liver triglycerides and had markers of increased fat metabolism. The authors speculate that this is a direct effect on gene expression from the excess short-chain fatty acids produced with the high-soluble-fiber diet (and show some convincing preliminary evidence to support this explanation). This could explain why the rate of obesity increases with lower fiber intake—a beneficial effect on metabolism from insoluble fiber. This also provides a warning against overdoing soluble fiber (whether through food sources or supplements).

The fact that this study was long-term (almost a year long, where the average life span of a mouse is about 2 years) is important because an amazing crossover in the effects was observed after about the 10-week mark. Early on, the benefits of soluble fiber seemed greater or the same as insoluble fiber. At the 10-week mark, insoluble fiber started to take over as the clear winner, and the effects kept magnifying over time. This might also explain why some studies show that soluble fiber is better: in the short term, it is (probably due to supporting growth of good bacteria). And it explains why prospective studies that look at long-term effects of diet show insoluble fiber to be more beneficial.

Soluble fiber is great for feeding our gut bacteria. And soluble fiber is the type that has been shown to have cholesterol-lowering properties. The short-chain fatty acids that are produced as a result of fiber fermentation are known to be very beneficial (so much so that they are being investigated as a possible supplement, called "postbiotics")—although too much of a good thing might be a problem (the cause of the changes in fat metabolism in the study we just looked at). What about insoluble fiber? Most types are still fermentable (at least moderately). Insoluble fiber is also one of the most important dietary factors suppressing ghrelin after a meal (ghrelin is the main hormone responsible for the feeling of hunger, and it is an important immune modulator—so having high ghrelin before we eat and then having very low ghrelin after we eat is very important; see page 90). Insoluble fiber binds toxins and surplus hormones in the gastrointestinal tract, facilitating their elimination from the body. Furthermore, bile salts are bound by soluble but not insoluble fiber, implying that insoluble fiber supports normal bile salt resorption (recycling) as well as fat digestion, and absorption of essential fatty acids and fat-soluble vitamins.

What about the different subtypes of fiber? As we looked at earlier on, there are many types of fiber, and the health effects are far more complicated than simply evaluating whether a type of fiber is soluble or insoluble. One recent study evaluated the effects of dietary fiber on pancreatic cancer risk and found that both soluble and insoluble fiber reduced cancer risk, but that the associations were strongest for cellulose and lignin. This study further showed that fruit and vegetable fiber reduced cancer risk, but not grain fiber.

This reduced risk might be explained, at least in part, by the phenolic content of lignin fibers. Another study showed that the phenols derived from lignin fibers reduced inflammation, decreased oxidative stress, and protected the kidneys of diabetic rats. Another study evaluating the effects of dietary chitin showed that this fiber is especially good at reducing the pro-inflammatory oxidized low-density lipoproteins (oxidized LDL) in particular (implicated in atherosclerosis), but didn't affect the good high-density lipoproteins (HDL). Lignin-derived phenols were even more effective than supplementation with olive oil extract.

Of course, this is contrasted by a study showing that both chitin and chitosan stimulate a subset of the adaptive immune system (Th1, or type 1 helper T cells that can help some immune and autoimmune diseases but make others worse). β-glucans, on the other hand, also stimulate a different subset of the adaptive immune system (Th2, or type 2 helper T cells this time). Pectins seem to have little to no effect on inflammation. Finally, a pair of studies show that hemicellulose supplementation dramatically reduces inflammation and disease activity in a mouse model of colitis.

Yes, the points seem to be adding up for insoluble fiber. But this isn't to say that soluble fiber isn't beneficial. Hundreds of studies have shown otherwise. This is more to say that soluble fiber isn't the only show in town, and that the often overlooked insoluble fiber (abundant in many vegetables and fruits) may be the true star.

There's also a strong argument to be made for whole-food sources of dietary fiber. Not only are diets rich in vegetables especially linked to reduced inflammation and lower risk of disease, as we've already seen in our discussion of micronutrients and phytochemicals, but there are complex ways that different fibers interact with the body (including the health of gut bacteria, gut motility, rate of macronutrient absorption, a variety of hormones, and the immune system). The best way to protect against possible negative effects of a specific fiber type is to increase variety through vegetable and fruit intake (which means avoiding supplements).

Whew! That was a lot to digest (pun intended). And now that we understand the importance of fiber (and all the hard work it does to support our health), it's easy to see why vegetables and fruits—which deliver a mixture of fiber types—are such valuable additions to our diets. Not only do they provide vitamins, minerals, and a stunning array of phytochemicals, but they're also our best vehicles to bringing fiber to our guts and affecting our health in countless ways.

Cooking breaks down fiber, which can make vegetables easier to digest but also potentially reduces some of the benefits of high fiber intake. As a general rule, some nutrients are enhanced by cooking whereas others are degraded, so eating a mix of raw and cooked vegetables is a good way to optimize their benefits (see page 143).

Another important factor to consider is that nonstarchy vegetables, while high in insoluble fiber, are also good sources of soluble fiber. They also tend to have outstanding amounts of essential vitamins, minerals, and phytochemicals. By focusing on nonstarchy vegetables as the foundation of your fiber intake and having moderate portions of fruit and starchy vegetables as well, you are able to easily reach the recommended intake without overconsuming calories or carbohydrates.

Recommended Fiber Intake

How much fiber do we need? The Recommended Dietary Allowance is 25 grams for women and 30 to 38 grams for men (and most of us don't get that: the average American intake is closer to 8 grams!). However, a variety of studies of hunter-gatherer diets show that most hunter-gatherers consume between 40 and 100 grams of fiber per day (with some populations eating as much as 250 grams per day!). And that's typically with only 35 to 55 percent of calories coming from plants.

It is exceedingly difficult to hit the 100-gram mark with the types of vegetables and fruits available to most of us. But 40 to 50 grams per day is pretty doable with a little awareness of which vegetables pack the best fiber punch and a focus on covering two-thirds to three-quarters of every plate of food in vegetables.

KNOWLEDGE BOMB *Eating grains to get more fiber is like eating carrot cake to get more vegetables. There is far more sugar in whole grains than in vegetables and even fruits.*

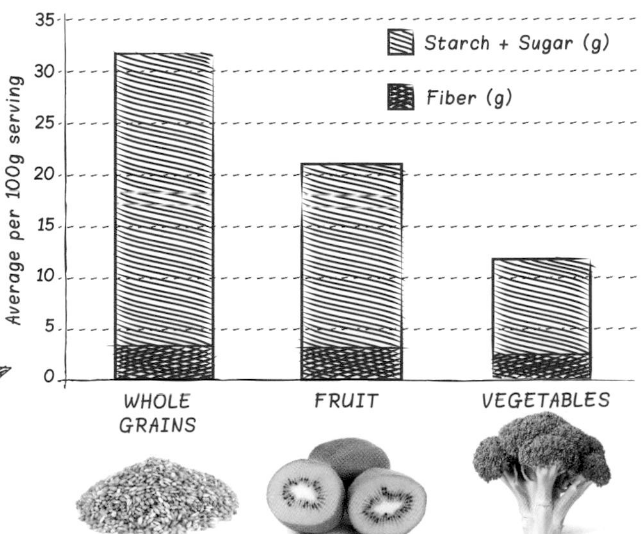

WHAT TYPE OF FIBER DO I NEED?

Does it matter which kind of fiber we eat? Most studies evaluating the impact of dietary fiber on human health do not differentiate between soluble and insoluble but show that fiber in general is beneficial. From the few studies that do differentiate between the two types, we know that a high intake of insoluble fiber reduces the risk of colon cancer, pancreatic cancer, and diverticulitis and correlates even more strongly with lower levels of C-reactive protein (a marker of inflammation) than soluble fiber (which also lowers inflammation). There is also evidence that insoluble fiber can improve insulin sensitivity, can help regulate blood sugar levels after eating, supports reabsorption of bile acids, and is essential for regulating hunger hormones, especially ghrelin.

However, a great many studies on animals evaluating the health benefits of fiber specifically look at inulin (which is a highly fermentable, fructose-rich soluble fiber found in sweet potatoes, coconuts, asparagus, leeks, onions, bananas, and garlic) and show that it reduces intestinal permeability and regulates the immune system. For this reason, soluble fiber gets a lot of attention. In contrast, studies also show that insoluble fiber can improve ulcerative colitis in animals, and there are studies suggesting potential negative health effects from very high intake of soluble fiber in the absence of insoluble fiber. It may be that the health benefits of fiber are derived from whether the fiber is fermentable (meaning that the bacteria in your gut can eat it) rather than whether it's soluble or insoluble. While soluble fiber typically is more readily fermentable, most soluble and insoluble fibers are prebiotics. The medical literature currently offers no clear answer as to whether soluble or insoluble fiber is more desirable. However, the wealth of studies showing health benefits to both imply that each is required for optimal health.

One important factor to consider is that nonstarchy vegetables tend to have a much higher fiber content per calorie than starchy vegetables, which tend to have a little higher fiber content per calorie than most fruit. Of course, all of these choices are better than grains, which contain a ton of sugar and starch and have a high glycemic load (see page 88) for relatively little vitamin, mineral, and fiber content (see page 23). We are accustomed to thinking that we have to eat "healthy whole grains" to get our dietary fiber, but the truth is that grains do not have any more or better fiber than fruits and vegetables.

THE PROBLEMS WITH SUPPLEMENTS

Why is it even important to get micronutrients from food? Can't we just take a good multivitamin and a fish oil supplement to cover our bases and then eat whatever we want? Unfortunately, no. There are several reasons why you can't supplement your way out of a bad diet.

First, the micronutrients in supplements tend to be poorly absorbed, and some synthetic forms of vitamins can't be readily used by our bodies. In the case of fish oil, the process of extracting the oils can damage them, and studies show that they benefit health for only about 4 to 6 weeks, beyond which point they either no longer provide a benefit or may even be detrimental. Second, supplements contain only nutrients that have been identified as the most essential and don't include other extremely important (although not technically essential) nutrients. Given how little we really know about what each nutrient does in our bodies, it seems a bit premature to try to extract them into pill form.

Another issue to consider is that many nutrients work synergistically: they need to be consumed in specific combinations in order to be most effective at enhancing health. At the same time, some nutrients compete with each other, either for absorption or for use (this competition is an important way in which the body regulates certain chemical reactions and protects against toxicity), so consuming those nutrients together in the same supplement means you may benefit from none of them. Our understanding of these relationships between nutrients is still limited, but we do know that whole foods tend to have the right combinations of nutrients to be effective. It is always better to get nutrients from whole foods. And it is always better to choose those foods that are abundant in nutrients.

Fiber supplementation, sometimes labeled as prebiotic supplements, is not recommended. There's a problem with fiber supplementation, whether concentrated inulin or the trendier potato starch as a source of resistant starch: when you supplement with one type of fiber, you are selectively feeding one type (or small group) of bacteria. (For more on resistant starch, see page 155.) Diversity of bacteria is the key to a healthy gut microbial community, and this requires feeding your gut bacteria a variety of substrates (that is, different types of fiber), which can be achieved only with whole-food sources. The best scenario is to focus on large servings (a minimum of eight per day) of a wide variety of vegetables.

NUTRIENT DENSITY QUICK-START GUIDE

When we consider the foods richest in essential vitamins and minerals, certain foods come up again and again as powerhouses of nutrition, especially liver and other organ meat, seafood (especially shellfish), and vegetables of all kinds, but notably leafy greens and vegetables from the cruciferous family (which includes cabbage, broccoli, and kale). One of the best things you can do to ensure that your diet is abounding with micronutrients is to eat these foods liberally.

Taking a nutrients-first approach to diet means eating organ meat, other high-quality meats, seafood (fish, shellfish, and sea vegetables), a wide variety of vegetables in large portions, and some fruit. When those foods form the foundation of our diets, we're guaranteed to consume all the nutrients our bodies need to thrive.

While there's lots of great information coming on the best foods to include in your diet, it's worth taking a moment to share three easy ways to up our nutrient intake.

1 Eat more organ meat!

In traditional cultures, organ meats were treated like gold reserved for the highest echelons of society—and they were definitely on to something! Organ meat is the most concentrated source of just about every nutrient, including important vitamins, minerals, healthy fats, and essential amino acids.

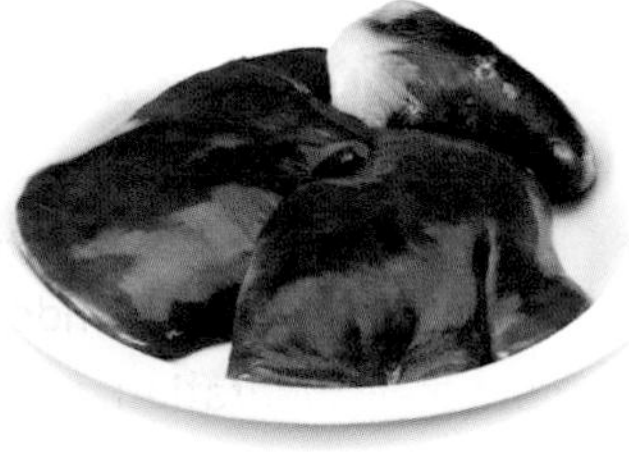

Organ meats are some of the most nutrient-dense foods available, and they provide essential benefits for the immune system, joint health, connective tissue health, cardiovascular health, hormone health, and digestive health. Yet most people who eat a Standard American Diet don't consume any organ meat at all, so they miss out on all of the amazing benefits packed into these fantastic foods!

If you're living on a tight budget, organ meat can be an excellent way to incorporate grass-fed meat into your diet while keeping your spending in check. Even grass-fed organ meat can be significantly cheaper than muscle meat. I recommend consuming organ meat at least twice a week, but the more you can incorporate this nutrient-packed protein, the better!

If you don't like liver or other organ meats, there are several recipes in this book designed to help you "hide" the flavor. The spices in these recipes do a nice job of masking the unique taste of these essential foods. And if organ meat is a complete nonstarter for you, consider adding encapsulated organ meat as a supplement to your diet.

2 Eat more seafood!

Seafood—including fish, shellfish, and sea vegetables—is some of the most nutrient-dense food available. Plus, it's just plain delicious! The amazing news is that varieties of seafood are nearly boundless, and each has unique nutritional benefits.

Fish is high in omega-3 fatty acids (specifically DHA and EPA; see page 158), easily digestible protein, vitamin D, vitamin A, iron, selenium, and many other essential nutrients that aren't as abundant in other foods. Wild-caught saltwater fish have the highest concentrations of vital nutrients, but farmed and freshwater fish are also excellent sources. If your diet includes rich sources of omega-6 fats (like lots of nuts), focus on oily, cold-water fish for their high omega-3 content. Fresh, frozen, and canned whole fish (such as sardines, tuna, and canned salmon, which are the cheapest options) are all great choices! Aim for three to five servings of fish per week as a start; there's no reason why you can't enjoy fish daily!

Many people are surprised to learn about the amazing nutritional benefits of shellfish. Bivalves, including oysters, clams, and mussels, are shellfish with a hinged, two-part shell. These tiny shellfish pack a nutrient punch that almost rivals that of liver! Oysters are a great source of vitamin D, vitamin B12, copper, zinc, and selenium. They support bone health as well as help with the production of red blood cells, maintain nerve cell and immune health, support thyroid function, and protect the body against damage from free radicals. Clams have particularly high levels of vitamin B12, iron, selenium, and manganese, which allows them to aid in nerve and blood cell health, treat or prevent iron-deficiency anemia, protect against cellular damage, form connective tissue and sex hormones, and support carbohydrate and fat metabolism. Scallops also have high levels of micronutrients that help synthesize DNA, enhance nerve and blood cell health, protect cells from free radical damage, boost immune health, and build healthy skeletal tissue. Mussels are great for supporting cellular health, DNA synthesis, fat and carbohydrate metabolism, connective tissue and bone health, and blood sugar regulation. Unless you have an allergy to them, bivalves are an amazing nutrient resource that you should tap into at least once per week.

While sea vegetables are rich in essential minerals and vitamins—iodine, calcium, magnesium, iron, potassium, chromium, selenium, zinc, B vitamins, vitamin C, vitamin E, and vitamin K, to name a few—the more compelling reason to include them in a nutrient-focused diet at least weekly is the dozens of additional trace minerals, many of which are depleted in modern soils and therefore insufficient in vegetables and fruit. If Seaweed Salad isn't your thing, try replacing salt both for cooking and at the table with one that includes sea vegetable flakes.

3 Eat tons (and tons and tons) of veggies!

While some vegetables are nutrient powerhouses, like kale, others contain a unique set of vitamins and minerals that often vary based on the color. A huge part of the Paleo diet is eating a variety of vegetables of all colors to maximize your nutrient intake and the health benefits of all these delicious veggies! So which veggies can help you scoop up which nutrients?

Carotenoids (including vitamin A) are antioxidants vital to immune system function. The vegetables richest in carotenoids include anything red, orange, yellow, or dark green, which includes carrots, beets, squash, sweet potatoes, bell peppers, kale, spinach, collard greens, and broccoli. Tomatoes (yes, I know they're a fruit!) are a great source of carotenoids, specifically lycopene. If you can eat nightshades like tomatoes, then they are a great source of vital antioxidants. Carrots, beets, and sweet potatoes are also rich in B vitamins, as are artichokes, asparagus, okra, broccoli, green peppers, leafy green vegetables, mushrooms, and cauliflower. B vitamins are great for cell metabolism, immune system health, and nervous system function. Many of these vegetables are also excellent sources of vitamins C and K, calcium, chromium, copper, iron, magnesium, manganese, potassium, sulfur, and zinc.

When it comes to committing to Paleo, eating a variety of vegetables is vital to getting the nutrients our bodies need. The best solution in the war against veggie boredom is to head to your local market and try a few new varieties! Kale, for instance, is a nutrient-packed superfood that can be enjoyed raw in a salad, chopped into a soup or stew, or even made into chips. Even your favorite vegetables can take on a whole new flavor with a different preparation. And make sure to "eat the rainbow" to enjoy a variety of essential nutrients. Simply incorporating a different vegetable into a meal can be a great start to upping your nutrient game!

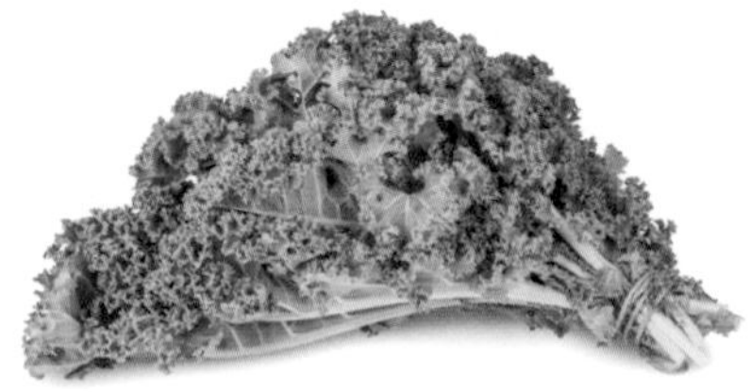

NUTRIENTS AND HEALTH

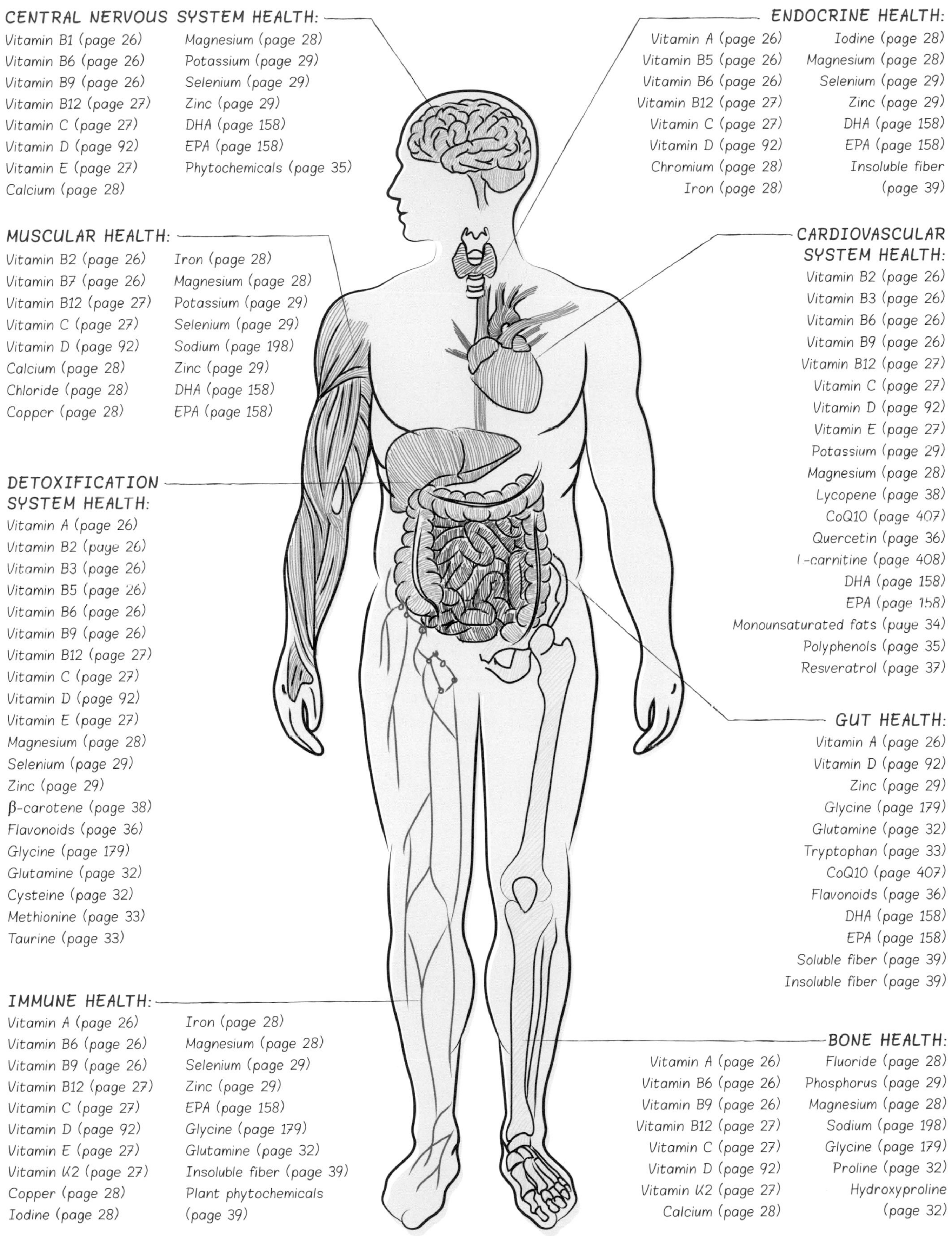

Chapter 2:
BALANCED MACRONUTRIENTS

Macronutrients are the nutrients we need in big ("macro") quantities: fat, protein, and carbohydrate (in contrast to micronutrients like vitamins and minerals that are even more vital for health, but which we need in smaller quantities). That's where the easy part ends! Defining an optimal dietary macronutrient ratio—what percentage of our calories should come from carbs versus fat versus protein—is a contentious issue in the nutrition world, and the debate often bleeds over into the Paleo community as well. In fact, there's a tendency for the media to misportray Paleo as being a low- or zero-carbohydrate diet, a high-fat diet, and/or a high-protein diet.

In reality, none of these labels is accurate. Multiple lines of research suggest that a relatively equal balance of macronutrients (30 to 40 percent fat, 30 to 40 percent carbohydrate, and 20 to 40 percent protein) is ideal for optimizing micronutrient intake and supporting human health. And this is the range into which a well-executed Paleo diet naturally tends to fall.

THE HISTORICAL ARGUMENT FOR BALANCED MACRONUTRIENTS

To understand why balanced macronutrients are part of the Paleo framework, we can start by looking at the fat, protein, and carbohydrate ratios of existing hunter-gatherers (who exhibit dramatically lower rates of chronic disease on their traditional, extremely nutrient-dense diets). Several studies have analyzed the macronutrient breakdowns of these groups, one of the most widely cited being Loren Cordain's 2000 publication "Plant-animal subsistence ratios and macronutrient energy estimations in worldwide hunter-gatherer diets." In this paper, Cordain and his team look at the ethnographic data for 229 hunter-gatherer societies (defined as relying solely on hunting, gathering, and/or fishing for their food) and estimate the average intake of fat, carbohydrates, and protein.

Not surprisingly, the intakes were pretty diverse! However, excluding outlier groups living in harsh climates (like the Inuit of the arctic north, whose diet is extremely atypical and a product of the sparse environment), the majority of hunter-gatherer diets fell within the following macronutrient ranges:

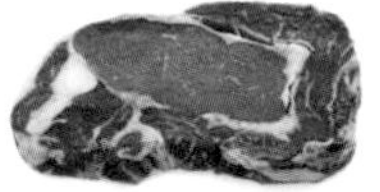

19% TO 35% PROTEIN

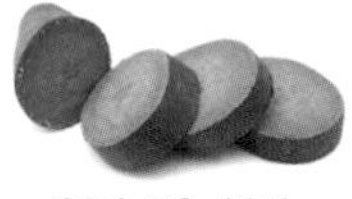

22% TO 40% CARBOHYDRATE

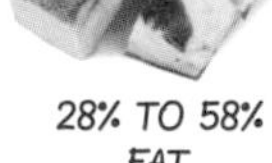

28% TO 58% FAT

In general, hunter-gatherers living close to the equator had higher carbohydrate intakes than populations living closer to polar regions, and virtually every group residing between 11 and 40 degrees north or south of the equator (equivalent to the range between Barranquilla, Colombia, and New York City) ate between 30 to 35 percent carbohydrates as a percentage of total calories.

Macronutrient data for all of these societies is estimated and prone to some error, however. For example, early ethnographers may have underestimated plant food and carbohydrate intake due to interacting more with male hunters than female gatherers. Fat intake may be overestimated due to most wild game being leaner than the grain-fattened (or even just grass-fed) animals raised on farms or may be underestimated due to hunter-gatherers often favoring certain parts of a carcass—especially organs, which tend to have a higher fat content—and, at least when food is abundant, discarding potentially edible parts of an animal instead of consuming the entire thing.

Even though measurements of hunter-gatherer macronutrient ratios can never be precise, it's safe to say that most populations subsisting on indigenous game, fish, and plants ended up with relatively balanced macronutrients.

Another interesting property of hunter-gatherer diets is seasonal changes in macronutrient ratios. In stark contrast to the Standard American Diet's year-round abundance of nearly every food, hunter-gatherer societies experience fluctuating availability of various plant and animal products—leading to seasonal changes in macronutrient ratios. For instance, the Hadza of Tanzania see a rise in meat consumption (and therefore fat and protein intake) during the dry season, when both humans and wild game start frequenting local watering holes. Various other tribes consume more carbohydrates when fruit, honey, and starchy roots are abundant and rely more on hunting and fishing when energy-dense plant foods are harder to find. This can be replicated in Western cultures by eating seasonally (see page 54).

Hunter-gatherers also experience cycles of feast and famine. As with fluctuating availability of different foods, fluctuating availability of food in general is an issue. On a day-to-day, week-to-week, and month-to-month basis, hunting and gathering successes can wax and wane. Periods of scarcity and hunger are interspersed with periods of feasting and abundance, leading to cyclical changes in energy consumption. While there may be advantages to intermittent or occasional short-term fasting for some people (see page 91), contemporary biology supports avoiding caloric excess (averaged over many days, which can mean that some days have fewer calories than you need to maintain your current body weight and other days contain more calories) as a primary property of a health-promoting diet.

OTHER SCIENTIFIC ARGUMENTS FOR BALANCED MACRONUTRIENTS

Of course, eating Paleo isn't simply about reenacting what early humans (or existing hunter-gatherers) ate! Additional science supports the idea that balanced macronutrients are more sustainable and health-supportive than macronutrient extremes (such as very low fat or very low carbohydrate). Another way to frame the issue is to determine how much of each macronutrient we need to avoid problems associated with either micronutrient deficiency or excess.

The Food and Nutrition Board of the Institute of Medicine has set Accepted Macronutrient Distribution Ranges (AMDR) for protein, fat, and carbohydrates based on evidence from interventional trials with support of epidemiological evidence that suggests a role in the prevention or increased risk of chronic diseases and based on ensuring sufficient intake of essential nutrients. While these percentages don't match up perfectly with hunter-gatherers, we see some alignment with AMDR for fat estimated to be 20 to 35 percent of total energy and protein estimated to be 10 to 35 percent of total energy for adults.

With carbohydrates, for example, consuming enough fiber is a high priority. Simple math shows that in order to meet current USDA fiber recommendations (25 to 38 grams per day), we need to eat a bare minimum of 50 to 76 grams of total carbohydrate, because the highest-fiber-per-calorie foods (leafy greens) have about a 1:1 ratio of fiber to nonfiber carbs. If we add other vegetables, starches, or fruit to the equation, that number quickly gets closer to 100 to 200 grams of carbohydrate (20 to 40 percent of calories on a 2,000-calorie diet), just to consume enough fiber! Likewise, carbohydrate-rich plant foods are our best sources of vitamin C, polyphenols, chlorophyll, carotenoids, isothiocyanates, and organosulfur compounds, all of which play various roles in disease prevention. And while the AMDR for carbohydrates as an estimated 45 to 65 percent of total energy (and below 25 percent from sugars) doesn't quite align with hunter-gatherer intakes, it does support the tenet that consuming too little carbohydrate can shortchange us in terms of fiber, vitamins, minerals, and phytochemicals.

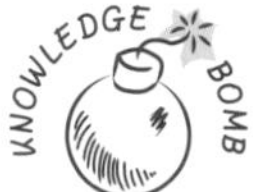

Low-carbohydrate diets make it extremely tough to meet fiber recommendations.

Current mainstream fiber recommendations are 25 grams per day for women and 30 to 38 grams per day for men. This is definitely less than what most Paleolithic and modern hunter-gatherers consumed (professors Boyd Eaton and Melvin Konner estimate 45.7 grams per day for a typical hunter-gatherer diet of 65 percent plant foods, and Dr. Jeff Leach estimates that some hunter-gatherers eat as much as 200 grams of fiber per day), but I'll use the USDA recommendations for the sake of illustration. If we look at nonstarchy vegetables with the highest ratio of fiber to nonfiber carbohydrates, we see that spinach comes out near the top, with roughly half of its carbohydrates coming from fiber. In order to get 25 grams of fiber per day from spinach, our minimum carbohydrate intake would be 50 grams. And for the record, we'd need to eat about 24 cups of raw spinach (almost 1½ pounds) to reach that level. That's pretty ambitious, even for those of us who love veggies!

Using this logic, a total carbohydrate intake of less than 50 grams per day (the upper limit for most low-carb diet recommendations) is almost guaranteed to shortchange us on fiber. And that's assuming we eat nothing but the highest-fiber carbohydrate sources available. When our diet includes starchier or more sugary carbohydrate sources like tubers and fruits, which have a lower ratio of fiber to nonfiber carbs (while also being denser fiber sources), the minimum total carbohydrates we need to eat to meet our fiber needs rises even higher. For example, you'd need only about 3½ cups of baked sweet potato to get 25 grams of fiber, but then, of course, you're looking at nearly 150 grams of total carbs.

Provided that your carbohydrates are coming from whole fruits and vegetables, the 100- to 200-gram range (20 to 40 percent of a 2,000-calorie diet) is probably adequate from a fiber consumption standpoint. Of course, if you're keen to emulate hunter-gatherer fiber intake, it would be incredibly challenging to do so without your total carbohydrate intake creeping up toward 300 grams or more.

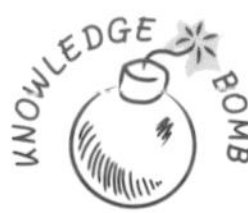

Think that a low-carb or low-fat diet is the magic bullet for weight loss? That's a myth! *See page 400.*

On the other hand, an extremely high carbohydrate intake (more than 70 percent of calories) leaves less room for dietary fat and protein, which creates its own set of problems. Inadequate fat can decrease our absorption of vitamins A, D, E, and K (which ultimately affect every system in our bodies, and which themselves tend to be most concentrated in fatty foods), as well as deprive us of essential fatty acids (especially omega-3) that play vital roles in cardiovascular health, inflammation regulation, cellular growth and repair, immune function, brain health, and cancer prevention—among many other roles! In fact, too little fat is associated with increased risk of coronary heart disease whereas too high of carbohydrate is associated with increased risk of obesity and complications of obesity like increased risk of coronary heart disease—just like Goldilocks, we're looking for that just-right middle ground.

Excessive fat intake is associated with increased risk of obesity, diabetes, cardiovascular disease, dementia, certain cancers, and even certain autoimmune diseases. Of course, it's not as simple as "go low-fat," which comes with its own health risks like obesity, diabetes, cardiovascular disease, depression and anxiety, certain cancers, depressions, and certain autoimmune diseases. (Yes, those lists are nearly identical! Mind blown, right?) It turns out that a huge variety of factors are at play here, like the type of fat, the overall quality of the diet, whether the diet includes excess calories, and whether the person is overweight. And even though many of these details still need to be worked out, the take-home message is clear: Goldilocks wins again.

Inadequate protein can cause muscle wasting, reduce immune function, and negatively affect bone mineral density. Although the human requirement for protein is relatively low for basic survival (the World Health Organization advises 0.8 gram of protein per kilogram of body weight), science consistently points to benefits from a higher intake—including greater thermogenesis (production of body heat, which burns calories), better preservation of lean muscle tissue (especially during weight loss), greater satiation after eating, better appetite regulation, a lower rate of weight regain after loss, better body composition, easier fat loss on reduced-calorie diets, improved blood glucose control, and greater bone density.

A special note on ketogenic diets before we move on. Extremely low-carbohydrate diets that induce ketosis have been gaining popularity (both for weight loss and for their neurological effects) and are sometimes associated with Paleo due to erroneous beliefs about carbohydrates being scarce during early human evolution, as well as the classic example of the hunter-gatherer Inuit subsisting on extremely low carbohydrate intakes. How does this square with the Paleo tenet of balanced macros?

For one, as I'll explain later, carbohydrates were anything but irrelevant in evolution (in fact, the consumption of starchy plants may have been a key factor in what made us human!). Two, the Inuit—along with being a true anomaly on the hunter-gatherer diet spectrum and not representative of typical carbohydrate intakes—have a special gene mutation that prevents them from entering ketosis (instead, they're able to burn long-chain fatty acids for energy, which may help increase their body temperature in their notoriously cold climate). The mutation occurs on the CPT1A gene and makes it so that any situation that would require relying on ketones (such as fasting or an extremely low protein intake along with low carbohydrates) becomes virtually lethal to the Inuit (this may be the cause of their higher infant mortality rate). It also solves the previous mysteries as to why no elevated ketone levels have been found among the Inuit and why they have normal glucose tolerance on their traditional diet (something not seen during ketosis due to the physiological insulin resistance that occurs). In other words, the Inuit are an extremely poor example of nutritional ketosis and shouldn't be used to argue that sustained ketosis is a defining feature of Paleo eating.

What's more, even if the Inuit didn't possess their unique gene mutation, their diet still wouldn't be ketogenic due to its super-high protein content (averaging 280 grams per day), since protein can be converted to glucose through the process of gluconeogenesis (and thus curtail ketosis) and due to some unique sources of dietary carbohydrates like the glycogen in whale blubber. In reality, we have no evidence of any hunter-gatherer society surviving on a ketogenic diet—even among the handful living in environments where it would theoretically be possible.

That being said, ketogenic diets have an amazing track record for treating epilepsy and certain other neurological conditions, and a growing body of evidence suggests that they might improve the outcome of brain cancers. For most of us, though, extremely low carb diets are neither necessary nor beneficial. Reported side effects include gastrointestinal disturbances, amenorrhea (loss of periods in women), impaired mood, hypoglycemia, kidney stones, increased susceptibility to infection, long QT intervals (a disorder of the heart's electrical activity that can cause dangerous arrhythmias in response to exercise or stress), hair loss, muscle cramps or weakness, impaired concentration, disordered mineral metabolism, increased fracture risk, and a shift toward atherogenic lipid profiles (high total cholesterol and LDL with low HDL, known to increase the risk of cardiovascular disease in the general population) in some people. Other potential issues require much more research before we fully understand the long-term effects of ketogenic diets and can declare them safe. In particular, the impact on the gut microbiota (gut health is strongly supported by fiber intake from carbohydrate-containing foods) and fertility in women without polycystic ovarian syndrome (the hormonal shifts seen in very-low-carbohydrate diets can be beneficial for women with PCOS but are problematic for those whose hormone levels are normal to begin with) are potential red flags.

Clearly, eating enough carbohydrate, fat, *and* protein is key for meeting a wide range of nutritional needs. That's why the Paleo template embraces a roughly balanced intake of all three.

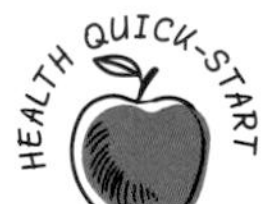

What does a balanced-macronutrients plate look like? About 6 to 8 ounces of meat or seafood, 1/2 to 1 cup of a starchy vegetable like sweet potato, 1 to 2 cups of nonstarchy veggies like broccoli or collards, and 1/2 cup of fruit for dessert. Go ahead and choose fattier cuts of meat or roast your veggies with a healthy fat (see Chapter 11), but don't go out of your way to add fat to your plate. (There's no need to douse your food in butter or salad dressing.) Scale up or down depending on your total caloric needs.

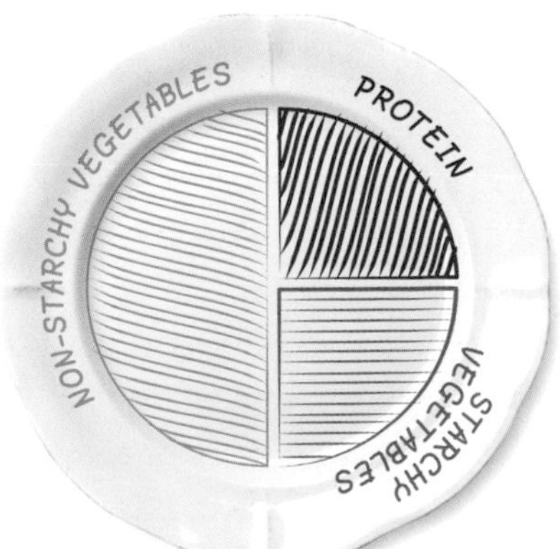

GUIDE TO EATING SEASONALLY

Eating seasonally simply means choosing only those fruits and vegetables that are in season, typically grown locally. Of course, this will vary depending on the climate you live in. For example, strawberries and asparagus are usually harvested beginning in late spring, peaches and cherries in summer, apples in fall, and citrus fruits and cruciferous veggies like kale and Brussels sprouts in winter. An easy way to eat seasonally (and eat the best-quality produce) is to do the bulk of your shopping at local farms and farmers markets. This may or may not be practical depending on where you live, so you may need (or want) to supplement with produce from the grocery store (in season, even if not grown nearby). Fruits and vegetables also tend to be cheaper when they are in season (since supply is high), which is great for anyone on a tight budget.

WHAT'S IN SEASON WHEN*?

SPRING

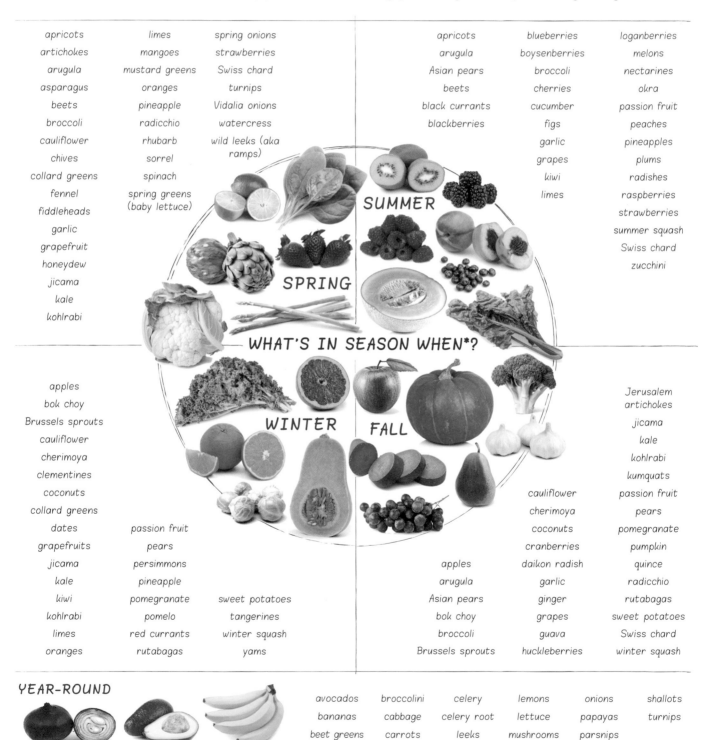

apricots
artichokes
arugula
asparagus
beets
broccoli
cauliflower
chives
collard greens
fennel
fiddleheads
garlic
grapefruit
honeydew
jicama
kale
kohlrabi
limes
mangoes
mustard greens
oranges
pineapple
radicchio
rhubarb
sorrel
spinach
spring greens (baby lettuce)
spring onions
strawberries
Swiss chard
turnips
Vidalia onions
watercress
wild leeks (aka ramps)

SUMMER

apricots
arugula
Asian pears
beets
black currants
blackberries
blueberries
boysenberries
broccoli
cherries
cucumber
figs
garlic
grapes
kiwi
limes
loganberries
melons
nectarines
okra
passion fruit
peaches
pineapples
plums
radishes
raspberries
strawberries
summer squash
Swiss chard
zucchini

WINTER

apples
bok choy
Brussels sprouts
cauliflower
cherimoya
clementines
coconuts
collard greens
dates
grapefruits
jicama
kale
kiwi
kohlrabi
limes
oranges
passion fruit
pears
persimmons
pineapple
pomegranate
pomelo
red currants
rutabagas
sweet potatoes
tangerines
winter squash
yams

FALL

apples
arugula
Asian pears
bok choy
broccoli
Brussels sprouts
cauliflower
cherimoya
coconuts
cranberries
daikon radish
garlic
ginger
grapes
guava
huckleberries
Jerusalem artichokes
jicama
kale
kohlrabi
kumquats
passion fruit
pears
pomegranate
pumpkin
quince
radicchio
rutabagas
sweet potatoes
Swiss chard
winter squash

YEAR-ROUND

avocados
bananas
beet greens
broccolini
cabbage
carrots
celery
celery root
leeks
lemons
lettuce
mushrooms
onions
papayas
parsnips
shallots
turnips

*Based on North American harvests. Varies regionally.

Chapter 3: DIVERSE OMNIVORISM

Another big-picture principle of the Paleo template is *diverse omnivorism*—eating a variety of high-quality foods from both the plant and animal kingdoms. Rather than being vegan or carnivorous, the Paleo diet maximizes nutrient density (and nutrient diversity!) by including food sources that fly, run, swim, grow on trees, and sprout from the ground.

The rationale for this Paleo tenet is rooted in evolutionary biology, basic anatomy, and human nutritional requirements. Despite seemingly endless controversy about whether humans are anatomical herbivores or carnivores, our need for (and adaptation to) both plants and animals is written all over our history, anatomy, and DNA. No matter which angle we approach it from, we're clearly omnivores. For starters, let's dive deep into history to see how both plant and animal foods played critical roles during human evolution.

THE EVOLUTION OF THE HUMAN DIET

Although there's no good reason to throw on a loincloth and try to replicate everything our early ancestors did, studying what they ate (and how their diet shifted over the course of thousands or millions of years) can tell us a lot about the forces that shaped the human genome and established our nutritional needs. When we view diet through this lens, our status as omnivores is clear as daylight.

One way scientists figure out what early humans ate is through something called *isotope analysis*. Basically, different foods leave different carbon and nitrogen "signatures" in our bones and teeth after they've been ingested and incorporated into our tissues. Plants that use the C3 pathway of photosynthesis (like temperate-climate fruits, berries, nuts, leaves, and grains that thrive in wet environments) leave a different carbon signature than plants that use the C4 pathway of photosynthesis (like dry-climate grasses, sedges, roots, seeds, grains, and starchy underground storage organs [things like tubers and bulbs]).

So scientists can gauge the ratio of C3 to C4 plants that early humans ate by looking at carbon measurements in fossilized remains. Eating animals that consume C4 plants, like grass-grazing ruminants, can leave a carbon signature similar to eating C4 plants directly—so scientists have to use other methods to get a sense of whether the carbon came from plant or animal foods. Those methods include looking at nitrogen isotopes, which tell us about protein intake; examining archeological sites for tools and food remains; analyzing dental wear and tooth structure; and studying coprolites (fossilized feces).

Carbon and nitrogen isotope analysis can also help us differentiate between land-based and marine protein sources and legume and non-legume foods, as well as tell us whether any animals consumed were herbivores or carnivores.

From these methods, scientists can paint a decent picture of what our ancient ancestors' diets looked like and how their eating patterns changed over the course of history:

FROM 4.4 MILLION YEARS AGO TO ABOUT 3.3 MILLION YEARS AGO:
The diet of our earliest ancestors (after splitting with our last common ancestor, the chimpanzee) was almost identical to that of modern primates: lots of C3 plants in the form of fruits, nuts, and leaves. There is virtually no evidence of C4 plant consumption.

1.95 MILLION YEARS AGO:
Our early ancestors were butchering and consuming aquatic animals such as turtles, crocodiles, and fish, as well as eating a variety of aquatic and shoreline plants.

1.5 MILLION YEARS AGO:
There's some sporadic (but inconclusive) evidence that early human populations started controlling fire (in which case, cooking would make a lot of sense as a contributor to increased brain size and decreased gut size), but the jury's still out until we have more evidence to draw from.

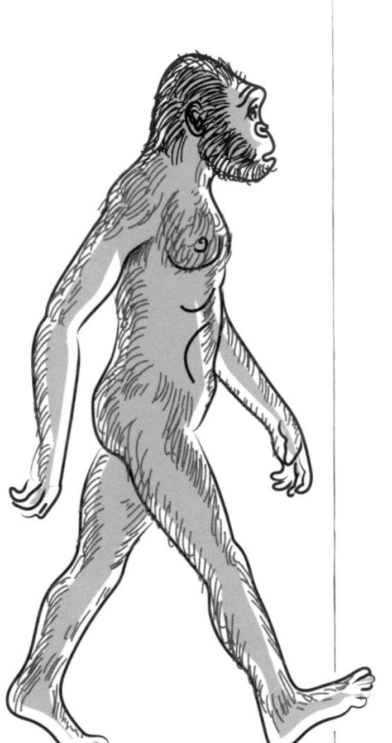

2.5 MILLION YEARS AGO:
We see the first strong indication of meat-eating, although we can't say for sure how much came from hunting versus scavenging.

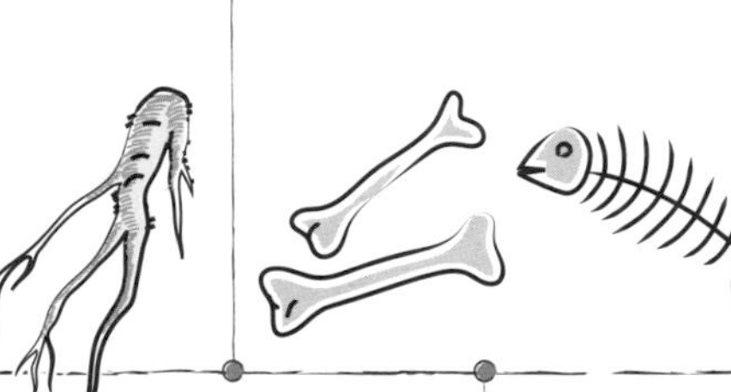

3 MILLION YEARS AGO:
Here we saw a major shift, where dry-climate C4 plants (and possibly the animals that grazed on them, but there isn't much evidence for that yet) entered the diet of our early ancestors. Basically, hominins stopped relying on forest resources and started eating more foods derived from grasses and succulents, such as seeds and roots.

2 MILLION YEARS AGO:
Some human ancestors engaged in "persistent carnivory"—that is, deliberately and frequently eating animal foods (which isn't to say that's all they were eating).

1.9 TO 1.8 MILLION YEARS AGO:
Homo erectus emerged and experienced a simultaneous increase in brain size and decrease in gut size that suggests some important dietary changes were happening—namely, an improvement in diet quality (foods that were denser, more calorie- and nutrient-rich, and easier to digest). Unfortunately, we don't know whether that improvement was from cooking, from advanced stone tool technology that made food processing easier, or both. And we don't know whether the increased energy density was from meat, from starchy plant foods like underground storage organs (USOs), or both. Since fire evidence, vegetation, and sticks used for digging up roots don't preserve very well in the fossil records, it's really hard to determine the role of plant foods versus meat in the dramatic physical changes of Homo erectus, and we'll probably be debating the issue for a long time.

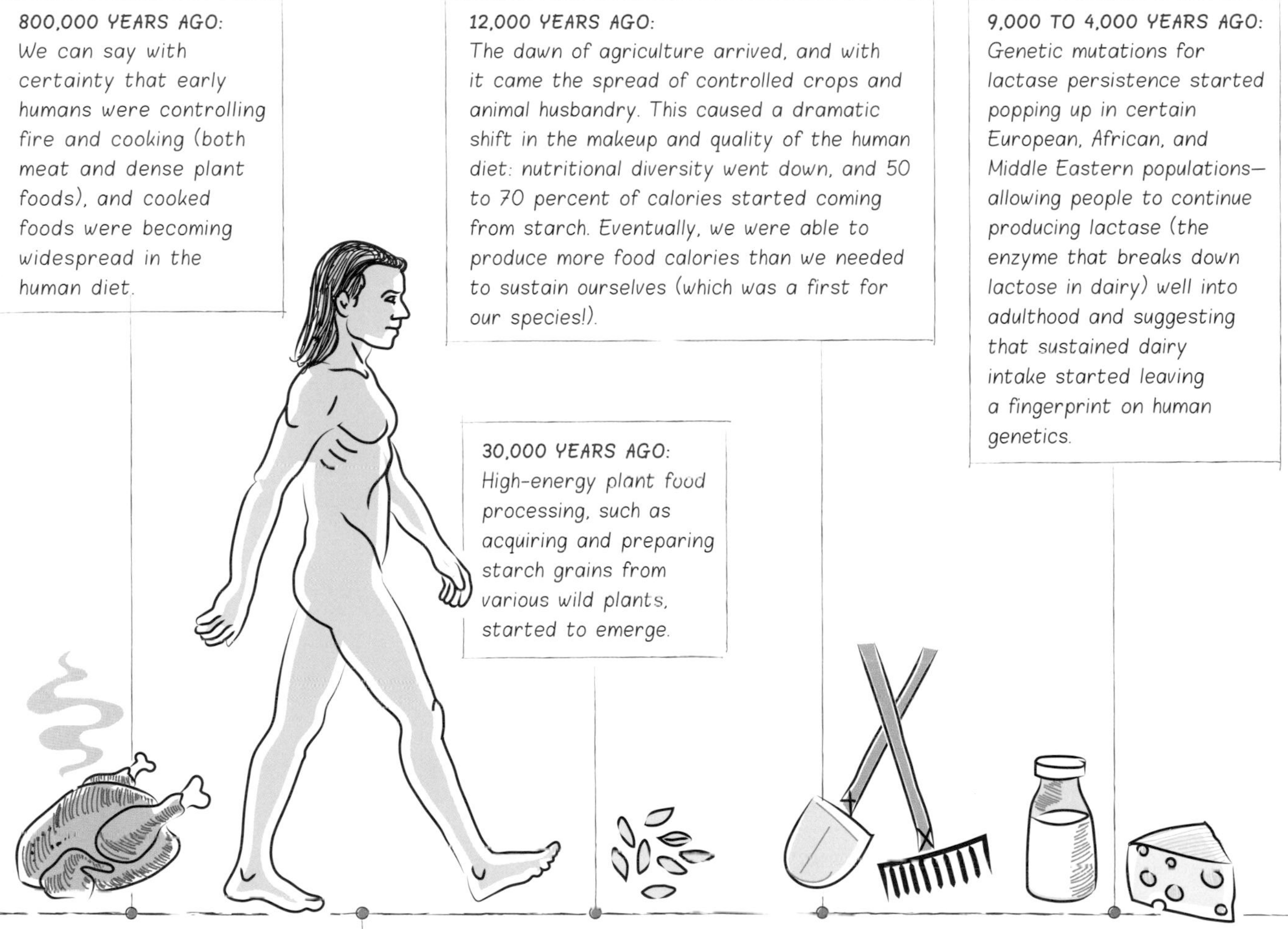

800,000 YEARS AGO:
We can say with certainty that early humans were controlling fire and cooking (both meat and dense plant foods), and cooked foods were becoming widespread in the human diet.
12,000 YEARS AGO:
The dawn of agriculture arrived, and with it came the spread of controlled crops and animal husbandry. This caused a dramatic shift in the makeup and quality of the human diet: nutritional diversity went down, and 50 to 70 percent of calories started coming from starch. Eventually, we were able to produce more food calories than we needed to sustain ourselves (which was a first for our species!).
9,000 TO 4,000 YEARS AGO:
Genetic mutations for lactase persistence started popping up in certain European, African, and Middle Eastern populations—allowing people to continue producing lactase (the enzyme that breaks down lactose in dairy) well into adulthood and suggesting that sustained dairy intake started leaving a fingerprint on human genetics.
30,000 YEARS AGO:
High-energy plant food processing, such as acquiring and preparing starch grains from various wild plants, started to emerge.

200,000 YEARS AGO:
Homo sapiens appeared, which is the species that you and I (and all modern humans) belong to.

What an amazing journey! Clearly, we can see that meat-eating has been a component of the human diet (and that of our pre-human ancestors) for *at least* 2.5 million years. At the same time, we can see that plant foods have long played an important and sustained role. The gut shrinkage seen with *Homo erectus* limited our ability to derive energy from seriously tough plant matter (like stems and twigs), but we still have colons chock full of bacteria that love fiber and other plant components, and for no extended period in history did we appear to eat animal foods exclusively. Our ancient ancestors thrived on plant *and* animal foods, which is one reason why Paleo embraces omnivory.

SCIENCE SIMPLIFIED

Humans have a long history of eating nutrient-dense plant and animal foods, which shaped our biology as we evolved. However, agriculture and the processing of grains go back only a little over 10,000 years. While we have partially adapted genetically to this dramatic dietary shift (see page 311), our physiology and nutritional needs are much more aligned with our ancient diets.

COMPARATIVE BIOLOGY: EVIDENCE FOR OMNIVORY

Despite the reality of our evolutionary history, arguments still abound that we must be herbivores (or carnivores) based on biology and physiology (such as analyses of other primates' diets, comparative anatomy, and other features that might help clarify our taxonomy—like teeth and length of the digestive tract). After all, just because we *choose* to eat both plants and animals doesn't mean that's what we're biologically suited for. We might choose to eat double-glazed donuts when they're sitting on the counter, too, but that doesn't make them good for us! So let's take a quick look at these arguments and see how, viewed objectively, they still support the concept of humans being omnivores.

From the vegan and vegetarian angle, a common justification for humans being herbivores comes from comparative anatomy with other primates—especially chimpanzees, one of our closest living relatives. The argument typically goes that: 1) the higher primates are essentially herbivores (with a trivial amount of insects on menu, but not enough to be nutritionally important) and 2) human anatomy is very similar to primate anatomy, so 3) the diet they eat resembles the one we're suited for. That *sounds* logical on the surface, but it doesn't hold up under scrutiny.

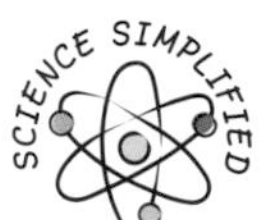

It's a myth that humans are natural herbivores and are better suited physiologically to vegetarian or vegan diets.

It's definitely true that chimpanzees love eating fruit, leaves, and other vegetation, and these foods comprise the bulk of their diet. But chimpanzees are actually far from pure herbivores. In every single site where chimps have been studied long-term, they've been observed to hunt and share meat—especially red colobus monkeys, which are their preferred prey. Their hunting strategy involves going out in groups, patrolling for smaller vertebrates, and deliberately chasing their future dinner over long distances (although chimps will also hunt spontaneously when a tasty opportunity arises). And it turns out that chimps are pretty impressive hunters: they have over a 50 percent success rate for their attempted kills!

Not only that, but certain groups of chimpanzees actually use tools to hunt—a behavior we used to think was exclusive to humans. Both male and female chimpanzees in Fongoli, Senegal, will whittle branches into sharp spears, which they use to capture and impale bush babies, mongooses, vervet monkeys, patas monkeys, bushbucks, and baboons. During one 10-year study, researchers observed a total of 308 instances of tool-assisted hunting (not counting the numerous other hunting instances that *didn't* feature tools). Both the frequency of hunts and the deliberation that goes into planning them (strategy-wise and tool-wise) implies that for chimpanzees, meat consumption isn't trivial, but an important part of their dietary ecology.

Evidence of meat-eating even shows up in chimpanzees' body tissues—which helps counter the argument that their meat consumption is an infrequent luxury rather than something nutritionally important (a claim sometimes put forth by proponents of the idea that chimpanzees are nearly vegan). In a 2013 study in Taï National Park, Ivory Coast, nitrogen isotopes in male chimpanzees' hair keratin (which reflects short-term protein intake) as well as their bone collagen (which reflects long-term protein intake) revealed levels that could be reached only with a regular intake of meat. Contrary to the longstanding belief that chimps get most of their protein from nuts and fruit, the researchers concluded that for the residents of this territory, "meat is a frequently sought-after protein resource."

Along with chimpanzees' meat intake, large-bodied great apes are well-known connoisseurs of another animal food: insects! Chimpanzees frequently consume ants, termites, caterpillars, bees, wasps, and beetle grubs; bonobos (which are about as close to us genetically as chimpanzees are) feast on larvae, termites, ants, earthworms, millipedes, and bees; orangutans love termites, ants, bees, crickets, caterpillars, and gall wasps; and mountain gorillas dine on ants, while western gorillas consume a wider variety of insects.

Despite insects' low calorie yield relative to other foods (like ripe fruit), many primate populations spend a disproportionate amount of time searching for insects to eat—and often go to great lengths to find them. In Senegal, male chimpanzees allot almost a quarter of their foraging and feeding time to finding termites, despite the fact that insects form only about 1 percent (by weight) of their total diet (that figure is similar for most chimpanzee and gorilla populations). Some primates even use tools to speed up the insect-catching process: wild Sumatran orangutans make tools out of twigs, sticks, and branches to extract and consume insects, while wild chimpanzees often use branch or twig "wands" to catch ants (along with digging sticks to excavate ant nests).

Plus, we have evidence that insects aren't just a "fallback food" when primates' preferred items are scarce. For instance, even when ripe fruit is dripping from the trees, researchers have observed chimpanzees of the Nimba Mountains of Guinea actively preying on ants—implying that they innately value insects regardless of whether other foods are abundant.

Some proponents of the "chimpanzees are herbivores" and "humans are herbivores by genetic proximity" argument make the mistake of assuming that because insects form a relatively small volume of the diet, they don't offer anything nutritionally significant. That couldn't be further from the truth! Nutritional analyses show that even at only 1 percent of food intake by weight, insects provide significant levels of protein, vitamin B12, iron, manganese, sodium, copper, and other nutrients that are low or absent in plant foods. Unlike vegetation (which contains limited amounts of certain amino acids), insect protein is composed of 46 to 96 percent easily digested essential amino acids, making them a valuable source of high-quality protein. Insects also supply amazing amounts of very healthy fatty acids, including essential fatty acids. For instance, termites are 49 percent fat, and nearly half of that fat is oleic acid, the heart-healthy monounsaturated fat that is thought to be a major contributor to the health benefits of olive and avocado oils.

And the great apes seem to have a knack for homing in on the absolute nutrient-richest insects they can find. In Cameroon, chimpanzees have been observed to choose insects higher in fat and protein (and pass over the insects that are lower in these nutrients), and in Tanzania, chimpanzees routinely pick only the insects that are richest in iron, manganese, and other minerals. Likewise, when some primates suffer the aftermath of eating too much laxative fruit, they appear to eat termites for their antidiarrheal properties (nature's version of Pepto-Bismol!).

So can we really call chimpanzees herbivores when they deliberately hunt meat, fashion tools specifically for catching animal foods, and consume large amounts of insects that supply nutrition sorely lacking in plants? The answer is a resounding no! And if genetic proximity is a valid argument, this could feasibly point to the importance of animal protein (and dare I say insects?) in human diets as well!

KNOWLEDGE BOMB *Not only are insects tremendous sources of protein, healthy fats, vitamins, minerals, and chitin fiber, but they are some of the most sustainable protein to grow from an environmental standpoint. For example, 100 pounds of feed will yield 60 pounds of cricket protein but only 5 pounds of beef protein. Likewise, it takes only about 1 gallon of water to raise 1 pound of crickets, compared to 51 gallons of water for a pound of beef. And crickets produce 100 times less greenhouse gas than cows. Think eating insects is weird? Eighty percent of the world's population, including the healthiest cultures on Earth, eat insects on a regular basis!*

There's still more to the "comparative anatomy" line of thinking, though. I've established that our closest living relatives are technically omnivores, but let's look at how much their diet informs the optimal one for us. We may share some impressive genetics, but how much *anatomically* do we have in common with other primates—and what do those similarities tell us about the human diet?

In a general sense, the "design" of our human digestive tract is similar to our great ape relatives: we all have the same gut anatomy that features a simple acid stomach, a small intestine, a small cecum, an appendix, and a colon. But that's where the similarities end. In humans, the greatest total gut volume (over 56 percent) is in the small intestine, whereas in other primates, the greatest total gut volume (over 45 percent) is in the colon. Basically, our colons are proportionately much smaller than those seen in other primates, who have giant hindguts perfect for breaking down woody seeds, seriously tough plant fiber, and other bulky material. The small-intestine-dominant guts of humans, on the other hand, suggest that we're adapted to higher-density foods (like meat and cooked starches) that are easier to digest than hardcore plant roughage.

Although we can't say for sure when this dramatic change in gut morphology occurred, the changes *do* suggest that we've adapted to a higher-quality omnivorous diet than our early ancestors and extant relatives. Both dense fat and protein sources (like meat) and dense unrefined carbohydrate sources (like starchy roots and tubers) likely allowed our intestinal anatomy to change into its current form over the few hundred thousand years (or more!) since our ancestors started routinely using fire for cooking. Of course, other components of our early ancestral diets can still benefit us, too: the rich micronutrient and phytochemical content of plant foods still demonstrate profound health benefits for us, and insects continue to be a part of indigenous human diets across the globe.

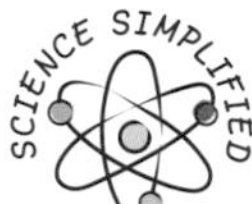

Not only do we have the digestive tracts of omnivores, but our digestive tracts are also adapted to energy-dense and easily digested foods like cooked meat and starchy vegetables.

More evidence of dietary divergence from other primates centers on α-amylase, an enzyme in saliva that breaks down starch into sugar (or more technically, hydrolyzes starch into maltose, maltotriose, and larger oligosaccharides). This enzyme is coded by the AMY1 gene, which can range from anywhere between two and fifteen diploid copies in humans. As a general rule, the more AMY1 copies we have, the more salivary amylase we'll produce (although lots of other factors can influence our levels at any given moment). As another general rule, populations with a long history of eating starch-rich diets (like the Japanese and Hadza) have higher average AMY1 copy numbers than populations consuming low-starch diets (like pastoralist tribes and arctic hunter-gatherers).

KNOWLEDGE BOMB

Unfortunately, it's not as simple as doing a genetic test to find out how many copies of AMY1 you have and then tailoring your carbohydrate intake accordingly. Inflammation, activity, sleep, and stress are profound influences on how our bodies respond to carbohydrates. *See Chapters 26 through 28.*

Chimpanzees and other nonhuman primates, on the other hand, have very few AMY1 copies and almost zero variation within their species. Chimpanzees universally possess only two diploid AMY1 copies, and bonobos have four (although their coding sequence is disrupted and those copies are probably only minimally functional, if not completely useless). In other words, humans are the only primates genetically equipped to handle larger starch loads.

So what does this tell us? Basically, at some point in our history (scientists are still trying to figure out exactly when), humans began facing selective pressure to digest starch-rich foods—possibly because of more plant underground storage units (like roots, tubers, and corms) making their way into our diet, or because cooking freed up starch sources that were previously unpalatable. As a result, our ancestors with less-than-efficient starch digestion were at a survival disadvantage, while those who could produce more salivary amylase had a better chance of staying in the gene pool. Over time, this led to the pattern we see today: much higher AMY1 copy numbers in humans relative to our great ape cousins, and particularly high numbers in populations that have traditionally relied on starch as a staple.

So how does this tie into the herbivore-carnivore-omnivore discussion? Well, it puts a giant nail in the coffin of the idea that humans are carnivores (with a nearly entirely carnivorous past). We have clear genetic evidence for a historical role of plant starch, significant enough to leave an imprint on our genome!

SCIENCE SIMPLIFIED

The Paleo diet is not a meat-heavy or all-meat diet as it is sometimes portrayed. It is a diet that puts heavy emphasis on vegetables while simultaneously endorsing meat consumption.

But our species' genetic quirks don't make the argument for herbivory, either. Humans are unique when it comes to lactase, the enzyme that breaks down the lactose in dairy. Whereas most mammals stop producing lactase after they're weaned, humans can exhibit the lactase persistence phenotype—the ability to digest lactose into adulthood. Lactase persistence is an inherited dominant trait that's widespread in populations with long histories of pastoralism and milk consumption (especially in Europe, the Middle East, and Africa). Basically, this phenotype lets many people obtain energy and nutrition from dairy products, when normally, the result would be gastrointestinal distress (as anyone with lactose intolerance understands!). If we were truly herbivores, we wouldn't have developed a genetic adaptation to a very specific animal food!

Finally, what about other elements of our anatomy? Some arguments for humans being herbivores or carnivores revolve around the shape of our teeth, jaws, and nails; our eating patterns; and other features that tend to be consistent among herbivorous or carnivorous animals. For example, some pro-vegan sources conclude that humans are herbivores because of our blunt nails, well-developed facial muscles, jaw position and motion, small mouth opening relative to our head size, broad and flattened incisors and molars, and blunt canines (to name a few!)—all of which are claimed to be features seen only in herbivores. Meanwhile, some pro-carnivore sources conclude that humans are carnivores because we have incisors on both jaws, intermittent feeding habits, vertical jaw movements, a lack of rumination behavior, a well-developed gallbladder, and a lack of stomach bacteria (among other things!)—all of which are claimed to be features seen only in carnivores. What to believe?

Actually, trying to understand the human diet based on general features of herbivores or carnivores is misleading from the get-go. For one, unlike every other species on the planet, we co-evolved with increasingly complex tools and processing methods that allowed our diets to expand without requiring us to have certain physical attributes. While many meat-eating species have powerful jaws, needle-sharp teeth, and claws that help them kill and chew prey, humans developed tools (such as spears and knives) that serve the same function. In other words, we do part of our "digesting" outside of our bodies!

And while many plant-eating species ruminate to obtain more nutrition from their food, have flat teeth for crushing vegetable matter, and have jaws that swing from side to side, humans found ways to process plant foods (through grinding, cooking, chopping, and so on) that bypass the need for those types of herbivorous attributes.

The end result is that general anatomical comparisons between humans and herbivores or carnivores are pretty much meaningless because they don't take into consideration the unique position humans are in—having co-evolved with big brains and tools that help us pre-process our food, lessen the burden on our digestive systems, and remove the need for specific physical traits used for acquiring and consuming plants or animals. Every other line of evidence points clearly at humans being omnivores, and that's why Paleo embraces plants *and* animals as elements of an optimal diet.

MY PALEO PLATE: HOW MUCH PLANT VERSUS ANIMAL?

This brings us to another important issue: we might be omnivores in a general sense, but what exactly does that mean? What does science say about our optimal ratio of plant to animal foods, and how is omnivory implemented in the Paleo framework?

One way to approach those questions is to look at data from hunter-gatherer populations that showcase what kinds of plant and animal food combinations can deliver health. The 2000 publication by Cordain et al that was discussed in Chapter 2—which helped gauge macronutrient ratios for 229 hunter-gatherer societies (as recorded in an ethnographic atlas)—also documented plant versus animal food ratios of those same societies. The vast majority of tribes ate between 45 and 65 percent of their diet as animal foods (as a percentage of total energy), with 35 to 55 percent of their diet coming from plants. (Tribes that fell outside those ranges were typically from polar regions [like the Inuit], where genetic mutations made it possible to thrive on an extremely high meat intake, or equatorial regions, where the greater bounty of nutrient-dense vegetables and fruits skewed the ratio more toward plant foods.) Because many of those 229 tribes were from North America (where hunting dominated) and relatively fewer were from Africa, Asia, Australia, and South America (where starchy or fatty plant foods were a frequent staple), the average proportion of plant foods might be a bit higher in reality than Cordain's analysis reflected. (For instance, the !Kung bushmen of southern Africa eat about 33 percent of their diet as meat and 67 percent as plant foods because they make use of the energy-dense mongongo nut in lieu of a higher animal food intake.)

So, as a ballpark figure, we could say that, calorie-wise, the average diet of hunter-gatherers is about half animal foods and half plant foods—with lots of wiggle room on either side. What's certain is that whenever both meat and vegetation are abundant, humans tend to gravitate toward a truly omnivorous diet that's about equal parts plants and animal rather than anything nearly herbivorous or nearly carnivorous. That ensures a broad micronutrient intake and plenty of fiber, phytochemicals, high-quality protein, and essential fats. For those of us who can hunt and gather only in the supermarket, 50/50 is still a pretty safe ratio to aim for.

But wait! Keep in mind that 50 percent of dietary *calories* coming from one type of food isn't the same as 50 percent of dietary *volume* (that is, how much space it takes up on a dinner plate) coming from that type of food. Meat and other animal foods tend to be much more energy-dense relative to most plant foods (as an extreme example, 1 cup of beef steak has 338 calories, whereas 1 cup of raw spinach has only 7 calories). That means a meal containing an assortment of vegetables plus a smaller portion of meat, fish, or eggs could easily come out to a 50/50 ratio of calories from plants to animals—even though it *looks* like more plant foods to the eye. While specific plants and animals vary in energy density (bone marrow is more dense than chicken breast, and a sweet potato is more dense than broccoli), it's typically safe to say that if we aim for a diet of approximately 50 percent plants and 50 percent animals, the plants will take up about two-thirds to three-quarters of our plate, while the animals will take up one-quarter to one-third.

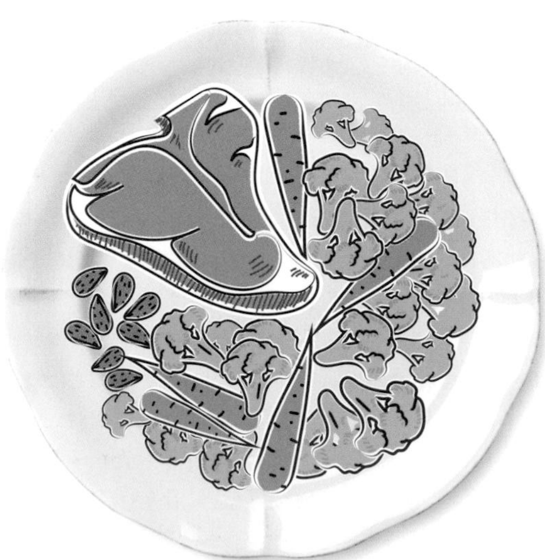

The 50/50 split between plant and animal foods is also supported by basic nutrition science. We get different nutrient needs met through animal foods versus plants. It's not a competition between these two kingdoms, where one is "better" or "worse" than the other; both play distinct but equally valuable roles. There's a huge spectrum of micronutrients and other beneficial compounds found mostly or exclusively in either plant foods or animal foods, such as:

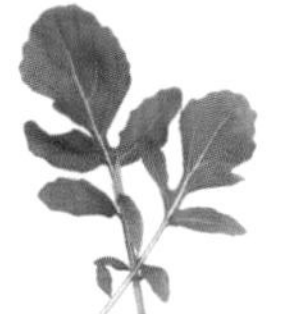 NUTRIENTS PREDOMINANTLY/ EXCLUSIVELY FOUND IN PLANT FOODS:	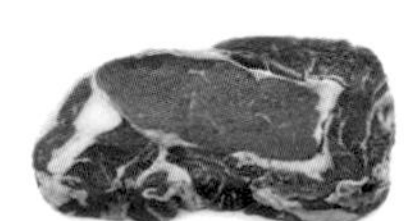 NUTRIENTS PREDOMINANTLY/ EXCLUSIVELY FOUND IN ANIMAL FOODS:
• Vitamin C	• Vitamin B12
• Carotenoids (lycopene, β-carotene, lutein, zeaxanthin)	• Heme iron
• Diallyl sulfide (from the allium class of vegetables)	• Zinc
• Polyphenols	• Pre-formed vitamin A (retinol)
• Flavonoids (anthocyanins, flavan-3-ols, flavonols, proanthocyanidins, procyanidins, kaempferol, myricetin, quercetin, flavonones)	• High-quality protein
• Dithiolethiones	• Creatine
• Lignans	• Taurine
• Plant sterols and stanols	• Carnitine
• Isothiocyanates and indoles	• Selenium
• Prebiotic fibers (soluble and insoluble)	• Vitamin K2
	• Vitamin D
	• DHA (docosahexaenoic acid)
	• EPA (eicosapentaenoic acid)
	• CLA (conjugated linoleic acid)

Ultimately, there are nutrients we can get only from plants and nutrients we can get only from animal foods: we need both to obtain the full complement of nutrients that our bodies need to be healthy.

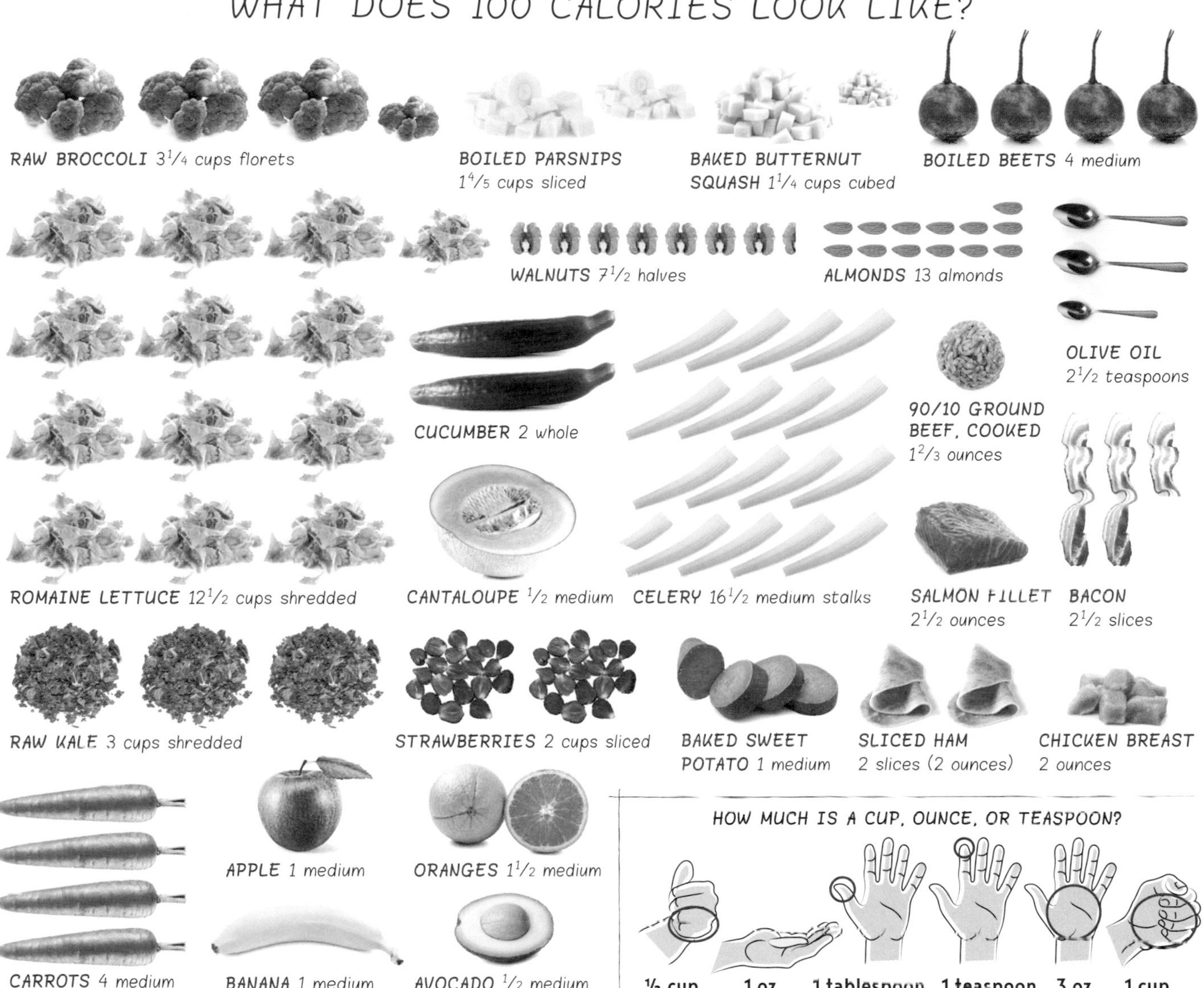

THE MEAT-CANCER CONNECTION

There's one more reason a roughly equal caloric ratio of plants and animals is optimal: these food sources, in many ways, work synergistically. A great example is the frequently discussed correlation between meat consumption and cancer. There really are a *lot* of studies out there linking meat consumption (especially red meat) to cancer—in human populations, in animal models, and even in some controlled trials focusing on precancerous changes in the human body. Hardly a month goes by without at least one of these studies popping up in the headlines and making the rounds on social media.

Despite a tendency for meat lovers (including some members of the Paleo community) to dismiss these studies because they did not use grass-fed and organic meat, researchers have uncovered several mechanisms linking cancer with components of meat that have nothing to do with an animal's diet or antibiotic exposure, including heme iron, specific proteins, other specific molecules, and heat-induced mutagens (a substance that can cause genetic mutation, which increases the risk of cancer). These things exist in meat whether it's conventional or grass-fed or wild game. That means that organic grass-fed meat, while it promotes health in other ways (better fats, more micronutrients), still has the capacity to increase cancer risk. So instead of dismissing the meat and cancer research as irrelevant, let's take the time to look objectively at how it affects us.

While this often gets framed as an argument for going vegetarian or vegan, it's actually a reflection of the importance of eating plenty of plant foods along with meat. When we take a closer look at these studies, we see something extraordinarily interesting: *the link between meat and cancer tends to disappear once the studies adjust for vegetable intake.* Even more exciting, when we examine the mechanistic links between meat and cancer, it turns out that many of the harmful (yes, legitimately harmful!) components of meat are counteracted by protective compounds in plant foods.

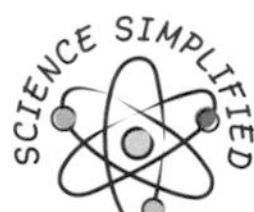

It's true that eating a lot of meat can increase cancer risk . . . if you also don't eat many vegetables!

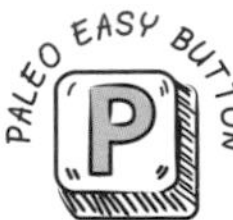

Always eat some vegetables, including at least one serving of a green vegetable, when you eat red meat.

One major mechanism linking meat to cancer involves heme, the iron-containing compound that gives red meat its color (in contrast to the nonheme iron found in plant foods). Where heme becomes a problem is in the gut: the cells lining the digestive tract (enterocytes) metabolize it into cytotoxic compounds (meaning toxic to living cells), which can then damage the gut barrier (specifically the colonic mucosa; see page 67), cause cell proliferation, and increase fecal water toxicity—all of which raise cancer risk. Yikes! In fact, part of the reason red meat is linked with cancer far more often than with white meat could be due to their differences in heme content: white meat (poultry and fish) contains much, much less.

KNOWLEDGE BOMB

Chlorophyll, the green molecule in plants that traps light for photosynthesis, and hemoglobin, the main protein in red blood cells that delivers oxygen throughout our bodies, have nearly identical structures. The difference? Chlorophyll is centered on a magnesium molecule, whereas hemoglobin is centered on an iron molecule.

Here's where vegetables come to the rescue! Chlorophyll, the pigment in plants that makes them green, has a molecular structure that's very similar to heme. As a result, chlorophyll can block the metabolism of heme in the intestinal tract and prevent those toxic metabolites from forming. Instead of turning into harmful by-products, heme ends up being metabolized into inert compounds that are no longer toxic or damaging to the colon. Animal studies have demonstrated this effect in action: one study on rats showed that supplementing a heme-rich diet with chlorophyll (in the form of spinach) completely suppressed the pro-cancer effects of heme. All the more reason to eat a salad with your steak.

Another mechanism involves L-carnitine, an amino acid that's particularly abundant in red meat (another candidate for why red meat seems to disproportionately increase cancer risk compared to other meats). When we consume L-carnitine, our intestinal bacteria metabolize it into a compound called trimethylamine (TMA). From there, the TMA enters the bloodstream and gets oxidized by the liver into yet another compound, trimethylamine-N-oxide (TMAO). This is the one we need pay attention to!

TMAO has been strongly linked to cancer and heart disease, possibly due to promoting inflammation and altering cholesterol transport. Having high levels of it in the bloodstream could be a major risk factor for some chronic diseases. So is this the nail in the coffin for meat eaters?

Not so fast! An important study on this topic published in 2013 in *Nature Medicine* sheds light on what's really going on. This paper had quite a few components, but one of the most interesting has to do with gut bacteria. Basically, it turns out that the bacteria group *Prevotella* is a key mediator between L-carnitine consumption and having high TMAO levels

PLANT CHLOROPHYLL
Magnesium at the center

HUMAN BLOOD HEMOGLOBIN
Iron at the center

in our blood. In this study, the researchers found that participants with gut microbiomes dominated by *Prevotella* produced the most TMA (and therefore TMAO, after it reached the liver) from the L-carnitine they ate. Those with microbiomes high in *Bacteroides* rather than *Prevotella* saw dramatically less conversion to TMA and TMAO.

Guess what *Prevotella* loves to snack on? Grains! It just so happens that people with high *Prevotella* levels tend to be those who eat grain-based diets (especially whole grain), since this bacterial group specializes in fermenting the type of polysaccharides abundant in grain products. (For instance, we see extremely high levels of *Prevotella* in populations in rural Africa that rely on cereals like millet and sorghum.) At the same time, *Prevotella* doesn't seem to be associated with a high intake of non-grain plant sources, such as fruit and vegetables.

So is it really the red meat that's a problem . . . or is it the meat in the context of a grain-rich diet? Based on the evidence we have so far, it seems that grains (and the bacteria that love to eat them) are a mandatory part of the L-carnitine-to-TMAO pathway. Ditch the grains, embrace veggies, and our gut will become a more hospitable place for red meat!

Yet another legitimate mechanism for the meat-cancer connection involves mutagens from cooking. Yes, a juicy steak on the grill tastes amazing. But what's *not* amazing is the molecular effect that high-temperature cooking has on meat. Harsh cooking methods like grilling and frying can generate compounds called heterocyclic amines, or HAs (formed from reactions between amino acids and creatine in muscle meat) and polycyclic aromatic hydrocarbons, or PAHs (formed when meat drippings hit open fire and cause PAH-containing flames to rise up, coating the meat with PAHs). Both of these compounds are known to be mutagenic, causing changes in DNA that may increase cancer risk. Plenty of animal experiments and human population studies point toward HAs and PAHs as being major players in the cancer correlations we see with meat.

Although we're not 100 percent sure how dramatically HAs and PAHs raise cancer risk in humans (it's really hard to measure people's exact intake and correlate it with disease incidence over time), it's safe to say that these compounds aren't harmless, and we should try to minimize our exposure to them. One way to do that, of course, is to stick with gentle cooking methods (hello, slow cooker!) instead of charring our meat to smithereens. But guess what else can counteract these grilled meat mutagens? It probably won't come as a surprise that the answer, *again*, is vegetables!

Multiple studies have shown that indoles, a class of phytochemicals abundant in cooked or crushed/chewed crucifers (like broccoli, cauliflower, Brussels sprouts, and cabbage), can suppress the tumors induced by PAHs and HAs, as well as totally change the way the body metabolizes these mutagens to make them less harmful. One study found that feeding people a diet containing 500 grams of crucifers per day (in the form of broccoli and Brussels sprouts) reduced the formation of toxic metabolites from a particularly dangerous HA called *2-amino-1-methyl-6-phenylimidazo[4,5-b]pyridine* (try saying THAT five times fast!). Basically, it looks like we can protect ourselves from some of the damage these mutagens cause by eating plenty of cruciferous vegetables. Let's fire up the barbecue (and make a shaved Brussels salad)!

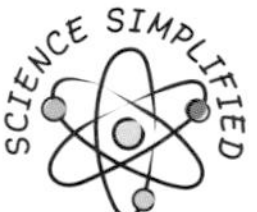

The antioxidants in cruciferous veggies like broccoli, cabbage, and kale protect against potentially cancer-causing chemicals created during high-heat cooking like barbecuing and frying. Veggies for the win!

So, although the "are we herbivores, carnivores, or omnivores?" issue is obviously a hot topic, it should be clear by now that we can truly put the question to rest. The Paleo framework embraces omnivory because every scientific avenue leads to the conclusion that we're omnivores—whether we approach it from an evolutionary angle, an ethnographic one, or comparative anatomy and physiology. Not only that, but by eating a diet that is about 50 percent plants and 50 percent animals, we can achieve tremendous dietary variety, maximize nutrient density, and obtain the protective effects of vegetables (whose absence or presence can mediate the carcinogenic effects of meat). That's a lot of points scored in favor of being an omnivore!

Chapter 4:
BIOLOGICAL SYSTEMS HEALTH

The various organs and tissues in the human body can be divided into twelve biological systems: the digestive and excretory system, skeletal system, nervous system, respiratory system, muscular system, endocrine system, reproductive system, immune and lymphatic system, cardiovascular and circulatory system, integumentary and exocrine system, renal system, and vestibular system. Each biological system (also called an "organ system" or "body system") is a group of organs and tissues that work together to perform certain tasks.

There is crosstalk between biological systems; the health of one system can impact the health of several or all of the others. As an extreme example, the digestive and excretory system is responsible for digesting food and eliminating waste from the body. When we can't absorb nutrients effectively (as can happen in pathologies of the gastrointestinal tract, like celiac disease and ulcerative colitis), the consequence is nutrient deficiencies that affect every other system in the body because every system requires specific nutrients to perform its functions. For the human body to experience health, each biological system needs to work effectively and efficiently on its own and in conjunction with other systems.

Biological systems health provides the chief arguments for avoiding those foods rejected by the Paleo diet. No, the Paleo framework is not simply derived from whether cavemen ate these foods, nor is choosing which foods to eat as simple as evaluating their nutrient density and our biological need for the nutrients they contain. Instead, we seek to understand how some foods can harm organs and tissues.

Some foods contain detrimental compounds that can undermine health, such as antinutrients, toxins, and carcinogens (see Chapters 5 and 17). Thus the food we eat affects our bodies beyond providing (or not providing) essential nutrients. Weighing "the good" versus "the bad" in each food is perhaps the most important metric for determining the role that food should play in our diets, be it foundational, occasional, or eliminated completely. "The good" in food is the nutrients that food contains. "The bad" is any compound that negatively impacts the health and functions of any of our biological systems.

I could write an entire book even thicker than this one about the functions of our biological systems, the nutrient requirements of each system, the compounds in foods that can interfere with each system, and the role that lifestyle plays. While this chapter reviews only those key biological systems and subsystems that are particularly susceptible to diet and lifestyle choices, at the end of the day it is important to remember three things:

- Our diet needs to provide the raw materials that each biological system needs to operate optimally.
- We must avoid consuming substantial amounts of foods that interfere with any of our biological systems.
- Our lifestyle choices must support biological systems health.

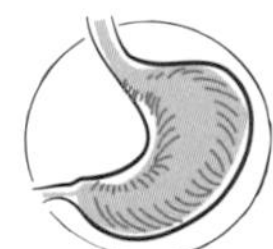 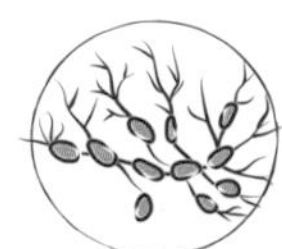 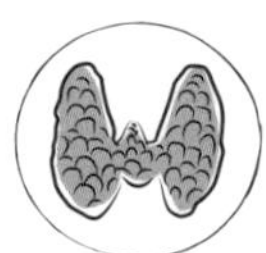 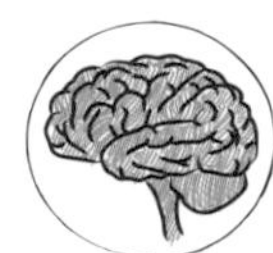 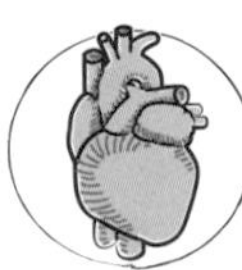 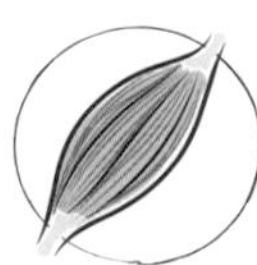 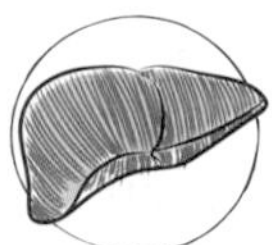

GUT HEALTH

Gut is the colloquial term for the gastrointestinal system, an organ subsystem composed of the esophagus, stomach, and small and large intestines. The gut is a major component of the digestive and excretory system—the biological system composed of the entire gut as well as the liver, pancreas, gallbladder, tongue, and salivary glands—which is responsible for digesting the food we eat, absorbing nutrients, and expelling waste.

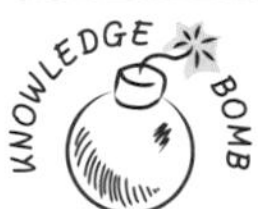

About 90 percent of all disease can be traced back to the health of the gut and gut microbiota.

The food we eat is digested inside the gut as it travels from one end of the gut to the other. Digestion is the chemical and mechanical breakdown of food, releasing nutrients for absorption into the body. Only relatively small molecules can cross the gut barrier (see below) to enter the body, which is why digestion is a prerequisite for nutrient absorption. Nutrients are absorbed by passing through the lining of the gastrointestinal tract (via several pathways) and into the circulation (either the blood or the lymphatic vessels, depending on whether the nutrient is water or fat soluble). Nutrients are then carried throughout the body.

Supplying nutrients to the body is clearly a very important job. Without the gut to accomplish this vital function, we could not survive. However, digestion is just the tip of the iceberg when it comes to the gut's contribution to our health!

The Gut Barrier

The gut is a barrier between the inside of the body and the outside world. Yes, as unintuitive as it may seem, the stuff inside the digestive tract is actually *outside* the body! But the gut is a unique, highly selective barrier. Its job is to let nutrients into the body while keeping everything else out. To achieve this function, the gut is equipped with an array of physiological defense mechanisms, including mucus, digestive enzymes, and acid. The gut also houses approximately 80 percent of our immune systems within the largest collection of lymphoid tissue in the body.

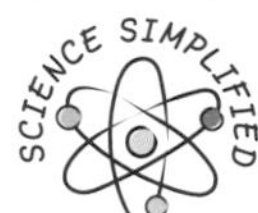

The gut barrier's job is to let nutrients into the body and keep everything else inside the gut, where it eventually gets eliminated as part of our poop. A leaky gut means that the gut barrier isn't doing a good job of keeping things out of the body that should stay in our poop.

Digestion of consumed food into small molecules is necessary for the proper functioning of the gut barrier. The gut barrier, also called the intestinal barrier, is semipermeable. It protects the body by being permeable to nutrients (small molecules) while blocking everything else—including compounds in foods that our bodies can't use as well as toxins, pathogens, and the trillions of bacteria that live in our guts. What we can't absorb from our food either becomes food for the bacteria that live in the intestines or is eliminated as waste.

How does the gut barrier work? The first line of defense against pathogens entering the body is digestion, with saliva, gastric acid and enzymes, and pancreatic enzymes all exerting a toxic action on these infectious microorganisms via the destruction of their cell walls. If a pathogen escapes degradation, two mechanisms prevent it from adhering to the wall of the gastrointestinal tract. *Peristalsis,* the coordinated contraction and relaxation of muscle tissues to propel the contents of the gut from one end to the other, limits the amount of time a pathogen has to adhere to, colonize (take up residence and multiply), or cross the intestinal barrier. The entire intestinal surface is lined with mucus, produced by specialized cells embedded within the intestinal wall (called goblet cells), that acts as a physical barrier to pathogens but also contains a variety of antimicrobial compounds to destroy any infectious microbes that may enter the mucus layer. The specialized cells that connect firmly to each other to form the majority of the intestinal wall, a type of epithelial cell called *enterocytes,* also form a physical barrier to large amounts of pathogens. Whatever makes it through these defenses is then confronted by the immune system.

Just inside the epithelial cell layer of the intestinal wall lies a vast array of resident immune cells acting as sentries, ready to protect the body from attack. Even in normal circumstances, a constant barrage of large molecules—including partially digested food particles, pathogenic organisms, and the normal microbiotic residents of our guts—cross into the body and must be identified and destroyed by the immune system. A variety of cell types accomplish this job, recognizing and cleaning up harmless substances, targeting harmful agents and mounting either a local or a systemic immune response, and remaining in a constant state of vigilance called "physiological inflammation."

Eighty percent of our immune systems are in our guts. So when compounds leak into our bodies across a leaky gut barrier, the immune system is revved up, causing inflammation that can spread to every part of the body, causing chronic diseases.

In the case of a leaky gut, or more technically "increased intestinal permeability," far more large molecules are getting across the gut barrier than normal, and far more than can be mopped up by the gut immune system. This happens when either the enterocytes or the complex structures that glue the enterocytes to each other, called junctions, are damaged. (There are four types of junctions between enterocytes: tight junctions, gap junctions, adherens junctions, and desmosomal junctions.) What leaks into the body is a variety of substances—like incompletely digested proteins, bacteria or bacterial fragments, infectious organisms, and waste products—all of which stimulate the immune system.

Some substances cause generalized inflammation, where the signal to the immune system within the gut tissues spreads throughout the body. For example, when bacterial toxins such as lipopolysaccharide (also called endotoxin) leak into the body, systemic inflammation is triggered. Other substances stimulate targeted attacks by the immune system. For example, a food intolerance or allergy could result from incompletely digested food proteins leaking into the body. The many symptoms and health conditions related to leaky gut are caused by this stimulation of the immune system. Importantly, an immune system that's chronically stimulated, as occurs in the context of a leaky gut, can end up attacking not just invaders like viruses and bacteria but also body tissues, which can contribute to chronic illnesses.

It is not an exaggeration to say that gut health is everything: the health of our guts has a profound effect on our overall health. As the connection between intestinal barrier function and health gains more recognition, the role that diet and lifestyle play is being examined more intensively.

Compounds in foods directly damage the gut barrier in two main ways: by adversely affecting the health of the cells that form the gut barrier or by interfering with how those cells bond together. Both cause the barrier to become permeable, or "leaky," hence "leaky gut syndrome," the umbrella term for chronic diseases associated with this problem.

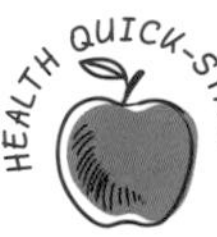

Ditch the grains. Beyond being nutritionally underwhelming, they are the biggest source of compounds that interfere with gut health in most Americans' diets. (See Chapter 19.)

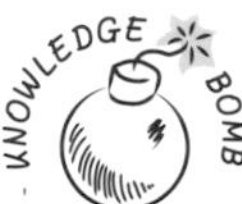

Grains are the starchy seeds of grasses and include barley, corn (aka maize), fonio, job's tears, kamut, millet, oat, rice, rye, sorghum, spelt, teff, triticale, wheat (all varieties, including einkorn, durum, and semolina), and wild rice.

Grains, legumes, dairy, and nightshades all contain substances that increase the permeability of the gut via direct damage both to enterocytes and to the junctions between them. These substances include prolamins (like gluten), agglutinins (like soy lectin), digestive enzyme inhibitors, glycoalkaloids, and phytic acid (all discussed in detail in Parts 3 and 4). Alcohol and sugar alcohols (like sucralose) also increase intestinal permeability via actions on the tight junctions. Some nutritional deficiencies are linked to leaky gut as well, including vitamins A and D. Of course, food isn't the only thing that affects gut barrier function: both acute stress (see Chapter 27) and overly strenuous activity (see Chapter 28) are known to increase intestinal permeability.

How harmful substances like gluten are to the gut barrier varies greatly from individual to individual. Certainly, genetics plays a factor. For example, 98 percent of all celiac disease sufferers have one of two variants of the human leukocyte antigen (HLA) gene: either DQ2 or DQ8. Celiac disease sufferers also produce exaggerated amounts of a protein called zonulin in response to gluten consumption. Zonulin is a protein that controls the formation of the tight junctions between enterocytes; when there is increased zonulin, those junctions open up, causing a leaky gut. There's some evidence that dysfunctionally high zonulin production is a consequence of having

THE LEAKY GUT GUIDE

WHAT IS A LEAKY GUT?

A leaky gut occurs when the cells that form the intestinal wall or the tight bonds between them are damaged. When this happens, the gut barrier loses its ability to regulate which molecules cross into the body.

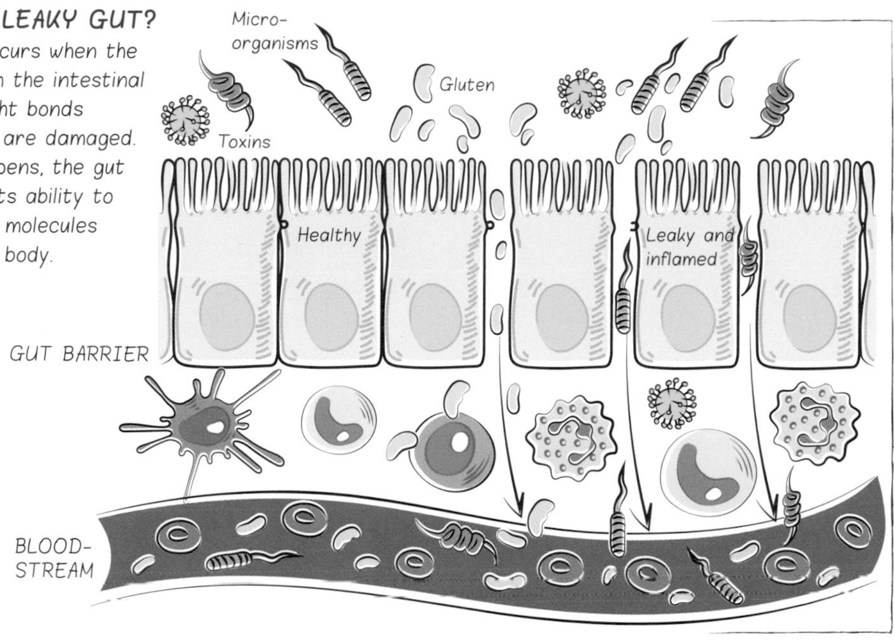

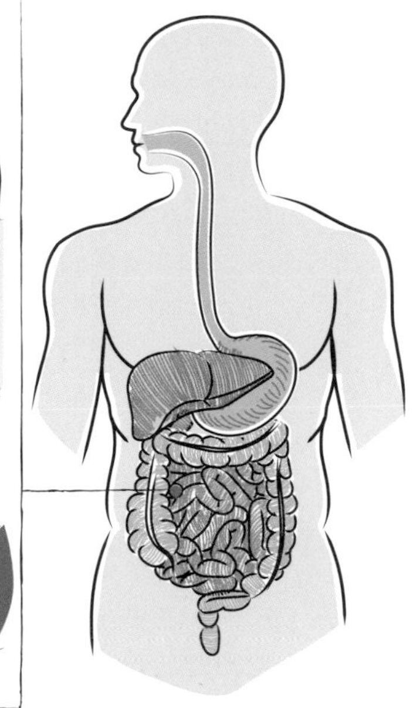

DEVELOPMENT OF A LEAKY GUT

1. A healthy gut barrier is resilient to some stressors and toxins. It is normal for some large molecules to cross into the body, and it's the immune system's job to deal with them while remaining well regulated. This is called mucosal or immune tolerance.

2. Minor intestinal permeability due to gut barrier defects results in an increased passage of large molecules into the body; however, homeostasis (the maintenance of a stable environment inside and outside the cells) is maintained.

3. Prolonged minor intestinal permeability results in an exaggerated immune response, causing damage to the gut barrier.

4. The passage of more and more large molecules into the body leads to inflammation and immune system activation, which may result in the destruction of tight junctions and enterocyte cell death, leading to even greater passage of large molecules. This becomes a vicious cycle.

5. Severe intestinal permeability develops and results in overactivation of the immune system, cell death, tissue damage, autoimmune disease, multi-organ system disorder, and chronic health problems.

WHAT CAUSES A LEAKY GUT?

- Advanced glycation end-products
- Antibacterial peptides
- Antibodies
- Antigens
- Dietary proteins and peptides
- Enzymes
- Infections
- Lipopolysaccharides
- NSAIDs (such as aspirin and ibuprofen)
- Stress
- Toxins
- Undigested food particles

SYMPTOMS OF A LEAKY GUT

GASTROINTESTINAL SYMPTOMS:

Abdominal pain
Bloating
Burping
Gas
Irregular stools (constipation or diarrhea)
Nausea/vomiting
Reflux/heartburn

NEUROLOGICAL SYMPTOMS:

ADD/ADHD
Anxiety
Brain fog
Depression
Fatigue, especially after eating
Headaches
Insomnia

SKIN SYMPTOMS:

Acne
Dry skin
Eczema
Hives
Itchy skin
Psoriasis
Rashes
Rosacea

OTHER SYMPTOMS:

Aches and pains
Autoimmune disease
Difficulty maintaining a healthy weight
Food sensitivities/allergies
Joint pain
Symptoms of malnutrition

DISEASES LINKED TO LEAKY GUT

Ankylosing spondylitis
Asthma
Atopic dermatitis
Cardiovascular disease
Celiac disease
Chronic fatigue syndrome
Chronic heart failure
Chronic inflammation
Crohn's disease
Depression
Eczema
Food allergy
HIV/AIDS
Inflammatory joint disease
Insulin resistance
Irritable bowel syndrome
Multiple organ failure
Multiple sclerosis
Non-alcoholic fatty liver disease
Obesity
Psoriatic arthritis
Psychological conditions
Rheumatoid arthritis
Stroke
Type 1 diabetes
Type 2 diabetes
Ulcerative colitis

either HLA-DQ2 or HLA-DQ8; for example, high zonulin production in response to gluten consumption is seen in people without celiac disease but with IBS who have HLA-DQ2. This link has led many experts to suggest that everyone with one of these two HLA variants—about 55 percent of the general population—should adopt a gluten-free diet.

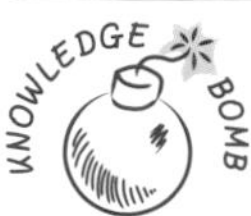

An estimated 55 percent of the general population has either the HLA-DQ2 or the HLA-DQ8 gene. These genes are believed to be linked to gluten sensitivity.

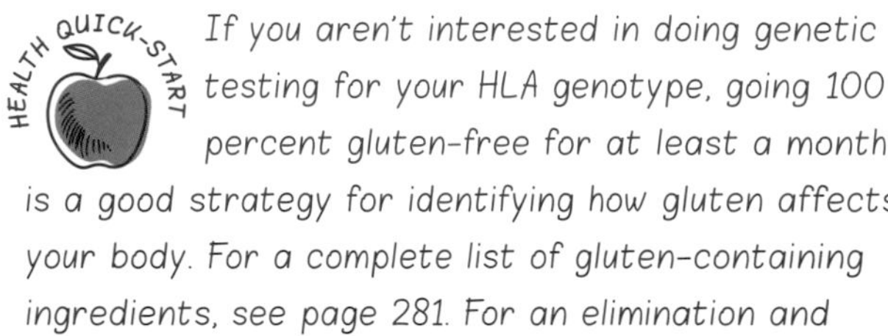

If you aren't interested in doing genetic testing for your HLA genotype, going 100 percent gluten-free for at least a month is a good strategy for identifying how gluten affects your body. For a complete list of gluten-containing ingredients, see page 281. For an elimination and reintroduction protocol, see Chapter 25.

Beyond genetics, your nutrient sufficiency, how much sleep you get, how much stress you're under, and how active you are all affect how strongly your body responds to suboptimal foods and how quickly you recover after eating them. However, with only a few exceptions, foods abundant in gut barrier-damaging compounds aren't nutrient-rich foods. If you're battling chronic illness, you may benefit substantially from removing all these foods from your diet (see Parts 3 and 4). If you're simply in search of optimal health, you have nothing to lose from cutting out these foods.

The Gut Microbiota

The gut is a biological niche, home to a diverse array of microbes that influence nearly all aspects of human biology through their interactions with our bodies. Every person's gut contains approximately 400 to 1,500 different species of microorganisms that are well adapted to survive in the gastrointestinal tract (with about 35,000 species total for all humankind), although about 99 percent of those microorganisms come from thirty to forty species of bacteria. Our guts are inhabited by other microorganisms besides bacteria, including archaea (similar to bacteria), viruses, and single-cell eukaryotes (like yeast). In fact, it is estimated that there are three to ten times as many microorganisms living in our guts as there are total cells in the entire human body! These microorganisms are collectively referred to as our *gut microbiota*, and we depend on them for health and survival. (*Microbiome* refers to the collective genome of the gut microbiota.)

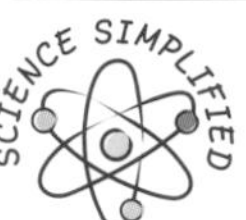

Our guts are home to trillions of beneficial bacteria that we need to be healthy. One major reason why eating a plant-rich diet is so important is that the fiber in vegetables and fruits is the best food for these bacteria.

Our gut microbiota help us digest food, produce chemicals that improve the health of the cells that form the gut barrier, and directly regulate the immune system, and they can even influence brain health by producing neuroactive chemicals that are absorbed into the bloodstream and travel to the brain. A healthy diversity of the right kinds of microorganisms in the gut is one of the most fundamental aspects of good health.

When the microbiota of people living in Western cultures were analyzed in comparison with those of people living in rural settings who had hunter-gatherer lifestyles and with those of wild primates like chimpanzees, Western-culture gut microbiota were found to be significantly lacking in both richness and biodiversity. This is directly attributable to diets high in industrially processed foods (which are also low in fiber), which don't supply enough nutrition for our microbiota to thrive. Interestingly, there is even less diversity of gut bacteria in obese people than in lean people: more food does not equal more nutrition, and the worse our diet, the more our gut microbiota suffer.

Diet is the single biggest influence on microbiota composition. In fact, diet is directly responsible for more than 60 percent of the variation in bacterial species in the gut. What's more, the population of microbes in the gut (types, total and relative quantities, and location) adapts quite rapidly to changes in diet, in a matter of a few days to a few weeks. That's good news!

It's not just a question of which kinds of bacteria our diet nourishes but also a question of bacterial metabolism. Just as a high-sugar diet causes oxidative stress in our bodies (see page 266), a high-sugar diet causes oxidative stress in our gut bacteria. Those bacteria adapt by altering their metabolism, which greatly affects our health.

Diet affects gut motility and colonic contractibility, which then influence gut microbiota composition.

However, diet also affects gut microbiota composition directly, which then affects gut motility and colonic contractibility. The impact of gut bacteria on transit (the passage of food through the digestive tract) largely depends on the amount and type (fermentable versus nonfermentable) of fiber in the diet. Generally, transit is well regulated when our diets are high in vegetables and fruits.

Another important factor is the role that the gut microbiota play in digestion, vitamin synthesis, and the body's ability to absorb certain vitamins and minerals. The nutritional value of our food is partly influenced by the community of bacteria in our gut. The relationship between diet, lifestyle (stress, sleep, circadian rhythms, and so on), and our gut microbiota is complex, and it's only beginning to be understood in the scientific

GALLBLADDER DISEASE AND GLUTEN

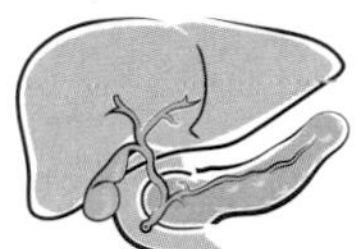

The gallbladder is a little pear-shaped sac nestled toward the front of and a little underneath the liver. It has a very simple job:

- store bile (which is produced by the liver) between meals
- concentrate bile by reabsorbing water
- release bile into the small intestine when food needs to be digested

Bile is composed of water, bile salts, bile pigments (products of red blood cell breakdown that are normally excreted in the bile), cholesterol, and various electrolytes. Bile salts are the only components of bile that actually have a digestive function. Bile salts are not the same as digestive enzymes (which are produced by the cells that line the stomach and by the pancreas). Instead, bile salts aid the actions of digestive enzymes and enhance the absorption of fatty acids and fat-soluble vitamins.

The most important action of bile salts is that of an emulsifier. In essence, bile salts break up fat globules in the small intestine into tiny droplets that are able to mix with water. The enzymes that break fat up into fatty acids (lipases) can then perform their function more effectively. Bile salts also aid in the absorption of fatty acids, cholesterol, and fat-soluble vitamins.

If the gallbladder is not functioning properly, fats cannot be properly digested (fats are essential for survival and health), and fat-soluble vitamins cannot be effectively absorbed, leading to micronutrient deficiencies. Gallbladder health is critical for digestive health and overall health.

Gallbladder problems can be directly linked to gluten intake. Approximately 60 percent of celiac disease sufferers are known to have liver, gallbladder, and/or pancreatic conditions. While some of these conditions may be a result of the malnutrition and/or directly linked to the gut damage that occurs in celiac disease, others are thought to share common genetic factors or have a common immunopathogenesis (that is, the condition originates from the same immune system attacks on the small intestine also attacking these organs). Specifically, primary biliary cirrhosis, primary sclerosing cholangitis, and autoimmune forms of hepatitis and cholangitis are thought to have a common immune system/inflammation origin as celiac disease itself—and that means gluten.

In celiac disease, gluten triggers an autoimmune response. The body's own immune system attacks the cells that line the small intestine, resulting in the characteristic shortening, or pruning, of the intestinal villi (microscopic, fingerlike projections of small intestine wall tissue made of columns of gut epithelial cells). As you can imagine, this creates a very leaky gut, which also stimulates the immune system, causes inflammation, and allows toxins and foreign proteins into the body. In the majority of celiac disease patients, the immune system does not limit its attack to the cells that line the small intestine; this is why second and even third autoimmune conditions are so common in people who have celiac disease.

When you eat, the cells that line the duodenum (the first segment of the small intestine) detect the presence of fat and protein and react by releasing a hormone called cholecystokinin, which stimulates both the release of digestive enzymes from the pancreas and bile from the gallbladder (see page 89). When the gut is damaged (whether from celiac disease or another gut pathology), duodenal enterocytes are less able to secrete cholecystokinin. This means there is not enough signal to the gallbladder that it's time to release bile salts into the duodenum. Reduced cholecystokinin release is reported in celiac disease and may be one of the key causes of the gallbladder malfunction that occurs concomitantly with celiac.

Importantly, the dominant gallbladder problems that might be caused by gluten sensitivity are cholecystitis (inflammation of the gallbladder) and malfunctioning gallbladder, not gallstones (reported in 20 percent of elderly celiac patients but only 2.5 percent of the more general celiac population). The frequency of liver and gallbladder conditions suffered by celiac disease patients has allowed researchers to make the converse argument. It is now recommended that those with unexplained liver and/or gallbladder symptoms be evaluated for celiac disease. If you have been diagnosed with gallbladder disease—especially if it is not gallstones, but don't rule out this possibility if it is—it is important to investigate gluten sensitivity or celiac disease as the possible cause.

community. However, research is starting to show that altering our gut microbiota can be a powerful way to improve immune function and control chronic disease—but doing so isn't as easy as supplementing with probiotics. We need to feed our gut bacteria the right food to encourage the growth of the right diversity and relative quantities of beneficial microorganisms.

PALEO EASY BUTTON

To support a healthy gut microbial community, start gradually increasing your consumption of vegetables until you reach at least eight servings per day. (See page 156 for what constitutes a serving.) If you're starting nowhere near that mark, try adding a half serving every few days. Also make sure to eat a variety of types and colors of veggies, including starchy roots and tubers, leafy greens, and cruciferous vegetables (see Chapter 8).

Beyond getting plenty of fiber from whole-food sources (that is, vegetables and fruit; see Chapter 8), it's important to avoid foods that promote the growth of the wrong kinds of bacteria. Grains, dairy, legumes, nightshades, and alcohol are all known to contain compounds that can hinder the growth of beneficial strains of bacteria while supporting the growth of undesirable strains, like *E. coli*. Hindrances to digestion, such as low stomach acid, inadequate pancreatic enzymes, and inadequate bile salts, are also a factor: any food that isn't easily digested (whether that's an inherent property of the food or our digestive system isn't up to par) can skew the types and numbers of gut microorganisms. When too many of the wrong types grow—a situation called *gut dysbiosis*—digestion is hindered, the health and function of the gut barrier becomes impaired, and the immune system is stimulated.

Having a healthy gut means more than just fixing a leaky one. It also means restoring gut microbiota to the appropriate diversity, numbers, and locations—different types of bacteria grow in different amounts in different parts of the gut. In general, this means consuming a moderate amount saturated fat, a balanced ratio of omega-3 to omega-6 polyunsaturated fats, and a diversity of fiber types from a wide range of fruits and vegetables. Choosing foods as well as engaging in lifestyle choices that support gut health is a major guiding principle behind the Paleo template. As you read Parts 2 through 4, you'll see gut health as a rationale for recommendations crop up again and again.

At-Home Gut Health Tests

A number of professional tests can help diagnose leaky gut; SIBO and other forms of gut dysbiosis; infections like *C. difficile* and *H. pylori;* parasite infection; inefficient digestion of fats, proteins, and/or carbohydrates; and of course, diseases of the gut, like diverticular disease, ulcerative colitis, and celiac disease. Certainly, if you're worried about a serious health issue, it's imperative to have a detailed conversation with your doctor. But what if you're just curious about how things are going in there? What if you're looking to understand the difference between meh, good, and amazing? Fortunately, there are a few tests you can do at home to gauge the state of your gut health and see if you have indications of a problem.

Fair warning: You're going to have to look at your own poop. A lot. In fact, visually inspecting every bowel movement is a great habit for keeping track of gut health.

Transit Time Test

"Bowel transit time" refers to how long it takes for the food you eat to pass through your digestive system and get eliminated in a bowel movement—in other words, the time from swallowing to pooping! This type of test can help diagnose constipation, which can indicate a gut microbiotic imbalance or a diet too low in fermentable substrates, as well as abnormally rapid transit times (which can indicate malabsorption of food) and certain diseases, like Crohn's.

In clinical settings, doctors monitor bowel transit time by having people swallow capsules filled with dyes or markers that show up on X-rays. But you can conduct a similar test at home by eating food that will be easily identifiable in a bowel movement. Any of the following foods will do the trick:

- Sesame seeds (a teaspoon to a tablespoon, mixed into a glass of water and swallowed whole)
- Corn kernels (a cup of cooked kernels eaten alone, at least an hour apart from other foods; this option is not technically Paleo)
- Red beets (a cup of cooked, or raw and shredded, beets, eaten alone)

Here's how it works: whichever food you use, simply note the time you eat it, and then watch and wait for it to "reappear" in a bowel movement. Sesame seeds or corn will be easy to spot, and beets will give your stool a distinct purple-red color. (Keep in mind that beets

LINKS BETWEEN GUT BACTERIA AND HEALTH

MOOD DISORDERS:
Bacteria in the gut activate neural pathways and central nervous system signaling systems. Gut dysbiosis, especially a lack of beneficial bacterial strains, is linked to depression and anxiety, with more than a third of depression sufferers also having a leaky gut.

SCHIZOPHRENIA:
Mice studies link a lack of normal bacteria with changes in brain development and schizophrenic behavior. Human infants born prematurely are known to lack biodiversity in their guts and be at a higher risk of schizophrenia.

CARDIOVASCULAR DISEASE:
Certain grain-loving bacteria are known to also convert L-carnitine, a protein rich in red meat, into an atherogenic compound called TMAO, raising the risk of cardiovascular disease (see page 64).

LIVER CANCER:
The same changes in microbial composition that are linked to obesity are known to increase the risk of liver cancer.

OBESITY:
Gut microbes can impact metabolism via signaling pathways in the gut, with effects on inflammation, insulin resistance, and deposition of energy in fat stores. A number of studies show specific microbial patterns associated with obesity.

INFLAMMATORY BOWEL DISEASES:
Abnormally high levels of certain undesirable strains of bacteria along with dysregulated immune responses to gut microbes may trigger the development and continuing symptoms of both Crohn's disease and ulcerative colitis.

IRRITABLE BOWEL SYNDROME:
There is a definitive link between IBS and an overgrowth of bacteria in the small intestines (SIBO).

COLORECTAL CANCER:
Lower levels of beneficial bacteria as well as higher levels of certain sugar-loving microbes in the gut are linked to increased risk and growth rates of colorectal cancers.

OBSESSIVE COMPULSIVE DISORDER:
Dysfunction of the gut microbiome, perhaps related to high stress and/or antibiotic use, is linked to OCD.

AUTISM:
Autism often co-occurs with gastrointestinal issues like leaky gut and irritable bowel syndrome.

PARKINSON'S DISEASE:
People suffering from Parkinson's have different microbial composition of the gut than healthy people.

MULTIPLE SCLEROSIS:
Dysbiosis and the resulting loss of balance in gastrointestinal immune responses are linked to the development of MS and may explain why MS symptoms can be mitigated with therapeutic diets.

ASTHMA AND ALLERGIES:
Low diversity of gut bacteria, especially early in life, is linked to increased risk of asthma and allergies.

DIABETES:
Diabetics have lower levels of beneficial strains of bacteria and skewed ratios of different strains, with lower numbers of gut microbes overall. Some compositional changes in gut microbiota appear to scale with glucose levels—that is, the higher a person's glucose levels, the fewer total microbes and the more undesirable species of bacteria are likely to be found in that person's gut.

RHEUMATOID ARTHRITIS:
Studies have found a link between low levels of probiotic bacteria and high levels of undesirable bacterial strains with autoimmune joint diseases like RA.

OTHER CANCERS:
Dysbiosis is linked to increased risk of gastric, esophageal, pancreatic, laryngeal, breast, and gallbladder carcinomas.

GOOD

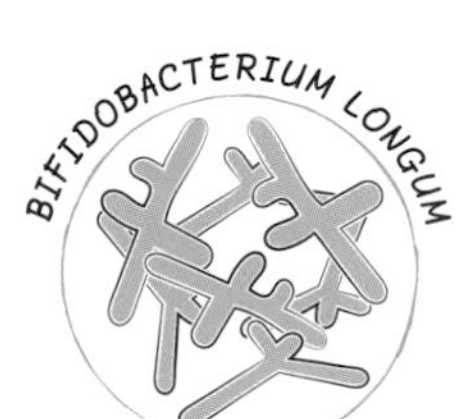

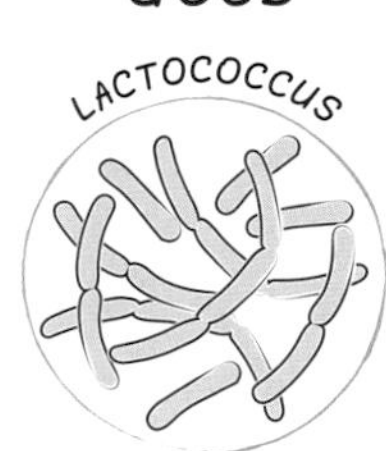

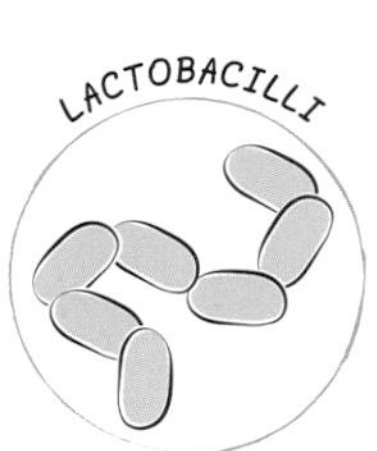

BAD

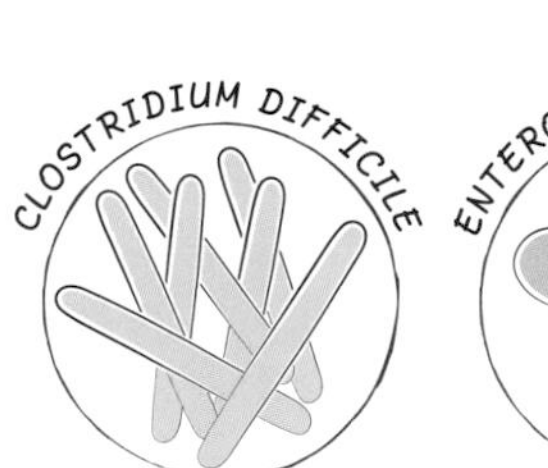

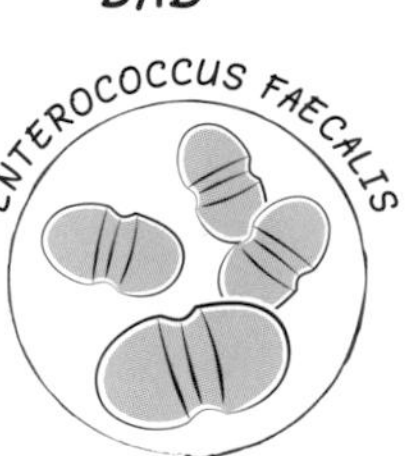

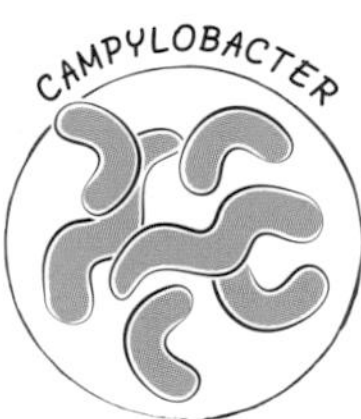

GUT HEALTH QUICK-START GUIDE

REMOVE THE BIGGEST OFFENDERS:

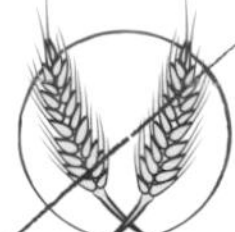
Grains (page 241)

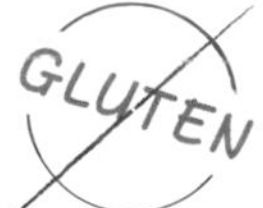

Gluten (page 242)

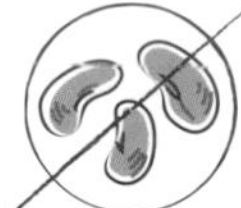
Legumes (page 249)

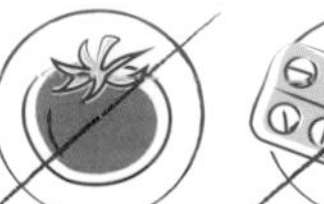
Nightshades (page 296)

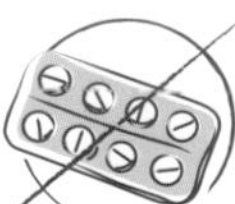
NSAIDs (page 115)

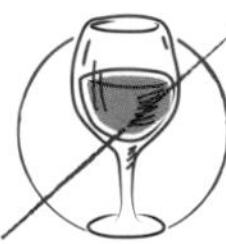
Alcohol (page 300)

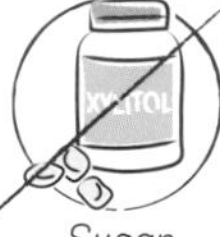
Sugar substitutes (page 276)

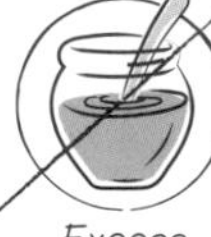
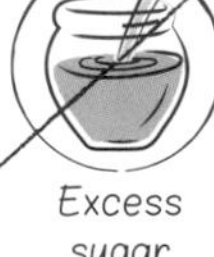
Excess sugar (page 266)

Processed and fast foods (page 259)

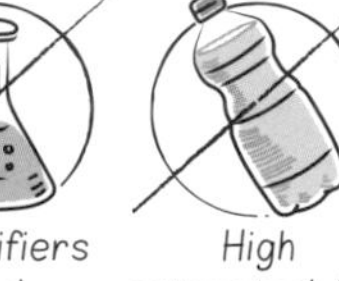
Emulsifiers and thickeners (page 235)

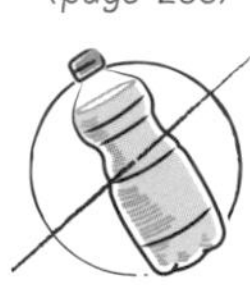
High saturated fat (page 186)

ANTIBIOTICS also cause damage to gut bacteria, so they should be used only when truly necessary, and not for the treatment of viral infections. For more information on antibiotic use, see page 116.

EAT MORE:

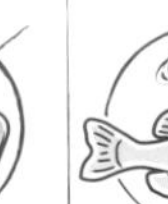
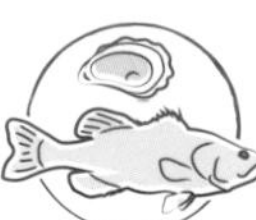
Seafood (page 158)

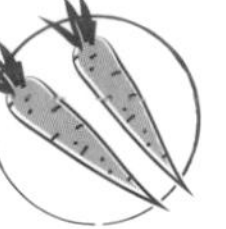
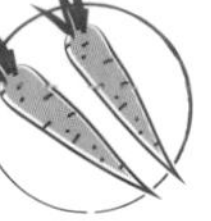
Starchy roots and tubers (page 153)

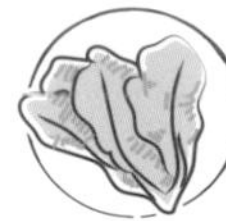
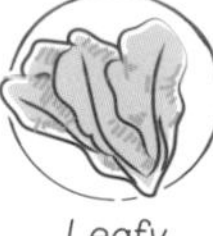
Leafy greens (page 137)

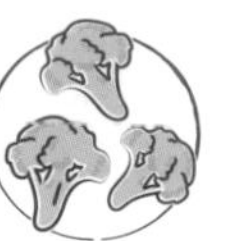
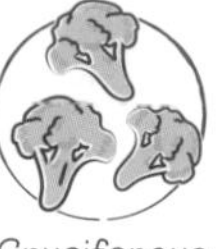
Cruciferous veggies (page 137)

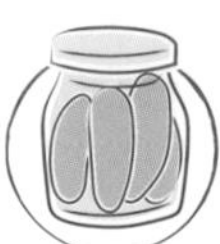
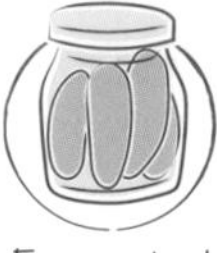
Fermented foods (page 190)

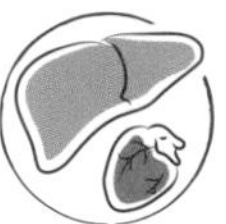
Organ meat (page 174)

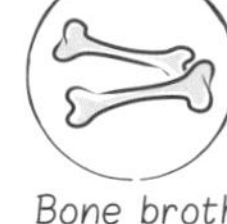
Bone broth (page 178)

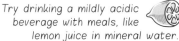

Aim for a 1:1 to 1:4 ratio of omega-3 to omega-6 polyunsaturated fats (see page 158). Avoid consuming more than 40 to 50 percent of calories from fat, and limit saturated fat intake to 10 to 15 percent of calories.

MEAL HYGIENE:

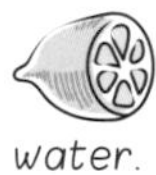
Try drinking a mildly acidic beverage with meals, like lemon juice in mineral water.

Avoid drinking too much with meals (but drink more between meals).

Drink plenty of water throughout the day.

Chew food thoroughly.

Don't eat when stressed or distressed.

Take your time eating; don't rush to finish your food or eat on the run.

Eat two or three distinct meals per day. Each meal should include a protein and two to four servings of a few different vegetables.

Avoid grazing and minimize snacking.

Don't get up and rush around immediately after a meal.

Avoid eating immediately before or after strenuous exercise.

NOTES ON FIBER AND FERMENTED FOODS:

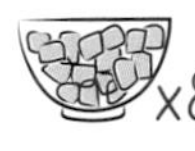

Aim for at least eight servings of vegetables per day.

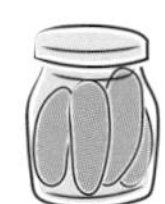
Choose some type of fermented food daily; mix it up!

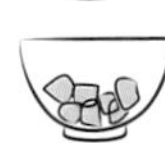
Ramp up your vegetable consumption slowly, adding half a serving of vegetables every few days until you reach eight servings.

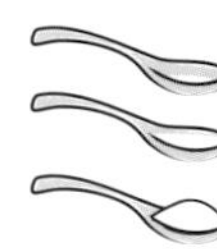
Ramp up your fermented food consumption slowly, starting with as little as half a teaspoon of fermented food and adding an additional teaspoon every few days until you reach a full serving.

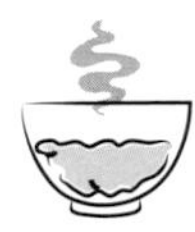
Opt for smoothies, puréed soups, and well-cooked veggies if high vegetable consumption causes gastrointestinal symptoms or poor stool quality.

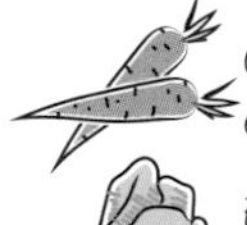
Choose more starchy tubers if you're experiencing loose stools.

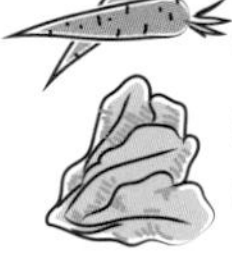
Eat more leafy greens and make sure you're well hydrated if your stools are too firm.

LIFESTYLE:

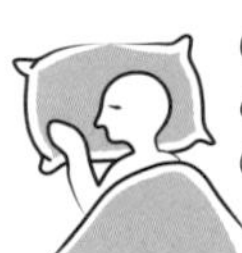
Get plenty of sleep (see Chapter 26).

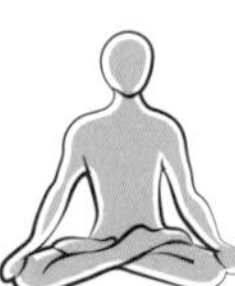
Reduce/manage stress (see Chapter 27).

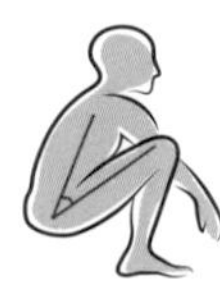
Assume a squatting position when using the toilet (a special footstool can help with this) to align your lower intestines properly for efficient defecation and to minimize strain.

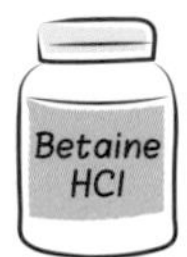

If necessary and not contraindicated, support digestion with supplements (see page 77).

can pigment urine as well, so don't worry if you see some pinkish pee!)

An optimal transit time is 12 to 48 hours. Longer than 72 hours indicates constipation and the possibility of other gut pathologies. Also, studies have shown that even when eating the same diet, men tend to have significantly faster transit times than women, so if you're female, you might be on the higher end of that range, while men can expect to be on the lower end.

Some foods naturally move more slowly or quickly through the digestive system depending on their fiber and water content, how hydrated you are, whether you've recently had caffeine or alcohol, and a variety of other factors. So it's recommended that you repeat this test three times (at different times of the day) to get a ballpark average of bowel transit time.

Bristol Stool Form Scale

A well-established gauge for the health of bowel movements is the Bristol Stool Form Scale. This visual aid, which classifies feces into seven different categories, was developed in the 1990s by researchers at the University of Bristol (United Kingdom) to help distinguish abnormal bowel movements from healthy ones.

Basically, the Bristol stool scale is another way to estimate bowel transit time (the longer poop stays in our bodies, the drier and harder it becomes; the faster it exits, the mushier and looser it is). But the chart can also be used to pinpoint gut disorders in a more specific way.

THE BRISTOL STOOL FORM SCALE

TYPE 1	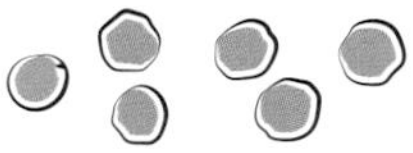 Separate hard lumps, like nuts (hard to pass)
TYPE 2	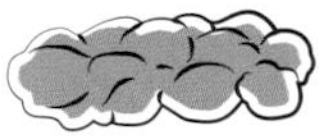 Sausage-shaped but lumpy
TYPE 3	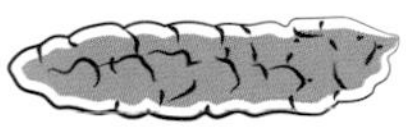 Like a sausage but with cracks on its surface
TYPE 4	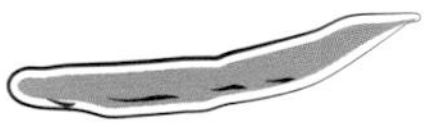 Like a sausage or snake, smooth and soft
TYPE 5	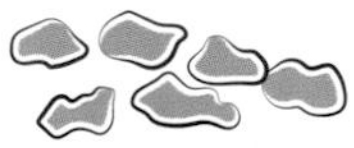 Soft blobs with clear-cut edges (passed easily)
TYPE 6	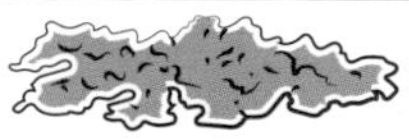 Fluffy pieces with ragged edges, a mushy stool
TYPE 7	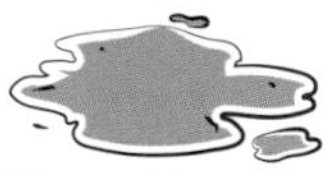 Watery, no solid pieces, ENTIRELY LIQUID

- Type 1 indicates problems with constipation from lack of fiber (such as attempting a zero-carb diet), low levels of beneficial gut bacteria, or a recent course of antibiotics.
- Type 2 can be a symptom of irritable bowel syndrome and can be associated with hemorrhoids, anal fissures, and long-term chronic constipation.
- Type 3 is considered normal but in some cases may indicate latent constipation and some of the problems associated with Type 2.
- Type 4 is optimal!
- Type 5 is considered normal for people who have two or three bowel movements per day, but it can indicate incomplete digestion of food (especially if food particles are visible) or insufficient amounts of fiber and other carbohydrates that feed gut flora.
- Type 6 suggests an abnormally fast bowel transit time and can be a result of excessive stress, laxative use, or certain gut disorders.
- Type 7 is classic diarrhea—the result of foodborne illness, the flu, Crohn's disease, or extreme gut irritation.

Frequently experiencing stools that match Type 1, 2, 6, or 7 may indicate a problem that should be investigated further.

Visual Inspection

Along with gauging bowel movements against the Bristol Stool Form Scale, a couple of other visual indicators can tell us a lot about our gut health.

"Floaters" (stools that float to the surface in the toilet) are usually caused by diet-induced gas but can also result from a bowel infection, lactose intolerance, pancreatic diseases, gallbladder diseases, and certain other health conditions. (Contrary to popular belief, undigested fat is not the cause of floating feces; this belief was debunked by experiments in the 1970s.) If no other symptoms are present, floaters usually don't indicate a problem. But when accompanied by gastrointestinal distress or other signs of gut dysbiosis, or when consistent, they might point to an underlying disorder or a gut microbe imbalance.

Undigested food particles in our stools can have a few different causes—some of them harmless, others indicating a potential problem. Not chewing thoroughly enough, gulping large amounts of liquid while eating, eating too quickly, and consuming hard-to-digest foods (like small seeds, nuts, corn, and the tough skins of certain fruits and vegetables) can all lead to unwanted food particle sightings. Undigested food—especially when the particles are from items that should have been digested thoroughly—can also suggest intestinal inflammation, poor absorption, low hydrochloric acid in the stomach, a deficiency in enzyme excretion in the pancreas, and more serious underlying health conditions. If undigested food is making frequent appearances in your stools, it's a good idea to find the root of the problem. Talk to your doctor!

Bowel Movement Frequency

Along with the previously mentioned tests, bowel movement frequency can tell us about the state of our gut health. Although there isn't a specific, ideal number of bowel movements a person should have every day (that "ideal number" will change a lot depending on diet), three times per day to three times per week is generally considered fine. More or less often than that could indicate problems with poor absorption or constipation, respectively.

If you find yourself on the lower end of the bowel movement frequency spectrum, it may be time to up your vegetable intake. Dr. Jeff Leach of the Human Food Project says, "I tell everybody if you're not having two to three bowel movements a day, then you need to go back and start over. And one of them should be a whopper. If you're not having that kind of bowel activity, then you're not fermenting enough—again, assuming you don't have other issues—and so you need to increase the diversity and quantity of fiber."

Symptom Checklist

Another simple way to tell if you might have a gut disorder is to look for symptoms that suggest abnormal digestive health. If you experience any of the following (especially if more than one of the following are relatively consistent complaints), an underlying gut disorder is a definite possibility.

- Gas, bloating, and belching after meals
- Frequent loose stools
- Alternating constipation and diarrhea
- Undigested food particles in stools
- Indigestion and heartburn
- Bad breath
- Chronic food sensitivities
- Mucus in stools
- Pain or straining while passing a bowel movement

If at-home tests suggest that your gut health is less than stellar, it's important to take steps to heal your gut (see pages 74 and 77). If a more serious condition seems to be at hand, professional testing by a health-care provider can help you identify the problem and figure out the best plan of action.

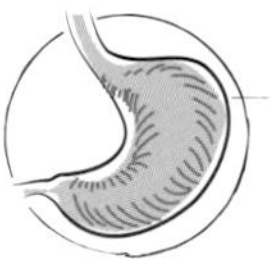

NUTRIENT SUPERSTARS FOR GUT HEALTH

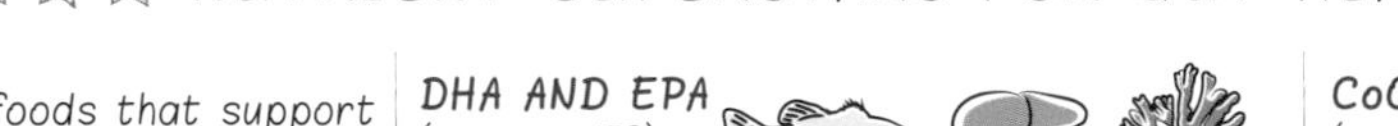

Choosing nutrient-rich foods that support gut barrier and microbiota health is an important tenet of the Paleo template.	**DHA AND EPA** (see page 158) Abundant in: 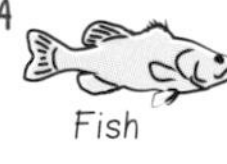 Fish 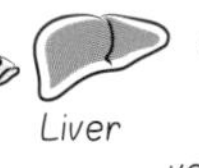 Liver 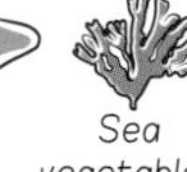 Sea vegetables	**CoQ10** (see page 407) Abundant in: 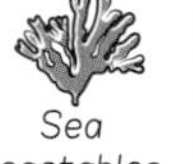 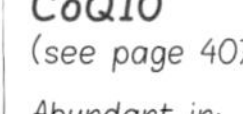 Fatty fish 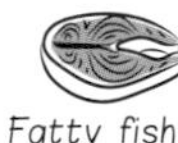 Heart 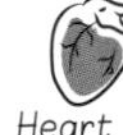 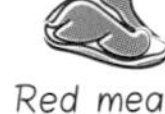 Red meat
VITAMIN A (see page 26) Abundant in: 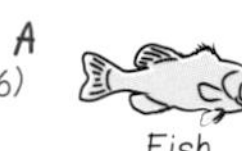 Fish 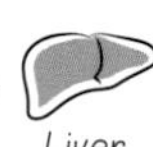 Liver 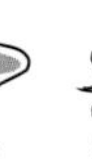  Shellfish	**GLYCINE** (see page 179) Abundant in: 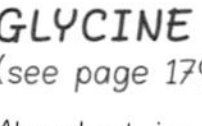 Bone broth 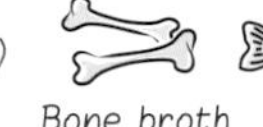 Fish 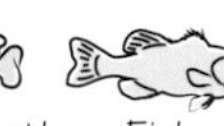 Red meat	**SOLUBLE FIBER** (see page 39) Abundant in: 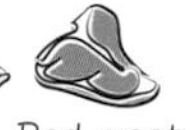 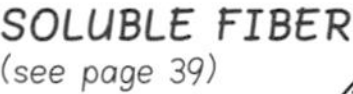 Root vegetables 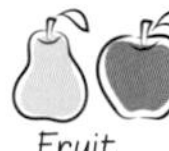 Fruit 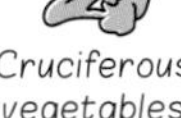 Cruciferous vegetables
VITAMIN D (see page 92) Abundant in: 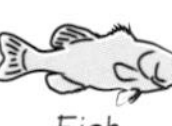 Fish 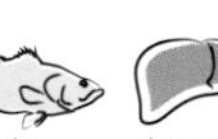 Liver 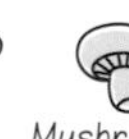 Mushrooms	**GLUTAMINE** (see page 32) Abundant in: 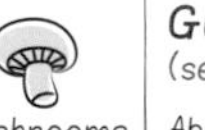 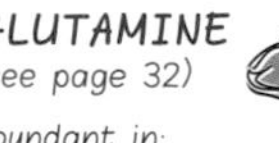 Meat 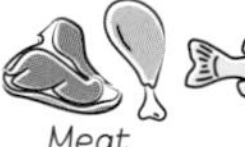 Fish 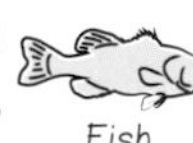 Shellfish	**INSOLUBLE FIBER** (see page 39) Abundant in:  Celery 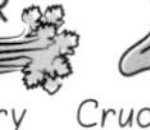 Cruciferous vegetables 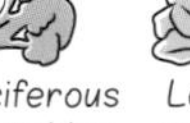 Leafy greens
ZINC (see page 29) Abundant in: 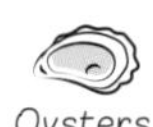 Oysters 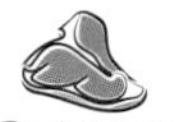 Red meat 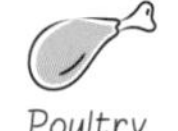 Poultry	**TRYPTOPHAN** (see page 33) Abundant in: 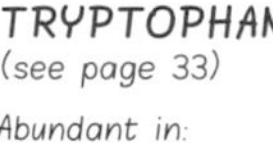 Shellfish  Poultry 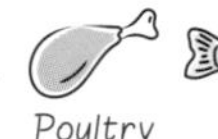 Fish	**FLAVONOIDS** (see page 36) Abundant in: 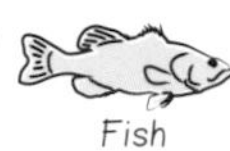 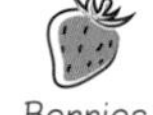 Berries 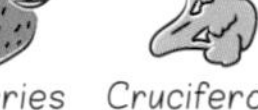 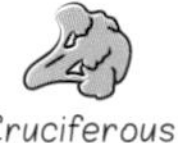 Cruciferous vegetables 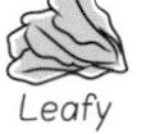 Leafy greens

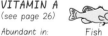

NATURAL SOURCES OF PROBIOTICS

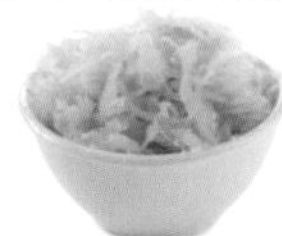

- Kombucha
- Kvass
- Milk kefir (can be made with coconut milk)
- Organic soil
- Raw lactofermented condiments (relishes, salsa)
- Raw lactofermented fruits (green papaya, chutney)
- Raw lactofermented vegetables (carrots, turnips, beets, pickles, kimchi)
- Raw sauerkraut
- Water kefir
- Yogurt (can be made with coconut milk or nut or seed milk)

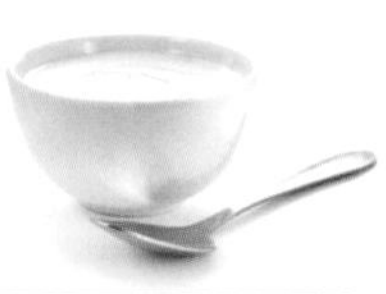

SUPPLEMENTS TO SUPPORT A HEALTHY GUT

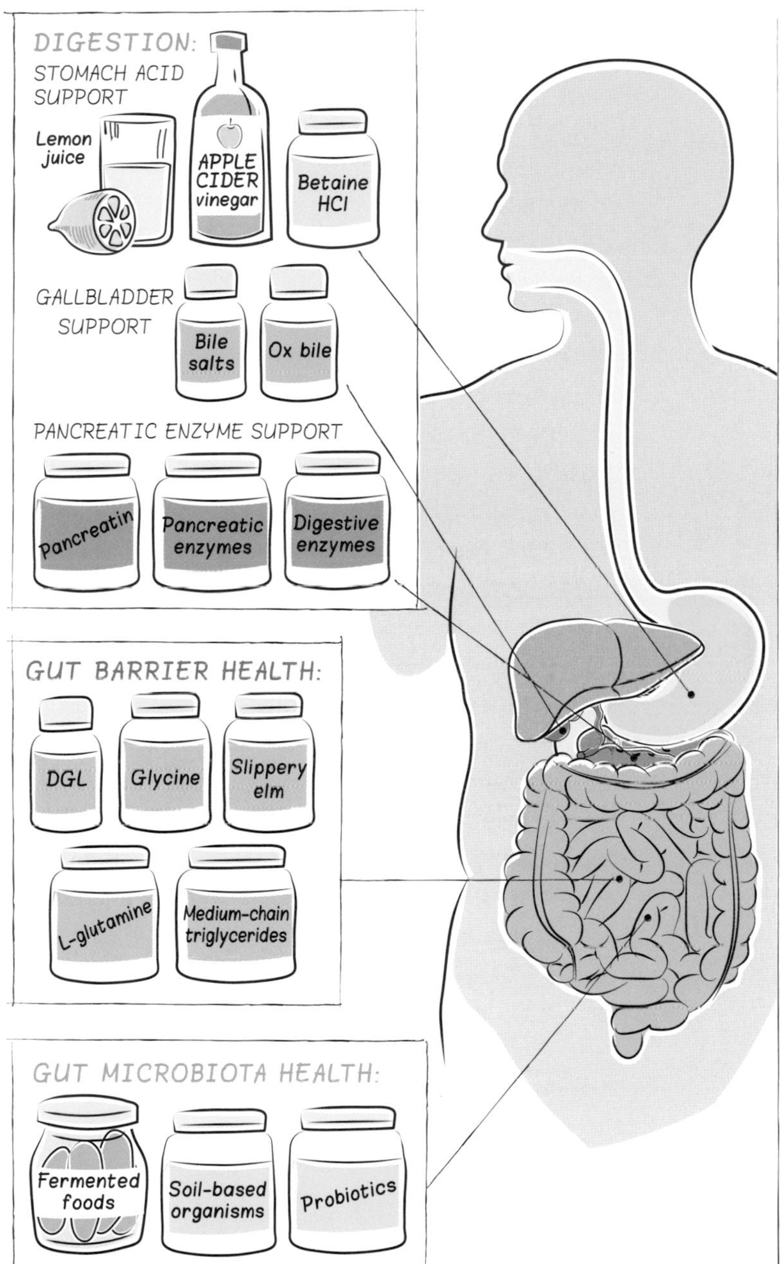

Stomach acid is critical in the initial phases of digestion and in signaling to the gallbladder to release bile and to the pancreas to release digestive enzymes. Addressing deficiencies in stomach acid can typically correct many gastrointestinal symptoms.

Digestive enzyme supplements are a good option for those with low stomach acid but for whom stomach-acid supplementation is contraindicated. They may be used to support digestion for those with severe gastrointestinal distress and may be equally beneficial for those with minor or no gastrointestinal symptoms but who want to optimize nutrient absorption.

Gallbladder support supplements are indicated if your gallbladder has been removed or if you've been given a diagnosis of any gallbladder disease or pathology, any liver disease or pathology (since the liver synthesizes bile salts), or any deficiencies in fat-soluble vitamins.

Always check with your doctor before using supplements.

OPTIMIZING STOMACH ACID WITH SUPPLEMENTS

Stomach acid supplementation is not recommended for anyone who is taking NSAIDs or corticosteroids, has a diagnosed blood-clotting disorder, has severe esophageal damage due to reflux (reflux esophagitis, esophageal strictures, or Barrett's esophagus), has diagnosed malformations of the lower esophageal sphincter, has or has a history of stomach ulcers, or has a disease affecting pancreatic health.

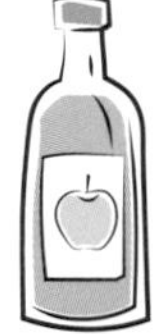

If you are using apple cider vinegar or lemon juice, simply dilute 1 to 2 tablespoons in 1 ounce of water and consume 10 minutes before starting a meal. If this is insufficient to alleviate symptoms, betaine HCl capsules are typically recommended.

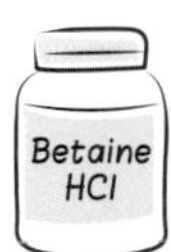

Optimizing your stomach acid dosing using betaine HCl may take days or even weeks. Don't rush this process: taking too much hydrochloric acid can damage your gastrointestinal tract.

1. Start by taking one pill right when you start eating or even after a few bites. Do not take betaine HCl with a meal that doesn't include animal protein.
2. After you have finished eating, notice whether you have any sensations in your abdomen, in particular warmth, heaviness, burning, or gastrointestinal distress.
3. Maintain this dose of one pill with each meal for two full days of meals. If you don't notice any abdominal sensations with any of those meals, increase the dose to two pills per meal.
4. Again, maintain two pills per meal for two full days of meals, paying attention to sensations in your abdomen after each meal.
5. Keep increasing the number of pills taken with each meal every two days until you notice some gastrointestinal discomfort or warmth as described in step 2.
6. Once you reach a dose that causes gastrointestinal discomfort or warmth, decrease the dose by one pill. This is your optimal dose.
7. If you reach a dose of 5,000 to 6,000 milligrams per meal without experiencing any sensations in your abdomen whatsoever, discuss the pros and cons of increasing your dose further with a qualified medical professional. Also discuss having your stomach acid levels tested if they haven't been tested already.

If you've found just the right dose of your stomach acid supplement, you should notice a rapid improvement in your stool quality.

IMMUNE HEALTH

The immune system works via the coordinated efforts of cells, antibodies, proteins, and chemicals to protect our bodies from pathogens, foreign invaders like viruses, bacteria, and parasites that can make us sick. It can be divided into two subsystems: the innate immune system (also called the nonspecific immune system) and the adaptive immune system (also called the specific or acquired immune system).

Inflammation is a broad term that describes the actions of the innate immune system. These actions include the activities of several cell types as well as many specific proteins that, together, form the body's first line of defense against infection and are essential for healing from injury. The innate immune system is quick to mobilize; however, the trade-off is that the innate immune system is not specific or targeted, meaning that its actions look pretty much the same regardless of the reason it is activated. And, perhaps more importantly, the innate immune system doesn't differentiate well between foreign invaders, damaged cells that need to be cleaned up, and healthy cells. So, while the innate immune system does have mechanisms for focusing its attacks, collateral damage occurs, such as to healthy cells adjacent to the site of injury or infection.

SCIENCE SIMPLIFIED *The immune system's job is to defend us from infections that can make us sick. But when the immune system isn't up to snuff, chronic inflammation can lead to diseases like cardiovascular disease, diabetes, and cancer.*

Sometimes the innate immune system can handle the whole job—for example, in healing from a scrape. But when the innate immune system is insufficient to deal with the infection or injury, the adaptive immune system becomes engaged. It then takes over, with an even more complex collection of cells and proteins, including antibodies, to effect a targeted and coordinated attack on the invaders.

Adaptive immunity is distinguished from innate immunity by its specificity for an invading organism. It also remembers invaders (this is called *immunological memory*) so that it can respond to subsequent infections more intensely and quickly. The adaptive immune system is why vaccines protect us against infection and why we get chicken pox only once. The adaptive immune system is responsible for recognizing enemies and distinguishing an antigen (what an antibody binds to) that is foreign from normal, healthy cells and proteins in the body. The adaptive immune system also tailors responses to eliminate specific pathogens or pathogen-infected cells in the most effective and efficient way possible.

When the adaptive immune system is activated, the innate immune system doesn't automatically turn off. Instead, the two work together to eliminate the pathogen, with the adaptive immune system orchestrating the efforts of the many cell types that comprise the immune system, in addition to antibodies, proteins, and chemicals that all have vital roles to play in a healthy immune response.

The immune system has two main jobs. The first is to attack whatever foreign invader is causing problems; the second is to keep the entire system reined in and, once the foreign invader is vanquished, to turn off the cells that attack invaders. We don't give enough credit to the types of cells that do the latter job, but they're essential. Without them, our immune system would turn on when we get a cold and never turn off again! Normally, immune system activation is an acute response. A cut or sliver triggers acute inflammation; exposure to a flu virus triggers acute activation of the adaptive immune system. The system stays restrained because, while some cells are attacking that flu virus, others are making sure that things don't get out of hand. In the case of chronic inflammation, though, our bodies lose the ability to balance attacking functions and regulating functions of the immune system.

In the context of chronic stress, persistent infection, some hormone imbalances, or a diet rich in pro-inflammatory foods, the signals to produce inflammation become chronic. Compounded with nutrient deficiencies and inadequate sleep, the regulatory functions of the immune system can become inefficient. In this case, inflammation can become bodywide and persistent. Although this inflammation is typically more diffuse, it can damage healthy tissue throughout the body on an ongoing basis.

In the case of chronic illness, the immune system is out of control, and our own tissues are innocent bystanders that are affected. Even worse, in the case of autoimmune diseases like multiple sclerosis and rheumatoid arthritis, there's a simultaneous failure on the part of the immune system that's supposed to differentiate between ourselves and foreign invaders, so the immune system targets our own tissues.

Inflammation is part of the pathology of every chronic illness. It might not always be the cause of the illness, but it contributes every single time. And this is where the Paleo template comes into play: how much inflammation we have is a direct result of how we eat, how much we sleep, how active we are, and how much stress we're under. So rather than mask symptoms with drugs that don't address the underlying problem (that doesn't include necessary, sometimes lifesaving medication, which is awesome!), it makes more sense to change our diet and lifestyle to reduce inflammation.

Yes, genetics certainly plays a role in disease, but it accounts for only one-quarter to one-third of our risk for autoimmune disease and most other chronic illnesses. Unlike with genetic diseases like cystic fibrosis and sickle cell anemia, which are directly caused by a single gene mutation, our specific genetic makeup only makes us more or less *susceptible* to developing nongenetic chronic illnesses, like cardiovascular disease, diabetes, obesity, and autoimmune diseases. Having some of the gene mutations that have been identified to increase the risk of nongenetic chronic illnesses is considered a *genetic predisposition*, which really just means that our bodies are not resilient to suboptimal nutrition, lifestyle choices, and environment. That makes understanding how the immune system is affected by nutrition and lifestyle even more important.

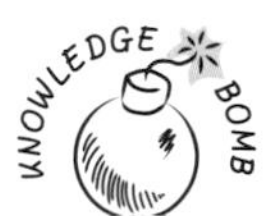

Having either the DQ2 or DQ8 variant of the HLA gene, discussed on page 69, is an example of having a genetic predisposition to autoimmune disease.

KEY IMMUNE SYSTEM CELL TYPES AND WHAT THEY DO

The immune system functions via the complex interplay of many immune cell types and chemical mediators, like antibodies and cytokines. Some key immune cell types that are mentioned throughout this book include the following:

Macrophages and dendritic cells are phagocytes ("eater" cells that destroy pathogens by engulfing them) that reside in various tissues of the body and act as sentinels. They produce cytokines that can kill pathogens, stimulate other phagocytes, and activate T-cells and B-cells.

Monocytes are white blood cells that are recruited to the site of infection to replenish macrophages and dendritic cells.

Neutrophils are phagocytic white blood cells that are recruited to the site of infection, where they rapidly engulf cells coated with antibodies and secrete cytokines that can kill pathogens and stimulate more macrophages and dendritic cells.

Natural killer cells are white blood cells recruited to the site of infection specifically to destroy virally infected cells in the body.

B-cells are lymphocytes (cells of the lymphatic system) produced in the bone marrow that circulate through blood and lymphatic vessels, patrolling the body for antigens. When they find an antigen, they become antibody factories, releasing thousands of antibodies into the blood or connective tissues.

T-cells are lymphocytes produced in the bone marrow and matured in the thymus gland that circulate through blood and lymphatic vessels, patrolling the body for antigens. There are many types of T-cells, including:

- **Cytotoxic T-cells** are specialized in attacking cells of the body infected by viruses and some bacteria. They release chemicals called cytotoxins, which cause its target cell to die by a process called apoptosis.
- **Helper T-cells** are the major driving force and main regulators of the adaptive immune defense. Th1, Th17, and Th22 cells release cytokines that recruit and stimulate macrophages, dendritic cells, and cytotoxic T-cells. Th2 and Th9 cells activate B-cells, which then divide rapidly and secrete antibodies.
- **Regulatory T-cells** suppress the activity of immune and inflammatory cells to shut down T-cell-mediated immunity toward the end of an immune reaction. They also suppress activation of dendritic cells and suppress the activity of any T-cells that recognize self and therefore have the ability to attack healthy cells within the body. Some helper T-cells perform a similar function, including Th3 cells.

Memory cells are a type of T-cell or B-cell produced in the bone marrow that circulate throughout the body, patrolling for antigens that match their antibodies/receptors in order to mount a faster response upon subsequent infection.

The immune system is a nutrient hog. It uses micronutrient resources like no other system in the body. And it needs a vast array of nutrients, including essential fatty acids, essential amino acids, vitamins, minerals, and plant phytochemicals, to do its work effectively. When the body is low on these nutrients, the first aspect of the immune system that suffers is the regulatory part, the part responsible for turning off inflammation when the job is done. When we're deficient in nutrients, our immune system doesn't do a good job of regulating itself and tends to get turned on and stay on.

Some foods are inherently inflammatory. It's quite surprising just how many ways foods can cause inflammation. Processed foods, fast food, foods made with processed "vegetable" oils, grains, and legumes are all high in omega-6 fatty acids, which control cell signaling that turns on inflammation via the production of specific paracrine and autocrine cell-signaling molecules. I discussed the ideal ratio of omega-3 to omega-6 on page 158. When that ratio is off-balance (as it often is when we eat these rich sources of omega-6s), omega-3s can't effectively counteract the inflammatory effect of omega-6s by producing different, less-inflammatory cell-signaling molecules.

In addition, both high blood sugar and high blood insulin levels propel inflammation, so all foods that are high in refined carbohydrates, sugars, and starches that hit the bloodstream quickly (owing to the absence of compounds in the food that slow the digestion of carbohydrates) are inflammatory. These foods also negatively impact many hormones, thanks to all the effects that insulin has in the body. Insulin is a hormone that affects many other hormones and organ systems, and having insulin in the happy-medium range is critical for health. Excess refined carbohydrates also negatively impact two other important hormones: leptin and ghrelin. These hormones help control appetite, metabolism, and the immune system. (Hormones are discussed in more detail on page 83.)

Okay, so there go processed foods, fast food, and junk food. But then those foods were already on the blacklist because they don't possess any nutritionally redeeming properties. What's less commonly known is that many foods considered to be healthy, like whole-wheat bread and low-fat dairy products, also spike blood sugar and insulin levels, and several compounds found in grains (even whole grains), legumes, and nightshades are inflammatory. Compounds called agglutinins (particularly wheat germ agglutinin, kidney bean lectin, soybean lectin, tomato lectin, and peanut lectin) and glycoalkaloids (found in nightshades such as tomatoes, potatoes, eggplants, and peppers) are such potent inducers of inflammation and stimulators of the immune system that several of these compounds have been investigated for use in chemotherapy or in vaccines as adjuvants (chemicals added to vaccines to ramp up the immune system; see Part 4). They're a necessary aspect of how vaccines work, but not a desirable property of food!

When you compound an immune system that isn't regulating itself well due to nutrient deficiency with inflammation stimulators, things aren't going to turn out well. Parts 3 and 4 go into much more detail on how some foods can cause inflammation, but food is only the tip of the iceberg. Stress causes inflammation. Not getting enough sleep causes inflammation. Being too sedentary causes inflammation. Participating in extremely intense exercise causes inflammation. Eating too much or too frequently causes inflammation. Exposure to toxins causes inflammation. Chronic and acute infections cause inflammation (a problem if your immune system doesn't regulate itself well). Not getting enough sleep further hinders the regulatory arm of the immune system. Too much stress hinders the regulatory arm of the immune system.

It may feel like we don't have any control over these factors (and some of them we genuinely can't control), but many of them are within our power to change, and making changes can mean great improvements to our health. Combine getting enough sleep, managing stress, and avoiding inflammatory foods with a super-nutrient-dense approach to food choices to create an internal environment that primes the immune system for success!

THE IMMUNE SYSTEM AT WORK

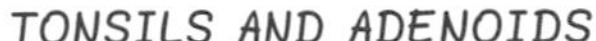

TONSILS AND ADENOIDS
As an early warning system, tonsils and adenoids can detect pathogens and food allergens especially quickly and activate the immune system.

THYMUS GLAND
T cells mature in the thymus, where they learn how to differentiate between our own cells and foreign invaders.

MALT
Other barrier tissues, like sinuses, lungs, bladder, and vagina, also contain lymphatic tissue acting as a sentinel for early detection of infections, referred to as mucosa-associated lymphoid tissue (MALT).

SPLEEN
The spleen stores red blood cells, immune cells like macrophages, T cells and B cells, and platelets for when needed. It also filters the blood, removing old red blood cells for degradation.

LYMPH NODES
Working like biological filter stations, lymph nodes contain different immune cells that trap pathogens and activate the production of specific antibodies in the blood.

GALT
A huge proportion of the immune system is housed in the tissues surrounding the gut, referred to as the gut-associated lymphatic tissue (GALT).

BONE MARROW
Most immune cells are produced in the bone marrow and then released into the bloodstream to reach other organs and tissues.

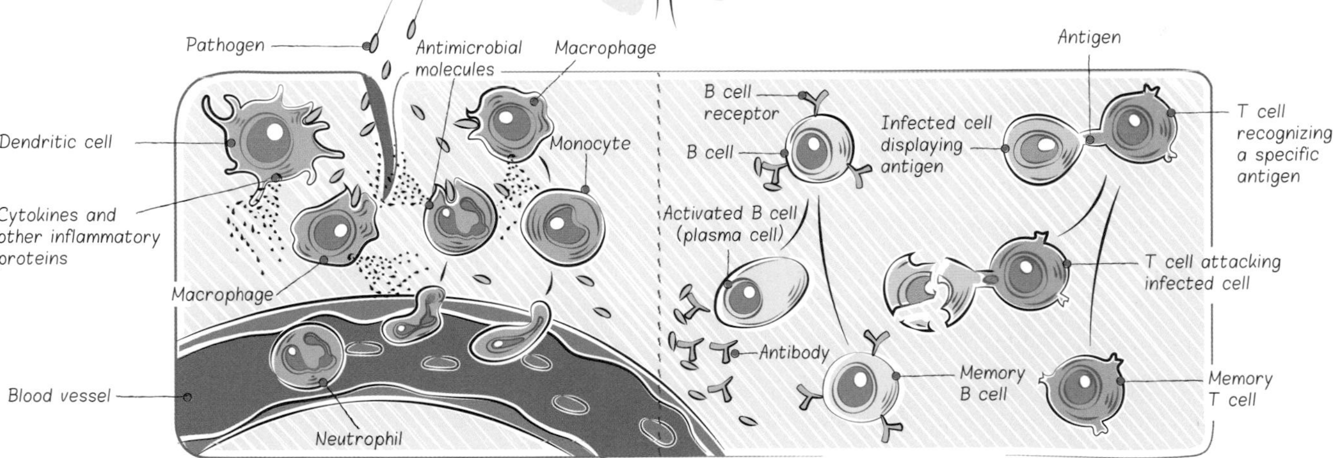

INNATE IMMUNE SYSTEM:
The innate immune system acts as a sentinel near entry points to the body, like skin, sinuses, lung tissues, and the gut. The system includes antimicrobial molecules (like the complement system) and phagocytic cells (cells that ingest and destroy pathogens, but also can alert the adaptive immune system about what they've found), like dendritic cells and macrophages. When the innate immune system gets activated, sentinel cells produce chemical messengers of inflammation (cytokines) that attract other immune cells to the area from blood vessels, like monocytes and neutrophils.

ADAPTIVE IMMUNE SYSTEM:
When the innate immune system presents antigens to the adaptive immune system, it kicks in to mount a targeted attack against the specific invader. B cells produce antibodies that bind to antigens, specific components unique to a given invader, and destroy the invader or mark it for attack by other cells. T cells recognize antigens. Some T cells help activate B cells, and others attack infected cells directly. T and B cells spawn "memory" cells that patrol the body and allow for a faster adaptive immune response on subsequent exposure to the same antigen.

INFLAMMATION IN CHRONIC DISEASE

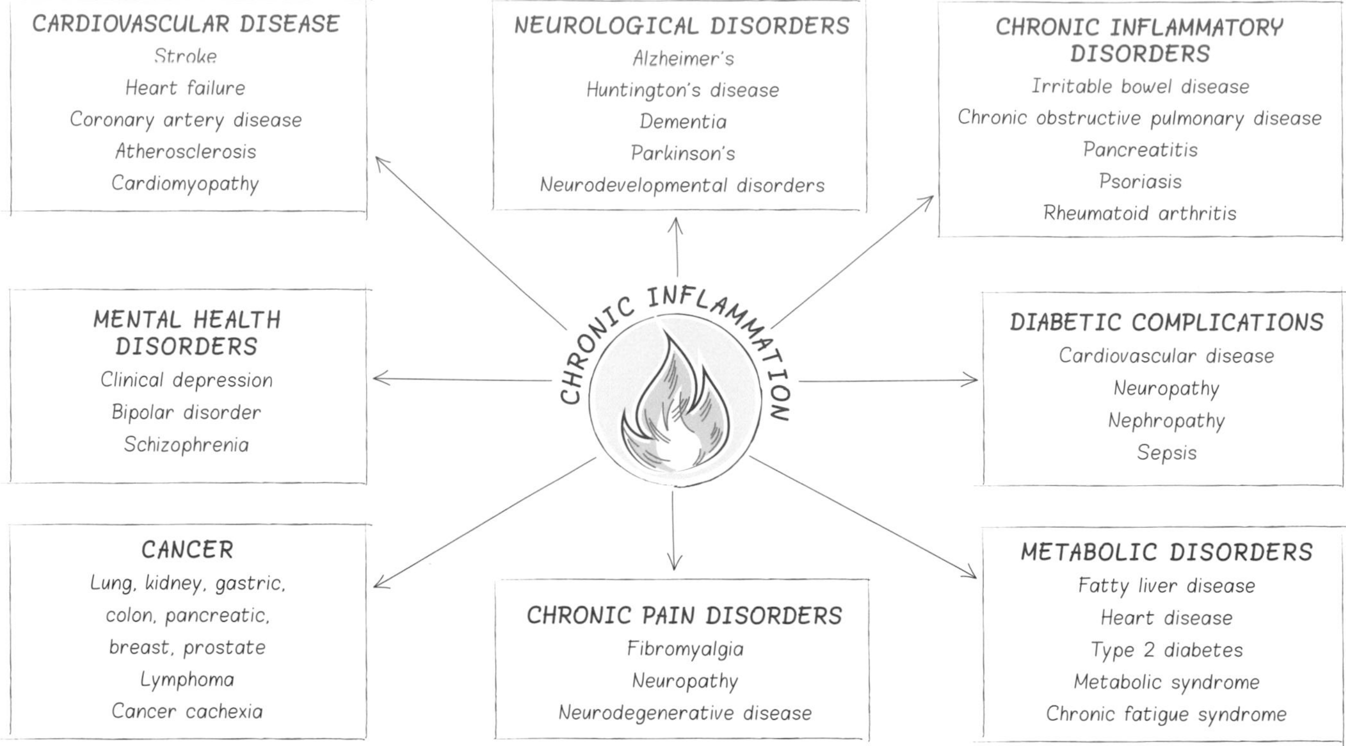

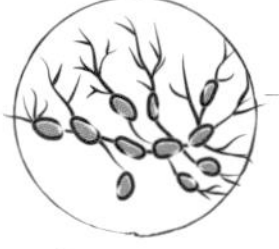

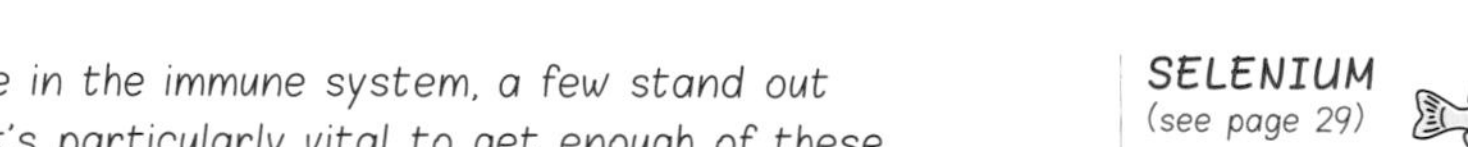

NUTRIENT SUPERSTARS FOR IMMUNE HEALTH

While every nutrient plays a role in the immune system, a few stand out as being especially important. It's particularly vital to get enough of these immune system superstars in your diet!

SELENIUM (see page 29)
Abundant in: Fish, Poultry, Red meat

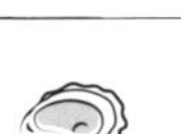

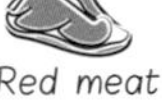

VITAMIN A (see page 26)
Abundant in: Fish, Liver, Shellfish

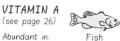

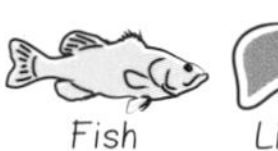
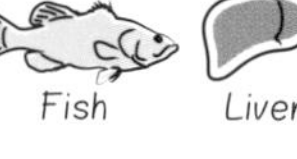
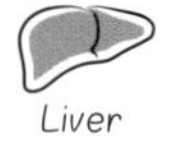

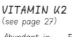

VITAMIN E (see page 27)
Abundant in: Avocados, Leafy greens, Fish

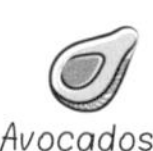
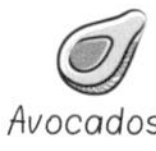
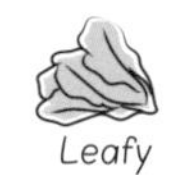
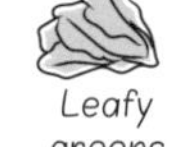
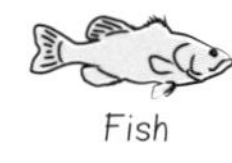
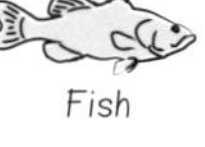
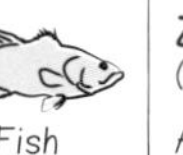

ZINC (see page 29)
Abundant in: Oysters, Red meat, Poultry

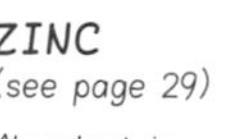
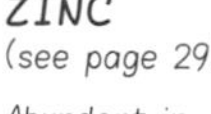
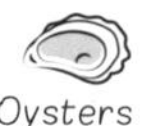
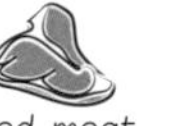

VITAMIN B6 (see page 26)
Abundant in: Leafy greens, Root vegetables, Red meat

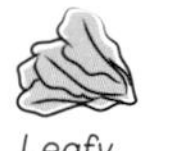

VITAMIN K2 (see page 27)
Abundant in: Fermented vegetables, Fish, Liver

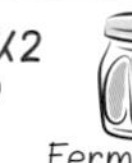
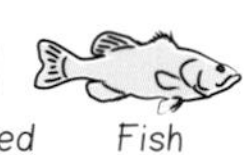
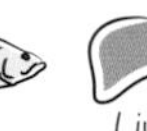

DHA AND EPA (see page 158)
Abundant in: Fish, Liver, Sea vegetables

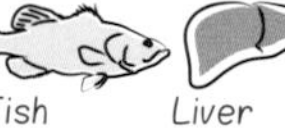
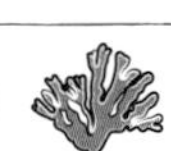

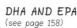

VITAMIN B9 (see page 26)
Abundant in: Avocados, Beets, Green vegetables

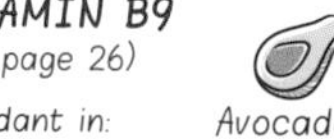
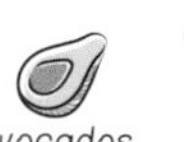

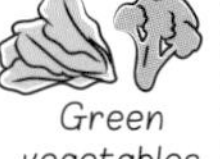

COPPER (see page 28)
Abundant in: Mushrooms, Organ meat, Shellfish

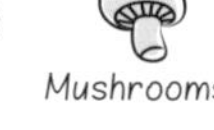
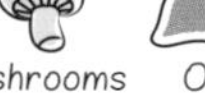
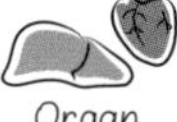

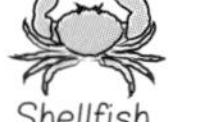

GLYCINE (see page 179)
Abundant in: Bone broth, Fish, Red meat

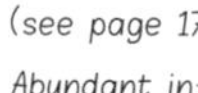
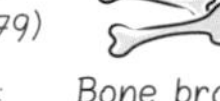
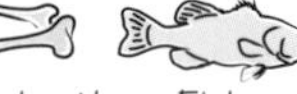
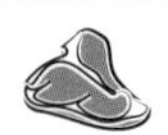

VITAMIN B12 (see page 27)
Abundant in: Fish, Shellfish, Red meat

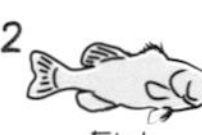

IODINE (see page 28)
Abundant in: Fish, Shellfish, Sea vegetables

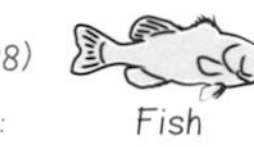

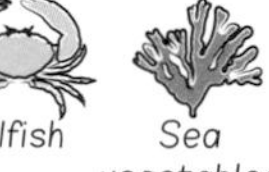
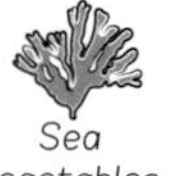

GLUTAMINE (see page 32)
Abundant in: Meat, Fish, Shellfish

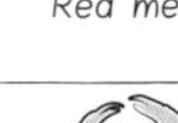
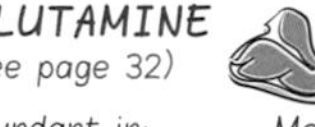
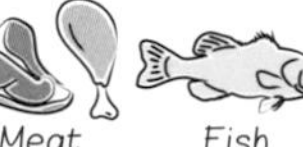

VITAMIN C (see page 27)
Abundant in: Berries, Citrus fruits, Dark leafy greens

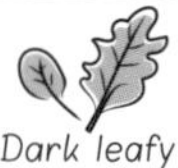

IRON (see page 28)
Abundant in: Dark leafy greens, Liver, Red meat

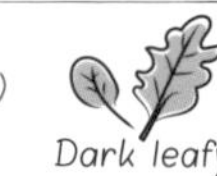
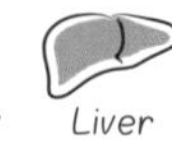
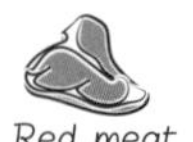

INSOLUBLE FIBER (see page 39)
Abundant in: Celery, Cruciferous vegetables, Leafy greens

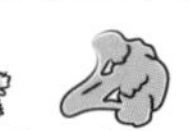

VITAMIN D (see page 92)
Abundant in: Fish, Liver, Mushrooms

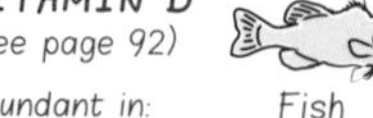
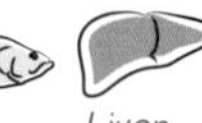
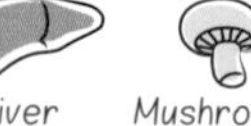
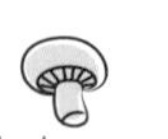

MAGNESIUM (see page 28)
Abundant in: Avocados, Green vegetables, Fish

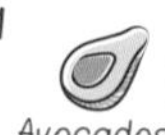
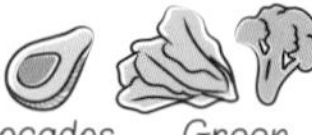
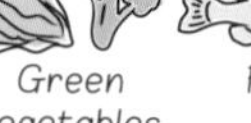
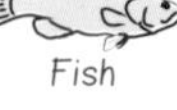

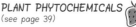

PLANT PHYTOCHEMICALS (see page 39)
Abundant in: Berries, Cruciferous vegetables, Leafy greens

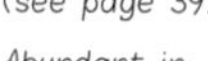
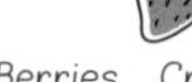

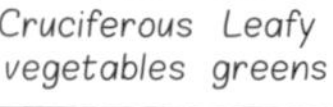

ENDOCRINE HEALTH

The endocrine system is made up of glands that secrete hormones into the circulatory system in order to reach target organs. Hormones are molecules produced by the endocrine organs; they act as chemical messengers that make contact with virtually every cell in the body, similar to a long-distance communication system. There are more than fifty different hormones sending out different kinds of signals, and the variety of functions they control is vast.

The endocrine glands include the pituitary gland, pineal gland, thyroid gland, hypothalamus, adrenal glands, parathyroid gland, pancreas, and ovaries or testes. Although the signaling role of the endocrine system is similar to that of the nervous system, the endocrine system's effects are initiated much more slowly and can last seconds to weeks (compared to the nervous system's extremely quick transmission time and very short-lived responses).

The endocrine system makes extensive use of negative feedback loops to maintain homeostasis (the maintenance of a stable environment inside and outside the cells). A good analogy here is a thermostat: when the temperature drops too low, the thermostat signals the heater to kick on to bring the temperature back up. When the desired temperature is reached, the thermostat tells the heater to turn off. This cycle repeats to keep the temperature within a comfortable range. Likewise, the endocrine system—particularly the pituitary gland and hypothalamus—is set up to increase hormone production when levels get too low and to inhibit hormone production once levels rise above a certain threshold. For instance, the hypothalamic-pituitary-thyroid axis uses a negative feedback loop to control thyroid hormone: the hypothalamus secretes thyroid-releasing hormone (TRH), in turn stimulating cells in the pituitary gland to secrete thyroid-stimulating hormone (TSH). TSH then binds to receptors in the thyroid and spurs the production of thyroid hormones. When levels of thyroid hormones in the blood rise above a certain threshold, the hypothalamus is inhibited from secreting TRH, and the process is diminished until levels drop. Another important example is the hypothalamic-pituitary-adrenal axis, discussed in detail in Chapter 27.

Maintaining a healthy endocrine system requires consuming a nutrient-dense diet that supports hormonal and glandular health, while avoiding foods and lifestyle factors that harm this critical but delicate system. Hormone systems vary in terms of the diet and lifestyle factors that influence them, and while hormone health in general is reliant on nutrient sufficiency, managed stress, adequate sleep, and an active lifestyle, it's worth delving into some specifics as they relate to the Paleo template.

Circadian Rhythm Hormones

The term *circadian rhythm* refers to the huge array of biological processes within the human body (and indeed all forms of life on earth) that cycle according to a 24-hour clock. The main hormones involved are cortisol and melatonin.

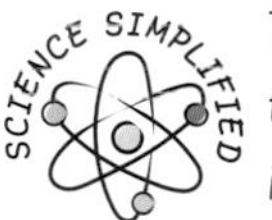

The hormones cortisol and melatonin cycle throughout the day and are the most important signals for the body's internal clock. Cortisol peaks in the morning, telling our bodies that it's time to get up and get going. Melatonin peaks in the evening, helping prepare our bodies for sleep.

Cortisol is a steroid hormone produced by the adrenal gland and released in response to stress (see page 340) and low blood sugar. (Cortisol's effects on sleep is covered in more detail in Chapter 26.) Melatonin is secreted by the pineal gland and is activated by the onset of darkness, helping regulate our sleep-wake cycle and synchronize our biological clock (it also works as a powerful antioxidant within the body).

Circadian rhythm allows the body to assign tasks to various organs and parts of the brain based on the time of day (and whether we are asleep)—for example, prioritizing tissue repair while we are sleeping and prioritizing the search for food, metabolism, and movement while we are awake. Circadian rhythm also influences a natural pattern of daily variations in body temperature, blood pressure, time-sensitive hormones, and digestion. Circadian rhythm is how our bodies know what time it is (like when it's time to get up in the morning), and a properly regulated circadian rhythm is critical for health.

The brain has a master clock, called the circadian clock, which is controlled by specialized cells in a region of the brain called the suprachiasmatic nucleus of the hypothalamus, or SCN. The SCN is connected to the retina of the eye, which makes our dependence on sunlight and darkness important for our circadian rhythm. We know that the SCN is critical for the sleep-wake cycle because damaging the SCN (which might happen after a traumatic brain injury, for example) eliminates regular, patterned sleep behavior based on time of day. This part of the brain is the conductor: it controls the ebb and flow of hormones that act as messengers throughout the body, communicating the time.

As cortisol and melatonin cycle throughout the day—cortisol peaking shortly after waking and melatonin peaking during the middle of the night—they tell all the cells in the body what "time" it is. Then the cells set their own internal clocks to the brain's clock, like us setting our watches to Greenwich Mean Time.

To have a healthy circadian rhythm, the circadian clock needs to be set to the right time. The circadian clock is set by a variety of external factors called *zeitgebers*—a German word for "time givers." The most important zeitgeber is light, because the relationship between the retina and the hypothalamus provides feedback for our circadian rhythm. This notion is supported by the fact that visually impaired people almost always (or at least 90 percent of the time) have circadian rhythm and sleep problems. Our activities throughout the day also send signals to the brain to help it interpret where in our circadian rhythm we are. Finally, hormones play a rather important role in regulating the circadian rhythm as well.

The vast majority of our hormones cycle during the day, meaning that the amounts in our blood vary throughout the day and can vary significantly even over a period of just a few minutes. Not only that, but the sensitivity of different types of cells to different hormones can also cycle. This cycling impacts every system in and many functions of the body, from the immune system to how well we digest food to how much insulin is released in response to sugar intake; all change based on the time of day.

This is why prioritizing circadian rhythm is so important: it not only helps regulate the levels of and sensitivity to different hormones, but even more importantly, it regulates the natural ups and downs that our hormones go through. And this is necessary for health. When our circadian rhythms are properly regulated, we sleep well, we have energy in the morning, our energy is constant throughout the day until it starts to gradually diminish in the evening, and our risk of chronic disease is reduced. Circadian rhythm is an incredible, finely tuned tool that our bodies use to tell time and function at our healthiest.

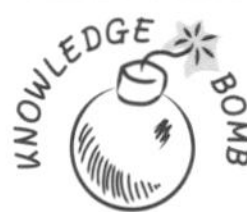

Fasting, low-calorie and low-carbohydrate diets, and alcohol consumption all can reduce the secretion of melatonin, causing sleep disturbances.

Maintaining a healthy circadian rhythm involves a combination of nutritional and lifestyle factors. Although light exposure is the most important synchronizer of melatonin production (as we experience darkness toward nighttime, melatonin secretion increases; exposure to bright light at night is a major disruptor of our circadian clock), various foods and nutrients also influence its production. The essential amino acid tryptophan is used to synthesize melatonin, and the availability of this precursor also impacts our levels of melatonin. Some evidence suggests that energy restriction (low-calorie dieting or fasting) reduces the nocturnal secretion of melatonin, and a very low intake of carbohydrate in particular seems to be the reason. (Some studies have shown that supplementing with glucose during short-term fasting returns melatonin concentrations to normal.) Certain foods, such as tomatoes, olives, rice, walnuts, milk, and coffee beans, contain non-trivial amounts of melatonin and can increase blood levels of melatonin after ingestion, although it's unclear whether this increase is due to the melatonin itself or to other vitamins and minerals present in these foods. Alcohol appears to reduce melatonin levels. Likewise, deficiencies in vitamin B6, vitamin B9, magnesium, and zinc have been linked to lower melatonin levels, likely because these nutrients are involved in both serotonin formation and the formation of melatonin from serotonin. Apart from light exposure, other health-related lifestyle factors, such as body fat levels, can affect melatonin production.

Cortisol is likewise influenced by a variety of nutrients and behaviors, but in a nutshell, inadequate nutrition (including extremely low carbohydrate intake, amino acid imbalance, dehydration, very-low-calorie diets, and micronutrient deficiencies) and excessive physical or psychological stress (including over-exercising and chronic low-grade stress) can elevate cortisol levels and increase our susceptibility to a variety of health problems.

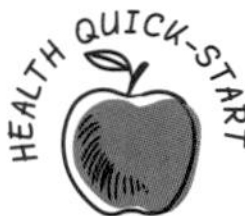

The two most important things we can do to regulate our circadian rhythms is get exposure to bright blue light (sunlight) during the day and keep lights dim and red in the evening. You can biohack this by placing a light therapy box on your desk during the day and by wearing amber-tinted glasses (also called blue-blocking or melatonin glasses) for the last 2 to 3 hours before bed.

Stress Hormones

When the brain perceives a stressful situation, the body reacts with a series of hormonal changes designed to help us survive—regardless of whether the threat could truly kill us (like a lion chasing us in the wild) or not (like a traffic jam). The process is known as the fight-or-flight response, and it occurs when the hypothalamus sets off an alarm that prompts the adrenal glands to release a surge of the stress hormones cortisol, epinephrine, and norepinephrine.

Cortisol is the main stress hormone, and it plays an important role in regulating blood sugar levels, immune responses, metabolism, inflammation, central nervous system activation, heart and blood vessel tone and contraction, and blood pressure and even assists with memory formation. In times of acute stress, cortisol is vital for maintaining blood pressure and fluid balance, as well as putting less immediately important functions on hiatus (such as reproductive drive, digestion, and growth). It also inhibits insulin production to help keep glucose available for immediate use by the muscles in case we need to run from the threat or roll up our sleeves and fight! However, chronically elevated cortisol that doesn't have a chance to return to normal levels (which many of us experience due to constant, non-life-threatening stress in our daily lives) can cause a cascade of problems, such as immune suppression, elevated blood sugar and blood pressure, impaired cognitive performance, decreased muscle mass, slow wound healing, reduced libido, weight gain (especially in the abdomen), sleep disturbances, and thyroid dysfunction. Chronically low levels of cortisol (which can happen in adrenal fatigue; see page 345) can also have negative effects, including hypoglycemia (low blood sugar), sleep disruption (thanks to its role as a circadian rhythm hormone, too), hypotension (low blood pressure), inflammation, and reduced immune function.

Epinephrine (also called adrenalin) is commonly known as the fight or flight hormone due to its role in the immediate reactions we experience during stress. It increases heart rate, respiration, pupil dilation, and sweat production and works to boost blood flow to the muscles, all of which prepare us to either face or flee the threat. Epinephrine is also used as a medication to treat anaphylaxis, a severe allergic reaction that can be fatal.

Norepinephrine is similar to epinephrine except that it is also a neurotransmitter that gets released from neurons (whereas epinephrine is produced only by the adrenal glands). Like epinephrine, norepinephrine helps redirect the body's resources toward immediate survival by increasing blood pressure and respiration and reducing digestive activity.

The effects of stress are discussed in more depth in Chapter 27. As with circadian rhythm hormones (which include cortisol), diet and lifestyle play a major role in maintaining optimal levels of stress hormones and avoiding the health conditions that can occur as a result of chronically elevated levels. Getting adequate sleep, avoiding controllable stressors like excessive high-intensity exercise and sleep deprivation, working on stress management by engaging in stress-relieving activities like walks in nature, yoga, and meditation, and consuming enough calories and micronutrients while avoiding excess caffeine and sugar can all promote stress hormone health!

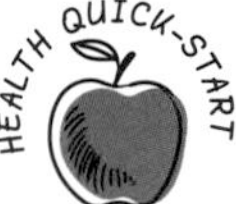

Ten to fifteen minutes of mindfulness meditation daily is clinically proven to greatly improve our resilience to stress. The easiest way to get started with mindfulness is to use one of the breathing techniques listed on page 354.

Insulin

Regulating blood sugar is a key feature of the Paleo diet. In fact, this may be the mechanism responsible for the clinically demonstrated benefits of a Paleo diet in managing diabetes (see page 128).

Diets high in refined carbohydrates or featuring very-high-carbohydrate meals can cause acute hyperglycemia (a notable rise in blood sugar after a meal—also called a glucose spike). Acute hyperglycemia occurs in everyone after eating a substantial amount of carbs. The difference between acute hyperglycemia in a healthy person and in a diabetic is how high blood glucose rises (and how exaggerated the spike is compared to the amount of carbohydrates consumed) and how quickly the body can bring the level back into a normal range.

Chronically elevated blood glucose is called chronic hyperglycemia, and it is a diagnostic criterion for diabetes. High blood sugar levels after eating are a major stimulator of reactive oxygen species (ROS), which are chemically reactive molecules that have important roles in cell signaling (the complex communication between and within cells) and in homeostasis. But ROS are also potent signals for inflammation, stimulating the production of pro-inflammatory chemicals called cytokines and injuring cells and tissue. As a result, chronically high blood sugar can cause serious damage throughout the body, including to blood vessels and vital organs, which is part of why diabetes is associated with a higher risk of stroke, heart disease, vision problems, kidney disease, deep vein thrombosis, and nerve damage.

Generally, blood sugar levels are well regulated when we focus on eating a variety of meat, seafood, eggs, vegetables, fruits, nuts, and seeds, but understanding the players involved in blood sugar regulation is important.

SCIENCE SIMPLIFIED *Keeping blood sugar levels within a healthy range is easy if we limit ourselves to whole-food sources of carbohydrates (like starchy root vegetables and whole fruits) and eat them as part of a meal that includes animal protein and nonstarchy veggies. For those with insulin resistance or diabetes, measuring carbohydrate serving sizes and keeping track of post-meal glucose levels is still advisable.*

When we consume carbohydrates, our blood sugar increases. In response to that rise in blood sugar, the pancreas releases the hormone insulin, which facilitates the transport of glucose into the cells of the body and signals to the liver to convert glucose into glycogen and triglycerides (molecules composed of three fatty acids and a glycerol) for storage. Using a wide array of enzymes, liver cells called hepatocytes first convert excess glucose into glycogen (which is stored in the liver and in muscle tissue) for short-term storage. When needed, that glycogen is rapidly converted back to glucose and released into the blood to maintain normal blood sugar levels and provide cells with energy between meals. There is a limit to the amount of glycogen the muscle tissue and liver can store, so whatever glucose is consumed beyond that amount is converted to triglycerides for longer-term storage in adipocytes (fat storage cells). This process is also stimulated by insulin. The liver releases triglycerides into the blood to circulate to adipose tissues (fat deposits), where they are taken up by adipocytes. So when we eat a high-carbohydrate meal, our blood glucose and blood triglycerides increase.

KNOWLEDGE BOMB *Insulin sensitivity refers to how sensitive the body is to the effects of insulin; if you have normal insulin sensitivity, your body needs less insulin to normalize blood glucose levels compared to someone who has impaired insulin sensitivity. We want to be insulin sensitive. Insulin resistance is a pathological condition in which cells fail to respond normally to the insulin; someone who is insulin resistant has low insulin sensitivity and needs more insulin to normalize blood glucose levels than someone who is not insulin resistant. Insulin resistance can lead to type 2 diabetes.*

Chronically elevated blood sugar levels stimulate adaptations within cells, rendering them less sensitive to insulin. These adaptations may include decreasing the number of receptors to insulin embedded within the cell membranes and suppressing the signaling within the cell that occurs after insulin binds to its receptor. This causes the pancreas to secrete more insulin to lower the elevated blood glucose levels. This is called insulin resistance or loss of insulin sensitivity, when more insulin than normal is required to deal with blood glucose. When normal blood sugar levels can no longer be maintained, you get type 2 diabetes.

Beyond its important action for the metabolism of fuels, insulin has an additional role as an adiposity signal to the brain—that is, it tells the brain whether we should eat and informs the brain about the body's energy status. There is a maximum amount of insulin that can cross the blood-brain barrier (blood vessels in the brain are specialized to restrict which substances in the blood can enter the brain, thereby protecting the

HEALTHY PALEO CARBS

GLYCEMIC INDEX (GI): LOW 0–55 · MEDIUM 55–70 · HIGH 70–100

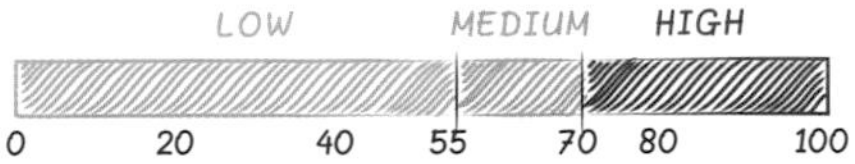

GLYCEMIC LOAD (GL): LOW 0–10 · MEDIUM 10–20 · HIGH 20–60

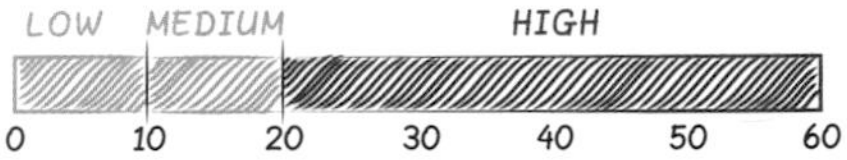

FRUITS

When carbohydrates come from whole fruits and vegetables, even the "carbiest" options tend to be packed with nutrients and fiber and have a low or moderate impact on blood sugar levels.

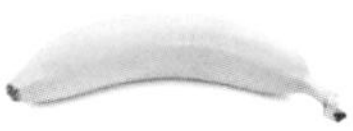

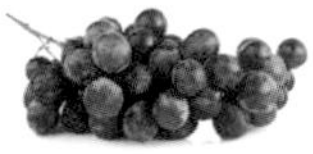

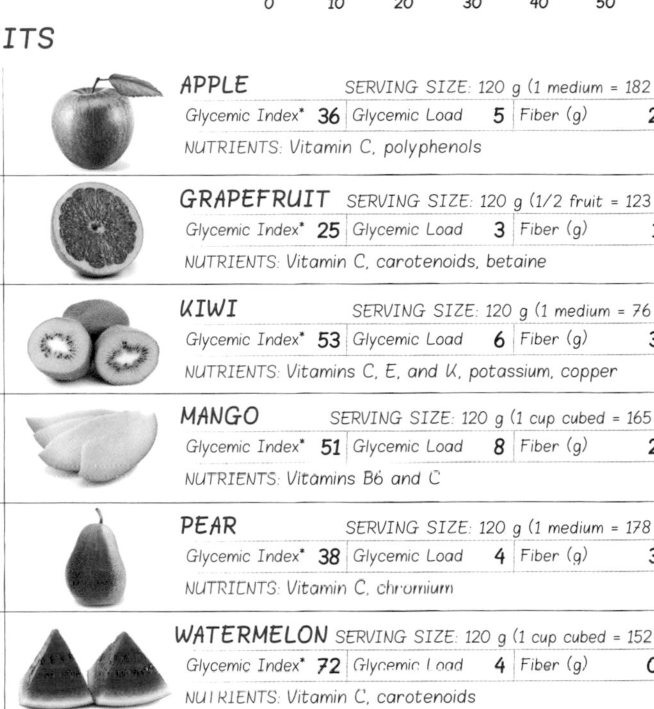

Food	Serving Size	Glycemic Index*	Glycemic Load	Fiber (g)	Nutrients
APPLE	120 g (1 medium = 182 g)	36	5	2.9	Vitamin C, polyphenols
BANANA	120 g (1 medium = 118 g)	48	11	3.1	Vitamins B6 and C, potassium, manganese
GRAPEFRUIT	120 g (1/2 fruit = 123 g)	25	3	1.9	Vitamin C, carotenoids, betaine
GRAPES	120 g (1 cup = 151 g)	59	11	1.1	Vitamins C and K
KIWI	120 g (1 medium = 76 g)	53	6	3.6	Vitamins C, E, and K, potassium, copper
ORANGE	120 g (1 medium = 130 g)	45	5	2.8	Vitamins B9 and C, betaine
MANGO	120 g (1 cup cubed = 165 g)	51	8	2.2	Vitamins B6 and C
PEACH	120 g (1 medium = 150 g)	42	5	1.8	Vitamin C
PEAR	120 g (1 medium = 178 g)	38	4	3.7	Vitamin C, chromium
PINEAPPLE	120 g (1 cup chunks = 165 g)	59	4	1.7	Vitamin C, magnesium, bromelain
WATERMELON	120 g (1 cup cubed = 152 g)	72	4	0.5	Vitamin C, carotenoids

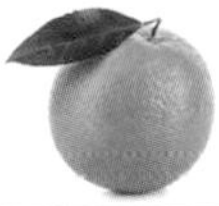

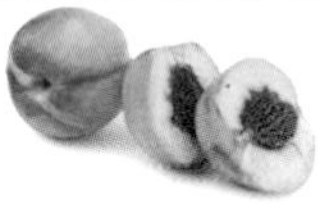

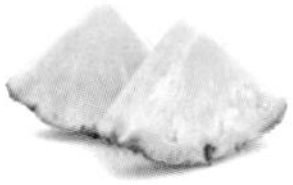

STARCHY VEGETABLES

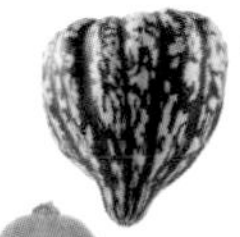

Food	Serving Size	Glycemic Index*	Glycemic Load	Fiber (g)	Nutrients
ACORN SQUASH**	150 g (1 cup cubed = 205 g)	75	6	5.3	Vitamins B1, B3, B5, B6, B9, C, and E, magnesium, potassium, phosphorous, copper, manganese
BEET	80 g (1/2cup sliced = 85 g)	64	5	3.4	Vitamin B6, manganese, betaine
BUTTERNUT SQUASH**	150 g (1 cup cubed = 205 g)	72	6	3.0	Vitamins B1, B3, B6, B9, C, and E, magnesium, potassium, manganese, carotenoids
CARROTS	80 g (1/2cup sliced = 78 g)	39	2	2.3	Vitamin K, carotenoids
CASSAVA, boiled	100 g (1 cup cubed = 206 g)	46	12	1.8	Vitamin C, manganese
GREEN PLANTAIN**	120 g (1 cup sliced = 154 g)	40	13	2.8	Vitamins B6 and C, magnesium, potassium, carotenoids
PARSNIP	80 g (1/2cup sliced = 78 g)	52	4	2.8	Vitamins B9 and C, manganese
POTATO, baked	150 g (1 small = 138g)	85	26	3.3	Vitamins B1, B3, B5, B6, B9, C, and E, magnesium, potassium, phosphorous, copper, manganese
POTATO, boiled	150 g (1/2cup chopped = 78 g)	54	15	3.0	Vitamins B1, B3, B5, B6, B9, C, and E, magnesium, potassium, phosphorous, copper, manganese
SWEET POTATO	150 g (1 cup cubed = 200 g)	61	17	3.8	Vitamins B6 and C, potassium, manganese, carotenoids
TARO	150 g (1 cup sliced = 132 g)	55	4	7.7	Vitamins B1, B6, C, and E, magnesium, phosphorous, potassium, copper, manganese
TURNIP	150 g (1 cup chopped = 144 g)	62	2	3.1	Vitamin C
RUTABAGA (swede)	150 g (1 cup cubed = 170 g)	72	7	2.7	Vitamin C, magnesium, phosphorous, potassium, manganese
YAM	150 g (1 cup cubed = 136 g)	54	20	5.8	Vitamins B1, B6, and C, potassium, copper, manganese

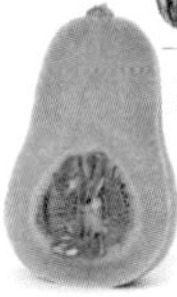

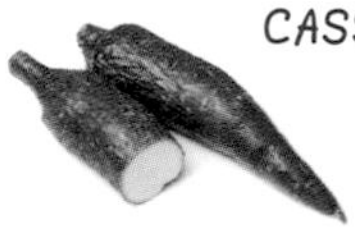

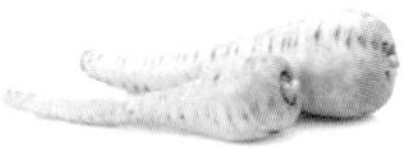

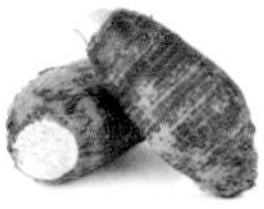

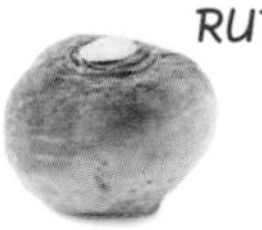

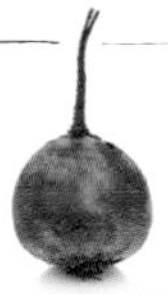

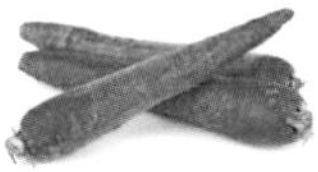

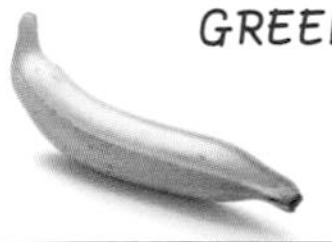

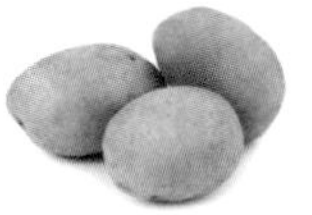

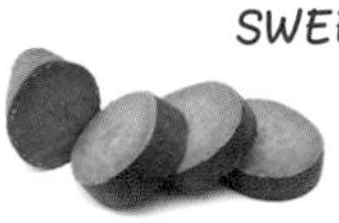

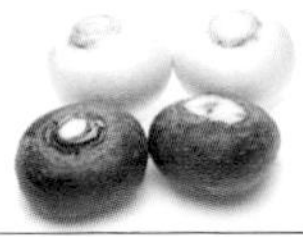

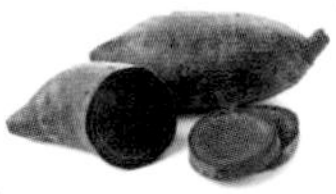

* Glucose = 100 ** Plantains and winter squash are technically fruits, but they cook like vegetables, which is why they are grouped with other veggies in this table.

brain from most toxins and pathogens). As the blood concentration of insulin increases beyond this level, no further signaling to the brain can occur. There's also the potential for decreased insulin receptors in the brain during insulin resistance, meaning that those high levels of circulating insulin don't decrease appetite the way they are supposed to.

KNOWLEDGE BOMB *It's important to differentiate between a food's glycemic index and its glycemic load. Glycemic index is a measure of how quickly the carbohydrates from a specific food impact blood sugar levels (the higher the glycemic index, the higher and faster blood sugar will rise after that food is eaten), but this concept doesn't take into account that food's carbohydrate density. Glycemic load measures how quickly the carbohydrates from a specific food impact blood sugar levels, adjusting for how many carbohydrates are likely to be consumed in a serving. Some foods have a high glycemic index but a low glycemic load: while the sugars in those foods are easily absorbed and cause a rapid impact on blood sugar, there aren't that many of them, so these foods are often still healthy choices (watermelon is a good example; see the previous page).*

Hunger Hormones

The feeling of hunger is regulated by a complex system of hormones that interact with neurotransmitters and neurotransmitter receptors within the hypothalamus region of the brain. These hormones essentially activate or deactivate specific neurons in the hypothalamus that control hunger. These neurons have receptors to neuropeptide Y (NPY), the essential neurotransmitter in regulating hunger. The hormones can increase or decrease hunger either through binding the receptors for NPY or increasing or decreasing NPY itself. Essentially, a hormone will increase hunger if it activates these NPY neurons, and a hormone will increase satiation if it deactivates the NPY neurons. The interplay between these hormones and the brain is complex and only partially understood. However, what scientists *do* know about these hormones can help inform our decisions and compulsions regarding diet and other lifestyle factors.

New hormones continue to be discovered, and their roles in regulating appetite, satiety, metabolism, and digestion continue to be studied. As the list of hunger hormones grows, understanding the complex interplay between them, the types of food we eat, and the amount of muscle and fat on our bodies quickly becomes overwhelming. The key players (at least as scientists currently understand them) include:

Hormones that tell the body it's hungry:

Ghrelin is considered the main hunger hormone. It is secreted by the cells that line the stomach when the stomach is empty and by the pancreas when it detects low blood sugar. Also, the liver secretes ghrelin when its glycogen storage runs low (and glucagon is high; see page 89). When ghrelin is released into the circulation, it directly activates NPY neurons to stimulate appetite. Increased levels of ghrelin are directly associated with the sensation of hunger. It is considered the counterpart of the hormone leptin (see page 90). Importantly, ghrelin is a potent stimulator of growth hormone (GH) secretion and regulates nutrient storage, thereby linking nutrient partitioning with growth and repair processes. Ghrelin activates several anti-inflammatory pathways in the body and promotes cell regeneration, thereby promoting healing, especially within the gastrointestinal tract. Ghrelin regulates glucose homeostasis through a direct action on the pancreatic islet cells (the cells that secrete insulin). It is also important for memory function and gut motility.

Cortisol is well known as a stress hormone (see page 85), but it has key roles in regulating metabolism and hunger. Cortisol levels determine whether the body uses glycogen stores or triglyceride stores for energy (stored carbohydrate or stored fat). Cortisol can also stimulate gluconeogenesis, the process of converting amino acids (proteins) and lipids (fats) into glucose in the liver. It is believed that cortisol directly influences food consumption by acting on NPY neurons in the brain as well as affecting the levels of NPY and leptin. Cortisol seems to have a particular effect on the desire to eat foods high in fat and sugar. This is why stress management (which really means controlling any factor that might mess with our natural cortisol levels) is so important.

Glucagon is a hormone secreted by the pancreas when it detects low blood glucose levels (typically between meals, but this can also happen as part of that "sugar crash" after eating something very high in carbohydrates). Glucagon signals the liver to convert stored glycogen into glucose, which is released into the bloodstream, a process known as glycogenolysis. When glycogen stores are low, high glucagon levels drive gluconeogenesis, the process of creating glucose from amino acids and fatty acids. Increased glucagon amplifies the hunger sensation.

Insulin is secreted by the pancreas in reaction to high blood glucose levels (see page 85). Insulin causes cells in the liver, muscle, and fat tissue to take up glucose (and fatty acids in the case of adipocytes) from the blood, storing it as glycogen. While insulin is released as a result of eating carbohydrates, it paradoxically increases hunger as opposed to decreasing it. This is caused by direct action on the NPY neurons and is the reason why eating a carbohydrate-rich meal is not as satiating as eating a meal that includes fats and proteins. It also explains how quickly we feel hungry again after a high-sugar snack.

Hormones that tell the body it's satiated:

Cholecystokinin (CCK) is secreted by the cells that line the duodenum (the first segment of the small intestine) when they detect the presence of fat. This causes the release of digestive enzymes from the pancreas and bile from the gallbladder. Increased levels of CCK signal to the stomach to slow the speed of digestion so the small intestine can effectively digest the fats. CCK is also a neuropeptide similar to NPY and has a direct action on neurons in the brain to signal satiety. This is the most immediate hunger-suppressing signal and is one reason eating fat with each meal is so important.

Oxyntomodulin is released in response to protein and carbohydrates in the stomach and signals a change in energy status to the brain. Oxyntomodulin enhances digestion by delaying gastric emptying and decreasing gastric acid secretion.

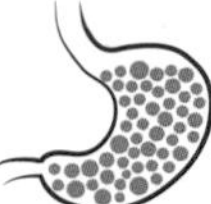

Peptide YY (PYY) is released by cells that line the jejunum, ileum (the next two segments of the small intestine), and colon in response to feeding and is especially sensitive to protein. PYY signals to the gallbladder and pancreas to stop producing digestive enzymes. PYY is important in increasing the efficiency of digestion and nutrient absorption after a meal by slowing down gastric emptying, slowing the speed of digestion, and increasing water and electrolyte absorption in the colon. PYY interacts directly with NPY receptors in the hypothalamus in an inhibitory fashion, thereby turning off hunger signals.

Glucagon-like peptide-1 (GLP-1) is secreted in the ileum in response to carbohydrate, protein, and fat. It rapidly enters the circulation and is one of the fastest and shortest-lived satiety signals. It inhibits acid secretion and gastric emptying in the stomach. GLP-1 also increases insulin secretion and decreases glucagon secretion. GLP-1 decreases hunger signals by reducing the amount of NPY.

Leptin plays a key role in regulating energy intake and energy expenditure, including appetite and metabolism. Leptin is released both by adipocytes (fat cells) and by the cells that line the stomach, so it signals both that the body is fed and that there is sufficient energy storage. This appetite inhibition is long term, in contrast to the rapid inhibition of eating by CCK and the slower suppression of hunger between meals mediated by PYY. Leptin both rapidly inhibits NPY production and deactivates NPY neurons in the brain to signal that the body has had enough to eat, producing a feeling of satiety. It is one of the most important adipose-derived hormones.

Adiponectin is secreted from adipose tissue into the bloodstream, where it signals decreased gluconeogenesis (the conversion of fats and proteins into glucose for energy), increased glucose uptake, lipid catabolism (breaking down of fats), triglyceride clearance (storage of fats), increased insulin sensitivity, and control of energy metabolism. Adiponectin acts directly on NPY neurons similarly to leptin but with additive effects.

These hormones have important roles both signaling to the brain whether we need to eat and in regulating aspects of digestion. Many are also critical in regulating blood sugar both after a meal and between meals (fed and fasted states). Some of these hormones also affect other systems in the body; for example, interacting with the immune system and controlling inflammation. Understanding how diet and lifestyle affect hunger hormones will help us make choices that regulate these hormones properly, allowing us to listen to our hunger cues and trust that the body knows what it's doing. Ultimately, regulating hunger hormones is a key part of healing and being healthy.

More on Leptin and Ghrelin

Leptin is secreted by adipocytes in direct proportion to the amount of stored body fat, in particular the amount of subcutaneous fat, as well as by cells that line the stomach in response to eating. Similar to insulin, circulating leptin enters the brain, where it binds to receptors, stimulating both a reduction in food intake and an increase in energy expenditure. The body can become leptin resistant, which is analogous to being insulin resistant, although leptin resistance can be a consequence of both overconsumption of food as well as fasting or consuming too few calories.

It was initially believed that leptin's dominant role was to tell the brain to stop eating. However, recent studies have shown that leptin also controls the adaptation to fasting. Fasting or consuming too few calories on a regular basis can decrease leptin sensitivity, which leads to increased hunger, cravings, and lack of energy. The reason it's so hard to keep weight off after going on a weight-loss diet is that reduced leptin sensitivity lowers metabolism and increases hunger—a nasty combination! There is also a link between leptin and cortisol release, potentially explaining both the normal increase in cortisol after meals and the cortisol spike that many people experience in response to intermittent fasting.

Leptin is not just a hunger hormone. It is also connected to the regulation of the reproductive, thyroid, and growth hormones, and the adrenal axes. Leptin promotes angiogenesis (the growth of blood vessels), regulates wound healing, controls hematopoiesis (the production of blood cells), and is an essential regulator of the immune system.

When it comes to understanding how diet influences leptin regulation, the key seems to be balance. Obesity, high-fat diets, high-carbohydrate diets, and hypercaloric diets in general all increase leptin and cause leptin resistance. However, the other extreme produces the same results: starvation, prolonged fasting, ketogenic diets, gross malnutrition, and severely calorie-restricted diets can all increase leptin and leptin resistance. Some micronutrient deficiencies have been associated with higher leptin levels, including vitamins A, C, and D and zinc.

There is a close connection between insulin and leptin. Leptin signaling directly impacts insulin release, and leptin resistance has been shown to increase insulin secretion and cause insulin resistance. Furthermore, chronic hyperinsulinemia causes an increase in leptin. Therefore, regulating blood glucose levels is crucial for regulating both insulin and leptin (levels and sensitivity). Other dietary factors that impact leptin include alcohol consumption, which increases leptin, and excessive fructose consumption, which causes leptin resistance.

In many ways ghrelin is the counterpart, or opposing hormone, to leptin. While leptin signals satiety, ghrelin signals hunger and is, in fact, considered the main hunger-stimulating hormone. Ghrelin is released into the circulation (it circulates throughout the body via the blood) by the cells that line the stomach and by specialized cells that line the small intestine when the stomach is empty (although 60 to 70 percent is released by the cells lining the stomach). It can also be secreted by numerous other cells and tissues in the body, including by the pancreas when blood sugar is low, and by the liver when glycogen stores are low. Ghrelin travels to the brain to stimulate the sensation of hunger; it peaks right before a meal (when we're feeling hungry) and drops quickly once we've eaten.

Increased ghrelin stimulates the production of growth hormone, which is essential to stimulating growth, cell reproduction, and cell regeneration, but also has critical roles in metabolism, including stimulating gluconeogenesis in the liver and stimulating lipolysis in adipocytes (release of free fatty acids from stored triglycerides in fat-storage cells). However, ghrelin seems to be quite the multitasker: it also contributes to regulation of gut motility, gastric acid secretin, gastric emptying, pancreatic function, glucose homeostasis (maintenance of normal blood glucose levels), cardiovascular function, blood pressure, immune function, the reproductive system, bone metabolism, secretion of a wide variety of hormones, sleep, anxiety, and even memory. Ghrelin also promotes intestinal cell proliferation and inhibits intestinal cell apoptosis (programmed cell death) during inflammatory states and oxidative stress. Its regenerative capacity and beneficial properties in the event of mucosal injury to the stomach imply that ghrelin regulation is very important for healing a damaged and leaky gut.

Ghrelin may also play a role in the adaptation to fasting. During a fast, ghrelin levels continue to rise, which may be essential for maintaining blood glucose levels needed for survival during prolonged nutrient restriction. This is achieved thanks to ghrelin's influence on catecholamines, cortisol, glucagon, growth hormone, insulin, and its effects on insulin sensitivity.

Regulation of ghrelin levels and ghrelin secretion appears to be a very complex process. There is an interplay between ghrelin and other hunger hormones; in particular, there is a link between ghrelin and insulin. Very low ghrelin levels are associated with elevated fasting-insulin levels and insulin resistance (which may be the link between overeating and diabetes). To support normal insulin responses and normal insulin sensitivity, ghrelin must be well-regulated, meaning both maximizing ghrelin before a meal and minimizing it after a meal.

SCIENCE SIMPLIFIED

Ghrelin and leptin are best regulated when we eat distinct meals well-spaced apart (it's important to feel hungry before a meal) that contain protein, fiber, and whole-food carbohydrate sources. They are also better regulated when energy deficiencies or excesses are low (meaning slow weight loss or weight gain, depending on our goals) and when we avoid fasting.

Ghrelin levels rise when the stomach is empty and when energy is low (including blood glucose, glycogen stores, and circulating triglycerides). This means that to maximize ghrelin, there must be sufficient time between meals. Ghrelin secretion is inhibited by the consumption of carbohydrates, especially glucose and dietary fiber, and protein. However, ghrelin is not inhibited by fructose, and excessive fructose consumption has been linked to chronically elevated ghrelin (which may be why overconsumption of fructose stimulates appetite). Ghrelin is less affected by dietary fats (more so by short-chain and medium-chain fatty acids, compared with long-chain fatty acids, but still much less than by carbohydrates and protein). There is also evidence that eating a high-protein, high-carbohydrate breakfast has big benefits in terms of regulating ghrelin (by decreasing it substantially).

Grazing, Fasting, and Breakfast

Hunger hormones are best regulated when we eat distinct, well-spaced, complete, and balanced meals that contain protein, slow-burning carbohydrates, moderate fat, and fiber.

The original studies that supported the assertion that grazing was healthier were correlative studies showing that the more frequently you eat, the more likely you are to be a healthy weight. However, this correlation evaporates once exercise is brought into the picture. Prospective studies have universally shown that increasing eating frequency yields no benefit in individuals of normal weight and results in a tendency toward weight gain and higher risk of diabetes in overweight people.

So what is optimal meal frequency? Analysis of hunter-gatherer and hunter-gatherer-farmer populations (modern and historical) shows that these populations typically eat one large meal in the afternoon or early evening. A small meal of leftovers is sometimes ingested in the morning, as are small amounts of food as it is gathered. Not only does this not look anything like the five to six small meals a day that are erroneously advocated for optimal metabolism, but it doesn't even look like the three "square" meals with which grazing is contrasted.

When we start to consider eating one meal a day (without restricting calories), there are some interesting research findings. One study showed that eating one meal a day in the absence of calorie restriction improves body composition and cardiovascular-risk factors and reduces cortisol. Another study showed that eating one meal a day reduces inflammation by preventing circulating white blood cells (specifically monocytes) from producing cytokines. And there is speculation that decreased meal frequency would result in decreased oxidative stress and increased leptin and insulin sensitivity. Although compelling, these studies do not make a strong case for one meal a day.

The concept of intermittent fasting has gained traction within the Paleo community, in part because some studies have shown that repeated short-term fasts (typically 16 to 24 hours long) improve our ability to handle stress (meaning that less cortisol is released in response to psychological stressors) and because intermittent fasting stimulates autophagy (akin to spring cleaning in every cell, with cells breaking down components that are not working properly to be recycled and rebuilt). However, when we skip breakfast (or breakfast and lunch), our bodies increase cortisol in order to stimulate glycolysis or gluconeogenesis to raise our blood sugar so that we have energy for the day. If cortisol levels and rhythmicity are not normal, this extra cortisol release to help regulate blood sugar can contribute to cortisol dysregulation or cortisol resistance.

Furthermore, there is evidence that autophagy is inhibited in those of us with chronic illness. This means the beneficial adaptations to fasting that healthy people enjoy are less likely to take place not just in people with chronic illness but in anyone dealing with chronic stress. In fact, repeated intermittent fasting (which is what eating one meal a day really amounts to) is used as a model of chronic stress in animal studies. In animals, fasting activates liver immune cells, increases fat accumulation in the liver, raises blood cholesterol, and accelerates the DNA damage in the liver and spleen caused by a high-fat diet. In humans, one study showed higher insulin resistance in people who ate only one meal a day. Furthermore, healthy women are more likely to experience lowered glucose tolerance in response to intermittent fasting than healthy men, so the jury is still out on whether intermittent fasting provides benefits to women at all.

A good argument can be made for eating breakfast. In fact, studies evaluating hunger and food cravings later in the day in relation to whether people ate or skipped breakfast imply that hunger hormones are much better regulated when breakfast is eaten. People who routinely skip breakfast are known to have greater risks of cardiovascular disease and obesity. This might not be directly related to any specific benefit of eating early in the day as much as to the fact that eating breakfast seems to make it easier to make healthy choices the rest of the day.

HEALTH QUICK-START *Make sure to have a protein-rich breakfast within an hour of waking up! Studies show that this sets you up for healthier choices throughout the day as well as improves your ability to reach a healthy weight.*

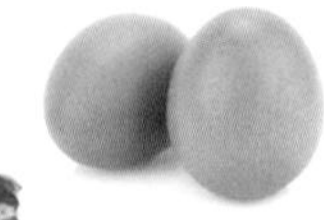

There must be a balance between eating frequently enough to encourage normal cortisol levels and insulin sensitivity but infrequently enough for ghrelin to become elevated between meals and leptin sensitivity maintained. For most people, this equates to two to four meals (or three meals and one snack) per day, the first being shortly after waking up and the last being 2 to 4 hours before going to bed. (There's a relationship between melatonin and insulin, and eating too late in the day disrupts sleep. In fact, clinical trials confirm that eating even a small snack within 1 hour of going to bed negatively impacts sleep quality.) Individual preference and a little trial and error will determine what works for you. The bottom line is that eating larger and less-frequent meals is far better than grazing or intermittent fasting.

Vitamin D

Despite being referred to as a vitamin, vitamin D is actually a steroid hormone (also called calcitriol). Vitamin D controls the expression of more than 200 genes and the proteins that those genes regulate. It is essential for mineral metabolism (it regulates the absorption and transport of calcium, phosphorous, and magnesium) and for bone mineralization and growth. It is also crucial for regulating several key components of the immune system, including the formation of important antioxidants. Very importantly, vitamin D has recently been shown to decrease inflammation and may be critical in controlling autoimmune and inflammatory diseases. Vitamin D is also involved in the biosynthesis of neurotrophic factors, regulating release of such important hormones as serotonin (required not only for mental health but also for healthy digestion!). Because it helps control cell growth, vitamin D is also essential for healing. In addition, it activates areas of the brain responsible for biorhythms. Scientists continue to discover new ways in which vitamin D is essential for human health; for example, it may help prevent cancer.

Our bodies synthesize vitamin D in response to sun exposure (see page 369). As we spend less and less time outdoors, dietary vitamin D becomes more and more important. The best dietary sources are organ meat, fatty fish, and egg yolks.

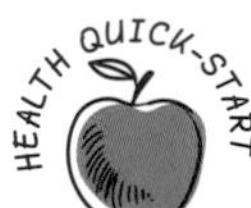

About 75 percent of Westerners are deficient in vitamin D, a key player not just in bone health but also in immune system health. Optimal serum vitamin D levels are between 50 and 70 nanograms per milliliter (ng/mL). It's important to ask your health-care provider to test your levels. If you're deficient, it can be tough to get enough vitamin D3 from foods (natural sources include grass-fed and pastured meats and seafood), so consider supplementing (your doctor may recommend anywhere from 500 IU to 5,000 IU daily to address deficiency) and recheck every three months to make sure you don't overshoot the mark. Vitamin D levels in excess of 100 ng/mL can also cause health problems.

Thyroid Hormones

The thyroid is a small but important gland that uses iodine (a mineral particularly abundant in seafood) to produce the tyrosine-based hormone triiodothyronine (T3) and its prohormone thyroxine (T4), which regulate metabolism. Under normal circumstances, the pituitary gland senses the level of thyroid hormone in the blood and releases thyroid-stimulating hormone (TSH) to tell the thyroid gland to produce more or less thyroid hormone to maintain the correct levels. This works through a closed-loop feedback process in which high levels of T3 and T4 in the blood inhibit the pituitary gland's production of TSH, while low levels stimulate greater TSH production. These hormones are then carried through the blood bound to plasma proteins, including thyroxine-binding globulin (TBG), transthyretin, and albumin.

Thyroid hormones affect numerous areas of the body, including the heart, eyes, intestines, brain, skin, and hair. As a result, thyroid hormone levels being either too high or too low can have a devastating effect on a person's health. Hyperthyroidism (including the autoimmune condition Graves' disease) occurs when excessive T3 and/or T4 are circulating and can cause symptoms such as rapid heartbeat, nervousness, irritability, anxiety, brittle hair, muscle weakness, sleep problems, heat intolerance, enlarged thyroid gland, weight loss, and diarrhea. Hypothyroidism (such as Hashimoto's thyroiditis) occurs when there's a deficiency of T3 and/or T4 and can cause symptoms such as cold intolerance, fatigue, depression, weight gain, constipation, poor concentration and memory, hair loss, low heart rate, hoarseness, cool extremities, shortness of breath, and heavy menstruation in women.

Triiodothyronine (T3) is the "true" thyroid hormone and is about four times more potent than its precursor, thyroxine (T4). It stimulates the body's oxygen and energy consumption (raising basal metabolic rate) and stimulates RNA polymerase I and II (promoting protein synthesis). T3 plays a role in cholesterol breakdown and increases LDL receptor activity, which is why low thyroid function is associated with higher LDL levels in the blood. In addition, T3 increases heart rate and the heart's force of contraction, which affects blood pressure.

Thyroxine (T4) is the less active form of thyroid hormone. Like T3, it helps control the body's basal metabolic rate, promotes protein synthesis, increases cholesterol breakdown and LDL receptor activity, and increases heart rate.

Diet and lifestyle can strongly impact thyroid health. For example, conditions that raise cortisol levels (such as stress and sleep deprivation) can negatively affect thyroid function because cortisol decreases TSH and inhibits the enzyme responsible for converting T4 to T3. Many chemicals can also harm thyroid hormone function and metabolism, including some food additives, herbicides, pesticides, dioxins, mercury and other heavy metals, BPA, benzene, arsenic, halogens (chlorine, bromine, fluorine, and perchlorate), and triclosan. Likewise, a variety of nutrients are needed for making thyroid hormone, TSH, and important enzymes:

- The nonessential amino acid tyrosine (and the essential amino acid phenylalanine, which is used to synthesize tyrosine in the body) is needed to produce thyroid hormone.
- Iodine deficiency can reduce the synthesis of thyroid hormone and cause thyroid enlargement, or goiter.
- Vitamin C and vitamin B12 are needed to help draw raw iodine into the thyroid gland.
- Zinc, magnesium, vitamin B12, and protein are required to make TSH. Deficiencies in any of these nutrients can impair the feedback loop that regulates the level of thyroid hormone in the blood.
- Selenium is needed for the enzyme that converts T4 to T3.
- Vitamins A and D are needed for T3 to activate cells to increase metabolic rate.

Sex Hormones

Sex hormones are steroid hormones that play central roles in reproduction, sexual development, and sexual function. They interact with the body's estrogen and androgen receptors and are produced by the gonads (the ovaries in women or the testes in men) and adrenal glands and can also be converted from other sex steroids in the liver or fat. Over the course of a lifetime, levels of sex hormone production and release can vary, increasing at puberty and declining in old age. The main classes of sex steroids are androgens, estrogens, and progestogens.

Androgens are involved in the expression of male sexual characteristics (although women also produce androgens) and include the hormones testosterone, androstenedione, dehydroepiandrosterone, and dihydrotestosterone. Androgens are important for development during puberty and play a role in sperm production, sex organ maturity, body hair growth, and fat and muscle distribution (promoting a reduction in excess fat and an increase in muscle tissue). Although testosterone is the most well-known androgen, the others also play critical roles: for instance, dihydrotestosterone contributes to male balding, sebaceous gland activity, and prostate growth.

Estrogens (the group of hormone compounds that includes estradiol, estriol, and estrone) are involved in female sex characteristics and reproduction. They help direct body fat distribution (particularly to the hips, thighs, and buttocks) and reduce facial hair growth. Most importantly, they're critical for the female reproductive process, helping regulate the menstrual cycle and preparing the uterus for pregnancy by thickening the endometrium. Estrogen is manufactured mainly in the ovaries by developing egg follicles, with smaller amounts produced by the liver, breasts, and adrenal glands. During a woman's reproductive years, estradiol is the main estrogen the body produces, and when total estrogen levels reduce after menopause, issues with reduced bone mineral density, vaginal dryness, memory problems, and fatigue can occur.

Progesterone is the main progestogen in the human body, and it is critical for regulating the menstrual cycle and maintaining pregnancy. (Men also produce some progesterone, but it plays a much smaller role in men's sexual health than in women's.) The female body produces progesterone right before ovulation to optimize the conditions for pregnancy (including an increase in vaginal mucus and a reduction in uterus contractions); after ovulation, progesterone levels drop off so that the uterine lining can be shed. If pregnancy occurs, progesterone brings about a reduction in the maternal immune response during sperm implantation to encourage the acceptance of the pregnancy and also inhibits lactation during pregnancy (the drop in progesterone level after giving birth helps trigger milk production in the mother). Progesterone also has a number of nonsexual roles in the body, including in blood clotting, immunity, inflammation, skin elasticity, bone strength, and thyroid health.

If any of these hormones is either overproduced or underproduced, sex hormone disorders can occur. Excessive androgens in women (which can result from polycystic ovarian syndrome, or PCOS) can result in menstrual irregularities, alopecia (hair loss), or extra hair growth. Insufficient testosterone in men can cause a reduction in libido, loss of muscle mass, loss of body hair, and erectile dysfunction.

Although sex hormone disorders can be genetic in nature, some factors are within our control for promoting optimal production of these steroid hormones. Consuming enough carbohydrate from whole-food sources, eating a high-fiber diet, avoiding long-term low-fat diets (which can reduce the production of sex hormones due to an effect on cholesterol, a sex hormone precursor), avoiding excessive high-intensity exercise and other physical stressors, and maintaining adrenal health (adrenal dysfunction can suppress the function of the pituitary gland and limit the availability of the necessary precursors for sex hormone production) can all help maintain healthy levels of these important hormones.

HORMONES AT A GLANCE

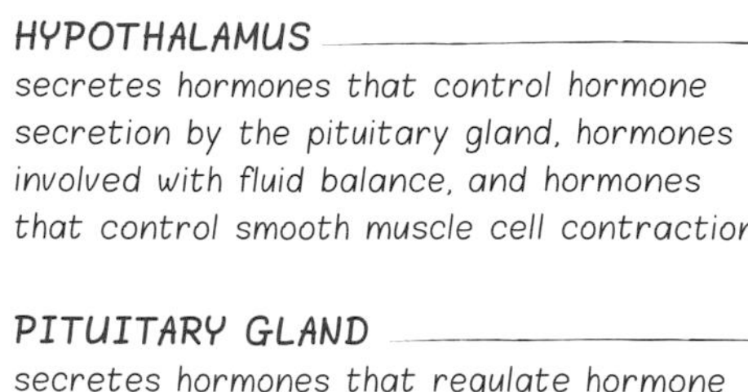

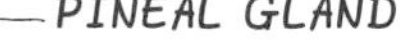

HYPOTHALAMUS
secretes hormones that control hormone secretion by the pituitary gland, hormones involved with fluid balance, and hormones that control smooth muscle cell contraction.

PINEAL GLAND
secretes melatonin, which affects reproductive function, gastrointestinal function, and sleep quality and establishes circadian rhythms.

PITUITARY GLAND
secretes hormones that regulate hormone secretion by other endocrine glands, including the adrenals, thyroid, and reproductive organs.

PARATHYROID GLAND
secretes a hormone important to the regulation of calcium ion concentrations in body fluids.

THYROID GLAND
secretes hormones that control metabolic rate and calcium ion concentrations in body fluids.

THYMUS
secretes hormones involved in immune system function.

HEART
secretes hormones that regulate blood volume.

PANCREAS
secretes hormones regulating glucose uptake and utilization.

ADRENAL GLANDS
secrete hormones involved in mineral balance, metabolic control, and reactions to stress and that establish circadian rhythms.

GUT
secretes hormones involved in regulating appetite, digestion, glucose metabolism, and immune function.

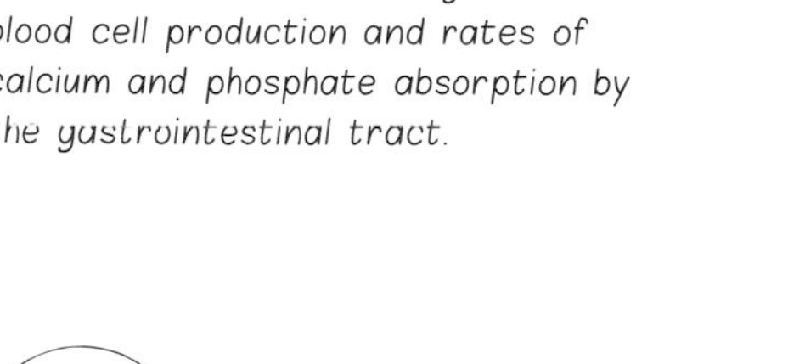

KIDNEYS
secrete hormones that regulate blood cell production and rates of calcium and phosphate absorption by the gastrointestinal tract.

GONADS
secrete hormones affecting growth, metabolism, and sexual characteristics, and that coordinate the reproductive system.

OVARY

TESTIS

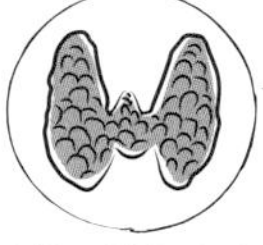

☆☆☆ NUTRIENT SUPERSTARS FOR ENDOCRINE HEALTH ☆☆☆

Nutrient	Abundant in:		
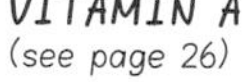 **VITAMIN A** (see page 26)	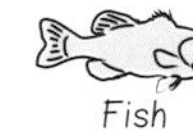 Fish	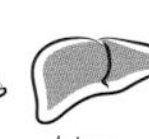 Liver	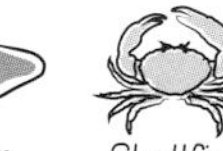 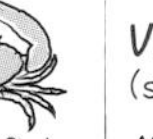 Shellfish
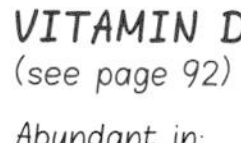 **VITAMIN D** (see page 92)	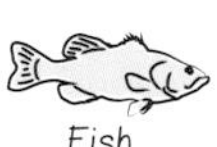 Fish	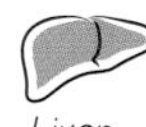 Liver	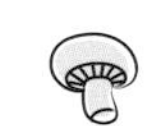 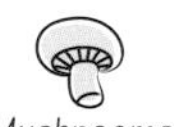 Mushrooms
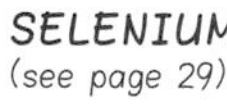 **SELENIUM** (see page 29)	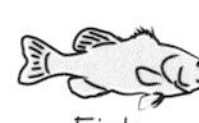 Fish	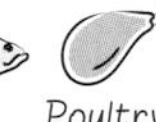 Poultry	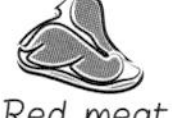 Red meat
VITAMIN B5 (see page 26)	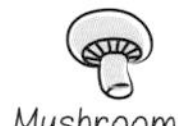 Mushrooms	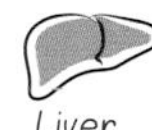 Liver	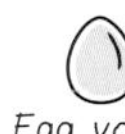 Egg yolks
CHROMIUM (see page 28)	 Shellfish	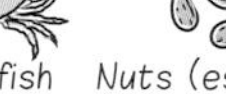 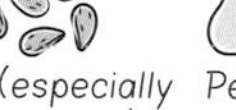 Nuts (especially Brazil nuts)	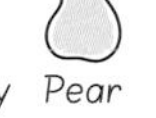 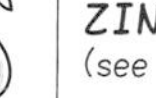 Pear
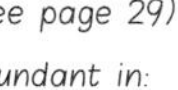 **ZINC** (see page 29)	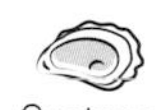 Oysters	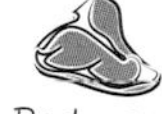 Red meat	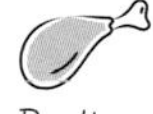 Poultry
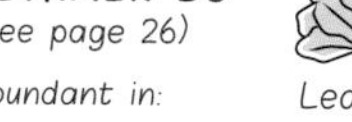 **VITAMIN B6** (see page 26)	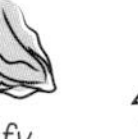 Leafy greens	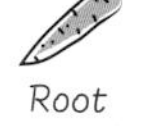 Root vegetables	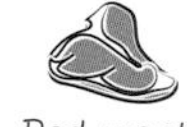 Red meat
IODINE (see page 28)	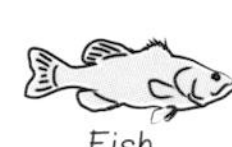 Fish	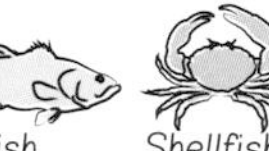 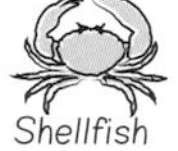 Shellfish	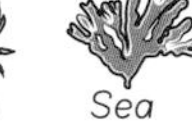 Sea vegetables
DHA AND EPA (see page 158)	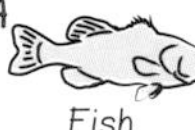 Fish	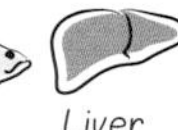 Liver	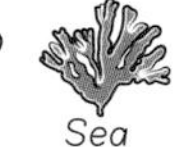 Sea vegetables
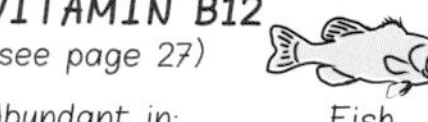 **VITAMIN B12** (see page 27)	Fish	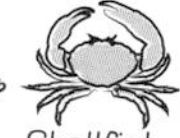 Shellfish	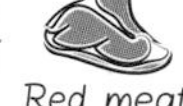 Red meat
IRON (see page 28)	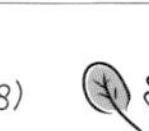  Dark leafy greens	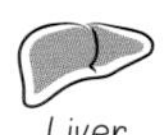 Liver	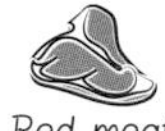 Red meat
INSOLUBLE FIBER (see page 39)	Celery	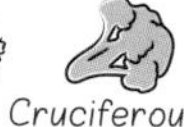 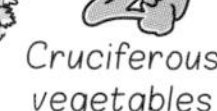 Cruciferous vegetables	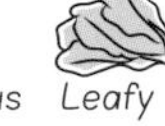 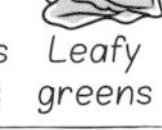 Leafy greens
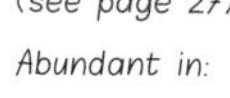 **VITAMIN C** (see page 27)	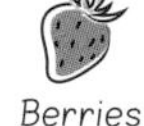 Berries	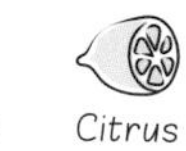 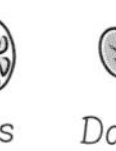 Citrus fruits	Dark leafy greens
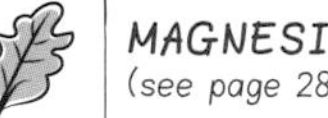 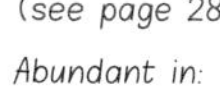 **MAGNESIUM** (see page 28)	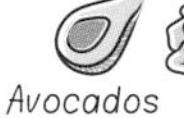 Avocados	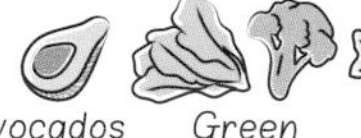 Green vegetables	Fish

NERVOUS SYSTEM HEALTH

The nervous system is the network of nerve cells and fibers that carry messages from the brain and spinal cord to different parts of the body. It includes the central nervous system (comprised of the brain and spinal cord) and the peripheral nervous system (containing nerves that connect the central nervous system to all other parts of the body). The peripheral nervous system is further divided into the autonomic nervous system, which governs the nerves of the inner organs that we don't consciously control (such as heartbeat and digestion), and the somatic nervous system, which picks up sensory information from distant organs and rapidly carries that information back to the central nervous system.

This complex and important system allows our bodies to process sensations, interact with our environment, move (through interactions with the muscular system), think, react, plan, speak, swallow, breathe, learn, remember things, digest food, and ultimately stay alive! When you think of it this way, it becomes a no-brainer (pardon the pun) that nervous system health is important for full-body health. But let's home in on three important links between diet, lifestyle, and the nervous system, as these form the backbone of the recommendations in the Paleo template geared toward nervous system health.

Gut-Brain Axis

The brain and digestive system communicate with each other by means of a complex system. Along with a hormonal component and a chemical/immunological component (collectively involving cortisol, melatonin, hunger hormones, and cytokines), there's also communication via the nervous system, specifically the enteric (gut) nervous system. This communication is why just thinking about food causes stomach acid and digestive enzymes to be released, and why insulin is released in anticipation of high blood sugar levels. If someone is nervous or stressed, their stomach may feel upset and their appetite may be suppressed. Very importantly, this communication goes both ways—the gut also sends signals to the brain. This multifaceted communication between the digestive system and the brain (including neural signals, hormonal signals, and chemical or immunological signals) is called the *gut-brain connection* or *gut-brain axis*, and problems in this link contribute to poor health.

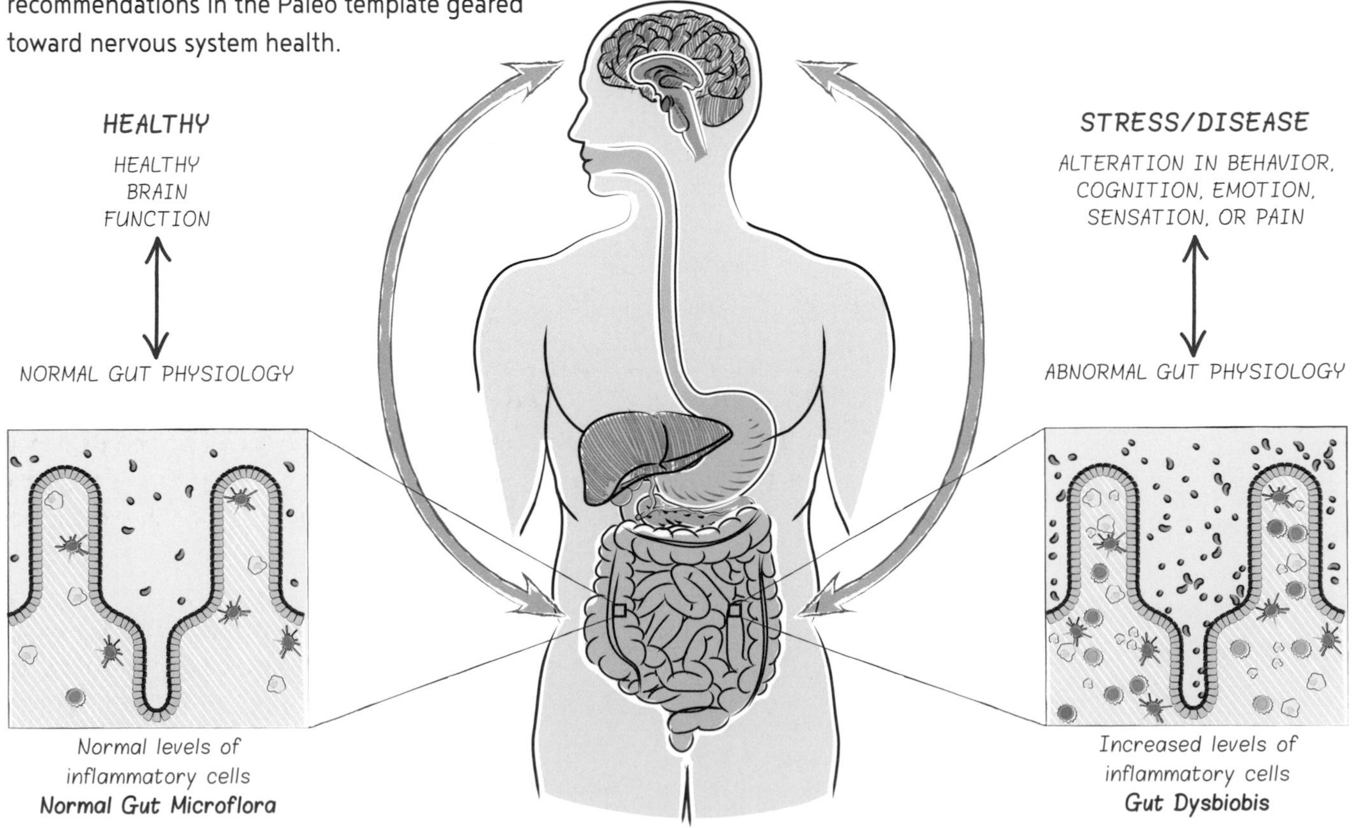

Normal levels of inflammatory cells
Normal Gut Microflora

Increased levels of inflammatory cells
Gut Dysbiobis

Embedded in its walls, an extensive network of neurons lines the entire gut—the esophagus, stomach, intestines, colon, and rectum. This is called the enteric nervous system, and it consists of more neurons than are present in either the spinal cord or the peripheral nervous system. This neural network is so extensive that it is often referred to as the "second brain." The enteric nervous system is responsible for regulating all aspects of digestion, from breaking down food to absorbing nutrients to expelling waste.

The brain sends signals to all the nerves in the body. These signals are essential for every action, from breathing to walking. A large portion of the brain's output is directed into the vagus nerve, which innervates (that is, branches into the nerves controlling) most of the thoracic and abdominal cavities, including the digestive tract. The vagus nerve thus controls a wide range of functions, from a heart beating to the secretion of digestive enzymes to the peristalsis of the digestive tract.

SCIENCE SIMPLIFIED *When we're stressed, depressed, or upset, digestion is inhibited, which can lead to bacterial overgrowth in the gut and to leaky gut. It's a two-way street, though: when our guts are inflamed or the gut microbial community isn't healthy, we may feel stressed or depressed or have mood issues. It's important to work on gut health and mental health together.*

Stress, anxiety, depression, and strong negative emotions decrease brain activity, which decreases activation of the vagus nerve. This has dramatic impacts on digestion, including reduced stomach acid production, reduced pancreatic enzyme secretion, poor gallbladder function, decreased gut motility, decreased intestinal blood flow, and suppression of the intestinal immune system. This is why it's important not to eat when we're upset. When reduced vagus nerve activation is persistent, as might happen during periods of chronic stress or clinical depression, the slowing of so many digestive functions can lead to small intestinal bacterial overgrowth (SIBO), which leads to a leaky gut and chronic inflammation. It's why people who are depressed often suffer from constipation or IBS as well.

Eighty percent of the fibers in the vagus nerve carry information from the gut to the brain, and not the other way around. This means that the gut (and even the gut microbiota) communicates directly with the brain, perhaps having a direct impact on emotions and moods. In fact, many of the beneficial effects of the probiotic bacteria in the gut are dependent on vagus nerve activation affecting brain function. The gut also utilizes chemical signaling to communicate directly with the brain. A variety of metabolites produced by probiotic bacteria in the gut are neuroactive, meaning that they affect neurons. These include short-chain fatty acids, a variety of neurotransmitters and neuromodulators (such as GABA, noradrenalin, serotonin, dopamine, and acetylcholine—yes, all can be produced by gut bacteria), and cytokines. Recent studies show that gut bacteria also affect the blood-brain barrier, controlling which types of substances can cross that barrier into the brain—yes, a leaky gut can lead to a leaky brain!

Chemical messengers of inflammation are called cytokines. When produced in substantial quantities, cytokines travel throughout the body (via the blood) and transmit their messages to virtually every cell, including cells in the brain. This is how inflammation that originates in the gut (or anywhere else in the body) can become generalized and systemic—that is, bodywide. When pro-inflammatory cytokines are produced in substantial quantities, as occurs in anyone with a leaky gut, they enter the bloodstream and travel to the brain. These cytokines cross the blood-brain barrier and activate the resident immune cells of the brain, called the microglia cells. Thus inflammation that starts in the gut can cause inflammation in the brain. As inflammatory signals from the gut persist, the inflammation in the brain increases. And an inflamed brain has less (and slower) nerve conduction, which manifests as stress, depression, or anxiety—which is why depression and mood-related symptoms are so often associated with chronic disease.

This communication between the brain and the gut is clearly related to chronic stress (see page 340). However, what makes the gut-brain axis worthy of discussion in other contexts is that once the microglia cells are activated in the brain, it can be very difficult to deactivate them—meaning that inflammation in the brain can be hard to turn off. And inflammation in the brain obstructs the healing of the gut because of decreased vagus nerve activation. It is, indeed, a vicious cycle.

Diet and lifestyle factors that support healthy communication between the gut and the brain involve all those that improve gut health, neural and mental health, immune health, and endocrine health.

Communication with the Immune System

Recent studies have established that the brain also communicates directly with the immune system and vice versa—also via the vagus nerve.

Under normal (healthy, uninjured) conditions, vagus nerve activation sends signals to the spleen that stimulate a subset of memory T cells residing in the spleen to release a neurochemical called acetylcholine. Acetylcholine then signals to other immune cells not to produce pro-inflammatory cytokines. But in the case of injury or infection, the nervous system is activated (by binding neuron receptors with cytokines, prostaglandins, and even pathogens themselves), and the signals not to produce pro-inflammatory cytokines get turned off. This is an early warning system, a way for the peripheral nerves to alert the brain to a developing threat long before it becomes severe enough to produce levels of inflammatory mediators (like cytokines) in sufficient quantities to enter the bloodstream and communicate with the brain chemically.

When the brain receives the neural signals that injury or infection has occurred, it activates the hypothalamic-pituitary-adrenal (HPA) axis (the stress axis which also modulates the immune system; see Chapter 27). Also, the output of the vagus nerve decreases. The resulting change in signal to the spleen stops the built-in inhibition of inflammatory signals; instead, the spleen releases large amounts of pro-inflammatory cytokines into the bloodstream. The pro-inflammatory cytokines signal the release of immune cells into the blood from the bone marrow, thymus gland, and spleen in search of an invader to neutralize or an injury to heal.

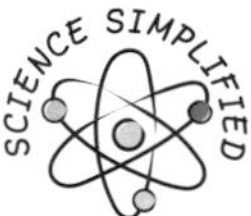

The brain is constantly putting the brakes on the immune system, but when the brain detects injury or infection, it releases the brake pedal so that the immune system can be quickly mobilized.

Nutrition-Neurotransmitter Link

Another way in which the food we eat can support (or harm!) our neurological health involves neurotransmitters. *Neurotransmitters* are chemicals released by nerve cells to send signals to other nerve cells. The most widely studied neurotransmitters include GABA (gamma-aminobutyric acid), dopamine, acetylcholine, glutamate, serotonin, epinephrine, and norepinephrine.

Nutrition can affect neurotransmitters in several ways. For one, diet influences the levels of neurotransmitter precursors in our blood (such as choline for acetylcholine, tryptophan for serotonin, and tyrosine for epinephrine, norepinephrine, and dopamine), which in turn influence the level of neurotransmitter precursors in the brain. These precursors regulate several things: the rate of synthesis for neurotransmitters, the concentration of neurotransmitters within nerve terminals, and the quantity of neurotransmitters released when neurons fire. Calcium plays an important role in neurotransmitter release. In addition, a variety of nutrients act as cofactors in neurotransmitter production (particularly vitamin B3, vitamin B6, vitamin B9, vitamin B12, vitamin C, zinc, copper, iron, and magnesium). Deficiencies in any neurotransmitter-related amino acids, vitamins, or minerals can impact neurotransmitter production (and consequently the wide number of functions they're involved in, including appetite regulation, activation of skeletal muscle in the somatic nervous system, regulation of motor behavior, emotional arousal, sleep regulation, memory and learning regulation, mood and behavior regulation, muscle contraction, body temperature regulation, alertness, and activation of the fight-or-flight response—to name just a few).

Link to Lifestyle

While diet obviously plays an important part in supporting neurological health, the role of lifestyle factors—particularly sleep and stress—can't be overstated. Sleep is one of the most critical times for body repair, including in the brain: during deep sleep, the brain cools and receives less blood flow, which likely boosts its function and allows for optimal repair. Even more importantly, sleep is prime time for the brain to undergo detoxification processes. The brain uses up to a quarter of the total calories we burn each day, resulting in a buildup of large amounts of toxic metabolic by-products. During sleep, brain cells shrink and the space between them widens so that those cellular waste products can be more effectively flushed away. Without adequate sleep, this detoxification process is impaired and the metabolic by-products continue to accumulate in the brain; as a result, cellular health, neurotransmitter systems, hormone systems, and neural communication are all negatively impacted. Additionally, sleep is vital for maintaining synaptic plasticity (the brain's ability to change), for the formation of memories, and for proper receptivity to dopamine. (For more on the role of sleep in our health, see Chapter 26.)

Stress, too, is a major problem when it comes to maintaining neurological health. Although the human body is well equipped to handle acute stress (when an immediate threat comes and goes and we can fully exhale afterward), chronic stress—during which stress hormones are elevated nonstop and we never get a chance to relax—has a much more damaging effect on the brain (among other body parts!). Stress increases the permeability of the blood-brain barrier, potentially allowing more toxins (like heavy metals) to enter. When levels of the stress hormone cortisol stay elevated, the result is a surplus of the neurotransmitter glutamate, and with it an increased formation of free radicals that can damage brain cells. Likewise, elevated cortisol can inhibit the production of a protein called brain-derived neurotrophic factor (BDNF), which helps keep existing brain cells healthy as well as stimulate the formation of new ones. Stress also tends to deplete levels of the neurotransmitters serotonin and dopamine, impacting mood, sleep, appetite, learning, and the pleasure-reward system. In fact, stress is consistently associated with a greater risk of developing several mental illnesses, including depression, anxiety, schizophrenia, post-traumatic stress disorder, and bipolar disorder, as well as alcoholism and drug addiction. It's also associated with a higher risk of other neurological conditions, like Alzheimer's disease and dementia. (For more information on the many effects of stress on health, including a deeper discussion of stress and the HPA axis, see Chapter 27.)

HEALTH QUICK-START

For optimal nervous system health, make sure to get a minimum of 8 hours of sleep every night and manage stress both by reducing stressors in your life and by incorporating activities that boost resilience to stress, like walking in nature and mindful meditation.

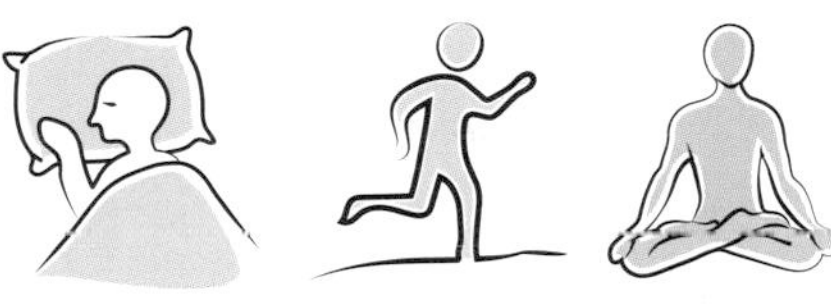

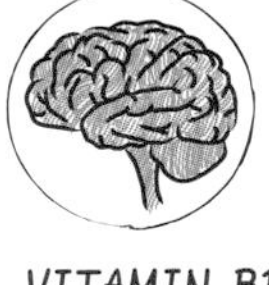

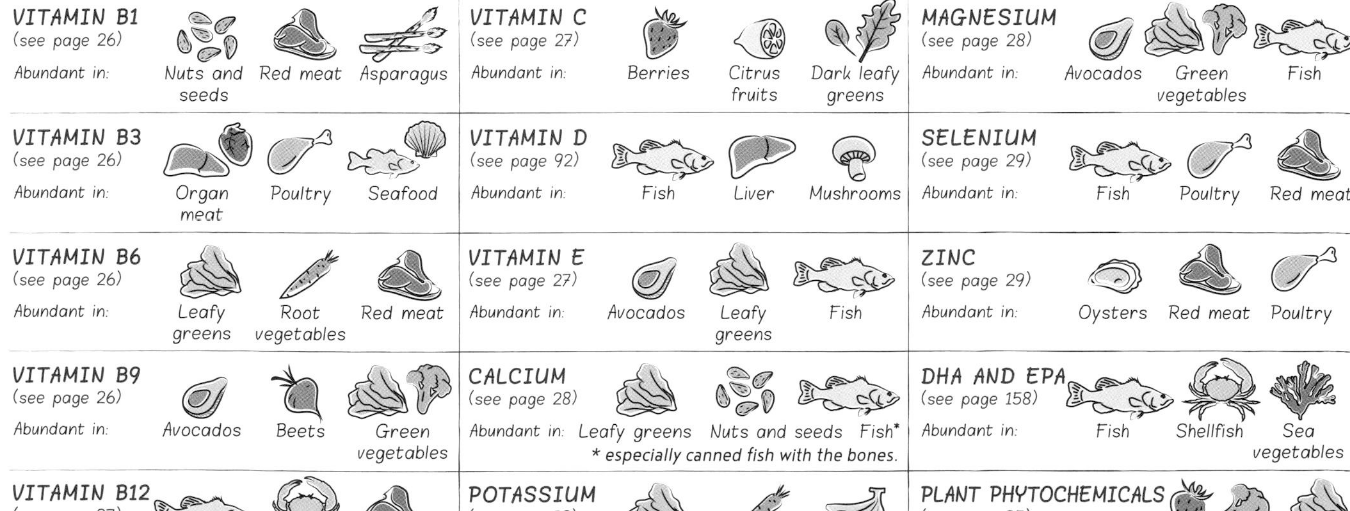

NUTRIENT SUPERSTARS FOR NERVOUS SYSTEM HEALTH

VITAMIN B1 (see page 26) Abundant in: Nuts and seeds, Red meat, Asparagus	**VITAMIN C** (see page 27) Abundant in: Berries, Citrus fruits, Dark leafy greens	**MAGNESIUM** (see page 28) Abundant in: Avocados, Green vegetables, Fish
VITAMIN B3 (see page 26) Abundant in: Organ meat, Poultry, Seafood	**VITAMIN D** (see page 92) Abundant in: Fish, Liver, Mushrooms	**SELENIUM** (see page 29) Abundant in: Fish, Poultry, Red meat
VITAMIN B6 (see page 26) Abundant in: Leafy greens, Root vegetables, Red meat	**VITAMIN E** (see page 27) Abundant in: Avocados, Leafy greens, Fish	**ZINC** (see page 29) Abundant in: Oysters, Red meat, Poultry
VITAMIN B9 (see page 26) Abundant in: Avocados, Beets, Green vegetables	**CALCIUM** (see page 28) Abundant in: Leafy greens, Nuts and seeds, Fish* * especially canned fish with the bones.	**DHA AND EPA** (see page 158) Abundant in: Fish, Shellfish, Sea vegetables
VITAMIN B12 (see page 27) Abundant in: Fish, Shellfish, Red meat	**POTASSIUM** (see page 29) Abundant in: Leafy greens, Root vegetables, Bananas	**PLANT PHYTOCHEMICALS** (see page 35) Abundant in: Berries, Cruciferous vegetables, Leafy greens

CARDIOVASCULAR HEALTH

The cardiovascular system is responsible for transporting oxygen, hormones, cellular waste products, immune cells, and nutrients throughout the body. This system includes the heart, blood vessels, and approximately 5 liters of blood (which the heart fully circulates once every minute!). The blood itself is made up of blood cells (white blood cells that are part of the immune system, red blood cells, and platelets) and plasma (which is 92 percent water and 8 percent proteins, glucose, hormones, carbon dioxide, and mineral ions). The cardiovascular system continuously adapts to the body's needs. For instance, the blood delivers more immune cells when an infection is present, and the heart pumps faster during exercise to deliver oxygen to muscle tissue.

For decades, cardiovascular diseases (mainly coronary heart disease and stroke) have been the leading cause of death in Westernized nations. Coronary heart disease occurs when white blood cells and dead cell remnants (including cholesterol and triglycerides) accumulate within the artery walls, forming plaques that can eventually narrow the coronary arteries, reduce the flow of oxygen in the blood to the heart, causing ischemic heart disease or heart attack, and rupture, causing a coronary thrombosis (a different kind of heart attack). Plaque rupture can also cause a stroke, which happens when an artery supplying blood to the brain becomes blocked.

Although some genetic factors increase a person's susceptibility to cardiovascular disease, diet and lifestyle are by far the biggest culprits. The Standard American Diet harms cardiovascular health in a number of well-documented ways. For example, inflammation plays a major role in all stages of cardiovascular disease progression (and high levels of the inflammation marker C-reactive protein, or CRP, are consistently associated with higher cardiovascular disease risk), so pro-inflammatory foods like refined vegetable oils, processed foods, grains, and refined sugar, along with pro-inflammatory lifestyle factors like chronic stress, sleep deprivation, and sedentary living, increase the risk of heart disease and stroke (see page 410). A high intake of omega-6 fats increases the susceptibility of LDL particles to oxidation, which makes them more likely to become incorporated into atherosclerotic plaques by the body's immune cells (which consume oxidized LDL particles and bloat into foam cells). Meanwhile, a low intake of omega-3 fats reduces the body's ability to control inflammation and is associated with higher triglyceride levels and a higher risk of heart disease and stroke. *Trans* fats (created from partially hydrogenating unsaturated oils like soybean oil) increase LDL ("bad") cholesterol and decrease HDL ("good") cholesterol, thus worsening the LDL/HDL ratio. A general pattern of energy excess and high refined carbohydrate intake tends to correlate with low HDL, high LDL and triglycerides, and a predominance of small, dense LDL particles, all of which raise the risk of cardiovascular disease. A low intake of fresh vegetables and fruit deprives the body of important micronutrients and fiber to support vascular health, including vitamin C, which enhances the flexibility of the arteries and reduces oxidative damage, and potassium, which helps reduce blood pressure.

KNOWLEDGE BOMB *It's well known that dietary cholesterol does not increase blood cholesterol or cause cardiovascular disease for most people (see page 186). Eggs are back on the menu!*

High blood pressure, or hypertension, is a major risk factor for both heart disease and stroke and is strongly linked to nutrient status and lifestyle. Blood pressure is the force of blood pushing against artery walls. When it's chronically elevated, blood vessels and arteries can become scarred and less flexible, predisposing them to blockages and ruptures. Blood pressure is strongly influenced by nutrition, particularly the balance of the minerals sodium, potassium, magnesium, and calcium.

By contrast, a Paleo framework provides ample nutrition and lifestyle adjustments to enhance heart and vascular function. A diet rich in minimally processed vegetables, fruit, nuts, seeds, red meat, poultry, seafood, and eggs provides vitamins and minerals that support muscle contraction (including the pumping of the heart muscle), vasodilation, red blood cell formation, waste product cleanup, blood pressure regulation, and oxygen transport. A lifestyle that involves plenty of sleep, stress management, nature connection, and gentle movement throughout the day likewise reduces numerous risk factors for heart disease and stroke. (Contrary to the ongoing myth, the saturated fat in natural animal products and some plant foods, like coconut, does *not* cause heart disease; see page 186.)

PALEO EASY BUTTON

While we don't need to go out of our way to add fats to our diet, we don't have to avoid them, either! For cooking and dressing food, focus on animal fats from grass-fed and pasture-raised sources, like grass-fed butter and tallow and pasture-raised lard. Healthy plant-derived fats include avocado oil, coconut oil, high-quality olive oil, and ethically sourced red palm oil.

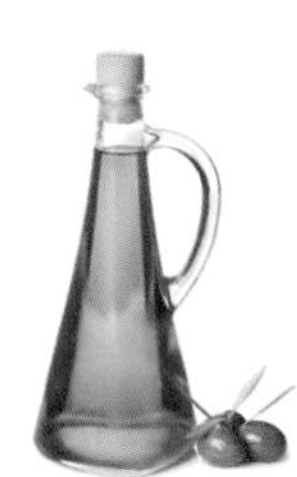

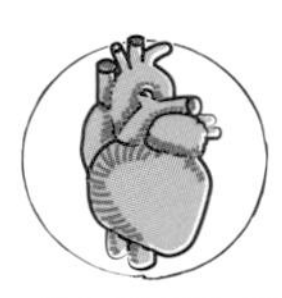

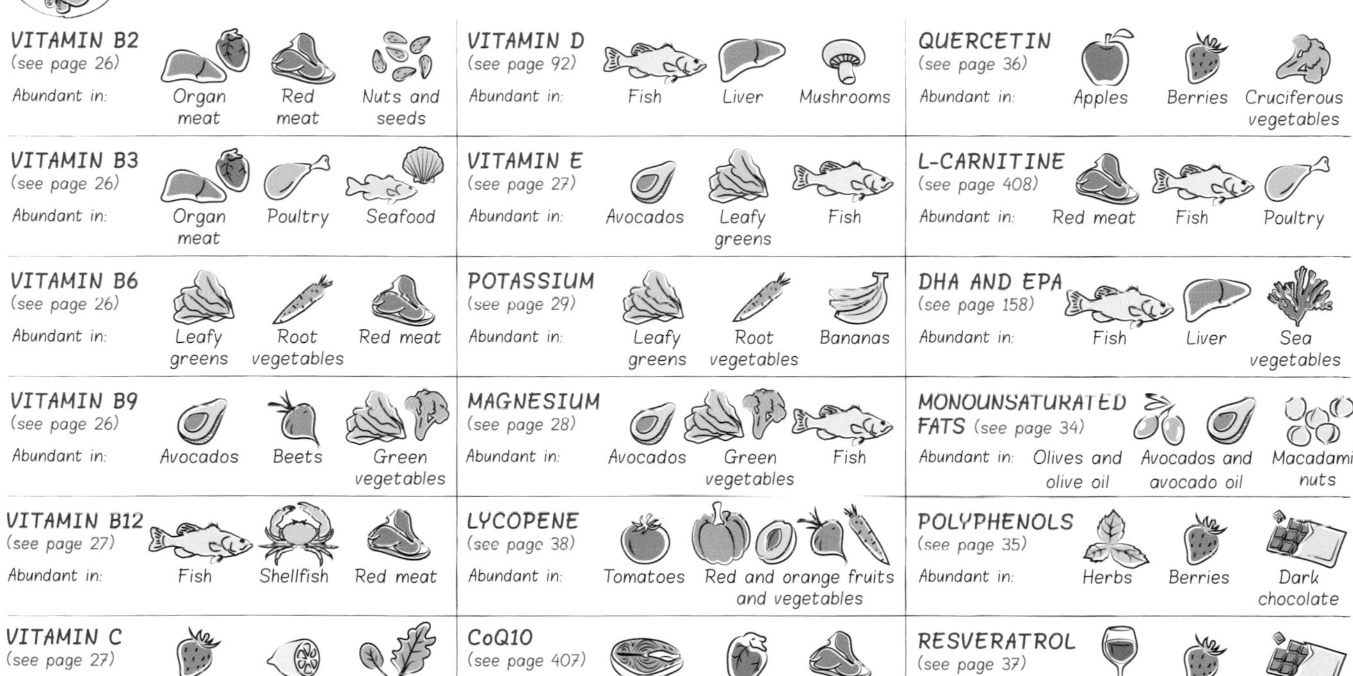

NUTRIENT SUPERSTARS FOR CARDIOVASCULAR HEALTH

VITAMIN B2 (see page 26) Abundant in: Organ meat, Red meat, Nuts and seeds	VITAMIN D (see page 92) Abundant in: Fish, Liver, Mushrooms	QUERCETIN (see page 36) Abundant in: Apples, Berries, Cruciferous vegetables
VITAMIN B3 (see page 26) Abundant in: Organ meat, Poultry, Seafood	VITAMIN E (see page 27) Abundant in: Avocados, Leafy greens, Fish	L-CARNITINE (see page 408) Abundant in: Red meat, Fish, Poultry
VITAMIN B6 (see page 26) Abundant in: Leafy greens, Root vegetables, Red meat	POTASSIUM (see page 29) Abundant in: Leafy greens, Root vegetables, Bananas	DHA AND EPA (see page 158) Abundant in: Fish, Liver, Sea vegetables
VITAMIN B9 (see page 26) Abundant in: Avocados, Beets, Green vegetables	MAGNESIUM (see page 28) Abundant in: Avocados, Green vegetables, Fish	MONOUNSATURATED FATS (see page 34) Abundant in: Olives and olive oil, Avocados and avocado oil, Macadamia nuts
VITAMIN B12 (see page 27) Abundant in: Fish, Shellfish, Red meat	LYCOPENE (see page 38) Abundant in: Tomatoes, Red and orange fruits and vegetables	POLYPHENOLS (see page 35) Abundant in: Herbs, Berries, Dark chocolate
VITAMIN C (see page 27) Abundant in: Berries, Citrus fruits, Dark leafy greens	CoQ10 (see page 407) Abundant in: Fatty fish, Heart, Red meat	RESVERATROL (see page 37) Abundant in: Grapes and red wine, Berries, Dark chocolate

MUSCULAR HEALTH

Muscle is a type of fibrous tissue with the ability to contract, resulting in movement. The human body contains more than 600 muscles, with functions as diverse as pumping blood to peristalsis of the digestive tract to moving our eyeballs to helping us lift heavy objects. Those many muscles fall into three basic categories:

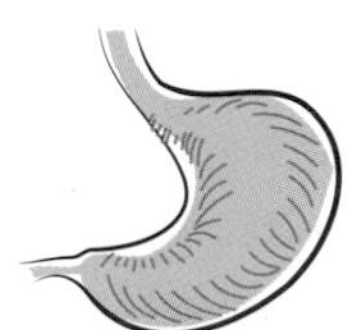

SMOOTH MUSCLES

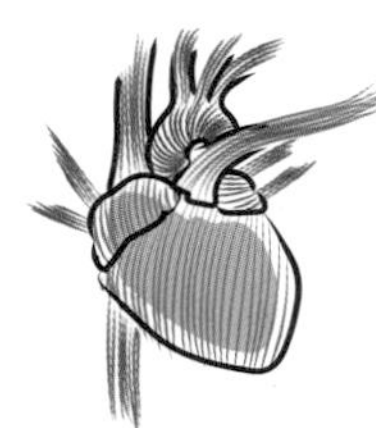

CARDIAC MUSCLE

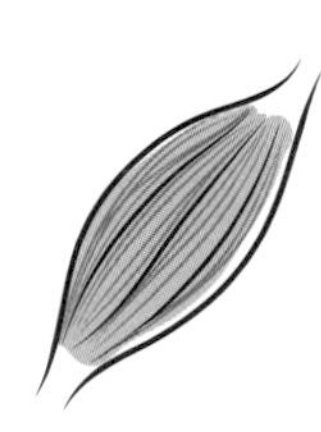

SKELETAL MUSCLES

- **Smooth muscles,** which contract involuntarily (without our conscious control) and are found in organs and structures like the stomach, esophagus, intestines, uterus, bladder, and blood vessels
- **Cardiac muscle** (the heart)
- **Skeletal muscles,** which we contract voluntarily to move our bodies and which stretch across joints and attach to bone (held in place with the help of tendons)

Skeletal muscle is further divided into three main types:

- **Type I,** or slow-twitch oxidative, which can carry more oxygen and is used for sustaining aerobic activity requiring low force and power production. (Think walking and maintaining posture, but these are also the primary fiber type found in endurance athletes.)
- **Type IIA,** or fast-twitch oxidative, which are used for sustained activates that require high power, force and/or speed, like most sports. They are more resistant to fatigue than Type IIX.
- **Type IIX,** or fast-twitch glycolytic, which contract powerfully and quickly, but get fatigued more easily—making them mostly used for short bursts of anaerobic activity (such as lifting heavy weights or sprinting).

Some forms of type II muscle fibers activate with progressively heavier loads and allow us to build greater muscle mass.

All forms of muscle are extremely important, and muscular and neuromuscular diseases (such as Parkinson's) can have devastating physical effects. Along with helping us move our bodies and keeping our organs functioning, muscle may help protect against insulin resistance and diabetes, especially in the form of higher skeletal muscle mass. One study found that with every 10 percent increase in the ratio between a person's skeletal muscle mass and total body weight, the risk of insulin resistance dropped by 11 percent and the risk of prediabetes or type 2 diabetes dropped by 12 percent. While resistance exercise itself helps lower blood sugar levels and improve insulin sensitivity (skeletal muscle takes up glucose when contracting), skeletal muscle serves as a storage tank for glycogen even when we're at rest. The more muscle we have, the more glucose we can store (versus letting it circulate in our blood or converting it into fat via lipogenesis).

KNOWLEDGE BOMB *Ever get leg or foot cramps in the middle of the night? These cramps are often caused by electrolyte imbalances or deficiencies. When our bodies are too low in sodium, potassium, magnesium, or calcium, our muscles can't properly contract and release. In particular, an imbalanced ratio of potassium (which opens or relaxes muscle) to sodium (which closes or constricts muscle) can lead to uncomfortable cramping while we're trying to fall asleep or when we're exercising (in which case electrolyte imbalance can be exacerbated by sweating and dehydration). Low levels of magnesium, which also facilitate muscle relaxation, are another common culprit in muscle cramps.*

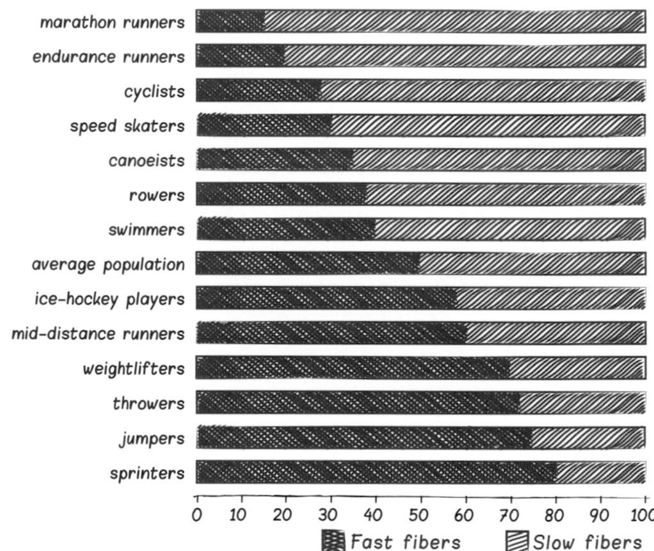

MUSCLE FIBER TYPE CHARACTERISTICS	TYPE I FIBERS	TYPE IIA FIBERS	TYPE IIX FIBERS
CONTRACTION TIME	Slow	Moderately fast	Very fast
SIZE OF MOTOR NEURON	Small	Medium	Very large
RESISTANCE TO FATIGUE	High	Fairly high	Low
ACTIVITY USED FOR	Aerobic	Long-term anaerobic	Short-term anaerobic
MAXIMUM DURATION OF USE	Hours	< 30 minutes	< 1 minute
POWER PRODUCED	Low	Medium	Very high
MITOCHONDRIAL DENSITY	High	High	Low
CAPILLARY DENSITY	High	Intermediate	Low
OXIDATIVE CAPACITY	High	High	Low
GLYCOLYTIC CAPACITY	Low	High	High
MAJOR STORAGE FUEL	Triglycerides	Creatine phosphate, glycogen	Creatine phosphate, glycogen

Protein is the most important nutrient when it comes to maintaining and building muscle, and it's part of the rationale for the Paleo diet's emphasis on a higher proportion of protein than the Standard American Diet (along with the other beneficial roles of protein, such as regulating appetite and increasing satiety). However, certain micronutrients are also critical for muscle health. The electrolytes calcium (found in leafy greens, small bone-in fish like sardines, and dairy), magnesium (found in dark green leafy vegetables, nuts, seeds, fish, avocados, and bananas), potassium (found in tomatoes, sweet potatoes, bananas, coconut water, spinach, acorn squash, and avocados), and sodium (found naturally in foods like celery and beets and in any salted food) are involved in muscle contraction. Vitamin D helps the body absorb calcium, thus it also plays a role in maintaining muscle health. Zinc (found in organ meat, muscle meat, pumpkin seeds, and shellfish) is key for helping our bodies utilize the protein we eat and facilitating muscle growth. Iron (rich in red meat, shellfish, and some leafy greens) is essential for the production of red blood cells, which carry oxygenated blood around the body, including to the muscles.

In conjunction with gentle activity that engages our muscles and helps increase lean mass, a micronutrient-rich, moderately high-protein Paleo diet is optimal for muscle health.

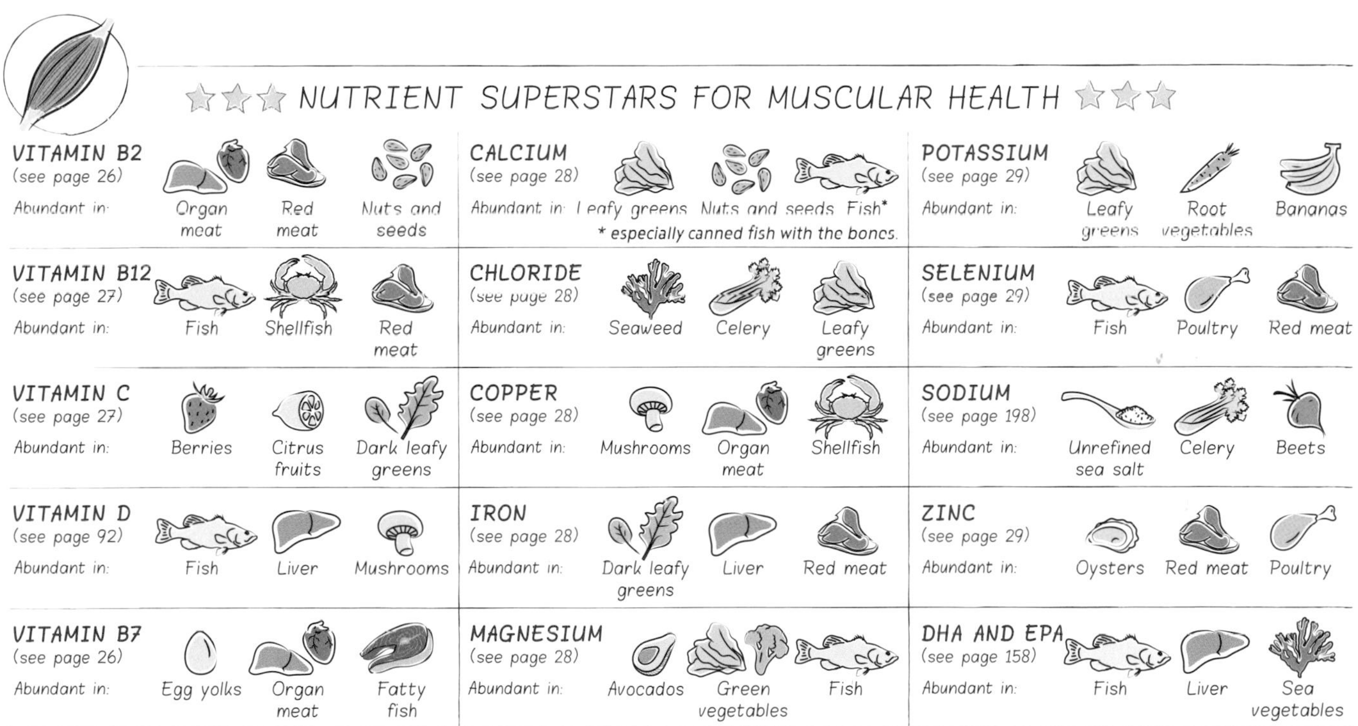

NUTRIENT SUPERSTARS FOR MUSCULAR HEALTH
VITAMIN B2 (see page 26) Abundant in: Organ meat, Red meat, Nuts and seeds
CALCIUM (see page 28) Abundant in: Leafy greens, Nuts and seeds, Fish*
* especially canned fish with the bones.
POTASSIUM (see page 29) Abundant in: Leafy greens, Root vegetables, Bananas
VITAMIN B12 (see page 27) Abundant in: Fish, Shellfish, Red meat
CHLORIDE (see page 28) Abundant in: Seaweed, Celery, Leafy greens
SELENIUM (see page 29) Abundant in: Fish, Poultry, Red meat
VITAMIN C (see page 27) Abundant in: Berries, Citrus fruits, Dark leafy greens
COPPER (see page 28) Abundant in: Mushrooms, Organ meat, Shellfish
SODIUM (see page 198) Abundant in: Unrefined sea salt, Celery, Beets
VITAMIN D (see page 92) Abundant in: Fish, Liver, Mushrooms
IRON (see page 28) Abundant in: Dark leafy greens, Liver, Red meat
ZINC (see page 29) Abundant in: Oysters, Red meat, Poultry
VITAMIN B7 (see page 26) Abundant in: Egg yolks, Organ meat, Fatty fish
MAGNESIUM (see page 28) Abundant in: Avocados, Green vegetables, Fish
DHA AND EPA (see page 158) Abundant in: Fish, Liver, Sea vegetables

DETOXIFICATION SYSTEMS HEALTH

The terms *toxin* and *detoxification* are frequently used in misleading ways, often to promote expensive supplements or detox diets that have no scientific basis. However, supporting the body's detoxification systems is vital for staying healthy and consequently is a key principle of Paleo.

From a scientific standpoint, a *toxin* is a poisonous substance produced by a living organism (whether plant or animal) that can cause disease or cellular injury. *Detoxification* is the process of transforming and clearing those toxic substances from the blood (like microorganisms, contaminants, drugs, alcohol, pesticides, and metabolic end-products). The body has several major detoxification hubs: the liver, kidneys, and skin (via sweating).

Liver Detoxification

First, let's look at the liver. No organ in the body really ever "slacks off" (at least not without dire consequences!), but when it comes to the liver, to say that it's hardworking is an understatement. Among its hundreds of functions, the liver stores vitamins and minerals, controls the production and removal of cholesterol, breaks down fat, manufactures triglycerides, helps regulate blood sugar, produces clotting and immune factors, releases bile, produces glycogen, metabolizes amino acids, and destroys old red blood cells. And of all our organs, the liver plays the most important role in detoxification.

Every day, we're exposed to toxins from a wide variety of sources. Some are external sources (like medications), and others are normal by-products of internal processes (like ammonia produced from protein metabolism) or from gut microbes (which can produce enterotoxins that we then absorb). No matter where the toxins come from, the liver has two important pathways for neutralizing them and eliminating them from the body. The first pathway, called Phase I, begins transforming dangerous chemicals into generally less-harmful substances as well as preparing them for easier excretion. The second pathway, called Phase II, involves attaching other molecules to the toxins, allowing them to be removed through bile or urine.

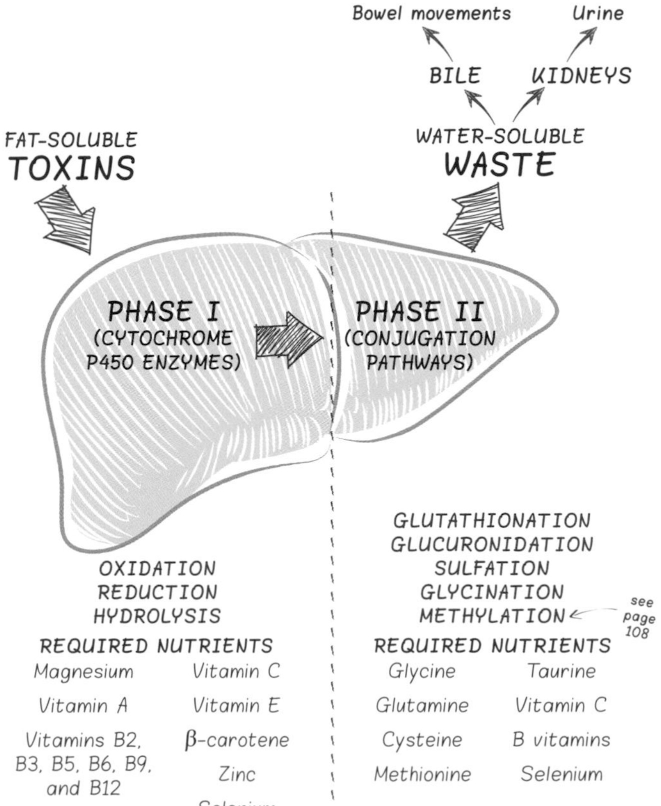

Phase I Detoxification

Because most of the harmful chemicals we encounter are fat-soluble (which means they can accumulate in our fatty tissues instead of being washed out through urine or bile), Phase I detoxification begins with chemically transforming them into water-soluble compounds in preparation for Phase II. The majority of the Phase I transformation reactions are performed by the cytochrome P450 family of enzymes, which change the molecular structure of toxins via oxidation, reduction, and hydrolysis reactions. Cytochrome P450 enzymes also help metabolize and activate prescription drugs and metabolize endogenous (produced in the body) compounds such as transforming testosterone to estradiol. Nutrient deficiencies, heavy metal toxicity, liver damage, and certain drugs can all impair Phase I by reducing the activity of these important P450 enzymes.

Several other enzymes contribute to Phase I, including flavin monooxygenases that detoxify the nicotine from cigarette smoke, alcohol and aldehyde dehydrogenases that metabolize alcohol, and monoamine oxidases, which break down several neurotransmitters.

Phase I requires a wide variety of nutrients for the cytochrome P450 enzymes to do their job. For starters, a too-low protein intake can hinder the activity of these enzymes, so it's a good idea to consume high-quality protein, particularly from animal products like seafood, chicken, beef, and eggs. Beyond that, the following vitamins and minerals are needed for the proper functioning of the various Phase I enzymes and to ensure that toxins are processed quickly enough to keep them from damaging our bodies:

- **Magnesium,** found in dark leafy greens, nuts, seeds, legumes, avocados, bananas, cocoa, and seafood
- **Vitamin A (retinol),** found in liver, eggs, and dairy
- **Vitamin B2 (riboflavin),** found in liver, beef, clams, portabella mushrooms, almonds, dairy, salmon, and eggs
- **Vitamin B3 (niacin),** found in tuna, poultry, salmon, lamb, beef, sardines, shrimp, asparagus, tomatoes, dark leafy greens, and avocados
- **Vitamin B5 (pantothenic acid),** found in brewer's yeast, cauliflower, kale, egg yolks, broccoli, tomatoes, organ meat, poultry, sweet potatoes, avocados, and salmon

- **Vitamin B6,** found in fish, organ meat, potatoes, sweet potatoes, sunflower seeds, spinach, and bananas
- **Vitamin B9 (folate),** found in dark leafy greens (like bok choy, lettuce, parsley, spinach, and turnip greens), broccoli, cauliflower, asparagus, and beets
- **Vitamin B12,** found in organ meat (especially liver), shellfish (especially clams), and other animal products, like meat, poultry, eggs, and dairy

On top of those, because Phase I relies heavily on oxidation to help transform toxins, free radicals are produced—making it imperative that the liver has plenty of antioxidants to draw from. In particular, the most important antioxidants for the liver are:

- **Vitamin C,** found in citrus fruits, cantaloupe, mangoes, papayas, bell peppers, berries, and pineapple (and many other fruits and vegetables)
- **Vitamin E,** found in nuts (especially almonds), seeds (especially sunflower seeds), avocados, beet greens, spinach, collard greens, and some seafood
- **β-carotene,** found in carrots, sweet potatoes, leafy greens, broccoli, squash, tomatoes, and most other orange, yellow, or green fruits and vegetables
- **Zinc,** found in oysters, crab, lobster, beef, poultry, pumpkin seeds, cashews, almonds, and legumes
- **Selenium,** found in Brazil nuts, organ meat, mushrooms, seeds (such as sunflower, sesame, and flax), broccoli, cabbage, spinach, seafood (especially tuna, salmon, halibut, sardines, and shrimp), ham, beef, and chicken

Phase I activity can get particularly ramped up from a high intake of alcohol, caffeine, drugs, or cigarette smoke, as well as a high absorption of enterotoxins due to compromised gut health. So both antioxidant and cofactor (those vitamins and minerals needed for cytochrome P450 enzymes to do their job) requirements increase when these substances are ingested in large quantities or with high frequency.

Phase II Detoxification

Phase II detoxification is all about *conjugation,* or linking things together. In this case, small molecules (sulfur or amino acids) are added to partially processed toxins to help neutralize them (especially because some intermediate metabolites from Phase I can be even more harmful than in their original state!). This also completes the process of turning them water-soluble so that the body can safely excrete them via fluids. The four major conjugation pathways in this phase are:

- **Glutathionation,** where glutathione (a combination of the amino acids cysteine, glutamine, and glycine) binds with toxic substances such as some drugs, foreign chemicals, carcinogens like aflatoxin, and toxic metals like mercury and lead.
- **Glucuronidation,** where glucuronic acid (a sugar acid derived from glucose) combines with foreign chemicals, pesticides, steroid hormones, NSAIDs, and other pharmaceuticals.
- **Sulfation,** where sulfate binds with artificial food colorings, steroid hormones, heterocyclic amines (produced from cooking meat at high temperatures), and other substances to make them water-soluble.
- **Glycination,** where the amino acid glycine binds with salicylates (like from aspirin), benzoic acids, and some decongestants and antihistamines.

Since Phase II involves attaching new molecules to toxins, the building blocks for those molecules are dietary must-haves. If they're in short supply, the liver can't adequately neutralize toxins and make them water-soluble enough to excrete! The most important players here are certain amino acids and sulfur, including:

- **Glycine** (to complete glycination), found in gelatin and bone broth, collagen, connective tissue attached to bones and meat, pork feet/skin/ears, pastrami, organ meat, crustaceans, and poultry.
- **Glutamine,** found in beef, pork, chicken, seafood, organ meat, spinach, and parsley. (Because glutamine is heat-sensitive, the most bioavailable sources are raw—such as sushi and raw spinach.)
- **Cysteine** (which contains sulfur), found in beef, chicken, seafood, pork, eggs, dairy, red bell peppers, garlic, broccoli, Brussels sprouts, and onions.
- **Methionine** (which contains sulfur), found in most animal-based foods (especially meat, but also fish and eggs), as well as Brazil nuts.
- **Taurine** (which contains sulfur), found in meat, fish, shellfish, eggs, and dairy.

If Phase I activity is high (and oxidation is rampant as a result), the liver's supply of glutathione gets used up to help neutralize free radicals. And that can leave Phase II without enough glutathione to complete its glutathionation pathway! That makes it really important to eat enough glutathione-building foods to support optimal liver function. Those are foods high in the sulfur-containing amino acids cysteine, methionine, and taurine.

Along with the building blocks for conjugation molecules, Phase II can be supported with other nutrients also used during Phase I, particularly certain B vitamins, vitamin C, and selenium.

If the Phase II pathway is impaired or overloaded, it can result in a buildup of fat-soluble toxins that get incorporated into fatty tissue (including in the brain and endocrine glands). That can lead to a wide variety of problems, including hormonal imbalances, recurrent infections, headaches and migraines, chemical sensitivities, and potentially a higher risk of cancer (if the chemicals are carcinogenic).

After toxins get processed through Phase I and Phase II and made water-soluble, they can be transported to the intestines with bile (and excreted through a bowel movement) or to the kidneys (and excreted through urine). Voilà! The liver just handled what could have been a danger to health and safely ushered it out of the body.

One of the most common misconceptions about the liver (and the reason some people are afraid of eating liver from other animals!) is the belief that it acts like a sponge, absorbing and accumulating toxins as it processes them. In fact, this is part of the rationale behind many "detox diets" that claim to clean out the liver (which is portrayed as getting gunked up with toxins from unhealthy eating and living).

KNOWLEDGE BOMB

Want to know what the best superfood is to support liver detoxification? It's liver! Yes, beef, bison, chicken, duck, lamb, and pork liver are amazing sources of the nutrients our livers need to work at their best! Many people are afraid of eating liver when they can't obtain it from grass-fed, organic, free-range animals. In this case, however, conventional liver is still better than no liver! Because a little liver goes a long way in terms of nutrition, and because the liver isn't actually hoarding more toxins than other parts of the body (it's a filter, not a sponge), the nutritional benefits of conventional liver outweigh any potential downsides as far as our health goes.

This couldn't be further from the truth. In reality, the liver acts more like a self-cleaning filter than a sponge: it processes and converts toxins to water-soluble products to be excreted, but it doesn't store them. What the liver *does* store are important nutrients, such as the fat-soluble vitamins A, D, and K; minerals like iron and copper; and vitamin B12. These are the nutrients it needs to perform its many functions, including detoxification.

Kidney Detoxification

Along with the liver, the kidneys play a vital role in removing toxins from the body. They're constantly at work filtering blood (about 150 quarts every day!), regulating the body's sodium and potassium balance, producing hormones, regulating blood pressure, controlling calcium metabolism, controlling red blood cell production, removing waste products and drugs from the body, and producing an active form of vitamin D.

Our two bean-shaped kidneys, each about the size of a fist, contain up to a million nephrons, which are functional units consisting of a glomerulus and a tubule. The glomerulus filters waste products out of the blood, and the remaining fluid passes through the tubule, where chemicals and water are either removed or added (the tubules also shuttle minerals back to the bloodstream as needed). The end product is urine, which flows from the kidneys to the bladder through ureters (two thin tubes of muscle) until we're ready to excrete it.

For the kidneys to do their job, the body needs a sufficient volume of water to carry away waste products. Therefore, staying fully hydrated is paramount. Few substances are more "Paleo" than water itself, and it should come as no surprise that drinking enough of it is key for optimal health!

The Importance of Drinking Water

How much water do we need? The classic recommendation of eight 8-ounce glasses (64 ounces total) per day is mostly a misconception. The latest research suggests that men should consume about 13 cups (102 ounces, or 3 liters) of fluid per day, and women should consume about 9 cups (74 ounces, or 2.2 liters)—but this includes *all* beverages, as well as the water content of the food we eat. We get up to 20 percent of our daily water from food, particularly fruits, vegetables, and soups! In addition to supporting kidney health, staying hydrated helps optimize digestion, neurological function, circulation, body temperature regulation, and muscle contraction.

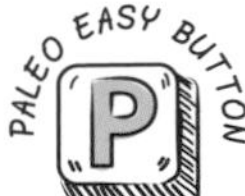

Aim for at least 9 cups for women and 13 cups for men of water and other beverages daily. Adding mineral drops to water is a great way to mimic the mineral-rich water sources of our Paleolithic ancestors.

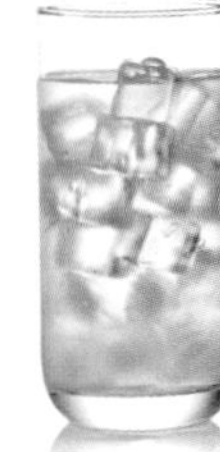

The quality of the water we consume is also important. Although most tap water and bottled water has a low mineral content, there's ample evidence that early humans consumed water containing non-trivial levels of sodium and other minerals. Natural freshwater sources (lakes, rivers, streams, and so on) contain some salt, and some have as much as 0.4 percent—which is quite a lot, especially knowing that the ocean is only about 9 times higher at 3.5 percent salt! Adding mineral drops to water before drinking it is one way to recreate its natural sodium content. (Read more about the effect of sodium on kidney health on page 201.)

What about fluoridated water? This is a hot (and highly controversial) topic, but the science is fairly clear-cut—at least when it comes to oral health. While there's significant evidence that topically applied fluoride (such as in toothpaste, foams, and gels) helps protect against cavities, systemic fluoride (ingested through water or foods) appears to have only a modest benefit for children and little to none for adults. Topical fluoride works by directly inhibiting demineralization inside the teeth, enhancing remineralization at the crystal surfaces of the teeth, and protecting against bacterial enzymes. Systemic fluoride, on the other hand, does not get incorporated into teeth and saliva in sufficient quantities to exert these effects, at least when consumed in nontoxic doses.

In a nutshell, fluoride is most beneficial when it makes prolonged contact with tooth surfaces rather than building up within the body. If we are using fluoridated toothpaste, drinking non-fluoridated water appears to pose no risk to oral health. Currently, most developed countries (including Japan and the majority of Western Europe) do not fluoridate their water.

Whether fluoridated water is harmful is another topic entirely, and the science here is much less settled. The EPA currently approves fluoride levels in water of up to 4 mg/L, while the Department of Health and Human Services recommends an upper limit of 0.7 mg/L (reduced in 2011 from a range of 0.7 to 1.2 mg/L). A 2015 Cochrane Review found that at fluoride levels of 0.7 mg/L, about 40 percent of the population develops some degree of dental fluorosis, a condition in which excess fluorine compounds cause discoloration and mottling of the teeth. Because people tend to drink more water (and therefore ingest more fluoride) when the weather is hot, dental fluorosis is more prevalent in warmer regions, even when the fluoride levels in the water are relatively low. Higher levels of fluoride (3 to 6 mg/L) can cause adverse changes in bone structure, and levels above 10 mg/L can cause crippling skeletal fluorosis.

Apart from known problems with fluorosis, much of the safety controversy surrounding water fluoridation stems from inadequate high-quality research. For example, some concerns exist with the type of fluoride used. Whereas the fluoride salts used in dentistry (like sodium fluoride and stannous fluoride) have been widely tested for safety, the silicofluorides added to drinking water (by-products of manufacturing phosphate fertilizers) haven't been the subject of many toxicology studies. And some studies have uncovered correlations between local water fluoride levels and lower IQ in children, leading to fears that fluoride, which can penetrate the blood-brain barrier in fetuses, negatively impacts early brain development. Overall, more research is needed to clarify the risks and benefits of water fluoridation for both children and adults.

Other Detoxification Pathways

Another major detoxification pathway happens through the skin: sweating. Research shows that some toxic chemicals and heavy metals are preferentially eliminated from the body through sweat, including bisphenol A (BPA), mono(2-ethylhexyl) phthalate (MEHP), persistent flame retardants, lead, cadmium, and mercury. Arsenic is also excreted through sweat, but in lower quantities than through urine. Historically, sweating was used as an effective treatment for sick mercury miners, and various sweat practices have been part of traditional cultures across the globe—such as Roman baths, Scandinavian saunas, Turkish baths, and Aboriginal sweat lodges.

Healthy sweat glands (meaning glands that aren't interfered with by chemical-laden antiperspirants) may help reduce oxidative stress, regulate immune function, and even reduce insulin resistance.

KNOWLEDGE BOMB *A number of factors can influence how efficient our bodies are at detoxification, and a major one involves the gene for methylenetetrahydrofolate reductase (MTHFR). Methylenetetrahydrofolate reductase is the rate-limiting enzyme in the methyl cycle, meaning that how quickly it works determines how quickly the whole cycle works. The methyl cycle is the process by which the body recycles methyl groups, which control the activity of a huge variety of proteins through the post-translational modification methylation. Some extremely important hormones (such as cortisol and melatonin) and some extremely important neurotransmitters (such as epinephrine and serotonin) are controlled through methylation. The methylation pathway is also critical for producing glutathione, one of the most essential cellular antioxidants in the body. Along with protecting against free radical damage, glutathione plays a role in the detoxification of certain carcinogens, heavy metals, and harmful chemicals, such as BPA.*

Defects in MTHFR activity, as occur in people with the C667T and/or A1298C variants of the gene for MTHFR, inhibit the body's ability to methylate and (by limiting glutathione production) detoxify. This is particularly true for homozygous mutation carriers, who can experience extreme reductions in MTHFR activity. These gene mutations can result in a buildup of the toxic nonprotein amino acid homocysteine, which can contribute to a variety of ailments, including cardiovascular disease, renal disease, neurodegenerative disease, osteoporosis, and cancer. In addition, by limiting glutathione production, MTHFR mutations can inhibit the detoxification of harmful carcinogens, metals, and chemicals.

You can learn whether you have a variant of MTHFR that reduces its activity through genetic testing; many functional medicine practitioners can order this for you. Ask your doctor about supplementing with vitamins B2 and B6 and methylated forms of vitamins B9 and B12.

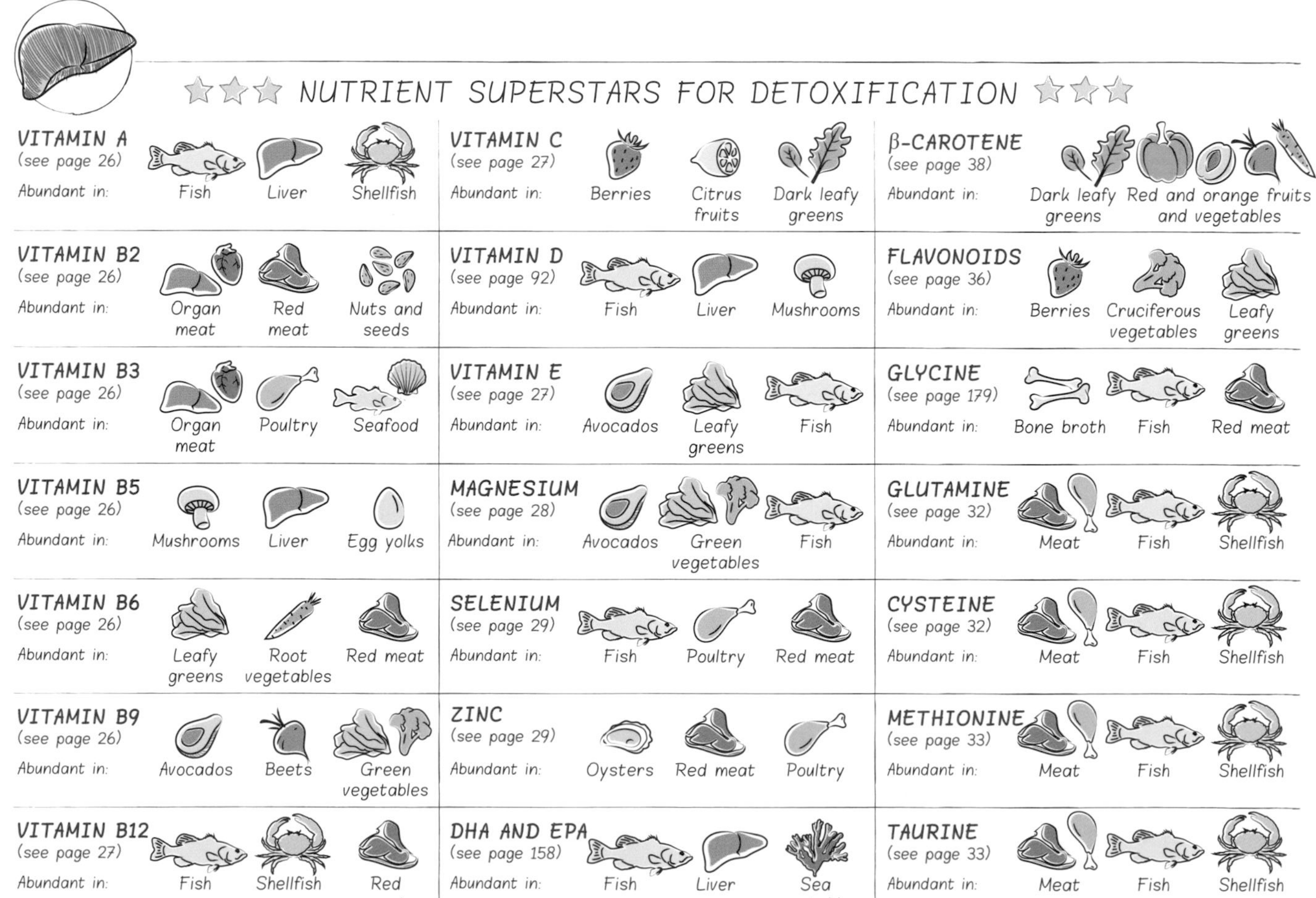

NUTRIENT SUPERSTARS FOR DETOXIFICATION

Nutrient	Abundant in	Nutrient	Abundant in	Nutrient	Abundant in
VITAMIN A (see page 26)	Fish, Liver, Shellfish	VITAMIN C (see page 27)	Berries, Citrus fruits, Dark leafy greens	β-CAROTENE (see page 38)	Dark leafy greens, Red and orange fruits and vegetables
VITAMIN B2 (see page 26)	Organ meat, Red meat, Nuts and seeds	VITAMIN D (see page 92)	Fish, Liver, Mushrooms	FLAVONOIDS (see page 36)	Berries, Cruciferous vegetables, Leafy greens
VITAMIN B3 (see page 26)	Organ meat, Poultry, Seafood	VITAMIN E (see page 27)	Avocados, Leafy greens, Fish	GLYCINE (see page 179)	Bone broth, Fish, Red meat
VITAMIN B5 (see page 26)	Mushrooms, Liver, Egg yolks	MAGNESIUM (see page 28)	Avocados, Green vegetables, Fish	GLUTAMINE (see page 32)	Meat, Fish, Shellfish
VITAMIN B6 (see page 26)	Leafy greens, Root vegetables, Red meat	SELENIUM (see page 29)	Fish, Poultry, Red meat	CYSTEINE (see page 32)	Meat, Fish, Shellfish
VITAMIN B9 (see page 26)	Avocados, Beets, Green vegetables	ZINC (see page 29)	Oysters, Red meat, Poultry	METHIONINE (see page 33)	Meat, Fish, Shellfish
VITAMIN B12 (see page 27)	Fish, Shellfish, Red meat	DHA AND EPA (see page 158)	Fish, Liver, Sea vegetables	TAURINE (see page 33)	Meat, Fish, Shellfish

Chapter 5:
AVOIDING TOXINS

The Paleo template addresses health from both sides of the equation: increasing health-promoting behaviors and foods while reducing or removing behaviors and foods that undermine health. Think of it this way: there's a whole lot less to gain from eating organic kale if you're smoking three packs a day. Not that we should give up on making healthy diet and lifestyle choices just because we may be having a hard time breaking bad habits or overcoming addiction, but we can't get the full benefits of our good choices if we're continuously exposed to more toxins than our detoxification systems can keep up with.

The catch-all term *toxin* may be hyperbolic when it comes to talking about antinutrients and phytohormones in foods, but the root of this principle is really about limiting exposure to all compounds that undermine health, including ingested problematic compounds in foods, environmental toxins, smoking, and substance abuse.

FOOD TOXINS

This may be an oversimplification, but we can lump together all the health-promoting nutrients in foods as "Good Stuff" and all the health-undermining compounds in foods as "Bad Stuff." When evaluating the merits of a food, we can weigh how much Good Stuff is in that food versus how much Bad Stuff it contains. Some foods have tons of Good Stuff and no Bad Stuff—these are definite "yes" foods (everything discussed in Part 2), and we can eat plenty of them without guilt. Other foods have tons of Bad Stuff and very little Good Stuff—these are definite "no" foods (everything discussed in Part 3) and should be avoided the vast majority of the time.

To make these distinctions, it's helpful to look at the many forms that Bad Stuff can take—collectively referred to here as "food toxins." These include antinutrients, carcinogens, endocrine disruptors, gut irritants, gut dysbiosis contributors, and immune stimulants—generally, all the types of substances that

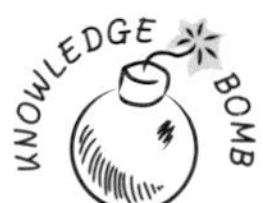

Some toxins are inherent to a food, meaning that even the organically grown non-GMO whole-food version still contains compounds that can undermine our health: for example, α-tomatine and α-solanine in tomatoes, gluten and wheat germ agglutinin in wheat, and soybean agglutinin in soy. Other food toxins are created during high-heat cooking, like heterocyclic amines and Maillard reaction products. Some food toxins come from food contamination, like mycoestrogens produced by molds and xenoestrogens that leach into foods from pesticide use and storage in certain plastics. Still other toxins are created in the processing and refining of foods, like D-amino acids, or are added to processed and refined foods to achieve texture or shelf stability, like carrageenan and BHT.

can interfere with biological systems health, discussed in Chapter 4. Part 3 includes expanded discussions on food toxins, but here is a brief summary:

Antinutrients are substances in food that interfere with the digestion or absorption of nutrients. They include prolamins, agglutinins, digestive enzyme inhibitors, saponins, glycoalkaloids, phytic acid, cyanogenic glycosides, glucosinolates, oxalic acid, purines, tannins, D-amino acids and lysinoalanine, emulsifiers, thickeners, stabilizers, oxidized sulfur amino acids, and Maillard reaction products. (See page 230.)

Carcinogens are substances with the potential to cause cancer in living tissue. A number of environmental carcinogens exist (including cigarette smoke, industrial chemicals, and UV exposure), but food can also contain carcinogens, such as heterocyclic amines (HCAs) and polycyclic aromatic hydrocarbons (PAHs) formed during high-temperature cooking. (See page 229.)

Endocrine disruptors are chemicals that can interfere with the body's endocrine system, such as by mimicking or blocking estrogens, androgens, or thyroid hormones. The most common endocrine disruptors in food are phytoestrogens, which include isoflavones (such as the genistein and daidzein found in soy) and lignans (found in flax seeds, sesame seeds, sunflower seeds, whole grains, and other plant foods). Mycoestrogens from food contamination as well as xenoestrogens from pesticides, plastics, and detergents are also a concern. Foods that spike blood sugar and therefore impair insulin regulation and sensitivity can also be categorized as endocrine disruptors. (See page 227.)

Gut irritants are substances that damage or irritate the gut and are particularly concentrated in grains and legumes. They include protease inhibitors, prolamins, agglutinins, and phytates. Other gut irritants include carrageenan, cellulose gum, capsaicin, excessive alcohol, and high fructose consumption. (See page 228.)

Gut dysbiosis contributors promote an imbalanced gut microbial community, including low levels of beneficial bacteria and high levels of pathogenic bacteria, as well as microorganisms growing in the wrong part of the gut (such as small intestinal bacterial overgrowth, or SIBO). These include antibiotic exposure, alcohol abuse, consumption of emulsifiers, thickeners, and stabilizers, excessive exercise, and a number of antinutrients (such as agglutinins, prolamins, digestive enzyme inhibitors, saponins such as glycoalkaloids, and phytic acid), as well as excessive sugar and fructose intake and inadequate intakes of fiber and omega-3 fats. (See page 229.)

Immune stimulators are substances that activate the body's immune system. They include components of spirulina and chlorella, the glycoalkaloids in nightshade vegetables, and the agglutinins in soybeans, peanuts, wheat, and grains and legumes in general. High intake of refined carbohydrates as well as high fructose consumption also increase inflammation. (See page 266.)

ENVIRONMENTAL TOXINS AND POLLUTANTS

A variety of environmental toxins and pollutants, workplace hazards, and other forms of chemical exposure have been linked to multiple chronic diseases, including autoimmune disease and cancer. Some environmental toxins occur naturally, like mercury, cadmium, lead, arsenic, radon, formaldehyde, and benzene. Others are man-made, such as phthalates and plasticizers like bisphenol A (BPA).

BPA and phthalates can seep into food or beverages from containers that contain them, such as some types of plastics and aluminum cans lined with BPA. Phthalates and BPA are xenoestrogens, discussed in the next section. In addition, while the long-term effects of BPA exposure remain controversial, there is concern about possible effects on brain health in fetuses, infants, and children. There is also a possible link between BPA exposure and high blood pressure.

Although some environmental toxins and pollutants are beyond our immediate control (such as air pollution), we can greatly minimize our exposure by being choosy about the products we use on our bodies and in our homes. Household cleaners, personal care products, and cosmetics are some of the most common sources of environmental toxins, particularly the following:

- **Formaldehyde** is classified as either a human carcinogen or a probable human carcinogen by different toxicology agencies, and it's also a skin, eye, and lung irritant. Formaldehyde and formaldehyde-releasing preservatives (FRPs) are common ingredients in keratin hair straighteners, nail polish, mascara, nail treatments, eye shadow, blush, and shampoo.
- **Phthalates** are endocrine disruptors that can enter the body through inhalation or skin contact. They're used in a number of fragranced household products, such as air fresheners, scented toilet paper, and dish soap.
- **Benzene** is considered both a carcinogen and an endocrine disruptor and is used to produce plastics and detergents. It is also found in some hair conditioners and styling products.
- **Perchloroethylene (perc)** is a neurotoxin and possible carcinogen, according to the EPA. It's found in dry cleaning solutions, carpet cleaners, upholstery cleaners, and spot removers.
- **Untreated or mildly treated mineral oils** are produced from crude oil and can act as carcinogens while contributing to skin, eye, and lung irritation. These oils are found in a wide variety of personal care products, such as lip gloss, lipstick, hair color, hair bleach, facial treatment, blush, concealer, moisturizer, eye shadow, and hairstyling gel. (Other names on ingredient labels include heavy mineral oil mist, paraffin oil mist, and white mineral oil mist.)
- **Coal tar** is a carcinogenic by-product of coal processing (typically associated with lung cancer, digestive tract cancer, kidney cancer, and bladder cancer). Its use in cosmetics is prohibited by the European Commission, although it is still allowed in the United States. Coal tar is found in hair dyes, dandruff treatment, rosacea treatment, and some shampoos. What's more, coal tar can contain other carcinogenic substances, such as polycyclic aromatic hydrocarbons (PAHs).

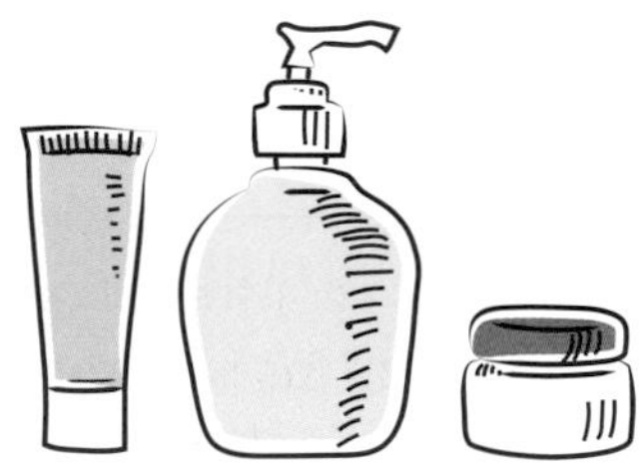

- **Crystalline silica** (also listed as cristobalite, quartz, tridymite, or tripoli on ingredient labels) is a known human carcinogen, most notably with links to lung cancer. It may also irritate the lungs and eyes through inhalation and skin or eye contact. Crystalline silica is found in many lipsticks, lip glosses, eye shadows, eyeliners, foundations, sunscreens, lotions, and shampoos.
- **Butylated compounds** such as butylated hydroxyanisole (BHA) and butylated hydroxytoluene (BHT) are endocrine disruptors with carcinogenic potential. They are also linked to organ system toxicity and reproductive toxicity. These compounds are typically used as preservatives in personal care products and are most common in hair products, lip products, makeup, sunscreen, fragrance, and antiperspirant and deodorant. They can also be used as preservatives in foods—for example, BHT is commonly added to breakfast cereal packaging to maintain freshness.
- **Talc** (or talcum powder) is a bulking and absorbent mineral that sometimes contains asbestos. It has been linked to ovarian cancer, gynecological tumors, and mesothelioma (a rare cancer affecting the protective tissues covering the lungs and abdomen). Although talc is banned from use in cosmetic products in the European Union, it's still used in some products sold in the U.S., like baby powder, face powder, and deodorant.
- **Methylisothiazolinone (MIT) and methylchloroisothiazolinone (MCIT)** are common preservatives with possible inhalation toxicity and neurotoxic effects. They are found in some brands of shampoo (including baby shampoo), conditioner, hair color, hairspray, shaving cream, mascara, makeup remover, lotion, and sunscreen.
- **Acrylates** (including ethyl acrylate, ethyl methacrylate, and methyl methacrylate) have the potential to act as carcinogens, cause reproductive and organ system toxicity, cause neurological damage, and irritate the skin, eyes, and throat. They're most commonly found in cosmetic artificial nails.
- **1,4 dioxane** is a carcinogen created when other ingredients react through a process called ethoxylation. It's found in products that create

suds (like bubble bath and shampoo). Although 1,4 dioxane isn't required to be listed on ingredient labels (since it's created through reactions rather than added to a product), it's generally found in products containing PEG compounds, sodium laureth sulfate, and any chemicals that include "xynol," "oleth," or "ceteareth."

- **Phenacetin** is a human carcinogen (including being linked to malignant mammary tumors) and is known to cause renal damage and anemia. This toxin is sometimes used as a stabilizer in hair color, facial hair bleach, and hair-removal products.
- **Ethanolamines** (including triethanolamine, DEA, cocamide DEA, myristamide DEA, DEA-cetyl phosphate, DEA oleth-3 phosphate, lauramide DEA, oleamide DEA, TEA, TEA-lauryl sulfate diethanolamine, cocamide MEA, linoleamide MEA, and stearamide MEA) are linked to liver tumors and organ system toxicity and, despite being banned by the European Commission, are still found in products in the U.S., such as soap, hair dye, shampoo, conditioner, shaving cream, makeup, fragrance, household cleaning products, waxes, lotions, and sunscreen.
- **Heavy metals** (including lead, mercury, arsenic, and aluminum) are found as both contaminants and deliberate ingredients in a variety of personal care products and cosmetics, such as whitening toothpaste, lipstick, eyeliner, nail polish, sunscreen, blush, concealer, eye drops, and moisturizer. In small amounts, some heavy metals (like zinc, chromium, and iron) are necessary for human health, but others are known carcinogens and can contribute to organ toxicity, developmental toxicity, and reproductive toxicity.

HEALTH QUICK-START

Start reading labels not just on foods but also on household and personal care products. While not all hard-to-pronounce ingredients are verboten (see page 285), a good place to start is to look for companies that specialize in products made from natural fats, essential oils, plant extracts, clays, probiotic bacteria, and natural food-based ingredients like vinegar and baking soda.

In all, hundreds of cosmetic, personal care, and cleaning products sold in the U.S. contain ingredients that have been banned in other countries. The Environmental Working Group (www.ewg.org) and the CDC's National Institute for Occupational Safety and Health (www.cdc.gov/niosh/) offer more exhaustive information about the many harmful chemicals lurking in everyday products. As with food, it's important to read the ingredient labels of the products we use in our homes or on our bodies to ensure that we aren't exposing ourselves to environmental toxins.

Estrogen Mimics

Environmental estrogens are estrogens or estrogen-mimicking compounds found everywhere in our environment. *Phytoestrogens* occur naturally in plants such as flax, soy, and other legumes. *Mycoestrogens* are common food contaminants produced by molds and other fungi. Meat, eggs, and dairy products from animals treated with hormones may contain high concentrations of estrogens. *Xenoestrogens* are a class of synthetic estrogens found in industrial products, such as pesticides, plastics, and detergents. *Metalloestrogens* are found in heavy metals. All these environmental estrogens are toxic to the immune system. While the effect of these substances on human health in general is still controversial and remains greatly under-studied, there is an established correlation between exposure to some environmental estrogens and the development of chronic illness.

You can limit your exposure to environmental estrogens by avoiding the most common sources. Reduce your use of plastic containers for food storage (and never heat food in plastic containers); stick to organically grown produce and organic, pasture-raised meat (see page 170); evaluate the estrogen-mimicking chemicals that may be present in household cleaning products, laundry detergents, and cosmetics; and reduce or eliminate foods that are high in phytoestrogens.

The foods highest in phytoestrogens include flax seed, soy, whole grains, corn, and meat or eggs from animals treated with hormones. Lesser sources of phytoestrogens include nuts and seeds (especially sesame seeds, pistachios, sunflower seeds, and chestnuts and, to a lesser degree, almonds, walnuts, cashews, and hazelnuts) and legumes (especially lentils, navy beans, kidney beans, pinto beans, and fava beans, but also chickpeas and split green and yellow peas). Many vegetables and fruits contain low levels of phytoestrogens as well, including winter squash, green beans, collard greens, broccoli, cabbage, and prunes. It is not necessary for most people to avoid these foods, although those with known reproductive hormone imbalances may benefit from consuming them in moderation. Alfalfa sprouts tend to be high in mycoestrogens because of contamination from a fungus that commonly grows on them.

Pesticides

Beyond being a source of environmental estrogens, many pesticides are known to negatively impact the immune system (although there remains an urgent need for more research on this topic). The effects of these chemicals can be broadly categorized as either suppression or inappropriate stimulation of the immune system—both of which can be hazardous to people with chronic illness.

The most immunotoxic class of pesticides is organochlorinated pesticides (many of which are now illegal, and some are even banned globally). These pesticides increase inflammation, decrease the ability of the immune system to regulate itself, suppress critical components of the immune system that are needed to detect and kill cancerous cells, and can even increase autoantibody production in people with autoimmune disease. While they are mostly being phased out of agricultural use, newer pesticides may also contribute to immune-function problems. Studies have linked organophosphates and carbamates (both widely used as insecticides) to changes in immune cell activities, stimulating some cell types while suppressing others. The widely used agricultural pesticide tributyltin chloride, an organotin pesticide, has been shown to cause cell death in the thymus gland (see page 81). Atrazine, another organotin pesticide, as well as the insecticide propanil are known to reduce numbers and activities of specific immune cell types.

As scary as this sounds, most of the studies evaluating the effects of pesticides on the immune system mimic occupational exposure rather than the much lower exposure that the majority of us would have simply by eating produce from crops treated with these chemicals. While large epidemiological studies on the correlation between insecticides and chronic disease have not been performed, the Women's Health Initiative Observational Study did show a positive correlation between insecticide use (as in, in your garden) and the risk of both rheumatoid arthritis and systemic lupus erythematosus. What effect the very small amounts of these chemicals that might be found on conventional produce causes either in a healthy person or in someone with chronic disease remains unknown.

While the benefits of eating a vegetable-rich diet almost certainly outweigh the health detriments from pesticides for those consuming exclusively conventionally grown produce, reducing pesticide exposure is very sensible. The easiest way to do so is to buy organically grown produce whenever possible. Certain food crops tend to have more residual pesticides than others, so familiarizing yourself with the "Dirty Dozen" is a good way to prioritize which foods to buy organic if budget is a concern. The Dirty Dozen is a list compiled every year by the Environmental Working Group of the foods that contain the highest amounts (and the most different types) of pesticides. (The EWG—www.ewg.org—also puts together a Clean Fifteen list of the fifteen crops with the least amount of pesticides.) As a general rule, apples, stone fruits, berries, and leafy greens are veterans of the Dirty Dozen list. Another way to lower your pesticide exposure is to peel fruits and vegetables before eating them. (For example, peeling apples removes the majority of the pesticides.)

Reduce your pesticide exposure by buying organic versions of the produce that appears on the Dirty Dozen list. The fruits and vegetables included in the most recent update are:

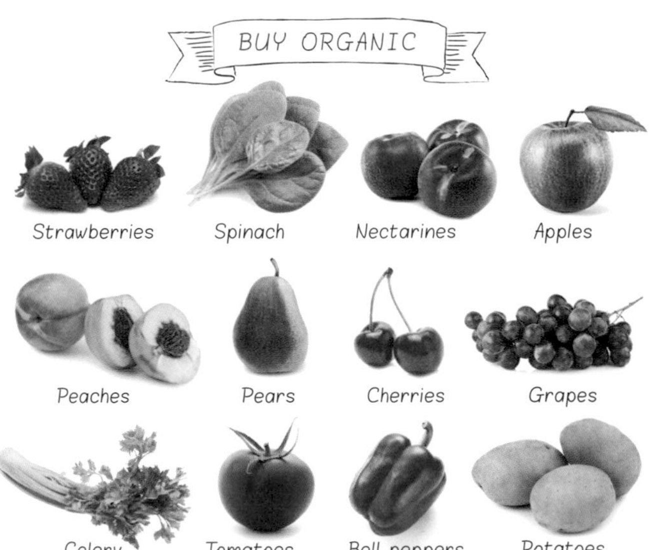
BUY ORGANIC
Strawberries
Spinach
Nectarines
Apples
Peaches
Pears
Cherries
Grapes
Celery
Tomatoes
Bell peppers
Potatoes

OVER-THE-COUNTER AND PRESCRIPTION DRUG USE

Just because some drugs don't require a prescription doesn't mean that they're always safe or healthful. It has become increasingly common to take medications (especially over-the-counter, or OTC, medications) without much concern other than the vague hope for immediate symptom relief. The ubiquity of drugs like aspirin and ibuprofen creates the illusion that they must be harmless. We also trust that drugs prescribed by our doctors, like steroids, statins, and proton-pump inhibitors, will help us.

However, many of the medications routinely taken for pain and inflammation are counterproductive when it comes to healing. Perhaps more insidious, many of these medications do reduce pain or decrease inflammation, resulting in less awareness (at least temporarily) of their detrimental effects on intestinal permeability, the immune system, and the gut microbiota. It's important to understand which medications are better to avoid, which are appropriate for certain circumstances, and which are lifesaving. Always talk with your health-care provider before taking, changing, or discontinuing any medication or supplement.

So which medications do more harm than good? As a general rule, any drug that lists gastrointestinal symptoms as a possible side effect is likely to harm gut health: constipation, diarrhea, nausea, abdominal pain, and vomiting are all fairly good indicators of damage or irritation to the gastrointestinal tract. Consequently, such drugs should be avoided if they're not critical for staying alive. In addition, drugs designed to manage symptoms while failing to treat (or worsening) the underlying cause of the disease are best avoided or greatly minimized. While the following list is by no means exhaustive, the biggest (and most commonly used) offenders are:

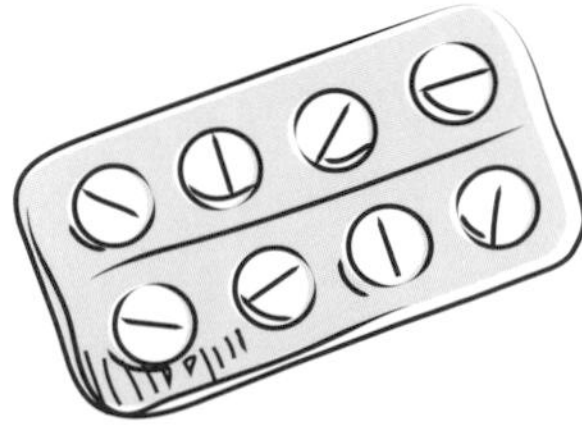

- **Immune-suppressing drugs,** including corticosteroids (such as prednisone) and DMARDs (such as methrotrexate). Corticosteroids work by binding to glucocorticoid receptors in immune cells, signaling the resolution of inflammation and immunity. However, they also flood the body with glucocorticoids (that is, cortisol), chemically mimicking severe chronic stress. This is why the side effects of glucocorticoids include weight gain especially in the trunk, restlessness and trouble sleeping, fatigue, and gastrointestinal symptoms. DMARDs suppress the immune system via a variety of mechanisms, and long-term use carries substantial risks of serious infection and cancer. Note, however, that these drugs are often prescribed in life-threatening situations, which is absolutely an appropriate time to take them!
- **Proton-pump inhibitors (PPIs), H2 blockers, laxatives, antidiarrheal drugs, and other drugs that interfere with digestion,** which are commonly designed to decrease stomach acid, increase gastrointestinal motility, or decrease gastrointestinal motility. PPIs include pantoprazole, omeprazole, and lansoprazole—more commonly known under the brand names Pantoloc, Nexium, and Prevacid; H2 blockers include famotidine and ranitidine, including the brands Pepcid and Zantac; laxatives include stimulant laxatives like bisacodyl and senna, castor oil, polyethylene glycol 3550, and, to a lesser extent, purely osmotic laxatives like milk of magnesia; and antidiarrheal drugs include loperamide and bismuth subsalicylate, as well as bulking agents like psyllium. Depending on the drug and the symptom(s) it was created to treat, the effects of short-term or long-term use can be impaired ability to digest and absorb nutrients, damage to epithelial cells lining the gut, and increased risk of infection by dangerous pathogens.
- **Nonsteroidal anti-inflammatory drugs (NSAIDs),** such as ibuprofen and naproxen, which are often prescribed to reduce pain and inflammation. In fact, NSAIDs are so pervasive and have such important consequences for our health that we'll look at them in more detail next!

Nonsteroidal Anti-inflammatory Drugs (NSAIDs)

NSAIDs include many familiar over-the-counter medications, the three most common of which are acetylsalicylic acid (aspirin), ibuprofen (Advil, Motrin, Nurofen, and so on), and naproxen (Aleve, Midol, and so on). These are routinely prescribed in higher doses to manage pain and reduce inflammation. However, they have a high incidence of gastrointestinal side effects. NSAIDs cause damage to the intestinal barrier, and chronic use carries significant risks of ulcers, hemorrhage, and perforation (a rip or tear in the intestine).

Even a single dose of an NSAID causes an increase in intestinal permeability, even in healthy people. NSAIDs do this in several ways.

The first discovered mechanism by which NSAIDs cause gastrointestinal injury is through the inhibition of an enzyme called cyclooxygenase. Inhibition of cyclooxygenase prevents the metabolism of arachidonic acid, which decreases the formation of prostaglandins and thromboxanes (see page 158). This is how NSAIDs achieve their anti-inflammatory, blood-thinning, and pain-relieving effects. However, it also damages the gut barrier, resulting in intestinal lesions (which can eventually become ulcers or worse). It turns out that cyclooxygenase is an essential enzyme for maintaining the integrity of the gut's mucous layer. Once this enzyme is disrupted, the gut is more susceptible to damage from other sources (such as toxins and exercise-induced intestinal barrier disruption).

Studies have also shown that NSAIDs inhibit production of the proteins that form the tight junctions between gut enterocytes, which causes the tight junctions to open. This might be because NSAIDs impair mitochondrial metabolism, which means that the gut enterocytes cannot produce enough energy to maintain their tight junctions. NSAIDs also weaken the gut barrier by causing changes in blood flow in the capillaries that supply blood to the tissues of and surrounding the gut. Furthermore, NSAIDs seem to increase the production of leukotrienes, causing the activation and recruitment of neutrophils from the blood, which have been implicated as contributing to the gastrointestinal damage caused by NSAIDs.

Unlike some other drugs, NSAIDs are rarely used as lifesaving necessities and are typically used for symptom relief. In these cases, NSAIDs are best avoided—they are just not worth the damage they cause to the intestinal barrier. The only exception is if NSAIDs are used as blood thinners. In some diseases, daily baby aspirin is often suggested to prevent blood clots (which can be life-threatening). It is exceptionally important to work with your doctor to be weaned off of aspirin if that is your goal, since removing blood thinners if you have a clotting disorder can be dangerous.

MEDICATION IS NOT FAILURE.

When making diet and lifestyle choices to take control of our health, it's tempting to want to make swallowing pills a thing of the past. However, going medication-free should not always be the goal. When organs are damaged as a result of disease, they need to be supported. This might mean taking insulin for a type 1 diabetic or thyroid replacement hormone for someone with Hashimoto's thyroiditis. Generally, in these conditions, going medication-free is counterproductive to health. For example, thyroid hormones control a vast array of functions in the human body, from metabolism to immune function. With inadequate thyroid hormone, the body is less responsive to diet and lifestyle changes. In this case, it's in our best interest to support the damaged organ through pharmaceuticals. And this is not failure.

Taking a medication, even for the rest of your life, does not make you a failure. It also doesn't mean that you don't have much to gain from diet and lifestyle changes. These changes can help prevent further damage to your body and prevent the development of additional chronic health problems.

HEALTH QUICK-START

If you take a daily medication that you think you're better off without, make sure to have your diet and lifestyle dialed in before discussing options with your doctor. For many medications, you'll need medical supervision to discontinue them safely. Also, some medications require you to wean slowly, which must be done under the guidance of a health-care professional.

Antibiotic Overuse

The word *antibiotic* literally means "against life" from its Greek roots. And that's exactly what antibiotics are designed to do: stop or slow down the growth of microscopic organisms (bacteria, fungi, and some parasites), in turn treating potentially dangerous infections.

First, let's make one thing clear: antibiotics are lifesaving medications, and there is definitely a time and a place for them. Before their advent and usage, a simple infection could easily turn deadly. In fact, for much of human history, infections were high-ranking killers that cut countless lives short. We're lucky to have access to medications that save us from diseases that plagued our ancestors.

However, the routine overuse of antibiotics has created a new, detrimental set of problems, and long-term courses of antibiotics can do more harm than good.

Why? One side effect of antibiotics is that, in addition to whatever infectious bacteria is making us sick, they can also kill the beneficial probiotic bacteria in our guts. (Some strains of probiotic bacteria are more susceptible to antibiotics than others, and different antibiotics kill different types of bacteria more readily.) Bacteria from the *Bacteroides* genus (one of the most dominant types of bacteria in a healthy gut) are particularly sensitive to a variety of antibiotics. Other heavily impacted probiotic genera include *Clostridium* and *Bifidobacterium*. When these "good guys" are killed off, other strains may grow disproportionately numerous, resulting in gut dysbiosis (see page 70). Furthermore, the use of antibiotics early in life has been associated with increased risk of asthma, attributable to a change in the gut microbiota.

Unfortunately, restoring the gut microbiota to its pre-antibiotic levels can take many weeks or months, and some evidence suggests that after heavy antibiotic use, the microbiota may never fully recover in terms of its original diversity. A large body of research shows that antibiotics not only destroy beneficial bacteria while they're being taken, but also alter the gut microbiota in ways that can be irreversible. Of course, antibiotics also cause a number of seriously unpleasant side effects—like diarrhea, rashes, nausea, vomiting, dizziness, headaches, taste alteration, abdominal pain, lethargy, and insomnia, just to name a few! What's more, overuse can result in resistant bacterial strains that no longer respond to drug therapy, leading to infections that are much harder to treat (like MRSA).

So how should we view antibiotics? The answer is context dependent. To preserve our gut microbiota and avoid contributing to the development of antibiotic-resistant strains of bacteria, it's smart to avoid antibiotics when they aren't necessary, such as for viral flus and colds. However, when it comes to certain infections (the ones that used to wipe out huge chunks of the human population, including things like "the morbid sore throat," aka strep throat), antibiotics can prevent serious complications and even save lives. The key here is avoiding antibiotic *over*use. It's also important to take the full course of antibiotics as prescribed to reduce the development of antibiotic-resistant bacterial strains. The take-home: don't take antibiotics if you don't truly need them, but when you do need them, go all in!

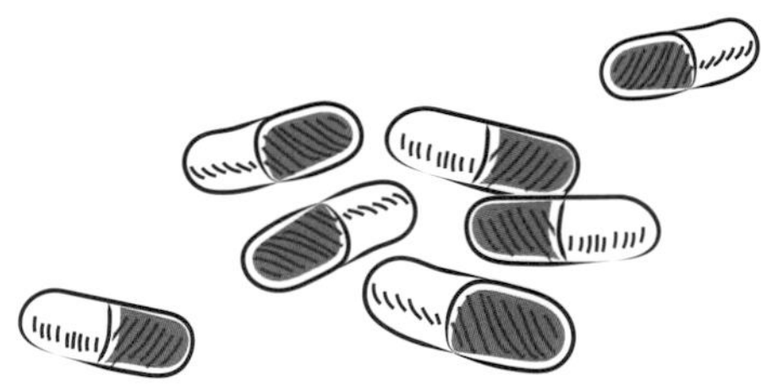

THE OBVIOUS: SUBSTANCE ABUSE

This book is all about laying a scientific foundation to inform your day-to-day diet and lifestyle choices for optimal health. But it's important to, at least briefly, address the elephant in the room: substance abuse. The most recent survey numbers show that approximately 17 percent of Americans smoke, a little over 9 percent of Americans engage in illicit drug use (recreationally or habitually), and nearly 25 percent of Americans are heavy or binge drinkers, with about 7 percent suffering from alcohol use disorder. A huge percentage of us are medicating our lives, destroying our health along the way.

Bottom line? If you're reading this book looking to improve your health, but you still smoke, abuse drugs, or drink excessively (or even regularly), then I want to emphasize that, while educating yourself on the best food choices is still a great idea, you've got bigger fish to fry. There is no evidence that a healthy diet and otherwise healthy lifestyle can fully counteract the harmful effects of substance abuse, and the risks are far too great to justify the presence of these destructive habits in anyone's life.

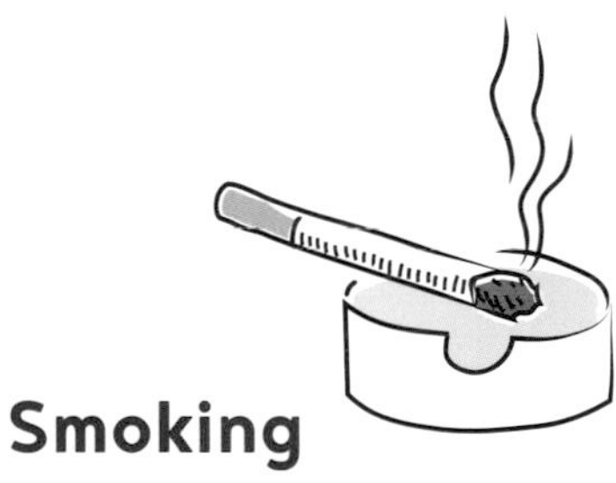

Smoking

There's a reason every credible health authority recommends stopping (or, better yet, never starting!) smoking cigarettes: smoking is harmful for practically every organ in the human body and raises the risk of multiple diseases more than any other diet or lifestyle factor. In the United States, smoking is responsible for about 90 percent of lung cancer deaths (it raises a person's risk of lung cancer twenty-five-fold) and 80 percent of all chronic obstructive pulmonary disease deaths, and it causes more deaths among women than breast cancer. In fact, smoking is the leading preventable cause of death in the U.S., causing nearly one out of every five deaths (nearly half a million people each year). According to the Centers for Disease Control and Prevention, that's more deaths than alcohol use, illegal drugs, HIV, car accidents, and firearm-related incidents *combined*. This one simple lifestyle factor also increases the risk of death from all causes for both men and women and, regardless of mortality, quadruples a person's risk of heart disease and stroke. If those figures sound scary, that's because they are!

How does smoking cause so much damage? First, tobacco smoke contains a mixture of more than 7,000 chemicals, including ammonia, formaldehyde, vinyl chloride, carbon monoxide, nitrites, nitrosamines, hydrocarbons, urethane, hydrogen cyanide, and heavy metals like chromium, arsenic, cadmium, and lead. At least 70 of those chemicals are known carcinogens and can reach any organ in the body via the bloodstream, dramatically raising cancer risk. Clinical studies show that smoking causes an immediate rise in white blood cell count, reflecting the body's fight against a perceived threat. Inhaling tobacco smoke induces other changes in blood chemistry as well, causing platelets to clump together, raising triglycerides, lowering HDL (good) cholesterol, and contributing to a faster heart rate and higher blood pressure (along with damaging blood vessels). All these changes contribute long-term to heart disease and stroke risk, but cigarette smoke can also trigger sudden blood clots, heart attacks, and strokes due to its immediate effects on the cardiovascular system. In addition, smoking can cause blood sugar to rise and increases the risk of type 2 diabetes (as well as making type 2 diabetes harder to control and making diabetics more likely to suffer from heart disease, kidney disease, retinopathy, and peripheral neuropathy). Smoking also interferes with immune function, which amplifies the carcinogenic potential of cigarette smoke by lowering the body's ability to fight off cancer. In fact, tobacco smoke can actually help tumors grow once they're established, so smoking after developing cancer is *extremely* dangerous.

Still not convinced that smoking is a bad idea? Let's consider the respiratory system. Many of the chemicals in cigarette smoke can damage and inflame the delicate linings of the lungs, reducing their elasticity and ability to exchange air (the classic coughing, wheezing, and excess mucus production seen in smokers are clear indicators of this damage occurring).

Not surprisingly, this increases the risk of lung diseases like emphysema (where the walls between the lung's air sacs lose their elasticity, leading to a reduced capacity to inhale oxygen and exhale carbon dioxide and eventually making it difficult to breathe) and chronic bronchitis (where the linings of the bronchial tubes swell, reducing air flow and causing mucus to build up).

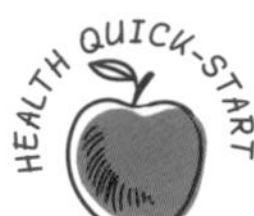

If you smoke, drink heavily, or do drugs, the very first place to start making health changes is breaking that habit!

The good news is that after quitting smoking, disease risk begins to slowly but steadily go back down: within 5 years of quitting, the risk of mouth cancer, throat cancer, esophageal cancer, and bladder cancer is cut in half. After 10 years, the risk of dying from lung cancer drops by half. The sooner you quit, the better chance your body has to heal.

Illicit Drugs and Alcohol

The mental and physical effects of substance abuse (including illicit drugs and alcohol) are indisputably devastating. Along with the very real possibility of death, substance abuse can lead to a weakened immune system, stroke, seizures, cardiovascular problems, kidney disease, liver damage or failure, extreme changes in appetite, global body changes, paranoia, impulsiveness, neurotransmitter changes, vomiting and nausea, impaired judgment, and birth defects in children born to mothers using illicit drugs. Once addicted, many users end up prioritizing drugs over every other aspect of life, including their families and careers. Depending on the drug, there can also be lasting physical damage after quitting (such as irreversible brain damage or the severe tooth decay and erosion associated with methamphetamine use). In a nutshell, illicit drugs have fully earned their negative reputation, and using them is one of the easiest ways to destroy your health and your life. Alcohol is discussed in more detail in Chapter 24.

Although even one-time use of many drugs can cause damage, the bigger threat is in their highly addictive nature that leads to a cycle of abuse (and ongoing, cumulative damage). Addictive drugs affect the reward circuit, which is part of the limbic system in the brain that controls our ability to feel pleasure. Although plenty of healthy activities also activate the limbic system (such as socializing and listening to music), illicit drugs hijack the reward circuit in an extreme way. These drugs change the way neurons (nerve cells in the brain) communicate information, sometimes by mimicking the structure of naturally occurring neurotransmitters (such as with heroin) or by forcing neurons to release huge amounts of natural neurotransmitters (such as with cocaine). Most addictive drugs work by flooding the reward circuit with dopamine, a neurotransmitter that regulates our perception of pleasure. The brain quickly learns to associate the drug with feelings of pleasure, and this reinforcement encourages a person to keep using. Even worse, over time, addictive drugs raise the level of dopamine that the brain needs to feel "normal." Because drugs can cause a dopamine response far beyond what any normal day-to-day activity can accomplish, the brain becomes accustomed to dopamine levels that only drugs can deliver, creating a vicious cycle of addiction.

While avoiding dietary and environmental toxins goes a long way in bolstering our bodies against disease, substance abuse is simply incompatible with good health. If you are currently struggling with this problem, seeking treatment should be your first step on the path toward wellness.

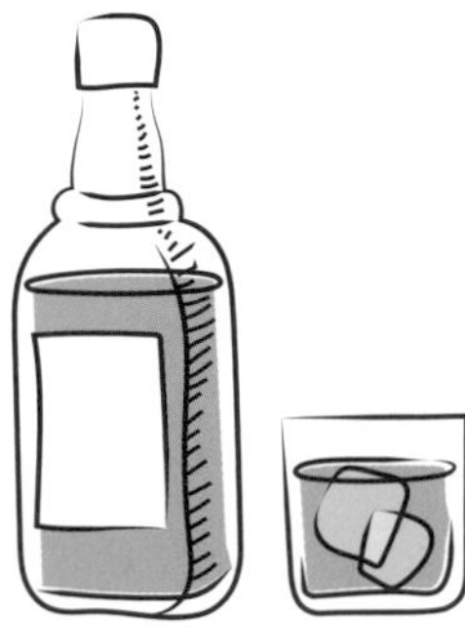

BEATING ADDICTION

Although addiction can feel like an impossible hurdle to overcome, there are steps anyone can take to regain control. In some cases, addiction rehab facilities or ongoing support may be needed to make a full recovery, but in other situations (like smoking or the less insidious but still problematic food addiction), going through the process of breaking harmful habits and forming new, healthier habits to replace them can help break the addiction cycle.

The following steps can serve as a guide for overcoming addiction:

1. Decide to make a change. Breaking free from addiction requires truly committing to recovery. It's normal to feel conflicted about living without a substance you're physically dependent on, but you can help yourself see the logical perspective by making lists of the pros and cons for quitting; keeping track of your use and associated expenses; writing down the things in your life that have been negatively affected by the addiction (such as your relationships, career, finances, or health); or asking a trusted friend or family member for an honest opinion about your addiction.

2. Set specific goals that you can measure, such as a start date for drug abstinence or limits on how much you will use. Concrete goals (such as "I will go two weeks without using drugs, beginning on Monday") are easier to stick to than more abstract goals that can't be measured or assessed.

3. Establish a new habit in place of drug use. During times you would normally engage in substance abuse (or any other time you feel tempted), exercising, learning or practicing an instrument, working on art, writing, socializing with supportive friends, or doing any other healthy and enjoyable activity will help keep your mind and body occupied.

4. Remove reminders of addiction from your environment (including your home and workplace). Facing constant reminders of the habits you want to abandon will only keep those habits in the front of your mind.

5. Limit your exposure to triggering people and places. This means temporarily or permanently cutting ties with friends who use (or who otherwise don't support your sobriety) and avoiding places you associate with drug use.

6. Find someone to hold you accountable. Telling a friend or trusted family member about your plan to stop using and asking them to check in with you and hold you to your commitment can increase your chances of following through.

7. Practice healthier ways of coping with stress. For many people, substance abuse is a way to escape life's challenges and stresses. Once drugs are gone as a crutch, it's important to have healthier methods of coping, such as yoga, meditation, exercise, hiking, walks in nature, listening to music, and other relaxing activities. (For more on stress management, see Chapter 27.)

8. Brace for withdrawal and learn what to expect. Due to the ways addictive drugs affect the brain and neurotransmitter levels, withdrawal symptoms (both physical and psychological) can occur during the recovery process and may be particularly intense early on. These symptoms can include insomnia, anxiety, cravings, muscle aches, sweating, and a runny nose or watery eyes. Be aware that unpleasant symptoms can arise, but they will pass.

9. Reach out for support. Recovery is much harder alone than with a support group. Close friends and family or a social group of sober, like-minded people can help you make it through the recovery process and avoid slipping back into old habits.

Chapter 6: BEYOND FOOD

I've mentioned it a few times: the food we eat isn't the only important thing to address in order to get healthy. There are a variety of known health risks—factors that increase the probability of illness, accident, and/or death—to consider. True, diet is a major player. For example, according to the World Health Organization (WHO), low fruit and vegetable consumption is responsible for approximately 1.7 million deaths worldwide each year, making it one of the top ten risk factors for global mortality. However, lifestyle factors and environmental exposures can be even more important. For example, each year 3.2 million deaths worldwide are attributable to physical inactivity; for tobacco use, the number is 7 million. According to WHO, 60 percent of risk factors for both death and loss of quality of life due to poor health are lifestyle factors. A further collection of health risks—high blood pressure, high blood sugar, and being overweight or obese are among the top five globally—are directly related to the combined effects of diet and lifestyle. For example, high blood pressure is responsible for 7.5 million deaths worldwide each year.

Since the goal of this book is to give you the knowledge you need to make the best day-to-day choices for your long-term health, it's important to tackle both the foods on our plates and the way we live. So let's expand Paleo principles beyond diet by homing in on the most important lifestyle factors. We can do so by 1) identifying those problematic behaviors that increase mortality and disease risk, 2) knowing the health-promoting behaviors of the healthiest, longest-lived peoples in the world, and 3) integrating our understanding of the biological mechanisms at play.

LEADING RISKS FOR MORTALITY

WHO has delved deep into the scientific research to identify the comparative impact of twenty-four risk factors, each of which must meet three criteria: 1) the risk must be something that occurs across the globe; 2) there must be data available to estimate how many people are affected by it; and 3) there must be a known way to reduce the risk. Understanding the role of these risk factors is important for developing clear and effective strategies for public health.

As identified by the WHO analysis, the leading risks for mortality in Western countries along with the percentage of total deaths attributable to each risk factor are:

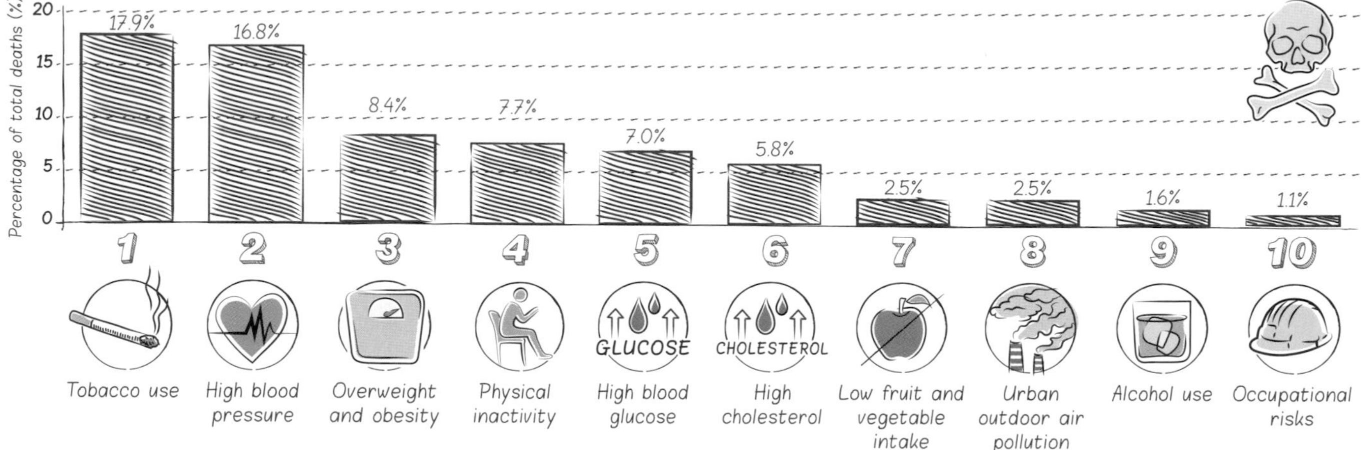

There are, of course, links between many of these health risks. For example, being physically inactive increases your chances of having high blood glucose and being overweight, and smoking increases your risk of having high blood pressure. And many of the same socioeconomic factors, environmental and community conditions, and individual behaviors underlie multiple risk factors. For example, routinely not getting enough sleep increases risk of addiction—including alcohol, illicit drug, and tobacco—as well as risk of high blood glucose and being overweight or obese. Poverty increases risk of tobacco use and eating too few vegetables and fruits. Men are twice as likely to suffer addiction as women and are much more likely to be subject to occupational health risks; but women are more likely to suffer from key nutritional deficiencies, including 80 percent of the deaths globally from iron deficiency. There's good news here, though, because the relationship between risk factors as well as the underlying causes of risk factors indicates that there are many ways to intervene and establish healthier behaviors.

The majority of the deaths attributable to these risk factors are deaths from chronic diseases, such as cardiovascular disease, diabetes, and cancers. They are considered preventable deaths because in the vast majority of cases, these diseases are tied to diet and lifestyle. Millions of preventable deaths could be averted by decreasing risk factors through educating and motivating people to make better diet and lifestyle choices. And we have real-world evidence for this fact: The reduction in tobacco use in the U.S. since 1964 is responsible for 30 percent of the increased life expectancy that has occurred since then. We can expect that further reduction in health risks will not only extend life expectancy further but also improve quality of life through lower incidence of chronic diseases. Let's take a closer look at each of these top-ten risk factors and their links to disease, diet, and lifestyle.

Tobacco use: Discussed in detail in the previous chapter, smoking increases the risk of lung and other cancers, heart disease, stroke, and chronic respiratory disease. Smoking can also harm others: 600,000 deaths globally each year are attributed to second-hand smoke.

High blood pressure: High blood pressure increases risk of stroke, heart disease, and kidney failure. High sodium intake (and not enough potassium; see page 198), alcohol consumption, lack of exercise, and obesity raise blood pressure, with the effects increasing with age.

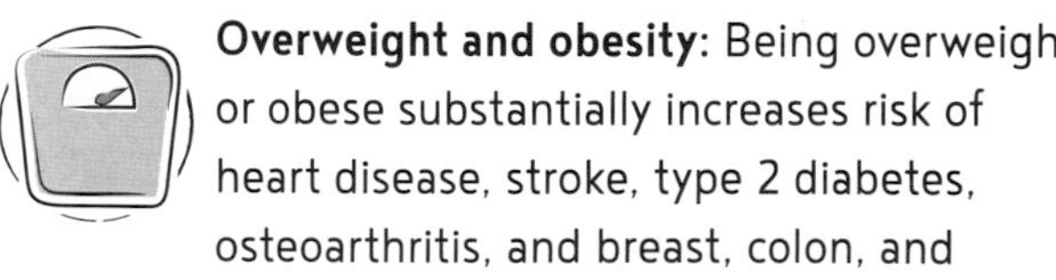

Overweight and obesity: Being overweight or obese substantially increases risk of heart disease, stroke, type 2 diabetes, osteoarthritis, and breast, colon, and prostate cancers. Risk steadily increases the higher your body mass index (BMI). See page 400.

KNOWLEDGE BOMB

Globally, overweight and obesity are responsible for 44 percent of diabetes, 23 percent of ischemic heart disease, and 7 to 41 percent of specific cancers. Physical inactivity is estimated to cause around 21 to 25 percent of breast and colon cancer burden, 27 percent of diabetes, and about 30 percent of ischemic heart disease burden.

Physical inactivity: Being active reduces risk of cardiovascular disease, some cancers, and type 2 diabetes while improving musculoskeletal health, helping to maintain a healthy body weight, and reducing symptoms of depression. See Chapter 28.

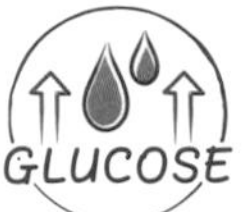

High blood glucose: Raised blood glucose increases risk of diabetes, heart disease, and stroke. Diet, stress, sleep, and activity all affect blood glucose levels and insulin sensitivity. See Chapter 4.

High cholesterol: Research shows that levels of low-density lipoproteins (LDL) and high-density lipoproteins (HDL) are more important for health than total cholesterol. Nevertheless, high total cholesterol increases the risks of heart disease, stroke, and other vascular diseases. See page 186.

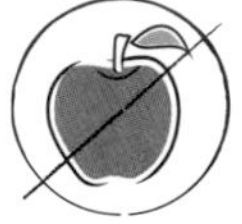

Low fruit and vegetable intake: Discussed in detail in Chapter 8, insufficient intake of fruit and vegetables increases risk of cancers, diabetes, and cardiovascular disease.

Urban outdoor air pollution: Of all the pollutants emitted from industry and vehicles, fine particulate matter, which mostly comes from fuel combustion, has the worst impact on human health. Fine particulate matter increases risk of a range of acute and chronic illnesses, including lung cancer and cardiopulmonary disease.

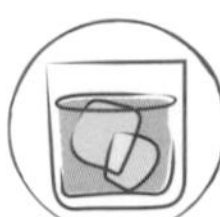

Alcohol use: Discussed in detail in Chapter 24, alcohol contributes to more than sixty types of disease and injury, including alcoholism, motor vehicle accidents, homicides, esophageal cancer, liver cancer, epilepsy, and liver cirrhosis.

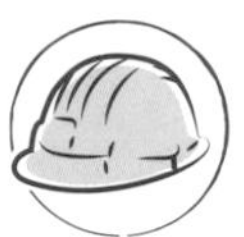

Occupational risks: People face numerous hazards at work, which may result in injuries, cancer, hearing loss, and respiratory, musculoskeletal, cardiovascular, reproductive, neurological, skin, and mental disorders. In addition, there is increasing evidence from industrialized countries to link coronary heart disease and depression with work-related stress.

Fortunately, adopting Paleo principles reduces nearly all of these health risks. (It doesn't help with urban air pollution or occupational risks, unfortunately.) Of course, limiting alcohol and eliminating tobacco use are also part of the Paleo framework, as is living an active lifestyle. But in addition, studies have shown that the Paleo diet beats out the American Heart Association dietary guidelines in reducing LDL ("bad") cholesterol and total cholesterol (as well as triglycerides). Paleo also beats out the American Diabetes Association dietary guidelines in terms of blood glucose control and insulin sensitivity. There are also several studies proving that the Paleo diet decreases blood pressure and promotes weight loss. And while there's no scientific study yet that proves you'll live a longer, healthier life when you adopt Paleo principles, the higher likelihood of doing so is implied by the reduction of eight of the top ten leading risk factors for mortality.

LIFESTYLE FACTORS THAT DECREASE DISEASE RISK

I want to flip this discussion around and consider behaviors that are associated with longevity and low rates of chronic disease. "Blue Zones" (including Sardinia, Italy; Okinawa, Japan; Loma Linda, California; Nicoya Peninsula, Costa Rica; and Icaria, Greece) are regions with a high rate of centenarians, low rate of chronic disease, and whose peoples enjoy many more healthy years of life than typical in other Western countries. Analyses of how these people eat and live have revealed some striking patterns. In terms of diet, they: consume moderate calories (they don't overeat) from whole, unprocessed foods; consume a lot of vegetables and fruit (so much so that they're labeled as semi-vegetarians); and consume only moderate amounts of alcohol, mostly wine. In terms of lifestyle, they: engage in moderate, regular physical activity; have low chronic stress; have a highly engaged social life including family life and spirituality; and have a life purpose.

THREE WAYS TO REGULATE INSULIN THAT HAVE NOTHING TO DO WITH DIET

To reduce the third-highest risk factor for mortality in Western countries, blood sugar regulation must be a major feature of any healthy diet. But blood glucose responses are impacted by more than just the quality and quantity of carbohydrates that we consume. In fact, there's emerging evidence that lifestyle factors may be equally important as, or perhaps even more important than, dietary choices when it comes to insulin sensitivity.

1. EXERCISE

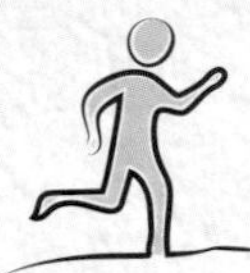

Exercise helps improve insulin sensitivity through a direct action on the glucose transport molecules (GLUT-4 receptors) in the individual cells of our muscles. On the flip side, sedentary behavior itself can induce insulin resistance. A series of studies performed in healthy adults, in overweight and obese adults, and in athletes have shown that even a relatively short period of inactivity (for example, 3 days of bed rest due to injury, illness, or volunteering for a clinical trial) induces insulin resistance. And, it's a pretty major effect: one study of healthy adults showed a 67 percent increase in insulin secretion following a glucose challenge test (meaning two-thirds more insulin was needed to regulate blood glucose levels) following 5 days of bed rest. And this inactivity-induced insulin resistance is paired with dyslipidemia, increased blood pressure, and impaired microvascular function—no wonder being inactive so dramatically increases risk of diabetes, obesity, and cardiovascular disease.

So, while exercise itself improves insulin sensitivity, we still need to avoid prolonged periods of inactivity, like sitting at a desk job. Fortunately, even short activity breaks regularly spaced throughout sedentary periods can dramatically improve glucose metabolism. One study of overweight and obese adults showed that a 2-minute movement break every 20 minutes of sitting time lowered post-meal glucose and insulin levels substantially. See Chapter 28 for more on movement and activity.

2. STRESS

Chronic stress causes insulin resistance, mediated directly via the actions of cortisol and indirectly via increased inflammation that is also a feature of chronic stress. In fact, many researchers have proposed that chronic stress may be a dominant contributor to the pathogenesis of metabolic syndrome, that nasty combination of obesity, insulin resistance and/or type 2 diabetes, dyslipidemia, and hypertension.

Epidemiological studies linking chronic stress with insulin resistance are now supported by mechanistic studies showing that chronically elevated cortisol is diabetogenic (meaning it can cause diabetes). Cortisol suppresses insulin secretion from pancreatic beta cells, impairs insulin-mediated glucose uptake in cells throughout the body (by inhibiting GLUT-4 translocation into the cell membrane), and by disruption of insulin signaling in muscle tissue. In addition, a growing list of inflammatory cytokines, such as TNF-α, which is induced by chronic stress, are known to cause insulin resistance.

Recent evidence shows that even acute stress causes hyperglycemia and insulin resistance. Liver insulin signaling is impaired following acute stress independent of cortisol. Plus, cortisol acutely suppresses insulin secretion by the pancreas as well as increasing glucose output by the liver. Mitigating stress and improving resilience to stress is a primary target for blood sugar regulation. See Chapter 27 for more on stress and resilience.

3. SLEEP

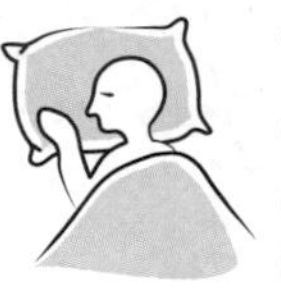

The health detriments of inadequate sleep are pervasive (see Chapter 26), affecting every system in the human body and increasing risk of nearly every chronic disease, including type 2 diabetes and insulin resistance. In fact, sleeping less than 6 hours per night (like an estimated 40 percent of Americans do) increases the risk of type 2 diabetes by 50 percent. And if we pool diabetes and impaired glucose tolerance together, that risk soars to a whopping 240 percent!

In fact, a variety of studies evaluating the effects of partial sleep (sleeping 4 to 5 hours per night, rather than the recommended 8 hours) demonstrate that inadequate sleep causes insulin resistance in healthy people. And while most studies show insulin sensitivity decreasing by 15 to 30 percent after 4 or 5 nights of partial sleep, one study showed that even a single night of partial sleep causes insulin resistance in healthy people (a 25 percent decrease in insulin sensitivity!). Sleep restriction also increases the measurable free fatty acids in the blood, a contributor to insulin resistance that plays a central role in the development of metabolic diseases. Getting 4½ hours of sleep per night compared to spending 8½ hours in bed increased serum free fatty acids in healthy men by 15 to 30 percent!

Even a modest sleep debt, getting a mere 30 minutes less per night than you need on weeknights, can have a big impact on insulin sensitivity. In a study of newly diagnosed type 2 diabetics, for every 30 minutes of weekday sleep debt, the risk of obesity 1 year later was 17 percent higher, and the risk of insulin resistance was 39 percent higher.

We see similar themes when we consider modern hunter-gatherers who also have very low rates of chronic disease and have a similar life expectancy to most Western countries despite lack of emergency medicine (once you account for high infant mortality rates). In terms of diet, hunter-gatherers tend to consume a high variety of vegetables and fruits along with moderate quantities of high-quality animal foods, while consuming moderate calories. In terms of lifestyle, hunter-gatherers engage in moderate, regular physical activity; have low chronic stress, live in sync with the sun and consistently get adequate sleep; and have strong social connections with family and tribe.

Scientific studies into the biological mechanisms of lifestyle factors further emphasize the importance to our long-term health of regular sleep, low chronic stress, living an active lifestyle, spending time outside and in nature, and nurturing strong social bonds. Of course, lifestyle factors that support health tend not to be controversial—everyone can agree that living an active lifestyle is beneficial—which is why a much larger proportion of this book is focused on diet. It's important to communicate the importance of lifestyle factors in addition to a healthy diet by way of motivation. Even though these small lifestyle changes may seem easy, we often put them off (and off, and off) because we don't realize the big impact they can have. So, when you dive into the detailed nutritional sciences in Parts 2 to 4, don't forget about the lifestyle factors discussed in Part 5. If you aren't seeing the improvement you're hoping for after making changes to your diet, chances are one of these lifestyle areas needs some work.

Sleep

Studies show that adults need 7 to 9 hours of sleep every single night. Getting enough sleep reduces the effects of stress on our bodies and has a tremendous positive impact on our hormones, metabolism, and insulin sensitivity. On the other hand, shortchanging our sleep by even a small amount, even a few times a week, can have terrible consequences on our health. The regulatory arm of our immune systems works primarily while we're sleeping, so just plain not getting enough sleep causes inflammation. Sleep is intricately tied to how our bodies respond to stress as well as insulin regulation—in fact, studies show that a single night of lost sleep may harm our insulin sensitivity as much as 6 months of bad diet does.

The importance of consistent adequate sleep cannot be underestimated. And while seven hours may seem like a doable minimum, if you're battling a chronic illness, chances are your body needs more than that.

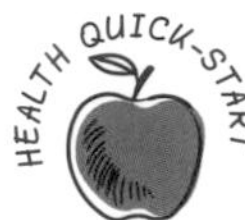

Set an alarm for yourself to signal that it's time to start winding down and preparing for sleep. After your alarm goes off, turn the lights down, turn off the TV and computer, put phones and tablets away, get into your jammies, and engage in quiet and peaceful activities. Aim to turn off your light and go to sleep at the same time every night.

The single best thing you can do to prioritize sleep is to have a regular bedtime—a bedtime that is early enough that you can get at least 8 hours of sleep (or more, if 8 hours isn't enough for you to wake up feeling refreshed and energized). Having a bedtime is such a simple thing, but it's one of the hardest things for adults to implement. Everything seems to be more important than sleep: going out with coworkers after work, watching that amazing new television show, checking social media, doing the laundry. But sleep must come first, not just in the initial healing phase of our health journeys but *for the rest of our lives.*

What else can we do to ensure that we get good sleep? Spend some time outside during the day and keep your indoor lighting dim in the evening—this helps maximize the production of melatonin, the hormone that regulates sleep, in the evening. Sleep in a cool, dark, quiet room. And avoid anything stimulating (such as work, exhaustive exercise, arguments, and emotionally intense, scary, or suspenseful TV shows and movies) in the last 2 hours before bed. It can also be helpful to avoid evening snacking. Chapter 26 dives into way more detail and offers sleep-supporting strategies.

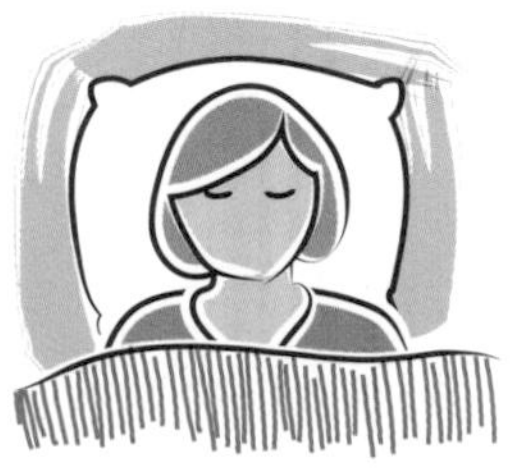

Stress Management

Stress has a direct impact on immune system function, nervous system health, and—via the gut-brain axis (see page 96)—gut health. Being under chronic stress (the kind that most of us struggle with) both increases inflammation and undermines the regulatory functions of the immune system. Chronic stress can inhibit digestion, encouraging the development of gut dysbiosis and leaky gut. And chronic stress can impact our endocrine system via effects on central nervous system function, blunting thyroid function and sex hormone production, and causing insulin resistance. Stress is a major contributor to chronic illness, and when stress is out of control, it worsens the prognosis. When it comes to stress management, there are two factors: stress reduction and resilience.

HEALTH QUICK-START *Getting enough sleep is probably the single most important thing you can do to improve your resilience to stress. You'll know you're getting enough when you wake up without an alarm and feel refreshed and ready for the day! (Of course, you can still set an alarm as a backup.)*

Reducing stress means removing things from our lives that are causing stress. Even if individual responsibilities aren't causing undue stress on their own, the sheer number of them on our plates may be creating stress. Whenever you can, say no, or ask for help to reduce stress. There are as many ways to reduce stress as there are stressed people—it's up to you to figure out what works for you. Take a critical look at everything you do and how it impacts your stress level, and determine where you can make small changes (or big ones!) to reduce stress.

Resilience refers to how the body responds to stressors. This is different from reducing stress—it's about implementing strategies so that the stressful aspects of your life just don't get to you as much. Activities that improve resilience include getting enough sleep, being physically active, meditating, forming social bonds, connecting with nature, laughing, and playing. Making time for these things can have a direct impact on both your health and your sense of well-being.

Chapter 27 discusses in detail the health impact of stress and suggests strategies for mitigating it.

Activity

We all know that we're supposed to exercise, but what is much less well known is that gentle movement throughout the day and daily weight-bearing exercise (like walking) has a bigger impact on overall health than a sweaty session at the gym five times per week. Yes, building muscle has all kinds of health benefits, and including some exercise sessions during the week is awesome, but when it comes to the immune system, it's more important to simply avoid being sedentary. That means not sitting all day!

KNOWLEDGE BOMB *When it comes to exercise, more isn't necessarily better. Exhaustive, strenuous, and overly intense exercise can actually undermine health by harming the immune system, gut health, and hormone health; see page 360.*

There are lots of ways to add movement to your day, but the simplest strategy is to set a timer to go off every 20 minutes during the part of the day when you typically sit (at work and in front of the television, for most of us). Whenever the timer goes off, get up and move around for 2 minutes. You can walk around, jump rope, do some push-ups, stand and stretch, or do some yoga poses—whatever works for you. Yes, studies show that just 2 minutes of movement for every 20 minutes of sitting is all it takes. Of course, you can ramp this up with a treadmill desk or bicycle desk if you have access to those sorts of things.

There are tremendous health advantages to one of the simplest and most accessible activities out there: walking. Walking helps build muscle, improves cardiovascular health, strengthens bones, helps improve resilience to stress, improves brain health (everything from mood to memory to cognition) and reduces the risk of problems like dementia, improves hormone health, and can even help us sleep better! If all you do is make time for a 30-minute walk every day (in addition to moving every 20 minutes throughout the day), you are doing great.

More-intense activity is awesome, too. If you love to lift weights, participate in a sport, or get your groove on at the gym, those activities are all worthwhile. It's important to emphasize, though, that even the hardest workout can't make up for damage that sitting all day does to your health. Even if you sweat up a storm for a couple of hours each day, moving around every 20 minutes the rest of the day is still essential for optimal health. The importance of activity, as well as why intense and strenuous exercise isn't a good choice, is discussed in detail in Chapter 28.

Nature and Sunlight

Exposure to nature and sunlight has been an integral part of human life since the very beginning of our existence. Only relatively recently have we transitioned to indoor lifestyles where we can go days—even weeks—without spending substantial time in the fresh air and sun.

HEALTH QUICK-START

Aim to spend 30 minutes to an hour (or more!) outside every day. We get the most benefits from being outside between late morning and early afternoon, when the sun is at its brightest. Get extra bang for your buck by going for a walk outside, which combines a resilience activity with a weight-bearing exercise.

Ample evidence exists that time outdoors has positive effects on the body and brain, whether we're strolling through the woods, walking barefoot in the backyard, or simply stopping to hear the sounds of nature (discussed in more detail in Chapter 29).

A major benefit of being outside is sun exposure. When exposed to ultraviolet light, our bodies produce vitamin D, which plays a critical role in health (vitamin D controls the expression of more than 200 genes and the proteins regulated by those genes; see page 369). The functions of vitamin D in our bodies include mineral metabolism, immunity, regulation of inflammation, cell growth, and biorhythm activation. In addition, cells throughout the body, including the skin and eyes, directly affect the pituitary gland and hypothalamus region of the brain when stimulated by blue light from the sun. As a result, sun exposure (and exposure to daylight in general) is vital for regulating our circadian rhythm (discussed in greater depth in Chapter 26).

Connection

An often-underrated lifestyle factor that directly impacts our health is community. Connecting with others, whether a spouse, child, friend, family member, or pet, helps regulate hormones and neurotransmitters that directly impact inflammation (discussed in more detail in Chapter 30). Plus, social bonding improves resilience to stress and generally improves mood, which makes every other change you're working on seem a bit easier.

There's a practical aspect to connection as well. When we have people in our lives whom we can depend on, we have resources to help us reduce stress and put other priorities, like getting enough physical activity and sleep, at the top of our to-do lists. And having a companion while we tackle the job of healing, whether it's a walking buddy, a friend to meet up with at the farmers market, someone to watch the kids while we exercise, or a family member to batch cook with on weekends, can make all the difference.

For some people, making community a priority requires effort and dedication. It can be easy to let social media sites provide us with the illusion of connection without having real, meaningful interactions with friends and family. It also can be easy to let every other item on our to-do lists supplant quality time with the people we care about. If you're struggling to find time for connection, think about how you might combine social interaction with other activities, like exercising, shopping, and even cooking.

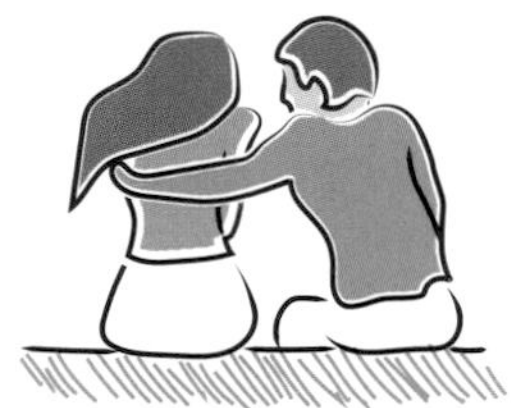

Chapter 7:
THE RESEARCH

Although we'll be zooming in on the details of the Paleo diet (and Paleo lifestyle tenets) to see how individual food components affect our health, let's start with the big picture: how do human beings fare when placed on Paleo-style diets?

A growing number of scientific papers have been published on the topic of Paleolithic nutrition, especially the potential for a Paleo-style diet to reduce risk factors for chronic disease and improve multiple areas of human health. Many of these papers are based on anthropological evidence, animal studies, or observational studies of populations. But while those forms of research provide great insight and invariably form the foundations of health described in this book, they can't definitively demonstrate that people become healthier by following Paleo principles.

That's where human trials come to the rescue! More and more human trials of the Paleo diet are being conducted each year, with ubiquitously positive results demonstrating wide-ranging benefits: improvements in blood lipids, body composition, glycemic control, satiation, insulin sensitivity, and various risk factors for chronic disease and obesity (among other things). Since there is no single "Paleo diet" (just a template of whole foods with a great deal of flexibility), some of these trials use interpretations of Paleo that differ slightly from the principles outlined in this book. For instance, some Paleo trials eliminate all added salt, while—as you'll see in Chapter 14—sea salt actually has a great deal of science-based value and is therefore espoused in this book. However, the core elements of these trials are generally very similar (no grains, legumes, refined sugar, or processed vegetable oils, and an abundance of vegetables, fruit, nuts, seeds, seafood, poultry, eggs, and other meats), so their results can be considered representative of whole-food Paleo diets in general.

Let's take a look at what the peer-reviewed scientific literature has to say about the effects of consuming Paleo-style diets in human beings, as of the printing of this book. For a summary of each study, see pages 129 to 133. Grouping studies by the particular health outcomes evaluated, we see some pretty impressive results!

Weight loss. Studies show that the Paleo diet is effective for healthy weight loss with concurrent reductions in total fat mass, liver fat, belly fat, BMI, waist circumference, and hip-to-waist ratio. And this success occurs with study participants eating as much as they want! In fact, Paleo beats out government dietary guidelines, weight control diets, and diabetes diets in terms of weight loss. Studies also go a long way to explaining why: the Paleo diet provides higher satiety per energy per meal, meaning that we feel fuller after consuming fewer calories. One study in men showed that participants reduced their caloric intake by about 400 calories per day without trying, and another study in postmenopausal women showed that participants reduced their caloric intake by 25 percent, also without trying! Multiple studies show that the Paleo diet reduces leptin levels (see page 90), which might explain why Paleo meals are so filling. Leptin reductions from Paleo are greater than those from following a Mediterranean diet.

Diabetes. Studies show that the Paleo diet is effective at improving type 2 diabetes. Multiple studies have shown that Paleo improves glucose tolerance on oral challenge, fasting blood sugar, insulin sensitivity, HbA1c (a measurement of average blood sugar levels over the last 3 months), C-peptide (a marker of insulin secretion), and HOMA indices (measures of insulin resistance and beta cell function). In fact, the Paleo diet outperforms the American Diabetes Association diet in terms of controlling glucose and restoring insulin sensitivity.

Cardiovascular disease. Studies show that the Paleo diet is effective at reducing cardiovascular disease risk factors, even in high-risk populations. Multiple studies have demonstrated that following a Paleo diet reduces systolic blood pressure, diastolic blood pressure, total cholesterol, LDL cholesterol, triglycerides, apolipoprotein B (a component of LDL and VLDL), apolipoprotein A1 (a component of HDL), plasminogen activator inhibitor-1 (PAI-1, related to intravascular clotting and linked to increased risk of diabetes and cardiovascular disease), BMI, waist circumference, and waist-to-hip ratio, as well as boosting HDL ("good") cholesterol and improving arterial distensibility (a measure of artery wall elasticity; low distensibility is a risk factor for cardiovascular disease). In fact, studies show that the Paleo diet beats out the American Heart Association dietary guidelines in terms of reductions in total cholesterol, LDL, and triglycerides and increases in HDL. Paleo reduces cardiovascular disease risk by 22 percent, comparable to the Mediterranean diet.

Cancer. One study that compared the Paleo diet to the Mediterranean diet in terms of cancer risk showed comparable reductions in all-cancer risk (Paleo reduced the risk of developing any cancer by 28 percent). Another study showed that the Paleo diet reduced risk of colorectal adenomas slightly more than the Mediterranean diet (Paleo reduced the risk by 29 percent, whereas the Mediterranean diet reduced the risk by 26 percent).

Inflammation. Multiple studies have shown that Paleo reduces C-reactive protein, a marker of inflammation easily measured by blood test. In fact, even over a 2-year span, Paleo is more effective at reducing C-reactive protein than the Mediterranean diet, although both Paleo and the Mediterranean diet reduce inflammation and oxidative stress.

Multiple sclerosis. Studies using the Paleo diet in conjunction with other therapies (including stretching, strengthening exercise, meditation, massage, and electrical stimulation) saw improvement in symptoms of both secondary progressing multiple sclerosis and relapsing remitting multiple sclerosis. Study participants experienced improvements in perceived fatigue, anxiety, depression, and cognitive function.

Inflammatory bowel disease. A recent study placed patients with active IBD on the Paleo autoimmune protocol (see page 412). Impressively, 73 percent of those patients were in full clinical remission after only 6 weeks.

Overall health and long-term safety. All-cause mortality is a measure of overall health and longevity. One large study showed that following a Paleo diet reduced all-cause mortality by 23 percent, comparable to the Mediterranean diet. Every single study of the Paleo diet has shown benefits to health markers. And studies of the Paleo diet have followed participants for as long as two years, with zero adverse events reported. Two years is considered ample time for any potential downsides to Paleo to turn up. At this point, there are none!

For scientific studies, the Paleo diet is typically defined as including lean meats, seafood, eggs, fruit, vegetables (including root vegetables), nuts, seeds, avocados, olive oil, coconut oil, and almond milk in place of cow's milk, plus complete avoidance of grains, legumes, and dairy. But there is variation from study to study, so it can be tricky to extrapolate the results of a particular study to different interpretations of Paleo eating. In fact, many of the studies performed so far have features that aren't embraced by mainstream Paleo (such as consuming canola [rapeseed] oil—even in small amounts—avoiding salt, and choosing only lean meats). However, while smaller details may differ among various interpretations of Paleo, the core elements are what really matter: micronutrient density, relatively balanced macronutrients, and a mixture of plant and animal foods. In that sense, the results of these studies can be expected to hold true for the Paleo framework at large.

For those of us who've experienced amazing healing, weight loss, and overall well-being from eating Paleo, the results of clinical trials might not seem that important. After all, we already know it works for us! But to the rest of the world (and because it's always a good idea to gain deeper understanding of how nutrition affects our bodies), clinical studies are important for helping Paleo gain legitimacy in the scientific community . . . and therefore reaching (and benefitting) even more people.

Even though we have *tons* of evidence that individual components of the Paleo diet are extremely health-promoting (like eating omega-3 fats from seafood, consuming high-quality protein, loading up on phytochemical-rich vegetables and fruits, getting plenty of fiber, and avoiding heavily processed foods low in nutrients), misleading news reports frequently claim that the Paleo diet is harmful and may even raise our risk of certain diseases or obesity. As a science-based diet, we should expect Paleo to make sense on both a mechanistic level and in terms of real-world evidence; it does!

SUMMARIES OF THE STUDIES

B. Bisht, W. G. Darling, R. E. Grossman, E. T. Shivapour, S. K. Lutgendorf, L. G. Snetselaar, M. J. Hall, M. B. Zimmerman, and T. L. Wahls. "A Multimodal Intervention for Patients with Secondary Progressive Multiple Sclerosis: Feasibility and Effect on Fatigue." *Journal of Alternative and Complement Medicine* 20, no. 5 (2014): 347-55. doi: 10.1089/acm.2013.0188.

This pilot study was the first of its kind to test how multiple sclerosis patients would respond to a modified Paleo diet (green leafy vegetables, sulfur-containing vegetables, intensely colored fruits and vegetables, plant and animal protein, seaweed, and nondairy milks) in combination with supplements, stretching, strengthening exercise, meditation, massage, and electrical stimulation. The six patients who were able to complete the 12-month study with full adherence saw a significant improvement in fatigue. (Their average Fatigue Severity Scale score dropped from 5.7 to 3.32 at the end of the year.) Given the small sample size and the multiple nondietary components of the study, the researchers concluded that further evaluation in the form of additional, larger studies is warranted.

H. F. Bligh, I. F. Godsland, G. Frost, K. J. Hunter, P. Murray, K. MacAulay, D. Hyliands, et al. "Plant-Rich Mixed Meals Based on Palaeolithic Diet Principles Have a Dramatic Impact on Incretin, Peptide YY and Satiety Response, but Show Little Effect on Glucose and Insulin Homeostasis: An Acute-Effects Randomised Study." *British Journal of Nutrition* 113, no. 4 (2015): 574-84. doi: 10.1017/S0007114514004012.

Researchers tested the immediate effects of Paleo foods by designing two Paleo-style meals based on fish and a variety of plants (selected because they were high in fiber and phytonutrients). Study participants were given the two Paleo meals as well as a third based on WHO guidelines, matched with one of the Paleo meals for total energy, protein, fat, and carbohydrate content, following a randomized crossover trial design (where participants eat each meal at separate times and are randomly assigned the order in which they go through the three meals). Compared to the WHO meal, both Paleo meals significantly increased satiety hormones glucagon-like peptide-1 (GLP-1) and peptide YY (PYY) over a period of 3 hours while significantly decreasing glucose-dependent insulinotropic peptide (GIP), a hormone that regulates digestion and stimulates insulin secretion. Both Paleo meals resulted in greater satiety scores. The changes in these gut hormones and satiety reports suggest that meals based on Paleo principles can have beneficial effects on appetite and may reduce the risk of obesity.

C. Blomquist, M. Alvehus, J. Burén, M. Ryberg, C. Larsson, B. Lindahl, C. Mellberg, I. Söderström, E. Chorell, and T. Olsson. "Attenuated Low-Grade Inflammation Following Long-Term Dietary Intervention in Postmenopausal Women with Obesity." *Obesity* (Silver Spring) 25, no. 5 (2017): 892–900. doi: 10.1002/oby.21815.

In this 24-month study, researchers assigned seventy obese postmenopausal women to either a prudent control diet (a higher intake of fruits, vegetables, legumes, whole grains, poultry, and fish, aiming for 15 percent of calories from protein, 30 percent from fat, and 55 percent from carbohydrates) or a Paleo-style diet (consisting of lean meat, fish, eggs, vegetables, berries and other fruits, avocados, nuts, and oils, aiming for 30 percent of calories from protein, 40 percent from fat, and 30 percent from carbohydrates). On both diets, participants were allowed to eat as much as they wanted. The Paleo group saw a significantly higher decrease in android fat (fat deposits in the abdomen and upper body, which lead to the characteristic "apple" shape that increases risk of cardiovascular disease and diabetes) and high-sensitivity C-reactive protein (a marker of inflammation).

I. Boers, F. A. Muskiet, E. Berkelaar, E. Schut, R. Penders, K. Hoenderdos, H. J. Wichers, M. C. Jong. "Favourable Effects of Consuming a Palaeolithic-Type Diet on Characteristics of the Metabolic Syndrome: A Randomized Controlled Pilot-Study." *Lipids in Health and Disease* 13 (2014): 160. doi: 10.1186/1476-511X-13-160.

In this study, thirty-two people with at least two criteria for metabolic syndrome spent 2 weeks on either a Paleo-style diet or an isoenergetic (equal-calorie) reference diet based on the guidelines of the Dutch Health Council. By the end of the study, the Paleo group saw notable improvements in cardiovascular disease risk factors, including lower systolic blood pressure, diastolic blood pressure, total cholesterol, and triglycerides, as well as higher HDL ("good" cholesterol) levels.

M. Fontes-Villalba, S. Lindeberg, Y. Granfeldt, F. K. Knop, A. A. Memon, P. Carrera-Bastos, Ó. Picazo, et al. "Palaeolithic Diet Decreases Fasting Plasma Leptin Concentrations More Than a Diabetes Diet in Patients with Type 2 Diabetes: A Randomised Cross-Over Trial." *Cardiovascular Diabetology* 15 (2016): 80. doi: 10.1186/s12933-016-0398-1.

These authors previously reported on a randomized crossover trial comparing a Paleo diet with a standard diabetes diet in diabetics (with thirteen patients enrolled and 3 months spent in each diet period). In this paper, the researchers reported on fasting plasma concentrations of glucagon (see page 89), insulin (see page 86), incretins (digestive hormones that regulate insulin secretion), ghrelin (see page 90), C-peptide (a marker of insulin secretion), and adipokines (signaling molecules released by fat cells) from the same study. The results showed that the Paleo diet was more successful than the diabetes diet at lowering plasma leptin levels, although there were no statistically significant differences in the other variables measured.

L. A. Frassetto, M. Schloetter, M. Mietus-Synder, R. C. Morris Jr., and A. Sebastian. "Metabolic and Physiologic Improvements from Consuming a Paleolithic, Hunter-Gatherer Type Diet." *European Journal of Clinical Nutrition* 63, no. 8 (2009): 947–55. doi: 10.1038/ejcn.2009.4.

In this metabolically controlled study, nine healthy, non-obese, sedentary volunteers spent 10 days consuming a Paleo diet consisting of lean meat, fruits, vegetables, and nuts. Compared with the participants' baseline diets, the Paleo diet resulted in significant improvements in arterial distensibility (a measure of artery wall elasticity; low distensibility is a risk factor for cardiovascular disease), insulin sensitivity and glucose tolerance, total cholesterol, LDL, and triglycerides. Although the trial was short-term, the researchers noted that the diet caused nearly consistent improvements in the status of circulatory, carbohydrate, and lipid metabolism and physiology.

A. Genoni, P. Lyons-Wall, J. Lo, and A. Devine. "Cardiovascular, Metabolic Effects and Dietary Composition of Ad-Libitum Paleolithic vs. Australian Guide to Healthy Eating Diets: A 4-Week Randomised Trial." *Nutrients* 8, no. 5 (2016): 314. doi: 10.3390/nu8050314.

Researchers randomly assigned thirty-nine healthy women to either the Australian Guide to Healthy Eating diet (whole grains, fruit, vegetables, low-fat dairy, and reduced quantities of high-sugar products and refined grains) or a Paleo diet (lean meats, fish, eggs, nuts, fruit, vegetables, olive oil, coconut oil, and almond milk in place of cow's milk; no grains, legumes, or dairy). By the end of the 4-week trial, the Paleo group had lost significantly more weight and saw a greater decrease in waist circumference.

T. Jönsson, Y. Granfeldt, C. Erlanson-Albertsson, B. Ahrén, and S. Lindeberg. "A Paleolithic Diet Is More Satiating Per Calorie Than a Mediterranean-Like Diet in Individuals with Ischemic Heart Disease." *Nutrition & Metabolism* 7 (2010): 85. doi: 10.1186/1743-7075-7-85.

In this 12-week study, twenty-nine male patients with ischemic heart disease, impaired glucose tolerance, or type 2 diabetes and a waist circumference greater than 94 centimeters were given either a Paleo diet (lean meat, fish, fruit, vegetables, root vegetables, eggs, and nuts) or a Mediterranean-style diet (whole grains, low-fat dairy products, vegetables, fruit, fish, and oils and margarines). On both diets, participants were allowed to eat as much as they wanted. The Paleo group reported being equally satiated, but while consuming fewer calories than the Mediterranean group (indicating the Paleo diet was more satiating per calorie). Leptin levels also decreased more dramatically in the Paleo group than in the Mediterranean group (by 31 percent versus 18 percent).

T. Jönsson, Y. Granfeldt, B. Ahrén, U. C. Branell, G. Pålsson, A. Hasson, M Söderström, and S. Lindeberg. "Beneficial Effects of a Paleolithic Diet on Cardiovascular Risk Factors in Type 2 Diabetes: A Randomized Cross-Over Pilot Study." ***Cardiovascular Diabetology*** **8 (2009): 35. doi: 10.1186/1475-2840-8-35.**

Thirteen patients with type 2 diabetes consumed a standard diabetes diet (whole grains, vegetables, fruits, berries, and lower total fat) and a Paleo diet (lean meat, fish, fruit, vegetables, eggs, and nuts) in a randomized crossover design, spending 3 months in each diet period. The Paleo diet resulted in larger drops in HbA1c (a measurement of average blood sugar levels over the last 3 months), triglycerides, diastolic blood pressure, weight, BMI, and waist circumference and boosted HDL levels. Overall, the Paleo diet was more successful than the diabetes diet in terms of improving glycemic control and multiple cardiovascular risk factors.

T. Jönsson, Y. Granfeldt, S. Lindeberg, and A. C. Hallberg. "Subjective Satiety and Other Experiences of a Paleolithic Diet Compared to a Diabetes Diet in Patients with Type 2 Diabetes." ***Nutrition Journal*** **12 (2013): 105. doi: 10.1186/1475-2891-12-105.**

This is a second publication based on Jönsson et al.'s study of a Paleo diet versus a standard diabetes diet in diabetic patients. The researchers found that compared to the diabetes diet, the Paleo diet resulted in greater satiety quotients for energy per meal (meaning that Paleo was more satiating on a per-calorie basis).

G. G. Konijeti, N. Kim, J .D. Lewis, S. Groven, A. Chandrasekaran, S. Grandhe, C. Diamant, E. Singh, G. Oliveira, X. Wang, B. Molparia, A. Torkamani. "Efficacy of the Autoimmune Protocol Diet for Inflammatory Bowel Disease." ***Inflammatory Bowel Diseases*** **(2017): epub ahead of print. doi: 10.1097/MIB.0000000000001221.**

Fifteen patients with active inflammatory bowel disease were placed on the Paleo Autoimmune Protocol following a 6-week gradual transition followed by a 5-week maintenance phase. (In fact, patients were given my first book, *The Paleo Approach*, as a resource for following the protocol.) Eleven of the fifteen participants (73 percent) achieved clinical remission by week 6, and they stayed in remission throughout the 5-week maintenance phase of the study.

J. E. Lee, B. Bisht, M. J. Hall, L. M. Rubenstein, R. Louison, D. T. Klein, and T. L. Wahls. "A Multimodal, Nonpharmacologic Intervention Improves Mood and Cognitive Function in People with Multiple Sclerosis." ***Journal of the American College of Nutrition*** **36, no. 3 (2017): 150–68. doi: 10.1080/07315724.2016.1255160.**

This trial assessed how patients with multiple sclerosis responded to a 12-month intervention (consisting of a modified Paleo diet, a stretching and strengthening exercise program, neuromuscular electrical stimulation (EStim), and stress management in the form of meditation and massage). Within just a few months, patients' anxiety and depression started to improve, followed by positive changes in cognitive function. Although the intervention as a whole was beneficial, the researchers noted that adherence to the modified Paleo diet seemed to be the most important factor for improving mood and cognition.

S. Lindeberg, T. Jönsson, Y. Granfeldt, E. Borgstrand, J. Soffman, K. Sjöström, and B. Ahrén. "A Palaeolithic Diet Improves Glucose Tolerance More Than a Mediterranean-like Diet in Individuals with Ischaemic Heart Disease." ***Diabetologia*** **50, no. 9 (2007): 1795–807. doi: 10.1007/s00125-007-0716-y.**

Twenty-nine patients with ischemic heart disease and either glucose intolerance or type 2 diabetes were randomly given either an Paleo diet (lean meat, fish, fruits, vegetables, eggs, and nuts) or a Mediterranean-style diet (whole grains, low-fat dairy products, vegetables, fruit, fish, and oils and margarines) for 12 weeks. On both diets, participants were allowed to eat as much as they wanted. Over the course of the study, the Paleo group saw a 26 percent decrease in glucose tolerance (compared to a 7 percent decrease in the Mediterranean group) and a trend toward a larger decrease of insulin resistance. The change in glucose tolerance was independent of changes in waist circumference.

U. Masharani, P. Sherchan, M. Schloetter, S. Stratford, A. Xiao, A. Sebastian, M. Nolte Kennedy, and L. Frassetto. "Metabolic and Physiologic Effects from Consuming a Hunter-Gatherer (Paleolithic)-Type Diet in Type 2 Diabetes." ***European Journal of Clinical Nutrition*** **69, no. 8 (2015): 944–48. doi: 10.1038/ejcn.2015.39.**

In this study, researchers compared the effects of a Paleo diet (fourteen participants) with a diet based on the recommendations of the American Diabetes Association (ten participants). The Paleo diet included lean meat, fruits, vegetables, and nuts (while excluding salt), and the ADA diet included whole grains, legumes, low-fat dairy, and moderate levels of salt. After 14 days on the test diets, both groups saw improvements in metabolic measures, but the Paleo diet group saw greater improvements in glucose control and lipid profiles. Moreover, the most insulin-resistant participants in the Paleo group experienced a significant increase in insulin sensitivity, whereas the ADA group saw no such benefit.

C. Mellberg, S. Sandberg, M. Ryberg, M. Eriksson, S. Brage, C. Larsson, T. Olsson, and B. Lindahl. "Long-Term Effects of a Palaeolithic-Type Diet in Obese Postmenopausal Women: A 2-Year Randomized Trial." *European Journal of Clinical Nutrition* 68, no. 3 (2014): 350–57. doi: 10.1038/ejcn.2013.290.

In this study, seventy obese postmenopausal women were assigned to eat either an ad libitum Paleo diet or a diet based on the Nordic Nutrition Recommendations (NNR) for 2 years. After 6 months, body fat mass had dropped significantly in both groups, but the loss was more pronounced in the Paleo diet group (although that difference equalized by the end of the study). Waist circumference and sagittal diameter (the distance from the small of the back to the upper abdomen, which measures the amount of fat in the gut region) also decreased in both groups, but the decrease was more pronounced in the Paleo group at the 6-month mark. Likewise, triglycerides had decreased significantly more at both 6 months and 12 months in the Paleo group than in the NNR group.

K. O'Dea. "Marked Improvement in Carbohydrate and Lipid Metabolism in Diabetic Australian Aborigines after Temporary Reversion to Traditional Lifestyle." *Diabetes* 33, no. 6 (1984): 596–603.

Published in 1984, this was one of the first studies to test the effects of ancestral diets. Ten diabetic, overweight Australian Aborigines switched from a standard Australian diet to eating only what they could hunt or gather in their native environment: kangaroo, crocodile, yams, figs, honey, turtle, crawdads, beef, and other local foods. Due to the leanness of wild animals, their diets ended up being high in protein (50 to 80 percent of calories), low in fat (an average of 13 percent of calories), and low to moderate in carbohydrates (5 to 33 percent), with a low overall calorie intake (1,200 per day). The participants also ended up engaging in more physical activity due to a lifestyle switch toward hunting and gathering. By the end of the study, the participants had lost over 17 pounds on average and saw major improvements in both fasting and post-meal glucose. (Fasting levels dropped from the diabetic range to normal by the seventh week!) The subjects' triglycerides and fasting insulin levels significantly improved as well.

M. Osterdahl, T. Kocturk, A. Koochek, and P. E. Wändell. "Effects of a Short-Term Intervention with a Paleolithic Diet in Healthy Volunteers." *European Journal of Clinical Nutrition* 62, no. 5 (2008): 682–85. doi: 10.1038/sj.ejcn.1602790.

This 3-week intervention placed twenty people (fourteen of whom successfully finished the study) on a Paleo diet, which included unlimited amounts of fresh or frozen fruits, berries, and vegetables except legumes; fresh or frozen seafood with no added salt; fresh or frozen unsalted lean meats and minced meat; unsalted nuts (except peanuts); fresh-squeezed lemon or lime juice; flax seed or rapeseed oil; coffee and tea (without sugar, honey, milk, or cream); and salt-free spices. Potatoes, dried fruit, salted seafood, honey, and cured meats were allowed in moderation, and dairy foods, legumes, grains, preserved meats, canned foods (except tomatoes), and foods with refined sugar were excluded. By the end of the intervention, mean weight, BMI, waist circumference, systolic blood pressure, and plasminogen activator inhibitor-1 (PAI-1, related to intravascular clotting and linked to increased risk of diabetes and cardiovascular disease) had all decreased.

J. Otten, A. Stomby, M. Waling, A. Isaksson, A. Tellström, L. Lundin-Olsson, S. Brage, M. Ryberg, M. Svensson, and T. Olsson. "Benefits of a Paleolithic Diet with and without Supervised Exercise on Fat Mass, Insulin Sensitivity, and Glycemic Control: A Randomized Controlled Trial in Individuals with Type 2 Diabetes." *Diabetes/Metabolism Research and Reviews* 33, no. 1 (2017): 10. doi: 10.1002/dmrr.2828.

This study featured thirty-two patients with type 2 diabetes who followed a Paleo diet for 12 weeks. One group followed standard exercise recommendations, and the other did one hour of supervised aerobic exercise and resistance training, three times per week. The Paleo diet was based on lean meat, fish, seafood, eggs, vegetables, fruits, berries, and nuts, while excluding cereals, legumes, refined fats, refined sugars, salt, and dairy. Over the course of the study, the standard exercise Paleo group lost 5.7 kilograms of body fat (compared to 6.7 kilograms for the supervised exercise group), improved insulin sensitivity by 45 percent (the same as the supervised exercise group), saw a 0.9 percent reduction in HbA1c (compared to 1.1 percent for the supervised exercise group), and saw a 62 percent decrease in leptin (compared to 42 percent decrease for the supervised exercise group). The researchers concluded that the Paleo diet improved fat mass and metabolic balance even without more vigorous aerobic and strength workouts, but supervised exercise helped preserve lean mass (at least in the male participants) while also improving cardiovascular fitness.

J. Otten, C. Mellberg, M. Ryberg, S. Sandberg, J. Kullberg, B. Lindahl, C. Larsson, J. Hauksson, and T. Olsson. "Strong and Persistent Effect on Liver Fat with a Paleolithic Diet during a Two-Year Intervention." *International Journal of Obesity* 40, no. 5 (2016): 747–53. doi: 10.1038/ijo.2016.4.

In this study, researchers tested an ad libitum Paleo diet against a standard low-fat diet over the course of 2 years, documenting changes in liver fat and insulin sensitivity. Seventy healthy, obese, postmenopausal women participated. By the 6-month mark, liver fat had decreased by 64 percent in the Paleo group compared to 43 percent in the standard diet group (although after 2 years, the margin of change was much narrower: a 50 percent decrease in liver fat in the Paleo group and a 49 percent decrease in the standard diet group). Insulin sensitivity also improved in the Paleo group during the first 6 months.

R. L. Pastore, J. T. Brooks, and J. W. Carbone. "Paleolithic Nutrition Improves Plasma Lipid Concentrations of Hypercholesterolemic Adults to a Greater Extent Than Traditional Heart-Healthy Dietary Recommendations." Nutrition Research 35, no. 6 (2015): 474–79. doi: 10.1016/j.nutres.2015.05.002.

Twenty volunteers between the ages of forty-two and sixty, all with diagnosed high cholesterol levels (hypercholesterolemia), followed an American Heart Association diet for 4 months, followed by a Paleo-style diet for another 4 months. After the Paleo period (but not the American Heart Association diet period), average total cholesterol, LDL, and triglycerides dropped significantly, while HDL rose. The improvements were independent of changes in body weight.

M. Ryberg, S. Sandberg, C. Mellberg, O. Stegle, B. Lindahl, C. Larsson, J. Hauksson, and T. Olsson. "A Palaeolithic-Type Diet Causes Strong Tissue-Specific Effects on Ectopic Fat Deposition in Obese Postmenopausal Women." *Journal of Internal Medicine* 274, no. 1 (2013): 67–76. doi: 10.1111/joim.12048.

Ten healthy, nonsmoking, postmenopausal women with BMIs greater than 27 were instructed to consume an ad libitum Paleo diet with relatively balanced macronutrients (30 percent protein, 30 percent carbohydrate, and 40 percent fat, mostly monounsaturated fat). Even without restricting their food intake, the women lost an average of 10 pounds in just 5 weeks and spontaneously reduced their calorie intake by 25 percent. In addition, the participants' waist-to-hip ratio decreased, their diastolic blood pressure went down, and they saw reductions in their fasting blood sugar, total cholesterol, triglycerides, LDL cholesterol, apolipoprotein B (a component of LDL and VLDL), apolipoprotein A1 (a component of HDL), urinary C-peptide (a marker of insulin secretion), and HOMA indices (measures of insulin resistance and beta cell function). Levels of intramyocellular lipids (fats stored in muscle cells and used for energy when we move) didn't change, but the women's liver triglyceride levels fell by 49 percent.

K. A. Whalen, M. McCullough, W. D. Flanders, T. J. Hartman, S. Judd, and R. M. Bostick. "Paleolithic and Mediterranean Diet Pattern Scores and Risk of Incident, Sporadic Colorectal Adenomas." *American Journal of Epidemiology* 180, no. 11 (2014): 1088–97. doi: 10.1093/aje/kwu235.

In this case-control study involving 2,301 people, researchers analyzed participants' risk of colorectal cancer based on how closely their eating habits matched a Paleolithic diet pattern or a Mediterranean diet pattern. The researchers calculated scores for each diet pattern by assigning point values to different foods (such as vegetables, fruits, lean meats, fish, and grains and starches) and then assessing which quintile rank each participant fell into for those foods. The calculations revealed that both diet patterns appeared to reduce the risk of colorectal adenomas.

K. A. Whalen, M. L. McCullough, W. D. Flanders, T. J. Hartman, S. Judd, and R. M. Bostick. "Paleolithic and Mediterranean Diet Pattern Scores Are Inversely Associated with Biomarkers of Inflammation and Oxidative Balance in Adults." *Journal of Nutrition* 146, no. 6 (2016): 1217–26. doi: 10.3945/jn.115.224048.

This pooled, cross-sectional study examined whether adherence to a Paleolithic diet pattern and/or a Mediterranean diet pattern was related to levels of inflammation and oxidative stress. After assigning scores to the diets of 646 adults based on how closely they matched the Paleo or Mediterranean pattern, the researchers found that both diet patterns were associated with lower levels of systemic inflammation and oxidative stress.

K. A. Whalen, S. Judd, M. L. McCullough, W. D. Flanders, T. J. Hartman, and R. M. Bostick. "Paleolithic and Mediterranean Diet Pattern Scores Are Inversely Associated with All-Cause and Cause-Specific Mortality in Adults." *Journal of Nutrition* 147, no. 4 (2017): 612–20. doi: 10.3945/jn.116.241919.

Using the results of food frequency questionnaires (checklists of foods and beverages with a response section for participants to report how often they consumed each item over a specified period), researchers analyzed a cohort of 21,423 people to see how closely their diets corresponded to a Paleolithic diet pattern or Mediterranean diet pattern. Over the course of an average of 6.25 years of follow-up, participants in the highest quintile of Paleo or Mediterranean diet scores had a lower risk of all-cause mortality, death from cancer, and death from cardiovascular disease. This study shows that you don't need to follow a Paleo diet to the letter in order to experience health benefits; however, those whose diets most closely resembled the Paleo template had a 23 percent reduction in all-cause mortality!

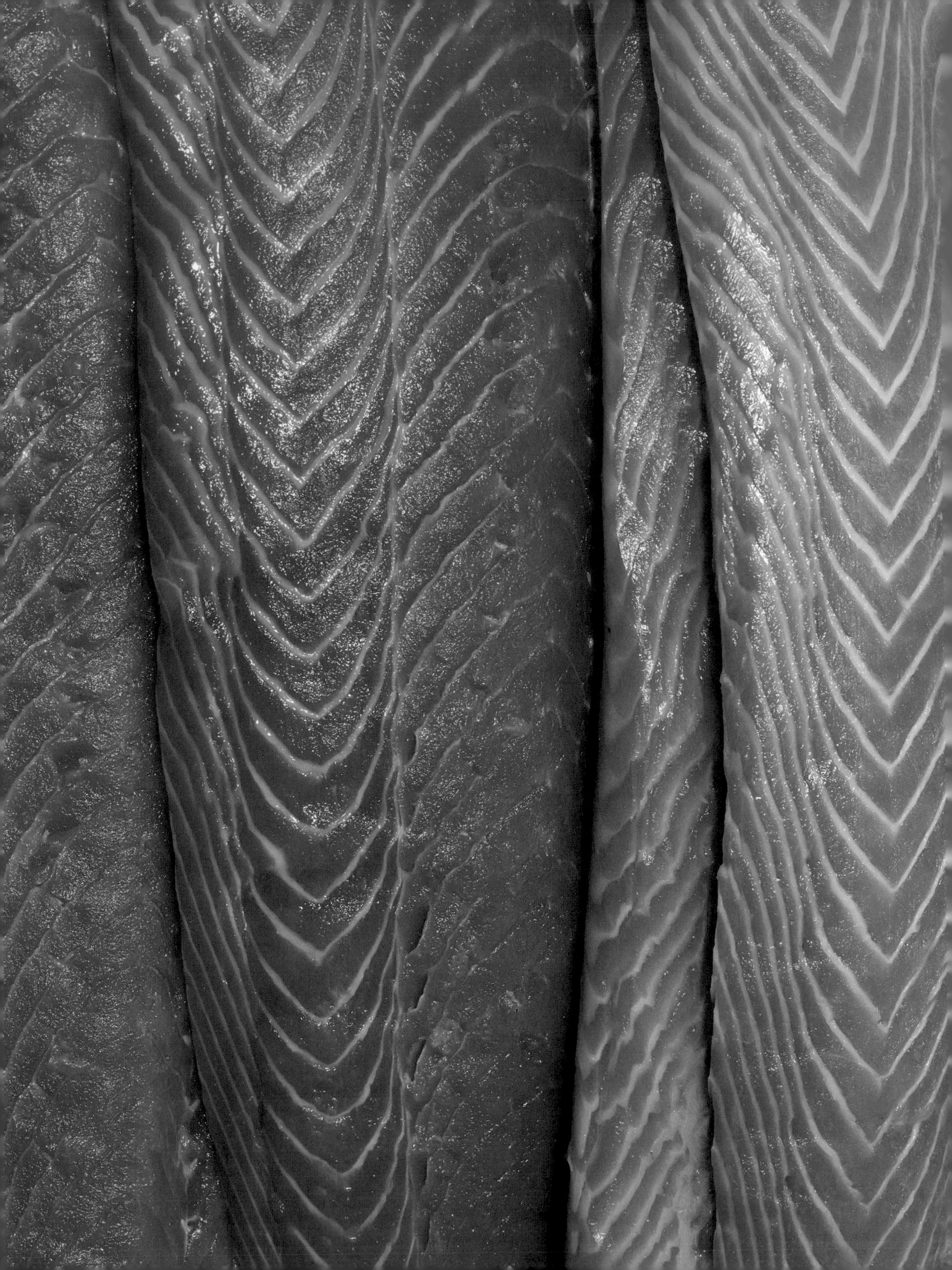

2.

THE SCIENCE BEHIND PALEO FOODS: WHAT TO EAT AND WHY

The Paleo diet has traditionally been defined by a list of foods that are omitted. However, it's not what we refuse to eat that makes a diet healthy—it's the foods we *do* eat that supply our bodies with vital nutrients, feed our gut microbiota, regulate our endocrine and immune systems, and support our overall health (or not!). When it comes to establishing an optimal human diet—that is, describing which foods to eat habitually to support health—this cannot be defined by a list of what's excluded.

Defining a diet based on which foods are avoided opens it up to criticism and misrepresentation. For example, you've likely heard news stories expounding that gluten-free diets provide inadequate nutrition, with medical professionals generally recommending that only those people with celiac disease, wheat allergies, or non-celiac gluten sensitivities follow a gluten-free diet. The most common argument against gluten-free diets is that store-bought gluten-free baked goods contain less fiber, less iron, and less B vitamins than their wheat-based counterparts. This argument is supported by studies showing that the most common nutrient deficiencies in celiac disease patients following long-term gluten-free diets are fiber and vitamins B3, B9, and B12. However, different gluten-free products vary greatly in nutrient content, due partly to the fact that only some companies add vitamins (analogous to the iron and B vitamins added to wheat flour to create "enriched wheat flour") and partly to the fact that different gluten-free flours offer inherently different nutrient values. In fact, some gluten-free products are *superior* to their wheat-based counterparts in terms of fiber and B vitamins.

More important in the argument against going gluten-free, an assumption is made that people will replace every gluten-containing food one-for-one with a commercially produced gluten-free version. The scientific evidence points to a different tendency: replacing at least a portion of the bread, pasta, muffins, and cookies that were consumed before going gluten-free with much more nutritious foods, such as vegetables, fruit, and meat. A recent study evaluating the nutrient intakes of children with celiac disease compared to their healthy non-gluten-sensitive counterparts found that the children with celiac disease consumed more calcium, vitamin B6, and vitamin B12 and substantially more zinc than those who ate gluten. Another recent study evaluated an even wider range of vitamins and minerals (this time in Australian adult celiac disease patients and compared to the general public) and found that patients with celiac disease following gluten-free diets consumed more calcium, magnesium, phosphate, zinc, vitamin B9 (folate), and vitamin C.

Gluten is not a nutrient. It is a difficult-to-digest protein found in wheat, rye, and barley that causes health issues for many people; it is discussed in more detail in Chapter 19. And grains in general are not nutritional powerhouses, contrary to what clever marketing might tell you. But going gluten-free (or grain-free) doesn't automatically mean that you are eating a healthier diet. It matters what you replace those wheat-based bagels and pasta with.

Remember, it's not about what you're *not* eating; it's about what you *do* eat.

When we define Paleo as "no grains, no dairy, no legumes, no refined or processed foods," critics think about what's missing. Just as is the case with gluten-free diets, many (erroneously) assume that not eating grains means we're missing out on B vitamins and fiber, and not eating dairy means we're missing out on calcium and vitamin D. But when we define a diet based on the incredible richness, diversity, and completeness of nutrients it contains, it's much harder to argue against it.

Even the healthiest whole grains can't compete with vegetables, fruit, seafood, or meat in terms of vitamin and mineral content (see page 23). When you choose a veggie side dish or a piece of fruit in place of a dinner roll, you're trading up substantially in terms of nutrients. And here's the crux of the Paleo diet: we trade up *all* the nutritionally underwhelming non-Paleo foods with nutrient-dense options. When our plates are teeming with a variety of veggies and rounded out with quality meats, fruits, seafood, nuts, and seeds, we are much more likely to get all the nutrients our bodies need.

A more insidious issue with focusing on omissions to define a dietary framework is that it can exaggerate the feeling of deprivation for those who follow it. How does it feel when someone says, "You can't have pizza," versus, "Let's eat steak and roasted veggies for dinner"? The latter is a decidedly more positive outlook on a meal! Another common criticism of the Paleo diet is that it's too hard to follow. This almost certainly stems from the negative way in which its tenets have been communicated in the past. It's actually not hard to follow (and you'll find tons of practical resources throughout this book to make sure of it!), but anytime you're forced to think about what you're missing, it's going to detract from what you could be enjoying.

I think it's paramount to reframe the Paleo diet in terms of what we *do* eat, which emphasizes the nutritive value of the Paleo framework while also being a psychologically healthier way to approach food choices. And while we can certainly create wonderful Paleo adaptations of pizza (see page 499), you're much less likely to think about pizza while you're eating a delicious steak. That's why this part of this book is all about the amazing variety of nutrient-dense foods that form the foundation of the Paleo template.

Chapter 8:
VEGETABLES AND FRUITS

Of all the foods and foodlike substances we could eat, vegetables and fruits are some of the only ones not mired in controversy: virtually every health authority agrees that they should have a place at the table. In fact, a high vegetable intake is the greatest common denominator among all diets that have scientific support for their health-promoting claims—the Paleo diet, the Mediterranean diet, plant-based diets, and indigenous diets from around the world. The body of evidence supporting a high intake of fresh, fibrous, low-energy-density plant foods is truly staggering.

Across the globe, Blue Zone areas (which boast a high concentration of centenarians and are frequently studied for longevity clues) are characterized first and foremost by their emphasis on eating vegetables. The Okinawans, who live on the Ryukyu Islands of Japan, consume a famously vegetable-heavy diet that includes mineral-rich gourds, bitter melon, local herbs and greens, and sweet potatoes. In Costa Rica, residents of the Nicoya Peninsula region, another longevity hotspot, consume abundant garden vegetables, squash, and tropical fruits (especially mangoes, papaya, and oranges). People living on the Greek island of Ikaria eat a diet rich in organic produce and herbs often grown and picked from their family gardens. Although Blue Zone diets are often described as plant-based, we should keep in mind that none of them is vegan, and only one community—the Seventh-Day Adventists of Loma Linda, California—is vegetarian.

High vegetable intake is also a hallmark of hunter-gatherer diets. Even the Inuit go to great lengths to collect nutrient-dense plant foods that provide a wide spectrum of micronutrients, prebiotics, and probiotics not available from meats and fish, including chlorophyll-rich seaweeds, berries, mosses, wild leafy greens, tubers, and the partially digested stomach contents of herbivorous animals.

Of course, the value of vegetables has been confirmed in more than just studies of homogenous populations (Blue Zone residents also partake in other health-promoting diet and lifestyle practices, which makes it hard to tease out the effect of vegetables alone). Study after study shows that consuming plenty of vegetables reduces the risk of disease—everything from diabetes to osteoporosis to diseases of the gastrointestinal tract to cardiovascular disease to autoimmune diseases to cancer. There are three likely reasons:

- Vegetables tend to be rich in important vitamins and minerals, including the most absorbable form of calcium (see page 264).
- Vegetables contain plenty of fiber to support a healthy diversity of gut microorganisms (see page 39).
- Vegetables are rich in thousands of beneficial plant phytochemicals. Recall that phytochemicals have abundant antioxidant, anti-inflammatory, and other health-promoting properties (see page 35).

All these components add up to serious benefits for people who include abundant vegetables in their diets.

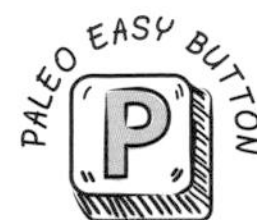

Eight servings of veggies per day (our minimum target) breaks down nicely to two servings at breakfast and three servings each at lunch and dinner. A serving is 1/2 cup for most cooked veggies, 1 cup for most raw veggies, and 2 cups for leafy greens.

THE BENEFITS OF A HIGH VEGGIE AND FRUIT INTAKE

When we look at the statistical relationship between vegetable and fruit consumption and mortality or disease risk, it becomes clear that the more of them we eat, the more protected we are. Every serving of vegetables or fruit reduces the risk of all-cause mortality (a measurement of overall health and longevity) by 5 percent, with the greatest risk reduction seen when we consume eight or more servings per day. That means eight daily servings of vegetables and fruits needs to be seen as a bare minimum for supporting health. It also means that the more we're able to increase our vegetable intake, the more health benefits we'll see.

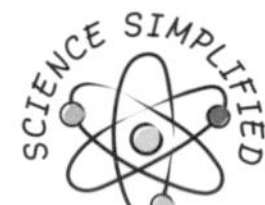

The more veggies you eat, the better. It's really as simple as that! Fruit is pretty great, too!

Even more exciting, those benefits extend to virtually every chronic disease afflicting modern society. For example, vegetables can be protective against all the following conditions:

· **Autoimmune disease:** Vegetables supply key nutrients for immune function while also providing multiple forms of fiber to boost gut health, consequently protecting against leaky gut, a precursor for autoimmunity. Eating plenty of cooked vegetables decreases the risk of rheumatoid arthritis; high vegetable and fruit consumption decreases the risk of inflammatory bowel diseases; and high vegetable and fiber intake decreases the risk of multiple sclerosis.

· **Cardiovascular disease:** Vegetables have a protective effect on the cardiovascular system by promoting healthy blood pressure (due to their abundance of potassium, calcium, and magnesium), reducing oxidative stress (due to their antioxidants), encouraging healthy body fat levels (by reducing the energy density of the diet and supporting weight loss), reducing LDL levels (through the actions of fiber binding to cholesterol in the intestines), and containing many micronutrients needed for vascular health. One study found that among more than 13,000 women, those consuming the most vegetables had a 38 percent reduced risk of dying from cardiovascular disease compared to the women eating the fewest vegetables.

· **Cancer:** The anti-cancer properties of many plant phytochemicals have been well documented (see page 35). In addition, the chlorophyll found in plant foods can help mitigate the potentially carcinogenic properties of heme iron (the form abundant in red meat), and certain fibers in vegetables and fruits appear to protect against colorectal cancer.

· **Diabetes:** Vegetables help reduce diabetes risk via a number of mechanisms, including supplying micronutrients necessary for blood sugar regulation, helping reduce the glycemic load of a meal, and containing fiber to slow glucose absorption. Vegetables can also reduce risk factors for diabetes by decreasing the energy density of the diet and encouraging weight loss. (Abdominal fat, especially around the organs, is a major contributor to diabetes in people who are genetically susceptible.) Not surprisingly, vegetable intake is frequently associated with lower diabetes risk, with one meta-analysis finding that each 0.2 serving per day increase of green leafy vegetable intake was associated with a 13 percent lower risk of type 2 diabetes. Yes, even one-fifth of a serving was able to lower diabetes risk that profoundly!

· **Obesity:** Along with helping people avoid micronutrient deficiencies associated with obesity (see page 406), vegetables are the lowest-energy-density foods in existence, adding bulk (fiber and water) to and reducing the overall energy density of our meals. This helps us naturally lower our caloric intake and makes it easier to reach a healthy body weight—especially because vegetables can displace foods that combine concentrated fats, carbohydrates/sugar, and salt in ways that encourage overeating.

· **Osteoporosis:** Vegetables supply an assortment of nutrients needed for bone health, including calcium, magnesium, phosphorus, chromium, and vitamin K. Berries have also been linked to higher bone density, potentially due to their phytochemicals and antioxidants. Among postmenopausal women, one study found that every 100-gram increase in vegetable and fruit intake was associated with a sizeable increase in bone mineral density. Additional studies show that high vegetable consumption is far better correlated with bone health than dairy consumption.

KNOWLEDGE BOMB *For every 1/3 cup or so of leafy greens you eat each day, you reduce your risk of type 2 diabetes by 13 percent. Eating at least five daily servings of veggies can reduce your risk of cardiovascular disease by 38 percent. And for every extra daily serving of vegetables or fruit, your bone mineral density increases markedly!*

Clearly, vegetables and fruits play many important roles in supporting our health. Vitamins, minerals, fiber, and an astounding spectrum of phytonutrients are packed into these fabulous plant foods! That's why they're a major component of the Paleo diet and should take up a large visual portion of each meal we eat. In fact, with two-thirds to three-quarters of every plate covered in vegetables and fruit, the Paleo template could be considered a plant-based diet.

Vegetables and fruits supply key vitamins and minerals as well as phytochemicals and fiber. Although some of these nutrients are also available in specific animal foods, plants tend to be the richest sources. Let's review some of the amazing nutrients that vegetables and fruits have to offer us that are either limited in or just aren't available from animal foods.

CAROTENOIDS: These potent antioxidants are important for immune system function. Vegetables and fruits rich in carotenoids include anything red, orange, or yellow (like carrots, beets, squash, sweet potatoes, cantaloupe, apricots, mangoes, and bell peppers) and anything dark green (like broccoli, collard greens, kale, and spinach). Tomatoes are particularly rich in lycopene.

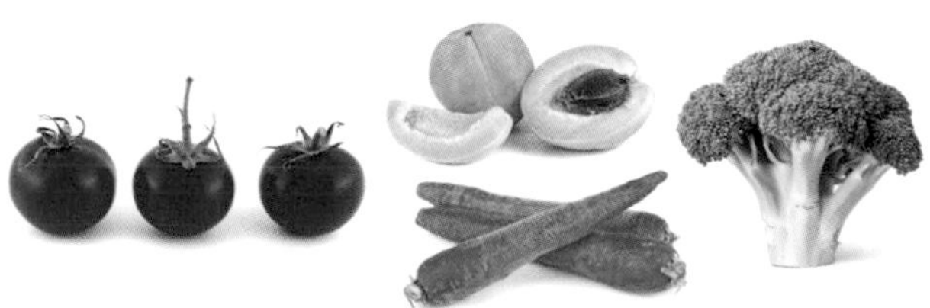

DIALLYL SULFIDE: A compound created and released by crushing garlic and other alliums. It has potent antimicrobial effects (including acting against the stomach bacteria *H. pylori*), reduces risk of cardiovascular disease, and may be responsible for garlic's protective effect against colorectal cancer. Foods containing diallyl sulfide include garlic, onions, chives, shallots, scallions, and leeks.

DITHIOLETHIONES: A class of cancer-protective compounds that also induce detoxification. Sources of dithiolethiones include cruciferous vegetables such as broccoli, cabbage, collard greens, and kale.

POLYPHENOLS: A class of chemical compounds with antioxidant properties, helping prevent cell damage from free radicals and potentially reducing the risk of heart disease and other chronic diseases. Rich sources include berries, citrus fruits, plums, brightly colored vegetables, and dark chocolate.

PLANT STEROLS AND STANOLS: With a similar chemical structure to animal cholesterol, these compounds can block the absorption of cholesterol in the small intestine and reduce levels of LDL ("bad") cholesterol in the blood without altering levels of HDL ("good") cholesterol. Sources of plant sterols and stanols include nuts, legumes, and most fruits and vegetables.

FLAVONOIDS: A class of more than 6,000 compounds with a range of health benefits, including reducing inflammation, protecting against smoking-related cancers, and reducing cardiovascular disease risk. Flavonoids also have antibacterial properties. Foods rich in flavonoids include parsley, berries (especially blueberries), citrus fruits, and cacao.

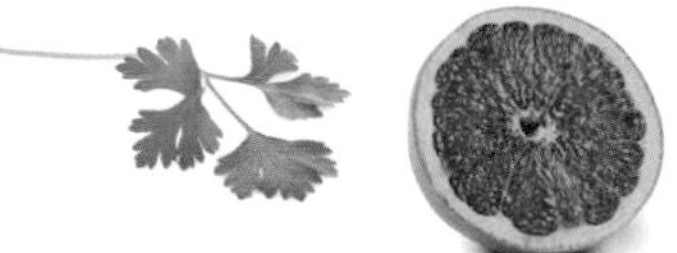

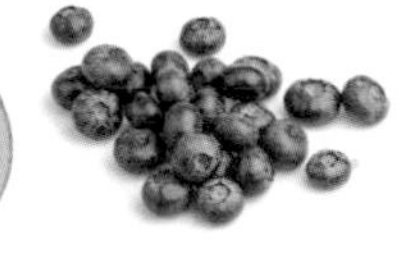

ISOTHIOCYANATES AND INDOLES: Sulfur-containing plant chemicals with strong anticancer properties due to their ability to help suppress tumor formation and eliminate carcinogens from the body. Foods with isothiocyanates and indoles include cruciferous vegetables such as broccoli, cabbage, cauliflower, kale, and Brussels sprouts, especially when eaten raw.

B VITAMINS: These vitamins are important for cell metabolism (including cell growth and division), immune system function, and nervous system function. Produce rich in B vitamins (except B12) include orange and red vegetables (like carrots, sweet potatoes, and beets), grapefruit, peaches, oranges, watermelon, bananas, many green vegetables (like artichokes, asparagus, okra, broccoli, and green bell peppers), leafy green vegetables, mushrooms, and cauliflower. Avocado is *very* high in several B vitamins.

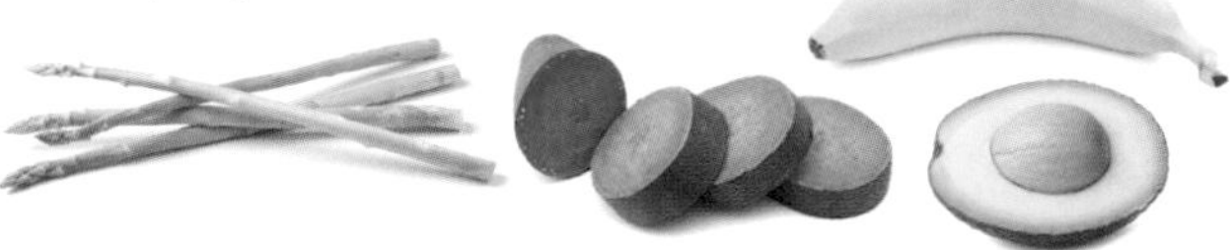

VITAMIN C: Vitamin C is a potent antioxidant, necessary for immune system function, cholesterol metabolism, and iron absorption. It is also essential for the function of several enzymes in the body, including some that help make collagen (a major component of connective tissue), which is why scurvy (the disease caused by vitamin C deficiency) includes symptoms like skin hemorrhages and bleeding in the joints. Vegetables and fruits rich in vitamin C include all citrus, kiwis, berries, papayas, pineapple, artichokes, asparagus, avocados, broccoli, carrots, cauliflower, cucumbers, green bell peppers, kale, mushrooms, onions, potatoes, spinach, squash, and sweet potatoes.

VITAMIN K: Vitamin K is critical for making proteins that are involved in blood clotting and metabolism. It is found in cruciferous vegetables (like broccoli, Brussels sprouts, cabbage, cauliflower, kale, and turnip greens) and leafy dark green vegetables.

CALCIUM: In addition to forming bone, calcium is essential to many processes within the cells, as well as neurotransmitter release and muscle contraction (including our hearts beating!). Some research suggests that our bodies absorb and use the calcium in vegetables much more readily than the calcium in dairy, likely one reason why high vegetable consumption protects against osteoporosis and hip fractures in the elderly. Vegetables and fruits rich in calcium include dark green vegetables, parsnips, papayas, kumquats, black currants, rhubarb, oranges, tangerines, figs, turnips, and butternut squash. Calcium is also found in nuts and seeds, especially sesame seeds.

CHROMIUM: Chromium is important for sugar and fat metabolism. Vegetable and fruits sources include broccoli, tomatoes, apples, bananas, onions, garlic, cabbage, carrots, mushrooms, parsnips, and leafy green vegetables.

COPPER: Copper is involved in the absorption, storage, and metabolism of iron and the formation of red blood cells. Vegetables and fruits containing copper include artichokes, avocados, pineapple, plums, dates, kiwis, lychees, cherries, parsnips, pumpkin, winter squash, and leafy green vegetables.

MAGNESIUM: Magnesium is necessary for cells to live. More than 300 different enzymes within our cells need magnesium to work, including every enzyme that uses or synthesizes ATP (the basic energy molecule in a cell) and enzymes that synthesize DNA and RNA. Vegetables and fruits rich in magnesium include berries, passionfruit, bananas, carrots, squash, sweet potatoes, and especially leafy dark green vegetables like spinach and kale.

MANGANESE: Manganese is necessary for enzymes that protect the body from and repair damage caused by free radicals. Vegetables and fruits high in manganese include sweet potatoes, raspberries, pineapple, grapes, kiwis, figs, bananas, leeks, eggplant, beets, cruciferous vegetables (like broccoli, Brussels sprouts, cabbage, cauliflower, kale, and turnip greens), and leafy dark green vegetables.

POTASSIUM: Potassium is critical for the function of every cell; it is necessary for nerve function, cardiac function, and muscle contraction. Vegetables and fruits rich in potassium include cruciferous vegetables (like broccoli, Brussels sprouts, cabbage, cauliflower, kale, and turnip greens), bananas, cantaloupe, avocados, guavas, kiwis, persimmons, apricots, many orange vegetables (like carrots, squash, and sweet potatoes), eggplant, and leafy dark green vegetables.

SULFUR: Sulfur is widely used in biochemical processes; it is a component of all proteins and is important for the function of many enzymes and antioxidant molecules. Cruciferous vegetables and alliums (onions, leeks, and garlic) are the best sources of sulfur.

ZINC: Zinc is important for nearly every function of the cell, from protein and carbohydrate metabolism, as well as the immune system. Most green vegetables are a good source of zinc, as are pomegranates and avocados.

FIBER: Fiber is a carbohydrate present in plant cell walls that our bodies can't digest. It provides us a variety of benefits by:

- feeding beneficial probiotic bacteria in the digestive tract
- binding with toxins, hormones, bile salts, cholesterol, and other substances in the gut to facilitate their elimination
- favorably regulating some hormones (like suppressing the hunger hormone ghrelin, which signals to the brain that you are full) and some neurotransmitters (like increasing melatonin, which helps control sleep)
- adding bulk to the stool, which improves the quality of bowel movements

KNOWLEDGE BOMB

Contrary to popular belief, insoluble fiber-rich foods like leafy greens and cruciferous veggies like broccoli are not abrasive to the gut and do not worsen gut pathologies like diverticular disease, inflammatory bowel disease, and irritable bowel syndrome.

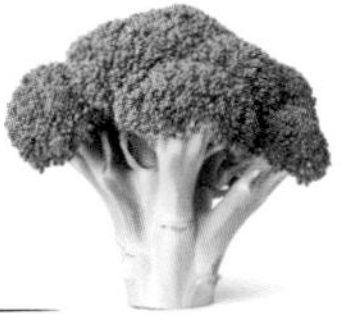

Diets rich in fiber reduce the risk of cardiovascular disease and many cancers (especially colorectal cancer, but also liver cancer, pancreatic cancer, and others) and promote lower inflammation. In fact, the higher your intake of fiber, the lower your inflammation. If you have kidney disease or diabetes, a high-fiber diet reduces your risk of mortality. High fiber intake can even reduce your chances of dying from an infection. Fiber is broadly categorized as soluble or insoluble (that is, whether or not it dissolves in water), and each class of fiber has different health benefits. In general, foods that are high in fiber include fruits (especially berries), vegetables (especially leafy green vegetables, root vegetables, and cruciferous vegetables), legumes, and nuts and seeds.

Soluble fiber forms a gel-like material in the gut and tends to slow the movement of material through the digestive system. Soluble fiber is typically readily fermented by the bacteria in the colon (although not all soluble fibers are fermentable), producing gases and physiologically active by-products like short-chain fatty acids, which yield a variety of health benefits, and vitamins. Soluble fiber also has cholesterol-lowering properties. Rich sources include apples, berries, pears, citrus fruits, and legumes.

Insoluble fiber tends to speed up the movement of material through the digestive system. Fermentable insoluble fibers also produce gases and physiologically active by-products like short-chain fatty acids and vitamins. Unfermentable insoluble fiber increases stool bulk, which is believed to be beneficial for regulating bowel movements and managing constipation. Insoluble fiber reduces inflammation. It also binds to toxins and surplus hormones in the gastrointestinal tract, facilitating their elimination from the body. Foods high in insoluble fiber include leafy green vegetables, bell peppers, cruciferous vegetables (such as bok choy, broccoli, Brussels sprouts, and cauliflower), celery, and carrots.

LIGNANS: A type of polyphenol-rich fiber that can be metabolized by intestinal bacteria into enterodiol and enterolactone, which may play a role in preventing osteoporosis, cardiovascular disease, and hormone-associated cancers (breast, endometrial, ovarian, and prostate). Foods high in lignans include flax seeds, sesame seeds, legumes, and cruciferous vegetables.

Clearly, some vegetables and fruits, like kale, are powerhouses of nutrition, but in order to get adequate amounts of all the necessary vitamins and minerals, eating a wide variety is key. Also keep in mind that vitamins are often linked to the color of a vegetable or fruit, so "eating the rainbow" is a good way to ensure nutrient diversity (see page 39).

HEALTH QUICK-START

What do you do if you have a condition like IBS or IBD and eating foods rich in insoluble fiber, like leafy greens, causes you increased gastrointestinal symptoms? What does it mean if you can see intact food particles in your stool after eating these high-insoluble-fiber foods? This is a reality for many people and one that helps perpetuate the myth that insoluble fiber should be avoided. But this isn't a case of insoluble fiber being the problem so much as it being a symptom—it's the big red flag indicating the need for digestive support and improvements to the gut microbiota.

The first step in improving digestion is always to follow good meal hygiene (see page 74). Next, consider digestive support supplements (see page 77). It is generally recommended for patients with gastrointestinal diseases to increase dietary fiber slowly. High-fiber foods are easier to digest when thoroughly cooked, fermented, and/or pureed. See also Chapter 34 for a discussion on food sensitivities.

A COMMON FIBER MYTH, BUSTED

Adequate intake of a diversity of whole-food sources of fiber is critical for the health of the gut microbiota (see pages 39 and 70), yet insoluble fiber gets a bad rap. Both conventional and alternative health-care providers typically warn those with gastrointestinal symptoms or diagnosed gastrointestinal conditions—inflammatory bowel disease (IBD), irritable bowel syndrome (IBS), diverticulitis, and leaky gut syndrome—not to consume foods rich in insoluble fiber because insoluble fiber is "rough and abrasive." It has been likened to eating sandpaper and supposedly causes damage to the gut as it scrapes its way through the digestive tract.

So what is the evidence? Diets rich in fiber reduce the risk of developing many gut pathologies. High-fiber diets (especially insoluble fiber) reduce the risk of diverticulitis and diverticulosis. Very few perspective studies have been performed to investigate dietary factors increasing the risk of IBS, but preliminary studies indicate that low fiber intake is a risk factor. High fiber and fruit intakes are both associated with a decreased risk of Crohn's disease. High vegetable intake is associated with a decreased risk of ulcerative colitis.

However, decreasing the risk of developing a disease is different from what happens when you eat insoluble fiber-rich foods like leafy greens after the disease has developed. So let's look at that scenario.

If insoluble fiber were irritating to the gastrointestinal tract, clinical trials in which patients with diseases such as IBD, IBS, and diverticulitis are supplemented with insoluble fiber should show exacerbation (or worsening) of their diseases. But the handful of studies that have investigated the effects of insoluble fiber in these severe gut pathologies have not borne this out.

The impact of insoluble fiber on disease activity is best understood with diverticular disease. In diverticular disease, tiny pouches form in the colon due to a weakening of the wall of muscles around the colon. These pouches are called *diverticula*, and the diagnosis when they are discovered is diverticulosis. When these pouches become inflamed, diverticulitis is diagnosed. When inflammation is severe, diverticula can bleed. Traditionally, a diagnosis of diverticulitis or diverticulosis comes with a lifetime ban on insoluble fiber-rich foods like corn, popcorn, nuts, and seeds, and low-residue (very-low-fiber) diets are often recommended. However, evidence supporting these recommendations has never actually existed. In fact, the opposite has been proven: high dietary fiber intake not only prevents new diverticula from forming but also reduces the risk of complications (such as bleeding and diverticulitis) in patients with diagnosed diverticular disease.

One fascinating prospective study looked at whether dietary fiber increased or decreased the risk of complications in patients with diagnosed diverticular disease. This study showed that a high intake of fiber from fruits and vegetables decreased the risk of complications, but not intake of cereal grain fiber. (The researchers were also able to show that it was the *fiber* in fruits and vegetables rather than other nutrients that made the difference.) The study further showed that a high *insoluble* fiber intake, especially cellulose (but also lignin and to a lesser degree hemicellulose; see page 43)—but not soluble fiber—correlated with the lowest risk of complications of diverticular disease. Even patients who

RAW OR COOKED?

Many people will tell you that cooking vegetables destroys their nutrients and beneficial enzymes. This is partially true. It's also true that cooking vegetables makes many of their nutrients easier for your body to absorb and use. So which is better—eating vegetables raw or cooked?

Prehistoric man mastered the art of cooking perhaps as early as 1.5 million years ago. This means that for the majority of human evolution, our ancestors have been eating cooked food. In fact, some believe that the advent of cooking may be one of the most important factors in our success as a species because it greatly increased the nutrition that could be digested out of our food for a lower energy expenditure (this is true for both meat and plant matter).

Some vitamins are volatile in heat. Vitamin C, for example, degrades with heat, dehydration, and prolonged storage. Polyphenols and allicin can be destroyed by the cooking process. Some beneficial enzymes are destroyed by cooking; for example, the enzyme myrosinase, whose activity forms sulforaphane, known to prevent cancer, is found in raw broccoli but is destroyed in cooking. While typical cooking procedures destroy only a portion of these nutrients, there is convincing evidence supporting the case for eating raw vegetables.

---

suffered such severe diverticulitis that the diverticula were bleeding benefited from a high insoluble fiber intake.

What about conditions affecting the small intestine rather than the large intestine, like Crohn's disease and irritable bowel syndrome? In one large study, patients with IBS were blindly and randomly assigned either a soluble fiber supplement (psyllium), an insoluble fiber supplement (bran), or a placebo. While soluble fiber significantly improved symptoms, insoluble fiber had only a marginal effect compared to a placebo—but it didn't make things worse. A study using chitosan and vitamin C supplementation in Crohn's disease patients showed no real benefit but also no detriment to disease activity.

This topic has been more thoroughly investigated in animal models than in humans (specifically animal models of ulcerative colitis). Hemicellulose supplementation has been shown to greatly improve disease activity in mice with colitis. Not only did hemicellulose supplementation reduce symptoms (like diarrhea), but it also accelerated repair of the mucosal barrier and reduced inflammation, attributable at least in part to improvements in the gut microbiota. Cellulose supplementation was also shown to improve colitis in mice. Again, these benefits were attributable to changes in gut microbiota; interestingly, when cellulose supplementation was stopped, the beneficial effects lasted only about 10 days before the disease started to worsen again.

No studies have been performed on the role that insoluble fiber may have in healing the gut in celiac disease patients. Celiac disease is hallmarked by a shortening (called pruning) of the intestinal villi (the fingerlike columns of gut epithelial cells that increase the surface area of the gut to maximize nutrient absorption). A study evaluating the effects of two types of insoluble fiber (one rich in both cellulose and hemicellulose versus one rich in lignin) on the morphology of the small intestine in piglets (not celiac, but rather the developing intestine, which is still very relevant) showed that insoluble fiber increases the height of the intestinal villi in both the jejunum and the ileum—and that's a good thing.

It's worth noting that within the relatively limited body of scientific literature evaluating the effect of insoluble fiber on the gut barrier, insoluble fiber has been shown to be potentially damaging in one situation: NSAID-induced small intestinal ulcers. In one study, cats were fed diets that differed in fiber content (high, low, normal) and type (either insoluble cellulose or soluble pectin) before being given very high doses of NSAIDs. The researchers found that the cats developed more ulcers if they received the high-fiber diet compared to the control group and fewer ulcers if they were fed the very-low-fiber diet. They also found that cats that received cellulose-enriched diets developed more ulcers, but cats that were fed pectin did not. The authors concluded that insoluble fiber contributes to the development of NSAID-induced ulcers. This may be an argument for a low-fiber diet in anyone taking large doses of NSAIDs. (See page 115 for why NSAIDs are not great for gut health in the first place.)

There is no evidence that insoluble fiber is abrasive to the gastrointestinal tract, and there is no scientific rationale for avoiding insoluble fiber for those with gut pathologies including IBS, IBD, and diverticular disease. In fact, eating plenty of fruits and vegetables will likely speed your healing.

While some nutrients are lost in cooking, we are compensated by the many other nutrients that are increased during cooking. Heat breaks down the thick walls of a plant's cells, which makes any nutrients bound to the cell walls or locked inside the cells available to our bodies for digestion. Typically, antioxidants are dramatically increased by cooking. For example, the bioavailability of many carotenoids increases (how well our bodies absorb and use them) when vegetables that contain them are cooked. Lycopene content increases when tomatoes are cooked or sun-dried. And some compounds require heat to be formed, such as indole, thought to prevent cancer, which forms when cruciferous vegetables (like broccoli, cabbage, Brussels sprouts, and kale) are cooked.

Scientific studies show no significant difference in terms of risk of all-cause mortality between eating raw and cooked fruits and vegetables. Instead, the scientific findings simply emphasize the importance of eating them.

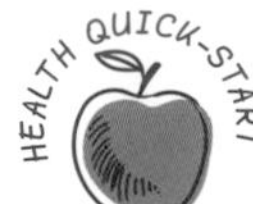

Both raw and cooked vegetables are advantageous, but it's good to mix it up. In addition to focusing on eating a variety of different veggies, switch up whether or not you cook them. Sometimes cook your carrots, sometimes eat them raw. Sometimes steam your broccoli (see page 548), and sometimes use it as a dipping veggie.

GREEN JUICES VERSUS SMOOTHIES

If you aren't used to eating large portions of vegetables, you may be wondering if it's okay to boost your vegetable intake with green juices or smoothies.

Green juices are not whole foods. The process of juicing removes the fiber from vegetables and fruits. This has the net effect of making some of the vitamins, minerals, and antioxidants more absorbable, although you also lose valuable nutrients in the pulp. Also recall that fiber is a crucial nutrient (see page 39) and an important signal for ghrelin (see page 90). Furthermore, removing fiber makes the sugars in vegetable juices much more absorbable, so they can have a substantial impact on blood sugar. Studies confirm that drinking liquefied carbohydrates causes a quicker and higher spike in blood sugar than consuming the same carbohydrates in solid form. This effect can be ameliorated by drinking green juice with a meal and limiting portion size.

Green smoothies may seem like a better alternative because the fiber is not removed. However, drinking your food can be hard on your digestive system because the simple act of chewing is an important signal to your body to increase stomach acid secretion, which in turn signals the secretion of digestive enzymes from the pancreas and bile from the gallbladder (see page 71). Because the same hormones that control these aspects of digestion also signal satiety to the brain, drinking a smoothie isn't as filling as eating the individual components (see page 213). If a smoothie replaces a meal, then your body's ability to digest the nutrients in that smoothie may be inhibited. This is made even worse by eating on the go, since the body does not prioritize digestion when it is moving or if you are stressed, as you may be during your commute. This effect can be counteracted by including green smoothies as part of a meal (and not make a smoothie a meal in itself) and by practicing good meal hygiene (see page 74).

Many people swear by green juices and smoothies to up their micronutrient intake. If you love them or struggle to get enough vegetables otherwise, then by all means go ahead and drink them—with meals. But there is no advantage to swapping them for whole vegetables.

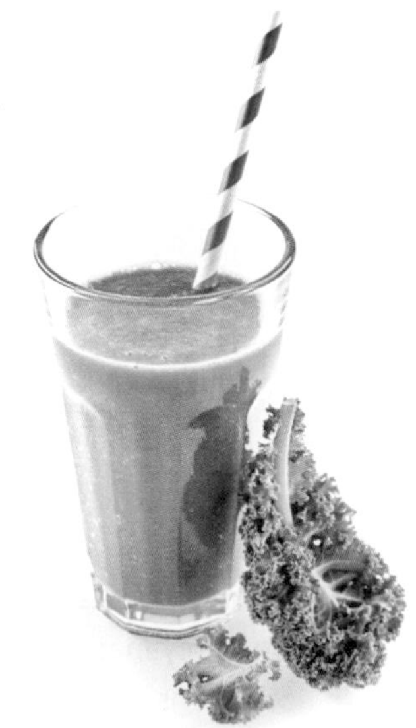

BUSTING THE CRUCIFEROUS VEGGIE AND HYPOTHYROIDISM MYTH

People with autoimmune thyroid disorders, such as Hashimoto's thyroiditis or Graves' disease, and with low thyroid function are often advised to avoid cruciferous vegetables, spinach, radishes, peaches, and strawberries because of their goitrogenic properties. Goitrogens are compounds that suppress the function of the thyroid gland by interfering with iodine uptake. Thyroid hormones play essential roles in metabolism and even in regulating the immune system, so supporting optimal thyroid function is important for healing and for general health (see page 93). But avoiding these foods is not well justified.

The cruciferous family, also called *Brassica*, comprises many of the most antioxidant-, vitamin-, and mineral-rich vegetables available, including:

- arugula (also known as rocket)
- bok choy
- broccoflower
- broccoli
- broccoli romanesco
- Brussels sprouts
- cabbage
- canola (also known as rapeseed)
- cauliflower
- Chinese broccoli
- collard greens
- daikon
- field pepperweed
- flowering cabbage
- garden cress
- horseradish
- kale
- kohlrabi
- komatsuna
- land cress
- maca
- mizuna
- mustard
- radishes
- rapini (also known as broccoli rabe)
- rutabaga
- tatsoi
- turnips
- wasabi
- watercress
- wild broccoli

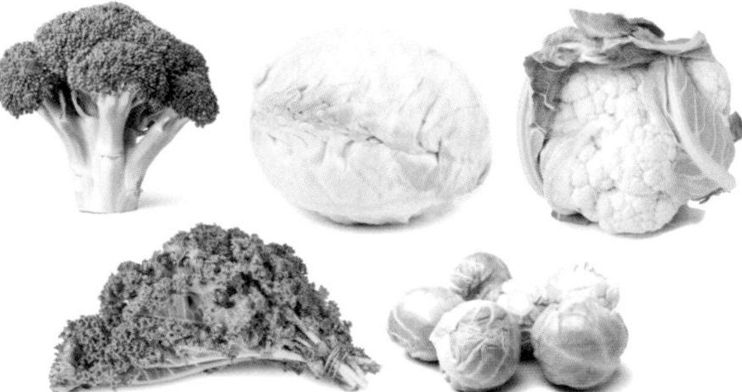

This family of vegetables is also a great source of sulfur-containing compounds called glucosinolates (see page 231). When these vegetables are chopped or chewed, the enzyme myrosinase in them breaks the glucosinolates apart (through hydrolysis) into a variety of biologically active compounds, many of which are potent antioxidants and prevent cancer. Two of these—isothiocyanates and thiocyanates—are also known goitrogens.

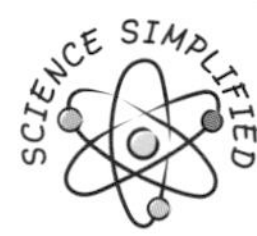

There's no reason to avoid eating cruciferous vegetables as long as you aren't deficient in iodine or selenium.

Isothiocyanates and thiocyanates appear to reduce thyroid function by inhibiting the enzyme thyroid peroxidase (thyroperoxidase, or TPO). During thyroid hormone synthesis, TPO catalyzes the transfer of iodine to a protein called thyroglobulin to produce either T4 thyroid prohormone (thyroxine) or the more active T3 thyroid hormone (triiodothyronine). When isothiocyanates or thiocyanates are consumed in large enough quantities, they interfere with the function of the thyroid gland.

There is no evidence of a link between human consumption of isothiocyanates or thiocyanates and thyroid pathologies in the absence of iodine deficiency: these substances have been shown to interfere with thyroid function only in people lacking adequate amounts of iodine. In fact, eating cruciferous vegetables correlates with diverse health benefits, including a reduced risk of cancer (even thyroid cancer!). In a recent clinical trial evaluating the safety of isothiocyanates isolated from broccoli sprouts, no adverse effects were reported, including no reductions in thyroid function.

Perhaps even more compelling, at low concentrations (like what you would get from including cruciferous vegetables in your diet), thiocyanates stimulate T4 synthesis, meaning that these vegetables labeled as goitrogens actually *support* thyroid function. There is also a strong synergy between isothiocyanates and selenium in the formation of the important antioxidant enzymes thioredoxin reductase and glutathione peroxidase. This means that consuming isothiocyanates, in conjunction with selenium, gives a tremendous boost to the body's antioxidant defense mechanisms and helps prevent cancer. So eat *more* rather than fewer of those cruciferous vegetables, even if you have autoimmune thyroid diseases, as long as you're not deficient in iodine and selenium.

SEAWEED

Seaweed is teeming with essential minerals, carotenoids, and even long-chain omega-3 fatty acids, making it a powerful addition to our diets. In fact, the benefits of seaweed are even greater than many land vegetables. Most of us are familiar with the nori that wraps sushi rolls, but the list of edible seaweeds doesn't end there. Common types of seaweed fit for human consumption include:

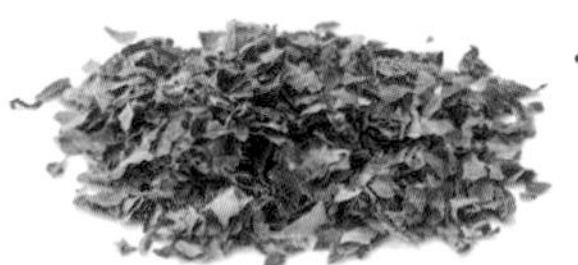

- **Dulse,** a salty red seaweed that can be eaten without soaking or cooking

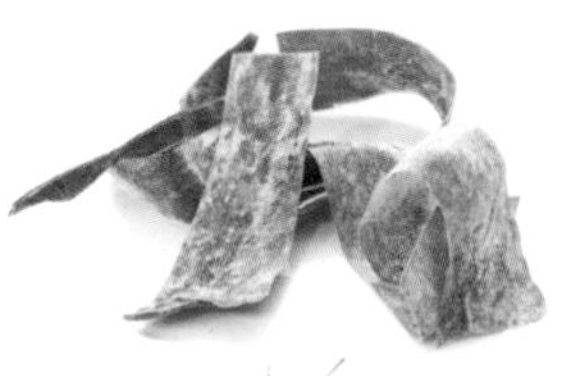

- **Kombu,** a thick seaweed often used as a flavor enhancer in broth and as a tenderizer for beans

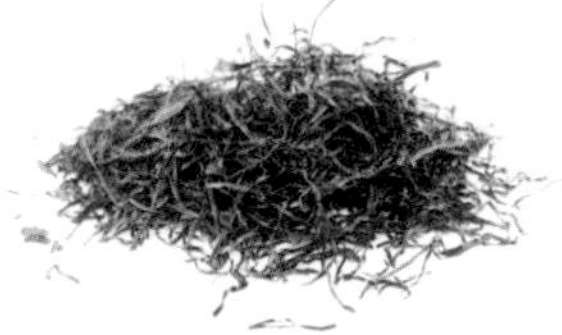

- **Arame,** a mild-flavored seaweed high in lignans

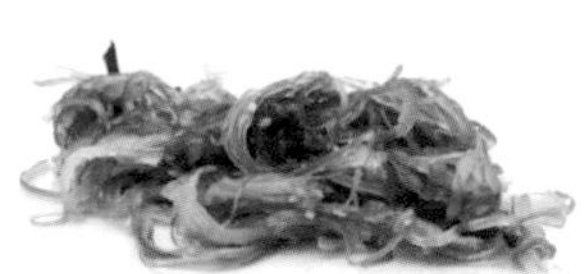

- **Wakame,** a subtly sweet seaweed often used in soups and salads (especially the seaweed salad found in Asian restaurants)

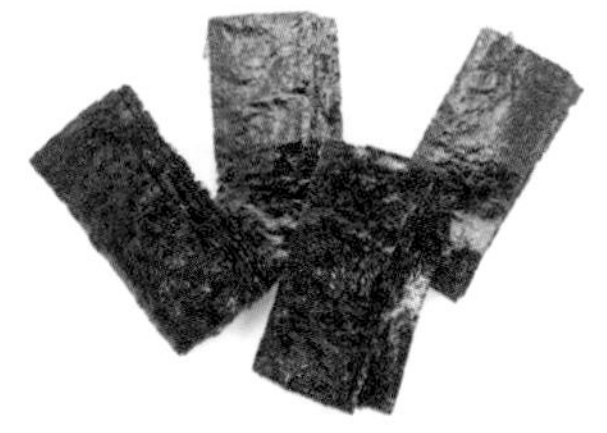

- **Laver,** a smooth, sheetlike red algae with a high iodine content (which makes its flavor similar to olives and oysters), used to make nori for sushi

KNOWLEDGE BOMB *Some green algae, such as chlorella and spirulina, may stimulate the immune system. Recent evidence suggests that the cell membrane of chlorella, a freshwater blue-green algae, contains lipopolysaccharide, the same toxic protein in the cell walls of Gram-negative bacteria. Chlorella has also been shown to increase inflammation and stimulate Th1 cells. Although spirulina, a blue-green algae that grows in saltwater lakes in Mexico and Africa, has a very different cell membrane than chlorella, studies show that it also activates the innate immune system and stimulates Th1 cells.*

Plenty of vegetables have impressive nutritional résumés, but seaweed takes the cake (er, the salad)! Although each variety of seaweed has a different nutrient profile, we can expect these foods to be rich in:

- Calcium
- Chromium
- Copper
- Iodine
- Iron
- Magnesium
- Manganese
- Phosphorus
- Potassium
- Selenium
- Zinc
- *Dozens* of additional trace minerals
- B vitamins (B1, B2, B3, B5, and B6)
- Vitamin C
- Vitamin E
- Vitamin K
- DHA (an omega-3 fat not found in many plant foods)

On top of all that, seaweed has some special components that aren't found in *any* land-based vegetables and may be responsible for some of its unique health benefits:

- **Fucoxanthin,** a type of carotenoid that gives seaweed a brown pigment and has potent anti-cancer properties, the ability to reduce liver fat and liver enzymes, and the potential to boost metabolic rate and assist in fat loss
- **Fucoidans and laminarins,** sulfated polysaccharides that have been shown to induce cell death of certain cancers (such as lymphoma), have antiviral and neuroprotective properties, help slow blood clotting, and may help modulate the immune system (although in most of these cases, more research in humans is needed)
- **Alginates,** cell-wall constituents of brown algae that may aid in weight loss, glycemic control, and appetite regulation

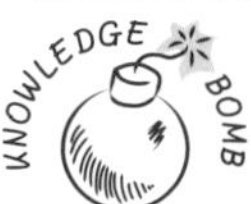

Some components of seaweed (particularly fucoxanthin) require dietary fat to be well absorbed, so consuming seaweed as part of a meal with a fat-rich food (like avocado, olive oil, or sesame oil) will enhance the nutritional perks.

Numerous studies have shown that some components in seaweed help fight inflammation. The fucoxanthin in seaweed is the biggie here: it reduces pro-inflammatory mediators (like inducible nitric oxide synthase (iNOS), cyclooxygenase-2 (COX-2), and the pro-inflammatory cytokines IL-1β, TNF-α, and IL-6) and helps reduce excessive inflammation in the body. Of course, that has a risk-lowering effect for the numerous conditions that stem from chronic inflammation.

Another of seaweed's many perks is the potential to improve cardiovascular health. The antioxidant and anti-inflammatory properties of fucoxanthin can help thwart multiple processes involved in the progression of heart disease while modulating immune function. Research has shown that many seaweeds have hypolipidemic (lipid-lowering) activity, helping reduce levels of triglycerides and LDL cholesterol. The DHA found in algae, algal oil, and some seaweeds can not only reduce triglycerides and LDL cholesterol but also raise HDL cholesterol—which, collectively, paints a more favorable picture for combatting heart disease.

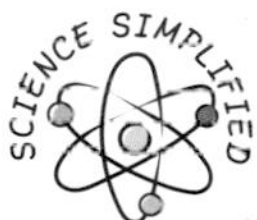

Eating seaweed reduces inflammation, cancer risk, and cardiovascular disease risk.

In Traditional Chinese Medicine and Japanese folk medicine, seaweeds have long been used to treat tumors, and Western science is beginning to discover why. Multiple studies have shown that seaweed can increase apoptosis (programmed cell death) of tumor cells, prevent the growth of new blood vessels that supply tumors, and inhibit tumor cell adhesion, which prevents metastasis. Even small amounts of seaweed seem to have a big effect. In one study of postmenopausal women, consuming just 5 grams of brown seaweed each day resulted in a 50 percent drop in a type of receptor that's overexpressed in cancer (urokinase-type plasminogen activator receptor, or uPAR, which is involved in multiple signaling pathways, cell adhesion, inflammation, immune function activation, tissue repair, and a number of other functions). The key players behind seaweed's anti-cancer effects may be its fucoxanthin content, its polyphenolic compounds, its sulfated polysaccharides (fucoidan and laminarin), its ability to increase the colon's protective mucus bilayer, and its ability to bind dietary toxins and carcinogens by increasing stool bulk.

In fact, the traditional use of seaweed in some parts of Asia, like Japan, may help explain why those areas have much lower rates of certain cancers, especially breast cancer, than most Westernized nations.

Another feature of seaweed is its antiviral potential. The sulfated polysaccharides in seaweed can block the interaction between many viruses and host cells—including important pathogens like HIV, herpes simplex, dengue virus, respiratory syncytial virus, and human cytomegalovirus. And seaweed appears to contain other antiviral components that are enhanced by light (especially UVA) and not only protect our cells but can directly inactivate the virus particles themselves.

Still, when it comes to seaweed, some of us may wonder about heavy metal toxicity. As with fish, there's some concern about seaweed accumulating heavy metals from polluted waters (see page 163). Fortunately, a number of researchers and seaweed manufacturers have begun testing seaweed samples to ensure safety and to identify high-risk species. Only one type of seaweed has consistently shown up as dangerous: hijiki, which frequently tests high for arsenic. Other types of seaweed—especially ones harvested or imported into the U.S.—generally contain such low levels of heavy metals that even an extremely high intake would be fine. But just to be safe, it's smart to buy seaweed from companies that regularly test their products to ensure low levels of dangerous contaminants.

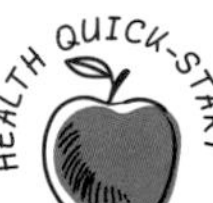

Here are some ways to incorporate more seaweed into your diet:

- *Make a delicious seaweed salad.*
- *Use dulse flakes as a salty, flavorful seasoning or mix into salad dressing.*
- *Put strips of seaweed such as kombu in soups and stews.*
- *Switch to a salt enriched with sea vegetables.*
- *Mix soaked, softened seaweed into land-vegetable salads for a unique flavor addition.*
- *Make your own sushi with nori.*
- *Choose seaweed snacks at the health food store (made with olive oil, not corn or canola oil—check the ingredients!).*

WILD EDIBLES

With so many vegetables and fruits available at most grocery stores, why would we bother foraging for food? Many of us have super-busy lives and limited time to prepare our food, much less go outside and gather it with our own hands! But collecting wild edibles is a rewarding experience, not only for the sense of accomplishment (and the perks that come from getting outside in nature; see Chapter 29), but also for the incredible nutritional benefits that foraged foods bring.

Studies of wild foods almost universally show that they're higher in micronutrients than their cultivated counterparts, especially when it comes to vitamin C, copper, calcium, sodium, potassium, and iron. In fact, hunter-gatherers and free-living primates (whose plant-food intake is 100 percent wild) can achieve intakes of certain vitamins and minerals that would be impossible for most of us to reach on a cultivated-food diet unless we were also taking supplements. For instance, even without dairy, it's estimated that early humans consumed about twice as much calcium as we do today, thanks in large part to a diverse intake of nutrient-dense foraged plants.

Plus, wild foods tend to be incredibly high in many phytochemicals (see page 35). Because wild foods don't have the assistance of external pesticides, herbicides, fungicides, greenhouses, or other man-made tools to protect them from predators, the plants are forced to ramp up their innate defense systems—including producing secondary metabolites like polyphenols, phenolic acid, flavonoids, organosulfur compounds, tannins, isothiocyanates, and other compounds that help protect them from pathogens and predators (while also hugely benefitting human health when we eat them).

So what easy-to-find wild foods can give us these micronutrient and phytochemical benefits? Here are some of the most common varieties:

WILD GREENS: The idea that we have to pay a lot of money for high-quality organic greens is a myth. In most regions, you only have to wander around the block to find a patch of delicious, nutrient-dense wild greens to throw into salads, pestos, side dishes, and other kitchen concoctions, for free. For example, check out these frequently spotted varieties:

- **Dandelion.** What do dandelions give us apart from extra yardwork? Tons of nutrition, for one! A single cup of dandelion greens contains 535 percent of the Recommended Dietary Allowance (RDA) for vitamin K, 112 percent for vitamin A (in the form of vitamin A precursors), 32 percent for vitamin C, and about 10 percent for vitamin E, calcium, iron, and manganese. And the buds and yellow flowers are edible, too. Not bad for a plant that most of us want to get rid of!

- **Nasturtium.** These plants have edible, peppery-tasting leaves and flowers and are a great addition to salads or pickled foods. Rich in vitamin C and iron, they frequently grow in city and suburban environments and are often used in gardens since they help protect other plants from predatory insects.

- **Clover.** Clover is a common sight in backyards and natural areas in most parts of the U.S. The entire plant—leaves, roots, and blossoms—is edible, although the flowers are the most palatable for most people. Clover is rich in calcium, magnesium, chromium, niacin, phosphorus, potassium, vitamin C, thiamine, and isoflavones. In fact, ongoing research is studying the effects of clover isoflavones on osteoporosis, menopausal symptoms, cancer, and cardiovascular disease.

- **Wood sorrel.** Wood sorrel is an edible weed often mistaken for clover; the main difference is that wood sorrel has heart-shaped leaves, like the iconic Irish shamrock, whereas clover has rounded leaves. Growing throughout most of North America, wood sorrel has a lemony flavor and an impressive vitamin C content. Some varieties of sorrel were used by sailors to avoid scurvy.

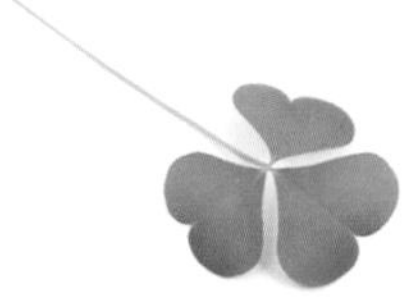

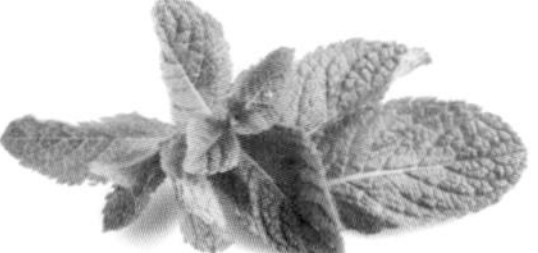

· **Mint.** Mint is a great wild edible because it's so easy to identify: rub a leaf between your fingers and take a whiff! Spearmint, peppermint, and other mint varieties are commonly found growing in yards, between rocks, on hillsides, in fields, and in both rural and urban areas in most regions of the country. And mint (especially peppermint) ranks high on the list of polyphenol-rich foods, enhancing its already impressive nutrient profile; iron, β-carotene, vitamin B9, vitamin C, calcium, and manganese are abundant.

· **Lamb's-quarter (wild spinach).** A common weed throughout moderate-climate regions, lamb's-quarter is one of the most nutritious leafy greens known—with even higher levels of β-carotene, lutein, fiber, vitamin C, calcium, zinc, copper, manganese, and vitamin B2 than its cousin, domesticated spinach. It's also up to four times higher in potassium than common green vegetables like Swiss chard and broccoli, with 1,286 milligrams per 100 grams by some analyses.

OTHER WILD VEGETABLES: The list of forage-worthy vegetables doesn't end with leafy dark greens. Other common wild vegetables include:

· **Wild garlic and onions.** Members of the *Allium* genus (and cousins of the familiar store-bought varieties), wild garlic and onions are a treasure to find outside—and often you can smell them before you see them! All parts of the plant are edible (the underground bulbs, the flowers, and the leaves), and, like other alliums, they're rich in anti-cancer allylsulfides and organosulfur compounds.

· **Cattails.** Cattails are a common sight in wetlands, pond edges, and even wet gutters along the side of the road. And they happen to be a great wild edible! Their starchy roots, called rhizomes, can be peeled, cooked, and eaten just like potatoes, and the corms (small stubs near the base) can be peeled and eaten either raw or cooked. Depending on the time of year, the shoots, flower heads, and hotdog-like pollen heads can also be consumed.

· **Nopales (prickly pear cactus).** Hot, dry climates might seem like hard places to forage, but even the desert is home to wild edibles—great news if you live in the southwestern United States or other arid areas! Nopales are a common cactus characterized by flat, oval-shaped pads and oblong fruit (typically reddish purple), with a high content of vitamin C, magnesium, calcium, fiber, copper, and potassium. Both the pads and the fruit are edible once they've been dethorned and peeled. Warning: Nopales are covered in needlelike spikes and smaller spines called glochids, so they're best gathered with thick gloves!

WILD MUSHROOMS: Any attempt at collecting wild mushrooms needs to come with a disclaimer! There are many poisonous look-alikes that resemble edible mushrooms, including those detailed below, and harvesting the wrong kind can quickly result in a hospital visit, a liver transplant, or worse (yes, I do mean death!). If you aren't an experienced collector who is 100 percent confident about distinguishing safe mushrooms from hazardous ones, there are mushroom-hunting clubs, expert-led expeditions, and even local classes that offer safe mushroom-hunting adventures without the risk of misidentification.

That said, wild mushrooms are rich in protein, fiber, micronutrients, and unique meaty flavors. Their distinctive tastes and versatility in the kitchen make them well worth the effort to collect. Favorites among mushroom hunters include:

· **Morels.** Morels are distinctive, spongy-looking mushrooms with a nutty, steak-like flavor. One hundred grams of raw morels contains the following RDA percentages: 25 percent of vitamin B3, 21 percent of vitamin B2, 13 percent of vitamin B5, 12 percent of copper, 12 percent of phosphorus, and 12 percent of potassium. Morels are available in almost every U.S. state except for Arizona and Florida and are typically ready to harvest in early spring before the trees leaf out.

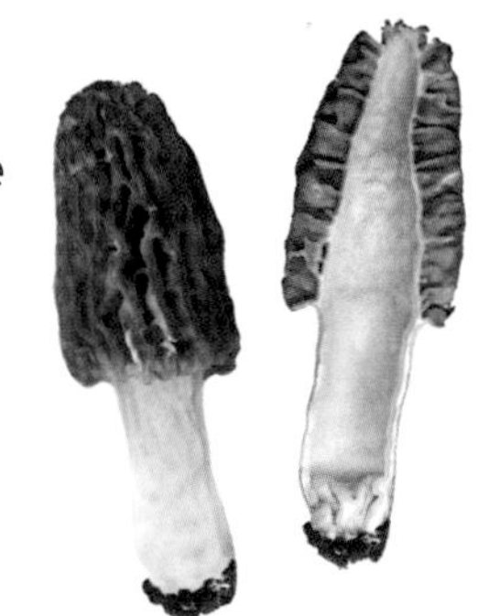

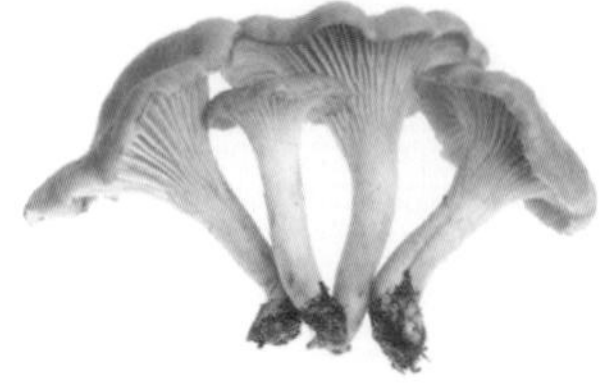

· **Chanterelles.** Chanterelles are highly prized yellow, trumpet-shaped mushrooms with a meaty texture and a distinctive flavor. When I was a child, my family would select late-summer campsites for vacations based on proximity to good chanterelle-collecting locations. They contain an impressive amount of vitamins B2, B3, and B5, as well as potassium, iron, copper, and fiber. They're also one of the richest sources of vitamin D that we know of, with concentrations of D2 as high as 212 IU per 100 grams of raw chanterelle. Chanterelles are available on the East Coast for most of the summer and into the fall and on the West Coast from September to February.

· **Oyster mushrooms.** Wild oyster mushrooms are a gold mine for micronutrients like vitamins B2, B3, B5, and B6, along with iron, phosphorus, potassium, copper, manganese, zinc, magnesium, and selenium. Typically found growing on dead hardwood trees in shelflike formations, these mushrooms are great for wild-edible beginners because they're easy to identify and don't have any poisonous look-alikes. Oyster mushrooms are available year-round and throughout most of the country but pop up most often in cooler weather.

· **Puffballs.** Puffballs earned their name because when they're ready to release their spores, the cap splits and a cloud of brown dustlike spores "puffs" out. (They're fun to step on when they're ready to release their spores!) Most puffballs are edible, though not all. The giant puffball, which grows unbidden in lawns, meadows, and deciduous woods across North America, especially where summers are humid, reaches a foot or more in diameter and is difficult to mistake for any other fungus. If collected before spores have formed, while the flesh is still white, puffballs have a delightful strong earthy flavor and can be cooked in a huge variety of ways. They are rich in heart-healthy oleic acid (a fatty acid), iron, magnesium, copper, potassium, selenium, zinc, B vitamins, vitamin K, and vitamin D2. Puffballs are another fall-harvest mushroom but are only good before the spores form inside the cap.

WILD FRUITS: Wild fruits are generally higher in glucose and fructose (as well as fiber) and richer in micronutrients than cultivated fruits, which tend to be sucrose-dominated. And because wild fruits tend to be smaller than their domesticated counterparts, they have a higher skin-to-pulp ratio—giving them greater levels of certain phytochemicals concentrated in the skin. When they're in season, they're fantastic foods to forage.

· **Wild berries.** The list of wild edible berries is a long one! Huckleberries, salmonberries, salal, strawberries, blackberries, blueberries, cranberries, mulberries, gooseberries, and raspberries are just a few. Depending on the region and the time of year, different berry varieties can be growing as weeds in the backyard (think blackberries), as ornamental shrubbery (like strawberries and salal), near swamps and marshes (like cranberries), along trails in the forest (like salmonberries and huckleberries), and in various other environments. Although the nutritional profile varies depending on the type, wild berries are generally higher in vitamins, minerals, and phytonutrients than cultivated berries. They also pack a punch of flavor that can't be beat!

· **Muscadine grapes.** These delicious (but seedy and thick-skinned!) grapes grow wild in well-drained lands, especially in warm, humid environments. They're rich in a variety of polyphenols, including resveratrol, quercetin, ellagic acid, kaempferol, flavan-3-ols, gallic acid, and proanthocyanidins. And they're super-high in manganese (100 grams of muscadines delivers over 100 percent of the RDA), along with some copper, potassium, magnesium, and calcium.

· **Crabapples**. Crabapple trees commonly line city streets and drop their bounty into backyards, covering the ground with small, tart fruit in late summer and early fall. Although they're not as sweet and juicy as cultivated apple varieties, crabapples are definitely edible! They are a good source of vitamin C, potassium, manganese, copper, and fiber, and due to their small size (and higher ratio of skin to pulp), they're richer than domesticated apples in quercetin, a flavonoid with antihistamine and anti-inflammatory properties.

Gathering wild edibles is *so* worth it! It's a great way to save money, spend time outdoors, and boost your diet with an incredible array of micronutrients and phytochemicals—which translates to enhanced disease protection, immunity, and overall better health.

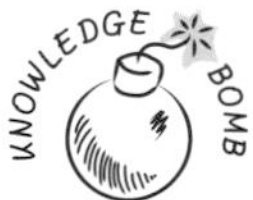

Wild mushrooms are awesome, but so are cultivated store-bought varieties! They provide good amounts of vitamins B1, B2, B3, B5, B6, C, and D, as well as chromium, copper, phosphorus, potassium, selenium, and sulfur.

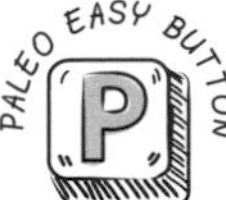

When it's time to forage, a huge number of field guides, online tutorials, and region-specific manuals await! Nearby woodlands, parks, forest trails, undeveloped land, vacant lots, marshes, roadsides, and even backyards are excellent places to find wild edibles. The website fallingfruit.org offers an interactive map with hundreds of thousands of wild fruit and vegetable locations across the world, making it easy to see what might be around the corner.

IS FRUIT JUST NATURE'S CANDY?

Even though fruit provides many of the same important vitamins, minerals, and phytonutrients as vegetables, should we be wary of eating too much fruit because of its sugar, especially fructose, content? This is a common concern that makes many people reluctant to consume fruit. With mounting research suggesting that fructose is a major player in chronic disease epidemics (see page 269), the resulting fructose phobia has caused many people to limit fruit or avoid it altogether.

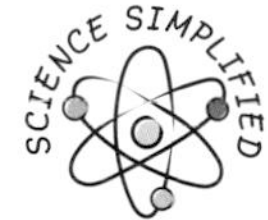

Whole fresh fruits are a healthy choice, provided that you limit your consumption to two to five servings per day.

Fructose increases blood triglyceride concentrations (increasing the risk of cardiovascular disease) and, when ingested in large amounts as part of a high-calorie diet, causes insulin resistance, stimulates appetite, and causes weight gain. In fact, the consumption of large amounts of fructose has been conclusively linked to obesity, type 2 diabetes, and cardiovascular disease. In addition, high sugar and/or fructose consumption causes micronutrient deficiencies, notably vitamin D, calcium, magnesium, chromium, and vitamin C. The health detriment of excessive fructose consumption is discussed in detail in Chapter 22.

But the fears surrounding fruit are almost all unfounded. Fruit is *not* a fructose bomb, and when consumed in reasonable amounts, its sugar content is not likely to be harmful.

Contrary to popular belief, fructose isn't the only type of sugar in fruit—and in some cases, it's not even the *main* type of sugar in fruit. All fruit contains a mixture of fructose, glucose, and sucrose (which is metabolized into equal parts fructose and glucose in our bodies). And each type of fruit has a different proportion of these sugars.

For example, papayas, grapes, and most berries are about half fructose and half glucose. Grapefruit is about a quarter fructose and a quarter glucose, with the rest coming from sucrose. And when we calculate total metabolic fructose (the fructose in the fruit when we eat it, plus the fructose that gets cleaved from sucrose molecules during digestion), most fruit yields roughly equal parts fructose and glucose.

This is great news! While fructose has to be processed in the liver, glucose is used directly by our cells for energy and doesn't pose the same metabolic consequences as extremely high fructose intake (nonalcoholic fatty liver, lipogenesis, and inflammation). But a little dietary fructose has some great health benefits, like improving glycogen repletion after a workout. Plus, fruit contains vitamins, minerals, and phytochemicals needed to process their sugars and mitigate potential damaging effects. Combined with the fact that fresh fruit is rich in fiber and water and takes up plenty of stomach space, it's hard to eat enough fruit to ingest the levels of fructose shown to cause harm in rodent studies and epidemiology. (The toxicity threshold is above 50 grams daily.)

In other words, eating multiple servings of fruit each day is nowhere *near* comparable to downing fast-

GUIDE TO FRESH FRUITS

Aim for less than 40 grams of fructose per day, and ideally between 10 and 20 grams. This generally equates to two to five servings of fresh fruit.

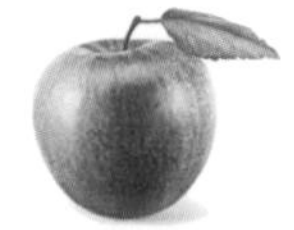

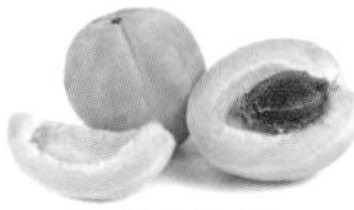

Fruit	Serving Size	Calories	Total Carbs (g)	Fiber (g)	Sugars (g)	Sucrose (g)	Glucose (g)	Fructose (g)	Total Metabolic Fructose (g)	Glycemic Load
APPLE	100 g (1 medium = 182 g)	52	13.8	2.4	10.4	2.1	2.4	5.9	6.9	3
APRICOT	100 g (1 cup halves = 155 g)	48	11.2	2.0	9.2	5.9	2.4	0.9	3.9	4
BANANA	100 g (1 medium = 118 g)	89	22.8	2.6	12.2	2.4	5.0	4.9	6.0	8
BLACKBERRIES	100 g (1 cup = 144 g)	43	10.2	5.3	4.9	0.1	2.3	2.4	2.4	3
BLUEBERRIES	100 g (1 cup = 148 g)	57	14.5	2.4	10	0.1	4.9	5.0	5.0	4
CANTALOUPE	100 g (1 cup diced = 156 g)	34	8.8	0.9	7.9	4.4	1.5	19	4.0	3
CHERRIES	100 g (1 cup pitted = 154 g)	63	16	2.1	12.8	0.2	6.6	5.4	5.4	5
GRAPEFRUIT, PINK	100 g (1/2 fruit = 123 g)	42	10.7	1.6	6.9	3.5	1.6	1.8	3.5	3
GRAPES	100 g (1 cup = 151 g)	69	18.1	0.9	15.5	0.2	7.2	8.1	8.2	6
HONEYDEW	100 g (1 cup diced = 170 g)	36	9.1	0.8	8.1	2.5	2.7	3.0	4.2	2
KIWI	100 g (1 medium without skin = 76 g)	61	14.7	3.0	9.0	0.2	4.1	4.4	4.4	4
MANGO	100 g (1 cup sliced = 165 g)	65	17	1.8	13.7	7.0	2.0	4.7	8.2	5
NECTARINE	100 g (1 medium = 143 g)	44	10.6	1.7	7.9	4.9	1.6	1.4	3.8	3
ORANGE, NAVEL	100 g (1 cup sections = 168 g)	49	12.5	2.2	8.5	4.3	2.0	2.3	4.4	4
PEACH	100 g (1 medium = 150 g)	39	9.9	1.5	8.4	4.8	2.0	1.5	3.9	3
PEAR	100 g (1 medium = 178 g)	58	15.5	3.1	9.8	0.8	2.8	6.2	6.6	3
PINEAPPLE	100 g (1 cup chunks = 165 g)	50	13.1	1.4	9.8	6.0	1.7	2.1	5.1	3
PLUM	100 g (one 2 1/8-inch-diameter fruit = 66 g)	46	11.4	1.4	9.9	1.6	5.1	3.1	3.9	3
RASPBERRIES	100 g (1 cup = 123 g)	52	11.9	6.5	4.4	0.2	1.9	2.4	2.5	2
STRAWBERRIES	100 g (1 cup halves = 152 g)	32	7.7	2.0	4.9	0.5	2.0	2.4	2.7	2
TANGERINE	100 g (1 medium = 88 g)	53	13.3	1.8	10.6	6.0	2.1	2.4	5.4	4
WATERMELON	100 g (1 cup diced = 152 g)	30	7.5	0.4	6.2	1.2	1.6	3.4	4.0	2

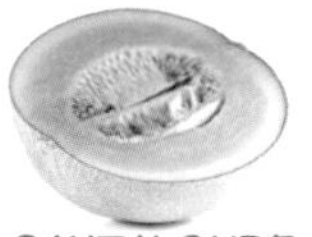

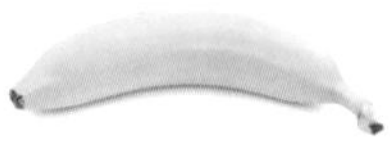

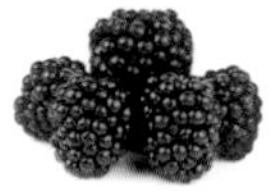

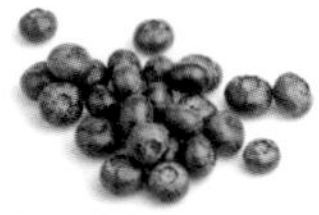

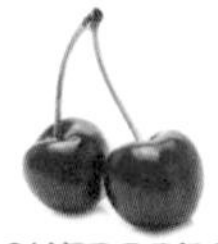

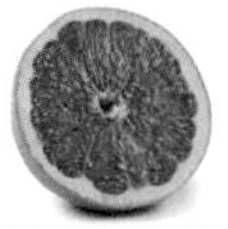

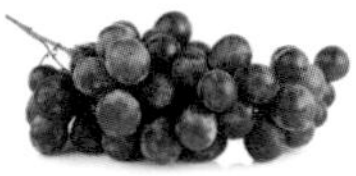

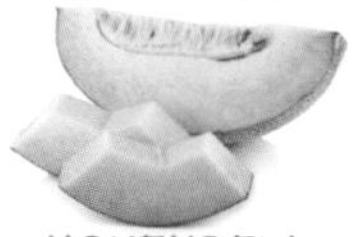

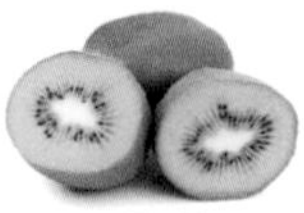

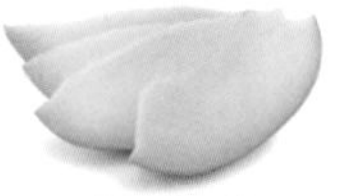

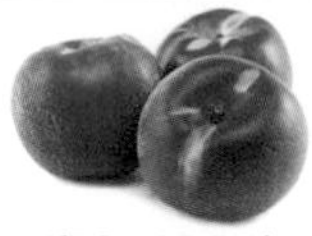

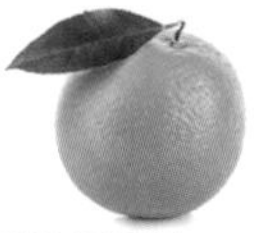

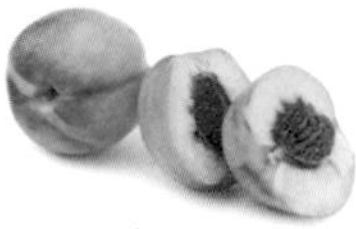

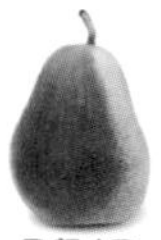

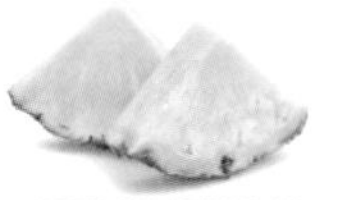

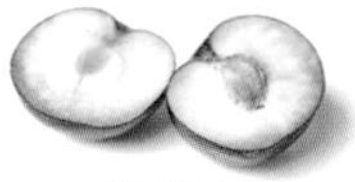

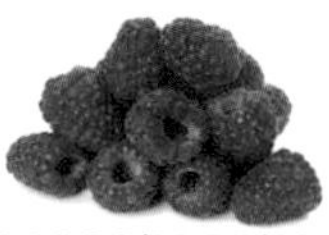

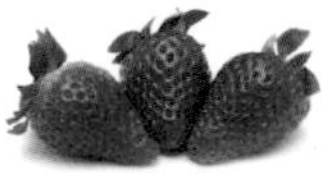

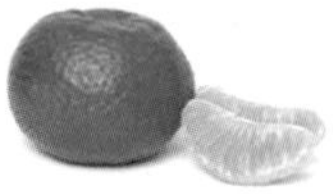

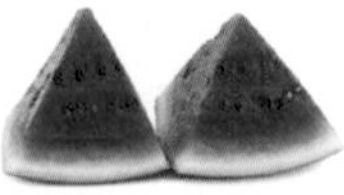

Source: USDA Food Composition Database

digesting high-fructose corn syrup-sweetened sodas and eating packaged foods loaded with fructose-rich sweeteners.

As I will discuss in detail in Chapter 22, less than 40 grams of fructose per day from whole-food sources is a great target. For reference, that's what you'd get from 1½ whole mangoes, 3½ apples, or 5½ cups of blueberries! Yes, two to five servings of fruit per day (closer to two if you choose higher-fructose-content fruits like mangoes versus five if you choose lower-fructose fruits like berries) is perfectly fine! (*Note:* Starchy veggies and fruits like plantains also contain some fructose. If you're worried that you might be eating too much, try keeping a food journal for a few days.)

PALEO EASY BUTTON

Berries are not only lower in sugar than other fruits, but they're also especially high in vitamins, minerals, antioxidant phytochemicals, and fiber. They're a great choice every day!

All that said, the optimal quantity of fruit for you depends on a host of factors: whether you're dealing with nutrient deficiencies (especially vitamin D); whether you're trying to lose or gain weight; whether you have fructose intolerance or gut dysbiosis that might require limiting high-FODMAP fruits (like mangoes, red apples, watermelon, and papaya; see pages 434 and 435); and whether fruit is satiating or is more like an appetite stimulant. This is serious one-size-does-*not*-fit-all territory, and as a result, there's no universal prescription for fruit intake. But one thing's for sure: there's no reason to avoid fruit on account of it being unhealthy, nutrient-poor, or worthless on the disease protection front. It's a fantastic carbohydrate source that deserves more love than it's been getting lately! And it certainly has a place within the Paleo framework as a health-promoting food.

PALEO STARCHES

It wasn't long ago that potatoes, yams, plantains, cassava, and other starchy foods were considered no-nos on the Paleo diet. This was due largely to the belief that high-starch foods spike blood sugar, promote weight gain, and contribute to chronic disease, along with the notion that such foods would have been scarce in the Paleolithic era and couldn't have made up a substantial portion of early human diets.

Fortunately, the Paleo framework continues to evolve in response to the latest science, and we now know that these beliefs are far from the truth! As it turns out, Paleo starches contain a special type of fiber called resistant starch (see page 43) while also providing some of the same phytochemicals as vegetables and fruits and serving as rich sources of certain micronutrients. Not only that, but some anthropological analyses position starches as central to human evolution!

Starches in Human History

Although meat gets plenty of attention for its role in human evolution, plant foods have also played an important and sustained part. One theory for the change in brain and gut size seen in *Homo erectus* (see page 56) has to do with the consumption of more starchy plant foods, especially in the form of underground storage organs (USOs).

Underground storage organs are starchy plant components like bulbs, tubers, rhizomes, and corms. They store water and carbohydrates for the plant to use but are also a highly nutritious and energy-dense food for humans. Our ancestors gathered and consumed USOs for a few million years before the dawn of agriculture, and USOs may have contributed to a significant plant-derived calorie intake even during the Paleolithic era.

Researcher Richard Wrangham is the leading voice for the theory that our crazy-big brains and relatively small guts developed not from eating more meat, but from eating more starchy USOs. And the evidence behind that theory is pretty interesting. Changes in our dental shape coincided with a shift toward using USOs as a fallback food, and the ecology of USOs suggests that they would have been plentiful in the environments that early humans inhabited. Homo fossils are often found near shallow-water or flooded habitats (where aquatic USO density is high) and where another brain-growth-spurring treat—aquatic creatures rich in DHA—frequently live. Collectively, the evidence suggests that even if animal foods played a significant role in our past, the claim that "meat is what made us human" (and we're therefore more aligned with carnivores) might not be accurate. It could be theorized that starches were critical in shaping our anatomical destiny.

Safe Starches

As discussed in Part 1, starchy roots and tubers are nutrient-dense sources of slow-burning low-glycemic-load carbohydrates and fiber. Another term for these types of foods that has gained plenty of scientific and anecdotal traction is "safe starches."

The term "safe starch" was introduced by Paul and Shou-Ching Jaminet in their book *Perfect Health Diet* and refers to any starchy food that, after being properly prepared, is low in fructose and relatively free from natural toxins, like lectins, saponins, and gluten and related proteins. Safe starches help supply energy in the form of slow-burning carbohydrates without exposing us to damaging plant proteins and other compounds implicated in certain health conditions, including leaky gut and autoimmunity. And it's not a novel concept: hunter-gatherer societies around the world consume starchy plant foods, and there's ample evidence that starchy underground storage organs played an important role in early hominid nutrition.

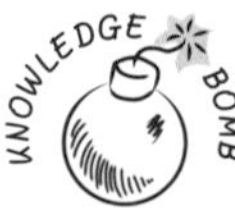

Studies show that including a serving or two of a starchy veggie with dinner can help improve sleep!

Safe starches include the following:

- *Cassava*
- *Plantains*
- *Sweet potatoes*
- *Tapioca*
- *Taro*
- *White potatoes (see page 298)*
- *White rice (see page 302)*
- *Yams*
- *Yuca*
- *Other heirloom tubers*

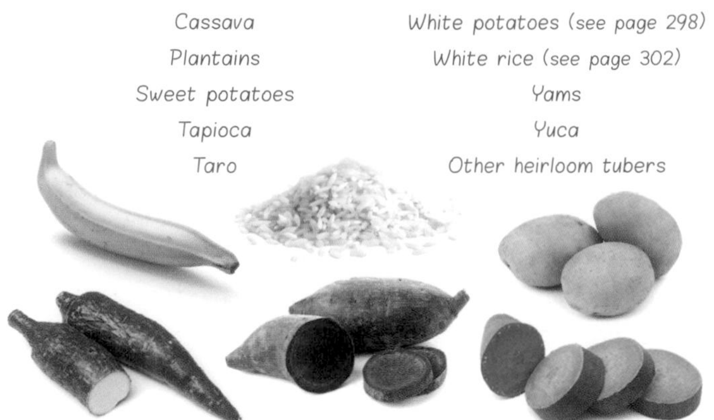

Note that white potatoes and white rice are middle-ground foods, discussed in more detail in Chapter 24. Non-rice grains and legumes are *not* considered safe starches due to their higher concentrations of lectins and other antinutrients (see page 230). And even though they do contain some starch, sweeter root veggies like carrots and beets are in a separate category.

So what are the benefits of safe starches? Consuming adequate amounts of these foods—the typical recommendation is about a pound of cooked safe starch per day, or about 400 calories' worth—helps us meet our physiological glucose needs, supports thyroid health (see page 93), supplies a range of micronutrients (see page 25), and can help us maintain adequate mucus production to lubricate our eyes, mouth, and intestines (mucus is made from glycoproteins, which can be broken down for gluconeogenesis when our carbohydrate intake is extremely low). In addition, Paleo starches provide a wide spectrum of nutrients, such as carotenoids (one medium sweet potato has over 400 percent of the RDA for vitamin A), vitamin C, potassium, magnesium, manganese, and a variety of B vitamins (see page 87 for more healthy Paleo carbs).

But there's another huge perk of safe starches: their potential impact on our gut microbiota (see page 70). Whole-food, Paleo-friendly starches are rich in fermentable fibers, including resistant starch (I'll get to that next), that bypass digestion in the small intestine and go directly to the hungry microbes in the colon. Certain bacteria strains then ferment these fibers into short-chain fatty acids (especially butyric acid) that are highly beneficial for our bodies and may even help reduce our risk of colon cancer. A huge body of research is confirming that the types of fiber in safe starches can have a positive effect on our gut health.

Many people are concerned that starchy veggies can raise blood sugar due to their higher glycemic index, but this doesn't seem to be the case. For one, glycemic load is a more important measurement of a food's impact on blood sugar and roots and tubers tend to have low to moderate glycemic loads (see page 88). We can also easily reduce the glycemic impact of starchy foods by including them in a meal with other ingredients (especially fat or protein), eating them with vinegar or other acidic foods, or increasing the fiber content of the meal (such as by adding some leafy greens). All these methods can reduce the post-meal blood glucose response to safe starches and keep blood sugar more stable. What's more, studies have found that certain safe starches (like potatoes) and their components (like resistant starch) score high on the satiety index and may even have an appetite-suppressing effect.

Except when specific health conditions are involved (like certain neurological conditions that benefit from nutritional ketosis, or diabetes, where carbohydrate intake may need to be closely monitored), it's clear that whole-food carbohydrates are beneficial. But some safe starches might not be safe for everyone. For example, white potatoes (and other nightshades) contain glycoalkaloids, especially solanine, that can trigger symptoms in people with certain health conditions, like autoimmune diseases or leaky gut. (I'll talk more about that on page 298.) White rice is more likely to be tolerated than other grains, and removing the hull eliminates most of the problematic antinutrients, but it can be gluten cross-reactive in some people with gluten sensitivity (see page 245). And the high oxalate content of sweet potatoes could aggravate joint pain in susceptible people, so it may be wise not to eat too many.

While "safe starch" might be the latest buzzword for Paleo sources of slow-burning carbohydrates, there's no doubt that starchy foods like roots and tubers (and potentially potatoes and white rice, if tolerated) are an important cornerstone for a nutrient-dense Paleo diet.

KNOWLEDGE BOMB *Heard of the trend of adding raw potato starch to your morning smoothie? Turns out it's not a good idea—it could increase tumor growth and feed gut dysbiosis. Instead, look for whole-food sources of resistant starch, like root veggies.*

Resistant Starch

Resistant starch is a type of insoluble fiber that, unlike most starches, isn't fully broken down in the small intestine. It "resists" the action of our digestive enzymes because of its molecular structure and instead becomes food for specific types of bacteria in the colon, which ferment it to produce beneficial short-chain fatty acids like acetic acid, propionic acid, and butyric acid. There are four main categories of resistant starch:

- **RS1** resists digestion because it's trapped by intact plant cell walls. It is found in legumes, grains, and seeds.
- **RS2** is protected from digestion because of its molecular structure and becomes accessible to human digestive enzymes only after being cooked. This one's found in raw potatoes, green bananas, and raw plantains.
- **RS3**, also called retrograded starch, forms when certain starchy foods, such as potatoes, rice, and other grains, are cooled after they've been cooked.
- **RS4** are chemically modified starches that don't occur in nature, but are created to resist digestion.

Recall that fiber (both soluble and insoluble) has been linked to reduced risk of diabetes, heart disease, and multiple cancers; can help quell inflammation; and helps protect against many gut pathologies (see page 39). However, resistant starch in particular—which is far more concentrated in tubers and other starchy plant parts—is unique in its effects on the gut microbiota and on health in general. Both human and animal studies have confirmed a number of legitimate benefits of resistant starch, including improved insulin sensitivity (and lower blood sugar responses after high-carb meals), reduced hunger/better satiation, improved blood lipids, and even better immunity (due to the influence of resistant starch on immune cell production and inflammatory compounds in the gut). In fact, the reduction in resistant starch-rich foods may be a major reason low-carbohydrate diets tend to alter the gut microbiota in unfavorable ways.

So far, the science suggests that resistant starch, especially RS2, exerts the most benefits when consumed with additional fermentable carbohydrates, soluble fibers that add fecal bulk, and perhaps other dietary components that enhance its positive effects. That means consuming resistant starch in the form in which it naturally occurs: whole foods! Although supplementing with resistant starch (typically in the form of raw potato starch) is becoming more popular, there's actually some science to suggest that supplementing with concentrated sources of resistant starch may enhance tumor growth and feed gut dysbiosis. The best solution? Eat resistant starch where it naturally occurs! Cooked and cooled potatoes, raw green bananas, plantains, yams, and other root vegetables provide not only resistant starch, but also a variety of other fibers and micronutrients that benefit health.

HOW MUCH IS A SERVING?

The standard vegetable and fruit serving size established by the World Health Organization in 2005, and used in most scientific studies evaluating benefits of high vegetable and fruit consumption, is defined as 80 grams raw, or just shy of 3 ounces. This roughly translates to:

1/2 cup cooked vegetables

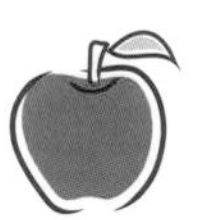

1 medium fruit (about the size of a baseball)

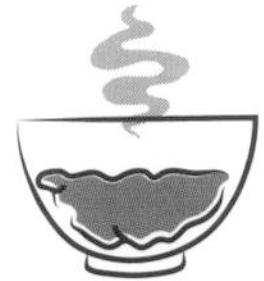

1/2 cup cooked fruit

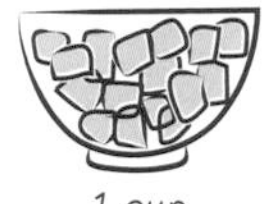

1 cup raw vegetables

80 GRAMS

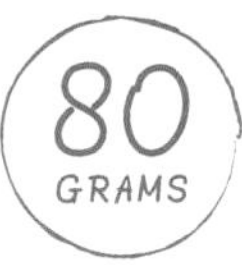

1/2 cup chopped fruit or whole berries

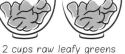

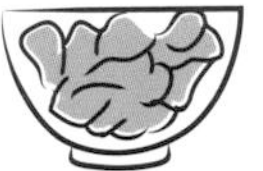

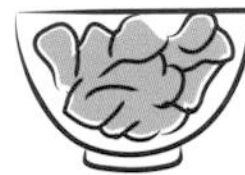

2 cups raw leafy greens

What About Potatoes?

For years, potatoes have had a reputation for being an empty-calorie, high-glycemic food, leading many people to limit their consumption or even avoid them entirely. Along with their perceived lack of nutrition, potatoes are often considered "not Paleo" due to their high starch content and naturally occurring toxins, especially glycoalkaloids. But potatoes aren't as bad as they're sometimes made out to be.

The belief that potatoes deliver empty calories probably stems from the fact that they're white and high in carbohydrates, similar to true "empty-calorie" foods like refined flour and refined sugar. But this claim couldn't be further from the truth. A single plain baked potato contains only 161 calories and boasts a huge array of micronutrients (in RDA percentages):

28% OF THE RDA FOR **vitamin C**

27% OF THE RDA FOR **vitamin B6**

26% OF THE RDA FOR **POTASSIUM**

19% OF THE RDA FOR **MANGANESE**

12% OF THE RDA FOR **MAGNESIUM**

12% OF THE RDA FOR **PHOSPHORUS**

12% OF THE RDA FOR **vitamin B3**

12% OF THE RDA FOR **vitamin B9**

10% OF THE RDA FOR **COPPER**

10% OF THE RDA FOR **IRON**

Smaller amounts of **vitamins B1, B2, B5, and K, ZINC, and CALCIUM**

That's actually more than *twice* as much potassium as a banana and more calcium than 3 cups of spinach. In terms of vitamin and mineral content, potatoes compare favorably to other root vegetables (like carrots, parsnips, rutabagas, and turnips).

Concerns about the glycemic index and glycoalkaloid content of potatoes (as well as other nightshades) *can* be legitimate, depending on the context. (For a more detailed look at these issues, see page 296.) For now, we can generalize that, barring certain health conditions, potatoes can be part of a Paleo diet, and the typical reason for avoiding them—their empty starchiness—is nothing to fear. Their micronutrient and resistant starch content makes them a valuable food for those who tolerate them.

Whether we're talking about potatoes or yams, cassava, plantains, or any other Paleo starch source, one thing is clear: we shouldn't fear these foods or minimize them on account of their carbohydrate content.

A NUTRIENT GUIDE TO VEGETABLES AND FRUITS

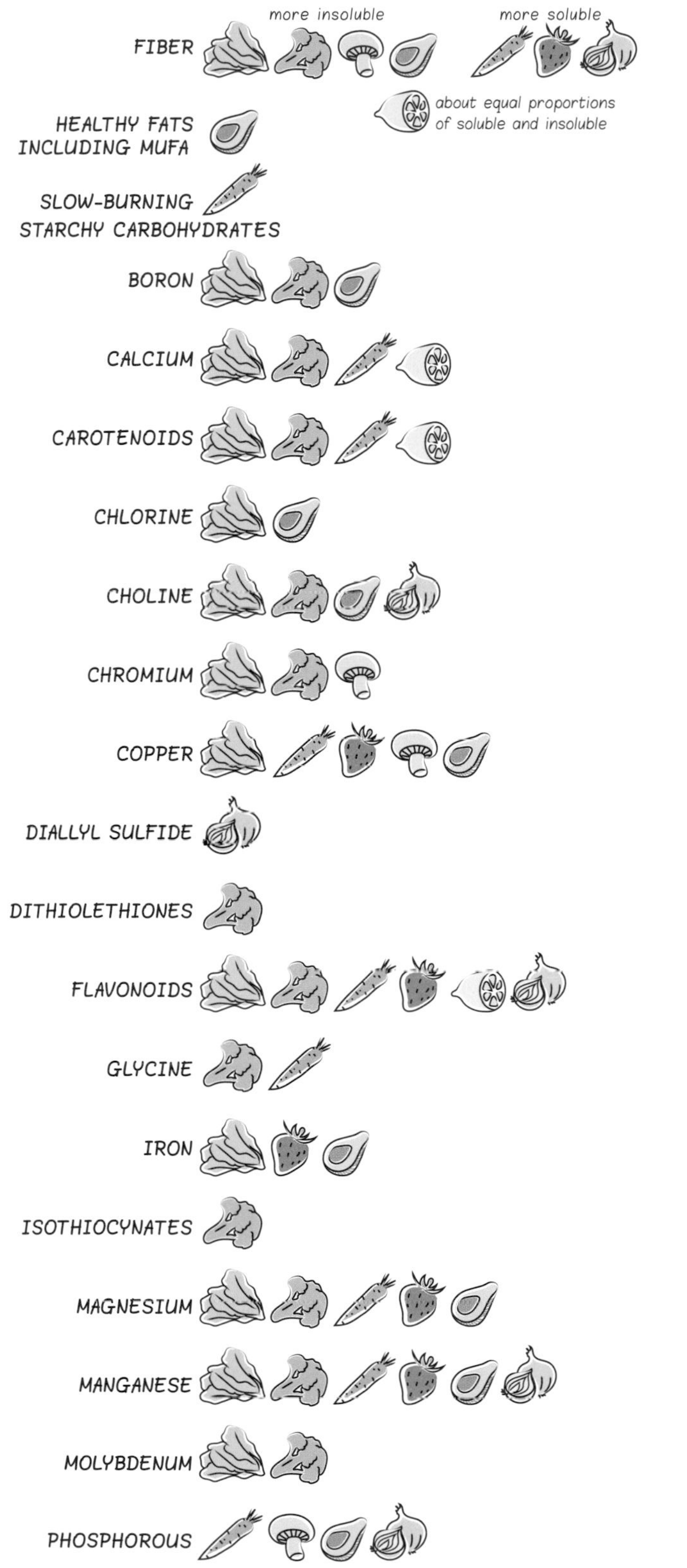

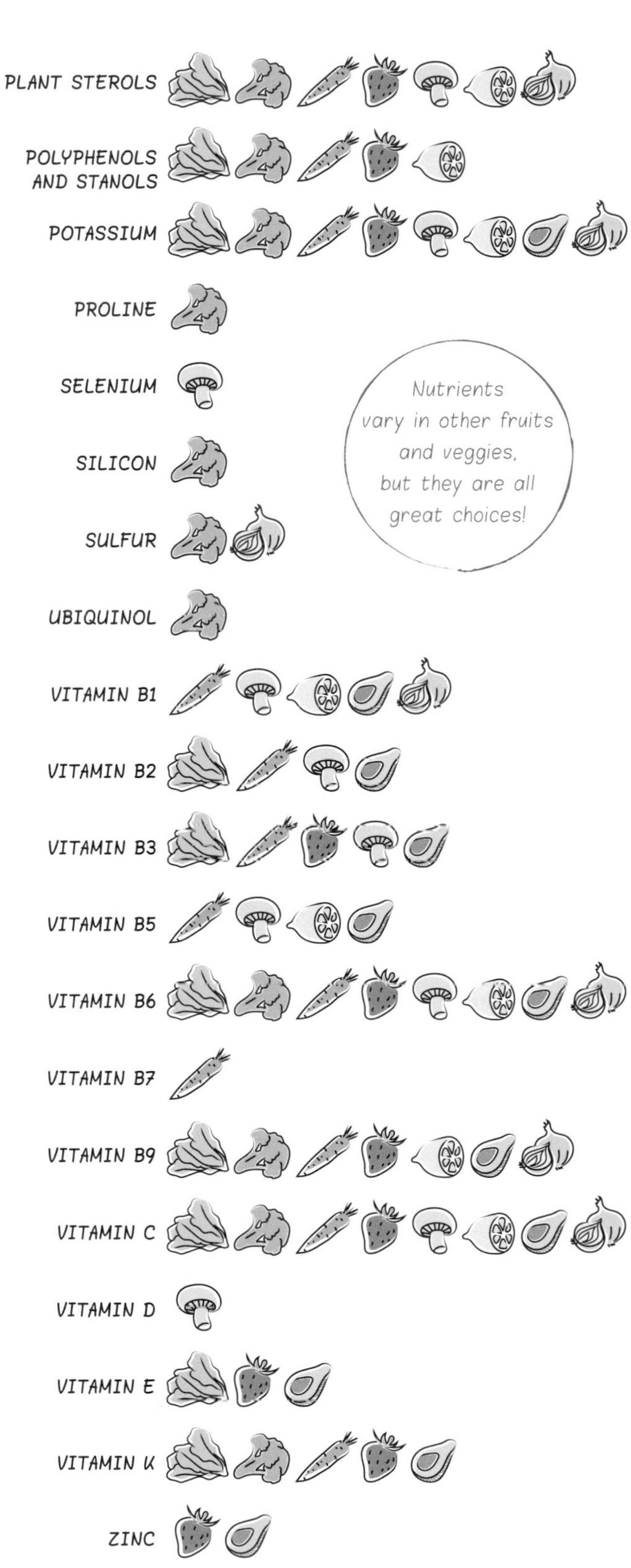

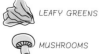

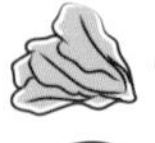
LEAFY GREENS

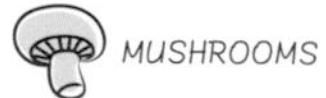
MUSHROOMS

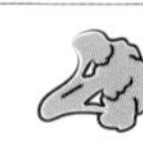
CRUCIFEROUS VEGETABLES

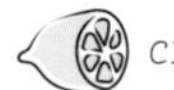
CITRUS FRUITS

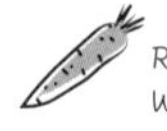
ROOT VEGETABLES AND WINTER SQUASH

OLIVES, AVOCADOS, AND OTHER HIGH-FAT FRUITS

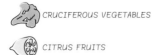

BERRIES

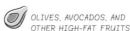

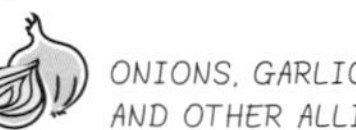
ONIONS, GARLIC, AND OTHER ALLIUMS

Chapter 9:
FISH AND SHELLFISH

Of all the animal products, seafood has one of the most consistently positive track records in the scientific literature. For one, fish and shellfish are the richest sources of the long-chain omega-3 fatty acids DHA and EPA, which block multiple inflammation pathways in our cells. Deficiencies in these anti-inflammatory omega-3 fats have been linked to dyslexia, violence, depression, anxiety, memory problems, Alzheimer's disease, weight gain, cancer, cardiovascular disease, stroke, eczema, allergies, asthma, inflammatory diseases, arthritis, diabetes, autoimmune diseases, and many others—so it's easy to see why getting enough of them is important. In fact, omega-3s have been confirmed in study after study to reduce our risk of many chronic diseases and chronic disease risk factors, such as high triglycerides.

Studies evaluating the role of dietary omega-3 fatty acids in human health show that the ratio of dietary omega-3 to omega-6 fats is far more important than the actual quantities of these fats, provided that we are eating enough fat to meet our basic needs. An ideal ratio is somewhere between 1:1 and 1:4. However, typical Western diets fall into a range between 1:10 and 1:25! This is largely thanks to processed vegetable oils, grains, and the higher levels of omega-6 fatty acids that are present in the meat and dairy from grain-fed animals.

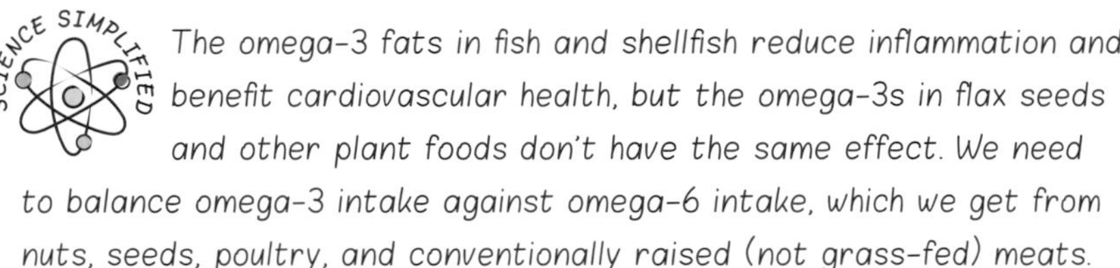

The omega-3 fats in fish and shellfish reduce inflammation and benefit cardiovascular health, but the omega-3s in flax seeds and other plant foods don't have the same effect. We need to balance omega-3 intake against omega-6 intake, which we get from nuts, seeds, poultry, and conventionally raised (not grass-fed) meats.

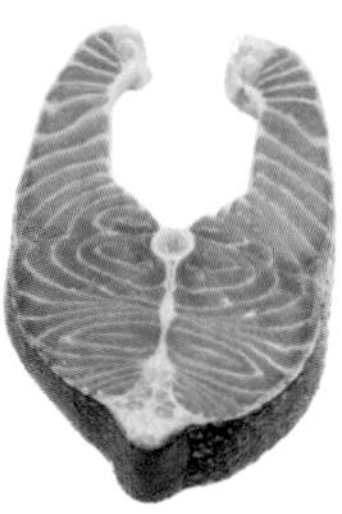

BENEFITS OF OMEGA-3 FATTY ACIDS AND OTHER NUTRIENTS IN SEAFOOD

The ratio of omega-3 to omega-6 fats is important because these two types of fat compete for many of the same functions in the body. In particular, the omega-6 fatty acid arachidonic acid (AA) competes against the omega-3 fatty acids DHA and EPA. Depending on which type of fat "wins," the effect is different. Within the outer membrane of every cell, various fatty acids and proteins are embedded, such as cholesterol molecules, receptors, and, yes, AA, DHA, and EPA. When incorporated into the membrane, DHA and EPA affect cell membrane properties, such as fluidity, flexibility, and permeability, and alter the activity of enzymes that are embedded in the membrane. These effects are beneficial to the health and function of the cell. And when needed, AA, DHA, and EPA can be internalized and metabolized into important signaling molecules (akin to short-distance hormones), called prostaglandins, thromboxanes, and leukotrienes, that control a variety of functions, including inflammation, clotting, vascular function and health, pain signaling, cell growth, kidney function, and stomach acid secretion.

HEALTH QUICK-START *Aim for three to five servings of fish or shellfish every week. This will not only help balance omega-3 to omega-6 intake, but also provide important fat-soluble vitamins and minerals that can be tough to get enough of from other foods.*

When diets contain predominantly omega-6 fatty acids, there is far more AA than DHA and EPA in the cell membranes. However, when diets are supplemented with omega-3 fatty acids, DHA and EPA can readily replace AA in the membranes of practically all cells. This is important because the prostaglandins, thromboxanes, and leukotrienes produced from AA are far more inflammatory and have other negative effects, like increasing pain, increasing thrombosis (clots forming in blood vessels, which can lead to things like deep vein thrombosis, stroke, and ischemic heart disease), and constricting blood vessels, which increases blood pressure. This is why fish oil supplements have proven so effective at reducing cardiovascular disease risk factors and reducing pain from diseases like rheumatoid arthritis.

The omega-3s that our bodies really need are DHA and EPA. The shorter-chain omega-3 fatty acid ALA, which is found in flax seeds, chia seeds, and walnuts, is not easily used by the body because it must (usually) first be converted to DHA or EPA, which is a very inefficient process. A 3½-ounce serving of oily coldwater fish like wild-caught salmon, sardines, albacore tuna, trout, or mackerel has more than 500 milligrams of DHA and EPA. Fish containing moderate amounts of DHA and EPA (150 to 500 milligrams per 3½-ounce serving) include most whitefish like bass, cod, haddock, hake, halibut, flounder, perch, and sole, as well as farmed salmon. Crab, oysters, and shrimp contain moderate amounts of DHA and EPA as well.

Why not just get DHA and EPA from fish oil supplements? These polyunsaturated fats are easily oxidized in response to heat or light and are not very shelf-stable, especially once isolated. Consuming oxidized omega-3 fats contributes to inflammation as opposed to reducing it. In fresh, frozen, or canned whole fish, the omega-3 fats are protected from oxidation, plus fish provides all the necessary cofactors for optimal absorption and use by the body.

Along with omega-3s, fish is high in protein, and research shows that the amino acids in fish are similarly bioavailable (our bodies can absorb and use them as readily) to those in beef, pork, and chicken. Fish also has balanced quantities of all the essential amino acids, giving the various types of fish high amino acid scores (a measure of protein quality).

Fish is also rich in two important minerals that can be challenging to get in sufficient quantities from other foods: iodine and selenium. Iodine (which is also rich in algae and seaweed) is vital for normal thyroid function (see page 93) but also extremely important for proper immune system function, wound healing, and fertility. Table salt is enriched with iodine due to rampant dietary iodine deficiency in the past (goiters were common before the advent of iodized salt). Since Paleo diets tend to be lower in salt—and many people switch to sea salt, which is not iodized—it is critical to consume food sources of this essential mineral.

Selenium is required for a class of enzymes called selenoenzymes, which are part of the body's natural protection against oxidants. Selenoenzymes are particularly important for protecting the brain against oxidative damage, but selenium deficiencies are also linked to thyroid disease, cardiovascular disease, and cancer.

Fish is also the best food source of vitamin D, which can also be found in organ meat but is generally hard to obtain from diet alone. People living far from the equator and/or in overcast climates may be particularly susceptible to vitamin D deficiency and incapable of obtaining enough of it through sun exposure, making dietary sources more important. Another way in which fish is an invaluable inclusion in our diet.

Which fish are best? Oily coldwater, wild-caught fish have the most omega-3 fatty acids and vitamin D. However, even freshwater whitefish are an excellent

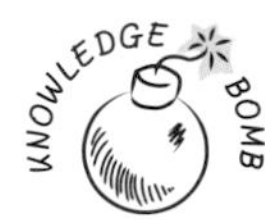

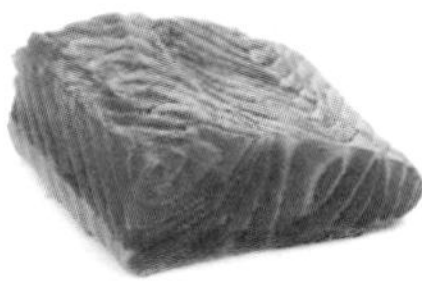

Fish supplies our bodies with some of the most digestible and bioavailable complete protein. In fact, all animal proteins are more easily digested than plant proteins (see page 169).

source of protein and omega-3s. The fish with the least favorable omega-3 to omega-6 ratio are farmed tilapia and farmed catfish, which have about a 1:1 ratio, as compared to a 300:1 ratio in salmon, but they still have that easily digested protein. And while fresh and frozen fish can be expensive, sardines, canned salmon, and other canned fish are great affordable options. Pickled herring and smoked kippers are often less expensive as well.

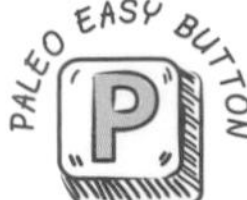

Canned fish is generally the most affordable, not to mention convenient—no cooking required and completely portable. Look for wild-caught varieties in BPA-free cans or pouches (see page 110).

SHELLFISH

Of course, finned fish aren't the only nutritious creatures from the sea. Shellfish—especially oysters, clams, and mussels—are among the most nutrient-dense foods on the planet. These foods are *bivalves,* a type of shellfish with a hinged two-part shell (called valves). They are found in both saltwater and freshwater environments and live everywhere from the tropics to the Arctic. They've been around since the early Cambrian Period (over 500 million years ago); today, more than 9,000 different species of bivalves live throughout the world.

From a biological standpoint, bivalves are fascinating creatures. They build their own ever-growing shells by secreting calcium carbonate, and some species have a retractable "foot" that helps them burrow into the ground or move around. They range in size from nearly microscopic to a whopping 4 feet long and 440 pounds: that honor goes to the aptly named giant clam. And they're comparable to organ meat as unbeatable sources of micronutrients!

In fact, bivalves have played an important role in the diets of coastal humans throughout history. When we look at their nutrient breakdown, it's easy to see why they've been such a prized, sought-out resource—and why they deserve a place of honor in the Paleo diet.

KNOWLEDGE BOMB

A mere 100 grams of oysters contains six times the RDA of zinc! Given that an estimated 73 percent of us aren't getting enough zinc and that it plays a fundamental role in our health (see page 27), a serving of oysters every week goes an incredibly long way toward supporting optimal health.

In general, bivalves tend to be rich in vitamin B12, highly digestible complete protein (as with fish), iron, zinc, copper, calcium, sodium, phosphorus, and selenium, as well as DHA and EPA. Some, like oysters, are a rich source of vitamin D, and others are off the charts for vitamin B12. (1,648 percent of the recommended daily allowance in clams? Yes, please!) But each bivalve has its own unique nutritional profile, so let's take a look at the most familiar ones—oysters, clams, scallops, and mussels—to a get a better sense of what these sea creatures have to offer.

OYSTERS:

Oysters are amazing sources of vitamin D, vitamin B12, copper, zinc, and selenium, making them a great food for supporting skeletal health, producing red blood cells, maintaining nerve cell and immune health, supporting thyroid function, and protecting the body against damage from free radicals.

Each 100 grams of raw eastern wild oysters contains:

672 MILLIGRAMS OF **OMEGA-3 FATS**

605% OF THE RDA FOR **ZINC**

324% OF THE RDA FOR **vitamin B12**

223% OF THE RDA FOR **COPPER**

91% OF THE RDA FOR **SELENIUM**

80% OF THE RDA FOR **vitamin D**

37% OF THE RDA FOR **IRON**

18% OF THE RDA FOR **MANGANESE**

14% OF THE RDA FOR **PHOSPHORUS**

12% OF THE RDA FOR **MAGNESIUM**

between 2% and 10% OF THE RDA FOR **vitamin A, vitamin C, vitamin E, vitamins B1, B2, B3, B5, B6, and B9, CALCIUM, POTASSIUM, and SODIUM**

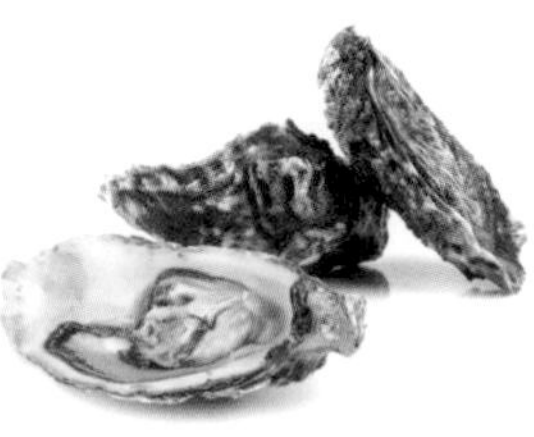

CALORIES: 68 FAT: 2 g CARBOHYDRATE: 4 g PROTEIN: 7 g

CLAMS:

A variety of edible clams are out there—hard-shell, soft-shell, razor clams, and surf clams, to name just a few—and they tend to be particularly high in vitamin B12, selenium, iron, and manganese. That makes them excellent for nerve and blood cell health, treating or preventing iron-deficiency anemia, protecting against cellular damage, forming connective tissue and sex hormones, and supporting carbohydrate and fat metabolism.

Each 100 grams of cooked clams (mixed species) contains:

396 MILLIGRAMS OF **OMEGA-3 FATS**	1,648% OF THE RDA FOR **vitamin B12**	155% OF THE RDA FOR **IRON**	91% OF THE RDA FOR **SELENIUM**
50% OF THE RDA FOR **MANGANESE**	37% OF THE RDA FOR **vitamin C**	34% OF THE RDA FOR **PHOSPHORUS**	34% OF THE RDA FOR **COPPER**
25% OF THE RDA FOR **vitamin B3**	18% OF THE RDA FOR **POTASSIUM**	18% OF THE RDA FOR **ZINC**	11% OF THE RDA FOR **vitamin A**
10% OF THE RDA FOR **vitamin B1**	between 4% and 10% OF THE RDA FOR **vitamins B5, B6, and B9, MAGNESIUM, CALCIUM, and SODIUM**		

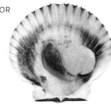

CALORIES: 148 *FAT:* 2 g *CARBOHYDRATE:* 5 g *PROTEIN:* 26 g

MUSSELS:

Have you ever seen oblong shellfish scattered along the beach or clinging to rocks or posts by the water? Who knew that these creatures were actually amazing nutritional resources? Mussels are teeming with vitamin B12, selenium, and manganese (offering over 100 percent of the RDA for each of them!), making them great for supporting cellular health, DNA synthesis, fat and carbohydrate metabolism, connective tissue and bone health, and blood sugar regulation.

Each 100 grams of cooked blue mussels contains:

866 MILLIGRAMS OF **OMEGA-3 FATS**	400% OF THE RDA FOR **vitamin B12**	340% OF THE RDA FOR **MANGANESE**	128% OF THE RDA FOR **SELENIUM**
37% OF THE RDA FOR **IRON**	28% OF THE RDA FOR **PHOSPHORUS**	25% OF THE RDA FOR **vitamin B2**	23% OF THE RDA FOR **vitamin C**
20% OF THE RDA FOR **vitamin B1**	19% OF THE RDA FOR **vitamin B9**	18% OF THE RDA FOR **ZINC**	15% OF THE RDA FOR **SODIUM**
between 3% and 9% OF THE RDA FOR **vitamin A, vitamins B5 and B6, CALCIUM, MAGNESIUM, POTASSIUM, and COPPER**			

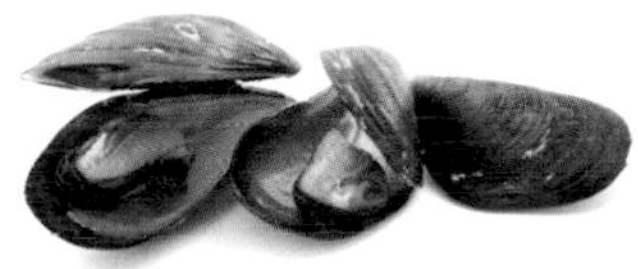

CALORIES: 172 *FAT:* 4 g *CARBOHYDRATE:* 7 g *PROTEIN:* 24 g

SCALLOPS:

Not only are scallops delicious, but they're also a solid source of a variety of micronutrients—particularly vitamin B12, selenium, zinc, and phosphorus. That means they're a great addition to our menus for helping synthesize DNA, enhancing nerve and blood cell health, protecting cells from free radical damage, boosting immune health, and building healthy skeletal tissue.

Each 100 grams of cooked scallops contains:

396 MILLIGRAMS OF **OMEGA-3 FATS**	40% OF THE RDA FOR **SELENIUM**	34% OF THE RDA FOR **PHOSPHORUS**	22% OF THE RDA FOR **vitamin B12**
20% OF THE RDA FOR **ZINC**	17% OF THE RDA FOR **IRON**	15% OF THE RDA FOR **COPPER**	14% OF THE RDA FOR **MAGNESIUM**
14% OF THE RDA FOR **POTASSIUM**	12% OF THE RDA FOR **CALCIUM**	11% OF THE RDA FOR **SODIUM**	
between 4% and 7% OF THE RDA FOR **vitamin A, vitamin E, and vitamins B1, B2, B3, B6 and B9**			

CALORIES: 112 *FAT:* 1 g *CARBOHYDRATE:* 0 g *PROTEIN:* 23 g

But what about toxins? Despite their incredible nutrient density, bivalves have a reputation for being unhealthy due to their "bottom-feeder" status (meaning that they eat near the bottom of an ocean, lake, or river). The logic goes that bottom-feeders consume the feces, parasites, decomposing animals, and various toxins that accumulate on the floor of a body of water, and therefore bivalves must contain unhealthy contaminants.

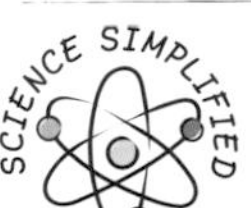

It's a myth that we should limit shellfish consumption over toxin concerns because they are "bottom-feeders." Shellfish actually have some of the lowest contaminant rates of all animal foods!

This is a misconception! Bivalves are generally filter-feeders, which means that they use their gills to draw in food (mostly phytoplankton and microscopic sea creatures) and filter out larger particles. (A few species are carnivorous and eat larger organisms, but they aren't the types of bivalves that humans usually consume—and you'll probably never find them on a restaurant menu.) This is much different than sea creatures that act as opportunistic scavengers, consuming dead animals and large debris, such as wild catfish.

Likewise, because most bivalves are so low on the food chain, they pose a minimal risk in terms of heavy metal contamination. Large-bodied, long-living sea creatures like swordfish and sharks tend to be higher in mercury because they accumulate heavy metals from their prey (which I'll talk about in the next section). By contrast, bivalves consistently rank as some of the lowest-mercury seafood available because the particulate matter they consume is nearly free from heavy metals.

As far as toxins go, the main legitimate danger with bivalves is the potential for one of four types of shellfish poisoning: amnesic, diarrheal, neurotoxic, and paralytic, distinguished by the specific toxin that causes the poisoning. When bivalves consume toxin-producing algae (from harmful algal blooms, or HABs, like red tide), they risk passing on marine biotoxins to the humans who eat them (namely domoic acid, okadaic acid, brevetoxins, or saxitoxin). Those toxins can cause a range of respiratory, gastrointestinal, and neurological symptoms and in some cases can be fatal (although this is rare). Those toxins aren't deactivated by heat, so simply cooking shellfish isn't enough to prevent poisoning. Shellfish poisoning is really a concern only if you're planning on harvesting wild shellfish yourself; you can protect yourself by checking with local authorities as to the presence of HABs before heading out on your hunt.

Of course, bivalves are not the only shellfish in town! Crab, shrimp, prawns, lobster, and crayfish belong to a different shellfish family: crustaceans. Crustaceans belong to the Arthropoda phylum (as do insects) and feature exoskeletons that molt as they grow, branched limbs, and a larval life stage. There are about 67,000 different species of crustaceans, mostly aquatic. And while not as impressive as bivalves in terms of nutrient content, crustaceans still provide substantial amounts of high-quality protein, omega-3 fats, and important vitamins and minerals.

SHRIMP:

With over 6 million tons produced annually, shrimp is the most commonly consumed seafood worldwide. One of the leanest protein sources available, shrimp is a fantastic source of selenium while also being low in mercury, making it great for supporting thyroid health, antioxidant systems, and detoxification. It also provides good amounts of vitamin B12 and iron.

Each 100 grams of cooked shrimp contains:

347 MILLIGRAMS OF **OMEGA-3 FATS**	57% OF THE RDA FOR **SELENIUM**	25% OF THE RDA FOR **vitamin B12**	17% OF THE RDA FOR **IRON**
14% OF THE RDA FOR **PHOSPHORUS**	13% OF THE RDA FOR **vitamin B3**	10% OF THE RDA FOR **ZINC**	10% OF THE RDA FOR **COPPER**

between 3% and 9% OF THE RDA FOR **vitamin A, vitamin C, vitamins B5 and B6, CALCIUM, MAGNESIUM, POTASSIUM, and SODIUM**

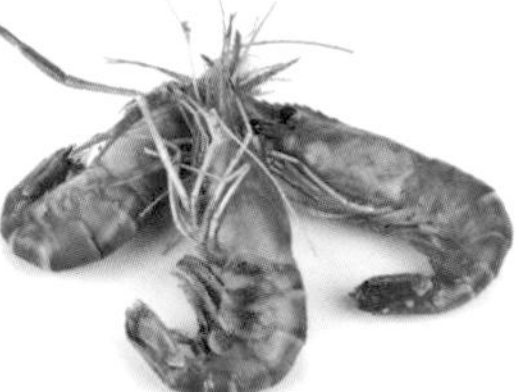

CALORIES: 99 *FAT:* 1 g *CARBOHYDRATE:* 0 g *PROTEIN:* 21 g

Prawns and crayfish boast similar nutrient profiles. Crayfish contains higher amounts of manganese and phosphorous and a good amount of vitamin B9.

CRAB:

From blue to Dungeness to king, crab is an impressively nutrient-packed lean protein and the obvious nutrition winner among crustaceans. With over 100 percent of the RDA of vitamin B12 and impressive amounts of most other B vitamins, crab is great for methylation, detoxification, and metabolism. It also contains impressive amounts of selenium, zinc, and copper, all essential nutrients for immune health.

Each 100 grams of cooked Dungeness crab contains:

407 MILLIGRAMS OF **OMEGA-3 FATS**	173% OF THE RDA FOR **vitamin B12**	68% OF THE RDA FOR **SELENIUM**	37% OF THE RDA FOR **COPPER**
36% OF THE RDA FOR **ZINC**	18% OF THE RDA FOR **vitamin B3**	18% OF THE RDA FOR **PHOSPHORUS**	15% OF THE RDA FOR **SODIUM**
14% OF THE RDA FOR **MAGNESIUM**	12% OF THE RDA FOR **POTASSIUM**	12% OF THE RDA FOR **vitamin B2**	10% OF THE RDA FOR **vitamin B9**

between 3% and 9% OF THE RDA FOR **vitamin C, vitamins B1, B5 and B6, CALCIUM, and MANGANESE**

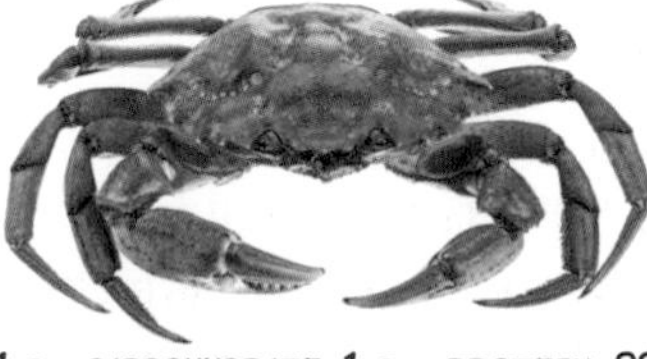

CALORIES: 110 *FAT:* 1 g *CARBOHYDRATE:* 1 g *PROTEIN:* 22 g

LOBSTER:

Lobster only became the culinary superstar that it is in the mid-nineteenth century. In my grandparents' time, lobster was considered a food for the poor, for servants, and was commonly served to prison inmates. In fact, it was common for servants to specify that they would not eat lobster more than twice per week in their employment agreements! Oh, how times have changed. Lobster is comparable to shrimp in nutrition, with high amounts of selenium, B12, and copper.

Each 100 grams of cooked lobster contains:

86 MILLIGRAMS OF **OMEGA-3 FATS**	97% OF THE RDA FOR **vitamin B12**	61% OF THE RDA FOR **IRON**	52% OF THE RDA FOR **SELENIUM**
19% OF THE RDA FOR **MANGANESE**	17% OF THE RDA FOR **vitamin C**	13% OF THE RDA FOR **PHOSPHORUS**	10% OF THE RDA FOR **COPPER**

between 3% and 9% OF THE RDA FOR **vitamin A, vitamins B5 and B6, CALCIUM, MAGNESIUM, POTASSIUM, and SODIUM**

CALORIES: 98 *FAT:* 0.6 g *CARBOHYDRATE:* 1 g *PROTEIN:* 21 g

OTHER SHELLFISH:

Squid, octopi, and cuttlefish are also shellfish! They belong to a family of shellfish called *cephalopods*, identified by their tentacles and internal shell, called a cuttlebone. Along with being yet another great source of easily digested protein and omega-3 fats, squid and octopi boast impressive levels of copper, selenium, phosphorous, and vitamins B2 and B12.

Each 100 grams of raw squid contains:

496 MILLIGRAMS OF **OMEGA-3 FATS**	95% OF THE RDA FOR **COPPER**	64% OF THE RDA FOR **SELENIUM**	24% OF THE RDA FOR **vitamin B2**
22% OF THE RDA FOR **vitamin B12**	22% OF THE RDA FOR **PHOSPHORUS**	11% OF THE RDA FOR **vitamin B3**	10% OF THE RDA FOR **ZINC**

between 3% and 9% OF THE RDA FOR **vitamins B5, C, and E, CALCIUM, MAGNESIUM, POTASSIUM, and IRON**

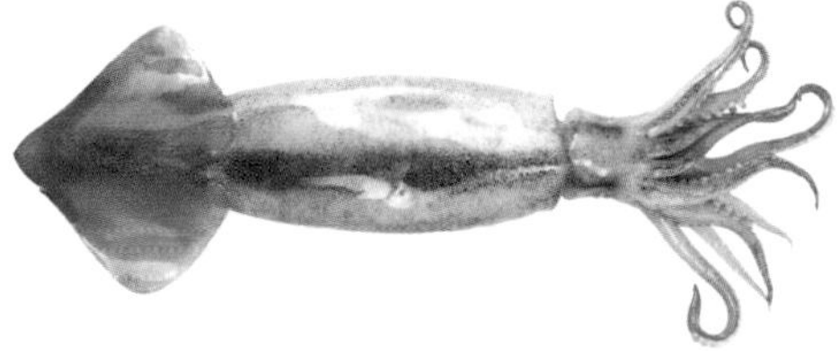

CALORIES: 92 *FAT:* 1 g *CARBOHYDRATE:* 3 g *PROTEIN:* 16 g

Shellfish, especially bivalves, rival organ meat in terms of nutrient density, and the consumption of shellfish is fundamental to any health-promoting diet. The exception, of course, is shellfish allergy, which affects approximately 2 percent of people. Fish, which is also a top-eight allergen, affects about one-fifth that number of people, at 0.4 percent of the population. In the presence of seafood allergies, it's even more important to incorporate organ meat into your diet.

Crustacean shells, like the exoskeletons of insects, are rich in minerals and a source of chitin fiber (see page 42). Eating deep-fried whole shrimp (deep-frying makes the shell easy to eat and gives it a pleasant, crunchy texture) and soft-shell crab is a great way to take advantage of this nutrient-packed, normally discarded part of these crustaceans.

MERCURY CONCERNS

We are often warned not to consume too much seafood due to the fear of mercury contamination in these foods building up in our systems and leading to mercury poisoning. Pregnant women are advised to limit seafood consumption to a measly two 6-ounce servings per week, the thinking being that mercury could cause brain damage in the developing fetus. It certainly sounds scary, but is this concern well founded?

Mercury is present in all foods. Concentrations in fruits and vegetables are quite low because mercury uptake by plants from the soil is low. In contrast, mercury levels can be quite high in certain types of fish because fish absorb mercury from the water and from the organisms they consume. Methylmercury, an organic form, is the predominant form of mercury in fish. It is concentrated in the muscle of the fish (not in the fat, which is why paying for low-mercury fish oil is pointless), and because it binds so tightly to certain proteins in fish, it accumulates over time. Fish at the lower end of the food chain tend to contain very low levels of methylmercury, but fish that eat other fish (that eat other fish . . .) tend to have higher concentrations of methylmercury. This process is called biomagnification.

The concern over consumption of methylmercury is that, when ingested, it is almost completely absorbed from the gastrointestinal tract and distributed to all tissues. (Elemental or inorganic forms of mercury are not easily absorbed, and some methylmercury is converted into elemental forms by our gut microbiota.) Methylmercury also readily crosses both the blood-brain barrier and the placenta. High levels of methylmercury are known to cause damage to the central and peripheral nervous system. The term "mad as a hatter" comes from feltmakers in the eighteenth and nineteenth centuries eventually going crazy due to chronic mercury exposure; mercury was used in the production of felt, which was a common material in hats. Yep, this definitely sounds scary.

SCIENCE SIMPLIFIED *For the vast majority of fish, mercury is not a concern. The selenium in seafood protects us from potential mercury contamination. In fact, the selenium in seafood can help protect us from mercury exposure from other sources, too.*

However, studies evaluating the effects of seafood consumption on the developing fetus have varied tremendously in their results. On one end of the spectrum is brain damage (albeit subtle) from methylmercury exposure, and on the other end is enhanced cognitive ability attributed to a maternal diet rich in omega-3 fatty acids (DHA in particular). So, should we eat more seafood or less? The answer lies in the selenium content of the seafood being eaten.

Selenium is a mineral that is required for activity of twenty-five to thirty different enzymes (selenoenzymes), whose job is to protect the brain from oxidative damage. Methylmercury irreversibly binds to selenium. This is bad if we're exposed to methylmercury because it renders selenoenzymes inactive. In fact, this is the mechanism through which methylmercury is believed to damage the brain and nervous system: by inhibiting the ability of selenoenzymes to protect these tissues from oxidants. Very importantly, most typically consumed varieties of ocean fish contain much more selenium than methylmercury. This is good for the fish (they don't die from mercury exposure) and even better for us. Selenium-bound methylmercury is not efficiently absorbed by our bodies. The methylmercury that is absorbed is already bound to selenium, so it can't interfere with our selenoenzymes.

Seafood that tends to contain very low levels of methylmercury include shellfish (including oysters, clams, scallops, mussels, crab, shrimp, lobster), salmon, trout, herring, haddock, pollock, sole, flounder, Atlantic mackerel, and lake whitefish. However, any fish that contains more selenium than methylmercury is perfectly safe to consume. This includes the vast majority of ocean fish and approximately 97 percent of freshwater fish. The only fish that we need to avoid are those that contain more methylmercury than selenium—a fairly short list. It includes king mackerel, marlin, pilot whale, shark, tarpon, tilefish, and swordfish, although some studies show that swordfish is okay. These recommendations are based on various small-scale studies.

Increasing our dietary intake of selenium is one way to protect ourselves from mercury exposure from food sources or environmental factors (broken compact fluorescent light bulbs or amalgam fillings, for example). Selenium is abundant in seafood, seaweed, mushrooms, onions, Brazil nuts, sunflower seeds, and meat and poultry (especially the liver). The vast majority of the fish we are likely to find in a store or restaurant are perfectly safe to eat. In fact, the dietary selenium we get from including fish and shellfish in our diet (not to mention all the good DHA and EPA omega-3 fatty acids, vitamin A, vitamin D, iodine, zinc, and very easily digested protein) will promote better health.

So, no, we don't need to worry about the mercury content of (most) fish. Actually, we should generally be increasing rather than decreasing our consumption of fish, even for pregnant women. Three to five 6-ounce servings of oily coldwater fish per week (on top of other varieties of fish and shellfish) will provide us with the recommended intake of DHA and EPA. And if we have unresolved inflammation, eating even more fish is a good idea.

There are two other pollutants—dioxins and PCBs—that may be of concern because of their carcinogenic properties. Although fish gets a bad rap, in general, it is much lower in these pollutants than other foods (including beef, chicken, pork, dairy products, and vegetables). Depending on the water it comes from, wild-caught fish is typically lower in dioxins and PCBs than farmed fish, but even in the case of farmed fish, the health benefits far outweigh the risks, especially in the context of the importance of DHA and EPA fats for overall health.

A NUTRIENT GUIDE TO SEAFOOD

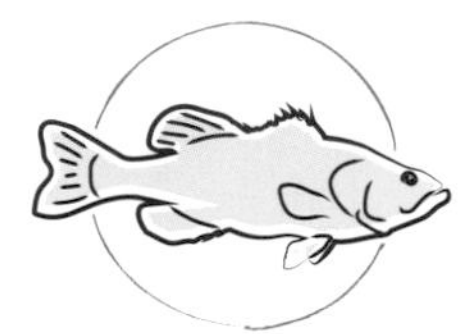

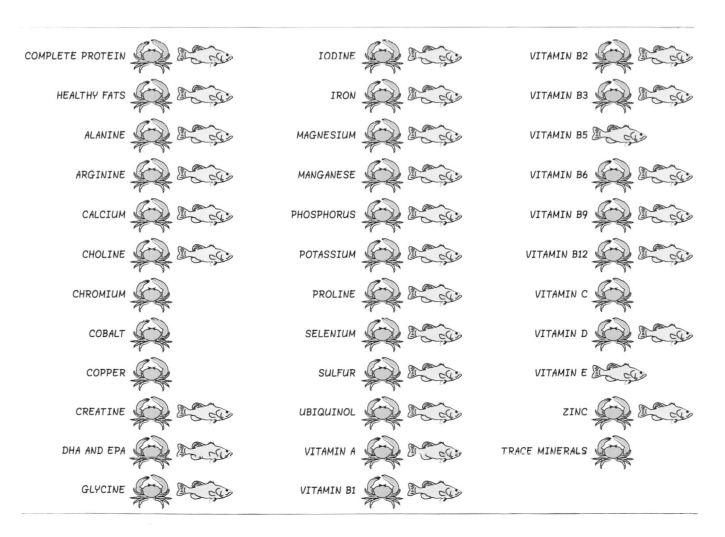

FISH

anchovy	conger	king mackerel*	plaice	swordfish*
Arctic char	crappie	lamprey	pollock	tarpon*
Atlantic croaker	croaker	ling	sailfish	tilapia
barcheek goby	drum	loach	salmon	tilefish*
bass	eel	mackerel	sardine	trout
bonito	fera	mahi mahi	shad	tub gurnard
bream	filefish	marlin*	shark*	tuna
brill	gar	milkfish	sheepshead	turbot
brisling	haddock	minnow	silverside	walleye
carp	hake	monkfish	smelt	whiting
catfish	halibut	mullet	snakehead	
cod	herring	pandora	snapper	
common dab	John Dory	perch	sole	

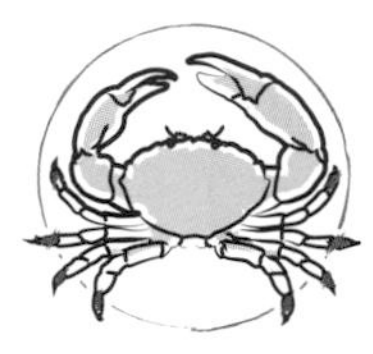

SHELLFISH

abalone	octopus
clam	oyster
cockle	periwinkle
conch	prawn
crab	scallop
crawfish	shrimp
cuttlefish	snail
limpet	squid
lobster	whelk
mussel	

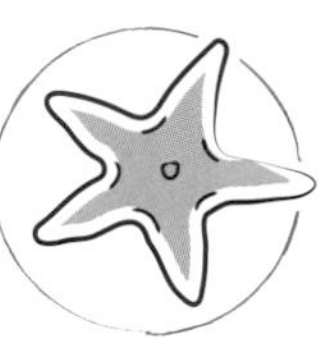

OTHER SEAFOOD

anemone
caviar/roe
jellyfish
sea cucumber
sea squirt
sea urchin
starfish

Nutrients vary in other seafood but they are all great choices!

*May contain higher levels of methylmercury than selenium.

Nutrient	Shellfish	Fish
COMPLETE PROTEIN	✓	✓
HEALTHY FATS	✓	✓
ALANINE	✓	✓
ARGININE	✓	✓
CALCIUM	✓	✓
CHOLINE	✓	✓
CHROMIUM	✓	
COBALT	✓	
COPPER	✓	
CREATINE	✓	✓
DHA AND EPA	✓	✓
GLYCINE	✓	✓
IODINE	✓	✓
IRON	✓	✓
MAGNESIUM	✓	✓
MANGANESE	✓	✓
PHOSPHORUS	✓	✓
POTASSIUM	✓	✓
PROLINE	✓	✓
SELENIUM	✓	✓
SULFUR	✓	✓
UBIQUINOL	✓	✓
VITAMIN A	✓	✓
VITAMIN B1	✓	✓
VITAMIN B2	✓	✓
VITAMIN B3	✓	✓
VITAMIN B5		✓
VITAMIN B6	✓	✓
VITAMIN B9	✓	✓
VITAMIN B12	✓	✓
VITAMIN C	✓	
VITAMIN D	✓	✓
VITAMIN E		✓
ZINC	✓	✓
TRACE MINERALS	✓	

Chapter 10:
MEAT AND EGGS

For years, many animal products have been unfairly maligned due to their saturated fat and cholesterol content as well as the tendency for red meat and processed meats to turn up unfavorably in epidemiological studies of cancer incidence. (Recall that we can easily counter their potential problems by eating more vegetables or being careful with cooking methods; see page 63.) Considering how many valuable nutrients meat and eggs contribute to our diet, their bad rap is a serious shame—and avoiding these foods, such as with vegetarian and vegan diets, results in a major drop in potential nutrient density and diversity, leading to problematic deficiencies. In this chapter, I'll share what science has to say about these foods and why they play a pivotal role in the Paleo diet.

First of all, let's make one thing clear: "red meat" includes a lot more than just beef and pork; "poultry" includes more than just chicken and turkey; and "eggs" includes a lot more than just chicken eggs! The foods in these categories are incredibly diverse—and admittedly not always easy to track down at the grocery store: antelope, beaver, boar, buffalo (bison), camel, caribou, deer, elk, goat, hare, horse, kangaroo, lamb, moose, rabbit, sea lion, seal, sheep, veal, duck eggs, quail eggs, turkey eggs, dove, duck, emu, goose, grouse, guinea hen, ostrich, partridge, pheasant, pigeon, and quail all belong on the list, too. Because diversity is a major goal of Paleo, the more of these foods we can include in our diet, the better.

In a nutshell, red meat, poultry, and eggs (along with seafood, which was discussed in Chapter 9) are our best sources of easily digestible protein. They also contain valuable fats and fat-soluble vitamins, among other micronutrients, including vitamins and minerals that we just can't get enough of from plant foods. Protein is necessary for building muscle, cartilage, skin, blood, bones, enzymes, hormones, and serving numerous functions that keep us alive, and a higher protein intake has been associated with greater thermogenesis (production of body heat, which burns calories), better preservation of lean muscle tissue (especially during weight loss), greater satiation after eating, better appetite regulation, a lower rate of weight regain after loss, better body composition, easier fat loss on reduced-calorie diets, improved blood glucose control, and greater bone density.

NUTRIENTS IN RED MEAT

What makes red meat red in color is an iron-rich protein called *myoglobin*. Myoglobin binds to oxygen similarly to hemoglobin, providing additional oxygen for muscles when demand is higher than what can be supplied by the blood—for example, during very intense exercise or when you hold your breath. The more myoglobin, the redder the meat when raw and the higher the iron content. The nutritional definition of red meat is any meat that contains more myoglobin than white meat, with white meat defined as being any non-dark meat from poultry or fish. Yes, even though you may have heard pork described as "the other white meat," scientifically speaking it's really red. The most common sources of red meat in Western countries are beef, pork, lamb, and bison. (I'm going to talk about poultry separately since it typically provides a mix of white and red meat.)

Recall from Chapter 3 that we get many nutrients predominantly or exclusively from animal foods; red meat is an excellent source of all these nutrients. Red meat provides easily digested protein, some heart-healthy and anti-inflammatory fats, and valuable vitamins and minerals. Red meat tends to be a great source of vitamins A and D, vitamin B12 and other B vitamins (including choline), chromium, cobalt, copper, iron (in the more absorbable heme form), magnesium, manganese, phosphorus, potassium, selenium, and zinc (see Chapter 1).

Nutrients in meat vary both by the cut and by the animal it comes from. For example, let's compare the nutritive value of three common cuts from three different animals.

GROUND BEEF:

Each 100 grams of raw 85/15 ground beef contains:

36% OF THE RDA FOR **vitamin B12**

30% OF THE RDA FOR **ZINC**

23% OF THE RDA FOR **SELENIUM**

23% OF THE RDA FOR **vitamin B3**

17% OF THE RDA FOR **vitamin B6**

12% OF THE RDA FOR **IRON**

between 2% and 10% OF THE RDA FOR **vitamin E, vitamin K, vitamins B1, B2, and B5, COPPER, MAGNESIUM, POTASSIUM, and SODIUM**

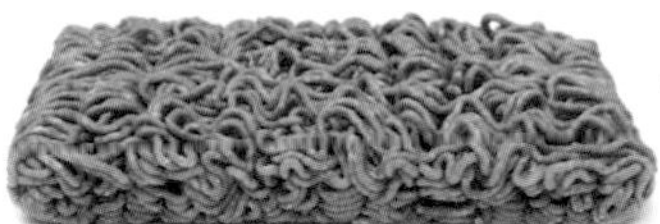

CALORIES: 215 *FAT:* 15 g *CARBOHYDRATE:* 0.4 g *PROTEIN:* 19 g

PORK LOIN:

Each 100 grams of raw boneless pork loin contains:

51% OF THE RDA FOR **vitamin B1**

46% OF THE RDA FOR **SELENIUM**

23% OF THE RDA FOR **vitamin B3**

21% OF THE RDA FOR **vitamin B6**

19% OF THE RDA FOR **PHOSPHOROUS**

15% OF THE RDA FOR **vitamin B2**

11% OF THE RDA FOR **POTASSIUM**

10% OF THE RDA FOR **ZINC**

between 2% and 10% OF THE RDA FOR **vitamin B5, COPPER, MAGNESIUM, IRON, and SODIUM**

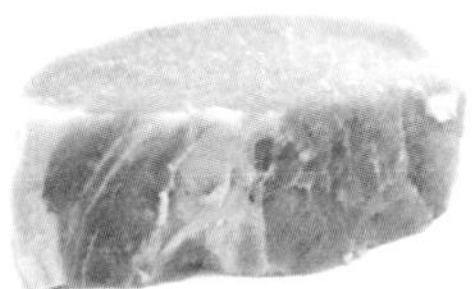

CALORIES: 211 *FAT:* 14 g *CARBOHYDRATE:* 0 g *PROTEIN:* 20 g

LAMB LOIN:

Each 100 grams of raw lamb loin contains

33% OF THE RDA FOR **vitamin B3**

29% OF THE RDA FOR **vitamin B12**

22% OF THE RDA FOR **vitamin B6**

19% OF THE RDA FOR **PHOSPHOROUS**

17% OF THE RDA FOR **vitamin B2**

17% OF THE RDA FOR **ZINC**

12% OF THE RDA FOR **SELENIUM**

11% OF THE RDA FOR **vitamin B1**

between 2% and 10% OF THE RDA FOR **vitamin B5, COPPER, MAGNESIUM, IRON, and POTASSIUM**

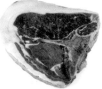

CALORIES: 203 *FAT:* 13 g *CARBOHYDRATE:* 0 g *PROTEIN:* 19 g

You can easily see that all three are great choices. Of course, offal is even more nutrient-dense, which I'll get to later in this chapter, but a mere 100-gram serving (3½ ounces) of red meat provides impressive amounts of essential nutrients. The vitamin B12, zinc, and iron content alone are sufficient rationale to include red meat in any health-promoting diet, but there's even more "Good Stuff" in red meat to consider!

Digestible Protein

Although plant protein has been getting a reputation boost recently, especially in the form of hemp protein, pea protein, brown rice protein, and other isolated products, animal protein remains king in terms of quality, digestibility, and density.

Protein is made up of long chains of amino acids—organic compounds that contain a carboxyl and an amino group. Even though about 500 different amino acids have been identified, only 20 are used to build the proteins in our bodies, and only 9 of those are considered essential, meaning that we can't synthesize them from other amino acids and have to get them from food. The essential amino acids are:

- Histidine
- Isoleucine
- Leucine
- Lysine
- Methionine
- Phenylalanine
- Threonine
- Tryptophan
- Valine

When we talk about a food being a "complete protein," it means that the food contains adequate portions of all nine essential amino acids. In general, animal foods supply complete protein, whereas plant foods tend to be low in at least one essential amino acid. That's why we see advice for vegetarian foods to be paired (or at least eaten on the same day) to fill in each other's gaps. Take, for example, the classic combination of rice and beans: beans are low in methionine but high in lysine, whereas rice is low in lysine but high in methionine.

But even the idea of complete protein can be misleading. Some amino acids (arginine, cysteine, glutamine, tyrosine, glycine, ornithine, proline, and serine) become essential in times of illness or stress. And even nonessential amino acids are important to consume, both because the process of synthesizing them can be inefficient (meaning that our bodies can't keep up with the demand, so we need to get nonessential amino acids from our diet) and because many of them play roles in the body that go beyond protein synthesis. Getting sufficient dietary protein is essential for our overall health.

On top of that, a protein's "completeness" doesn't reflect its bioavailability (how well our bodies actually digest and absorb its amino acids). That's where protein *quality* becomes important.

A number of methods have been used to assess protein quality, but the newest and most comprehensive one (promoted by the Food and Agriculture Organization of the United Nations) is the Digestible Indispensable Amino Acid Score (DIAAS). This method measures the digestibility of individual amino acids by analyzing fecal matter at the end of the small intestine (in contrast to the previous protein ranking standard, the Protein Digestibility Corrected Amino Acid Score [PDCAAS], which measures absorption throughout the digestive system and doesn't take into account protein absorption by gut bacteria). The DIAAS score is calculated based on individual amino acid digestibility, the original amino acid content of the food, and human amino acid requirements. The higher the score, the higher

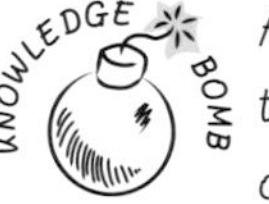

Americans consume more meat per capita than almost any other country, at a little over 270 pounds of meat per person per year. We consume only a little over 16 pounds of seafood per person per year, but over 600 pounds of dairy products. This intake of animal foods is more than necessary to meet our nutritional demands—somewhere around three-quarters to a pound of animal foods per day is about right for most of us—but our average intake is skewed too heavily toward meat and dairy at the expense of seafood.

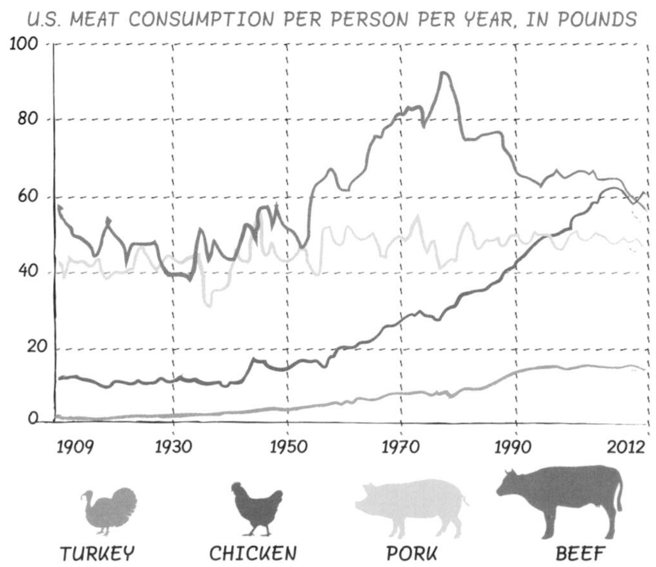

the protein quality. While DIAAS scores have been calculated for only a limited number of foods so far, here are some protein quality measurements of common foods and protein supplements:

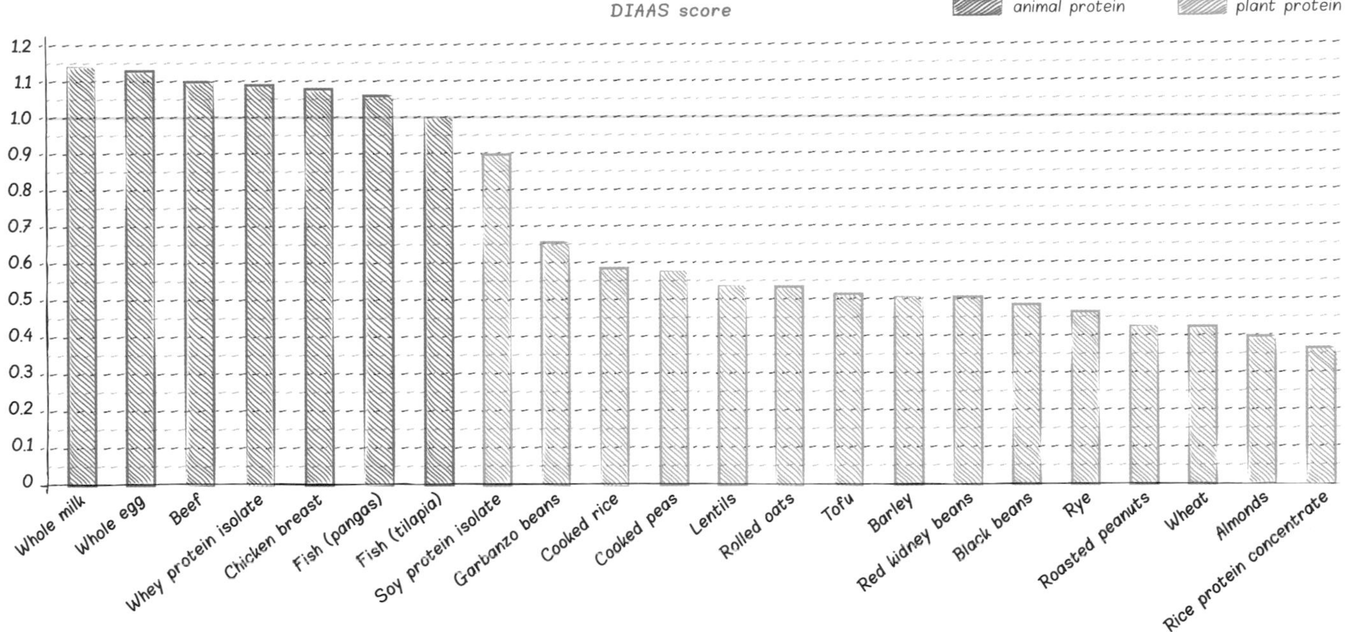

Clearly, not all of these foods are fully endorsed by the Paleo template, but this list helps to emphasize just how valuable animal foods are: they dominate the top of the chart when it comes to protein quality. Also note that while dairy and eggs score well in terms of protein quality, there are other concerns with regard to these foods that place them in the middle-ground category (see Chapters 21 and 24).

Another reason why animal protein in meat and eggs is superior involves *density.* Along with antinutrients that inhibit absorption (which lower protein quality scores), even the highest sources of plant protein come packaged with carbohydrates (including fiber) that dilute the protein per bite we can get from those foods (unless the food is processed and refined into smithereens and sold as a protein powder—but in that case we're talking about supplements, not nutrient-dense whole foods). Conversely, animal products tend to be extremely protein dense, and the vast majority of calories in lean meats (as well as seafood) are in the form of protein. For example, chicken breast is 80 percent protein and light tuna is 94 percent protein.

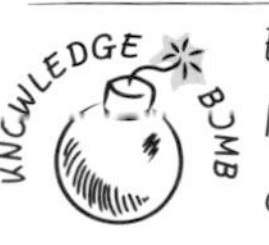

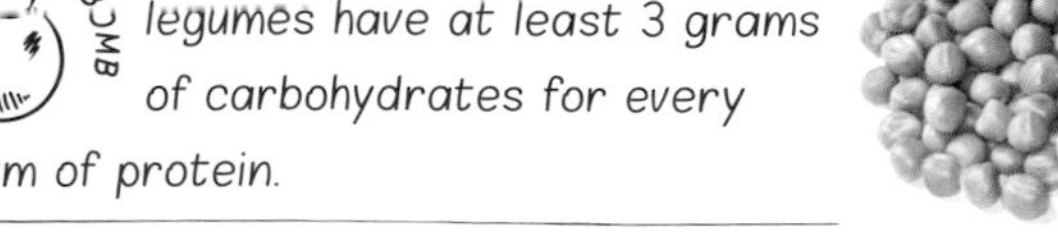

Even the highest-protein legumes have at least 3 grams of carbohydrates for every gram of protein.

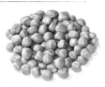

Fats and Fat-Soluble Nutrients

The fat in animal products is also extremely valuable. I'll talk more about healthy fats in Chapter 11, but for now, let's just consider the fact that fat is essential for cell construction, nerve function, digestion, and the formation of hormones that regulate everything from metabolism to circulation. The membranes of every cell in our bodies are composed of fat molecules. And we need to eat fat in order to absorb vitamins A, D, E, and K. (Incidentally, these vitamins are present in a number of animal products—including the often-vilified egg yolk, which is actually a nutrition powerhouse and should *not* be avoided on the basis of cholesterol fears! As a matter of fact, dietary cholesterol has a neutral effect on most people's blood cholesterol due to the body's ability to downregulate cholesterol synthesis and absorption in response to its presence in our diet.) Although meat has somehow become synonymous with saturated fat, the fat from red meat tends to be about half monounsaturated fats. Many high-quality meats, like grass-fed beef, also contain some omega-3 (the fabulous fat that makes seafood famous) and conjugated linoleic acid (CLA), known to reduce inflammation, promote healing, and even fight cancer.

CLA is a special family of naturally occurring *trans* fats that we can get only from meat and dairy products from ruminants such as beef and lamb. That's because CLA is created from linoleic acid (an omega-6 fat found in most plant foods) by the bacteria in the stomachs of these herbivorous animals. CLA performs diverse actions in the human body, reducing the risk of obesity, cancer, cardiovascular disease, diabetes, and osteoporosis. Specifically, CLA

- improves body composition by increasing fat metabolism, decreasing fat storage, stimulating the death of fat cells (adipocyte apoptosis), increasing muscle mass, and decreasing leptin (see page 90)
- blocks the growth and metastatic spread of tumors via effects on arachidonic acid metabolism (impacting prostaglandin, thromboxane, and leukotriene formation; see page 158) and modulation of apoptosis (programmed cell death) and cell cycle control
- prevents atherosclerosis by activating a group of proteins called PPARs that regulate genes involved in lipid metabolism, carbohydrate metabolism, vascular health, and inflammation
- prevents diabetes through improvements in body composition and PPARs' actions on carbohydrate and lipid metabolism
- improves bone formation by enhancing the absorption of dietary calcium and stimulating differentiation (maturation) of bone-forming cells called osteoblasts
- reduces inflammation by reducing the expression of pro-inflammatory cytokines like TNF-α and IL-1β while increasing levels of the anti-inflammatory cytokine IL-10

With CLA having so many beneficial effects, you might think to run to the supplement store. Once again, dietary sources win out over capsules—overdoing CLA by loading up on supplements may have some negative effects, such as fatty liver and spleen, colon carcinogenesis, and hyperproinsulinemia (where insulin is not sufficiently processed before it is secreted from the pancreas).

MEAT QUALITY

Of course, when it comes to meat and eggs, quality *definitely* matters. Ironically, conventionally raised meat is anything but! This misleading term refers to factory farming, where animals are raised indoors, typically in small pens with little or no room to move, and fed fattening grain-based diets and dosed with antibiotics and hormones. While conventional meat still provides invaluable nutrition, seeking out quality meat is worthwhile for a number of reasons.

Just like eating our natural diet makes us healthier, the same is true for animals. Cows, sheep, and bison are ruminates; their natural diet is grasses and leaves (not grains!). Chickens and turkeys are omnivores; their natural diet includes grains, grasses, and bugs (they're not vegetarians!). Pigs are also omnivores; their natural diet includes plants of all kinds, bugs, small animals, and carrion. Animals are also healthiest when they are raised outdoors with plenty of space to move around. Improved living conditions and a natural diet for animals raised for meat is not only more humane and environmentally protective, but it also improves the nutrient content of the meat produced from these animals. This quality meat is called *grass-fed* if it comes from an herbivore (such as beef, bison, and lamb) and is called *pasture-raised* if it comes from an omnivore (such as chicken, turkey, and pork).

There are many excellent reasons to choose grass-fed or pasture-raised meat over conventional meat. From an animal welfare standpoint, grass-fed animals are treated better, are happier, and are healthier. The frequency of *E. coli* contamination of grass-fed meat is extremely low compared to conventional meat (in large part because pastured cows have healthy intestines!) in spite of the fact that while antibiotic use is routine in factory farming, antibiotics are not used at all in grass-fed animals. Pasture-raised pigs and chickens are healthier, too, with far lower rates of contamination with antibiotic-resistant strains of bacteria (notably salmonella and *E. coli*). From an environmental impact standpoint, eating grass-fed and pasture-raised means supporting smaller, often local and family-owned farms, thereby reducing fuel costs to get the meat to us. And by avoiding non-organic grains in any part of our personal food chain (we'll see why this is so important in Chapter 19), we avoid supporting large factory farms that degrade topsoil and leach fertilizers and pesticides into our rivers, lakes, and oceans.

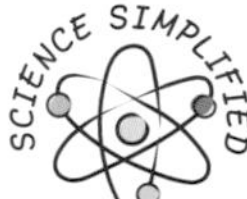

Grass-fed meat is superior because it's leaner, its fats are healthier, and it has more of some important nutrients while typically having a smaller carbon footprint and being raised free of hormones and antibiotics.

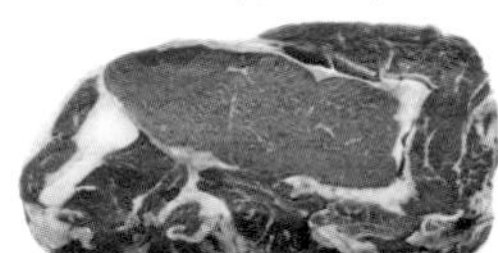

But it is the superfood status of grass-fed beef (or lamb or bison or goat—any ruminant) that justifies its higher cost. Red meat is typically recommended due to its high (complete, easily digested) protein content, as well as its being a good source of iron, zinc, and many B vitamins (it is a particularly valuable source of vitamin B12). This is, of course, still true for grass-fed meat. Grass-fed beef is an excellent source of vitamin A (ten times more than grain-fed) and vitamin E (three times more than grain-fed) and is higher in B vitamins, calcium, magnesium, and potassium. So, while grain-fed meat certainly isn't devoid of nutrients, grass-fed meat is far superior in terms of its nutritional profile.

Grass-fed meat also tends to have a much lower water content and is much leaner than conventional meat, which means that it is higher in protein. Plus, the fats that it does contain are healthier. While the amounts of saturated, monounsaturated, and omega-6 fatty acids are similar, grass-fed meat contains approximately four times more omega-3 fatty acids (in the useful DHA and EPA forms) than grain-fed meat. (Seafood is still a far better source of omega-3s.) While this improved omega-3 to omega-6 ratio is often cited as the most important reason to choose grass-fed, given that the total polyunsaturated fat content of red meat is pretty low no matter the quality, the more compelling reason is the fact that meat (and dairy) from grass-fed cows is the richest known source of CLA. Grass-fed beef contains about double the CLA found in conventional beef.

Pasture-raised pork is also more nutritious than conventional pork. The meat from pigs raised on pasture tends to be leaner overall and to contain more omega-3 fats and less omega-6 fats. This is because foraged grass is high ALA; when pigs are fed diets rich in ALA, their meat is enriched with DHA and EPA (see page 158). Pasture-raised pork is also much lower in saturated fat, higher in monounsaturated fat, and higher in protein. Pasture-raised pork is also higher in vitamins B1 and B2, vitamin E, and antioxidant phenolic compounds and tends to be higher in zinc, copper, and iron.

One quick word of warning when shopping for grass-fed meat: grass-fed means that the animals eat only grass for their entire lives. It can also be described as "grass-fed and grass-finished." Some producers "grain-finish" their meat in order to increase the size of the cattle and can be somewhat cagey about this fact. Also note that organic beef or lamb is not the same as grass-fed; although grass-fed meat may also be organic, organic meat is not usually grass-fed. Some producers supplement with grain so the animals are "mostly grass-fed," which is an improvement over conventional meat, but it's hard to quantify just how much of an improvement. So, whether you're buying from a local farmer or a butcher, it's worth asking whether the meat is grass-*finished*.

Of course, grass-fed and pasture-raised meat tends to be more expensive. Grass-fed ground beef typically runs at least $6 per pound, which is about 50 percent more than conventional beef. The tips for incorporating grass-fed meat into our diets are the same as for buying anything on a budget: shop around, keep an eye out for coupons and sales, and, when possible, buy in bulk. Many farmers will sell customers a quarter or half butchered cow or pig, and while the initial investment (and freezer space requirement) is fairly steep, the price per pound can be as low as $2!

It's even more important to opt for grass-fed and pasture-raised when buying cheaper, fattier cuts (like 80/20 ground beef, a nicely marbled steak, or pork shoulder), since toxins are stored in fat and to take full advantage of the healthier fats and higher levels of fat-soluble vitamins in high-quality meat. So, when working with a tight budget, go ahead and buy leaner cuts (such as strip steaks, chicken breast, or pork tenderloin) from conventional sources. That being said, when we can't afford to have all our meat come from grass-fed, pastured, and wild sources (or can't access these products where we live), even conventional meat provides essential nutrition that we can't do without. See page 446 for a quality guide to help you prioritize within your budget.

A PRIMER ON POULTRY

Let's take a moment to discuss the role of birds in the Paleo diet. Domesticated fowl like chicken and turkey are favored in mainstream nutrition due to being relatively lean and low in calories, but for those of us who don't fear natural animal fats, other meats may be more popular choices (hello, sizzling rib-eye!). One reason is flavor (skinless chicken breast isn't known to make most people salivate), but another has to do with poultry's reputation for being nutritionally inferior to other meat sources, especially its relative abundance of omega-6 fats. But does poultry in general deserve a place on our menus? Let's take a look at what poultry can and can't offer.

As mentioned earlier, one of the most legitimate concerns with poultry involves its fatty acid profile. Poultry is the richest source of omega-6 of any animal food: conventional chicken fat is almost 20 percent omega-6 as a percentage of total energy, which is more than canola oil (19 percent omega-6) and not too far behind peanut butter (22.5 percent). In fact, chicken contributes an average of 13 percent of the omega-6 content to the average American diet! Recall that an overabundance of omega-6 fats (and an under-abundance of omega-3s) plays a major role in chronic disease, and minimizing foods that tilt the balance too far in favor of omega-6s is typically smart.

Chicken has more omega-6 fats as a percentage of total energy than canola oil, with a typical omega-3 to omega-6 ratio of 1:40 or worse!

Simply giving poultry access to the outdoors (which allows the meat to be labeled "free-range") isn't always enough to turn the fatty acid tables. Research focusing on the effects of different poultry farming methods (caged versus free-range) and diets (conventional, organic, or pasture access) have had mixed results and suggest that the labeling we associate with higher-quality chicken doesn't guarantee a better fatty acid profile for the birds. Some studies of cereal-fed chickens with or without access to pasture show no difference in omega-3 to omega-6 ratio, unless the birds' intake of cereal grains is deliberately restricted (which sometimes increases their levels of the omega-3 fats eicosapentaenoic acid, docosapentaenoic acid, and docosahexaenoic acid). Likewise, meat from chickens that pasture-graze in the spring but not in other seasons tends to have higher levels of omega-3 fats. And some studies of free-range versus conventional chicken have shown that free-range breast and thigh meat has a *lower* omega-3 to omega-6 ratio than the same meat from conventionally raised birds!

What *does* seem to make a difference isn't so much the "free-range" or "conventional" distinction, but other particulars of the birds' diets. One report by the American Pastured Poultry Producers Association found that among pastured chickens, those that were fed soy-containing diets had an omega-3 to omega-6 ratio of 1:8, while those fed soy-free diets had a much improved ratio of 1:3. Another study of chickens raised predominantly on grasshoppers showed that those chickens had an omega-3 to omega-6 fatty acid ratio of approximately 1:7, and studies of chickens supplemented with large amounts of flax seeds were able to achieve a 1:1 ratio of omega-3 to omega-6 (although a high percentage was ALA as opposed to DHA and EPA; see page 158). For comparison, a chicken labeled "organic free-range" had a typical ratio of 1:11.6, and a chicken labeled "non-organic free-range" had a ratio of 1:11.3. Studies of turkey have shown similar omega-3 to omega-6 patterns related to diet and forage access.

Unfortunately, that level of detail isn't usually available on meat labels at the store (though befriending the local poultry vendor at the farmers market is one way to get the scoop!). But here's the good news: reducing our omega-6 intake from poultry doesn't require knowing every detail of the birds' lives. In general, leaner meat (particularly breast) has less omega-6 than fattier parts (like legs and wings), and the skin—even though it's pretty delicious—is a highly concentrated fat source. Choosing lean poultry and removing the skin will automatically reduce our omega-6 intake, regardless of how the birds were raised and fed.

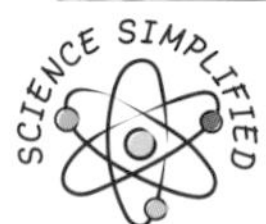

The fats in poultry tend not to be particularly healthy, but poultry does have some redeeming nutritional features; it contains a lot of vitamin B3 and is a great source of protein. Balance chicken and turkey consumption with seafood for a better overall dietary fat intake.

Apart from fatty acid content, how does poultry measure up to other meat sources on the micronutrient front? Although the exact nutritional profile depends on the specific cut of poultry meat, which bird we're eating (chicken, turkey, duck, goose, pheasant, and so forth all have slightly different nutritional profiles), and what the birds were fed, we can still get a ballpark idea by comparing poultry to other meats of similar quality.

For example, let's look at the daily value (DV) percentages for 100 grams of conventional chicken breast and 100 grams of conventional top round beef:

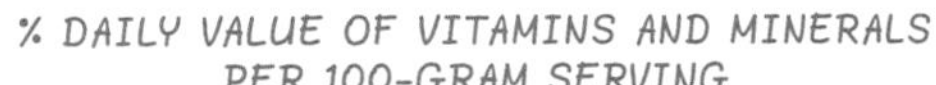

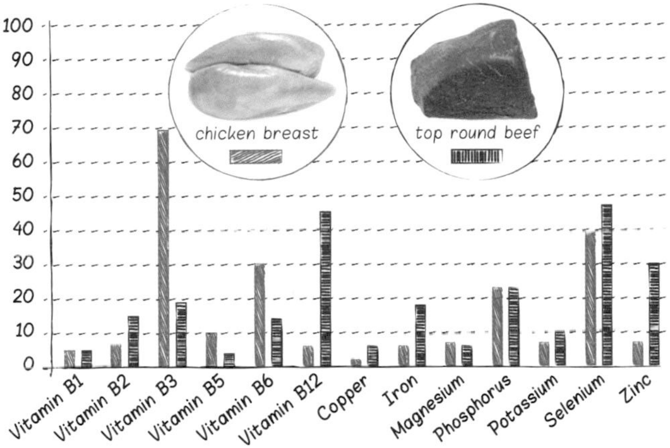

As you can see, beef is the clear winner when it comes to iron, zinc, and vitamin B12, but chicken comes out ahead for vitamins B3, B5, and B6, and many of the other nutrients are comparable between these two meat sources. But what about other meats? Here's chicken compared side by side with another Paleo favorite, pork chops!

% DAILY VALUE OF VITAMINS AND MINERALS
PER 100-GRAM SERVING

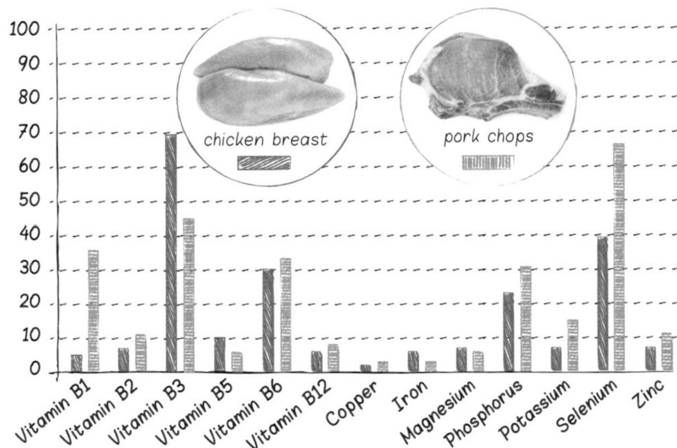

Pork is a much better source of selenium and vitamin B1, but chicken wins for vitamin B3 and is relatively neck-and-neck with pork for most other nutrients.

So we can safely say that when it comes to vitamins and minerals, chicken (and poultry in general) is far from empty calories. In particular, poultry's high concentration of vitamin B3 can assist with energy production as well as digestive, skin, and nervous system health; its vitamin B6 content helps the body manufacture neurotransmitters; its phosphorus plays a big role in skeletal health; and its selenium helps maintain thyroid function and protect against free radical damage.

Overall, there's no reason to avoid poultry, even though it may be wise to limit consumption of conventionally raised varieties. It's a great way to diversify an omnivorous diet and enhance the quantity and scope of our micronutrient intake. But we shouldn't rely exclusively on poultry to meet our animal-food needs. Consuming plenty of omega-3-rich seafood, like salmon and mackerel, can help balance out any excess omega-6 we get from poultry, and most of us could benefit from the iron and zinc found in higher concentrations in other animal products, like beef and shellfish. Bottom line: we can definitely enjoy poultry as part of a varied and delicious Paleo diet.

THE LOWDOWN ON EGGS

It's worth taking a moment to mention the pros and cons of eggs. Eggs are often vilified as a source of saturated fat and dietary cholesterol, but now that we know these aren't a health concern for most people (see page 186), we can appreciate eggs for their bountiful essential nutrients. Eggs, especially those from pasture-raised birds, can be an incredible source of B vitamins (especially vitamin B2); they are also one of the best sources of biotin and choline. They boast impressive amounts of iodine, molybdenum, sulfur, and selenium as well as modest amounts of calcium, iron, phosphorous, potassium, zinc, and the fat-soluble vitamins A, E, D, and K2 while providing an easily digested protein. Eggs from pasture-raised hens or hens fed a diet rich in flax seeds (the latter are typically labeled as "omega-3 eggs") are a good source of DHA and EPA as well. It's important to emphasize that most of this nutrition comes from the yolk and not the white—so much for egg white omelets!

On the con side, egg whites contain lysozyme, which can be problematic for some people, and eggs are a top-eight allergen; this is discussed in more detail in Chapter 24.

THE IMPORTANCE OF VARIETY

It is important to include as much variety as possible, in terms of both the animal your protein comes from and the cuts of meat from that animal. This is because different cuts of meat and different animals provide slightly different nutrients, in different quantities and ratios. Variety is the best way to ensure that you're getting all the nutrients you need.

In general, your protein will come from the following categories:

OFFAL. Offal, or organ meat, is the most nutrient-dense protein. Organ meat and other non-muscle cuts should be consumed at least four or five times a week. If possible, offal should come from grass-fed and pasture-raised or wild-game sources (but note that some organs from wild game are toxic to humans, like bear liver). If you're buying offal that comes from conventionally raised animals, lamb and calf are the preferred sources.

SEAFOOD. Fatty fish, such as salmon, sardines, mackerel, and trout, should be consumed at least three times a week—or more often if grass-fed and pasture-raised meats are not affordable for you. Seafood is very nutrient-dense and is your best dietary source of EPA and DHA omega-3 fatty acids (discussed in more depth in Chapter 9). The proteins in seafood are also highly digestible. You can include fatty fish, whitefish, and shellfish as often as you want. The more variety, the better.

RED MEAT. Red meat is likely to become the staple of your diet after you meet a minimum intake of offal and seafood. Grass-fed and pasture-raised meats and wild game are preferable, especially for fattier cuts. If you're buying conventional meat, stick with leaner cuts of beef and pork.

EGGS. While egg white contains a compound that may be problematic for some people (see pages 294 to 296), thanks to the nutrient-dense yolks, eggs are a rich source of valuable nutrients and stand out for their B vitamin, iodine, molybdenum, sulfur, and selenium content.

POULTRY. Pastured poultry and game birds are preferable. Limit your consumption of conventional poultry (because of its high omega-6 fatty acid content) unless you also eat a large amount of seafood.

Animal protein at every meal provides our bodies with necessary nutrients that we just can't get from plants (see page 62). That doesn't mean Paleo is an all-meat diet, though! As you read in Chapters 2 and 3, the Paleo template focuses on balanced and complete nutrition, meaning that our plates are piled with veggies but also feature quality animal protein.

OFFAL

Although it technically falls under the umbrella of meat, offal is so unique in its benefits that it really deserves a section of its own.

First of all: what the heck *is* offal? Offal, also called organ or variety meat, refers to animal organs and "miscellaneous" parts: things like liver, kidney, tripe (stomach), heart, and even brain. What do these meats have that the muscle meat we're used to eating doesn't have? The answer is *a lot!* Organ meat is the most concentrated source of just about every nutrient, including important vitamins, minerals, healthy fats, and essential amino acids.

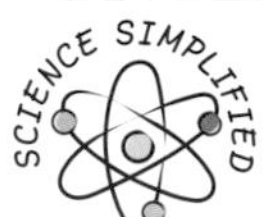

Organ meat is quite simply the most nutrient-dense food on the planet. Not only that, but it's high in many nutrients in which we tend to be deficient, so eating more organ meat is one of the most expedient ways to improve health.

Compared to muscle meat, organ meat is more densely packed with just about every nutrient, including heavy doses of vitamins B1, B2, B6, B9, and the very important B12. Organ meat is also loaded with minerals like phosphorus, iron, copper, magnesium, iodine, calcium, potassium, sodium, selenium, zinc, and

A NUTRIENT GUIDE TO ORGAN MEAT, RED MEAT, POULTRY, AND EGGS

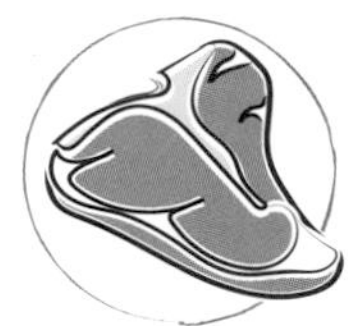

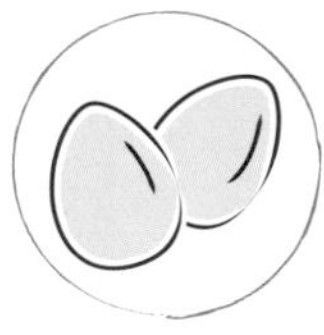

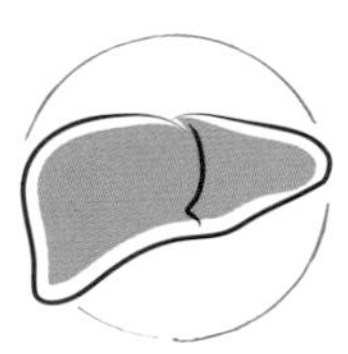

RED MEAT AND POULTRY:

antelope, bear, beaver, beef, bison/buffalo, boar, camel, caribou, chicken, crocodile, deer, dove, duck, elk, emu, frog, goat, goose, grouse, guinea hen, hare, horse, kangaroo, lamb, moose, mutton, ostrich, partridge, pheasant, pigeon, pork, quail, rabbit, sea lion, seal, snake, turkey, turtle, whale

EGGS CAN COME FROM:

chicken, duck, emu, goose, quail, turkey

OFFAL INCLUDES:

blood, bones (marrow bones or they can be ground or used to make broth), brain, chitterlings and intestines (used to make natural casings), fats and other trimmings (tallow and lard), fries (testicles), head meat (used to make head cheese or cuts like cheek), heart, kidneys, lips, liver, melt (spleen), rinds (skin), sweetbreads (the thymus and the pancreas), tail, tongue, tripe (stomach)

COMPLETE PROTEIN

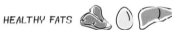

HEALTHY FATS

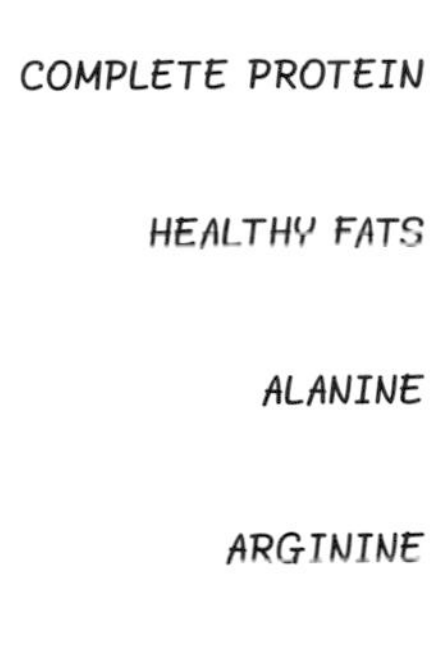

ALANINE

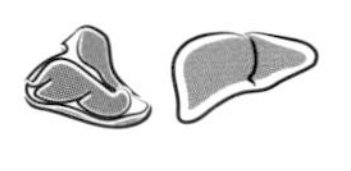

ARGININE

CALCIUM

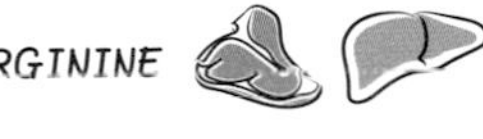

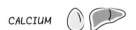

CHLORINE

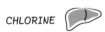

CHOLINE

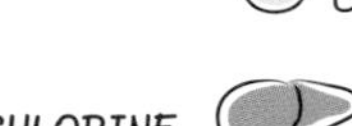

CHROMIUM

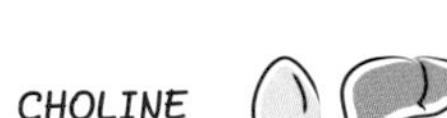

CLA *

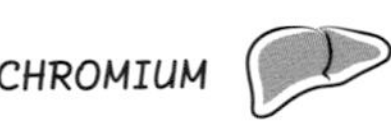

COBALT

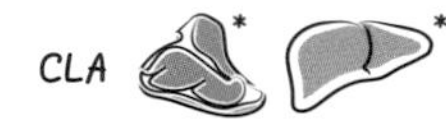

COPPER

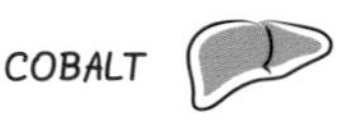

CREATINE

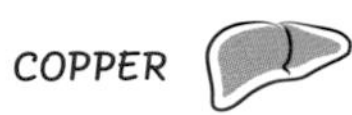

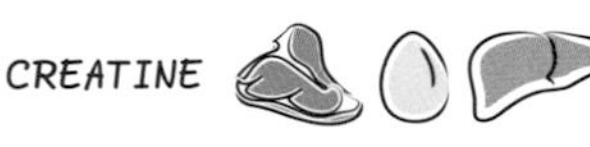

DHA AND EPA * ** *

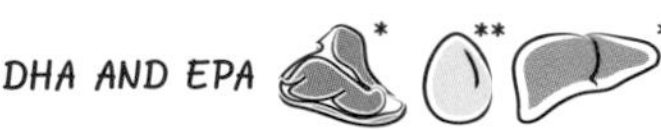

GLYCINE

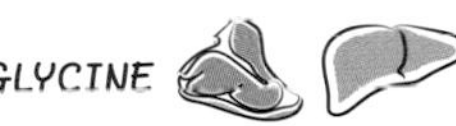

IODINE

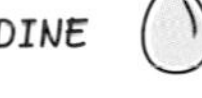

IRON

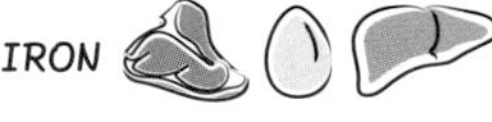

MOLYBDENUM

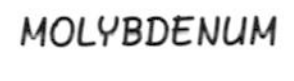

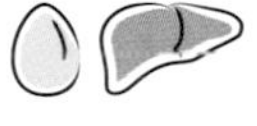

PHOSPHORUS

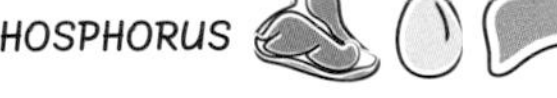

POTASSIUM

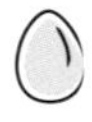

PROLINE

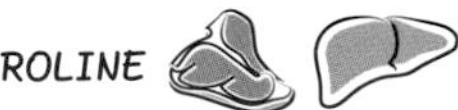

SELENIUM

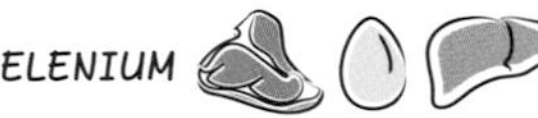

SULFUR

UBIQUINOL

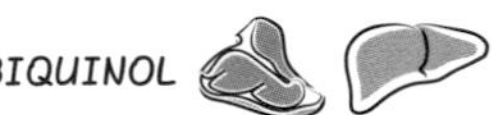

VITAMIN A

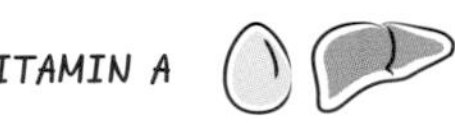

VITAMIN B1

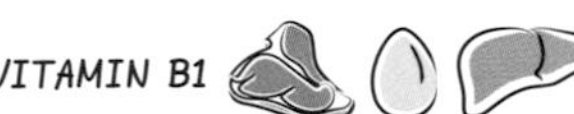

VITAMIN B2

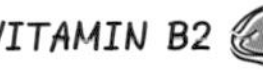

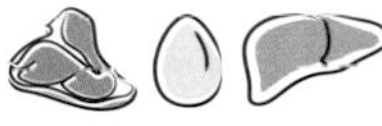

VITAMIN B3

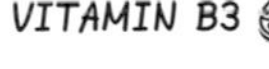

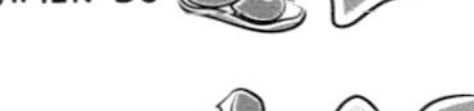

VITAMIN B5

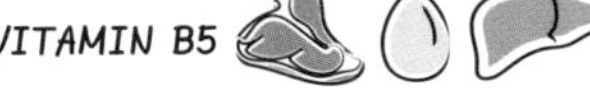

VITAMIN B6

VITAMIN B7

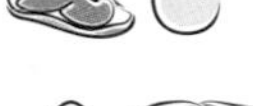

VITAMIN B9

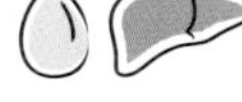

VITAMIN B12

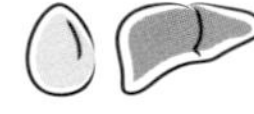

VITAMIN C

VITAMIN D

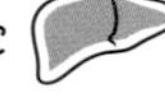

VITAMIN E

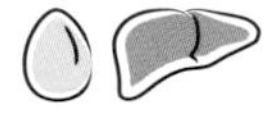

VITAMIN K

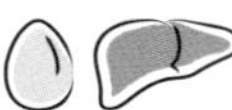

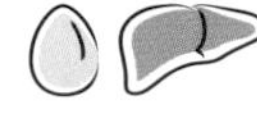

ZINC

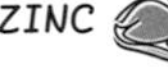

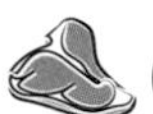

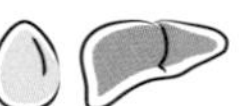

* when grass-fed

** when pastured or labeled as omega-3 eggs

manganese and provides the important fat-soluble vitamins A, D, E, and K. Organ meat is known to have some of the highest concentrations of naturally occurring vitamin D of any food source. Organ meat also contains high amounts of essential fatty acids, including arachidonic acid and the omega-3 fats EPA and DHA.

Liver is one of the most concentrated sources of vitamin A of any food. In addition to containing dozens of important vitamins and minerals, it is an outstanding source of vitamin D, vitamin B12 (and other B vitamins), copper, potassium, magnesium, phosphorous, manganese, and iron in the heme form that is readily absorbed and used by the body. Kidney is particularly high in vitamin B12, selenium, iron, copper, phosphorus, and zinc. Even though heart is technically a muscle, it also is a superfood. Heart is a concentrated source of the supernutrient coenzyme Q10 (CoQ10, important for cardiovascular health and also rich in kidney and liver) and contains an abundance of vitamin A, vitamin B9, vitamin B12, iron, selenium, phosphorus, and zinc. It's the number-one food source of copper. Heart also contains twice as much collagen and elastin than regular muscle meat (which means that it is rich in the amino acids glycine and proline), which are essential for connective tissue health, joint health, and digestive health. (I'll expand on that in the section on bone broth later in this chapter.)

KNOWLEDGE BOMB

This might be a great time to emphasize that it takes only a few weeks for our taste buds to adapt to big shifts in our diets. Studies looking at taste adaptation to one of a low-sugar, low-salt, or low-fat diet have shown that over the course of a few weeks (4 to 12, depending on the study), participants develop a preference for the healthier foods they've been eating. This is attributable to our taste buds becoming more sensitive. Food familiarity and flavor association with positive experiences (e.g., feeling good physically, the food tasting good, or eating in a positive social environment) is another key driver of food preference. Studies show that with repeated exposure to foods that we innately dislike, we can not only lose our aversions to those foods but actually develop a preference for them. In fact, we can learn to like new flavors after trying them as few as four or five times. What does this mean? If you aren't enjoying the new healthy foods you're adding to your diet, don't give up! The more of these healthy foods you eat, the more you'll enjoy them!

Studies of modern hunter-gatherers show a great preference for organ meat, which is often given to the most prized members of the tribe (be it hunters, elders, or sometimes pregnant women). In some hunter-gatherer cultures, muscle meat is given to the dogs or thrown away and left for scavengers in times of plenty. And some of the healthiest hunter-gatherer populations are those that eat predominantly organ meat. However, when food is scarcer, we see snout-to-tail consumption, meaning that every part of the animal is consumed and nothing is wasted. This translates to eating a ratio of organ meat to muscle meat that's similar to the animal's own ratio.

How much is that? Approximately 54 percent of an industrially produced steer and 58 percent of an industrially produced hog is considered edible. (The remaining percentage includes parts that are used in other ways or discarded, such as the hide and bones.) This edible portion includes edible by-products (or offal) and muscle meat, which is sold as cuts of meat and ground meat or processed into deli meats and sausages. Typically, offal accounts for approximately 12 percent of the live weight of cattle and 14 percent of the live weight of hogs (when pork rinds [skin] are included as offal and not discarded). Converting this to a ratio, we get:

- 22 percent of the edible portion of a steer is offal
- 24 percent of the edible portion of a hog is offal

How representative are these percentages? Well, pastured pork is leaner, so the percentage of organ meat to muscle meat will be slightly higher. But even in wild game, such as elk and mule deer, the percentage of body weight that is organ meat versus muscle meat is fairly consistent. The bottom line is the same: about one-fifth to one-quarter of the meat we eat should be offal (that is, not steak and burgers!). If you eat fish several times a week and meat the rest of the time (and you eat three meals a day), this translates to about four meals of offal per week.

HEALTH QUICK-START

Ramp up your organ meat consumption until you reach four or five meals a week. Remember, it's okay to incorporate organ meat into dishes in a way that disguises the flavor!

TIPS AND TRICKS FOR EATING OFFAL

Organ meat isn't the most familiar food to most of us, and it's not always the most palatable animal part, so here are some tips for maximizing our intake without having to pinch our noses with every bite:

EAT HEART. Heart is a muscle and actually has a familiar flavor. Ground beef heart is nearly indistinguishable from ground beef—the flavor is a bit richer, so some people even like it better!—and can substitute for ground beef in any recipe. To get the best texture, grind it in a countertop meat grinder or use the meat grinder attachment for your stand mixer. Heart can also be ground in a food processor, although the texture is not quite the same. Heart generally tastes like the animal it comes from, so beef heart tastes like beef, lamb heart tastes like lamb, and so on.

EAT TONGUE. Tongue can be a little disconcerting to cook because it looks like, well, a disembodied tongue, but once again, because it is a muscle, the flavor is very familiar. Once cooked, tongue can be shredded and used for carnitas (very traditional), sliced and added to salads, or served with gravy.

IT'S OKAY TO HIDE LIVER. If using a mild-flavored liver like bison, lamb, or chicken, you can use a 1:1 to 1:2 ratio of liver to ground meat (meaning to add 1 to 2 pounds of ground meat for every 1 pound of liver). With stronger-flavored livers like beef and (blech!) pork, I recommend diluting the liver even more and going with a 1:3 to 1:5 ratio. If using strong seasonings, such as when making tacos or chili, meatloaf, or 50/50/50 burgers, err on the side of more liver. When combining it with milder flavors (in a spaghetti sauce, for example), err on the side of a little more ground meat. And if you really can't stand the taste, use even less liver.

LEARN WHICH ANIMAL HAS AN ORGAN THAT YOU PREFER. Organs taste different from one animal to the next. Even the texture is different. You may find liver unpalatable in one species but delicious in another. Tasting a variety of organs from a variety of species can help you identify your preferences.

BROTH IS SIMILAR TO OFFAL. Sometimes people get so fixated on not liking organ meat that they forget some far more commonly enjoyed animal parts. Bone broth—preferably broth that is simmered until the bones crumble easily in your hands—is highly nutritious. Marrow is ridiculously delicious, as are pork rinds. Cuts of meat like cheek and jowl are considered offal even though they're still muscles. There's amazing nutrition in all of these parts, and even though eating plenty of them still doesn't let us off the hook when it comes to eating organ meat, it's a good entry point.

TRY MAKING LIVER PILLS. You can do this with any organ meat, although people usually use liver. Cut the liver into pill-sized pieces (whatever looks like an easy size to swallow). Freeze the pieces on a cookie sheet, and then, once frozen, move them to a freezer-safe bag or container. Keep frozen for at least 2 weeks (this kills pathogens). Then take a palmful of frozen liver pills with some water every day.

TRY ADDING JUST A WEE BIT Even a tiny bit of offal is better than none. Try adding a teaspoon of liver (cooked or raw, as long as it was frozen for at least 2 weeks to kill pathogens) to a smoothie or to any baking recipe where the batter goes in the blender, or blend some with a little water and use it to thicken a stew.

OFFAL IS NOT AWFUL. The average taste bud lasts for up to 2 weeks. This means our taste buds are constantly regenerating and will adapt to changes in our diet. Just because you don't like it now doesn't mean you won't like it in the future! Keep trying it. This will actually increase future enjoyment.

DON'T GET STUCK ON JUST ONE KIND OF OFFAL. It's important to eat a variety of foods, and this goes for offal as well. Aim to eat different cuts/organs from different animals. Think snout to tail. Yes, this means sometimes eating tripe, sweetbreads, chitterlings, or Rocky Mountain oysters. You also get to experiment with how you prepare offal, what flavors and cooking techniques you use, whether you hide the flavor or embrace it. Be adventurous!

DON'T STRESS ABOUT IT. Eating a nutrient-dense diet is one of the absolute best things we can do for our health. But remember that reducing and managing stress is also super important. If eating liver is so repulsive that it is causing you psychological stress, then don't. If you've figured out how to include heart in your diet, but cooking tongue gives you the heebie-jeebies, then don't. But don't use this as an excuse not to try to figure out ways to consume offal. And remember that many nutrients help make us more resilient to stress.

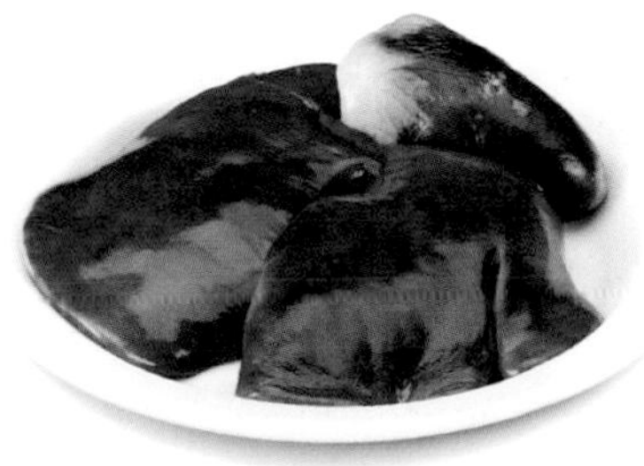

What About Toxins in Liver?

One of the most common misconceptions about liver (and the reason some people are afraid of eating it) is the belief that this organ acts like a sponge, absorbing and accumulating toxins as it processes them. In fact, this is part of the rationale behind many "detox diets" that claim to clean out the liver, which is portrayed as getting gunked up with toxins from unhealthy eating and living.

This couldn't be further from the truth! In reality, the liver acts more like a self-cleaning filter than a sponge: it processes and converts toxins into water-soluble products to be excreted, but it doesn't serve as a storage space for them. What the liver does store is the full array of nutrients needed to perform its many functions, including detoxification; for example, the fat-soluble vitamins A, D, and K; minerals like iron and copper; and vitamin B12. Liver is a ridiculously nutrient-dense food (arguably the most nutrient-dense food!) because it's a vital, hardworking, multitasking organ (see page 104)!

In fact, because of liver's extreme nutrient density, the biggest risk with consuming it isn't the ingestion of toxins like pesticides or heavy metals, but excessive intake of certain nutrients like vitamin A (or iron, for people with iron overload disorders) if very high quantities of liver are eaten on a regular basis, and in the context of other nutritional deficiencies like vitamin D deficiency. That's why it's good to eat a wide variety of organ meats as well as seafood and vegetables to ensure a broad and balanced micronutrient intake.

What's more, because the liver has so much enzymatic equipment to break down toxins (and because of its relatively low fat content, making it less likely to store fat-soluble chemicals and other contaminants), it may actually be one of the *safest* organs to eat.

BONES AND BONE BROTH

Bones offer some unique benefits, especially when used to make bone broth (the liquid made from boiling bones in water). There's a reason broth has been prized across numerous cultures and traditional societies, and not just because it's so delicious! Bones (and the broth made from them) contain several health-promoting nutrients that are hard to get elsewhere, making them a valuable addition to the Paleo framework.

HEALTH QUICK-START *You can easily incorporate broth into meals by using it to braise meats and veggies, in mashed root veggies, and as a base for soups and stews. It's also delicious on its own in a mug! Aim to have a serving of broth at least once a week or up to every day. See page 486 for recipes.*

Virtually any animal bones can be used to make bone broth: turkey, chicken, beef, bison, lamb, and even fish bones all create flavorful, nutritious broth. Typically, the bones have some connective tissue, like joints and tendons, and some meat attached. There are a number of different cooking techniques for broth, but in general, bones are boiled for anywhere from a few hours to 40 hours (or more) to liberate their nutrients and create a yummy liquid. In contrast, meat broth is cooked for a much shorter period (1 hour or more) from very meaty bones, like a whole chicken. While meat broth certainly has health benefits, it has a lower nutrient content than a long-cooked bone broth.

What's the difference between broth and stock? Stock is meat or bone broth that has veggies and/or herbs added for flavor (and nutrients!). In the Paleo community, we tend to use the term *bone broth* to refer to either bone broth or stock made from bone broth.

From a nutritional standpoint, bone broth offers two important things: minerals and amino acids (the building blocks of protein, used in every cell in our bodies). Keep in mind that the nutrient profile of bone broth is highly variable and depends on the type of bones used, how long they're cooked, how much they disintegrate, and which other ingredients are added (like vegetables and herbs, which contain their own vitamins and minerals that can seep into the broth). But enough analyses have been performed on bone broth to give us a ballpark idea of what it contains. A recent test performed by Covance Laboratories in Wisconsin, using long-cooked bones from organically raised chickens as well as vegetables added during cooking, found that 8 ounces of broth contained the following:

MINERALS:

Calcium: 6.14 mg
Copper: less than 0.03 mg
Iron: less than 0.12 mg
Magnesium: 52 mg
Manganese: 0.02 mg
Phosphorus: 19.50 mg
Potassium: 94.30 mg
Sodium: 57.50 mg
Zinc: 0.05 mg

Another analysis from way back in 1934, using chopped veal bones simmered in water and a little vinegar for 4 to 9 hours, showed similar mineral values.

AMINO ACIDS:

Alanine: 773.33 mg
Arginine: 696.67 mg
Aspartic acid: 553.30 mg
Cystine: less than 24.03 mg
Glutamic acid: 1013.33 mg
Glycine: 1773.33 mg
Histidine: 93.67 mg
Isoleucine: 131.67 mg
Leucine: 276.33 mg
Lysine: 303 mg
Methionine: 96.33 mg
Phenylalanine: 192.33 mg
Proline: 986.67 mg
Serine: 242.67 mg
Threonine: 214 mg
Tyrosine: 76.33 mg
Valine: 181 mg

That's a long list, but really, just a few key nutrients are behind broth's main benefits. Along with containing small amounts of important minerals (including electrolytes) that support various biological processes and skeletal health, bone broth is rich in two valuable amino acids that tend to be underrepresented in most diets: glycine and proline (see page 28). Both of these amino acids are found in connective tissue (the biological "glue" that holds our bodies together) and play major roles in healing. But each amino acid also supports some unique functions. And even though they're technically nonessential (meaning that our bodies can produce them if we don't get enough from our diets), consuming glycine and proline from food is much more efficient than manufacturing them internally and helps ensure that we get their maximum health benefits.

SCIENCE SIMPLIFIED

The nutrients in a long-cooked bone broth are great for connective tissue and immune health. They're tough to get enough of from other foods but can be found in seafood and organ meat.

Glycine is the smallest amino acid, but that doesn't mean it's not important! Along with being required for synthesizing DNA, RNA, and numerous proteins in the body (which makes it critical for digestive health, nervous system health, and wound healing), glycine is converted into the neurotransmitter serine—which improves memory, alertness, mood, and relaxation. And in the brain, glycine produces a calming effect by inhibiting excitatory neurotransmitters. In other words, this amino acid helps us feel good and think clearly.

Glycine also plays a role in blood sugar regulation by helping control gluconeogenesis (the manufacturing of glucose in the liver) and enhances muscle repair and growth by regulating the secretion of human growth hormone (HGH) and increasing creatine levels. In case all that isn't enough, glycine is an amazing helper for detoxification (it's required to produce the "master antioxidant" glutathione) and digestion (it regulates the synthesis of bile salts and the release of gastric acid). Whew! And the best part? Bone broth is one of the best sources of glycine, since this amino acid is richest in connective tissue.

Proline also plays significant roles, including in regulating gene expression, protein synthesis, cellular metabolism, wound healing, and immune responses. Proline has an interesting property: it can scavenge free radicals, making it a valuable antioxidant. Like glycine, it is a major component of collagen, so it's important for cardiovascular health, bone health, and gut health.

Even though proline is officially classified as nonessential, some research shows that when people are placed on a proline-free diet, their plasma proline levels fall by 20 to 30 percent—suggesting that our bodies might not be able to produce as much as we need. It would be a huge bummer to get shortchanged on such an amazing amino acid, so dietary sources really are vital.

A quick note on calcium: Although rumors abound that bone broth contains as much calcium as milk, this actually isn't true. Multiple analyses of bone broth from different sources show that one 8-ounce serving contains less than 10 milligrams of calcium, compared to about 300 milligrams in the same amount of cow's milk. The low level of calcium in broth holds true even after longer cooking times and when vinegar is added during cooking, which is sometimes advocated as a way to increase calcium extraction. Studies show that the addition of vinegar, even in larger amounts than typically used when making broth, doesn't have a significant effect on how much calcium is pulled out of the bones. This might be due to the collagen and other protective colloids encasing bone, which could act as a buffer against acids.

But that doesn't mean bone broth isn't still helpful for our bones! It does contain some magnesium, phosphorus, and copper, which also support skeletal health, among many other things.

Broth Fears Put to Rest

When it comes to bone broth, many people are concerned that it has high levels of glutamate—especially *free* glutamate. The logic goes that cooking bones for long periods breaks down naturally occurring amino acids and increases the concentration of free glutamate, causing some of the same problems associated with monosodium glutamate (MSG) and other unbound glutamate sources. As the theory goes, adding vinegar to broth (a common technique believed to help break the bones down faster) raises the free glutamate content even higher by hydrolyzing the existing proteins.

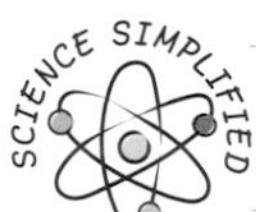

The various articles warning against bone broth are not well founded.

There are a few problems with this idea. First, analyses of the amino acid content of bone broth found that 8 ounces contained only about 1,013 milligrams of glutamic acid. To compare, a fillet of salmon contains 12,940 milligrams of glutamic acid, a roasted chicken breast contains 8,620 milligrams, 1 cup of boiled lobster contains 5,060 milligrams, 3 ounces of roasted turkey breast contains 4,120 milligrams, 3 ounces of broiled ground beef contains 3,280 milligrams, ½ cup of unsalted tomato paste contains 1,930 milligrams, and 1 ounce of walnuts contains 1,420 milligrams. Some articles warning that bone broth is dangerous have named glutamic acid in general as a problem with long-cooked broths. But clearly, if we should be suspicious of broth on the basis of its total glutamic acid content, then there are plenty of other Paleo-friendly foods that we should be even more concerned about.

More importantly, we have no idea whether the glutamic acid measured in bone broth is bound (making it theoretically less harmful) or free (making it behave similarly to MSG). Existing studies have reported only total glutamic acid content, without separating bound and unbound sources. Even people promoting the idea that bone broth could be harmful due to its free glutamate content acknowledge that it's only speculation that glutamate gets freed up in broth and that we don't know how much is actually released.

By contrast, we *do* know the free glutamate content of some other foods. Per 100 grams, Parmesan cheese has 1,200 milligrams, walnuts have 658 milligrams, fresh tomato juice has 260 milligrams, peas have 200 milligrams, red grapes have 184 milligrams, and potatoes have 102 milligrams. Even if cooking bones for extended periods does release some free glutamate, the levels probably don't exceed those of many of these foods (especially given the lower levels of glutamic acid as a starting place). So again, if we were going to single out free glutamate as a health danger, then a lot of other nutritious foods would have to get blacklisted, too!

Another common belief about bone broth is that adding vinegar to the broth water causes protein to hydrolyze, releasing even more free glutamate from the bones. One way chemists hydrolyze protein into free amino acids is by boiling the protein in a strong acid for 24 hours. By the end of that period, the free amino acids and peptides have been liberated from the original protein source. So it's certainly true that long-term exposure to high acidity and heat can help break down proteins and lead to the formation of free amino acids, including free glutamate.

But that's only part of the story! When making bone broth, we aren't boiling bones in high concentrations of a strong acid like they do in a lab. Not only is vinegar only 5 percent acetic acid (a very weak acid compared to hydrochloric and sulfuric acid), but the vinegar is diluted in large amounts of water during cooking (typically 1 tablespoon of vinegar per gallon or two of water). As a result, the amount of acid that ends up in the broth is extremely small! Likewise, while strong acids are used for fully hydrolyzing proteins into individual amino acids, weak acids are mostly capable of cleaving proteins at aspartic acid residues—which isn't the same as releasing free amino acids like glutamates.

So even though we don't have exact data on how the addition of vinegar influences protein breakdown from bones (and the level of free glutamate that ends up in the broth), we can use logic and basic math to conclude that the effect is probably trivial. If it takes 24 hours of boiling protein in a strong, highly concentrated acid to release all the free amino acids, then using liquid that's only 0.01 percent weak acid (the amount from mixing a tablespoon of vinegar with a gallon of water) probably isn't going to do much!

Another common argument against bone broth involves heavy metals. Because heavy metals bind to apatite, the primary mineral component of bones and teeth, there is some concern that bones sequester heavy metals and contain dangerously high levels (which, in turn, could seep into broth!). This is especially true for bones from animals that are exposed to heavy metals in their environment or their feed. This fear seemed to be confirmed by a 2013 analysis, which found that organic chicken bones did indeed release lead into the water in which they were boiled (concentrations of 9.5 mcg/L and 7.01 mcg/L, respectively, for broth made from chicken skin and cartilage versus broth made just from chicken bones).

But here's the catch! Those numbers mean nothing without context. As it turns out, the amount of lead in the bone broth was still well below the Environmental Protection Agency's safe upper limit for lead in drinking water (15 mcg/L) and wouldn't feasibly be high enough to cause harm. And a number of other nutrients abundant on a real-food Paleo diet can help protect against lead toxicity: B vitamins, vitamins C and D, calcium, and iron. That makes lead exposure from broth an even less likely problem in the context of a healthy diet.

Based on the evidence, there's no reason to fear heavy metal poisoning from bone broth! But to make extra-sure that our broth is free from contaminants, the best bet is to use bones from 100 percent pastured animals raised on small-scale farms away from industrialized areas (to minimize their environmental exposure to heavy metals), as well as making broth at home with filtered water (instead of using store-bought brands).

A Word of Caution: Skim the Fat

Despite its benefits, there's a valid concern when it comes to bone broth: oxidized fats. You might be tempted to save that delicious layer of fat that rises to the top for cooking (or even to slurp it down with the broth), but could the prolonged exposure to heat and oxygen cause some of that fat to oxidize and become harmful?

Unfortunately, there aren't any studies measuring how much oxidation occurs in the fat rendered from bone broth. However, we can apply what we know about oxidative rancidity, the composition of different animal fats, and the broth-making process to get a sense of what's likely going on.

As discussed on page 31, saturated, monounsaturated, and polyunsaturated fats are distinguished by the number of double bonds in their carbon chains: saturated fats have no double bonds, monounsaturated fats have one double bond, and polyunsaturated fats have multiple double bonds. Because these double bonds are essentially missing hydrogen atoms, they're molecularly unstable and can easily oxidize—undergoing a series of reactions leading to free radical production and rancidity in the presence of heat, light, and air. The oxidation rate for a fatty acid increases with the number of double bonds it has. So, while saturated fats are relatively stable, monounsaturated fats are slightly more oxidation-prone, and polyunsaturated fats can be *extremely* oxidation-prone given the right conditions (such as during cooking!).

So how does this apply to the ingredients in bone broth? Although animal fat is sometimes thrown under the umbrella of "saturated fat," this is a massive oversimplification. All animal fats contain a mixture of saturated and unsaturated fatty acids, including some linoleic acid (the type of polyunsaturated fat abundant in vegetable oils). The unsaturated fat content in animal fat is at risk of oxidation during prolonged, oxygen-exposed, or high-temperature cooking. For example:

- **Beef fat:** 37 percent saturated, 61 percent unsaturated (2 percent linoleic acid)
- **Chicken or turkey fat:** 29 percent saturated, 65 percent unsaturated (20 percent linoleic acid)
- **Lard:** 40 percent saturated, 59 percent unsaturated (11 percent linoleic acid)

To make broth, we simmer bones at a temperature just below boiling (typically 200°F/94°C). Although this temperature won't cause fats to oxidize as rapidly as high-temperature cooking methods like frying, damage still does occur—especially because broth simmers for such a long time (the cooking process can last more than 40 hours). Studies show that highly unsaturated oils like corn oil, olive oil, and mixed-seed oil (canola, sunflower, and safflower) begin showing signs of oxidation after only 40 minutes at 176°F (80°C), with oxidation increasing during longer cooking times and at higher temperatures. So, especially when making a long-cooked broth from bones from animals with a higher polyunsaturated fat content, like chicken and other poultry, we would expect to see a similar process occur. This is particularly true because the fat rises to the top of the broth and can spend many hours, or even days, exposed to both heat and air. Hello, oxidation!

So how do we reduce our exposure to potentially oxidized fat without forgoing bone broth entirely?

- The easiest route is to skim the fat off the top of the broth and discard it instead of eating it. You can scoop off the fatty layer while the broth is simmering or remove it after refrigerating the broth when the fat hardens and turns whitish or yellowish. (Keep in mind that animal fat can easily gunk up plumbing, so put the fat in a waste receptacle and not down the sink.)
- Use bones from animals with a higher saturated fat content (more heat-stable) and a lower polyunsaturated fat content (think beef and lamb bones rather than chicken or turkey bones).
- Use bones from animals raised in non-industrial-polluted areas that are free from heavy metal contaminants. Along with being harmful to the human body when consumed in excess, certain heavy metals—especially copper and iron—promote oxidation and can increase the oxidation rate of fragile fats.
- Avoid eating broth fat that tastes "off." Rancid fat has a distinctly unpleasant taste!
- Make broth in a pressure cooker in order to limit the fat's exposure to oxygen.

With these tips in mind, we can reap the benefits of bone broth without ingesting harmful oxidized fats!

INSECT PROTEIN: THE THING NO ONE WANTS TO TALK ABOUT

In recent years, consuming insects has gained wider acceptance in the West for both economic and nutritional reasons, and in case you're wondering: yes, it's definitely Paleo! (Of course, insects remain an important part of other cuisines around the globe and are a much-loved food among primates; see page 58) Insects are a fantastic source of protein and, thanks to their exoskeletons, are the only animal protein source that also includes fiber (see page 42). What's more, they're incredibly rich in micronutrients, including iron, calcium, copper, magnesium, potassium, manganese, zinc, and vitamin B12, while also providing omega-3 fatty acids.

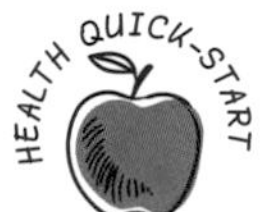

Challenge yourself to try cricket flour in a smoothie or protein bar. They're tastier than they sound!

The easiest way to incorporate insect protein into your meal plan is cricket flour! Surprisingly tasty, with a mild nutty flavor, cricket flour is hitting the shelves in many stores as well as increasingly appearing as an ingredient in food bars and other specialty food products. Cricket protein is made from milling whole crickets, resulting in a nutrient-rich, high-protein powder that can be used in baking and other forms of cooking. Along with containing more protein than beef, cricket flour is extremely sustainable: crickets require only a fraction of the resources used by traditional livestock farming—one-sixth of the feed and one-tenth of the water. There's one major catch: people with allergies to crustaceans (like shrimp) may react to crickets as well and should avoid consuming cricket flour and other cricket products. For everyone else, though, insect protein can be a fantastic addition to a Paleo diet.

Edible insects include:

agave worm	*cicada*	*earthworm*	*locust*
ant	*cockroach*	*fly pupa*	*mealworm*
bamboo worm	*cricket*	*grasshopper*	*sago worm*
bee larva	*dragonfly*	*hornworm*	*silkworm*
centipede	*dung beetle*	*june bug*	

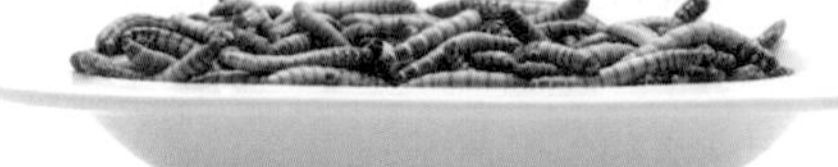

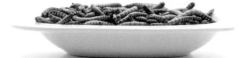

Chapter 11:
HEALTHY FATS

I've already established that the Paleo framework should settle around roughly balanced macronutrients; 30 to 40 percent fat is a healthy and comfortable zone for many people. But apart from meat, seafood, and certain plants, like coconuts and avocados, where should this fat come from—especially when it comes to cooking and flavoring food?

In a nutshell, excellent choices include cold-pressed olive oil, coconut oil, avocado oil, and palm oil, butter (preferably grass-fed), rendered (clarified) ghee, lard, tallow, and duck fat (preferably pastured). Although whole-food fats (those naturally occurring in meat, eggs, seafood, nuts, seeds, avocados, coconuts, olives, and dairy, if tolerated) are generally superior to isolated fats and oils in terms of micronutrient density, these cooking fats also have an important place in the Paleo diet. Monounsaturated fats, saturated fats in reasonable quantities, and omega-3 fats are all excellent for supporting numerous functions in our bodies and assisting with the absorption of the fat-soluble vitamins A, D, E, and K, so oils composed primarily of one or more of these fats are ideal—the less refined, the better for additional nutrient retention.

Recall that adequate fat intake is necessary for health (see page 31), with saturated fats, monounsaturated fats, and polyunsaturated fats playing various roles. Chapter 9 looked at the role of anti-inflammatory omega-3 fats, and we'll be looking more closely at omega-6 fats when we discuss the reasons to avoid processed vegetable oils in Chapter 20. The main takeaways when it comes to fat intake are:

- Moderate saturated fat intake is healthy.
- Monounsaturated fats have lots of health benefits.
- It's important to balance omega-3 with omega-6 fatty acid intake, which means anywhere from a 1:1 to a 1:4 ratio.
- An unrefined, minimally processed fat or oil contains more vitamins and other nutrients.

KNOWLEDGE BOMB *Contrary to 40 years of anti-saturated fat propaganda, saturated fat is actually healthy, provided that intake is moderate (see page 186).*

Rendered animal fats are rich in fat-soluble vitamins and are delicious for cooking. It's best to use fats from grass-fed and pasture-raised animals to take full advantage of their higher levels of nutrients and healthier fat profile. Animal fats are generally equally rich in saturated fat and monounsaturated fat and, when they come from grass-fed and pastured sources, typically have a good ratio of omega-3 to omega-6 fats.

Some plant oils are also great for cooking. Unlike the seed or grain oils that are generally called vegetable oils, like soybean, corn, and canola oils (in which the oil is extracted using solvents or a mechanical process called extrusion, which involves high heat and pressure), these healthy plant oils can easily be isolated from fatty fruits and nuts using a process called *cold pressing*.

Coconut and palm oils are rich in medium-chain triglycerides (MCTs), which are a special type of "short"-chain saturated fat (unlike the longer saturated fatty acid chains typically found in animal fats). MCTs do not require bile salts for digestion. They diffuse passively from the intestines into the blood and do not have to be modified before they can be used as energy for our cells, and they are metabolized extremely easily, even by people without a gallbladder. Their chemical structure includes chains that are much shorter than those in most animal fats, and after being absorbed, they can be rapidly converted into ketone bodies by the liver (ketone bodies are water-soluble molecules normally produced as intermediates or by-products when the body accesses fat stores). Ketone bodies can be readily used as fuel by every cell and are the brain's preferred fuel source in the absence of glucose or in the presence of insulin resistance. In fact, supplementing with MCT oil has been shown to be highly beneficial for neurodegenerative disorders such as Alzheimer's disease.

Also, because MCTs are a saturated fat, they do not oxidize easily or produce free radicals, which makes MCT-rich fats like coconut oil good for cooking. Coconut oil is approximately 60 percent MCTs. It is very stable and will keep at room temperature for long periods. And coconut oil has diverse microbial properties and therefore may be useful for people with bacterial or yeast overgrowth.

Some less-saturated plant oils are excellent for lower-temperature cooking as well. Avocado oil can be used for high-temperature cooking due to its predominance of monounsaturated fat (as opposed to highly oxidation-prone polyunsaturated fats). It is also fantastic for salad and vegetable dressings and for marinating meat. Walnut, hazelnut, and macadamia nut oils are delicious and have good fatty acid profiles for lower-temperature cooking. Although some can be high in omega-6 polyunsaturated fat, all nut oils can be used in moderation to add delightful flavor to salads and veggies.

THE QUINTESSENTIAL OLIVE OIL

Who could forget olive oil? Every pantry should be stocked with high-quality olive oil due to its health benefits and culinary usefulness. In fact, due to its popularity (as well as some myths that surround it), olive oil deserves a much deeper discussion than the other Paleo-friendly oils. Let's take a closer look at this fantastic fat.

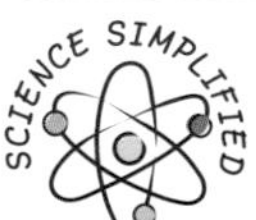

The only olive oil that is suitable for cooking is high-quality extra-virgin olive oil—fresh, cold-pressed, and rich in polyphenols.

Olive oil is one of the oldest and most revered edible oils out there, with culinary uses dating back to at least 1000 BC and other uses (such as anointing priests and kings) dating back even further. Not to mention that it's versatile and delicious. (Olive oil ice cream, anyone? See page 586.) Combined with mounting research suggesting that olive oil is cardio-protective, it's no wonder that this is one of the least controversial fats out there—given the green light by the Paleo community, vegans, vegetarians, low-carbers, the Harvard School of Public Health, and even the USDA. Not many foods can claim such widespread acceptance!

But there is one area of ongoing debate when it comes to olive oil: cooking. Because it's composed mostly of unsaturated fat (which is less chemically stable than saturated fat), many voices in the health community are claiming that olive oil can become damaged when heated and lose its famed health benefits. In fact, some of the more extreme claims are that heated olive oil becomes legitimately toxic and can contribute to heart disease and cancer.

Along with its high monounsaturated fat content, olive oil contains 1.4 grams of polyunsaturated fat (PUFA) per tablespoon, mostly in the form of linoleic acid—about 10 percent of its total fat content. Like all polyunsaturated fats, linoleic acid has multiple double bonds that are vulnerable to oxidation, especially when exposed to high temperatures, like when frying foods. Likewise, monounsaturated fat contains a single double bond, which makes it less heat-stable than saturated fats (though a definite step up from PUFAs).

So, in theory, we might expect olive oil to get damaged when we expose it to heat on the stove. And with reports of olive oil's smoke point being as low as 250°F (121°C), this would seem to provide corroborating evidence that olive oil should never be heated. The molecular damage from heating olive oil would erase many (if not all) of its beneficial properties and make it somewhat hazardous to consume (since oxidized lipids in the diet can contribute to oxidized lipids in the blood—a big factor in heart disease).

A number of studies have been conducted on olive oil to assess the effects of cooking on its structure and nutritional content, as well as what happens in the human body after olive oil is ingested. Across the board, the research shows that even with a fair amount of heat exposure, extra-virgin olive oil resists oxidation better than many other cooking oils. In one study, it took over 24 hours of frying before the olive oil generated enough polar compounds to be considered harmful. In another study, even after 36 hours of cooking, the olive oil had retained most of its beneficial vitamin E content.

In fact, high-quality (low-acid) extra-virgin olive oil can have a smoke point as high as 410°F (210°C). That's higher than most cooking applications and makes olive oil (at least the good stuff) more heat-stable than many of our other go-to cooking fats.

The magic words here, though, are "extra-virgin": refined olive oil (the kind with a low smoke point) starts to degrade in heat faster than its unrefined counterpart and overall is more susceptible to oxidation. The reason is extra-virgin olive oil's high content of antioxidants that protect the oil from damage in the face of heat or other oxidants. High-quality olive oils are rich in at least thirty phenolic compounds with antioxidant activity—particularly oleuropein, hydroxytyrosol, and tyrosol—as well as α-tocopherol, an important form of vitamin E. It turns out that olive oil's phenolic acid content helps stabilize vitamin E in the presence of heat, explaining why even sustained cooking times don't obliterate the oil's nutritional value.

In fact, those same beneficial compounds that protect olive oil from oxidation also help protect human LDL particles from damage. A number of trials have shown that after consuming olive oil, LDL from people's serum takes longer to oxidize and is more resistant to oxidation, suggesting a major benefit for heart disease risk. So whatever potential harm could come from olive oil's relatively less-stable structure (compared to saturated fats like ghee and coconut oil) appears to be more than compensated by its awesome phytonutrient content.

To get olive oil's powerful antioxidant properties (and therefore avoid some of the hazards of its more delicate chemical structure), quality is key! Unfortunately, obtaining high-quality olive oil isn't always straightforward. Even brands labeled "extra virgin" can vary wildly in freshness, phenol content, and linoleic acid level, and the olive oil industry is notorious for deceptive labeling.

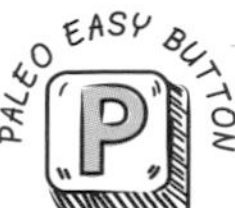

How do we choose the best olive oil? A few simple tips can help:

- *Look for brands that list a harvest date on the bottle, which will tell you when the olives were picked. The more recent the date, the better (no more than 12 to 18 months)!*
- *Always choose oils in dark glass bottles—never plastic or clear ones.*
- *Oils imported from other countries are more likely to be deceptively labeled (and even cut with non-olive vegetable oils—yikes!), so look for more local oils, especially ones from California, or choose oils from domestic companies that are transparent about their Mediterranean sources and production practices.*
- *The oil should taste pungent and peppery, even stinging the back of your throat a bit—that's a sign of a high polyphenol content.*
- *Make sure that the label says "extra-virgin" and not "refined."*
- *Fresher is better. Unlike vinegar or wine, olive oil does not get better with age.*

Equally important is taking care of the olive oil so that it doesn't oxidize before it's even consumed! For best results, store olive oil in a cool, dark place (for example, in the pantry instead of on the counter next to the stove). Even high-quality, properly stored olive oils can start to degrade after 4 to 6 months, so purchase oils in smaller bottles to ensure that you finish each one while it's still fresh. And even though olive oil may be relatively stable when heated, keep in mind that any fat will eventually get damaged by high temperatures (and that high-temperature cooking can destroy nutrients in the other ingredients in the meal)—so limit frying in favor of gentler cooking methods, like sautéing.

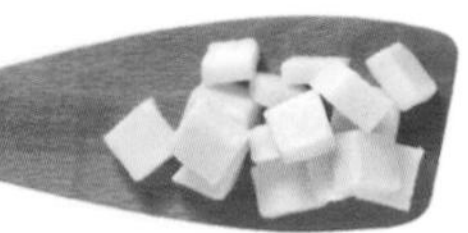

THE SATURATED FAT CONTROVERSY

Many whole foods and oils embraced by the Paleo diet are rich in saturated fat. When eaten in normal quantities (the amounts we get from whole foods, plus reasonable portions of cooking oils), saturated fat is unlikely to be a problem. But there are some issues—and plenty of controversy—involving saturated fat that we should be aware of.

For decades, we've been warned that saturated fat is a dangerous substance capable of raising our cholesterol, clogging our arteries, and sending us to an early grave. Official guidelines told us to swap out animal fats for high-omega-6 vegetable oils to stay healthy (blech!). So natural sources of saturated fat, like butter and coconut oil, were shunned from our menus . . . without actually resulting in improvements to public health.

But the tide is finally turning. Recent meta-analyses have cast substantial doubt on the idea that saturated fat is a major player in heart disease and suggest that the link is either very weak or nonexistent. A major 2010 paper pooled the available research and found "no significant evidence" for the saturated fat/heart disease connection that we've been taught for decades. Awareness that saturated fat is highly resistant to oxidation has also boosted its reputation. As a result, saturated fat has been making a major comeback, with fatty cuts of meat and saturated cooking fats no longer being feared.

So let's get one thing clear: saturated fat, in the amounts present in whole-food animal products and certain plant foods (like coconut), is unlikely to be harmful. Paleo foods high in saturated fat should certainly not be feared or avoided. But some people have taken the "saturated fat isn't bad for you" idea one step further and believe that eating more (and more and more!) saturated fat is health-promoting. In particular, some members of the low-carb and Paleo communities are striving to get as much saturated fat as possible into their diets, above and beyond what would have been possible during most of human history (before we could run to the store and stock up on bricks of grass-fed butter).

Are high intakes of saturated fat really safe, much less beneficial? One of the less-known issues with saturated fat is its potential impact on gut health (which plays a huge role in immunity, disease protection, mental health, obesity, allergies, and countless other conditions). A number of studies have shed light on the ways saturated fat can interact with our gut microbiota, and the news isn't always good. In mice, diets containing high amounts of saturated fat (from palm oil) cause an overflow of fat into the ileum (the last segment of the small intestine) and large intestine, leading to an increase in the *Firmicutes*-to-*Bacteroidetes* ratio, which is associated with obesity. Even though we're not mice, a similar effect likely occurs in humans, leading to harmful changes in mucosal gene expression. In fact, some research in humans has correlated gut dysbiosis and obesity-promoting gut microbes with diets high in saturated fat and low in fiber.

Additional rodent studies show a similar effect from high-saturated-fat foods. One experiment fed mice diets rich in either lard (high in saturated fat) or fish oil (low in saturated fat) for 11 weeks and found that the lard diet raised the animals' levels of *Bilophila, Turicibacter,* and *Bacteroides* while they simultaneously developed metabolic diseases. The change in microbe proportions appeared to increase inflammation through activation of immune molecules called Toll-like receptors (namely TLR4).

In humans and other animals, a very high intake of saturated fat can also induce endotoxemia (raised levels of endotoxins in the blood). Endotoxins (also called lipopolysaccharides, or LPS) are found in the outer membrane of certain bacteria and can trigger strong immune responses and inflammation in our bodies. In fact, endotoxemia is increasingly being viewed as an activator of metabolic diseases and other inflammation-related conditions. In multiple trials using different types of fat (fish oil, cod liver oil, coconut oil, butter, olive oil, and vegetable oils), saturated fats clearly triggered the release of endotoxins from the gut and into the bloodstream. Researchers are still figuring out exactly why, but possible explanations are the tendency for high-saturated-fat diets to increase the abundance of Gram-negative bacteria in the gut (the type of bacteria with endotoxin-containing membranes, an example being *E. coli*), and increase the transport of endotoxins across the gut barrier (using a cellular structure called lipid rafts). It does look like there might be ways to offset the endotoxemic effect from saturated fat: at least in rodents, the addition of prebiotics like oligofructose lowers the endotoxin response, and certain fibers and phytochemicals appear to do the same. Yay for yet another imperative for consuming veggies with our meat!

Too much saturated fat might also cause less-restful sleep. A recent study published in the *Journal of Clinical Sleep Medicine* found that higher saturated fat intake was associated with lighter, less restorative, more disruptive sleep (waking throughout the night). This is a fascinating finding, and we need more research to explore why this connection exists and what mechanism is behind it.

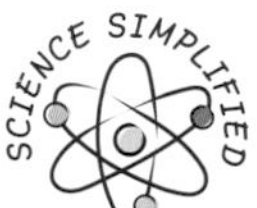

Eating too much saturated fat can both cause the wrong types of bacteria to thrive in our guts and increase the amount of gut bacterial toxins getting inside our bodies.

In addition, even though saturated fat has pretty much been redeemed on the heart disease front, there's one subset of the population that might genuinely need to limit their intake for the sake of heart health: ApoE4 carriers. The ApoE lipoprotein (coded by the ApoE gene) plays a major role in metabolizing and transporting cholesterol and saturated fat. All of us have two copies of the ApoE gene, which can be a combination of any of three variants: ApoE2, ApoE3, or ApoE4. While ApoE2 and ApoE3 carriers generally don't have a noteworthy response to eating saturated fat, ApoE4 carriers are a different story!

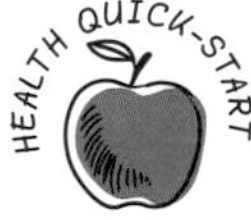

To find out whether you're an ApoE4 carrier, a number of genetic testing services are available, including from www.23andme.com. Your doctor may be able to order an ApoE test for you as well, especially if you have a family history of heart disease and Alzheimer's. If you have one or two copies of ApoE4, it's best to reduce your saturated fat intake.

A number of studies show that compared to the other variants, ApoE4 carriers see a much higher spike in LDL ("bad") cholesterol from eating large amounts of saturated fat (without a corresponding rise in HDL or "good" cholesterol). And they're the group most likely to benefit from lower-saturated-fat diets, since decreasing saturated fat intake causes a sharp decline in LDL cholesterol and an improvement in the HDL/LDL ratio (non-E4 carriers usually don't see that ratio improve from going on a low-fat diet).

The scary news about ApoE4 is that for people who are born with at least one copy (about 20 percent of the population), the risk of heart disease (as well as Alzheimer's) is much higher than the rest of the population. So managing heart health should be on the forefront of these people's minds . . . which means being conservative with saturated fat intake and not going gung ho on things like butter coffee (bulletproof coffee) and bacon.

Even some non-ApoE4 carriers seem to react to extremely high-saturated-fat diets with skyrocketing LDL cholesterol. Some health leaders, such as Peter Attia, MD, have witnessed patients' blood lipid profiles become disconcerting after they embarked on ketogenic diets high in saturated fat (see page 53 for more on ketogenic diets). And we're not just talking LDL concentrations that went up because the particles became big and fluffy: some people exhibited LDL particle counts of more than 3,500 nmol/L (more than could be measured by the NMR machine!), along with increased levels of inflammation, as measured by C-reactive protein. Some of those patients were able to drop their LDL and CRP to less-risky levels simply by replacing most of the saturated fat they were eating with monounsaturated fat. Although this reaction won't happen in everyone, it is important to realize that some people may be "hyper-responders" to saturated fat and are better off moderating their intake.

Several studies have measured the effects of meals rich in different types of fat (saturated versus unsaturated) on the function of endothelial cells, the cells that line all the blood vessels in our bodies. The results? Not looking good for saturated fat! One experiment found that flow-mediated dilation (an artery's ability to relax in response to sheer stress) was impaired after people spent 3 weeks on a high-saturated-fat diet (in the form of butter). That diet also increased levels of adhesion molecules in the subjects' blood (molecules that both endothelial cells and white blood cells use to connect with each other, allowing the white blood cells to leave the bloodstream and move into the tissue as part of an inflammatory response) relative to people who were eating monounsaturated fat-rich or polyunsaturated fat-rich diets. Another study found that a high-saturated-fat meal impaired endothelial function of the arteries and reduced the anti-inflammatory potential of HDL—both bad for cardiovascular health. (Fortunately, some of these effects might be mediated by other components of the diet, such as vitamin E intake.)

When there's any type of bad news about animal foods, people often complain: "But the meat (dairy, tallow, lard, and so on) they used wasn't grass-fed and organic!" After all, most of our research is done on meat and dairy from conventionally raised animals that eat terrible diets, are exposed to extra hormones and antibiotics, and are generally sick and unhealthy. Could that explain some of the negative effects we see from eating lots of saturated fat?

The answer is most likely no. The major concerns with saturated fat are due largely to its chemical structure, which isn't affected by what the animal it came from ate (although the amount of the animal's fat that is saturated is certainly affected). And some of the studies done on saturated fat have used coconut oil or palm oil rather than animal products, with the same results. So this really isn't something we should consider irrelevant just because we shop at farmers markets and eat higher-quality animal foods.

So what constitutes a reasonable (and safe) intake? One clue comes from hunter-gatherers. Even though most contemporarily studied hunter-gatherers get more than half of their calories from animal foods and, in rare cases like the Inuit, as much as 58 percent

PALEO FATS AND OILS

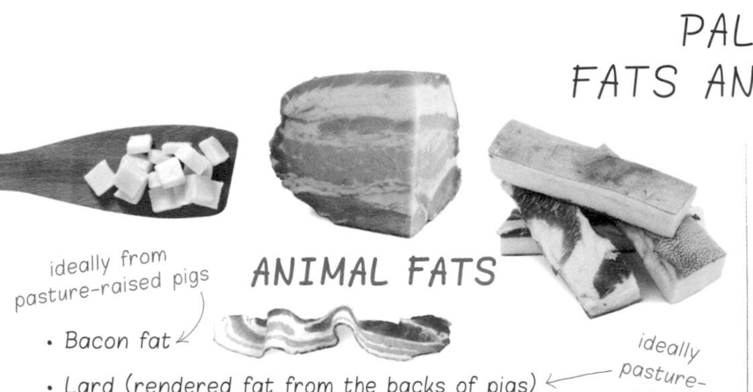

ANIMAL FATS

- Bacon fat (ideally from pasture-raised pigs)
- Lard (rendered fat from the backs of pigs) (ideally pasture-raised)
- Leaf lard (rendered fat from around pigs' kidneys and other internal organs)
- Poultry fat (typically duck, goose, or emu)
- Salo (rendered fat from cured slabs of pork fatback)
- Schmaltz (chicken or goose fat)
- Strutto (clarified pork fat)
- Tallow (rendered fat from beef, lamb, or mutton) (ideally grass-fed)

ideally pasture-raised (Salo, Schmaltz, Strutto)

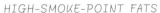

Generally, animal fats are used for cooking, but they can also be used to flavor baked root veggies and steamed vegetables.

HIGH-SMOKE-POINT FATS

—any fat with a smoke point higher than your cooking temperature; think 350°F and above for typical applications—are ideal for cooking. They each impart a different flavor and nutrition profiles, so it's best to mix it up!

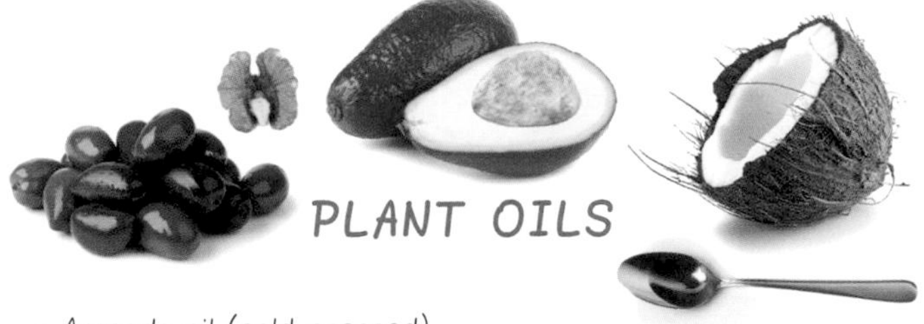

PLANT OILS

- Avocado oil (cold pressed)
- Coconut oil (typically extra-virgin, expeller pressed, but also naturally refined)
- Macadamia nut oil
- Olive oil, extra-virgin and virgin
- Palm oil (not to be confused with palm kernel oil)
- Palm shortening
- Red palm oil
- Sesame oil (regular or toasted)
- Walnut oil

look for ethically and sustainably sourced (Palm oil, Palm shortening, Red palm oil)

Plant oils are typically used for dressings, although coconut oil, palm oil, red palm oil, and palm shortening are all solid at room temperature.

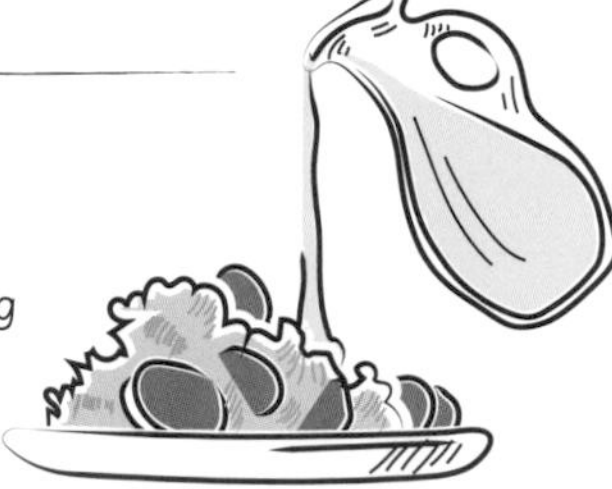

Nut and seed oils, avocado oil, and olive oil are liquid at room temperature and work well for salad and vegetable dressings.

of their calories from fat, the average caloric intake from saturated fat among these populations is only 13 percent. Surprised? Wild game meat is much lower in saturated fat than industrially produced (grain-fed) meat, in addition to being lower in fat overall. (In fact, depending on the source, the fat can be up to about 50 percent monounsaturated and 30 percent polyunsaturated, compared to about 50 percent saturated in some fats from grain-fed animals.) And while fish and shellfish do contain saturated fat, the dominant fats in seafood are monounsaturated and long-chain omega-3 polyunsaturated fats. Add the fact that most plant sources of fat are monounsaturated and polyunsaturated, the 13 percent calories from saturated fat number starts to make sense.

HEALTH QUICK-START *Aim for 10 to 15 percent of your total caloric intake to come from saturated fat; that equates to a quarter to a half of all fat consumed being saturated if you're aiming for 30 to 40 percent total caloric intake from fats. That's pretty easy to accomplish when you stick to quality whole foods and modest amounts of healthy fats for cooking and dressing foods.*

All that said, while eating excessive amounts of saturated fat doesn't seem to be a good idea, going out of our way to avoid it isn't wise, either. Along with assisting in the absorption of fat-soluble vitamins, saturated fat is found in many foods that have additional health-promoting compounds. Consuming a variety of plant and animal foods (without deliberately trying to increase saturated fat intake) will naturally land most of us in a healthy intake range.

SMOKE POINTS OF VARIOUS FATS AND OILS

FAT/OIL	TEMPERATURE
Almond oil	420°F
Avocado oil, refined	520°F
Avocado oil, virgin	375°F
Butter	350°F
Coconut oil, extra virgin	350°F
Coconut oil, refined	450°F
Flax seed oil	225°F
Ghee	485°F
Hazelnut oil	430°F
Lard	370°F
Leaf lard	370°F
Macadamia nut oil	410°F
Olive oil, extra-virgin	250°F–450°F*
Olive oil, virgin	375°F
Palm oil	450°F
Palm shortening	450°F
Poultry fat/schmaltz	375°F
Red palm oil	425°F
Salo	370°F
Sesame oil, semirefined	450°F
Sesame oil, unrefined	350°F
Strutto	370°F
Tallow	400°F
Walnut oil, semirefined	400°F
Walnut oil, virgin	320°F

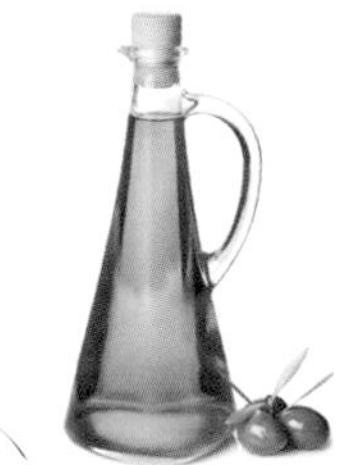

*The smoke point of olive oil varies depending on the quality. A fresh cold-pressed olive oil (one that has a press date instead of a best by date on the bottle) typically has a very high smoke point thanks to its polyphenol content. If you aren't sure how good your olive oil is and the manufacturer doesn't specify on the bottle, it's best to assume 250°F and reserve for dressings.

FAT PROFILES OF VARIOUS ANIMAL FATS AND PLANT OILS**	TOTAL FAT IN 100g SERVING (g)	SATURATED FAT (g/100g)	MONOUNSATURATED FAT (g/100g)	POLYUNSATURATED FAT (g/100g)	OMEGA-6 FATTY ACIDS (g/100g)	OMEGA-3 FATTY ACIDS (g/100g)
Almond oil	100.0	8.2	69.9	17.4	17.4	0.0
Avocado oil	100.0	11.6	70.6	13.5	12.5	1.0
Beef tallow	100.0	49.8	41.8	3.1	0.6	0.0
Butter	55.1	34.3	15.9	2.0	1.2	0.8
Coconut oil	100.0	86.5	5.8	1.8	1.8	0.0
Duck fat	99.8	33.2	49.3	12.9	11.9	1.0
Flax seed oil	100.0	9.4	20.2	66.0	12.7	53.3
Ghee	99.5	61.9	28.7	3.7	2.2	1.5
Hazelnut oil	100.0	7.4	78.0	10.2	10.1	0.0
Lard	100.0	39.2	45.1	11.2	10.2	1.0
Mutton tallow	100.0	47.3	40.6	7.8	5.5	2.3
Olive oil	100.0	13.8	73.0	10.5	9.7	7.6
Schmaltz (chicken fat)	99.8	29.8	44.7	20.9	19.5	1.0
Sesame oil	100.0	14.2	39.7	41.7	41.3	0.3
Walnut oil	100.0	9.1	22.8	63.3	10.4	52.9

**Data is for conventional and industrially produced non-organic products. Higher-quality products like grass-fed tallow and fresh estate olive oil will have slightly different fat profiles. The biggest differences between conventional and higher-quality animal fats are the ratio of omega-3 to omega-6 fat and the concentration of fat-soluble vitamins. The biggest difference with plant oils is in phytochemical and vitamin content. Remember that the omega-3 fatty acids from plant oils are predominantly ALA, which is converted very inefficiently into DHA and EPA, the main forms of omega-3 used by the body. The omega-3 fatty acids in animal fats are DHA and EPA.

Chapter 12: PROBIOTIC AND FERMENTED FOODS

Most of us are familiar with at least a handful of fermented foods (like sauerkraut and yogurt), but the history, variety, and benefits of fermentation are much more extensive than many people realize. In fact, more than 5,000 types of fermented foods have been documented across the globe, and they include nearly every edible thing you can think of—meats, fish, cereal products, legumes, vegetables, fruits, beverages, nuts, and seeds. Especially before refrigeration was widespread, fermentation was ridiculously useful for preserving foods and extending the shelf life of perishable items. That's why populations around the world have used fermentation in their traditional cuisines for thousands of years.

Just because we have refrigerators now doesn't mean that fermentation isn't still a valuable practice. In fact, fermented foods offer some amazing benefits that can't be obtained from other nutrient-dense foods. Including them in our diet can be a major plus for our health—and not to mention, they're delicious!

FERMENTATION

Fermentation is the process of biochemically modifying a food by using microorganisms and their enzymes. It is a type of preservation, allowing a food to be shelf-stable without rotting or degrading. Different types of bacteria (especially *Lactobacillus* and *Acetobacter* species), mold (including *Penicillium* species used for cheeses), and yeast (including the *Saccharomyces* family) are used to produce different types of fermented foods. In contrast to food getting contaminated by pathogenic organisms (which is bad!), only "safe" microbes are involved in the fermentation process.

Typically, when we talk about foods that are rich in probiotics, we're referring to foods that have been bacterially fermented. Mold fermentation can create health-promoting foods (such as some types of cheese and tempeh, a type of fermented soy), but it generally doesn't supply the types of probiotic organisms that benefit our guts the most. Some forms of yeast, especially in the *Saccharomyces* family, are also considered to have probiotic effects.

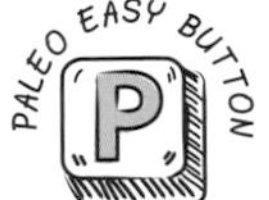

When buying kombucha, water kefir, or sauerkraut, look for "raw" or "unpasteurized" on the packaging. Pasteurization applies high heat to a food in order to kill bacteria (pathogenic contaminants and probiotics). While this process extends shelf life, it also kills all the wonderful microbes that make these foods uniquely beneficial.

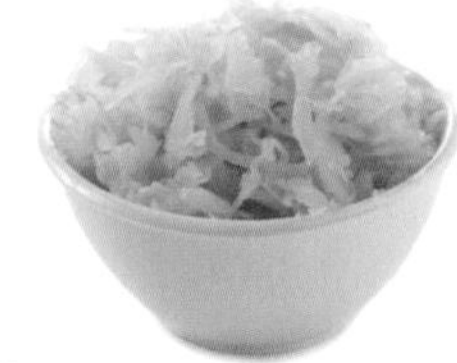

PROBIOTIC BENEFITS

In a nutshell, probiotics are living microorganisms that are beneficial to the host who eats them (that's us!). We don't yet fully understand how they exert all those benefits (partly because there are about 35,000 species of probiotic bacteria out there, only a tiny fraction of them have been characterized, and each strain seems to have a unique effect on the body). But we can say with confidence that probiotics can have a profound effect on the immune system, can decrease the populations of less favorable bacteria in the gut (helping improve gut dysbiosis), and may directly and indirectly impact a number of health conditions, ranging from autoimmune diseases to obesity to diabetes.

When we consume fermented foods (raw, unpasteurized, and still teeming with friendly microbes), we get the benefits of these probiotics along with the additional micronutrients and helpful compounds found in whole foods. So it's no surprise that fermented foods have repeatedly turned up as protective in the scientific literature. Fermented dairy containing *Lactobacillus bulgaricus* and *Streptococcus thermophilus* (yes, there are probiotic species in the *Streptococcus* genus, and no, they won't give you strep throat) has been shown to deactivate etiologic risk factors for colon cancer—increasing the excretion of components that harm colon cells and induce oxidized DNA bases. (Even for people sensitive to dairy, other foods fermented with *Lactobacillus* strains may have a similar effect.) Foods fermented with *Bifidobacteria* have shown up as protective against gastrointestinal disorders. Studies of yeast-fermented foods containing the *Saccharomyces* family suggest that they may reduce some symptoms of irritable bowel syndrome (IBS). A variety of lactofermented foods have been linked to improved intestinal tract health, reduced symptoms of lactose intolerance, and reduced risk of certain cancers.

TYPES OF PROBIOTICS AND FERMENTED FOODS

As previously mentioned, there are tens of thousands of probiotic species, and we've only scratched the surface in terms of characterizing them and researching their effects. But a few main types of probiotics have been extensively studied, and their specific health effects are well documented.

***Lactobacillus* strains** (rich in fermented veggies, dairy, and meats):

In general, improve lactose digestion (and decrease symptoms of lactose intolerance) and boost mucosal immune function (gut, lung, sinuses, and so on)

- ***Lactobacillus acidophilus*** can reduce cholesterol levels and protect against urogenital infection; in animal models, it decreases colon polyps, colorectal adenomas (precursors to cancerous colon tumors), and colon cancer
- ***Lactobacillus plantarum*** can reduce pain, constipation, bloating, flatulence, and inflammation in inflammatory bowel disorders
- ***Lactobacillus reuteri*** shortens episodes of diarrhea and acute gastroenteritis
- ***Lactobacillus rhamnosus*** can enhance cellular immunity
- ***Lactobacillus salivarius*** has been shown to suppress and eradicate *H. pylori* in animal models and tissue cultures

***Bifidobacteria* species** (rich in fermented veggies, dairy, and meats):

- Can help prevent and treat gastrointestinal disorders such as colonic transit disorders, colorectal adenomas, colon cancer, and intestinal infections
- May prevent or improve gastroenteritis (infectious diarrhea)
- Tentative evidence of protective action against carcinogenic activity of intestinal flora

Saccharomyces boulardii (rich in kefir and kombucha, but also in fermented veggies, dairy, and soy):

- Reduces occurrence of *difficile* infection
- Reduces duration of acute gastroenteritis
- In irritable bowel syndrome, may decrease functional diarrhea

Although probiotic supplementation can be useful in a lot of circumstances, we can get a much broader range of probiotics (including the ones listed above and the less well characterized but still very beneficial ones) by eating fermented foods. When you ferment your own vegetables at home, the probiotic strains will vary from batch to batch, thereby providing far greater diversity than you can garner from supplements. For example, an analysis of different sauerkraut fermentations yielded a total of 686 probiotic bacterial strains. By contrast, most probiotic supplements contain between two and nine strains. The most common probiotic strains in sauerkraut are bacteria from the genera *Lactobacillus, Leuconostoc, Weissella,* and *Pediococcus.*

FERMENTATION IS GREAT FOR FOOD STORAGE, TOO!

Other perks of fermentation aren't even nutritional. One of the oldest (as in thousands of years old) known benefits of fermentation is its ability to extend the shelf life of food. By increasing acidity, fermentation can kill off many pathogenic organisms (including ones that cause spoilage and food poisoning, like *E. coli*) and prevent food from going bad. In that way, fermentation serves a similar function to canning, pasteurization, dehydration, and other food preservation methods—but with a huge list of additional perks!

As a result, fermentation is a great method to use on fresh fruits and vegetables that would otherwise be available only in season, allowing us to enjoy them year-round. Did you buy too many summer cucumbers at the farmers market? Pickle them! Did you go blackberry picking and end up with more buckets than you can possibly eat? Ferment the ones you don't want to freeze—and within a few days you'll have a tart and bubbly treat, packed with probiotics, micronutrients, antioxidants, and flavor.

Fermented beverages, such as kombucha and kefir, contain beneficial strains of yeast in addition to probiotic bacteria. Kombucha and kefir both typically contain the beneficial yeast *Saccharomyces boulardii.* Kombucha typically contains probiotic bacteria from the *Acetobacter* genus. Both coconut milk kefir and water kefir typically contain probiotics from the genera *Lactobacillus, Leuconostoc, Acetobacter,* and *Streptococcus.* Kombucha and kefir cultures regularly contain upward of forty probiotic strains.

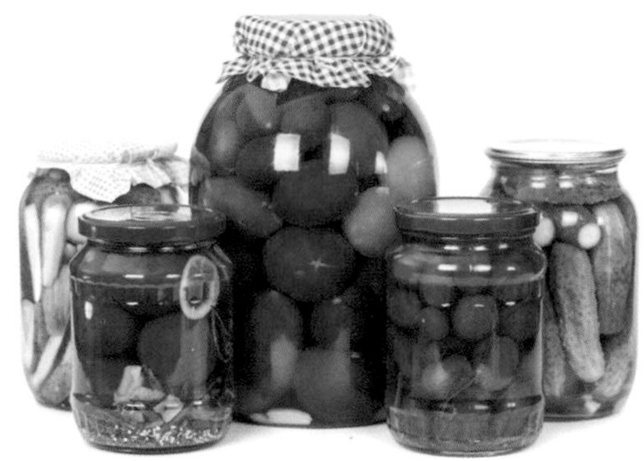

What can we load our plates with? Let's start with some of these:

- Raw, unpasteurized fermented vegetables (sauerkraut, kimchi, pickles, beets, carrots)
- Raw, unpasteurized fermented fruits (chutneys, jams, green papaya, pickled jackfruit)
- Kombucha
- Raw, unpasteurized fermented condiments ("real" ketchup, relishes, salsas, pickled ginger)
- Water kefir
- Coconut milk kefir
- Coconut milk yogurt
- Beet kvass
- If you tolerate quality dairy (see Chapter 24), raw, unpasteurized yogurt or kefir
- If you tolerate soy, natto, miso, tempeh, and tamari (fermented soy is also rich in vitamin K2, but keep in mind that fermentation doesn't reduce the phytoestrogen content of soy foods, so these products still contain very high levels of potential endocrine-disrupting chemicals)

Want to make your own fermented foods? See page 491 for a recipe for homemade sauerkraut and page 492 for a recipe for homemade kombucha. Once you've got those mastered, a great resource to challenge your home fermentation skills is the book *Fermented* by Jill Ciciarelli.

MORE THAN HELPFUL MICROBES: NUTRIENT BIOAVAILABILITY, CONVERSIONS, AND PRESERVATION

While the probiotic content of fermented foods is reason enough for us to include them in our diets, fermentation offers a number of other perks. One is enhancing the bioavailability of nutrients. As a nutrient geek, this excites me even more than the probiotic benefits.

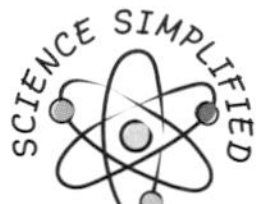

Not only do fermented foods provide beneficial bacteria and other microbes, but they tend to be nutritionally enhanced, containing more vitamins and minerals.

Bioavailability refers to the proportion of a nutrient within a food that gets digested, absorbed, and used/metabolized by the body. Cooking enhances the bioavailability of many fiber-bound foods, for example, by breaking down cellulose (the main component of plant cell walls) and making nutrients more accessible to digestive enzymes. But it just so happens that fermentation does something similar, without the nutrient destruction that comes from high temperatures or heavy processing. In fact, some probiotic microbes produce cellulase, an enzyme that degrades cellulose without needing heat. Tomatoes illustrate this perfectly: cooking is known to increase their lycopene and β-carotene content, but lactic acid fermentation has the same effect—increasing bioavailable lycopene from 3.70 to 5.68 milligrams per 100 grams and β-carotene from 0.28 or 0.89 milligrams to 1.14 milligrams per 100 grams, depending on the tomato variety.

In their unprocessed state, many foods contain antinutrients that bind to minerals and inhibit their absorption. Phytates (antioxidant compounds found in grains, legumes, nuts, and seeds) are a common example, and their presence can limit the absorption of iron, zinc, and manganese (and to a lesser extent, calcium). But some microbes involved in fermentation can produce phytase enzymes, which hydrolyze phytate and grant our bodies greater access to the minerals in the food we're eating. By some estimates, fermentation can remove at least 90 percent of existing phytate from corn, cassava, cowpeas, lima bean, sorghum, soybeans, and cocoyam. As an added bonus, organic acids produced during fermentation, including citric acid, malic acid, and lactic acid, can potentially enhance mineral absorption as well, especially for iron and zinc.

A similar effect happens with polyphenols—plant chemicals that are widely considered beneficial for their antioxidant properties but can also reduce the bioavailability of certain minerals. Because fermentation increases the acidity of a food, it can create the optimal pH conditions for polyphenols to be enzymatically degraded. For example, a study on cocoa pods found that fermentation (done by piling cocoa beans between layers of banana leaves for 6 days) increased the beans' copper content by about 100 percent, due in part to reducing levels of tannin—a type of polyphenol—that naturally occurs in cocoa.

Along with increasing bioavailability, fermentation can convert some micronutrients into new forms. This happens through the process of biosynthesis, where certain bacteria help synthesize new beneficial compounds. A great example is the conversion of menaquinones (vitamin K2) by *Bacillus subtilis*, the strain of bacteria used to ferment natto (a traditional Japanese soybean product). Even though fresh soybeans don't contain vitamin K2, fermentation with *Bacillus subtilis* causes the resulting product to be one of the highest sources of vitamin K2 of any food in existence, due to it being synthesized by bacteria during fermentation. In fact, most of the Paleo rationale against eating soy is no longer valid once we start talking about these nutrient-dense, more easily digested fermented versions of soy. Those of us who don't have an overt sensitivity to soy and don't have sex hormone imbalances might find natto or tempeh to be a good addition to our diet (even if other soy-based foods are off-limits).

Chapter 13:
NUTS AND SEEDS

Nuts and seeds are typically regarded as nutritious, health-promoting foods. Since they were around before humans even existed, it's hard to argue that they're not really Paleo!

A mere 20 grams of tree nuts per day is associated with substantially reduced risk (think 20 to 70 percent) of cardiovascular disease, cancer, neurodegenerative disease, kidney disease, diabetes, infections, and mortality from respiratory disease. Even three 1-ounce servings a week can lower all-cause mortality risk by a whopping 39 percent, meaning that eating nuts on a regular basis can not only improve health, but potentially extend life span, too.

Nut consumption is also known to decrease markers of inflammation (see page 78), including C-reactive protein (CRP, a common indirect measure of inflammation that your doctor can test for with a simple blood test), the pro-inflammatory cytokines IL-6, TNF-α, and IL-18 (messenger molecules that drive immune responses), and some endothelial markers of inflammation (molecules like ICAM-1 that mediate the interaction between endothelial cells, the cells that form blood vessels, and activated immune cells as the latter leave the blood and enter inflamed tissues). There's emerging evidence of beneficial effects on oxidative stress, vascular reactivity (how a blood vessel responds to changing stimuli, like a change in blood pressure due to exertion), and hypertension. Numerous studies show that people who regularly eat nuts tend to have more favorable blood lipid profiles, and one meta-analysis of twenty-five clinical studies showed that nut consumption had a dose-response cholesterol-lowering effect, meaning that the higher the nut consumption, the bigger the improvement in cholesterol. Interventional studies consistently show that increasing nut intake has a cholesterol-lowering effect, even in the context of a healthy diet. Plenty of research suggests that, despite their energy density, nuts and seeds don't contribute to weight gain, and they may even protect against obesity and diabetes.

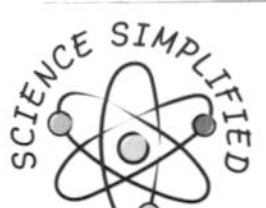

A palmful of nuts or seeds per day is associated with many health benefits. However, more is not better, and there are good reasons to limit nut and seed consumption to about an ounce per day.

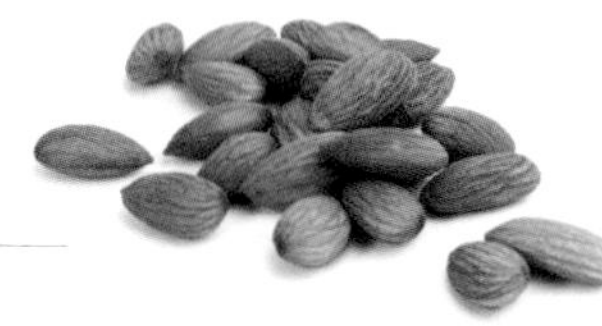

The health benefits of consuming nuts and seeds can be attributed to their nutritional content. They are rich in antioxidant vitamins and essential minerals and are a major dietary source of magnesium, dietary fiber, and L-arginine. Some nuts contain high levels of heart-healthy monounsaturated fats and the omega-3 fatty acid α-linolenic acid. Brazil nuts are a fantastic source of selenium (a relatively hard-to-get antioxidant mineral), pistachios are rich in prebiotic fiber, walnuts are high in anti-inflammatory omega-3 fats, and nuts and seeds in general tend to be good sources of copper, manganese, vitamin B1, vitamin B9, tocopherols (vitamin E), phytosterols, and phenolic compounds. In fact, nuts are often rich in the same minerals that Paleo adherents tend to be low in (especially people who don't eat much organ meat) and, in that sense, are a valuable addition to the menu to help ensure nutritional adequacy.

KNOWLEDGE BOMB

Peanuts are not actually a tree nut, but rather a legume! In fact, they are one of the most inflammatory legumes owing to their peanut lectin content, which is discussed in more detail on page 251. Unlike nuts, peanuts have a soft, porous shell, so contaminants—fertilizers, pesticides, and molds—can permeate them. Because mold is a common problem for peanut farmers, peanuts are some of the most heavily sprayed crops, with more than 99 percent of U.S. peanut farms using pesticides, including fungicide. Unfortunately, when it comes to peanuts, going organic is a little like going from the frying pan into the fire: the same mold that makes organic farming of peanuts so challenging contaminates them with the carcinogen aflatoxin. That gives us three good reasons to switch to nut butter alternatives like almond butter, cashew butter, and sunflower seed butter.

KNOWLEDGE BOMB

The botany of nuts is fascinating! Most common nuts aren't actually nuts at all, but rather the seeds of drupes, a type of fleshy fruit with a hard stone or pit. The stone or pit is what we call a "nut." Almonds, cashews, pecans, pili nuts, pistachios, walnuts, and coconut are all the seeds of drupes. A true nut, on the other hand, is a hard-shelled, uncompartmented fruit that does not split to release seeds once mature. True nuts include chestnuts and hazelnuts. Pine nuts are from yet another botanical category, called nutlike gymnosperm seeds; Brazil nuts and macadamia nuts fall into the botanical category nutlike angiosperm seeds.

BUT DON'T "GO NUTS"

The health benefits of nut and seed consumption do not continue to increase beyond about 20 grams per day, and there's some evidence that consuming large amounts of nuts daily can increase disease risk (at least for stroke). That means we get benefits with about a palmful of nuts or seeds per day, but eating more than that won't do us any favors (and may potentially undermine our health).

Tree nuts are among the most allergenic foods, with true allergies (meaning the body produces IgE antibodies against proteins in nuts) estimated at about 1 percent of the population. Some preliminary scientific studies show that nut intolerance (meaning the body produces IgG antibodies against proteins in nuts) may affect a whopping 20 to 50 percent of us. There are two ways to diagnose allergy and intolerance to nuts. The first is to do food allergy and sensitivity testing (a blood test that looks for IgE and IgG antibodies and sometimes IgA and IgM antibodies against various food antigens), and the second is to follow an elimination protocol (see Chapter 25). If you aren't sure, tree nuts may be worth avoiding (at least temporarily), especially if you have a digestive or autoimmune disorder.

HEALTH QUICK-START

To be sure you aren't intolerant or allergic to nuts, consider getting food intolerance and allergy testing (a simple blood test that looks at IgE and IgG antibodies against foods) before including them as part of your regular diet.

Nuts and seeds also contain phytates, which inhibit nutrient absorption by binding to minerals—typically iron, calcium, and magnesium—in the small intestine (although soaking nuts prior to eating them can reduce the phytic acid content). Our gut bacteria can liberate some of these valuable minerals from phytates for us, but their capacity is limited, which might partially explain why we cease to see benefits from nut consumption beyond 20 grams daily.

Likewise, nuts and seeds typically contain large amounts of polyunsaturated fats, usually the pro-inflammatory omega-6 fatty acids (see page 158). Even the nuts that contain the highest amounts of omega-3s (like walnuts) still have ratios of omega-3 to omega-6 fatty acids in the neighborhood of 1:3, and many nuts and seeds contain only trace omega-3 fatty acids. Although their omega-6 content is often used as a rationale for limiting nut and seed consumption, most evidence suggests that when these foods are consumed in moderate amounts in their whole form (opposed to highly processed oils stripped of most micronutrients and phytochemicals), their net effect is anti-inflammatory due to the presence of other beneficial compounds, such as vitamin E, dietary fiber, L-arginine, and phenolic compounds. In other words, their omega-6 content alone doesn't appear to be a reason to cut out nuts and seeds completely and instead reinforces the concept of moderate consumption.

What's more, two exceptions to the omega-6 concern are coconut and macadamia nuts, both of which contain a very low percentage of their fats as polyunsaturated fats. The fat in coconut is largely medium-chain saturated fat. The fat in macadamia nuts is predominantly monounsaturated fat. (These two nuts also have some of the lowest levels of phytates.)

Overall, nuts and seeds can definitely fit within a Paleo framework but are best consumed in moderation (1 ounce per day) and should be avoided by people with nut or seed allergies or sensitivities.

One study showed that cashews are one of the most common nuts to which people have intolerances, affecting upwards of 50 percent of the study participants. In comparison, incidence of intolerance to almonds was about 28 percent, Brazil nuts was 23 percent, and walnuts was 3 percent. Note that this study included people with gastrointestinal symptoms and did not represent the general population.

PALEO EASY BUTTON

It's easy to overdo it with nuts and seeds. If you have trouble moderating portion size, try thinking of them as a condiment—perhaps sprinkling them on salads or veggies—instead of eating of them as a snack food or base for baked goods. For example, 1 cup of almond flour contains about 90 whole almonds, or nearly 4 ounces. Nut butters can add up quickly, too: 2 measly tablespoons is more than an ounce for most nut butters.

COCONUT

Coconut is a very unique nut. It's generally not considered a tree nut because it is the seed of the coconut palm fruit, a type of plant that is more closely related to grass than to other trees, although co-allergies with tree nuts do occur. Unlike most nuts and seeds, coconut does not contain much omega-6 fatty acid. Instead, coconut is rich in medium-chain triglycerides (MCTs), a very special "short"-chain saturated fat with diverse health benefits. Approximately 60 percent of the fat in coconut is MCTs.

Coconut is also a rich source of manganese, a mineral necessary for enzymes that work to protect the body from and repair damage caused by free radicals. Copper, iron, and selenium are also found in good quantities in coconut, as are calcium, magnesium, phosphorous, potassium, and zinc to a lesser degree. Coconut is a fairly good source of many B vitamins, including vitamins B1, B2, B3, B5, B6, and B9. Coconut also provides vitamins C and E, phytosterols, and fiber. In fact, it contains a lot of inulin fiber, a highly fermentable soluble fiber that the beneficial bacteria in our guts love. Inulin fiber is one of the most heavily studied functional fibers (see page 39).

Coconut has long been recognized for its ability to boost the immune system and act as an antibiotic, antiviral, antibacterial, antifungal, and antimicrobial (basically, small things that might make you sick don't like coconut). It is even believed that a daily dose of coconut is one of the best ways to restore healthy gut flora (I don't think there are any studies proving this, though). Note that coconut does contain some phytic acid (although much, much less than most tree nuts), which can be a problem for some people and does suggest that coconut too should be consumed in moderation.

Coconut oil also has diverse antimicrobial properties. Dietary MCTs have been shown to radically reduce the production of a variety of pro-inflammatory cytokines (meaning that they reduce inflammation), increase activity of the histamine-clearing enzyme diamine oxidase (great for histamine sensitivity and allergy), increase mucus production (great for gut barrier health), and support gut-barrier healing (by increasing cell turnover rate in the gut). However, MCTs can also increase the secretion of IgA antibodies in the gut (specifically in the Peyer's patches), generally considered a marker of a healthy immune system but which may be problematic for people whose secretory IgA antibody levels are already high, despite all the other benefits. If you have a reaction to coconut oil, switch to other healthy fats for cooking.

NUTS AND SEEDS

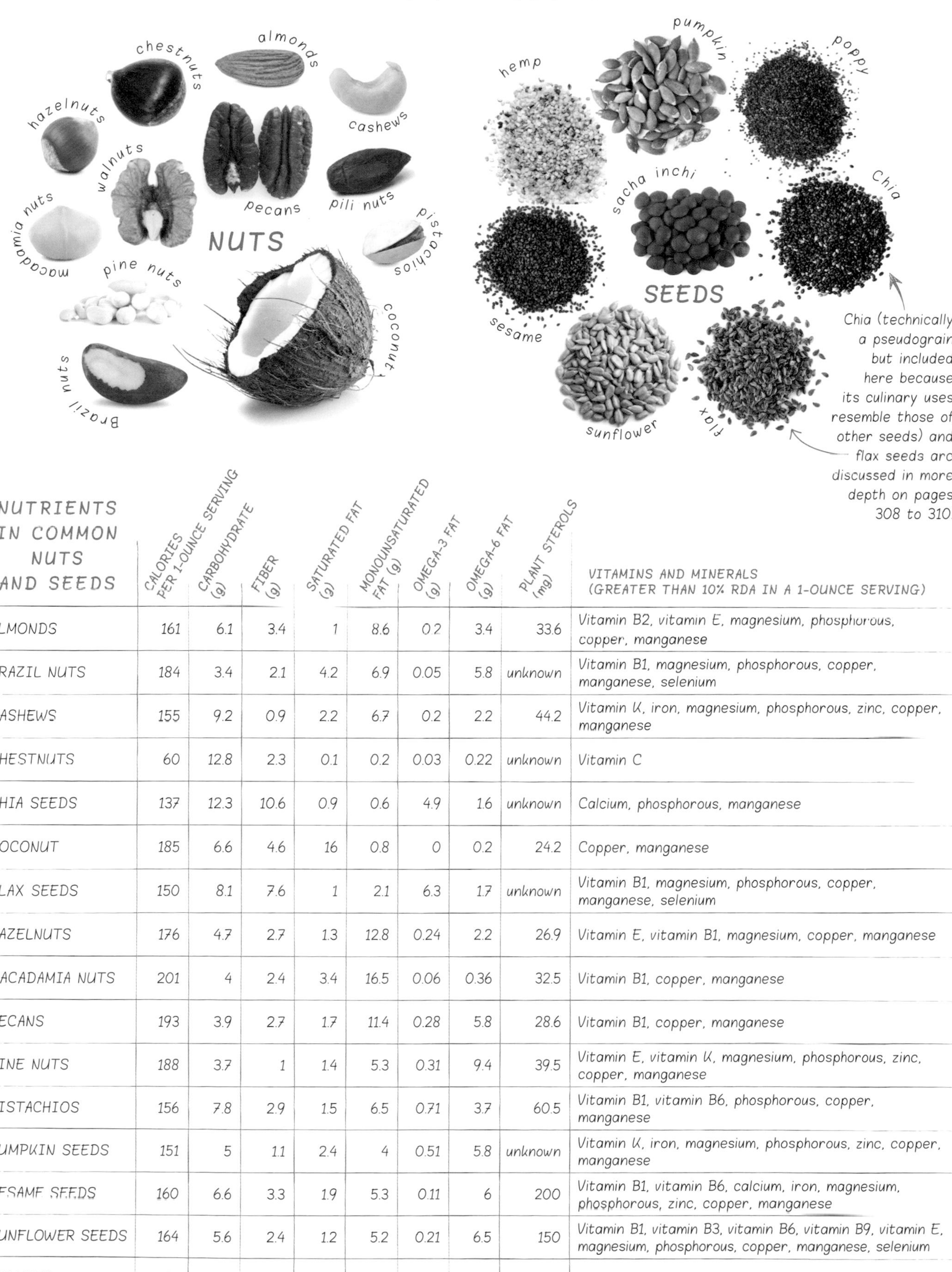

Chia (technically a pseudograin but included here because its culinary uses resemble those of other seeds) and flax seeds are discussed in more depth on pages 308 to 310.

NUTRIENTS IN COMMON NUTS AND SEEDS	CALORIES PER 1-OUNCE SERVING	CARBOHYDRATE (g)	FIBER (g)	SATURATED FAT (g)	MONOUNSATURATED FAT (g)	OMEGA-3 FAT (g)	OMEGA-6 FAT (g)	PLANT STEROLS (mg)	VITAMINS AND MINERALS (GREATER THAN 10% RDA IN A 1-OUNCE SERVING)
ALMONDS	161	6.1	3.4	1	8.6	0.2	3.4	33.6	Vitamin B2, vitamin E, magnesium, phosphorous, copper, manganese
BRAZIL NUTS	184	3.4	2.1	4.2	6.9	0.05	5.8	unknown	Vitamin B1, magnesium, phosphorous, copper, manganese, selenium
CASHEWS	155	9.2	0.9	2.2	6.7	0.2	2.2	44.2	Vitamin K, iron, magnesium, phosphorous, zinc, copper, manganese
CHESTNUTS	60	12.8	2.3	0.1	0.2	0.03	0.22	unknown	Vitamin C
CHIA SEEDS	137	12.3	10.6	0.9	0.6	4.9	1.6	unknown	Calcium, phosphorous, manganese
COCONUT	185	6.6	4.6	16	0.8	0	0.2	24.2	Copper, manganese
FLAX SEEDS	150	8.1	7.6	1	2.1	6.3	1.7	unknown	Vitamin B1, magnesium, phosphorous, copper, manganese, selenium
HAZELNUTS	176	4.7	2.7	1.3	12.8	0.24	2.2	26.9	Vitamin E, vitamin B1, magnesium, copper, manganese
MACADAMIA NUTS	201	4	2.4	3.4	16.5	0.06	0.36	32.5	Vitamin B1, copper, manganese
PECANS	193	3.9	2.7	1.7	11.4	0.28	5.8	28.6	Vitamin B1, copper, manganese
PINE NUTS	188	3.7	1	1.4	5.3	0.31	9.4	39.5	Vitamin E, vitamin K, magnesium, phosphorous, zinc, copper, manganese
PISTACHIOS	156	7.8	2.9	1.5	6.5	0.71	3.7	60.5	Vitamin B1, vitamin B6, phosphorous, copper, manganese
PUMPKIN SEEDS	151	5	1.1	2.4	4	0.51	5.8	unknown	Vitamin K, iron, magnesium, phosphorous, zinc, copper, manganese
SESAME SEEDS	160	6.6	3.3	1.9	5.3	0.11	6	200	Vitamin B1, vitamin B6, calcium, iron, magnesium, phosphorous, zinc, copper, manganese
SUNFLOWER SEEDS	164	5.6	2.4	1.2	5.2	0.21	6.5	150	Vitamin B1, vitamin B3, vitamin B6, vitamin B9, vitamin E, magnesium, phosphorous, copper, manganese, selenium
WALNUTS	183	3.8	1.9	1.7	2.5	2.5	10.7	20.2	Magnesium, phosphorous, copper, manganese

Chapter 14: SEASONINGS

Seasonings include any salt, herbs, or spices we add to food to enhance its flavor. Along with being among the most important intricacies of any meal we cook, they form the backbone of regional cuisines around the globe (think of the distinctive herb and spice blends that characterize Italian food, Thai food, Mexican food, Indian food, French food, and so on). In fact, seasonings have been part of human history for thousands of years, and the quest to obtain them inspired some of humankind's earliest global trade routes.

But as delicious as they may be, not all seasonings are created equal. They range from having proven medicinal qualities to being likely autoimmune triggers in susceptible individuals (in fact, some seasonings fit both those categories simultaneously). Let's take a closer look at salt, herbs, and spices individually to understand how each one fits into a Paleo framework.

SALT

Salt doesn't really taste like anything, yet it is the ubiquitous seasoning, enhancing the flavor of just about everything. Salt accomplishes this amazing feat in two ways. First, by helping some molecules in foods more easily release into the air, salt heightens a food's aroma; smell is essential to our perception of taste. Second, salt reduces our perception of bitter flavors. Our taste buds detect five distinct flavors: sweet, sour, bitter, salty, and umami. Most aromatic foods (like herbs and green vegetables) are bitter, so by suppressing our bitter taste buds, salt enhances our ability to taste sweet, sour, and umami, making most foods more palatable.

Yet, along with saturated fat, few nutrients have gotten as much flak over the years as salt! The belief that salt (or more specifically, sodium) raises blood pressure and contributes to disease risk is still common. But despite the controversy and misconceptions, salt absolutely has a science-based place within the Paleo framework.

Salt has a remarkably simple molecular structure, being made predominantly of just two elements: sodium and chloride (pure salt is the molecule sodium chloride, NaCl).

Sodium is an essential nutrient: living in a moderate climate and not sweating much, the human body would need about 115 milligrams per day just to stay alive (the safe lower limit is generally given as 500 milligrams per day). Sodium is vital for cellular function, nutrient absorption in the digestive tract, kidney health, adrenal function, and cardiac health. And because sodium is an electrolyte (a special type of mineral that carries an electrical charge), it also plays a role in maintaining a normal blood pH, regulating the amount of water in the body, conducting nerve impulses, and controlling muscle contractions (including those of the heart!).

While "low-sodium diet" has reached buzzword status, it's important to discuss the other half of the salt molecule, which is chloride. Chloride (the ionic form of chlorine—that is, a single chlorine atom with a net electrical charge due to the loss of an electron) is required for the production of hydrochloric acid in the stomach and is important for electrolyte balance, as well as fluid balance in the body. The effects of excess chloride have not been studied extensively (although we could argue that all studies looking at high salt intake are really looking at what happens when we eat both too much sodium *and* too much chloride). There's an interesting interplay between chloride levels and potassium levels, which may explain some of the effects of high chloride intake, such as increasing the hypertensive effects of high sodium intake but decreasing the kidney damage associated with high sodium intake.

Salt in Hunter-Gatherer Diets

When forming theories about what's best for our bodies, looking at our evolutionary diet is a great place to start. While there's no evidence that early humans actively mined and collected salt in the way we do today (the oldest salt mine dates back about 6,500 years), chances are good that salt was available and at least occasionally consumed.

One clue comes from wild animals. A huge variety of creatures—including moose, African elephants, mountain goats, deer, bats, woodchucks, squirrels, porcupines, tapirs, and a number of non-human primates—regularly flock to mineral licks (deposits of salt and other minerals) to supplement their diets with sodium and other nutrients. Herbivores in particular seek out salt licks because inland plant foods generally don't supply enough sodium to meet their nutritional needs.

While it's *possible* that humans are one of the few mammals that never capitalized on salt licks encountered in the wild, it seems unlikely. For one, there is evidence that Paleolithic humans scavenged mammoth bones from natural salt licks (where mammoths flocked!), so humans clearly interacted with salt-rich areas in the past.

Likewise, given the tendency for early humans to cluster around coastal and other aquatic regions, salt from the water probably made it onto the menu unintentionally. There's evidence that, when near the coast, Paleolithic man ate seaweed, which is rich in salt and other valuable minerals.

Natural sources of drinking water also provided a valuable source of salt in ancient diets. Water from lakes, rivers, and streams contains as much as 0.4 percent salt, which is a nontrivial one-ninth the concentration of ocean water, which is 3.5 percent salt.

Our early ancestors might not have had access to as much salt as we do today, but salt was definitely present in the Paleolithic era.

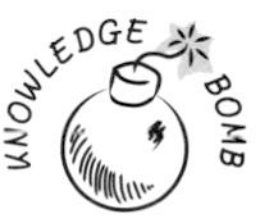

Salt has been mined (and cherished) for thousands of years across the globe. It was once so valuable that the Roman legions were paid with it (hence the word salary, which comes from the word salt). We could even argue that salt made modern civilization possible: it gave us the ability to preserve food without refrigeration—allowing us to store (and trade) perishable items, prevent meat from rotting, travel long distances with a secure food supply, and release our dependence on seasonal eating.

Salt, Potassium, and Blood Pressure

The most common criticism against salt is that too much of it raises blood pressure, in turn elevating our risk of heart attack or stroke. But this isn't exactly true! Research shows that reducing sodium has only a modest impact on blood pressure (and cardiovascular outcomes).

A 2014 Cochrane Review using eight different trials found that salt restriction had no significant benefit for overall mortality and only a weak benefit for cardiovascular events and deaths. The researchers noted that the "benefit" was due almost entirely to a single trial of retirement home residents, which drove the results when all eight studies were pooled together. In fact, a 2011 Cochrane Review on the same topic, this one using seven different studies, showed "no strong evidence of any effect of salt reduction" on cardiovascular disease mortality for either hypertensive people or people with normal blood pressure.

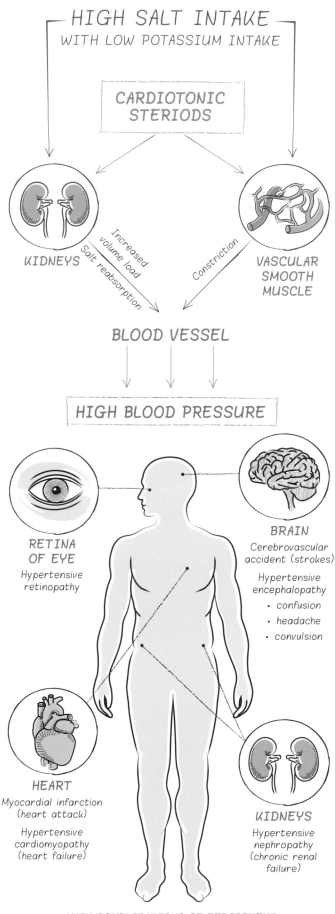

HIGH SALT INTAKE
WITH LOW POTASSIUM INTAKE

CARDIOTONIC STERIODS

KIDNEYS

VASCULAR SMOOTH MUSCLE

Increased volume load

Salt reabsorption

Constriction

BLOOD VESSEL

HIGH BLOOD PRESSURE

RETINA OF EYE
Hypertensive retinopathy

BRAIN
Cerebrovascular accident (strokes)
Hypertensive encephalopathy
- confusion
- headache
- convulsion

HEART
Myocardial infarction (heart attack)
Hypertensive cardiomyopathy (heart failure)

KIDNEYS
Hypertensive nephropathy (chronic renal failure)

MAIN COMPLICATIONS OF PERSISTENT
HIGH BLOOD PRESSURE

When we talk about minerals that influence blood pressure, sodium usually steals the spotlight. But potassium plays a significant role in regulating blood pressure and protecting against cardiovascular disease risk. For example, an analysis of nineteen clinical trials found that potassium supplementation significantly reduced both systolic and diastolic blood pressure—to a greater degree than most salt-restriction trials show.

SCIENCE SIMPLIFIED *High sodium intake increases blood pressure only if you're also deficient in potassium. It's probably much more important to increase potassium consumption than it is to lower sodium.*

More recent research has confirmed that the sodium-to-potassium ratio may be more important than sodium or potassium intake alone. A trio of papers published in the *New England Journal of Medicine* in 2014 pointed toward an interaction between sodium and potassium, where higher sodium intake was mostly harmful in the presence of low potassium intake (as measured by excretion levels of both minerals). An editorial accompanying the papers summarized, "The authors suggested that the alternative approach of recommending high-quality diets rich in potassium might achieve greater health benefits, including blood-pressure reduction, than aggressive sodium reduction alone."

So which foods have potassium? Here's where eating a nutrient-dense Paleo diet comes in handy! A number of tasty plant foods (which we've already established are a critical component) are high in potassium, including:

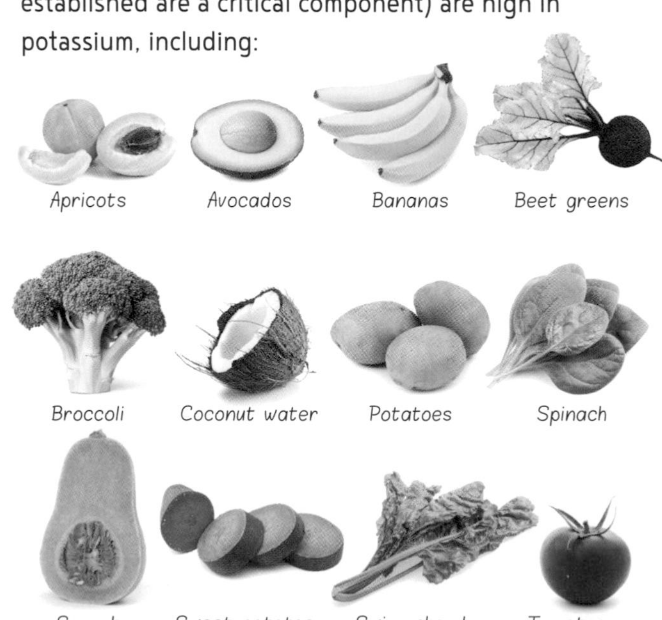

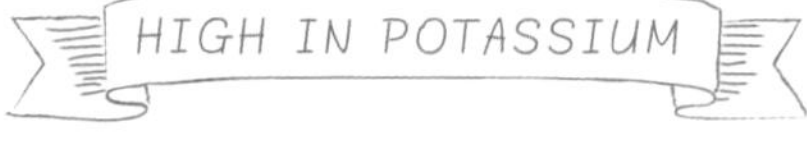

Salt and Kidney Disease

High salt intake has long been known to worsen kidney disease, and there's evidence that it also increases the risk for *developing* kidney disease. Why is there a link? The kidneys are responsible for maintaining the balance between water and electrolytes (like sodium!) in the body, as well as for removing water-soluble waste products (which are excreted in urine). In the production of urine, the kidneys remove water from the blood via osmosis (meaning that the water moves from an area of low concentration of electrolytes across a semipermeable barrier of cells to an area of high concentration of electrolytes, sodium and potassium being especially important for regulating this filtration process). A high-salt diet alters the gradient of sodium concentration, causing the kidneys to have reduced function and remove less water, resulting in higher blood volume (and therefore blood pressure). Strain on the kidneys comes not just from hypertension and a reduced ability to perform their filtering job, but also from direct tissue damage from high sodium levels.

Contrary to what the high salt-kidney disease correlations imply, long-term adoption of a reduced-salt diet (whether that's defined as less than 3 grams daily or less than 5 grams daily) does not improve mortality from or progression of chronic kidney disease. However, it does improve the response to several drug options for mitigating kidney disease and is still a recommendable option for anyone battling kidney problems.

Because kidney function has a direct effect on bone mineralization (due to pH balance), one would expect high salt intake (and therefore hindered kidney function) to be correlated with incidence of osteoporosis and/or hip fracture. However, even at intake levels of 9 grams per day, studies show no clear link between high salt intake and bone health.

Salt and the Immune System

High salt intake stimulates the immune system. Seminal research from 2013 revealed that the higher the concentration of salt in the diet, the greater the number of Th17 cells (a major culprit in autoimmune disease; see page 79) that are activated and the greater the amount of pro-inflammatory cytokines that are secreted by those Th17 cells, causing generalized inflammation. In a study of mice with multiple sclerosis, mice that were fed a high-salt diet had significantly exacerbated symptoms, directly attributable to increases in Th17 cell differentiation (maturation), proliferation (division), and activation. Subsequent research showed that females are more susceptible to this effect than males, at least in mice.

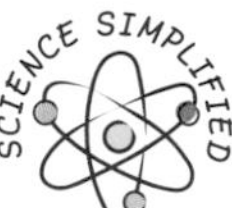

High salt intake increases the risk of kidney disease and may cause inflammation.

Very recent research expands the link between high salt intake and inflammation by showing that high dietary salt also activates macrophages (resident immune cell sentinels present in nearly every tissue in the human body). It appears that high salt intake primes the immune system to attack. However, there is a paucity of human data on this subject. One recent study showed that high salt intake increased the risk of rheumatoid arthritis in smokers, but not non-smokers. And asthmatics are more likely to have exercise-induced attacks if they eat a high-salt diet and see improvements in their symptoms with a low-sodium diet.

In people, high salt intake is considered above 9 grams per day. That's 4 teaspoons! Importantly, these studies—both animal and human—don't compare high salt intake to an absence of salt, but rather to standard low-sodium recommendations. For humans, that's 2.4 grams, or 1 teaspoon, of salt per day.

Salt and Cancer

Any factor that influences how the immune system works is also a candidate for increasing cancer risk. Some research suggests that cancer incidence rises with very high salt intake—this is especially true of stomach (gastric) cancer. For instance, a meta-analysis of seven prospective studies encompassing almost 270,000 people found that both "high" and "moderately high" salt intakes were associated with a significantly increased risk of stomach cancer over the span of at least 4 years of follow-up.

What explains this association? As it turns out, salt can play multiple roles in the etiology of stomach cancer. First, it tends to affect both the risk and the outcome of *H. pylori* infection (a bacteria that grows in the intestinal tract that can attack the stomach lining), which is a major risk factor for stomach cancer. Gut barrier damage from salt can increase the susceptibility to *H. pylori* infection, and *H. pylori* reacts to high-salt environments with altered cell morphology and increased growth, survival, and virulence—all of which result in a more aggressive infection that becomes an even stronger promoter of stomach cancer. In addition, rodent models show that for *CagA+ H. pylori* strains (CagA, or cytotoxin-associated gene A, is a bacterial oncoprotein that can bind to and deregulate proteins), a high-salt diet leads to increased expression of a pro-inflammatory protein called interleukin-1β in gastric cells, more-severe stomach inflammation, higher gastric pH, and an upregulation of CagA synthesis—all of which suggest that a high-salt diet increases the carcinogenic effects of certain *H. pylori* strains.

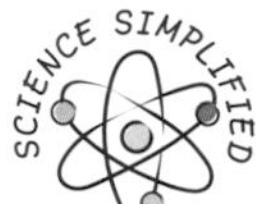

High salt intake increases stomach cancer risk because salt increases the growth and destructive abilities of H. pylori, a bacteria associated with ulcers and stomach cancer.

Apart from the role of *H. pylori*, salt can increase stomach cancer risk through two other avenues: increasing exposure to gastric carcinogens such as nitrates and causing inflammation that leads to increased cell proliferation and mutation (which boosts the risk of cancer developing). This happens because a high salt intake can alter the quality of the stomach's mucous barrier, leading to direct exposure to harmful compounds and making the stomach more susceptible to mucosal damage.

There's some evidence that a high salt intake can increase overall cancer risk as well. For instance, a 2015 study found that older men who reported "always" adding salt to their food were 20 percent more likely to die of cancer-related causes over the course of a 12½-year (on average) follow-up, compared to men who reported "never" adding salt to their food. In absolute terms, 21.3 percent of men who always added salt and 16.8 percent of men who never salted their food had died of cancer-related causes by the end of the study. (Although the researchers tried to adjust for other contributors to cancer risk, like smoking, we can't rule out the possibility that the men who never added salt to their food had other protective dietary or lifestyle factors working in their favor.)

Theoretically, one reason salt could increase overall cancer risk involves its effects on intracellular electrolytes and pH. In several studies, dietary salt loading increased intracellular sodium and calcium, decreased intracellular potassium and magnesium, and lowered intracellular pH—all factors that may support cancer progression.

Note that all these correlations are with *high* salt intake. And these effects are highly dependent on the level of other electrolytes in the diet. For example, although salt loading can decrease intercellular pH, potassium loading has been shown to *increase* it, thus counteracting the salt's potential pro-cancer effects. Likewise, the sodium/potassium and calcium/magnesium ratios will vary based on the dietary intake of all minerals involved, not just sodium from salt.

Another component of salt—iodine, found in large amounts in iodized salt and in smaller amounts in unrefined salts—may actually reduce the risk of thyroid cancer. So the relationship between salt intake and cancer is highly context-dependent and more complex than first meets the eye.

The Happy Medium of Salt Intake

It's true that in studies of salt consumption, very high intakes were associated (albeit modestly, in most cases) with a higher risk of certain cardiovascular events, cancer, and death. But how high is too high? A recent survey across all European Member States (plus Norway and Switzerland) showed that daily sodium consumption is between 8 and 12 grams per day, and these are the levels at which we start to see statistically significant correlations between salt intake and health problems in large epidemiological studies. The cusp for negative health impacts of sodium (in the context of the Standard American Diet, since the effects of high salt intake have never been studied in more nutrient-dense [potassium-rich] anti-inflammatory diets, like the Paleo diet), is about 7 grams per day. This daily level of 3 to 4 teaspoons of salt is much higher than the World Health Organization's recommended target of 5 to 6 grams per day and much, much higher than the low-sodium diet's target of 3 grams. At these more modest amounts—which equate to 1 to 2 heaping teaspoons of salt per day—salt consumption is not linked to health problems.

KNOWLEDGE BOMB *Table salt is roughly 40 percent sodium and 60 percent chloride by weight. So it works out that there's about 2.4 grams of sodium in 1 teaspoon of salt (which weighs about 6 grams). Unrefined salt has less sodium per teaspoon (thanks to sodium being displaced by other minerals), but it varies.*

For people eating the Standard American Diet (the population studied in many salt trials), the biggest source of salt is processed foods. In fact, according to the U.S. Centers for Disease Control and Prevention, the three biggest sodium contributors are bread/rolls, processed and cured meats, and pizza—not exactly Paleo staples, as we'll see in Part 3. Over 75 percent of the sodium that most people consume comes from packaged store-bought foods and restaurant meals. By contrast, only 11 percent of dietary sodium comes from salt added at home during cooking *and* at the table. If we do the math, anyone who cooks their own food from whole-food ingredients automatically lands in the low-sodium-diet category.

When we ditch the heavily processed, low-nutrient foods that dominate most Western diets, our salt intake will naturally go way down—and as we eat more tasty vegetables and fruits, our potassium intake will tend to go up. As our taste buds adjust to the more diverse and subtler flavors of whole plant and animal foods, we may find ourselves wanting to add less salt to our meals than we used to. In other words, it's pretty hard to eat dangerous levels of salt on a Paleo diet unless you *really* try! Most of us naturally find ourselves under 3 to 5 grams per day.

This begs the question: If low-sodium is good, is no-sodium better? Because studies show benefits from low sodium intake, will giving up salt altogether make us even healthier?

As it turns out, eating too *little* salt can be just as detrimental as eating too much! We find time and time again with nutrients that there's a happy medium in which we thrive, and both too much and too little can cause problems.

HEALTH QUICK-START *Aim for between 1 and 2 teaspoons of salt per day. If you're cooking all your own meals using whole foods, this is an easy target to achieve. So go ahead and season your food to taste!*

Research has shown that restricting salt too much can *increase* the risk of death. Another 2014 meta-analysis found that salt intake and mortality formed a U-shaped curve, with all-cause mortality increasing with both very low and very high salt intake. A 2011 study that analyzed sodium excretion (a more accurate way to assess sodium intake than recall surveys and food-frequency questionnaires) found that excretion of more than 7 grams or less than 3 grams per day were both associated with worse health outcomes—in the case of less than 3 grams, higher rates of cardiovascular death and hospitalization for congestive heart failure.

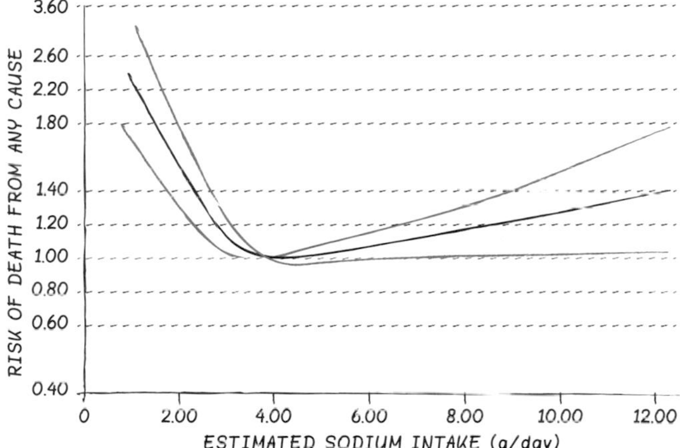

Thinking of 3 grams per day as a minimum healthful amount of salt to consume raises new questions in the context of a whole-foods diet like Paleo. While most people eating the Standard American Diet won't have to worry about their salt intake dipping too low, this can be a problem for people who eliminate processed/packaged foods and don't use much salt in their cooking (which can definitely include Paleo adherents).

Hyponatremia is the technical term for having too little sodium in the blood, and it can result in symptoms such as nausea, vomiting, confusion, fatigue, muscle weakness, spasms, vertigo, fainting, and headaches. Hyponatremia becomes even more likely if we're sweating heavily from heat or exercise, if we're sick and losing fluids through vomiting or diarrhea, if we have an underactive thyroid, or if we're taking diuretics or certain antidepressant medications. Worst of all, hyponatremia can be life-threatening if left untreated—making it imperative to watch out for early symptoms!

To lower the risk of hyponatremia on a Paleo diet, it's best to consume *some* salt (rather than none).

The Best Salt

Although regular table salt is unlikely to be harmful in moderate amounts, we can get even more benefits by opting for unrefined salts—like Himalayan pink salt or "dirty" (French *sel gris*, or Celtic) sea salt—that contain naturally occurring trace minerals. Himalayan pink salt, for example, contains 84 minerals—including magnesium, calcium, chromium, manganese, iron, potassium, copper, zinc, cobalt, selenium, bromine, strontium, molybdenum, iodine, sulfur, phosphorus, scandium, and dozens of others. The exact micronutrient content varies, depending on the type of unrefined salt and where it was mined.

Although the Paleo framework emphasizes getting nutrition from whole foods, it's also true that hunter-gatherers (both ancient and still existing) had a much higher micronutrient intake than most of us do today. Nutrient depletion in farmed soils, less access to truly wild/nutrient-dense plant foods, consumption of produce that's been transported long distances and picked prematurely, and a variety of other factors all result in us having less-nutritious food at our disposal, even when we're eating the best of the best. In addition, hunter-gatherers typically consumed some dirt with their food—which might sound gross, but it's another source of micronutrients (and probiotics!) that we've lost due to food washing.

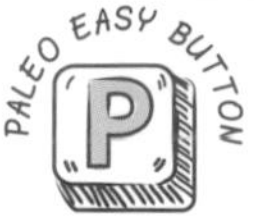

The best choices for salt are unrefined sea salts, including Celtic sea salt, Himalayan pink salt, and sel gris.

For these reasons, unrefined salt can be valuable for the trace minerals it provides, helping us achieve an intake that's more optimal for our health. Another great option is seaweed flakes, which are rich in many minerals and a great natural source of salt.

So does salt belong on a Paleo diet? The answer is absolutely yes! As long as we're eating a moderate amount (3 to 7 grams of sodium per day), consuming a wide variety of potassium-rich foods (magnesium and calcium, too), and choosing good-quality salts for the extra trace minerals, there's no reason to avoid salt (or actively worry about consuming too much). The literature reinforces the fact that salt and health risk form a U-shaped curve, with too little being just as harmful as too much. Our best bet is to keep some in our diet and enjoy both the flavor and micronutrient boost it gives our food.

HERBS AND SPICES

In technical terms, herbs are the leaves of herbaceous (non-woody) plants, and spices come from roots, bark, flowers, fruits, berries, or seeds. So ingredients like thyme, sage, basil, mint, parsley, oregano, and marjoram (all leaves) are considered herbs, while ginger (root), cloves (flower bud), cumin (seed), vanilla (undeveloped fruit), and cinnamon (bark) are considered spices—to name just a few examples! Herbs and spices are the backbone of flavorful meals, and most of them are perfectly acceptable within a Paleo framework.

First, the good news: many herbs and spices are concentrated sources of micronutrients, including vitamins, minerals, and phytochemicals. As explained in Chapter 8, *phytochemicals* is an umbrella term for a huge array of helpful plant-derived compounds that aren't necessarily needed for survival but support our health in a number of ways. For instance, many dried herbs and spices are rich in polyphenols, a type of phytochemical with potent antioxidant properties (see page 35).

HERB OR SPICE	POLYPHENOLS PER 100 g
Cloves	15,188 mg
Dried peppermint	11,960 mg
Star anise	5,460 mg
Dried cocoa	3,448 mg
Dried oregano	2,319 mg
Celery seed	2,094 mg
Dried sage	1,207 mg
Dried rosemary	1,018 mg
Dried spearmint	956 mg
Dried thyme	878 mg
Capers	654 mg
Dried sweet basil	322 mg
Dried ginger	202 mg

These herbs and spices are rich in polyphenols when fresh, too, but their polyphenol content becomes more concentrated when they're dried due to the removal of water. Even if you use a few teaspoons to flavor a dish, the polyphenol contribution to your diet is substantial.

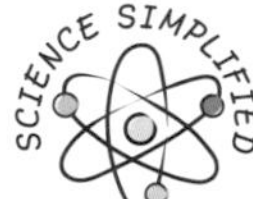

Herbs and spices have some of the highest concentrations of beneficial phytochemicals of any plant food. So go ahead and use them liberally!

In addition, several herbs and spices have been studied for their unique benefits beyond antioxidant activity, and scientists have clarified their role in supporting our health:

Basil contains the flavonoids orientin and vicenin, which appear to protect cell structures (as well as our chromosomes) from oxidative damage and radiation. Likewise, the volatile oils in basil (containing estragole, linalool, cineole, eugenol, sabinene, myrcene, and limonene) have strong anti-inflammatory and antibacterial properties and can inhibit the growth of a variety of pathogenic bacteria, such as *Listeria monocytogenes, Staphylococcus aureus, Escherichia coli* O157:H7, *Yersinia enterocolitica*, and *Pseudomonas aeruginosa*. Basil is also extremely rich in vitamin K and contains manganese, copper, carotenoids, vitamin C, calcium, vitamin B9, and iron.

Cayenne pepper contains a compound called capsaicin, which is responsible for the "heat" we taste when eating cayenne (a result of capsaicin coming into contact with mucous membranes). According to a variety of studies, capsaicin may also inhibit substance P (a neuropeptide associated with inflammatory processes), reduce cholesterol and triglyceride levels, reduce platelet aggregation, reduce oxidation of blood lipids, and reduce the spread of prostate cancer cells. Cayenne has also been shown to improve insulin sensitivity during meals and boost immune function. Plus, cayenne contains high amounts of the carotenoids β-carotene, β-cryptoxanthin, lutein, and zeaxanthin, as well as some vitamin B6, vitamin C, vitamin E, vitamin K, and manganese. (See also page 296.)

Cinnamon is rich in tannins, flavonoids, glycosides, terpenoids, phytosterols, coumarins, and anthraquinones and also contains calcium, manganese, and chromium. In numerous studies, it's been shown to help lower blood sugar levels by improving insulin sensitivity and inhibiting α-glucosidase, slowing the rate of carbohydrate digestion in the small intestine. Cinnamon also helps improve blood lipids, reduce inflammation, and reduce blood clotting (by preventing unwanted clumping of platelets). These effects are apparently due to three components in the oils of its bark: cinnamaldehyde, cinnamyl acetate, and cinnamyl alcohol.

Cloves are rich in a compound called eugenol, which may help prevent cancers of the digestive tract, reduce joint pain and inflammation, and protect against toxicity from certain environmental pollutants. They also contain vitamin K, iron, calcium, and magnesium.

Ginger has a long track record for treating nausea (whether from morning sickness, chemotherapy, seasickness, or other causes) and also possesses strong anti-inflammatory and anti-arthritis properties owing to compounds called gingerols.

Peppermint (particularly its oil) has been shown to reduce IBS-associated indigestion, dyspepsia, and pain during bowel movements (by relaxing the smooth muscles in the colon), most likely due to its menthol content. Some compounds in peppermint, such as perillyl alcohol, also show the potential to reduce tumor growth in pancreatic, liver, and mammary cancer, though the evidence thus far is limited to animal models.

Sage is not only rich in vitamin K, but also contains compounds (particularly rosmarinic acid) that reduce inflammation by changing the concentrations of inflammatory messaging molecules, such as leukotriene B4. Several well-designed placebo-controlled studies have shown that the volatile oils in sage can also improve memory, specifically immediate recall.

Turmeric contains a huge number of special compounds (more than 100 different components have been isolated so far) that play different roles in supporting our health and protecting against disease. It's by far the most-studied spice, with the widest range of health benefits discovered to date. In fact, well over 3,000 scientific publications exist on this spice, just from the last 30 years or so. And when we look at all the amazing micronutrients in turmeric, it's easy to see why it's been the focus of so much research. This spice deserves a longer discussion to fully understand!

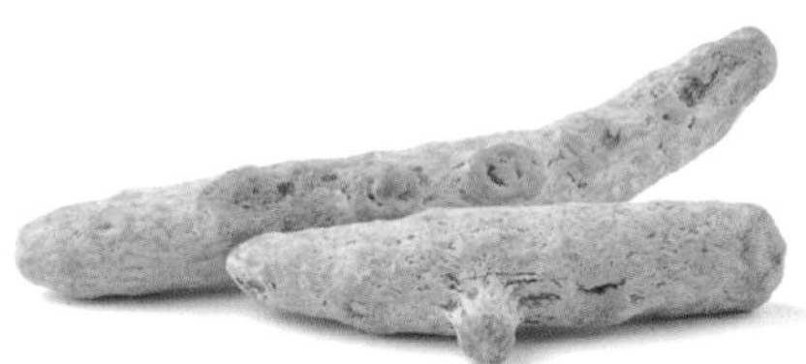

Turmeric: A Rock Star Spice

Turmeric is probably best known for giving curry its characteristic vibrant yellow color. But there's a lot more to this spice! Turmeric (also known by its scientific name, *Curcuma longa*) is an herbaceous perennial plant belonging to the ginger family. It has been used in India (where it's native) for nearly 4,000 years, and it's also used in local cuisines, as dye, and as medicine throughout other parts of Asia where it grows. The plant's rhizomes (an underground portion of the stem) are what get harvested to produce turmeric spice. The rhizomes are typically boiled or steamed and then dried out to produce the yellow powder many of us are familiar with.

Among turmeric's many beneficial compounds, curcumin (technically known as diferuloylmethane) steals the spotlight. Curcumin, a natural phenol, is one of three different curcuminoids present in the plant (the others are demethoxycurcumin and bisdemethoxycurcumin). It was first discovered about 200 years ago by researchers who isolated the "yellow-coloring matter" from the turmeric rhizome and named it curcumin.

SCIENCE SIMPLIFIED *Many scientific studies show health benefits to turmeric; however, it's not all good news, particularly in high doses. The take-home message: go ahead and cook with turmeric, but supplement only under medical supervision.*

So what can curcumin do? It's a pretty long list! Chiefly, this compound has potent anti-inflammatory effects that make it comparable to non-steroidal anti-inflammatory drugs, or NSAIDs. (In fact, studies have been done comparing curcumin to phenylbutazone in rheumatoid arthritis patients and people healing from hernia surgery, and they found that curcumin was just as effective as the NSAID treatment.) Curcumin works by helping regulate a number of transcription factors, protein kinases, adhesion molecules, cytokines, and enzymes involved in inflammatory processes. There's also some evidence that curcumin works as a cyclooxygenase (COX)-2 inhibitor by acting at the transcriptional level and possibly post-translational level. (We'll talk more about this a bit later, since it's actually a double-edged sword.) And the fact that inflammation is so central to many chronic illnesses, like heart disease, metabolic diseases, neurodegenerative diseases, and cancer makes curcumin (and the turmeric that contains it) a potentially helpful substance for disease prevention.

Curcumin happens to be a powerful antioxidant as well; it can reduce lipid peroxidation by supporting antioxidant enzymes (such as superoxide dismutase, catalase, and glutathione peroxidase). There's also evidence that curcumin can directly scavenge oxygen free radicals (like superoxide anions and hydroxyl radicals) and nitric oxide involved in the initiation of lipid peroxidation.

The list doesn't end there! Other studies show that curcumin may have antibacterial activity, as well as the potential to lower LDL ("bad") cholesterol and triglycerides (and improve HDL ("good") cholesterol to total cholesterol ratio). It's been shown to boost brain-derived neurotrophic factor, which may play a role in combating neurodegenerative diseases and depression. A number of studies also suggest that curcumin may inhibit tumor proliferation, making it a potentially useful adjunct to cancer treatment.

Apart from all that, curcumin has strong and somewhat complicated effects on the immune system. It can play a role in the activation of many immune cell types, including T cells, B cells, macrophages, neutrophils, natural killer cells, and dendritic cells, making it an important immune modulator.

Although demethoxycurcumin is less frequently discussed, this curcuminoid has a number of benefits as well. Like curcumin, demethoxycurcumin possesses strong antioxidant activity, has tumor-suppressive effects, and can help reduce inflammation. In all cases, though, it's slightly less powerful than curcumin.

Ground turmeric is a surprising source of micronutrients. A single tablespoon provides 26 percent of the Recommended Dietary Allowance (RDA) for manganese and 16 percent of the RDA for iron. Manganese is essential for helping the body form connective tissue, synthesize clotting factors and sex hormones, develop bone tissue, regulate blood sugar levels, and regulate fat and carbohydrate metabolism. Meanwhile, iron (as a component of hemoglobin) helps transport oxygen throughout the body while also helping neurotransmitters function properly.

On top of that, a tablespoon of turmeric contains 6 percent of the RDA for vitamin B6 and smaller amounts of vitamin C, magnesium, phosphorus, copper, potassium, calcium, vitamins B1, B2, B3, and B9, vitamin K, and vitamin E. It contains 1.4 grams of fiber and a small amount of awesome anti-inflammatory omega-3 fatty acids.

That said, the compounds in turmeric (especially curcumin) are *really* poorly absorbed when it is eaten on its own. (Curcumin is rapidly metabolized in the liver and intestinal wall, so very little of it actually makes it into the bloodstream.) That means simply adding turmeric to a meal here and there might not be enough to reap its potential rewards. But there are some proven tricks for enhancing its absorption and getting the most out of this spice. For example:

- Piperine (an alkaloid that gives black pepper its pungent flavor) can inhibit the detoxifying enzymes responsible for breaking down curcumin. Consuming black pepper along with turmeric can increase the absorption of curcumin by 2,000 percent.
- Curcumin is fat-soluble, so cooking turmeric-containing meals with a source of fat will greatly enhance its bioavailability (ability to be absorbed and used by the body). Traditional curries are great because the dairy fat in Indian curries or the coconut milk in Thai curries naturally helps increase the absorption of turmeric's active components.

The Downsides of Spices

And now the bad news: some herbs and spices can be double-edged swords depending on the context—level of intake and whether a person has existing health conditions, in particular. For example, let's look at turmeric again. Despite its huge list of valid benefits and the evidence supporting its various components, eating extremely high amounts could backfire—and so can supplementing with only small amounts for medicinal purposes! Why? It turns out that the effects of turmeric (and in particular curcumin) aren't linear. There's some evidence that at both low and excessive levels, it stops becoming anti-inflammatory and actually becomes either *pro*-inflammatory or immune-suppressive—increasing pro-inflammatory cytokine production (immune messenger molecules), enhancing antibody responses (at low concentrations), suppressing the immune system, and even causing DNA damage to mucosa cells and lymphocytes at high concentrations.

Although the role of curcumin as a COX-2 inhibitor is still being researched, there's a risk that high doses of curcumin can have an impact on the gut that is similar to that of NSAIDs (which are also COX-2 inhibitors)—which is to say, not good! NSAIDs are known for damaging the gut barrier and causing intestinal lesions (which can become ulcers), since cyclooxygenase, the enzyme they inhibit, plays an essential role in maintaining the integrity of the gut's mucous layer. The result is a gut that becomes far more susceptible to damage from other sources, like dietary toxins and exercise-induced intestinal barrier disruption (see page 360).

In fact, some research supports the possibility that turmeric can have the same negative gut effects as NSAIDs: clinical trials on ulcers found that healing was worse in the turmeric groups compared to placebo or antacid groups—suggesting that turmeric might actually be ulcerogenic and delay the rate of healing in peptic ulcer disease. Although only a few studies have been done on humans, some rodent studies have found that curcumin supplementation was capable of inducing gastric ulcers after 6 days. So supplementing with curcumin is *strongly* discouraged for anyone with a history of ulcers or who's dealing with an ulcer.

On top of that, excessive curcumin may produce additional negative side effects. One study found that high doses might cause neurotoxicity and aggravate morphine tolerance by inhibiting the expression of anti-apoptotic cytokines and neuroprotective factors. Several clinical studies using daily curcumin supplements of 3.6 to 8 milligrams resulted in nausea and diarrhea in some participants. Other studies have shown that eczema can occur when turmeric is used externally. And there's a possibility that curcumin can interfere with certain drugs, such as antiplatelet agents (since curcumin can inhibit platelet aggregation), as well as be a problem for pregnant women when taken in medicinal doses, since it can increase uterine contraction.

And turmeric isn't the only spice with potential problems. For people with autoimmune diseases and/or

A TOUR OF PALEO HERBS AND SPICES

Herbs and spices offer impressive, well-documented health benefits and can greatly enhance the micronutrient and phytochemical content (not to mention flavor!) of a Paleo diet. While herbs are generally safe for everyone, some spices (especially those derived from seeds, berries, fruit, and nightshades) should be viewed with caution when autoimmunity, various gut pathologies, or nightshade sensitivity is involved. See Chapter 25 for how to identify food sensitivities via elimination and challenge.

HERBS:

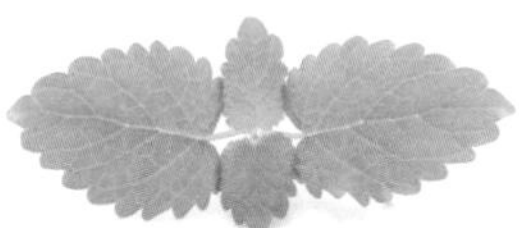
BALM (LEMON BALM): Leaf of *Melissa officinalis L.*

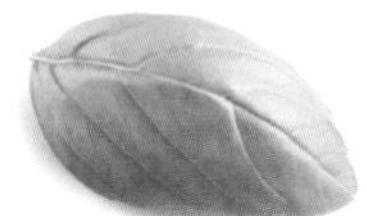
BASIL LEAF (sweet): Leaf of *Ocimum basilicum*

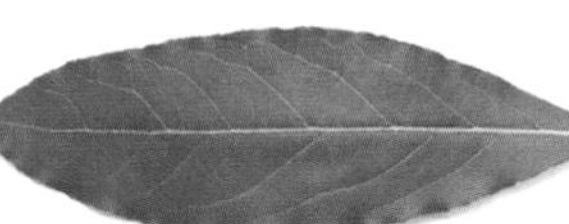
BAY LEAF (laurel leaf): Leaf of *Laurus nobilis*

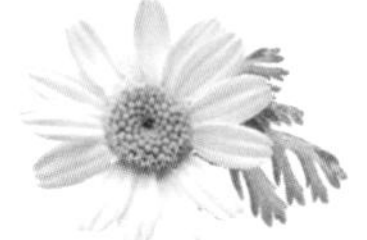
CHAMOMILE: Flower of *Anthemisnobilis L.* or *Matricaria chamomilla L.*

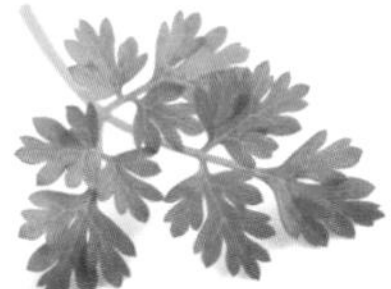
CHERVIL: Leaf of *Anthriscus cerefolium*

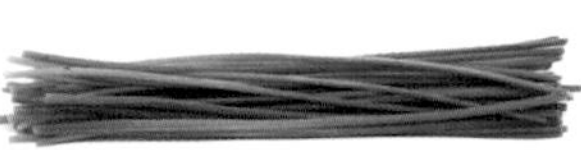
CHIVES: Leaf of *Allium schoenoprasum*

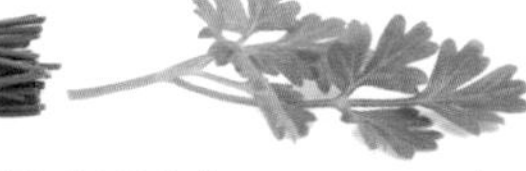
CILANTRO (coriander leaf): Leaf of *Coriandrum sativum*

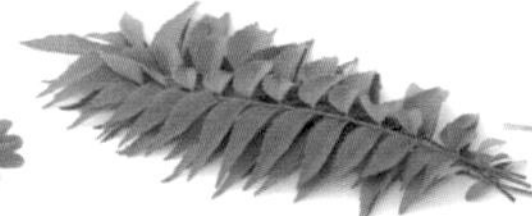
CURRY LEAF: Leaf of *Murraya koenigii*

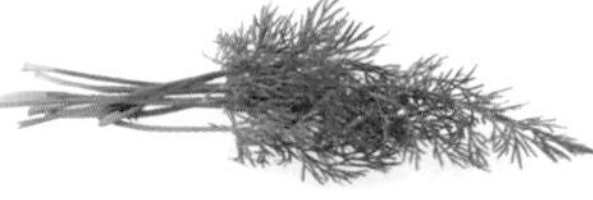
DILL WEED: Leaf of *Anethum graveolens/Anethum sowa*

EPAZOTE: Leaf of *Dysphania ambrosioides*

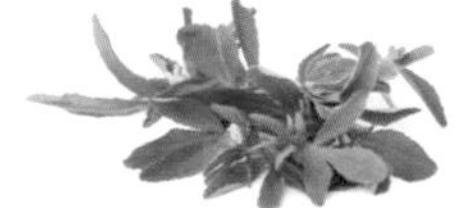
FENUGREEK LEAF: Leaf of *Trigonellafoenum-graecum*

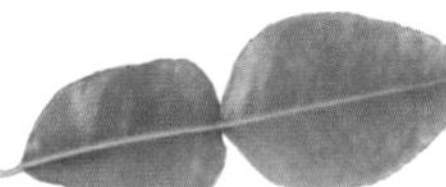
KAFFIR LIME LEAF: Leaf of *Citrus hystrix*

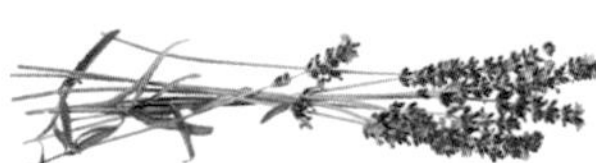
LAVENDER: Flower of *Lavandula officinalis Chaix*

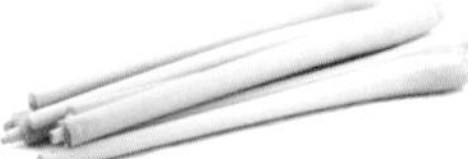
LEMONGRASS: Leaf of *Cymbopogon* genus

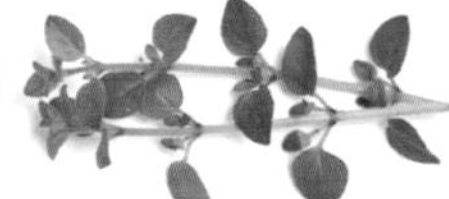
MARJORAM LEAF: Leaf of *Majorana hortensis Moench*

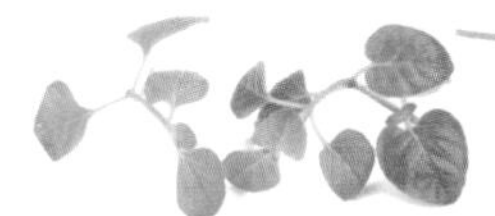
OREGANO LEAF: Leaf of *Origanum vulgare/Lippia spp.*

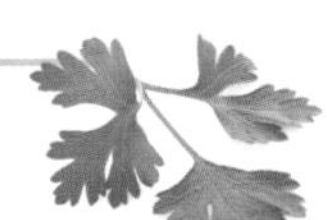
PARSLEY: Leaf of *Petroselinum crispum*

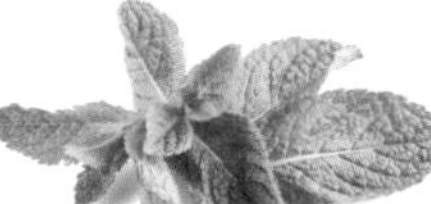
PEPPERMINT: Leaf of *Mentha piperita*

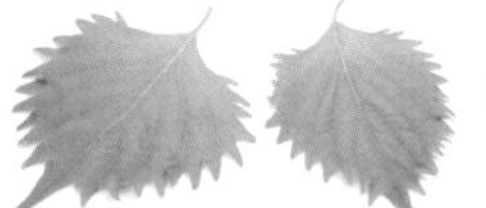
PERILLA LEAF (beefsteak leaf): Leaf of *Perilla frutescens*

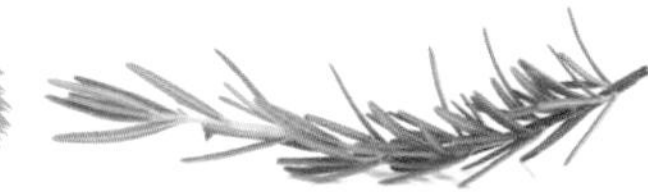
ROSEMARY: Leaf of *Rosmarinus officinalis*

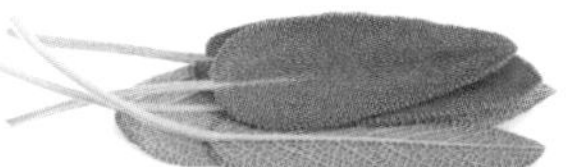
SAGE: Leaf of *Salvia officinalis/Salvia triloba*

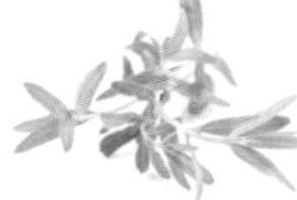
SAVORY LEAF: Leaf of *Satureia montana/Satureia hortensis*

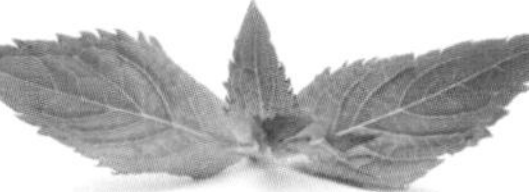
SPEARMINT: Leaf of *Mentha spicata*

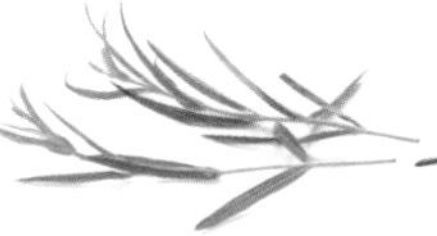
TARRAGON: Leaf of *Artemisia dracunculus*

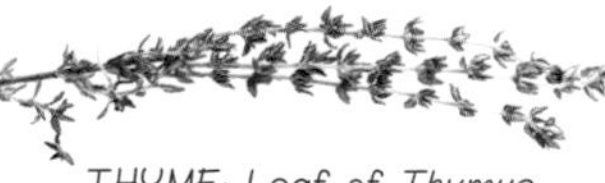
THYME: Leaf of *Thymus vulgaris/Thymus serpyllum/Thymus satureioides*

MINERALS:

Celtic sea salt
Himalayan pink salt
Sea vegetable salt
Sel gris
Truffle salt

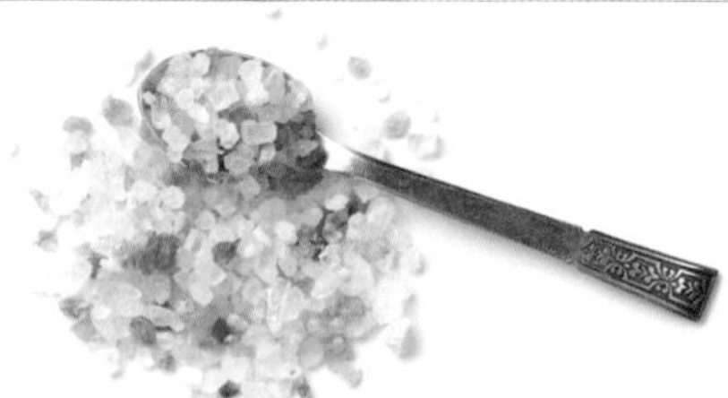

gut pathologies, certain spices can aggravate symptoms due to their lectin and phytic acid content (as is the case with seed spices; see pages 254 and 412) or their saponin content (as is the case with spices from the nightshade family; see page 296). Whether spices will be tolerated without harm depends on the particular spice and the particular person.

SPICES:

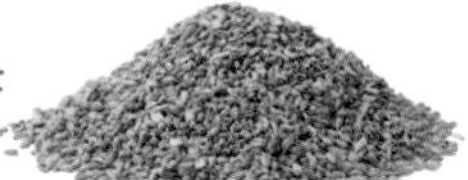

AJWAIN: Fruit of *Trachyspermum ammi*

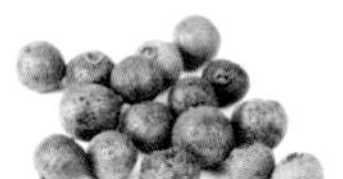

ALLSPICE: Berry of *Pimenta officinalis*

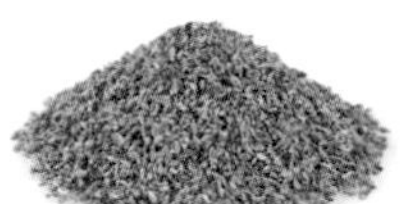

ANISE SEED: Seed of *Pimpinella anisum*

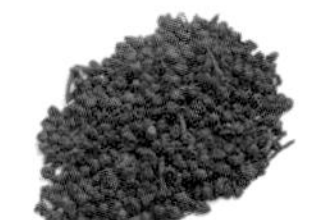

ANNATTO SEED: Seed of *Bixa orellana*

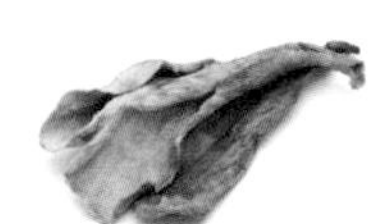

AMCHUR (mango powder): Made from dried unripe green mangoes

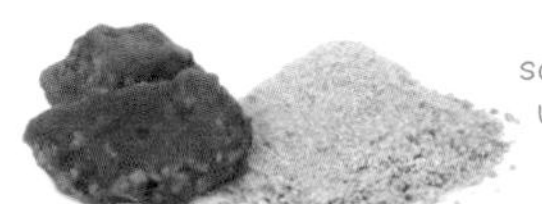

*Frequently sold mixed with wheat starch

*ASAFETIDA: Dried gum oleoresin exuded from the rhizome of a species of *Ferula*

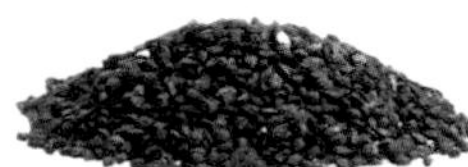

BLACK CARAWAY (Russian caraway, black cumin): Seed of *Nigella sativa*

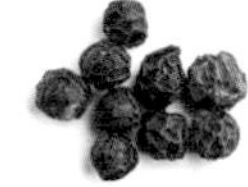

BLACK PEPPER: Berry of *Piper nigrum*

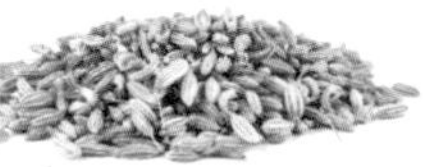

CARAWAY: Fruit of *Carum carvi Maton*

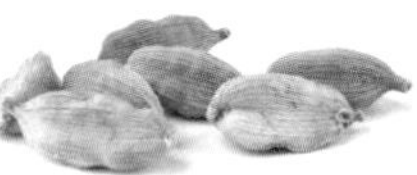

CARDAMOM: Fruit of *Elettariacardamomum*

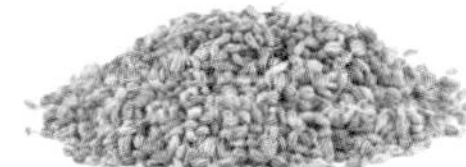

CELERY SEED: Seed of *Apium graveolens*

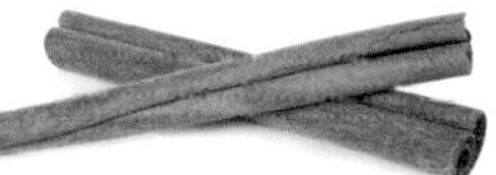

CINNAMON/CASSIA: Bark of *Cinnamomum spp.*

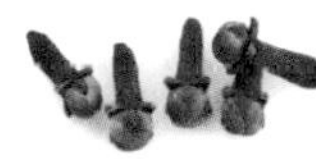

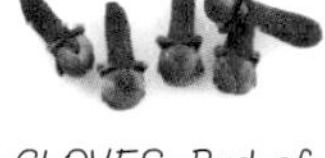

CLOVES: Bud of *Syzygium aromaticum*

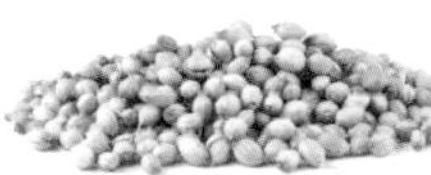

CORIANDER SEED: Seed of *Coriandrum sativum*

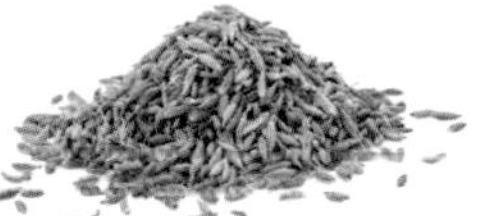

CUMIN SEED: Seed of *Cuminum cyminum*

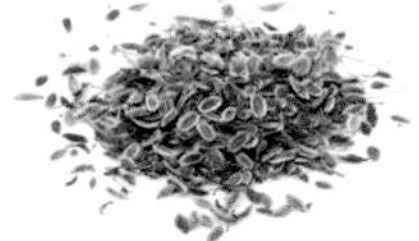

DILL SEED: Seed of *Anethum graveolens/Anethum sowa*

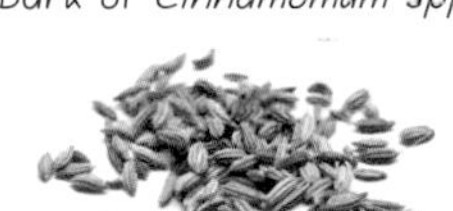

FENNEL SEED: Seed of *Foeniculum vulgare*

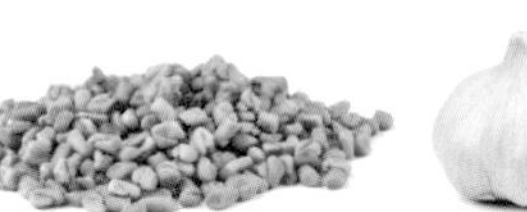

FENUGREEK: Seed of *Trigonellafoenum-graecum*

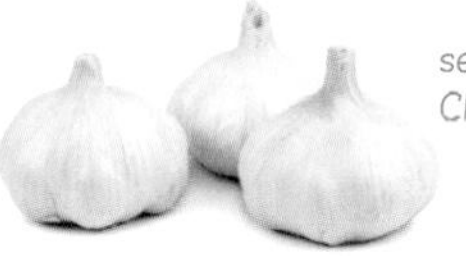

see also Chapter 8

GARLIC: Bulb of *Allium sativum*

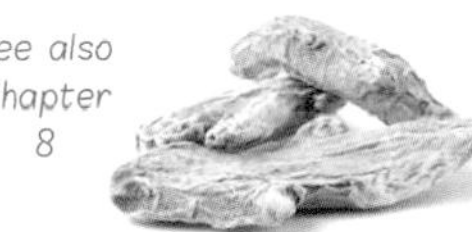

GINGER: Root of *Zingiber officinale*

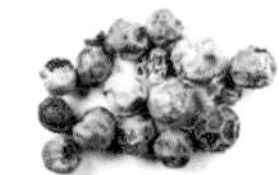

GREEN PEPPERCORN: Berry of *Piper nigrum*

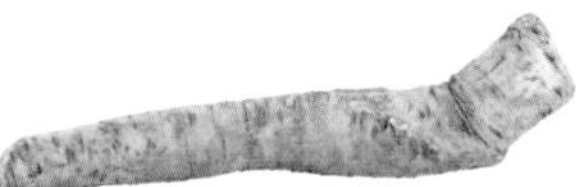

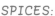

HORSERADISH: Root of *Armoracialapathfolia Gilib.*

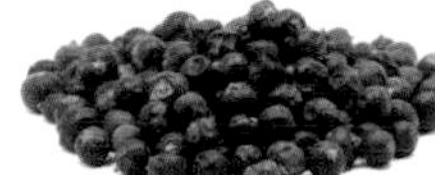

JUNIPER: Berry of *Juniperus communis*

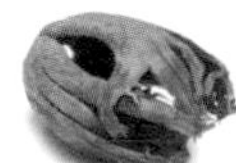

MACE: Aril of *Myristica fragrans*

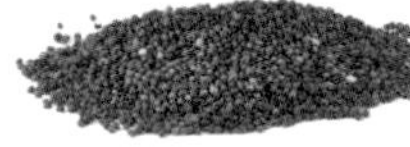

MUSTARD SEED: Seed of *Brassica juncea/ B. hirta/B. nigra*

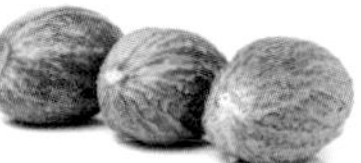

NUTMEG: Seed of *Myristica fragrans*

see also Chapter 8

ONION: Bulb of *Allium cepa*

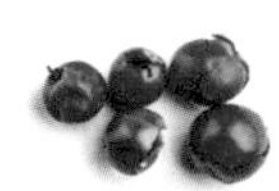

PINK PEPPERCORN: Berry of *Schinus terebinthifolius*

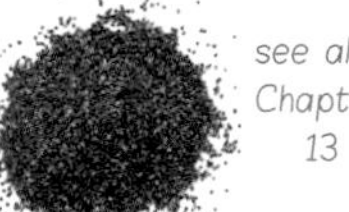

see also Chapter 13

POPPY SEED: Seed of *Papaver somniferum*

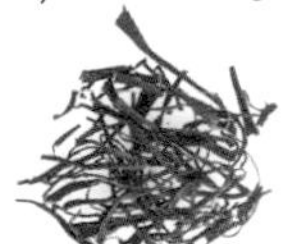

SAFFRON: Stigma of *Crocus sativus*

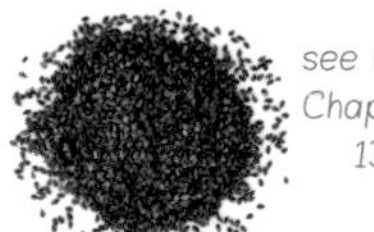

see also Chapter 13

SESAME SEED: Seed of *Sesamum indicum*

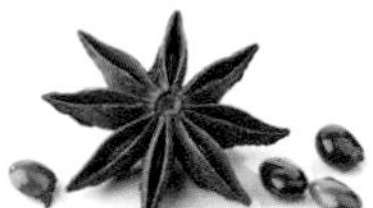

STAR ANISE: Fruit of *Illicium verum Hook*

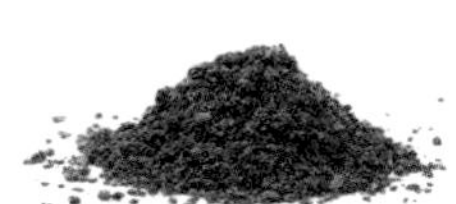

SUMAC: Drupe of *Rhus genus*

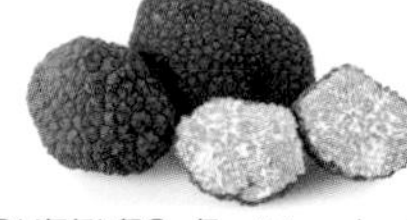

TRUFFLES: Fruiting body of a subterranean *Ascomycete fungus*

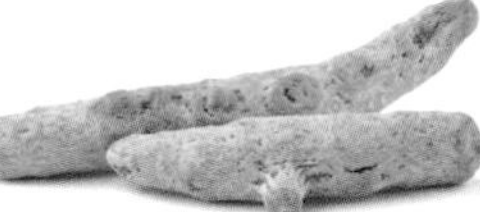

TURMERIC: Root of *Curcuma longa*

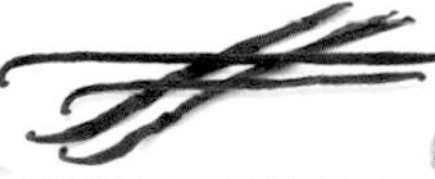

VANILLA BEAN: Fruit of *Vanilla planifolia/ Vanilla tahitensis*

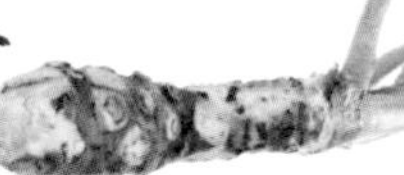

WASABI: Stem of *Eutrema japonicum*

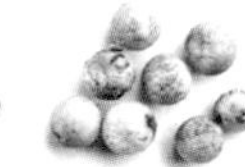

WHITE PEPPER: Berry of *Piper nigrum*

SPICES FROM THE NIGHTSHADE FAMILY (see page 296):

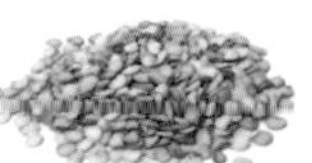

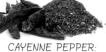

CAPSICUM: Seed of *Capsicum spp.*

CAYENNE PEPPER: Fruit of *Capsicum annuum*

CHILI PEPPER FLAKES: Many varieties; fruit of *Capsicum genus*

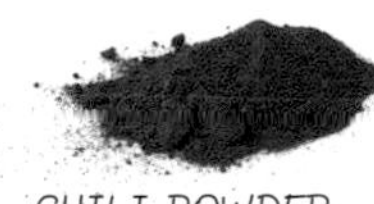

CHILI POWDER: Blend of fruit of *Capsicum genus*

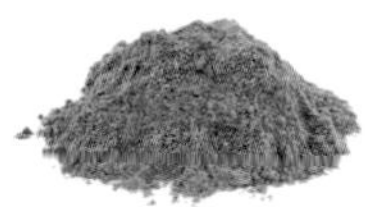

CURRY POWDER: A blend that typically contains coriander, cumin, fenugreek, and red pepper

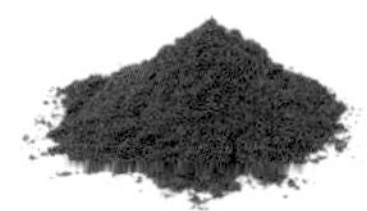

PAPRIKA: Fruit of *Capsicum spp.*

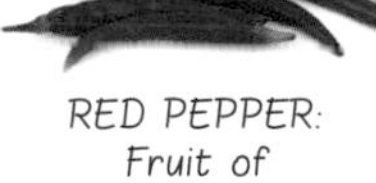

RED PEPPER: Fruit of *Capsicum annuum*

Flavor Characteristics of Herbs and Spices

The primary function of herbs and spices is to provide aroma, color, flavor, or texture to food. Here are the fifteen most common flavor/sensory characteristics used to describe the taste and aroma profiles of spices.

Note that herbs and spices can have multiple flavor characteristics. For example, cumin is earthy, nutty, and spicy, while thyme is bitter, floral, herbaceous, and piney.

BITTER:

ajwain, bay leaf, celery, clove, cumin, epazote, fenugreek seeds, horseradish, juniper, lavender, mace, marjoram, oregano, savory, star anise, thyme, turmeric

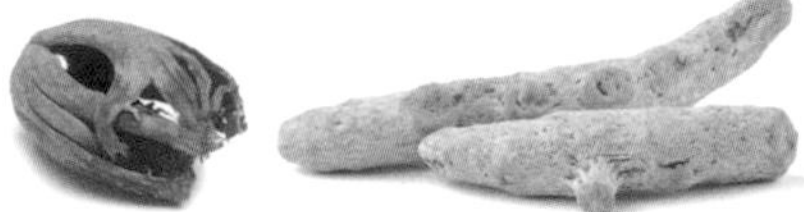

COOLING:

anise, fennel, sweet basil

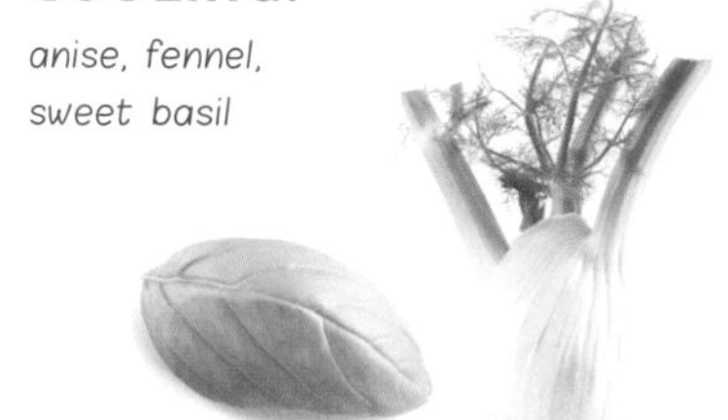

EARTHY:

annatto, cumin, saffron, truffle, turmeric

FLORAL:

coriander, lemongrass, saffron, sweet basil, thyme

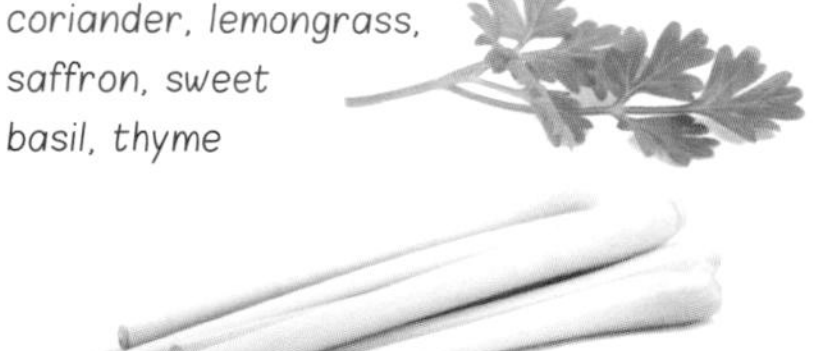

FRUITY:

anise, fennel, nigella, savory, star anise

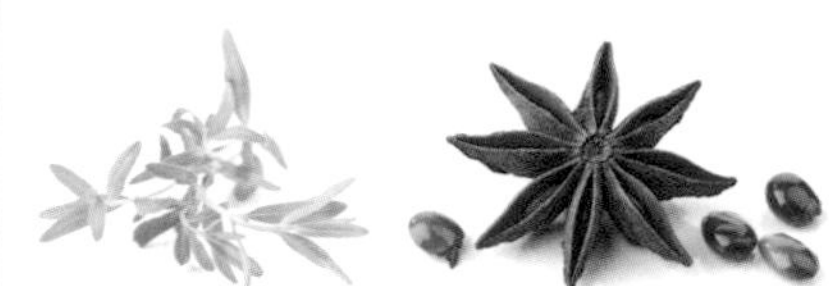

HERBACEOUS:

dill weed, lavender, oregano, parsley, rosemary, sage, savory, tarragon, thyme

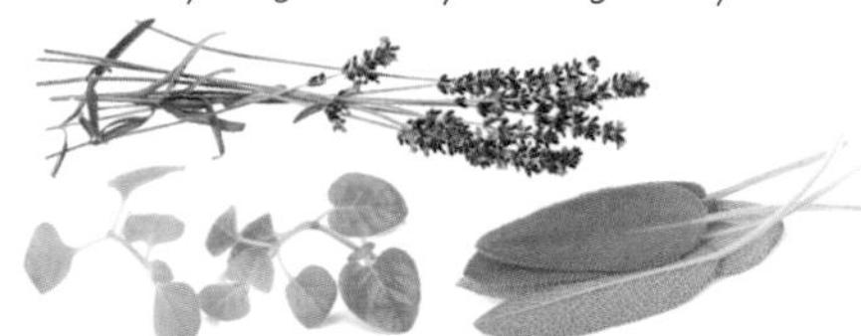

HOT:

black pepper, chilies, ginger, horseradish, mustard, wasabi, white pepper

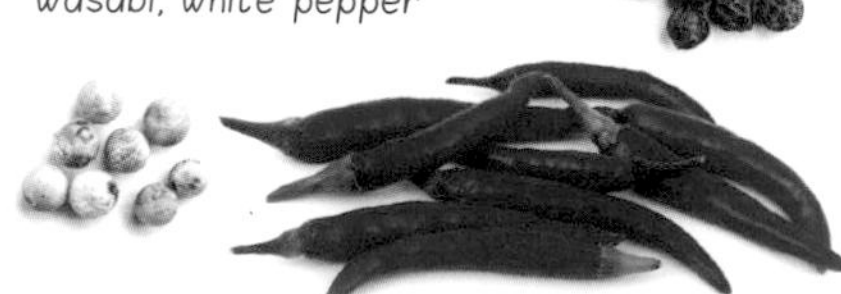

NUTTY:

ajwain, cardamom, coriander seed, cumin seed, fenugreek seed, mustard seed

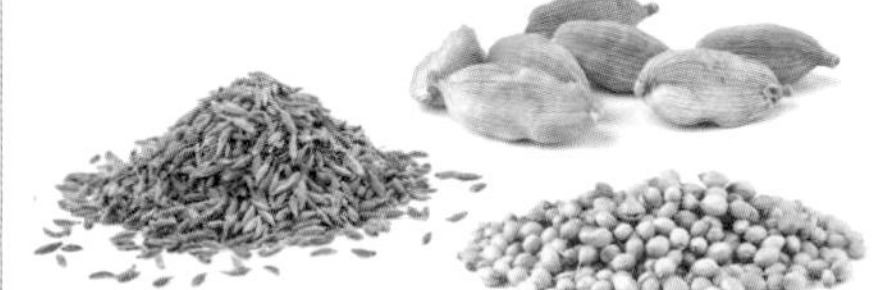

PINEY:

bay leaf, rosemary, thyme

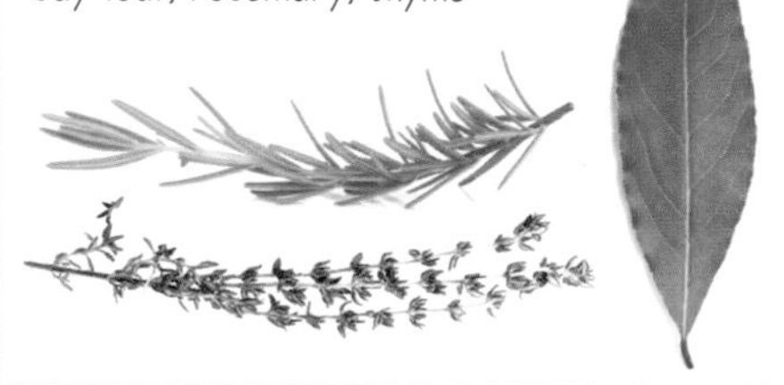

PUNGENT:

allspice, epazote, garlic, ginger, horseradish, marjoram

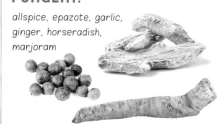

SOUR:

amchur, pomegranate, sumac

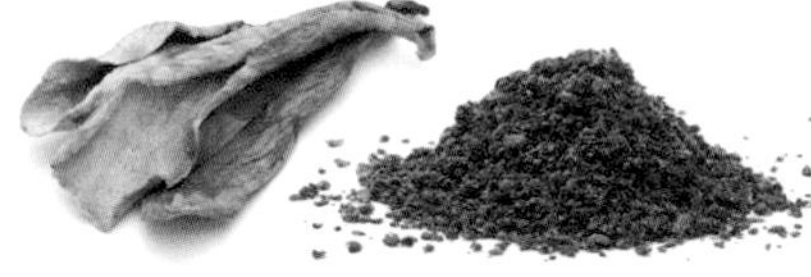

SPICY:

allspice, bay leaf, cardamom, cinnamon, cloves, coriander, cumin, curry leaf, ginger, marjoram, nutmeg

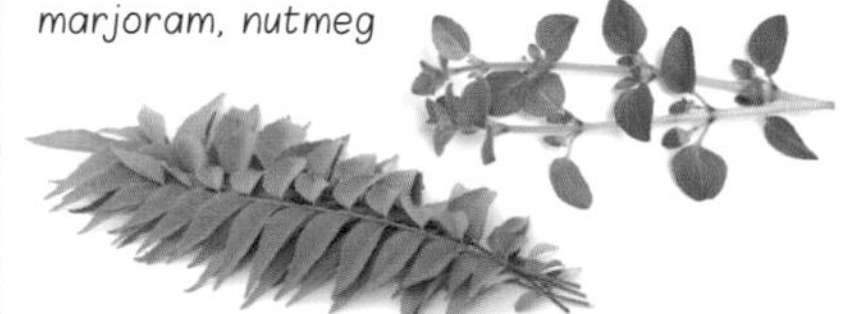

SULFURY:

asafetida, chives, garlic, onion

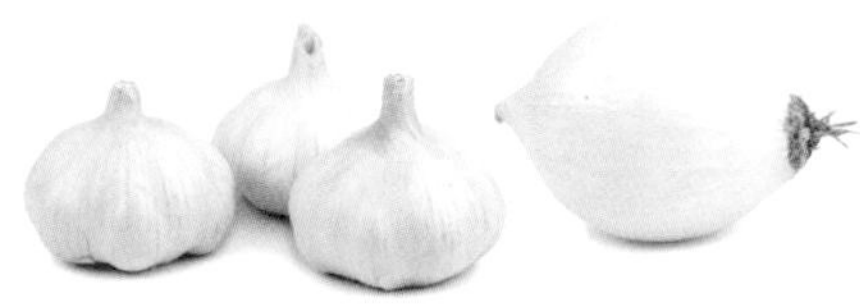

SWEET:

allspice, anise, caraway, cardamom, chervil, cinnamon, cloves, dill seed, fennel, nutmeg, poppy seed, star anise

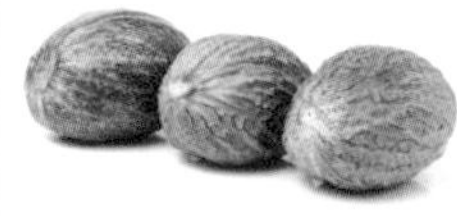

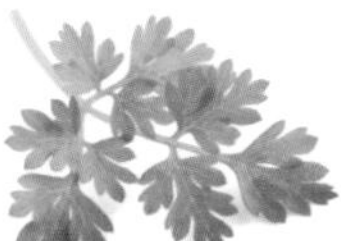

WOODY:

cardamom, cinnamon, clove, juniper, lavender, rosemary

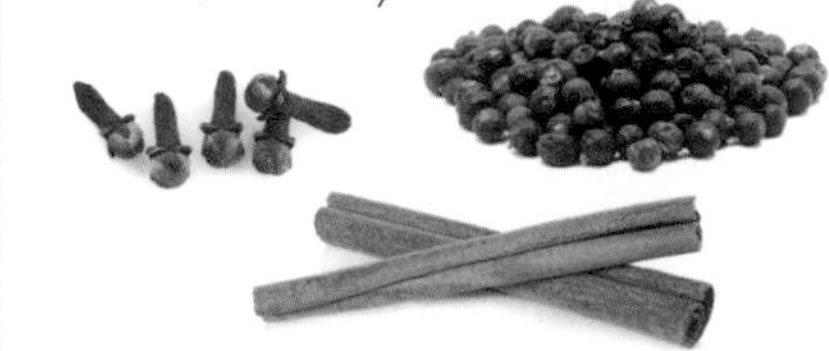

Chapter 15:
BEVERAGES

The importance of hydration for optimal health (not to mention for simply staying alive!) cannot be overstated. Along with enabling the kidneys to properly filter and excrete waste products from the body (see page 106), water helps regulate body temperature, lubricates joints, helps transport nutrients, impacts cognitive performance, and plays a role in gastrointestinal function (dehydration is one cause of constipation). Although humans can survive for several weeks or more without food, most people would die after only a few days without water.

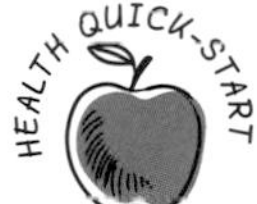

Men should consume about 13 cups (104 ounces) of total fluid per day, and women should consume about 9 cups (72 ounces) per day.

The Paleo framework includes a wide array of beverages that provide the hydration we need to stay alive and, in some cases, micronutrients or probiotics to support health in additional ways.

WATER

Water: Water is the only beverage we truly need, and filtered or spring water is generally the best choice. Natural sources of drinking water from streams, rivers, and lakes provide small amounts of minerals from the soil (including as much as 0.4 percent salt and trace levels of calcium, magnesium, potassium, sulfate, chloride, and silica), which would have contributed to the mineral content of early human diets. When spring water or other mineral-containing water isn't an option, an alternative is to add mineral drops to the water we drink. (For more information on the hot topic of fluoridation, see page 107.)

Carbonated and sparkling water: Carbonated water is more acidic than regular water (meaning it has a lower pH). Consequently, it may improve the digestion of meals for people with low stomach acid. However, in sensitive individuals, it may irritate the gut if consumed between meals.

Soda water: Soda water is more acidic than regular water but slightly more alkaline than sparkling water (meaning it has a higher pH). As a result, it offers some of the same digestion-boosting benefits during meals (and some of the same gut-irritating risks on an empty stomach) as carbonated water.

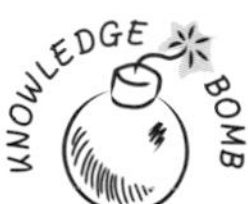

Alkaline water is a buzzword in alternative health communities, but the claims have not been substantiated with scientific studies. Neutralizing stomach acid with any strongly alkaline food or drink can have detrimental effects on digestion.

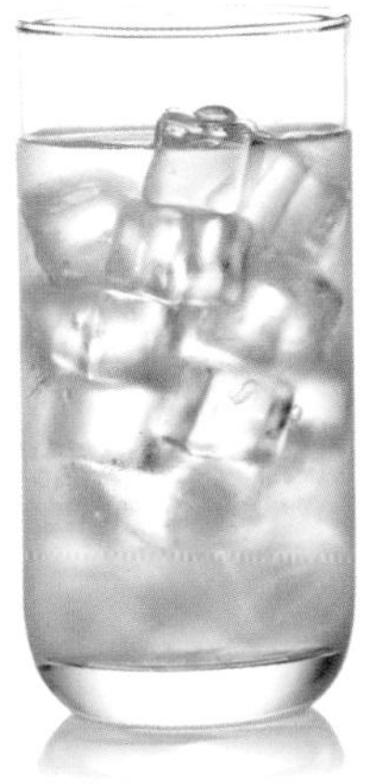

NUT AND SEED MILKS

Almond milk: It can be tough to find prepackaged almond milk that is free of emulsifiers (see page 235), but it's one of the most universally enjoyed dairy substitutes that fits into the Paleo framework. You can make it at home by following the recipe on page 481.

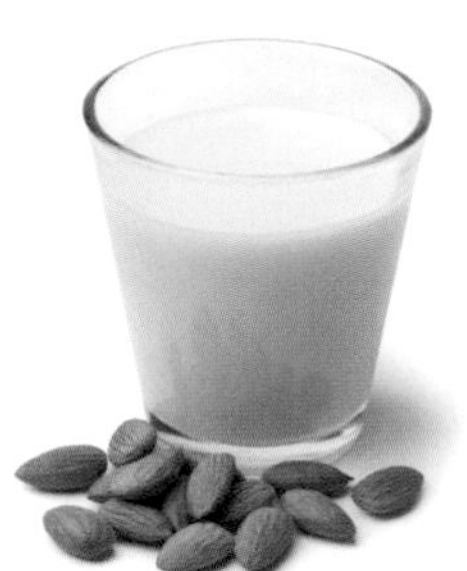

Other nut and seed milks: You can make a milky beverage from just about any nut or seed by soaking your choice of nut or seed in water for several hours and up to overnight. Drain and rinse the nuts and seeds well, then combine them with four parts water (so 4 cups of water for every 1 cup of unsoaked nuts or seeds). Blend in a high-speed blender on high for several minutes, then filter out the pulp with a nut-milk bag or several layers of cheesecloth. The flavors and nutrient profiles vary, and certainly some nutrients are lost in the pulp (which you can repurpose to make crackers or flour).

COCONUT MILK AND WATER

Coconut milk: Light and full-fat coconut milk fits into a Paleo framework, as long as it's free from emulsifiers (see page 235). It contains manganese, copper, phosphorus, iron, magnesium, potassium, and selenium and smaller amounts of zinc, vitamins B3 and B9, and vitamin C, and it's rich in beneficial medium-chain triglycerides, particularly lauric acid. Make your own at home by using the recipe on page 480.

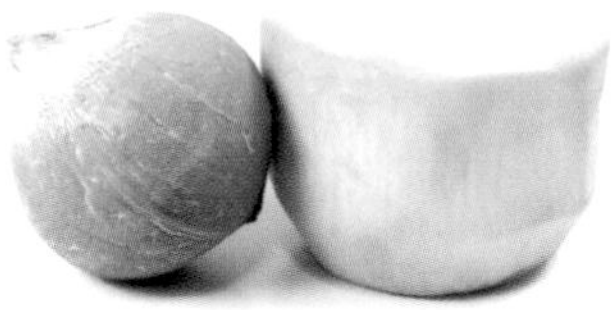

Coconut water: Coconut water is known for its electrolyte content (potassium, sodium, magnesium, and calcium), but it also contains small amounts of vitamins B1, B2, and B6, vitamin C, copper, iron, manganese, and phosphorus. Because of its sugar content, coconut water is best consumed in moderation. It can be used as a natural sports drink to replenish electrolytes during and after exercise.

PROBIOTIC BEVERAGES

Coconut milk kefir: Coconut milk kefir is made with milk kefir grains (which are living organisms) grown in coconut milk, resulting in a yogurt-like beverage rich in probiotics.

Water kefir: Water kefir is made with water kefir grains (which are living organisms) grown in juice, sweetened herbal teas, coconut water, or sweetened flavored water. The kefir eat the sugars in the liquid and produce a sparkling, fermented, probiotic-rich beverage.

Kombucha: A kombucha SCOBY (Symbiotic Colony Of Bacteria and Yeast, also called a mushroom or mother) is grown in sweetened green or black tea. When the SCOBY eats the sugar in the tea, it produces a sparkling, fermented, probiotic-rich beverage.

Beet or other vegetable kvass: Vegetables are wild or lactofermented (as with making sauerkraut) and then juiced. The result is an acidic, mildly sweet, and mildly salty beverage rich in probiotics.

JUICES AND SMOOTHIES

Vegetable juices: Vegetable juices (in moderation) can fit into a Paleo framework, particularly for people who have severe gastrointestinal damage or have a hard time digesting even cooked vegetables. Vegetable juices are no longer whole foods, but the removal of fiber from the vegetables during the juicing process has the net effect of making many vitamins, minerals, and antioxidants much more absorbable (although some nutrients are lost in the pulp). However, juicing also makes natural sugars much more absorbable, so it's best to consume vegetable juices with a meal to slow digestion. Fruit juices are very high in sugar and are best avoided.

Green smoothies: Green smoothies (vegetables blended with a liquid base and/or fruit) can be an alternative for increasing vegetable intake while still consuming the fiber naturally found in plant foods (in contrast to vegetable juices, which remove this fiber). However, drinking our food can still be hard on the digestive system because the simple act of chewing signals to the body to increase stomach acid secretion, which prompts the pancreas to secrete digestive enzymes and the gallbladder to secrete bile. In fact, studies have confirmed that consuming liquefied protein or carbohydrates doesn't fill you up as much as consuming the same foods in solid form and that blood sugar spikes earlier and higher following the consumption of liquefied carbohydrates as compared to solids. Ideally, a green smoothie should be consumed as part of a meal to ensure optimal digestion.

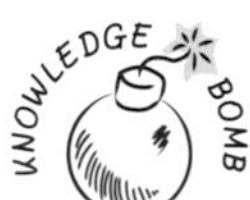

While drinking a smoothie leaves you feeling hungrier than you would be if you had consumed the individual components of the smoothie without blending them, one recent study showed the opposite effect when it came to soup. In this study, participants consumed chicken, vegetables, and a glass of water or the same foods pureed into a soup. Not only did the soup keep participants fuller longer, but it also improved digestion—the soup caused slower gastric emptying and greater gallbladder contraction.

TEA

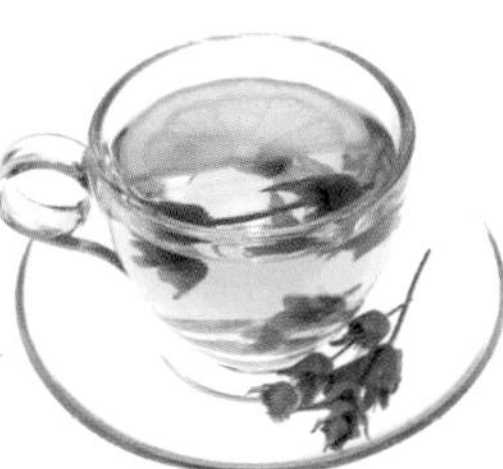

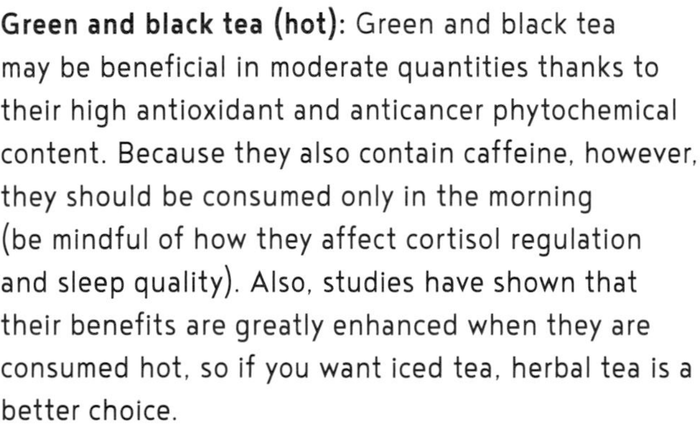

Green and black tea (hot): Green and black tea may be beneficial in moderate quantities thanks to their high antioxidant and anticancer phytochemical content. Because they also contain caffeine, however, they should be consumed only in the morning (be mindful of how they affect cortisol regulation and sleep quality). Also, studies have shown that their benefits are greatly enhanced when they are consumed hot, so if you want iced tea, herbal tea is a better choice.

Herbal teas (hot or cold): Herbal teas are made from infusions of herbs, spices, or other plant parts. Unlike "real" tea (made from the leaves of the tea bush), they typically don't contain caffeine while still boasting impressive levels of antioxidant phytochemicals. With some exceptions (noted below), herbal teas are an acceptable and often beneficial addition to the Paleo framework.

Common herbal teas include:

Chamomile

Chicory

Cinnamon

Citrus rind (often combined with other teas)

Clover

Dandelion root

Dried fruit (often combined with other teas)

Ginger (which is a fantastic digestive aid and may help modulate the immune system by inhibiting activated T cells and B cells)

Greek mountain

Hibiscus (caution: hibiscus tea can lower blood pressure)

Honeybush

Lavender

Lemon balm (caution: lemon balm extract is a known immune stimulator)

Lemon verbena

Marshmallow root (may help repair the damaged gut mucosa)

Milk thistle (supports liver detoxification; see page 104)

Mint (caution: mint tea relaxes the upper gastroesophageal sphincter and can exacerbate acid reflux)

Nettle

Olive leaf

Rooibos (contains potent antioxidants, may help promote regulatory T-cell production, and has been shown to improve colitis in animal models)

Rosehip

Sage

Sea buckthorn

Turmeric (caution: has potent anti-inflammatory properties but in large doses may suppress regulatory T-cell activity; see page 79)

Herbal teas, typically those that have medicinal properties or are marketed as antioxidant, immune supportive, or energizing, are made with herbs known to be immune modulators or stimulators or sometimes adaptogenic herbs (see page 348). These herbs or herbal extracts typically stimulate subsets of the immune system or influence adrenal function in a way that is counterproductive for those with autoimmune disease (see page 412) or adrenal fatigue (see page 345). While the effects of these teas would be greatly diluted compared to the extracts used in scientific studies, caution should be used when consuming them, including astragalus, ashwagandha (a nightshade; see page 296), echinacea, American ginseng, grapeseed, licorice root, panax ginseng, and maitake, reishi, and shiitake mushrooms.

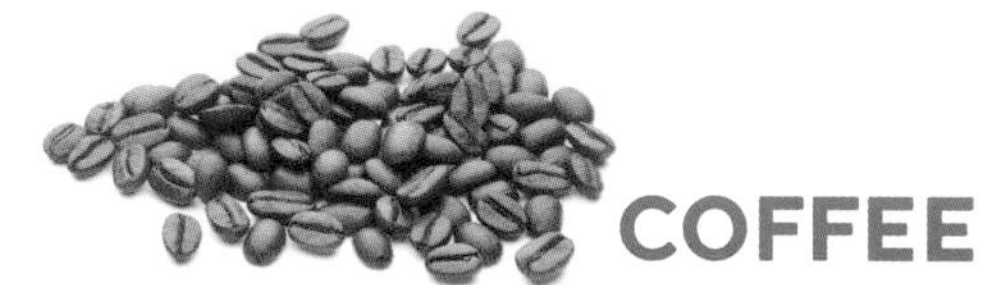

COFFEE

A number of research studies show that drinking coffee in moderation could provide a range of health benefits, including reduced risk of certain cancers, stroke, diabetes, Parkinson's disease, Alzheimer's disease, cardiovascular disease, gout, gallstones, and depression, along with protection against antibiotic-resistant bacterial infections and cirrhosis of the liver. It can even reduce muscle soreness after a workout! There are studies that show coffee drinkers are plain old less likely to die from any cause. In fact, a 2014 meta-analysis found that drinking 4 cups of coffee per day was associated with a 16 percent reduction in all-cause mortality, as well as a 21 percent reduction in cardiovascular disease mortality.

Some of these effects are owed to the antioxidants, polyphenols, and bioactive compounds in coffee (including some with insulin-sensitizing and anti-inflammatory properties). And some of the health benefits of coffee are directly attributable to its caffeine content (which is why drinking tea—which is rich in antioxidants and polyphenols while also containing caffeine—is also associated with good health). This is partly why many of the health-protective effects of regular coffee are not seen with decaf coffee. In addition, the decaffeination process tends to strip the coffee of many of its antioxidants and polyphenols, potentially leaving behind a few of the more harmful substances that can be found in coffee.

Despite many potential benefits, coffee can be a double-edged sword. For one, coffee is made from a seed (not a legume, but the pit of the coffee fruit). Right away, this should put us on alert, as seeds tend to contain protective compounds to prevent digestion and thereby ensure the survival of the plant species. A large percentage of people report that coffee upsets their stomach or gives them heartburn. This happens because coffee stimulates the secretion of the main gastric hormone gastrin, resulting in excessive secretion of gastric acid and speeding up gastric peristalsis (even decaf coffee has this effect). Coffee also stimulates the release of the hormone cholecystokinin (CCK), which stimulates the release of bile from the gallbladder. In a healthy individual, this release of bile is likely sufficient to neutralize the highly acidic chyme (the mix of food, beverages, and stomach acid that empties from the stomach into the small intestine). However, deficiencies in gallbladder function are associated with metabolic syndrome. In the case of reduced gallbladder function or excessive coffee consumption, non-neutralized chyme travels through the small intestine, where it irritates and inflames the lining. This is clearly a good argument for consuming coffee with food.

Although caffeine does have benefits in many cases, people who are genetically slow caffeine metabolizers (involving reduced activity of the CYP1A2 enzyme) may not receive the heart-protective benefits of coffee, but instead experience high blood pressure and an *increased* risk of heart attack. Due to caffeine's disruptive effects on sleep, consuming caffeinated coffee late in the day can have a negative impact on sleep quality. Another of the detrimental effects of consuming caffeine (whether from coffee, tea, chocolate, or energy drinks) is the effect that it has on cortisol. Caffeine acts to increase cortisol secretion by elevating the production of adrenocorticotropic hormone by the pituitary gland. Excessive cortisol production can lead to a variety of health issues, including an overactive immune system, disrupted sleep, impaired digestion, and depression. When you consume caffeine, your cortisol level rises (depending on what your cortisol management is like to begin with and how much caffeine you consume) and can stay elevated for up to 6 hours. With daily consumption, your body will adapt somewhat and not produce quite as much cortisol, but complete tolerance to caffeine does not occur. Very importantly, if you are a habitual consumer of caffeine, your cortisol will increase more dramatically in response to stress (like that guy cutting you off in traffic) than someone who doesn't consume caffeine. If you have difficulty managing stress as it is, caffeine is not helpful to you.

One key study showed that moderate coffee consumption in healthy individuals correlated with increased markers of inflammation in their blood. People who drank more than 200 milliliters of coffee (that's one large cup in my house) every day—equivalent to about 37 milligrams of caffeine—had increased circulating white blood cells and several key inflammatory cytokines (chemical messengers of inflammation, usually restricted to the site of injury or infection). Cytokines circulating in the blood cause low-level inflammation everywhere in the body. This chronic systemic inflammation is exactly one of the situations we are trying to prevent with the adoption of a Paleo diet! These increases in markers of inflammation persisted even after adjusting for other health and lifestyle factors, such as age, sex, weight, activity level, and smoking.

Several compounds in coffee (namely cafestol and kahweol) have cholesterol-raising effects and can cause higher LDL ("bad") and total cholesterol in some individuals (although they may also have a protective effect on the liver and help explain the association between coffee consumption and reduced risk of liver cancer). These compounds are largely removed via paper filtration, so whether they are present depends on how the coffee is prepared.

In a nutshell, coffee offers a variety of pros and cons that are extremely context dependent. For many people, coffee is a fine addition to a Paleo diet—especially when consumed in moderation, in filtered form, early in the day, and with a meal rather than on an empty stomach. People with gallbladder problems, who metabolize caffeine more slowly, or who simply experience adverse side effects like an upset stomach or heartburn should proceed with caution where coffee is concerned.

ALCOHOLIC BEVERAGES

Our gene to process alcohol goes back about 18 million years, long before humans were humans. Seeking out riper fruit gave us an evolutionary advantage: in addition to its higher alcohol content, riper fruit also has more vitamins and minerals. It's likely that Paleolithic man overindulged (in the form of fermenting fruit), perhaps by accident, once in a while toward the end of the season when overripe fruit was abundant. We are adapted to alcohol in small to moderate quantities. The bacteria in our guts also produce about 3 grams of ethanol per day.

Alcohol consumption is a double-edged sword, with some scientific studies touting benefits and many others showing increased risk of disease. Alcohol is psychoactive (that's why we get drunk when we drink enough of it) and addictive. It's also hepatotoxic (that is, it damages liver cells, which is why cirrhosis of the liver and fatty liver disease are consequences of alcoholism), and there are several ways in which alcohol can harm gut health (both increasing permeability and causing gut dysbiosis); this should be especially concerning to anyone battling chronic illness. While occasional moderate consumption is likely harmless for most people based on the scientific evidence, alcoholic beverages cannot be fully endorsed as part of a healthful diet. This is discussed in further detail in Chapter 24.

If you choose to drink alcohol, wine, non-grain-based spirits like tequila and rum, and cider are your best bet. Steer clear of grain-based drinks that can also include gluten, such as beer, bourbon, gin (some brands are distilled from grain-based alcohol), grain-based vodka, and whiskey.

Chapter 16:

THE PALEO DIET QUICK-START

Before we launch into the foods eliminated on the Paleo diet and the foods for which the science is less than conclusive, let's review the amazing variety of health-promoting foods that form the basis of an optimal human diet.

FOODS TO EAT

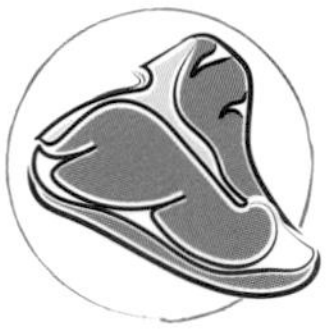

RED MEAT

antelope
bear
beaver
beef
bison/buffalo
boar
camel
caribou
deer
elk
goat
hare
horse
kangaroo
lamb
llama
moose
mutton
pork
rabbit
sea lion
seal
whale
(essentially, any mammal)

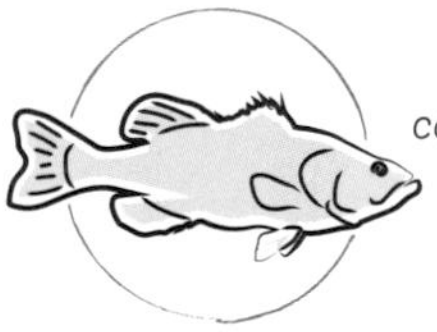

FISH

anchovy
Arctic char
Atlantic croaker
barcheek goby
bass
bonito
bream
brill
brisling
carp
catfish
cod
common dab
conger
crappie
croaker
drum
eel
fera
filefish
gar
haddock
hake
halibut
herring
John Dory
king mackerel*
lamprey
ling
loach
mackerel
mahi mahi
marlin*
milkfish
minnow
monkfish
mullet
pandora
perch
plaice
pollock
sailfish
salmon
sardine
shad
shark*
sheepshead
silverside
smelt
snakehead
snapper
sole
swordfish*
tarpon*
tilapia
tilefish*
trout
tub gurnard
tuna
turbot
walleye
whiting

**May contain higher levels of methylmercury than selenium (see page 163); consume in moderation*

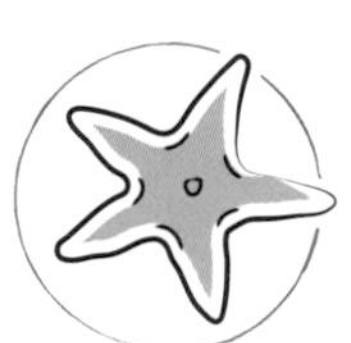

OTHER SEAFOOD

anemone
caviar/roe
jellyfish
sea cucumber
sea squirt
sea urchin
starfish

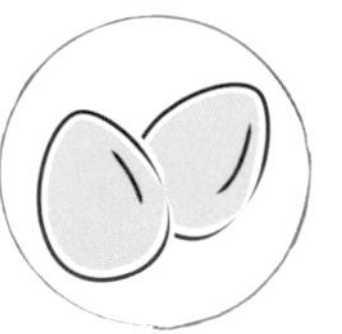

POULTRY AND EGGS

chicken
dove
duck
eggs (chicken, duck, goose, quail, and so on)
emu
goose
grouse
guinea hen
ostrich
partridge
pheasant
pigeon
quail
turkey
(essentially, any bird)

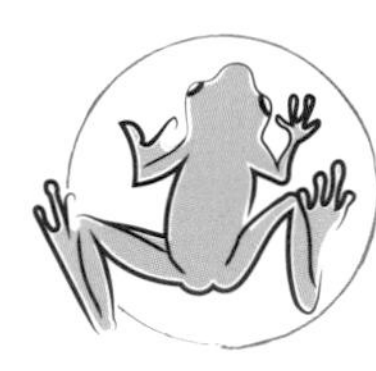

OTHER ANIMAL FOODS

crocodile
frog
snake
turtle

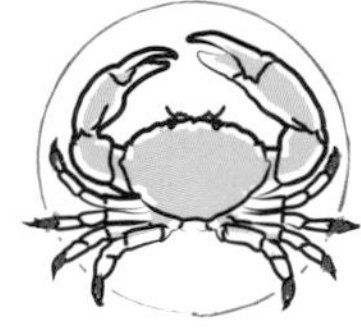

SHELLFISH

abalone
clam
cockle
conch
crab
crawfish
cuttlefish
limpet
lobster
mussel
octopus
oyster
periwinkle
prawn
scallop
shrimp
snail
squid
whelk

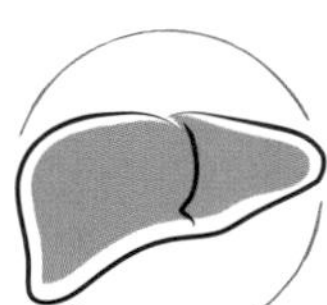

OFFAL

blood
bone broth
bone marrow
brain
chitterlings and natural casings (intestines)
fats and other trimmings (tallow and lard)
fries (testicles)
head meat (cheek and jowl)
heart
kidney
lips
liver
melt (spleen)
rinds (skin)
sweetbreads (thymus gland or pancreas)
tail
tongue
tripe (stomach)

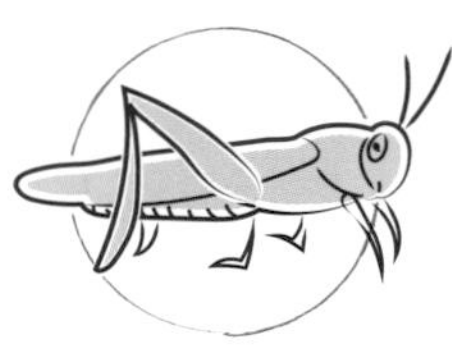

EDIBLE INSECTS

- agave worm
- ant
- bamboo worm
- bee larvae
- centipede
- cicada
- cockroach
- cricket
- dragonfly
- dung beetle
- earthworm
- fly pupa
- grasshopper
- hornworm
- June bug
- locust
- mealworm
- sago worm
- silkworm

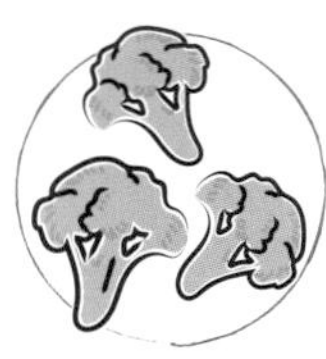

CRUCIFEROUS VEGETABLES

- arugula (rocket)
- bok choy
- broccoflower
- broccoli
- broccoli rabe (rapini)
- Brussels sprouts
- cabbage
- canola (rapeseed)
- cauliflower
- Chinese broccoli
- collard greens
- daikon
- field pepperweed
- flowering cabbage
- garden cress
- horseradish
- kale
- kohlrabi
- komatsuna
- land cress
- maca
- mizuna
- mustard
- radishes
- Romanesco
- rutabaga
- tatsoi
- turnips
- wasabi
- watercress
- wild broccoli

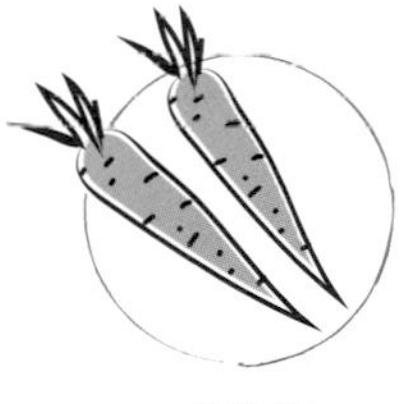

ROOT VEGETABLES AND WINTER SQUASH

- acorn squash
- ambercup squash
- arracacha
- arrowroot
- bamboo shoot
- banana squash
- beet root
- broadleaf arrowhead
- burdock
- butternut squash
- calabaza
- camas
- canna
- carnival squash
- carrot
- celeriac
- Chinese artichoke
- daikon
- delicata squash
- earthnut pea
- elephant foot yam
- Ensete
- ginger
- gold nugget squash
- Hamburg parsley
- horseradish
- Hubbard squash
- Jerusalem artichoke
- jicama
- kabocha squash
- lotus root
- maca
- mashua
- parsnip
- pignut
- prairie turnip
- pumpkin
- salsify
- scorzonera
- skirret
- spaghetti squash
- squash, winter (all varieties)
- swede
- sweet potato
- taro
- ti
- tiger nut
- turban squash
- ulluco
- water caltrop
- water chestnut
- yacón
- yam
- yuca (cassava, manioc, tapioca)

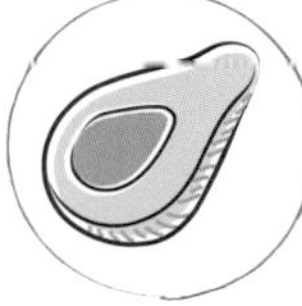

HIGH-FAT FRUITS

- avocado
- olives (green and black)

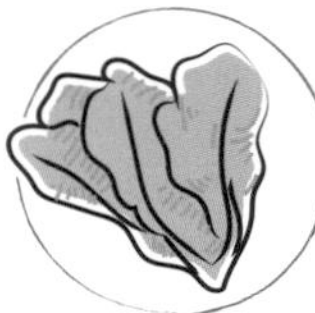

LEAFY GREENS AND SALAD VEGGIES

- amaranth greens
- beet greens
- borage greens
- carrot tops
- cat's-ear
- celery
- celtuce
- Ceylon spinach
- chickweed
- chicory
- Chinese mallow
- chrysanthemum leaves
- cress
- dandelion greens
- endive
- fat hen
- fiddlehead
- fluted pumpkin leaves
- Good King Henry
- greater plantain
- komatsuna
- Lagos bologi
- lamb's lettuce
- land cress
- lettuce
- melokhia
- New Zealand spinach
- orache
- pea leaves
- poke
- pumpkin sprouts
- radicchio
- radish sprouts
- sculpit (stridolo)
- sorrel
- spinach
- squash blossoms
- summer purslane
- sunflower sprouts
- sweet potato greens
- Swiss chard
- water spinach
- winter purslane

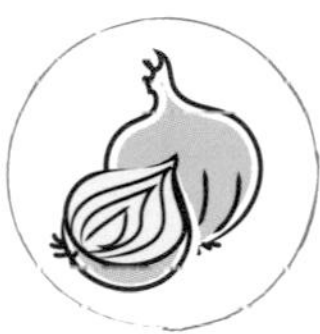

ONIONS, GARLIC, AND OTHER ALLIUMS

- abusgata
- chives
- elephant garlic
- garlic
- kurrat
- leek
- onion
- pearl onion
- potato onion
- scallion
- shallot
- spring onion
- tree onion
- wild leek (ramp)

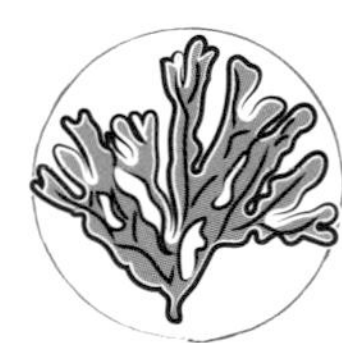

SEA VEGETABLES

- aonori
- arame
- carola
- dabberlocks
- dulse
- hijiki
- kombu
- laver
- mozuku
- nori
- ogonori
- sea grape
- sea kale
- sea lettuce
- wakame

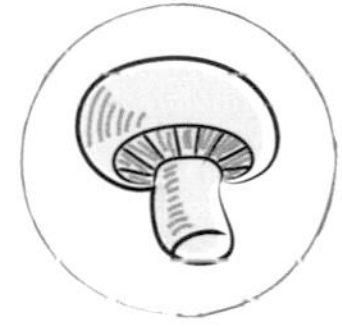

MUSHROOMS AND OTHER EDIBLE FUNGI

- beech mushroom (shimeji)
- boletus, many varieties
- button mushroom, many varieties (includes portobello and crimini)
- cauliflower mushroom (Sparassis crispa)
- chanterelle, many varieties
- field blewit
- gypsy mushroom
- hedgehog mushroom (sweet tooth fungus)
- kefir (includes both yeast and probiotic bacteria)
- king trumpet mushroom
- kombucha (includes both yeast and probiotic bacteria)
- lion's mane mushroom
- maitake
- matsutake
- morel, many varieties
- oyster mushroom, many varieties
- saffron milk cap
- shiitake (oak mushroom)
- snow fungus
- straw mushroom
- tree ear fungus
- truffle, many varieties
- winter mushroom (enokitake)
- yeast (baker's, brewer's, nutritional)

BERRIES

açaí
bearberry
bilberry
blackberry
blueberry
cloudberry
cranberry
crowberry
currant
elderberry
falberry
gooseberry
grape
hackberry
huckleberry
lingonberry
loganberry
mulberry
Muscadine grape
nannyberry
Oregon grape
raspberry
salmonberry
sea buckthorn
strawberry
strawberry tree
thimbleberry
wineberry

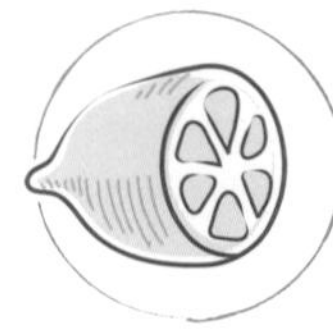

CITRUS

amanatsu
blood orange
Buddha's hand
cam sành
citron
clementine
fernandina
grapefruit (many varieties)
kaffir lime
key lime
kinnow
kiyomi
kumquat
lemon (many varieties)
lime (many varieties)
limetta
mandarin
Meyer lemon
orange (many varieties)
orangelo
oroblanco
pomelo
pompia
ponkan
rangpur
shonan gold
sudachi
tangelo
tangerine
tangor
ugli
yuzu

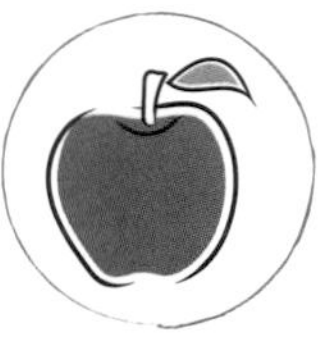

OTHER FRUITS AND VEGGIES

abiu
acerola
ackee
African moringa
ambarella
apple
apricot
artichoke
asparagus
babaco
banana
biriba
bitter melon (bitter gourd)
camucamu
canary melon
canistel
cantaloupe
capers
cardoon
casaba
celery
ceriman
Charentais
chayote
cherimoya
cherry
chokeberry
chokecherry
Christmas melon
coco plum
coconut
crabapple
Crenshaw melon
cucumber
custard apple
date
derishi
dragonfruit
durian
edible flowers (such as carnation, clover, dandelion, gladiolus, hibiscus, honeysuckle, lavender, marigold, nasturtium, pansy, primrose, scented geranium)
fennel
fig (many varieties)
Florence fennel
Galia
gambooge
granadilla
greengage
guanabana
guava (many varieties)
guavaberry
hawthorn
honeydew
horned melon
ilama
ivy gourd
jackfruit
jujube
karonda
kiwi
korlan
kumquat
lizard's tail
longan
loofa
loquat
lychee
mamey sapote
mango
mangosteen
maypop
medlar
melon pear
muskmelon
nance
nectarine
net melon
nopal
ogen melon
okra
papaya
passion fruit
pawpaw
peach
peanut butter fruit
pear
pepino melon
Persian melon
persimmon
pineapple
plantain
plum
pomegranate
Prussian asparagus
pulasan
quince
rambutan
rhubarb (only the stems are edible)
riberry
rose apple
rose hip
rowan
Russian melon (Uzbek melon)
safou
salak
samphire
santol
sea beet
sea kale
service tree
serviceberry
sharlyn
shipova
soursop
squash blossoms
star apple
star fruit (carambola)
sugar apple
sweet melon
tinda
ugni
wampee
watermelon
West Indian gherkin
winter melon
zucchini

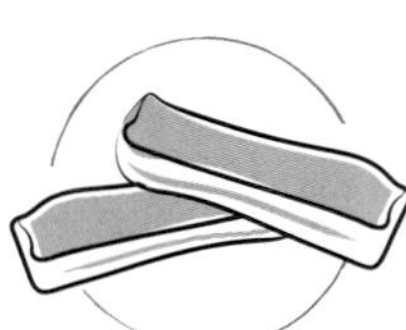
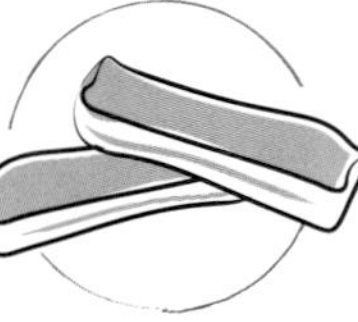

ANIMAL FATS*

bacon fat
lard
leaf lard
poultry fat
salo
schmaltz
strutto
tallow
pan drippings

**Ideally from grass-fed or pasture-raised animals*

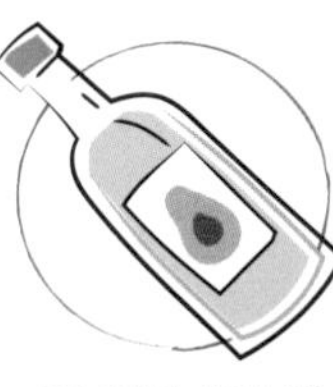

PLANT OILS*

avocado oil
coconut oil
macadamia nut oil
olive oil
palm oil
palm shortening
red palm oil
sesame oil
walnut oil

**Ideally cold-pressed, unrefined, organic, and ethically sourced*

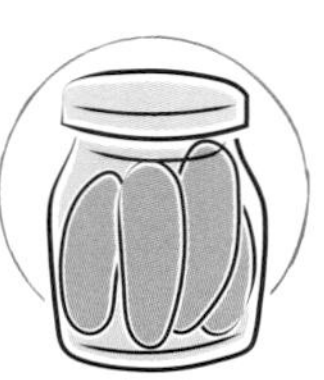

PROBIOTIC FOODS

beet and other vegetable kvasses
coconut milk kefir or yogurt
kombucha
raw, unpasteurized, lactofermented condiments (relishes, salsas)
raw, unpasteurized, lactofermented fruits (green papaya, chutneys)
raw, unpasteurized, lactofermented vegetables (kimchi, beets, carrots, pickles)
raw, unpasteurized sauerkraut
water kefir

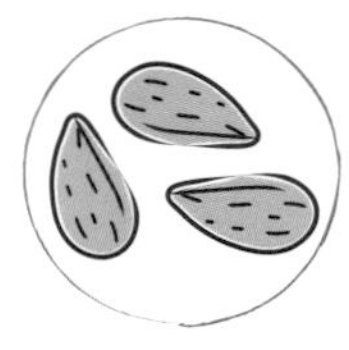

NUTS*

almonds
Brazil nuts
cashews
chestnuts
coconut
hazelnuts
macadamia nuts
pecans
pili nuts
pine nuts
pistachios
walnuts

*Limit nut consumption to 1 ounce per day

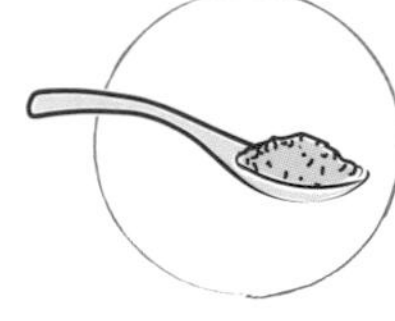

MINERALS

Celtic sea salt
Himalayan pink salt
sea vegetable powder (or salt)
sel gris
truffle salt

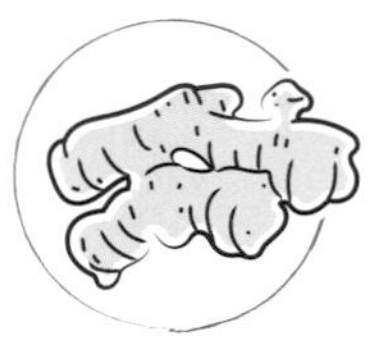

SPICES

ajwain
allspice
amchur (mango powder)
anise seed
annatto seed
asafetida*
black caraway
black pepper
caraway
cardamom
celery seed
cinnamon
cloves
coriander seed
cumin seed
dill seed
fennel seed
fenugreek seed
garlic
ginger
green peppercorns
juniper
mace
mustard seed
nutmeg
pink peppercorns
saffron
star anise
sumac
truffles
turmeric
vanilla bean
wasabi
white pepper

*Frequently sold mixed with wheat starch; check ingredients.

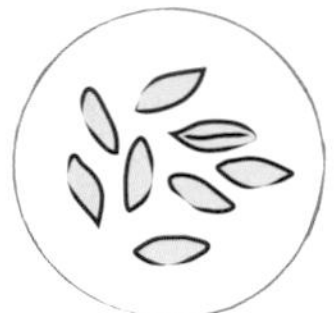

SEEDS*

cacao (chocolate)
chia (see page 256)
flax (see page 308)
hemp
poppy
pumpkin
sacha inchi
sesame
sunflower

*Limit seed consumption to 1 ounce per day

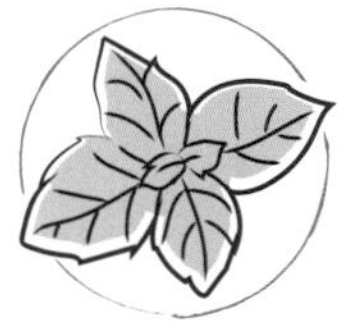

HERBS

balm (lemon balm)
basil leaves (sweet)
bay leaves (laurel leaves)
chamomile
chervil
chives
cilantro (coriander leaf)
curry leaves
dill weed
epazote
fenugreek leaves
Kaffir lime leaves
lavender
lemongrass
marjoram
oregano
parsley
peppermint
perilla leaves (beefsteak leaves)
rosemary
sage
savory
spearmint
tarragon
thyme

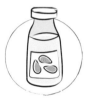

BEVERAGES

almond milk (emulsifier-free)
beet and other vegetable kvasses
carbonated or sparkling water
coconut milk (emulsifier-free)
coconut milk kefir
coconut water
coffee (in moderation)
kombucha
lemon or lime juice
mineral water
nut and seed milks (emulsifier-free)
soda water
tea (green, black, or white)
tea, herbal (including chamomile, chicory, cinnamon, citrus rind, clove, dandelion root, dried fruit, ginger, Greek mountain, hibiscus, honeybush, lavender, lemon balm, lemon verbena, marshmallow root, milk thistle, mint, olive leaf, rooibos, rose hip, sage, sea buckthorn, turmeric, and yerba mate)
vegetable juices and green smoothies (in moderation)
water
water kefir

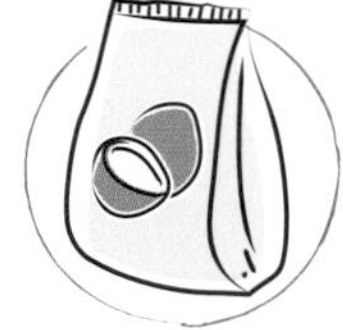

PANTRY ITEMS AND FLAVORING INGREDIENTS

agar agar
almond flour
anchovies or anchovy paste*
apple cider vinegar
arrowroot powder
baking soda
balsamic vinegar
bonito flakes
capers
carob powder**
cassava flour
chestnut flour
chocolate (dark)
chutneys*
coconut aminos (a great soy sauce substitute)
coconut butter (aka creamed coconut, coconut cream concentrate)
coconut cream
coconut flour
coconut milk
coconut water vinegar
cream of tartar
dried fruit**
fish sauce*
gelatin
green banana flour
honey**
jams and jellies*,**
kuzu starch
maple syrup**
molasses**
nutritional yeast (caution: common sensitivity)
nuts and seeds
olives
plantain flour*
pomegranate molasses**
red wine vinegar
sea vegetables
shrimp paste*
sunflower seed flour
sweet potato flour or starch
tamarind paste
tapioca starch
truffle oil* (made with extra-virgin olive oil)
truffle salt*
truffles
umeboshi paste
unrefined cane sugars
vegetable powders (such as pumpkin, sweet potato, spinach)
water chestnut flour
white wine vinegar

* Check ingredients. **In moderation.

MEAT VERSUS PLANTS

As a reminder, approximately half of our calories should come from animal foods and half from plant foods, but that doesn't mean half of the plate will be steak and half will be salad. Animal foods tend to be much more energy dense than plant foods (nuts, seeds, and fatty fruits like avocados being the exceptions), so this generally translates to about two-thirds to three-quarters of the plate being vegetables with some fruit, nuts, and seeds in moderation and the other one-quarter to one-third being meat or seafood. See page 61.

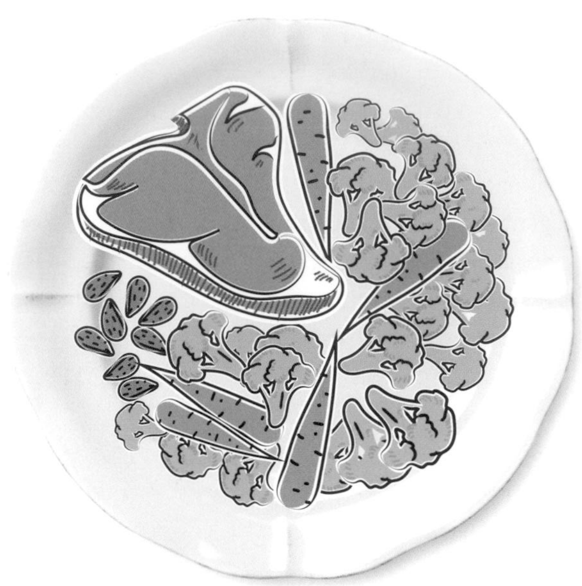

VARIETY, VARIETY, VARIETY

The single best way to ensure that we are getting the nutrition our bodies need is to eat as much variety as possible. This means variety in both the plant foods and the animal foods we are eating.

By now, you know that different foods contain different nutrients. When it comes to eating plants, it's important to "eat the rainbow" (see page 39). An easy way to accomplish this is to aim to consume at least two different-colored vegetables with every meal.

Just as it's important to eat a diversity of colors when choosing plant foods, it's important to switch up foods within a particular color category. Even within one color of the rainbow, the nutrients you get from different plants can be very different. In fact, it may surprise you to know just how different closely related foods can be when it comes to nutritional features. Kale and collard greens are both dense, slightly bitter leafy greens from the cruciferous family of vegetables. They are often prepared in similar ways, and you might see them as interchangeable in cooking. But while they substitute nicely for each other in recipes, they contribute slightly different nutrients to your diet. For example, kale has more vitamin C and K, but collards contain more vitamin B5 and B9.

The same rule holds true for animal foods: variety ensures a greater breadth of nutrition. You might look at ground beef and ground lamb as being interchangeable. Both are red meat, after all, and you can easily substitute one for the other when making meatloaf, burgers, and meat sauces. But beef has more potassium and zinc, whereas lamb contains more vitamin B3 and selenium.

Nutrition doesn't just vary by the animal; it also varies by the cut of meat. A beef rib-eye steak has more than double the vitamin B12 of a beef sirloin steak. And absolutely no muscle meat can compare to the nutrient density of any organ meat. Organs are powerhouses of nutrients and should find their way onto your plate at least four times per week.

The animal food version of eating the rainbow is to eat "snout to tail." This means eating every edible part of the animal (see page 177). You can achieve this in one of two ways: you can make a concerted effort to buy different cuts of meat and source organ meat whenever you go shopping, or you can buy meat by the whole or substantial fraction of an animal (such as a whole pig or half a cow) and get everything the meat processor or butcher will give you.

Just as it's super-important to eat every part of the animal, it's important to eat a variety of animals, including red meat, poultry, fish, and shellfish. The difference in nutrition between different types of animals can be substantial, not just in terms of vitamins and minerals but also in relative quantities of various amino acids and essential fatty acids. Too-limited food choices can lead to nutrient deficiencies and excesses, neither of which are helpful when we're trying to achieve optimal health.

Incorporating seafood into our diet is especially important, in part because of the complementary nutrition that fish and shellfish have to meat from land animals. Seafood is our best source of a variety of essential vitamins and minerals, like vitamins A and D, zinc, and selenium; it is our best source of essential long-chain omega-3 polyunsaturated fatty acids (well, unless you're eating brain); and it provides the most digestible protein available. And don't forget sea vegetables, which are some of the most nutrient-dense plants and the only plant sources of long-chain omega-3 polyunsaturated fatty acids (see page 146).

It's also important to vary how and whether we cook our foods. Cooking depletes some nutrients and causes others to form. Cooking improves the digestibility and bioavailability of many nutrients (how well our bodies actually digest, absorb, and use them) but inactivates some beneficial enzymes, kills probiotic organisms, and changes the quality of the fiber in foods. And different cooking techniques have different effects. For example, high-heat cooking can cause undesirable compounds to form (let me clarify: undesirable from a health standpoint because they are potential carcinogens, but typically very desirable from a taste standpoint). Boiling vegetables can cause nutrients to leach into the water. (Of course, if you're making soup, that's not an issue because you're going to drink that nutrient-rich liquid.) Fermentation also changes the nutritional value of foods, typically increasing it (see page 193). The way to get the best of all worlds is to vary your cooking techniques as much as you vary the types of foods you eat: sometimes steam broccoli, sometimes eat it raw, sometimes ferment vegetables, sometimes roast your meat, sometimes slow-cook it, sometimes eat sashimi.

When it comes to food choices, the more different ones we make within the food lists given earlier in this chapter, the better. Variety is the key to getting all the nutrients we need in synergistic quantities for optimal health.

FOOD QUALITY GUIDE

It's probably obvious to say that the higher the quality of your food, the better off you are. Higher-quality food provides more nutrition while containing fewer potentially problematic substances.

In general, it's best to consume whole and fresh foods, which means foods made from unprocessed, unmanipulated ingredients and foods in their most natural state and as close to harvest as possible. Processing and storing foods depletes their nutrients. It's okay to stock the pantry and have a variety of flavoring ingredients in the door of the fridge, but the vast majority of the foods we cook with should look as close as possible to how they look while growing or roaming in the wild. And when farm-fresh isn't an option, buying frozen is typically just as good.

For red meat and poultry, high-quality means grass-fed if the animal is an herbivore (like a cow, buffalo, or lamb), pasture-raised if the animal is an omnivore (like a pig, turkey, or chicken), or wild if the animal is a game animal, regardless of natural diet (like deer and boar). The meat from these animals tends to be leaner and richer in vitamins and minerals, with healthier fats (most notably a better ratio of omega-3 to omega-6 fats, but also some other health-promoting fats, like conjugated linoleic acid), while never being treated with antibiotics or hormones. For more on meat quality, see Chapter 10.

For seafood, high-quality means wild, caught from the ocean or from unpolluted lakes, rivers, and streams. However, farmed fish is still a great option (and far better than not eating fish at all); it provides high levels of beneficial long-chain omega-3 fatty acids, highly digestible protein, and a plethora of vitamins and minerals that are essential for thyroid and immune function.

For produce, the ideal is to consume fresh, locally grown, organic, and in-season vegetables, fruits, and herbs. If you don't have easy access to farm-fresh produce, there are many delivery options available, including regional services and nationwide services like Farmbox Direct. Whatever produce you can source from local farmers or grow in your backyard will be more nutrient dense than organic produce purchased from a grocery store. Frozen organic vegetables and fruits are the next best thing to fresh, since they are frozen very soon after being harvested and are harvested ripe at the peak of the season. For mushrooms, the ideal is to consume wild mushrooms. For dried herbs and spices, the best choice is organic.

Animal fats should come from grass-fed and pasture-raised animals or wild game. Plant fats like coconut oil and olive oil should be cold pressed and ideally completely unrefined and as fresh as possible. If you're going to splurge on one high-quality ingredient, make it your cooking fat. If you're going to splurge on two high-quality ingredients, make the second one your salad dressing fat.

High-quality foods are more readily available than ever. Major retailers like Costco, Kroger, Sam's Club, Target, Trader Joe's, and Walmart carry awesome options like grass-fed beef, wild-caught seafood, eggs from pastured hens, and organic produce. Eating the best-quality foods you can source is very important, but if you can't afford high-quality ingredients or you just don't have access to them where you live, it's not a nonstarter. Even buying all your food from your regular neighborhood grocery store will have you feeling better when you know how to choose the best options available to you. (See also Chapter 31.)

If budget is an issue, the following lists will help you prioritize which foods are worth spending a little more on and which ones are okay to purchase in the conventionally produced, non-organic varieties.

MEAT AND SEAFOOD PRIORITIES

BEST 

Organ meat from grass-fed and pasture-raised animals: Organ meat is densely packed with just about every vitamin and mineral, and the fat content is also extremely healthy.

Wild-caught fish and shellfish: Wild-caught fatty fish can be found fresh, canned, or frozen. Look for sales in the late summer and early fall.

Grass-fed beef, bison, lamb, venison, and goat: Ground meat is always the cheapest. Some local farmers sell bulk meat at a steep discount.

Wild game: You can buy wild game if you do not hunt.

GOOD

Organic meat and conventionally raised lamb and veal: These animals do spend some time in pasture and eat at least some grass.

Lean cuts of beef: Marbled steaks typically contain ten to fifteen times more omega-6 than omega-3 fatty acids; leaner cuts limit your intake of these omega-6 fats.

Lean pork: Usually, the lighter colored the meat, the lower the fat content.

BETTER

Organ meat from organic and conventionally raised animals: The fat profile is less favorable, but the organs still contain denser nutrition than muscle meat.

Farmed fish and shellfish: Even farmed fish contains extremely beneficial fats and is rich in amino acids, vitamins, and minerals that aren't as easy to get from meat and poultry.

Pasture-raised pork and free-range poultry: Look for meat from animals that are not fed soy.

MODERATE OR AVOID 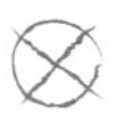

Fatty cuts of conventional beef and pork: Ideally, these cuts would be only an occasional treat.

Conventional chicken and turkey: Conventionally raised chicken can have some of the highest omega-6 levels of any meat.

VEGETABLE AND FRUIT PRIORITIES

BEST 

Wild edibles: Wild varieties of mushrooms, alliums, leafy greens, and berries are some of the most nutrient-dense foods on the planet. Learn which edible plants grow near you so that you can forage (or get to know a local farmer who forages and sells the bounty at a nearby farm stand or farmers market). Be careful of wild mushrooms; misidentifying them can be very dangerous.

Local, organic, in-season fresh produce: Next to wild plants, this is the most nutrient-dense produce you can get. Look for a farmer who is passionate about soil quality.

Homegrown vegetables, fruits, and herbs: Even if your space is limited, many edible plants grow well in flowerpots. You'll notice the savings just from growing fresh herbs.

Organic frozen produce: Picked at the peak of ripeness and frozen soon after harvest, organic frozen produce can be more nutrient dense than fresh.

Organic fresh herbs and spices: Herbs and spices tend to pack quite a nutrient punch. Including more herbs in your cooking, in salads, and even in green smoothies is a great way to increase nutrient density.

BETTER

Local, non-organic, in-season fresh produce: Local, in-season produce is still nutrient dense even if it is not certified organic or naturally grown. Avoid non-organic produce from the Environmental Working Group's Dirty Dozen list (see page 113) unless you can talk to the farmer about pesticide policies. Some farms use pesticides very sparingly, but enough that they are unable to be certified organic. Produce from these farms is usually a good option.

Organic fresh or frozen produce off the Dirty Dozen list: When buying produce off the Dirty Dozen list, buy organic whenever possible, preferably in season (see page 54 and 113).

Conventional fresh or frozen produce off the Clean Fifteen list: When buying off the Clean Fifteen list, conventional produce, preferably in season, is a great option (see page 113).

Organic dried or frozen herbs and spices: While fresh herbs are packed with phytochemicals and flavor, dried organic herbs and spices are still great options. Using frozen herbs is a great way to get the flavor of fresh herbs in your cooking while preserving nutrients. You can freeze your own when herbs are in season (see page 453).

GOOD

All other conventional produce: It's important to eat lots of vegetables, even if your budget or location limits you to conventional store-bought options. Peeling fruits and vegetables is a very good way to limit your exposure to pesticides and produce waxes (some of which contain soy or gluten). If you are limited to conventional produce, choose those on the Dirty Dozen list less often, wash thoroughly, and peel if possible.

Additive-free vegetables and fruits in BPA-free cans: Canning does preserve nutrients, though not as well as freezing. As long as these products don't contain preservatives or other additives, they are good options.

Non-organic herbs and spices: As already mentioned, fresh herbs are nutrient-dense foods. Using frozen herbs is a great way to get the flavor of fresh herbs in your cooking while preserving nutrients. You can freeze your own when herbs are in season. Dried spices are also great options for flavoring foods and are great to include in your diet even if you can't afford or source organic versions.

MODERATE OR AVOID 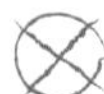

Conventional produce off the Dirty Dozen list: If you do buy conventional produce off the Dirty Dozen list, wash it thoroughly and peel it whenever possible.

Canned vegetables or fruits with preservatives, additives, or added sugars or salts or in BPA-lined cans: Many of the additives and preservatives in canned vegetables and fruits are antinutrients or gut irritants.

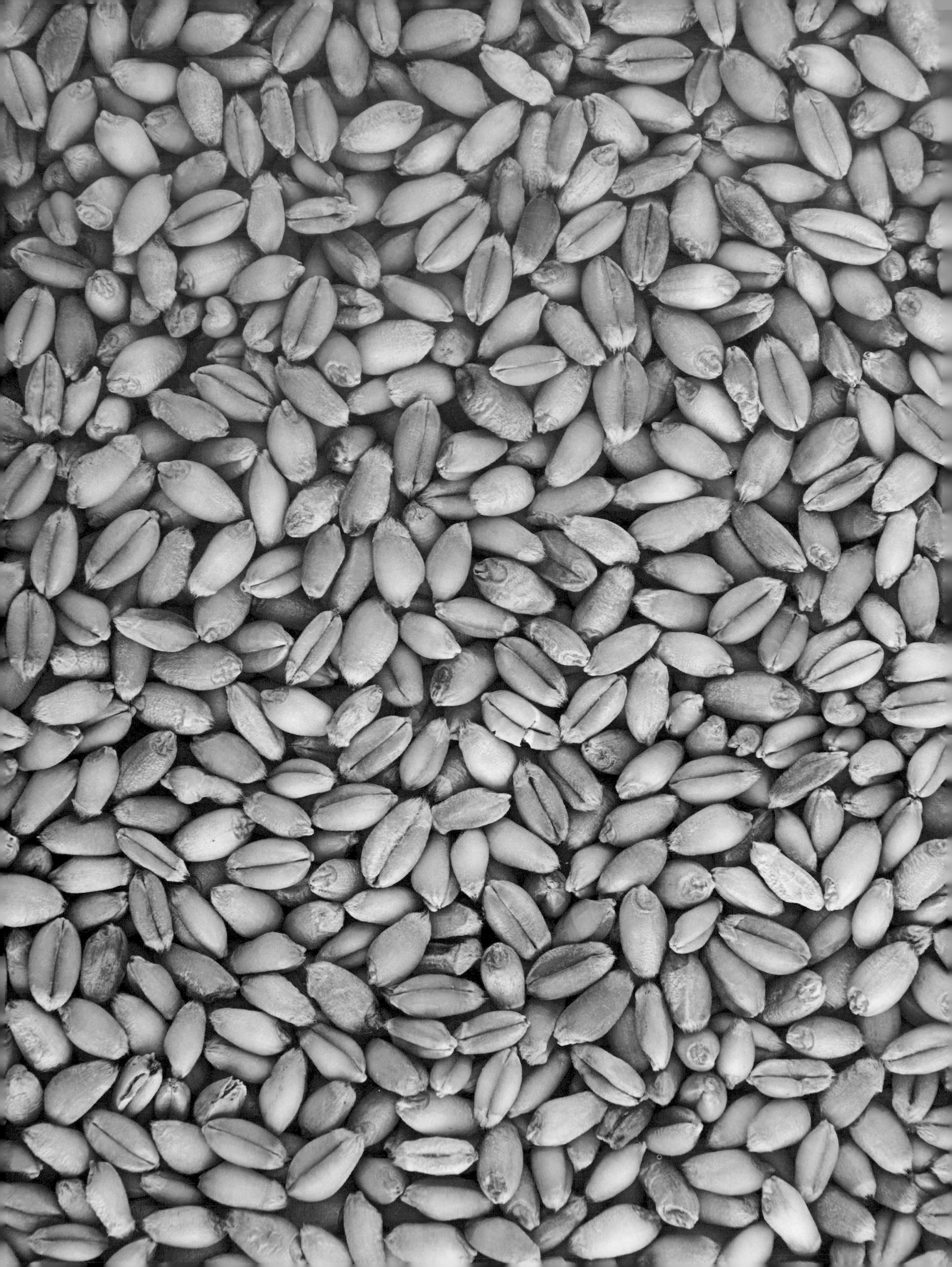

3.

THE SCIENCE BEHIND PALEO ELIMINATIONS: WHAT TO AVOID AND WHY

The word *food* is defined as any nutritive substance that we eat or drink. That means food must provide our bodies with essential nutrients to qualify as food! The sad fact is that grocery store shelves are filled with foodlike substances that provide very little in the way of nutrients but contain compounds that may undermine our health. Of course, you won't be surprised to learn that potato chips, candy bars, and soda fall into this category, but it may come as a bit of a shock to know that many foods marketed as healthy really shouldn't be called food, either. These items provide adequate amounts of only a couple of nutrients while interfering with biological systems health owing to the presence of problematic compounds.

This may be one of the biggest differences between the Paleo diet and other dietary approaches that focus on micronutrient sufficiency. The Paleo diet goes beyond ensuring that our bodies have the resources they need to be healthy and omits problematic foods as well—meaning any food that has the capacity to undermine health by increasing inflammation, damaging the gut, negatively affecting hormones, or causing other problems. A healthy diet isn't just about eating more of the good; it's also about avoiding the bad.

Most of us aren't used to thinking of food in these terms. Certainly, we understand that fast food and junk food might make us gain weight or raise our cholesterol levels, but we don't typically think of them as contributing to our diagnosed health conditions. Type 2 diabetes is likely the only exception: most of us recognize that diabetes is linked to food choices (although we probably fail to see the true extent of that link). The fact is, an alarming number of compounds in common foods are known to negatively impact health. And unfortunately, most diets and nutrition guidelines do not take them into account.

For example, some foods are inherently inflammatory. It's actually quite surprising how many different ways foods can cause inflammation. Processed foods, fast food, foods made with processed "vegetable" oils, grains, and legumes are all high in omega-6 fatty acids, which control cell signaling that turns on inflammation (via the production of specific paracrine and autocrine cell-signaling molecules; see page 158). When the ratio of omega-3 to omega-6 (see page 34) is off-balance—as it often is when we eat these rich sources of omega-6s—omega-3s can't effectively counteract the inflammatory effect of the omega-6s by producing different, less-inflammatory cell-signaling molecules.

In addition, both high blood sugar and high insulin levels propel inflammation, so foods that are high in refined carbohydrates, sugars, and starches that hit the bloodstream quickly (owing to the absence of compounds in those foods that slow the digestion of carbohydrates) are inflammatory. These foods also negatively impact many hormones thanks to all the effects that insulin has in the body (see page 85). Excess refined carbohydrates also negatively impact the hormones leptin and ghrelin, which help control appetite, metabolism, and the immune system (see page 90).

Okay, so there go processed foods, fast food, and junk food. But those foods were already on the blacklist because they don't possess any nutritionally redeeming properties. What's less commonly known is that many foods considered to be healthy, like whole-grain bread and low-fat dairy, also spike blood sugar and insulin levels, and several compounds found in grains (even whole grains), legumes, and nightshades (see pages 296 to 299) are inflammatory. Compounds called *agglutinins* (particularly wheat germ agglutinin, kidney bean lectin, soybean lectin, tomato lectin, and peanut lectin) and *glycoalkaloids* (found in nightshades such as tomatoes, potatoes, eggplants, and peppers) are such potent inducers of inflammation and stimulators of the immune system that several of these compounds have been investigated for use in chemotherapy or in vaccines as adjuvants (chemicals added to vaccines to ramp up the immune system). They're a necessary aspect of how vaccines work, but not a desirable property of food!

This part of the book talks about the manufactured and naturally occurring foods that aren't doing us any favors. These foods are best avoided or consumed only sporadically.

Chapter 17: TOXINS IN FOODS

There are two main elements of healthy eating. The first is nutrient sufficiency, meaning that we consume ample amounts of all the nutrients our bodies need. The second is avoidance of problematic foods, meaning any food that has the capacity to undermine health, whether by increasing inflammation, damaging the gut, negatively affecting hormones, or creating other undesirable effects.

Chapter 5 looked briefly at some of the toxins found in foods and in the environment that the Paleo template strives to reduce or eliminate in order to promote health and healing. Now let's dive in for a more detailed look at the types of problematic compounds in foods and how they can harm us.

ENDOCRINE DISRUPTORS

Endocrine disruptors are chemicals that can interfere with the body's endocrine system (see page 83) in a number of ways, including by mimicking estrogens, androgens, or thyroid hormones; binding to receptors within cells and blocking hormones from binding; and interfering with the way natural hormones and/or hormone receptors are made or controlled (such as in the liver). As a result, these chemicals can cause problems with development, reproduction, neurological health, and the immune system.

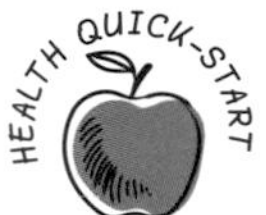

Keep fructose consumption from all sources (vegetables, fruit, and added sugars) below 40 grams per day. See page 269.

The biggest dietary sources of endocrine disruptors are phytoestrogens, including isoflavones (such as genistein and daidzein, found in soy) and lignans (found in flax seeds, chia seeds, sesame seeds, sunflower seeds, whole grains, and other plant foods); for more on estrogen mimics, see page 112. Some grains and legumes like alfalfa sprouts can also be contaminated with fungi that produce mycoestrogens, particularly zearalenone, zearalenol, and zearalanol.

Phytoestrogens

Scientific studies have identified both pros and cons of phytoestrogen consumption. The jury is still out on whether it increases the risk of breast cancer or prevents it, but there appear to be some measurable benefits to bone and cardiovascular health. Phytoestrogens also can mitigate undesirable symptoms of menopause, a main selling point for soy and other phytoestrogen-rich foods. On the con side, a high intake of phytoestrogens can interfere with the ovulatory cycle by suppressing circulating estrogen and progesterone levels and attenuating the pre-ovulatory surge of luteinizing hormone (LH) and follicle-stimulating hormone (FSH). They can negatively impact behavior, including decreasing libido, increasing aggression, and increasing anxiety. High phytoestrogen intake can interfere with oxytocin release in response to estrogen (see page 375). And significant phytoestrogen exposure early in life can lead to many problems, including malformations in the ovary, uterus, and mammary glands or prostate, early puberty, reduced fertility, disrupted brain organization, and reproductive tract cancers.

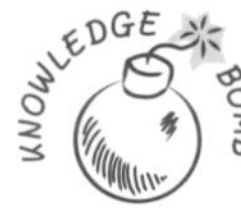

Edamame (raw green soybeans) contains 128.9 milligrams of isoflavones (60.1 milligrams of genistein and 61.7 milligrams of daidzein) per 100 grams. Flax seed contains 305 milligrams of lignans, and chia seed contains 114 milligrams per 100 grams. Of course, many plant foods contain some phytoestrogens, just at much lower levels. For example, broccoli contains 1.3 milligrams of lignans and 0.25 milligrams of isoflavones per 100 grams, levels unlikely to cause problems.

Sugar

Another dietary endocrine disruptor is excess sugar. Sugar disrupts the endocrine system in two different ways: one involving cross-talk between insulin, leptin, and cortisol; and the other involving endotoxin (also called lipopolysaccharide or LPS) and its effects on the hypothalamic-pituitary-adrenal (HPA) axis (see page 340).

Consuming large quantities of refined sugar (a common occurrence on the Standard American Diet) causes abnormal spikes in insulin, beyond what the body is accustomed to handling from natural carbohydrate sources like tubers and fruit. These insulin spikes can subsequently impact leptin and cortisol levels (see pages 90 and 85, respectively), disrupting the body's finely tuned hormonal orchestra. Similarly, a high intake of fructose, a sugar naturally found in fruit, can induce leptin resistance and act as an endocrine disruptor through that pathway.

A high intake of fructose can cause lipopolysaccharide to leak out of the gut into the bloodstream, activating different levels of the HPA axis. Lipopolysaccharide is found in the outer cell membrane of Gram-negative bacteria residing in the gut. When it enters the bloodstream, it triggers the release of inflammatory chemicals (cytokines) from immune cells, which then stimulate corticosteroid-releasing hormone (CRH) production in the hypothalamus and adrenocorticotropic hormone (ACTH) in the pituitary. The ability of fructose to increase intestinal permeability and usher endotoxin into the bloodstream (a finding that's been shown across animal models and in humans) makes it a potent endocrine disruptor when consumed in large quantities (quantities typical in the Standard American Diet).

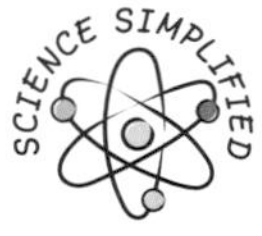

Too much fructose can cause bacterial toxins in the gut to leak into the bloodstream, causing inflammation and triggering a stress response.

GUT IRRITANTS

Gut irritants are substances that cause damage or irritation to the gut. Particularly concentrated in grains and legumes, they exist in a variety of forms within our food supply, including:

- **Digestive enzyme inhibitors:** Substances designed to help seeds escape digestion by blocking the activity of our digestive enzymes that cause gastrointestinal inflammation.
- **Prolamins:** Lectins that aren't fully broken down by digestive enzymes, resulting in prolamin fragments crossing the gut barrier largely intact, damaging the barrier, and causing leaky gut. Gluten is the best-known prolamin.
- **Agglutinins:** Lectins that can interact with the cells that form the gut barrier, increasing intestinal permeability.
- **Phytates and phytic acid:** Substances that can limit the activity of digestive enzymes, including trypsin, pepsin, amylase, and glucosidase. In large quantities, they act similarly to digestive enzyme inhibitors.
- **Carrageenan (derived from seaweed):** A substance that causes gastrointestinal inflammation, ulcerations, and colitis-like disease in animals.
- **Cellulose gum:** A common food additive that causes damage and inflammation in the small intestinal mucus barrier.
- **Capsaicin:** One of the chemicals that gives peppers "heat"; also acts as a gut irritant.
- **Excessive alcohol:** Damages the mucosal lining of the gut.

GUT DYSBIOSIS CONTRIBUTORS

Gut dysbiosis is an imbalance of microbiota in the gastrointestinal tract, with low levels of beneficial bacteria and high levels of pathogenic bacteria (and/or yeasts and parasites), as well as microorganisms growing in the wrong part of the gut (such as small intestinal bacterial overgrowth, or SIBO). A variety of dietary and environmental factors can contribute to gut dysbiosis, including antibiotic exposure, alcohol abuse, excessive exercise, and a number of substances most abundant in grains, pseudograins, legumes, dairy, nuts, seeds, and nightshades (namely agglutinins, prolamins, digestive enzyme inhibitors, saponins such as glycoalkaloids, and phytic acid). In addition, inadequate intake of fiber and omega-3 fats can contribute to gut dysbiosis.

PALEO EASY BUTTON

Because nuts and seeds can be relatively high in phytates and digestive enzyme inhibitors, limit consumption to 1 ounce, or about a palmful, per day. Soaking and sprouting nuts can reduce their phytate content.

Some common emulsifiers, thickeners, and stabilizers (often added to processed and shelf-stable foods) are also known to promote gut dysbiosis. Guar gum has been shown to increase the growth of a toxic strain of *E. coli* in the small intestine. Carrageenan can increase intestinal permeability. Xanthan gum can potentially increase the growth of pathogenic fungi and bacteria. Cellulose gum is known to cause massive bacterial overgrowth, damage to the mucus barrier of the small intestine, and inflammation in the small intestine in animals, all hallmarks of Crohn's disease.

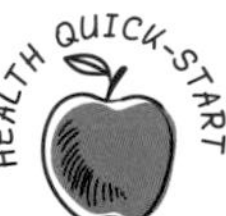

The simple act of eating a diet focused on whole vegetables and fruits and quality meats will eliminate most foods that cause gut dysbiosis while providing the fiber and nutrients that feed a healthy diversity of gut microorganisms.

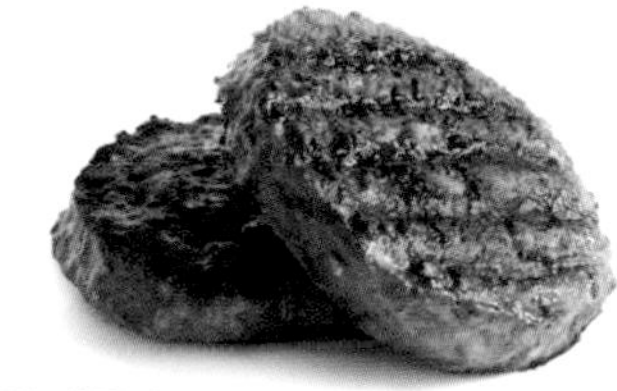

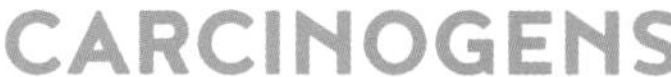

CARCINOGENS

Carcinogens are substances that can cause cancerous changes in living tissue, such as by directly damaging DNA or causing cells to divide faster than normal (increasing the chances of DNA changes). A wide variety of environmental factors can be carcinogenic (such as certain industrial chemicals, cigarette smoke, or excessive UV exposure), but diet can also expose us to carcinogens. Carcinogens in foods and beverages include aflatoxins (which are produced by the mold *Aspergillus flavis*, found most frequently on peanuts and corn, and can cause liver cancer), acetaldehyde from alcoholic beverages, nitrates and nitrites found in deli meats, and dioxins (also found in alcoholic beverages).

The most common dietary carcinogens come from meats cooked at high temperatures. Yes, a juicy steak off the grill tastes amazing, but the molecular effect that this harsh cooking method has on protein-rich animal foods is most certainly not. High heat from grilling and frying can generate compounds called *heterocyclic amines*, or HAs (formed from reactions between amino acids and creatine in muscle meat) and *polycyclic aromatic hydrocarbons*, or PAHs (formed when meat drippings hit the open fire and cause PAH-containing flames to rise up, coating the meat with PAHs). Both compounds are known to be mutagenic, meaning that they cause changes in DNA that may increase the risk of cancer. Plenty of studies point to HAs and PAHs being major players in the cancer correlations we see with meat consumption.

It's important to note that cooking techniques are the problem here: PAHs and HAs don't occur naturally in unprocessed animal foods. To limit the formation of carcinogens in foods, use gentler, lower-temperature cooking methods, such as stewing, poaching, and steaming, rather than high-heat methods like grilling and frying. Also see page 63 for why a high vegetable intake can be protective for those times when you just have to fire up the grill.

ANTINUTRIENTS

Any compound that interferes with the digestion or absorption of nutrients is an antinutrient. Broadly speaking, antinutrients fall into two categories: naturally occurring and synthetic.

The most problematic naturally occurring antinutrients lay the foundation for the elimination of grains and legumes from the Paleo diet. These include:

- **Agglutinins:** A class of problematic lectins in grains and legumes. Wheat germ agglutinin (WGA) is a prime example. Along with being difficult to digest, these proteins are characterized by their ability to induce clumping of red blood cells (called agglutination).

- **Prolamins:** Prolamins are a family of lectins rich in the amino acid proline, and they include gluten. These lectins are abundant in grains, legumes, and pseudograins (see page 242). Prolamins are difficult for human digestive enzymes to break apart, meaning that they are likely to cross the intestinal barrier (either intact or partially digested), as well as disproportionately feeding bacteria in the gut and contributing to gut dysbiosis.

- **Digestive enzyme inhibitors**: Part of a seed's natural defense system. Digestive enzyme inhibitors, found in particularly high concentrations in grains, pseudograins, and legumes, can survive cooking and resist digestion. When consumed, they can cause increased intestinal permeability and gut dysbiosis (along with potentially activating the innate immune system; see page 251).

- **Saponins:** Compounds with detergent-like properties that are often concentrated in seeds, especially legumes, pseudograins, and vegetables from the nightshade family. They're designed to protect plants from being eaten by microbes and insects, and they work by dissolving the cell membranes of potential predators. In humans, saponins can enter the bloodstream (either through a direct influence on intestinal permeability or because of the presence of an already leaky gut) and, when concentrations are high enough, cause hemolysis (the destruction of red blood cell membranes).

- **Glycoalkaloids:** A particularly toxic subset of saponins concentrated in the flowers, fruit, and foliage of nightshade plants. Some of the most well-studied glycoalkaloids include α-solanine and α-chaconine in potatoes, α-solanine in eggplant, and α-tomatine in tomatoes. These lectins can have adjuvant activity, such as α-tomatine stimulating cytotoxic T cells. Glycoalkaloids also inhibit a key enzyme, acetylcholinesterase, which is required to conduct nerve impulses.

However, it isn't necessary to avoid all dietary antinutrients; in fact, many antinutrients have health benefits when consumed in moderate amounts. For example, our gut bacteria can process moderate amounts of phytates and oxalates, liberating the bound minerals and making them available for us to absorb, adding valuable nutrients to our diets. Saponins in the quantities and types found in most fruits and vegetables (excluding nightshades) may aid in nutrient absorption. These dietary antinutrients are typically toxic at very high levels, but consuming toxic quantities is nearly impossible when eating whole Paleo foods. Naturally occurring antinutrients that are okay in moderate amounts include the following:

- **Cyanogenic glycosides:** Hydrogen cyanide, which is highly toxic, is released from cyanogenic glycosides when plants that contain them are chewed and digested (through an enzyme that is also present in the plant). Cassava (also called manioc, yuca, and tapioca and a major ingredient in fufu flour), as well as almonds, bamboo, cashews, chickpeas, corn, lima beans, sorghum, yams (but not sweet potatoes), stone fruits (like peaches and apricots), and fruits from the apple family, are all food sources of cyanogenic glycosides. In most cases, the amounts of these compounds can be greatly reduced by using traditional preparation methods, which involve soaking (often grinding and then soaking) or fermenting followed by thorough cooking. Excess cyanide residue from improper preparation is known to cause acute cyanide intoxication and goiters (because cyanide

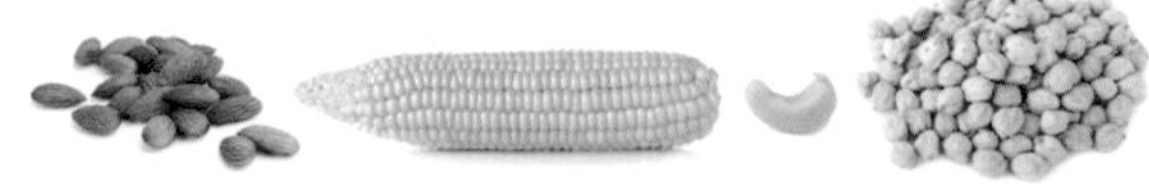

binds to iodine and depletes it from the body—hence cyanide's status as an antinutrient). It has been linked to ataxia, a neurological disorder affecting a person's ability to walk, as well as to tropical calcific pancreatitis, leading to chronic pancreatitis. You can minimize your exposure to cyanogenic glycosides by not eating the pits or seeds of stone fruits and fruits from the apple family, eating only canned bamboo shoots (in BPA-free cans) if you eat bamboo, and properly preparing fresh cassava.

- **Glucosinolates:** Glucosinolates are a class of sulfur-rich compounds found in almost all plants from the *Brassicaceae* family, which includes all cruciferous vegetables (such as broccoli, Brussels sprouts, cabbage, cauliflower, kale, and turnips). Glucosinolates prevent the uptake of iodine by the thyroid, so very high doses (especially in combination with an iodine deficiency) can affect thyroid function (see page 93), thus they are considered goitrogens (substances that suppress thyroid hormone production by inhibiting iodine uptake in the thyroid gland). Diverse health benefits, including cancer prevention, have also been correlated with diets high in glucosinolates. These compounds are discussed in more detail on page 145.

- **Oxalic acid and oxalates:** Oxalic acid and its salts, oxalates, are present in many plants, particularly in members of the spinach family but also in radishes, berries, grains, and legumes. Oxalic acid binds to minerals, most notably calcium (which then forms calcium oxalate), and thus prevents their absorption by the body. Because the most common type of kidney stone is composed largely of calcium oxalate, avoiding foods containing oxalates or oxalic acid is traditionally recommended for kidney stone sufferers (and gallstone sufferers as well). However, this recommendation is not supported by the scientific literature, which shows that increasing consumption of oxalate-rich foods actually *hinders* the formation of kidney stones. See also page 416.

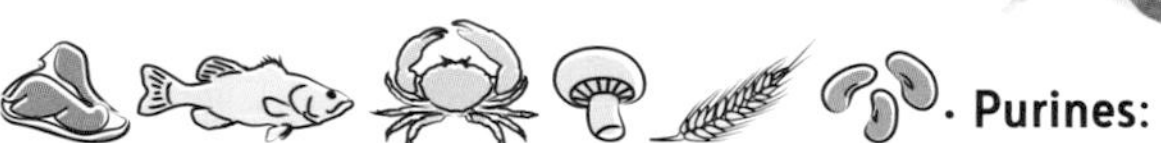

- **Purines:** Purines are uricogenic nucleic acids—that is, nucleic acids (components of DNA and RNA) that elevate uric acid levels in the blood. Purines are considered antinutrients because they bind to iron. High-purine foods include meat, fish, shellfish, asparagus, cauliflower, spinach, mushrooms, grains, and legumes. Low-purine diets have traditionally been recommended for those with gout and hyperuricaemia (high blood levels of uric acid); however, more recent research shows that refined sugar, and especially fructose, is the more likely culprit. It is clearly more complicated than "fructose causes gout," which is not the case: obesity and alcohol consumption are the dominant risk factors in gout. But consumption of vegetables high in purines is known to decrease the risk of gout, and so is the consumption of red meat. Regulating blood sugar is by far the most important aspect of gout management. See also page 271.

- **Phytic acid and phytates:** All seeds (and other plant parts as well, though in much smaller quantities) contain antinutrients called phytates. Phytates are the salts of phytic acid—that is, phytic acid bound to minerals—typically calcium, magnesium, iron, potassium, and zinc. Within the seed, the primary function of phytic acid is to store phosphorus, but it also serves as an energy store, as a source of cations (positive ions) for various chemical reactions in the plant, and as a source of a cell wall precursor called myoinositol. Because phytates are formed when phytic acid binds to minerals, these minerals are then unavailable to be absorbed by the gut. Therefore, consuming phytate-rich foods like grains and legumes can cause mineral deficiencies, especially when these phytate-rich foods displace other mineral-rich foods in the diet. See page 254.

- **Tannins:** Tannins are water-soluble polyphenolic compounds found in grains, legumes, green and black tea, wine, smoked foods, nuts, and some types of fruit (most notably grapes and berries). Tannins are known antimicrobial compounds and have been linked to some health benefits, most likely because of their powerful antioxidant properties. However, tannins can bind to and precipitate proteins (so the proteins clump together and are no longer water-soluble) and therefore can reduce amino acid digestibility. It appears that tannins interact primarily with proline-rich proteins (like lectins), so these compounds are another factor that hinders the digestion of grains and legumes.

In contrast to naturally occurring antinutrients, antinutrients that arise from the processing of foods or that are added to processed foods are generally harmful. The following are just a few of the antinutrients found in processed foods:

- **D-amino acids and lysinoalanine:** Exposing food proteins to heat or alkaline treatments, as is common in the production of many processed foods, results in two major chemical changes: the concurrent formation of D-amino acids (which are essentially mirror images of the normal L-amino acids found in food and in our bodies, and which are generally not usable by our bodies) and lysinoalanine (LAL). These compounds are found in high levels in pasteurized dairy products, mature cheeses, products made with wheat flour and corn (such as crackers and corn tortillas), textured soy protein, powdered egg whites, and cured bacon. D-amino acids and LAL are considered antinutrients because they impair protein digestibility. LAL is also a strong chelator of (meaning it binds to) minerals, including calcium, copper, iron, and zinc, and therefore reduces the absorption of these minerals.
- **Oxidized sulfur amino acids:** The sulfur-containing amino acids methionine and cysteine are essential for life. However, they may become oxidized during heat and alkaline food processing (treating foods with a high-pH chemical during processing or processing a food with a naturally high pH), rendering them nutritionally unavailable (or reducing their bioavailability). These compounds are commonly found in pasteurized and heat-processed foods, such as dairy, powdered egg whites, soy products, and cornmeal.
- **Emulsifiers, thickeners, and stabilizers:** This category includes a vast variety of food additives, including xanthan gum, guar gum, carrageenan, cellulose gum, and lecithin. These difficult-to-digest polysaccharides are used to emulsify (make fat and water mix) and typically to thicken as well. They are derived from a variety of sources: guar gum comes from guar beans; carrageenan is a derivative of red seaweed; xanthan gum is secreted by a specific bacteria; and lecithin is typically isolated from soy but may be isolated from eggs or sunflower seeds. These chemicals are considered antinutrients because they reduce the absorbability of dietary minerals, such as calcium. Furthermore, concerns have been raised over the safety of some emulsifiers. For example, carrageenan has been shown to cause gastrointestinal inflammation, ulcerations, and colitis-like disease in animals. Both carrageenan and guar gum have been shown to increase intestinal permeability. Xanthan gum (commonly contaminated with gluten because the bacteria are grown in a medium that frequently contains wheat, corn, or soy) is a highly efficient laxative and can cause intestinal bloating and diarrhea. Cellulose gum (more technically carboxymethylcellulose) is known to cause massive bacterial overgrowth and inflammation in the small intestine in animals. Gut microbiota metabolites of lecithin have been linked to increased risk of cardiovascular disease and atherosclerosis, probably by promoting inflammation. These are discussed in more detail starting on page 235.
- **Maillard reaction products:** The Maillard reaction is a chemical reaction that occurs when foods undergo thermal processing, like pasteurization, browning, searing, or frying. The chemical reactions that take place when food is browned are complicated, and the Maillard reaction is just one type. (For example, caramelization, which looks and tastes similar, is a different process.) The Maillard reaction, which happens in stages, essentially occurs when certain sugars react with the amino acid lysine to modify the lysine into a biologically unavailable form. Some Maillard reaction products (various stages of the modification of lysine) have powerful antioxidant and cancer-preventing properties, while others (by promoting glycation reactions) have been associated with increased risk of disease, including cardiovascular disease and Alzheimer's. They are broadly considered antinutrients because some Maillard reaction products reduce the digestibility of proteins (which is an argument against eating deep-fried foods). In terms of reducing protein digestibility, one of the most affected proteins is pasteurized dairy protein (another argument against consuming pasteurized dairy). The Maillard reaction is a step in the formation of advanced glycation end-products.

Chapter 18: THE BIGGEST CULPRIT: REFINED AND MANUFACTURED FOODS

When we look at diets that have a track record of improving people's health in clinical trials (such as the Paleo diet or the Mediterranean diet) or for supporting healthy communities for many generations (such as the Okinawan diet; see page 134), there's always one common denominator. Ditching the junk food is what all healthy diet templates have in common. And while the Paleo template incorporates a bigger focus on nutrient density as well as lifestyle factors, simply focusing on whole foods and keeping micronutrients in mind (see page 24) are the two most important steps most people can make to improve their health.

Current estimates are that upwards of 70 percent of the calories consumed by the average American comes from processed, refined, and manufactured foods. That means the average American gets only 30 percent of calories from real, whole foods. What's more, 57 percent of calories come from *ultra*-processed foods, defined in a paper published in *BMJ Open* as "formulations of several ingredients which, besides salt, sugar, oils, and fats, include food substances not used in culinary preparations, in particular, flavors, colors, sweeteners, emulsifiers and other additives used to imitate sensorial qualities of unprocessed or minimally processed foods and their culinary preparations or to disguise undesirable qualities of the final product." Gross!

Processed and manufactured foods cause problems in two ways:

1) through direct damage to the endocrine system, cardiovascular system, immune system, digestive system, and other body systems, and

2) by displacing more-nutritious foods and lowering the overall nutrient density of our diet.

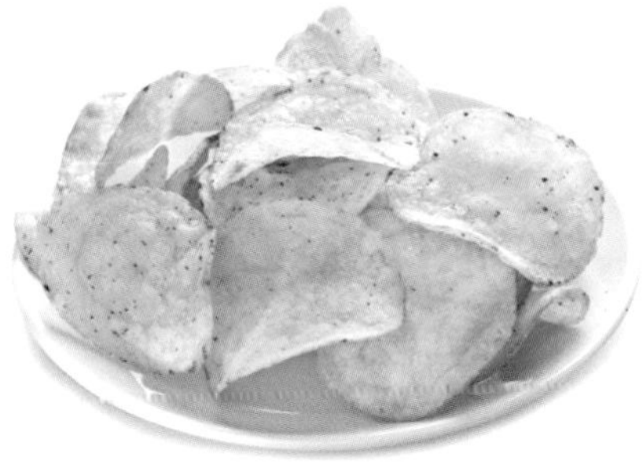

DIRECT DAMAGE TO THE BODY

When we consume processed and manufactured foods (such as potato chips fried in vegetable oil, meals from fast-food restaurants, snacks from vending machines, microwave dinners, commercial breakfast cereals, and candy), we're usually ingesting some of the most harmful ingredients in the modern food supply. These include refined grains, high-fructose corn syrup (or other empty-calorie sweeteners), vegetable oils prone to molecular damage and oxidation, excessive sodium, and additives and dyes. So how can these ingredients cause damage? Here's a quick rundown:

- **Refined carbohydrates:** Consuming large quantities of low-fiber, fast-digesting carbohydrates (namely refined grains and sweeteners) interferes with blood sugar regulation and satiety signaling, causing blood glucose and insulin spikes and often encouraging overeating (see page 241 for more on grains and page 266 for more on sweeteners). Along with taxing the endocrine system, these foods can feed the wrong bacteria in the gut and have a negative effect on the immune system. Refined wheat flour (often one of the first ingredients in processed foods) has the added problem of negatively affecting the gut and immune system due to the effects of gluten and wheat germ agglutinin (see Chapter 19).

- **Damaged fats:** The types of fats used in manufactured foods are generally cheap vegetable oils, rich in omega-6 fats and highly prone to oxidation. These fats can become damaged before consumption (from exposure to air, heat, or light) or after they're inside our bodies, digested, and incorporated into cells (when cell membranes have a higher proportion of polyunsaturated fats from our diet, they're more susceptible to free radical attack and damage within the body). Regardless of how they become damaged, the fats in processed foods can harm the cardiovascular system and even increase the risk of cancer. See Chapter 20 for more on these unhealthy fats.

- **Excessive salt:** In normal quantities, there's nothing wrong with salt. In fact, sodium is an essential nutrient, and high-quality salts provide other trace minerals that can benefit our health (see page 198). However, processed foods tend to be extremely high in sodium chloride (table salt) without providing enough potassium to maintain an optimal ratio of electrolytes, leading to micronutrient imbalances that can impair fluid regulation and kidney function.

- **Additives and dyes:** The list of potential additives and dyes in processed foods is vast, but in short, this class of ingredients is known to cause a number of short-term and long-term health problems. These include contributing to gut dysbiosis and leaky gut and increasing the risk of hyperactivity and cancer (particularly with certain food dyes). These additives and dyes are discussed next.

What's more, combinations of these ingredients (refined carbs, refined fats, and excessive salt) tend to be "hyperpalatable," triggering reward centers in the brain and compelling us to eat more than our bodies need. Some research suggests these ingredient combinations affect the brain in ways that resemble addiction. As a consequence, manufactured foods are a major culprit behind weight gain and the obesity epidemic, providing excess energy without satiation.

KNOWLEDGE BOMB *Monosodium glutamate (MSG) is a flavor enhancer used in many packaged goods (especially canned soups and processed meats), fast foods, and some restaurant foods (like Chinese). Researchers have yet to identify a mechanism underlying MSG reactions—sufferers report a wide range of symptoms, including flushing, headaches, hives, fatigue, chest pain, numbness or tingling, nausea, and feeling weak—and double-blind studies in patients with self-reported sensitivity to MSG show very inconsistent results. Even if MSG sensitivity remains hypothetical, there are some compelling reasons to ban this chemical from your life. One recent study linked MSG with obesity; MSG decreases secretion of glucagon-like peptide-1 (GLP-1; see page 89) and is toxic to enteroendocrine cells (the cells in the gut responsible for secreting hormones that regulate digestion, metabolism, and hunger signals), even at levels that are easy to get from diet. Mice that are injected with MSG develop obesity and endocrinological dysfunction—including effects on sex hormones, metabolic hormones, and cortisol—attributable to MSG's effects on the hypothalamus region of the brain.*

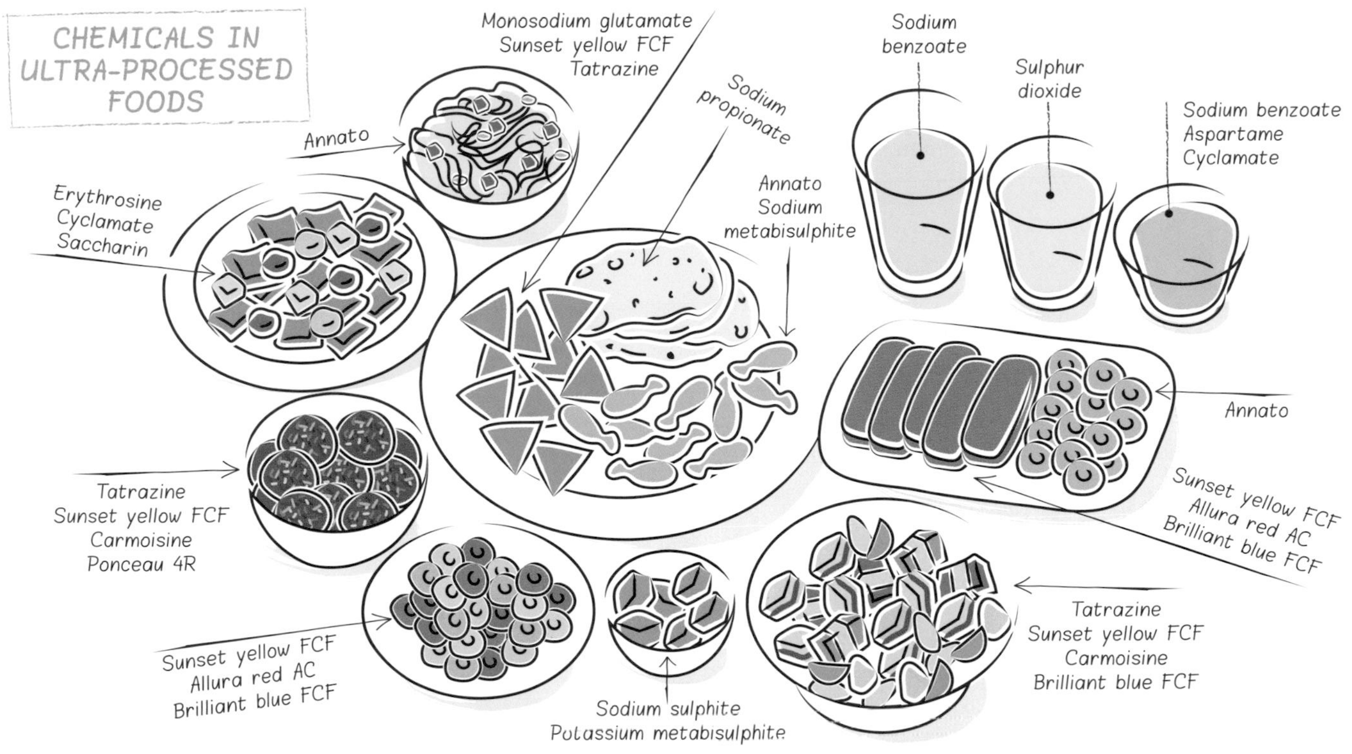

EMULSIFIERS, THICKENERS, AND STABILIZERS: WHAT ARE THEY?

This category of food additives includes a vast variety of ingredients. Some of the most common are xanthan gum, guar gum, cellulose gum, carrageenan, and lecithin. They all share the properties of emulsifying, thickening, and stabilizing, which is why they are considered a single category of food additives. I'll refer to them collectively as emulsifiers, since emulsifying (making fat and water mix) is their primary property. As secondary properties, they typically thicken and act as stabilizers and binders. Which additive is chosen for a particular purpose depends on the exact chemistry of that additive and the desired effect in the food product to which it's being added.

Let's look into these chemicals and ingredients in detail, in part to emphasize the scourge that is processed and manufactured foods but also because some of them are finding their way into packaged goods catering to the Paleo community—and that's not a good thing!

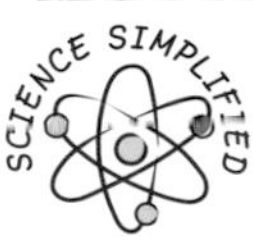

There just aren't any good choices when it comes to additives, although lecithin may be okay. Avoid ingredients with the word gum in the name, along with carrageenan.

Xanthan gum, guar gum, cellulose gum, carrageenan, lecithin, and other members of this food additive category are polysaccharides, or complex sugar molecules. They are all difficult to digest (which technically makes them types of fiber), and they have detergent-like properties, meaning that they are used to emulsify. The term "detergent-like" shouldn't be categorically scary, though. Simply being an emulsifier isn't the problem; mustard seeds and egg yolks are also emulsifiers. But there's a big difference between whole foods that contain nutrients and these manufactured food additives.

These emulsifiers are derived from a variety of sources:

- **Guar gum** comes from guar beans (yes, a legume). The guar beans are split and husked, and then the endosperm is milled and screened to obtain the gum. The by-products of this manufacturing process are turned into animal feed for Concentrated Animal Feedlot Operations (CAFO).
- **Carrageenan** is derived from edible red seaweed. The seaweed is dried, ground, sifted, and then washed prior to being chemically treated with a hot alkali solution

(typically potassium hydroxide, also known as caustic potash, which is used to make batteries and biodiesel as well!). The carrageenan is separated out by centrifugation and filtration and then dehydrated back into a powder.

- **Xanthan gum** is secreted by a specific bacteria called *Xanthomonas campestris*, which causes a variety of plant diseases, such as leaf spot. This bacteria is grown in a liquid containing glucose, sucrose, and/or lactose (typically derived from wheat, corn, soy, and/or dairy). After the bacteria ferments the sugar, the xanthan gum is extracted by precipitation from the liquid (the growth medium) using isopropyl alcohol. It's then dried and ground into a fine powder.

- **Cellulose gum** (more technically called carboxymethyl cellulose) is extracted from wood pulp and cotton cellulose. The cellulose is chemically modified to make it water-soluble, by treating it with sodium hydroxide (also called caustic soda, or lye, which is used to make soap and detergents) and then with chloroacetic acid. (Not-so-fun fact: Exposure to chloroacetic acid can be fatal if more than 6 percent of a person's body surface area is exposed.) Impurities are then removed with an aqueous solvent.

- **Lecithin** is a by-product of soybean oil production, but it can also be derived from eggs, canola seeds, or sunflower seeds. During soybean oil production, oilseeds are screw-pressed and solvent extracted to obtain crude oil, but this creates a gummy deposit that can coat the machinery. The degumming process was invented to render these gums insoluble so that they could be separated by centrifugation. Originally considered a waste product, this gummy stuff is now additionally processed to make lecithin. In addition to polysaccharides, lecithin contains phospholipids and glycolipids, triglycerides, sterols, free fatty acids, and carotenoids.

Knowing how these food additives are manufactured is probably enough to make most people wary of consuming them. None of these emulsifiers can be considered a whole food, and none would have been found in the diets of our Paleolithic ancestors (whole seaweed, *yes*; seaweed treated with the goo found inside alkaline batteries, *no*). But that fact alone isn't enough to exclude a food from our diet. It's important to look at the contemporary biology and ask how these additives affect health.

Concerns over the safety of some emulsifiers have been raised in the medical literature, with some scientists calling for their banishment from the food supply. In fact, some of these food additives are banned, at least for specific uses, in other countries. For example, the use of carrageenan in infant formulas is banned in the European Union.

- **Guar gum** has been shown to increase intestinal permeability (at least in rats), although the mechanism has not been studied. Guar gum has also been shown to increase the growth rate of a toxic strain of *E. coli* in the small intestine. In piglets fed a diet containing added guar gum, this overgrowth of *E. coli* led to increased large intestine weight and overall stunted growth. Another study showed that adding guar gum to milk increased the survival rate of pathogenic bacteria in milk through high-heat pasteurization. It remains unknown whether guar gum can increase the survival of pathogens in the digestive tract, but the increased growth rate of enterotoxigenic *E. coli* suggests that it can.

- **Carrageenan** increases intestinal permeability. In fact, extensive research has shown that carrageenan causes gastrointestinal inflammation, ulcerations, and colitis-like disease in animals. Furthermore, the products of carrageenan degradation through normal digestion are known carcinogens. Carrageenan is actually used to cause cancer in animal models of various tumor types. There is so much evidence demonstrating that carrageenan is unsafe for consumption that many researchers are blowing the whistle on it.

- **Xanthan gum** is a highly efficient laxative and can cause intestinal bloating and diarrhea. It was found to be the culprit behind an increased rate of necrotizing enterocolitis in infants after it was introduced to formula (the FDA has since banned its use in formula). While direct effects on intestinal permeability have not been studied, xanthan gum has been shown to be one of the best choices for growing fungi and bacteria in petri dishes in laboratory environments. Added bonus: Xanthan gum is commonly contaminated with gluten because the bacteria are grown in a medium that frequently contains wheat, corn, or soy.

- **Cellulose gum** is known to cause massive bacterial overgrowth, damage to the mucus barrier of the small intestine, and inflammation in the small intestine in animals, all of which are hallmarks of Crohn's disease. Here's a quote from a 2009 paper in the journal *Inflammatory Bowel Diseases:* "[carboxymethyl cellulose] is an ideal suspect to account for the rise of IBD in the twentieth century."

Lecithin is the only emulsifier on this list that is not a major gut irritant or contributor to gut dysbiosis, but that doesn't mean lecithin is off the hook! TMAO, a gut microbiota metabolite of lecithin, has been strongly linked to increased risk of cardiovascular disease and atherosclerosis, probably by promoting inflammation (see page 64). How diet might affect this risk by influencing the type of bacteria growing in the gut remains unknown.

PALEO EASY BUTTON *Read labels! Just because a product's label says Paleo doesn't mean that it's made with healthful ingredients. Just like the word natural, the use of the term Paleo on product labels is not regulated (with the exception of the "Paleo Approved" certification). And as more and more companies want to get in on the Paleo community market share, there are more and more examples of products made with non-Paleo ingredients being marketed toward Paleo peeps. Your only defense is to educate yourself and be a smart shopper!*

Plus, all these emulsifiers are considered antinutrients because they reduce the absorbability of dietary minerals, such as calcium.

A few of these emulsifiers have found uses in the medical industry. For example, cellulose gum is a major component of an adhesion barrier called Seprafilm that is used in abdominal surgeries to prevent postoperative adhesions. (It also appears to cause cell damage.) Xanthan gum and guar gum have been shown to have utility in the creation of ophthalmic liquids for drug delivery (prescription eye drops). Several emulsifiers have been investigated as diet aids; because they expand so prodigiously in the bowel, they create a feeling of fullness that may encourage people to eat less.

Lecithin is the only emulsifier shown to have any properties that might be considered beneficial. It lowers blood cholesterol. However, it does so by interfering with enterohepatic circulation, which is ultimately undesirable since it also interferes with fat-soluble vitamin absorption and the normal recycling of bile salts. Because of lecithin's ability to bind with cholesterol, it has been investigated as a supplement to help dissolve gallstones. Between two studies, only one patient experienced a reduction in gallstone size, which is pretty underwhelming evidence for a beneficial effect. Lecithin is also being investigated as a therapy for ulcerative colitis (efficacy has not yet been determined, but a phase two clinical trial is underway), so there's a glimmer of hope.

Ultimately, when it comes to their effect on our health, there's a long list of cons to these additives—and few, if any, pros.

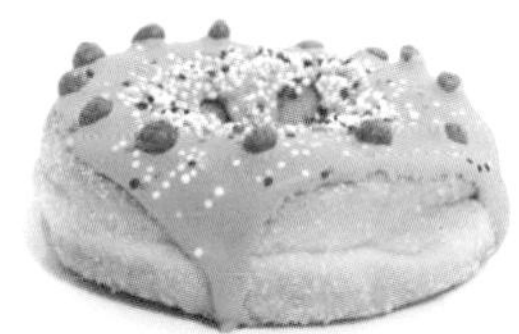

FOOD DYES

What do cupcake sprinkles, movie theater popcorn, and bright orange macaroni and cheese have in common? Food dyes! While some manufacturers are moving toward natural food dyes to meet consumer demand, synthetic and artificial food dyes are still found in thousands of products on grocery store shelves. Some food dye-laden foods are obvious, like breakfast cereals, candy, snacks, beverages, vitamins, and other colorful products marketed to children. Others are less obvious, like some canned soups, flavored yogurts, and pickles; even some oranges are dipped in dye to brighten them.

Synthetic food dyes are derived from petroleum, and food manufacturers (and even some chefs) use them to alter or enhance the color of foods. On ingredient labels, these dyes have names like Red 40, Yellow 5, Blue 1, and sometimes just "artificial color." (Keep in mind that synthetic food dyes are different from natural food pigments, like beet extract and grape skin extract, which can also be used to color foods.)

Synthetic food dyes are often lumped in with other artificial additives as ingredients to avoid when eating Paleo. But why exactly are they harmful? Dyes are definitely worth a closer look so that we can understand exactly how they affect our health and why they're excluded from the Paleo framework based on the scientific literature.

Over the years, the FDA has banned the use of many dyes due to evidence of harm. But nine artificial dyes are still approved for use in food—Blue 1, Blue

2, Citrus Red 2, Green 3, Orange B, Red 3, Red 40, Yellow 5, and Yellow 6—and there's a great deal of concern about whether these dyes are truly safe.

As with any ingredient, it's hard to study the long-term effects of synthetic food dyes in humans, since we can't create rigorous, controlled studies that last for years and years. But multiple lines of evidence suggest that even the FDA-approved dyes are bad news. In rodent studies, a number of artificial dyes have been shown to induce malignant cell transformation, increase tumor incidence, damage DNA in the stomach and colon, and increase total mortality (depending on the dye and the species and strain of rodent). One study found that the soaking liquid from commercial red ginger pickles induced DNA damage in the rodent colon, glandular stomach, and bladder. Blue 2 has resulted in a statistically significant increase in brain gliomas (a type of tumor) in male rats, and Red 3 has been shown to act as a thyroid carcinogen. And for Red 2, Red 40, and Yellow 5, DNA damage in mouse gastrointestinal organs happens even at low doses close to the acceptable daily intake.

When we look at the molecular properties of artificial dyes, it's not hard to see why they could contribute to cancer in mammals. Some of the most widely used food dyes—particularly Red 40, Yellow 5, and Yellow 6, which make up 90 percent of the dyes used in foods in the U.S.—contain benzidine, a chemical carcinogen that doesn't occur in nature. Although the FDA tests for levels of free benzidine in food dyes and factors those into safety assessments, bound benzidine (which can be released by our intestinal enzymes and contribute to our total exposure) isn't documented. So consuming certain dyes may result in higher exposures to this carcinogen than generally believed! That means the FDA's acceptable daily intake levels (which are based on intakes at which no adverse effects are observed) could be higher than they should be for certain food dyes—in other words, even lower levels could be harmful.

In 2010, the Center for Science in the Public Interest (CSPI) published a report called "Food Dyes: A Rainbow of Risks" that questioned the safety of dyes still approved for human consumption. The report noted that along with seven of the FDA-approved dyes contributing to cancer in lab animals, four dyes are linked to uncommon but severe allergic reactions. Yellow 5 has been shown to exacerbate asthma in certain people (especially those with cross-sensitivity to aspirin), and some studies suggest that dyes may contribute to behavioral problems, including impaired performance in hyperactive children, increases in aversive behavior, ADHD, restlessness, and sleep disturbance.

Likewise, many of the existing safety studies on food dyes suffer from design flaws, including rodent studies lasting only 2 years and therefore missing the diet-related cancers that don't show up until their third year of life; studies using relatively few animals; and lack of testing of combinations of food dyes versus individual dyes, since mixing them could compound certain adverse effects. And the FDA doesn't currently require food dyes to be tested for developmental neurotoxicity, so their safety for growing children is a question mark. In other words, existing studies on food dyes aren't strong enough to confirm their safety—especially in light of their known carcinogenic properties and potential neurological effects!

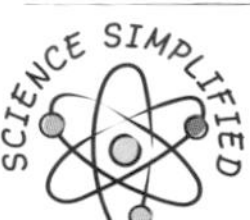

Artificial food dyes are not healthy! In fact, many of them are linked to health problems, including behavioral problems in kids. Why do we need to color our foods, anyway?

Considering the levels of artificial dyes that many people ingest, all of the above should be major concerns. Due to the increase in processed foods in the Western diet over the decades, our intake of food dyes is now *five times* as high as it was 60 years ago. Manufacturers put over 15 million pounds of artificial dyes into the U.S. food supply each year! And sometimes those dyes end up in less-than-obvious places—like in sausage coatings and orange peels, which are sometimes colored with Citrus Red No. 2. (By contrast, many other countries use plant-based colorings instead of artificial petroleum-based dyes. For example, in Britain, McDonald's strawberry sundaes are colored with real strawberries, while the same item in the U.S. uses Red 40. And in Europe, most foods with artificial dyes are required to carry a warning label saying that the dye "may have effects on activity and attention in children.")

Considering that artificial food dyes contribute no nutrition to our diets and are totally unnecessary for health, there's really no reason to consume them. But is there anything we can do if we want to color foods in a Paleo-friendly way? Fortunately, there is! Natural (non-petroleum-based) food colorings are available: beet juice can impart a red or pink color, cacao powder can tint foods brown, and various spices can act as food colorings, without any of the risks associated with artificial dyes.

PRESERVATIVES

A number of health concerns surround the chemicals commonly added to manufactured and processed foods to increase their shelf life. Preserved foods in general increase the risk of some cancers. Excessive nitrites (commonly added to processed meats) are linked to higher rates of cancer due to their ability to react with secondary amines and form nitrosamines—although the nitrates that occur naturally in foods like vegetables appear to be fine (due to the antioxidants these foods naturally contain, which prohibit nitrosamine formation). Sodium benzoate, a microbial agent commonly used in soft drinks, has been shown to increase hyperactivity in children and forms a carcinogen, benzene, when it combines with vitamin C. Phosphates (used as preservatives in meats, dairy, and seafood and as flavoring agents, acidifying agents, and emulsifiers in processed foods) are linked to kidney disease.

Sulfites are another problematic class of preservatives. These are widely used to prevent discoloration or browning of foods through preparation, storage, and distribution. Sulfites include sodium sulfite, sodium bisulfite, sodium metabisulfite, potassium sulfite, potassium bisulfite, potassium metabisulfite, and sulfur dioxide. Although sulfites have been used in traditional winemaking for centuries, cases of severe reactions started increasing dramatically when these preservatives gained popularity with the food and beverage industries in the 1970s and 1980s. Eventually, the FDA prohibited their use on fresh fruits and vegetables (sulfites were used to keep the produce looking fresh), but sulfites continue to be used routinely on fresh potatoes and some shrimp, in beer and wine, and in many processed and packaged foods.

Sulfites are implicated in asthma symptoms that range from mild wheezing to potentially life-threatening reactions. While breathing difficulties are the most common symptom, other possible symptoms include atopic dermatitis (eczema), hives, flushing, hypotension (low blood pressure), abdominal pain, diarrhea, and anaphylaxis. While some people react to sulfites when tested for allergies, sulfite sensitivity reactions are generally not mediated through IgE antibody production. A test called an oral metabisulfite challenge may be performed, in which lung function is monitored while the patient is given increasing doses of metabisulfite. Elimination diets may also be used to diagnose sulfite sensitivity.

The precise mechanisms of sulfite sensitivity remain unknown. However, sulfites have been shown to impact the immune system, which may be the cause of both asthmatic and allergy-like symptoms. In particular, when studied in cell-culture systems, sulfites suppress some aspects of the adaptive immune system (Th1). While this hasn't been tested in humans, it is believed to lead to exaggerated responses by other aspects of the adaptive immune system (Th2). This combination of immune effects causes an increased likelihood of allergic and immune responses to allergens, thereby increasing susceptibility to immune diseases, such as allergies, asthma, and eczema.

In most countries, sulfites must be labeled if they are added to foods as preservatives but not necessarily if they are used in food processing but not explicitly for food preservation. Foods that may contain significant quantities of sulfites include:

- **Alcoholic and nonalcoholic cider**
- **Bottled lemon and lime juices and concentrates**
- **Canned and frozen fruits and vegetables**
- **Condiments (such as horseradish, pasteurized pickles, and pasteurized sauerkraut)**
- **Deli meats, hot dogs, and sausages**
- **Dried fruits and vegetables (for example, apricots, coconut, raisins, and sweet potatoes)**
- **Dried herbs, spices, and teas**
- **Fish and shellfish**
- **Fruit and vegetable juices**
- **Gelatin**
- **Guacamole**
- **Jams, jellies, preserves, and marmalade**
- **Molasses**
- **Vinegar and wine vinegar**
- **Wine and sparkling wine**

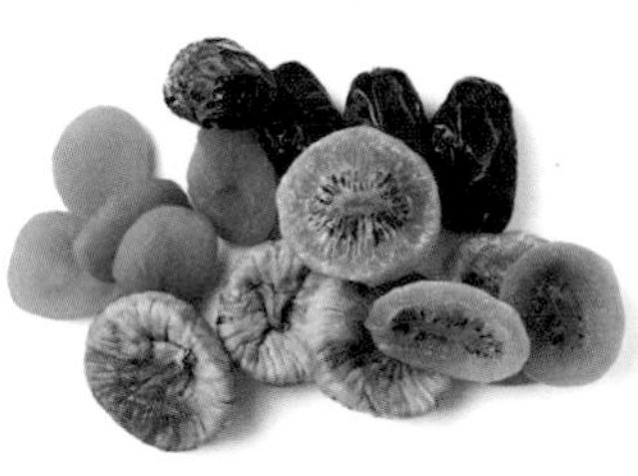

Sensitivities to various other preservatives are common as well. While studies specifically evaluating their effects on existing health conditions (such as autoimmune diseases) have not been performed, there is enough information in the scientific literature to suggest that avoiding foods that contain these additives is a good idea.

PROCESSED FOOD CHEMICALS AND INGREDIENTS

By purchasing whole vegetables and fruits, quality meats and seafood, eggs, nuts, seeds, healthy fats, and herbs and spices, you naturally avoid processed food chemicals and ingredients. But even the most devout Paleo enthusiast still buys some packaged goods. So it's best to be able to identify undesirable ingredients on food labels so that we can avoid them.

THESE INGREDIENTS ARE ALL BEST AVOIDED: ACRYLAMIDES; ARTIFICIAL FOOD COLOR; ARTIFICIAL AND NATURAL FLAVORS; AUTOLYZED PROTEIN; BROMINATED VEGETABLE OIL; EMULSIFIERS (CARRAGEENAN, CELLULOSE GUM, GUAR GUM, LECITHIN, XANTHAN GUM); HYDROLYZED VEGETABLE PROTEIN; MONOSODIUM GLUTAMATE; NITRATES OR NITRITES (NATURALLY OCCURRING ARE OKAY); OLESTRA; PHOSPHORIC ACID; PROPYLENE GLYCOL; TEXTURED VEGETABLE PROTEIN; TRANS FATS (PARTIALLY HYDROGENATED VEGETABLE OIL, HYDROGENATED OIL); YEAST EXTRACT

\+ ANY INGREDIENT WITH A CHEMICAL NAME THAT YOU DON'T RECOGNIZE (but see page 285 for ingredients that sound scary but aren't)

HIGH IN ENERGY, LOW IN NUTRITION

The importance of nutrient density is discussed in Chapter 1, but this concept is worth revisiting in order to understand the damage caused by manufactured foods. Every bite of energy-rich, low-micronutrient processed foods displaces the green leafy vegetables, seafood, organ meats, fruit, nuts, seeds, sea vegetables, and other delicious nutrient-dense foods that *could* be taking up space on our plates. A diet based on processed foods stands an extremely low chance of meeting our micronutrient needs. Considering the prevalence of vitamin and mineral deficiencies in developed countries like the United States, this should set off some serious alarm bells!

Hundreds of thousands (and in some cases, literally millions) of Americans fail to consume adequate levels of vital nutrients like vitamin E, magnesium, calcium, vitamin D, vitamin A, vitamin C, vitamin B6, vitamin B9, and zinc. These deficiencies can impair immune function and increase our susceptibility to a wide range of both chronic and acute illnesses. Even without considering the direct harm caused by common ingredients in processed foods, the fact that these items push aside nutrient-dense foods is concerning.

The food we eat is one of many factors that affect our health, but it permeates every aspect of health. Our bodies simply cannot function efficiently and effectively without all the nutrients our systems need to form tissues and do their jobs, and the only way to get all those nutrients is to choose micronutrient-dense foods. Neither can we be healthy if the foods we eat cause inflammation, disrupt our hormones, or damage our guts. It's preposterous that we even call substances that undermine our health to this extent "food." And while the next few chapters focus on why grains and grainlike seeds (like buckwheat and quinoa), legumes, processed vegetable oils, industrially produced dairy, refined sugars, and food additives are not doing us any favors, step one is to ditch the junk.

HEALTH QUICK-START

Processed foods can be addictive, and it's hard to make healthy choices when battling intense cravings. To help yourself give them up for good, commit to going at least a month without processed foods and simultaneously focus on getting lots of sleep, reducing stress, and getting some exercise. This will help your body adapt to dietary changes and mitigate cravings.

Chapter 19:
GRAINS, LEGUMES, AND PSEUDOGRAINS

The idea that grains, legumes, and pseudograins are not healthful foods is one of the most fundamental tenets of the Paleo diet—and one of the most surprising for those coming from a mainstream nutrition background, where whole grains and dried beans in particular are frequently lauded. But the Paleo rationale for avoiding grains and legumes is often misunderstood. It is sometimes oversimplified to the idea that because early humans didn't have access to significant quantities of these foods, we shouldn't eat them, either (an argument that's hardly scientific and easy to refute).

Actually, a large body of literature (as well as basic physiology and biochemistry) sheds light on how grains, legumes, and pseudograins can harm us and why replacing them with nutrient-dense Paleo foods can be a boon to our health. This chapter summarizes what you need to know!

Before we jump in, let's briefly review which foods fall under the grain, legume, and pseudograin categories.

Grains, also called *cereal grains*, are the starchy seeds of grasses and include many frequent flyers of the modern global food supply, including wheat, oats, rice, and corn. (For a more complete list, see page 280.) Domestication of grain crops goes back about 12,000 years and represents a major turning point in human history; the ability to store food spurred the shift from nomadic hunter-gatherer to settled agricultural societies, eventually leading to civilization. Wheat and corn especially have found their way into the majority of manufactured foods offered on grocery store shelves (see Chapter 18). Breakfast cereals, breads, muffins, pizza, cookies, doughnuts, granola bars, and pasta are all made with grains.

Legumes are the fruits or seeds of plants from the *Fabaceae* (also called *Leguminosae*) family. Soy is the most pervasive legume in our modern food supply, but other common examples include peanuts, lentils, and all varieties of dried beans. (For a more complete list, see page 280.) Some legumes are rife with the problematic compounds discussed in this chapter, but others contain much lower amounts, so those legumes that are considered middle-ground foods are discussed in Chapter 24.

Pseudograins are similar to grains in cooking applications but are the starchy seeds of broad-leaf plants instead of grasses; the best-known examples are quinoa and chia. Pseudograins are discussed in detail on page 256.

Grains, legumes, and pseudograins contain many of the same compounds that are known to be inflammatory, increase intestinal permeability, and/or feed gut dysbiosis. For these reasons (and not because cavemen didn't eat them), they are omitted from the Paleo diet.

A PRIMER ON LECTINS

Grains, legumes, and pseudograins have particularly high concentrations of lectins, which are a class of proteins that are present in all plants to some degree. The gluten in wheat is a famous example. Not all lectins are bad, but two subclasses are of particular concern for human health: prolamins (like gluten) and agglutinins (like wheat germ agglutinin). While the term is a little hyperbolic, these problematic subclasses of lectins are often referred to as *toxic lectins* to differentiate them from the harmless members of this protein family. These toxic lectins are part of a plant's natural defense system against predators and pests and are usually concentrated in the seeds (which is why grains and legumes, which are seeds, contain so much lectin). To defend themselves, the seeds from these plants either deter predators (like insects or humans) from eating them by making us sick or resist digestion completely—or both.

The grains and legumes that have become a part of the human diet since the Agricultural Revolution occurred 10,000 years ago aren't toxic enough to make most of us severely ill immediately after eating them; otherwise, humans never would have domesticated them! Instead, their effects are more subtle and can take years to manifest as life-threatening disease.

Toxic lectins are not broken down during the normal digestive process for three reasons:

- Their structure is not compatible with our bodies' digestive enzymes.
- Toxic lectins can directly inhibit certain digestive enzymes.
- The foods that contain lectins also contain digestive enzyme inhibitors (see page 251).

Prolamins and agglutinins (or predictable peptides resulting from the partial digestion of these lectins) can enter the body intact in a variety of ways. While in transit across the gut barrier, they may cause changes inside the enterocytes (the cells that form the wall of the intestine) that either kill those cells or render them ineffective at their job, which can lead to increased intestinal permeability (leaky gut). Plus, once inside the body, these lectins activate the immune system. All this can set the stage for many health conditions, including cardiovascular and autoimmune diseases.

Because avoiding grains is such a central tenet of the Paleo diet—and one of the most hotly debated by skeptics—it's worth discussing these mechanisms in more detail.

Prolamins

Prolamins (also called glutenoids) are found in abundance in grains, legumes, and pseudograins. They function as storage proteins in plants and are the major source of important proteins for seed germination. In fact, prolamins account for about half of the total protein in grains. A variety of prolamins exist, including gliadin (a protein fraction of gluten) in wheat, hordein in barley, secalin in rye, zein in corn, kafirin in sorghum, orzenin in rice, and avenin in oats, all of which are characterized by their high content of the amino acid proline.

SCIENCE SIMPLIFIED

Gluten is a protein in wheat that is very good at getting across the gut barrier and into the body, potentially damaging the gut, feeding the wrong kinds of bacteria in the gut, and causing inflammation. Most of the ways in which gluten can be harmful occur only in people with certain genetic susceptibilities or gluten intolerance. However, gluten can undermine health in ways that likely occur, at least to a degree, in all of us. Other grains contain proteins similar to gluten that may act similarly in our bodies, although more studies are needed. This class of proteins is called prolamins.

Most of what we know about the effects of prolamins—especially how prolamins cross and damage the gut barrier—comes from studying gliadin, a component of gluten. We know from a large body of research that gliadin fragments can cross the gut barrier through a paracellular (between the cells that line the gut) and two transcellular (through the cells that line the gut) pathways, stimulate the immune system, and inhibit the activity of three important digestive enzymes.

HOW GLUTEN CROSSES THE GUT BARRIER

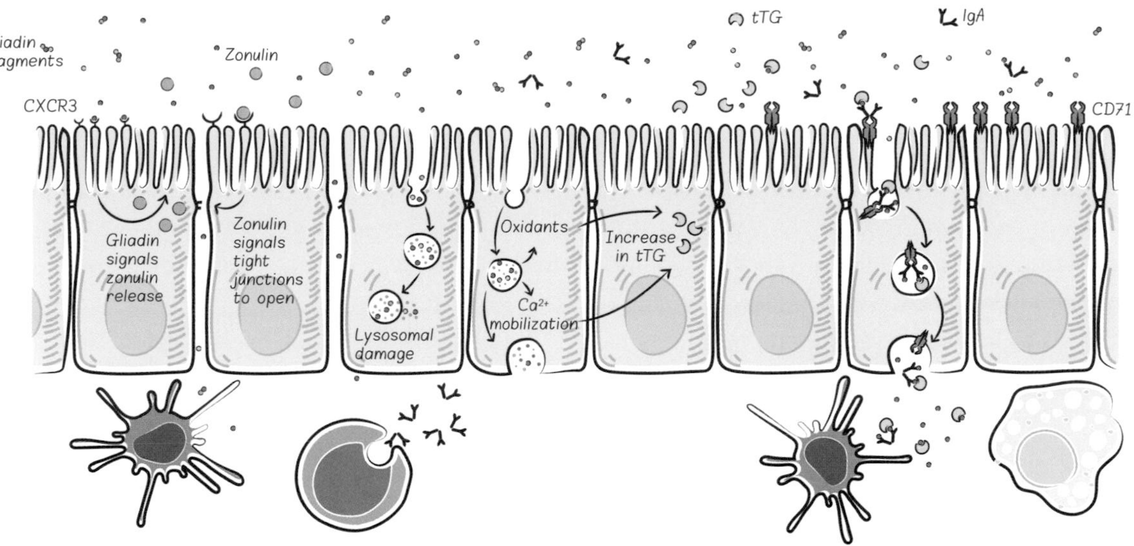

Gluten is known to open up the tight junctions between enterocytes, at least in genetically susceptible individuals (see page 67); this is the paracellular pathway from the gut into the body. This occurs through an increase in zonulin production by the enterocytes, stimulated by exposure to gluten (more specifically, gliadin). Recall that zonulin is a protein secreted into the gut by the enterocytes that regulates the rapid opening and closing of tight junctions to allow for the absorption of specific nutrients in healthy individuals. People with celiac disease are known to have increased zonulin levels, stimulating the opening of more tight junctions and probably keeping them open longer. When these tight junctions are opened, the contents of the gut can cross the gut barrier helter-skelter and then encounter gut-associated lymphoid tissue, causing generalized inflammation and immune activation. Recall that inflammation is part of the pathogenesis of every chronic illness (see page 78)—when compounds in foods stimulate the immune system, not only do we get inflammation and higher probabilities of food intolerances, but the ability of the immune system to protect us from pathogens is diminished.

HEALTH QUICK-START *Ditching gluten-containing foods is a great first step toward improving health! And don't worry: going gluten-free doesn't mean you'll miss out on any important nutrients (see page 135). But contrary to Paleo dogma, not everyone needs to be 100 percent gluten-free to be healthy. If you aren't sure whether gluten is a problem for you, try a four-week elimination and challenge (see Chapter 25 for the protocol). For a list of ingredients that contain gluten, see page 281.*

Another way in which gliadin can negatively impact gut health and cause inflammation is by exploiting a normal recycling pathway meant to protect the cells of the gut barrier from damage by infectious organisms—this is one of the transcellular pathways from the gut into the body. IgA, a type of antibody produced in gut-associated lymphoid tissue, is secreted into the gut, where it performs a variety of functions, including what is called *immune exclusion*—the interference with the ability of antigens (including viruses, bacteria, bacterial toxins, and enzymes) to adhere to and penetrate the gut barrier. These antibodies are then recycled back into the body via a process called retrotranscytosis, where they can present the antigens to the immune system. This both prepares the immune system to defend the body against pathogens and directly protects the gut enterocytes from viral and bacterial infection (because when the pathogens are bound to the IgA antibodies, it's harder for them to infect the cells). When IgA antibodies bind to gliadin fragments in the intestines, they form a stable complex that fits perfectly into a specific receptor called the transferrin receptor (which is normally used for the absorption of iron) in the membrane of the enterocytes. The complex is retrotranscytosed, which causes intact gliadin fragments to be transported into the body, where they can activate the immune system. Gluten intolerance (forming antibodies against gluten) is a prerequisite, and iron deficiency ramps up this pathway.

Even in healthy, nongenetically sensitive individuals, gliadin fragments are taken up by enterocytes through a process called endocytosis—this is the other transcellular pathway from the gut into the body. Endocytosis is a normal function of all cells in the body by which the cells absorb molecules (such as long proteins that can't enter the cells through the cell membrane or through specific transporters embedded in the cell membrane) by engulfing them in a membranous structure—sort of like a bubble. These "bubbles" are called *endosomes*, and they allow the cells to sort and recycle proteins in a targeted way. (Protein recycling is an important function for every cell because it allows proteins to be reused, which is more efficient than building new proteins.)

Within the enterocyte, endocytosed proteins are held within a type of endosome called a *lysosome*. Lysosomes contain enzymes (called lysosomal-acid proteases) that can break proteins apart into individual amino acids. Lysosomes travel across the cell, where their contents can be exocytosed (secreted out of the cell, with the lysosome membrane being reintegrated into the outer cell membrane—the opposite of endocytosis). In many healthy individuals, gliadin peptides can be fully digested within the lysosomes, but this is not the case for those with celiac disease.

There is also evidence that lysosomal damage may occur in response to gliadin fragments. (Interestingly, casein, a milk protein, has the same effect.) If a lysosome is damaged, not only do the still-intact gliadin fragments enter the cell cytoplasm, but so do the enzymes within the lysosome, which can then attack proteins within the cell, damaging and potentially killing the cell. Basically, if a lysosome is damaged while digesting and transporting proteins across the cell, the release of the contents of the lysosome within the cell can cause the cell to die. A damaged or dead cell opens up a hole through which other compounds in the gut can leak into the body and activate the immune system. This is one mechanism by which gliadin (and casein) can cause leaky gut, even in healthy individuals who have no gluten sensitivity or intolerance. It is unknown if a dietary threshold exists for this lysosomal damage to occur or whether such a threshold could vary depending on genetic or other factors.

An additional effect of the lysosomal pathway is the stimulation of inflammation through the production of oxidants. The accumulation of specific gliadin fragments within the lysosomes causes an increase in the production of reactive oxygen species (oxidants) without damaging the lysosomes. Although not all the details of this process are understood, some of the signaling pathways have been uncovered, and it appears that some gliadin fragments stimulate signals known to drive inflammation. The production of oxidants can also cause damage to the cell, which may alter cell morphology (or cell shape, which also affects cell function) and cell division and may affect cell viability and cause apoptosis (programmed cell death). Again, enterocyte damage or death leaves a hole in the gut barrier.

Another damaging effect of lysosomal transport of gliadin fragments is the mobilization of intracellular calcium ion stores, which causes endoplasmic reticulum stress (because the endoplasmic reticulum contains the highest concentration of calcium ions within the cell and the cell cannot function properly if it loses them). The endoplasmic reticulum is the organelle within every cell that is responsible for protein synthesis, lipid and carbohydrate metabolism, and detoxification. When it is stressed, it can't do its job efficiently, and when endoplasmic reticulum stress is severe or prolonged, cell death (via apoptosis) occurs. Again, this causes a hole in the gut barrier. As in the case of lysosomal damage, it is unknown whether dietary thresholds or genetic predisposition are factors in endoplasmic reticulum stress; however, both of these mechanisms appear to apply to the general population.

The prolamin gliadin can cross and damage the gut barrier in many ways, even in people without a genetic susceptibility to a leaky gut and without a diagnosed

WHAT ABOUT WHOLE GRAINS? AREN'T THOSE BETTER?

You may be wondering how much of this discussion applies to refined grains versus whole grains, so often touted as a dietary necessity. A whole grain is any grain product that uses the entire grain, including the bran, the germ, and the endosperm. Refined grains are milled to remove the bran and the germ. It's true that much of the fiber, vitamins, and minerals are concentrated in the bran and the germ, so whole-grain products have more nutritive value than refined grains. Unfortunately, the problematic compounds discussed in this chapter also happen to be concentrated in the bran of the whole grain. This doesn't make refined grains a valuable food, either—beyond being empty calories with a high glycemic load, they contain sufficient quantities of lectins, digestive enzyme inhibitors, saponins, phytates, and omega-6 fats to be problematic. As you will read in this chapter, "healthy" whole grains are anything but.

gluten sensitivity. Inflammation is triggered by gliadin fragments that cross the gut barrier, as previously noted, as well as by other partly digested food proteins, gut bacteria, bacterial fragments, and waste products or toxins crossing over if gliadin damages enterocytes. This further activates the immune system, causing a vicious cycle of inflammation and gut barrier damage.

How important is genetic susceptibility? Certainly it is involved in the zonulin response to gliadin. Although the role that genetic factors play in enterocyte damage caused by transport through the enterocytes remains unstudied, genetic predisposition may explain the variability in the severity of the damage caused by wheat consumption. It is likely that some damage to the gut barrier occurs in everyone who consumes wheat, but genes might explain why some people suffer from severely leaky gut or autoimmune disease in response to wheat consumption while others seem to tolerate wheat without experiencing overt health issues.

Not only are prolamins inherently difficult for our bodies to digest, but they interfere with important digestive enzymes in the intestine. In particular, gliadin is known to inhibit the activity of three important enzymes: lactase, sucrase, and dipeptidyl peptidase 4. These enzymes are important for breaking down sugars into monosaccharides and proteins into amino acids for transport across the enterocyte barrier. (Lactase breaks apart lactose; sucrase breaks apart sucrose; and dipeptidyl peptidase 4 has diverse functions related to digestion, metabolism, and immune regulation.) The inhibition of these enzymes may have a profound effect on gut microbiota—stimulating overgrowth in particular—because it means more food for gut bacteria farther down the digestive tract. Prolamin-rich foods feed only certain species of gut bacteria, so only certain strains increase in number, leading to an imbalance. In fact, studies show that mice fed a gluten-containing diet show much higher (too high!) levels of gut bacteria than mice fed a gluten-free diet.

Although there haven't been comprehensive studies evaluating the effects of all food sources of prolamins, there is a great deal of structural and functional similarity (due to similarity in amino acid sequences) between the prolamins of different grains and legumes. So it's highly probable that the effects of gliadin also apply, at least to a degree, to other prolamins. For example, studies show that the prolamins in quinoa, corn, and oats can damage the gut and stimulate the immune system in celiac sufferers in a manner analogous to gliadin.

Gluten is especially insidious because parts of this protein closely resemble many proteins in the human body. When our bodies produce antibodies against gluten (the hallmark of gluten allergy or intolerance, the difference being which type of antibody is produced), it is likely that some of those antibodies will also target other cells, setting the stage for autoimmune disease.

One commonly formed antibody triggered by gluten exposure is against transglutaminase, an essential enzyme in every cell of the body. It makes important modifications to proteins as they are produced inside the cell, and it also stimulates wound healing. But the playing field changes if antibodies have formed against it! When damaged cells secrete transglutaminase in inflamed areas of the small intestine (or any other damaged tissue in the body), the immune system sees those areas as targets rather than helping to heal the surrounding tissue. This is yet another mechanism linking gluten with leaky gut. Importantly, when antibodies form against transglutaminase, every cell and organ in the body becomes a potential target.

Because an exaggerated sensitivity to gluten is the cause of celiac disease, which affects at least 1 in 133 people, its effects on the gut have been the most frequently studied. Scientists still don't know which of the many ways in which gluten can harm the body apply to all prolamins and which are specific to gluten.

Gluten Where You Least Expect It

Once you've mastered recognizing ingredients that are derived from wheat and indicate the presence of gluten (see page 281 for a detailed list), it's important to know that other foods may be contaminated with gluten or may be misidentified as gluten by your body.

Gluten cross-reactivity is of particular concern for anyone whose body produces antibodies against gluten, technically considered a gluten allergy or intolerance. Essentially, when our bodies create antibodies against gluten, those same antibodies also recognize proteins in other foods, such as dairy and soy. When we eat those foods, even though they don't contain gluten, our bodies react as though they do.

We can do a fantastic job of remaining gluten-free but still suffer all the symptoms of gluten consumption—because our bodies still think we are eating gluten.

To understand gluten cross-reactivity, it helps to know a little bit more about antibodies and how they recognize and bind to specific proteins.

Antibodies Drive Targeted Immune Responses

Proteins are made up of long chains of amino acids; small proteins may be only 50 amino acids long, whereas large proteins may be 2,000 amino acids long. The specific sequence of these amino acids determines which kind of protein is formed. These amino acid chains are folded, kinked, and buckled in extremely complex ways, which gives a protein its "structure." This folding/structure is integral to the function of the protein.

An antibody is a Y-shaped protein produced by immune cells in the body. Each tip of the Y contains the region of the antibody (called the paratope) that can bind to a specific sequence of amino acids (called the epitope) that are a part of the protein that the antibody recognizes or binds to (called the antigen). The classic analogy is that the antibody is like a lock and a fifteen- to twenty-amino acid section of a protein/antigen is the key.

There are five classes (or isotypes) of antibodies, each with distinctive functions in the body:

- **The IgE class** is responsible for allergic reactions; for example, when someone goes into anaphylaxis after eating shellfish.
- **The IgG and IgA classes** protect us from invading pathogens but also are responsible for food sensitivities/intolerances. IgG and IgA antibodies are secreted by immune cells into the circulation (that is, into the blood to be transported throughout the body), the lymphatic system, various fluids of the body (like saliva), and tissues themselves. Both of these antibodies are found in high concentrations in the tissues and fluids surrounding the gut—this is partly why the gut is considered our primary defense against infection.
- **The IgD and IgM classes** function as antigen receptors on the surface membrane of B cells, so they help B cells detect pathogens and then help activate other immune cells to ramp up the immune response. IgM antibodies can also be secreted by B cells, similarly to IgG and IgA.

The way the adaptive immune system can target a specific pathogen (like a flu virus) is thanks to antibodies binding to an antigen from that specific foreign invader, signaling to immune cells, "Here's the thing we need to attack!" Antibodies are produced by B cells; when they are released and bind to their antigens, they signal to phagocytes (immune cells that destroy pathogens by engulfing them) to come and destroy the foreign invader they've bound to.

The formation of antibodies against an antigen (whether it is an invading pathogen or a food) is an extremely complex process. When antibodies are being formed against a protein, the antibodies recognize specific (and short) sequences of amino acids in that protein. Depending on how the antigenic protein is folded, certain amino acid sequences in that protein are more likely to be the targets of new antibody formation than others, simply because of the location of those sequences in the structure of the protein. Certain sequences of amino acids are more antigenic—that is, more likely to stimulate antibody formation—than others. This is another part of the reason why certain foods have a greater potential to cause allergies and sensitivities.

Understanding that antibodies recognize short sequences of amino acids and not an entire protein is key to understanding the concept of cross-reactivity. It also is the reason why many different antibodies can be formed against one protein. This redundancy is important for protecting us from pathogens—if the antibodies we produce when we get sick with a flu virus also bind to another virus, we won't get sick when we're exposed to that other virus.

Gluten Cross-Reactivity

So what happens in gluten cross-reactivity? First, this is something that can happen only if you have a food allergy or intolerance to gluten, meaning that your body produces an antibody against it. In this case, the amino acid sequence in gluten that the antibody recognizes is also present in another protein in another food. There are only twenty amino acids, so while there are millions of possible ways to link various amounts of each amino acid to form a protein, there are certain amino acid sequences that tend to repeat in biology.

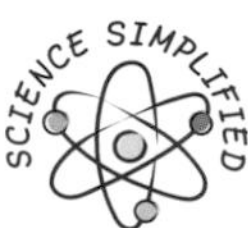

Gluten cross-reactivity means that other foods, like dairy and soy, may trigger the same reaction in the body as gluten for people with gluten intolerance. You may choose to avoid these foods altogether; do an elimination and challenge with each of them (see Chapter 25); or get tested for IgE, IgG, and IgA antibodies against these other potential trigger foods.

A recent study evaluated the potential cross-reactivity with gluten of twenty-four food antigens using a lab test called an ELISA (in this case, Cyrex Labs' gluten cross-reactivity blood test, aka Array 4) to identify the foods most likely to be additionally problematic for those with gluten intolerance or celiac disease. The tested food antigens included rye, barley, spelt, Polish wheat, oats, buckwheat, sorghum, millet, amaranth, quinoa, corn, rice, potato, hemp, teff, soy, milk (α-casein, β-casein, casomorphin, butyrophilin, whey protein, and whole milk), milk chocolate, brewer's/baker's yeast, coffee (instant, latte, espresso, and imported), sesame seeds, tapioca (aka cassava or yuca), and eggs.

The researchers did not find cross-reactivity with all these foods, but they did find that their anti-gliadin antibodies (antibodies that recognize the protein fraction of gluten) cross-reacted with all dairy, including whole milk and isolated dairy proteins (casein, casomorphin, butyrophilin, and whey); this may explain the high frequency of dairy sensitivities in celiac patients. They also identified cross-reactivity with oats (but only one of two cultivars tested), brewer's/baker's yeast, instant coffee (but not fresh coffee), milk chocolate (attributable to its dairy proteins), millet, soy, corn, rice, and potato.

It's important to emphasize that not all people with gluten sensitivities will also be sensitive to all these potential gluten cross-reactors. Nonetheless, these foods should be highlighted as high risk for stimulating the immune system. Just as trace amounts of gluten can cause a reaction in those with celiac disease (the threshold for a reaction has not been tested in non-celiac gluten sensitivity), even a small amount of these foods can perpetuate inflammation and immune responses. This is important when we think of the small amounts of corn used in so many foods, and even the trace milk proteins that can be found in ghee.

The take-home message: Depending on which antibody or antibodies we form against gluten, it/they may or may not cross-react with other foods. So not only are we sensitive to gluten, but our bodies now recognize non-gluten-containing foods as being one and the same as gluten. Who needs to worry about this? Any of the estimated 20 percent of people who are gluten intolerant or have celiac disease—that is, anyone who has formed antibodies against gluten.

The foods to be wary of if you have a gluten sensitivity are:

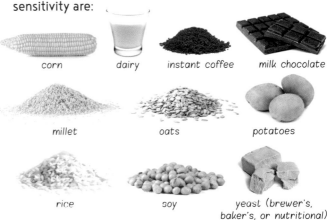

Gluten Contamination

Gluten contamination is common in our food supply, and many grains and flours that are inherently gluten-free may still contain gluten once processed. Commonly contaminated grain products include:

- buckwheat flour
- millet
- sorghum flour
- soy flour
- white rice flour

As these are common ingredients in commercial gluten-free baked goods, extreme caution should be exercised.

So for people with autoimmune disease (which has a high correlation with gluten sensitivity), celiac disease, or gluten sensitivity, one or all of the foods described in this section may be the culprit. We have the choice to either cut these foods out of our diets and see if we improve (see page 432) or get tested to see if our bodies produce antibodies against these foods.

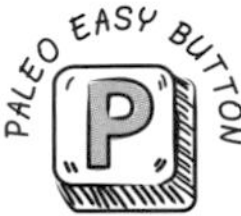

It just so happens that most of the foods that can act as gluten cross-reactors are not Paleo foods anyway! The only additional food to avoid is nutritional yeast, plus some middle ground foods like cider and wine, rice, grass-fed dairy, and potatoes. See Chapter 24.

Gluten and Obesity

In case the preceding information didn't give you reason enough to avoid gluten, here's one more point to consider: emerging research suggests a link between gluten and weight gain. An intriguing study in mice, published in 2016, offers the biggest clue yet for how gluten could be contributing to the obesity epidemic.

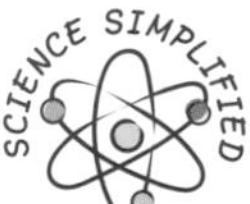

Partially digested fragments of gluten can cross the gut barrier intact. New science indicates that once in the body, those fragments can bind with receptors in liver and fat cells, causing inflammation and cellular metabolism changes that can lead to weight gain.

The study investigated the effects of gluten on metabolism and fat storage. (Previously, the same team showed that mice fed gluten-free diets gained less weight than mice fed the same number of calories in the form of gluten-containing foods.) Over the course of eight weeks, the mice were fed one of four diets: a gluten-free control diet (standard rodent chow), a gluten-free high-fat diet (designed to produce obesity in mice), and those same two diets with 4.5 percent added gluten. (Although the researchers didn't provide much detail on other elements of the diets, keep in mind that high-fat diets in rodent studies bear little resemblance to high-fat human diets: the rodent diets are typically composed of lard, casein, sugar, soybean oil, and other purified ingredients rather than anything resembling whole food.) From there, the animals' food intake, energy expenditure, and gluten absorption and distribution throughout the body were monitored, with fat tissue changes measured after euthanization.

The results? As expected, the mice eating high-fat diets gained more weight than the mice eating standard rodent chow. But here's where it gets interesting. Even though the addition of gluten didn't alter the mice's energy intakes, the gluten-eating mice ended up with 20 percent higher body weight (and 30 percent higher fat deposits in both visceral and abdominal tissue) than their respective controls. Further analysis showed that the gluten-eating mice had lower basal oxygen consumption in their fasting state (resulting in lower total energy expenditure), pro-obesity changes in certain thermogenesis-linked proteins in brown adipose tissue and subcutaneous adipose tissue, and increased expression of the pro-inflammatory cytokines IL-6 and TNF in the mice eating standard chow, indicating a higher inflammatory profile. On top of that, radiolabeled gluten was found in the mice's blood and peripheral organs, including visceral fat, suggesting the potential for gluten to act directly on fat tissue and induce harmful changes in cell metabolism.

It's worth emphasizing here that this study confirms gluten's ability to cross mammalian gut barriers and enter the body without genetic predisposition. Gluten—or, more specifically, gliadin fragments—can enter the human body via several mechanisms (see page 242). And while certain mechanisms appear to require a genetic factor, like the increased zonulin production seen in celiac sufferers and others with DQ2 and DQ8 variants of the HLA gene, gluten appears to be able to enter all of our bodies in several ways, at least to some degree. However, it remains unknown how much gluten can pass through a healthy human gut and exactly what role it might play once inside the body. This study does give us a clue, though: the sequestering of radiolabeled gluten in liver and fat tissues strongly suggests binding with a receptor. The authors of this study postulate that receptor-binding is what triggers the metabolic changes conducive to weight gain, and their research will now focus on this line of investigation to improve our understanding of exactly how gluten is affecting liver and fat cells.

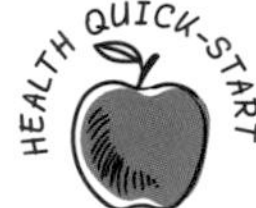

If one of your health goals is to lose weight, new science suggests that going gluten-free will help!

So what does this mean for us? While we can't extrapolate the results of a rodent study directly to humans (that's what controlled clinical trials are for!), this study explains—for the first time—some mechanisms that could underlie a link between gluten and obesity. And it's very possible that those mechanisms are relevant to us. For one, the mice's gluten intake (4.5 percent of their diet by weight) was high, but a human eating a wheat-based diet could feasibly reach that same intake. So the mice's gluten exposure is similar to what some people face on a daily basis. We know from previous research that gluten can increase intestinal permeability in both celiac and non-celiac individuals, so it's not outside the realm of possibility that gluten peptides could enter the circulation, travel to peripheral tissues, and influence gene expression in cells in ways that promote fat gain in humans (which is what happened with the mice).

Other mechanisms uncovered in this study, such as the effect of gluten on proteins in brown fat and subcutaneous fat, could play out differently in humans, who have proportionately less brown fat than mice, as well as differences in gene expression in various types of fat tissue. Determining whether gluten decreases energy expenditure as dramatically in humans as it does in mice requires further research. And considering that the high-fat-diet mice in this study tended to react more dramatically to gluten than the standard-chow mice, dietary context might play an important role in how gluten interacts with animal bodies—which raises even more questions for future studies to tackle.

Another study also shows that gluten can inhibit leptin from binding with its receptor. Recall that leptin is an important hunger hormone and adiposity signal (see page 90) and that leptin resistance is a primary risk factor for obesity. This is yet another potential mechanism linking gluten with obesity. And, at least in mice, gluten-free diets reduce weight gain, inflammation, and insulin resistance.

For the 1 in 133 people who have celiac disease, avoiding gluten is a no-brainer. It may even be a no-brainer for the estimated 55 percent of us with HLA-DQ2 or HLA-DQ8 (see page 68). But for everyone else, the evidence against gluten is mounting. Interactions between gluten, different dietary components, and human genes point to a potentially harmful effect of gluten on gut health, immunity, inflammation, and fat regulation, even in otherwise healthy people. And there's no nutrient found in gluten-containing foods that can't be obtained—typically at much higher levels!—from nutrient-dense plant and animal foods on a Paleo diet (see page 135).

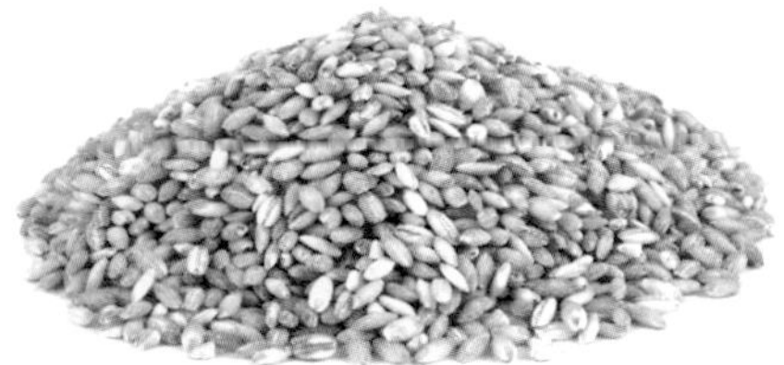

Agglutinins

The other subclass of lectins, agglutinins, are characterized by their ability to induce clumping (agglutination) of red blood cells. In plants, agglutinins help protect seeds from fungal infection and possibly from insect predation as well. In fact, genetically modified industrial grain crops generally have higher levels of agglutinins to help protect them from pests—including wheat germ agglutinin (WGA), which is so powerful at resisting insects that the gene for WGA has been added to genetically modified corn! Although most other agglutinins haven't been studied as thoroughly as WGA, we know that many types, such as peanut agglutinin, soybean agglutinin, and nettle agglutinin, have significant effects on intestinal permeability, and can stimulate both the innate and adaptive immune system.

In comparison to gluten, WGA is a close second in terms of negatively impacting our health; it has the added effect of stimulating inflammation. This is another reason why the simple act of removing wheat from our diets can make a profound difference. In the concentrations we would typically derive from food, WGA is not directly toxic to gut enterocytes, but it's good at interacting with the brush border of the intestine and in doing so increases intestinal permeability. In fact, its activities in the gut qualify it as a biologically active protein, which is not normal (or healthful!) for proteins in food.

SCIENCE SIMPLIFIED *Wheat germ agglutinin is so good at getting across the gut barrier and into the body intact that it's been investigated as an oral drug-delivery molecule. WGA is also extremely inflammatory!*

The outer membrane of every cell is composed of a double layer of fat molecules called the lipid bilayer, with various proteins (receptors, for one) embedded within the layer that perform a variety of functions. Some of the fats and proteins within the membrane have sugar molecules (which are important for a variety of normal membrane functions) attached to the outside of the membrane. These membrane carbohydrates constitute 2 to 10 percent of a cell's membrane and include any of eight sugars: glucose, galactose, mannose, fucose, xylose, N-acetylgalactosamine, N-actetylglucosamine, and

N-acetylneuraminic acid. WGA binds specifically to N-acetylglucosamine and N-acetylneuraminic acid, which happen to be membrane carbohydrates in all animal cells and form key parts of the glycocalyx of gastrointestinal cells. WGA binds at a high rate to human intestinal cells via these membrane carbohydrates, and WGA is rapidly internalized into the enterocytes, probably via endocytosis.

One of the membrane glycoproteins to which WGA binds (by binding to the carbohydrate component of the glycoprotein) is the epidermal growth factor (EGF) receptor. The EGF receptor is known to promote what's called receptor-mediated endocytosis and may be the reason WGA is so readily internalized by gut enterocytes. Even more important, the EGF receptor regulates the paracellular permeability of epithelial cells—meaning that when the EGF receptor is activated (such as by binding with WGA), signals are sent throughout the cell that result in the opening of the tight junctions between enterocytes. It's believed that the EGF receptor plays an important physiological role in maintaining epithelial tissue organization and permeability, thereby maintaining the integrity of the gut barrier.

Very low concentrations of WGA (very possible to achieve from dietary sources) increase epithelial cell permeability, meaning that WGA causes the tight junctions between epithelial cells to open up sufficiently for molecules to cross (at least scientists have measured this in isolated cells studied in the lab). WGA accumulates in lysosomes (whether this damages the lysosomes, as in the case of gliadin, has not been studied), and some of the WGA crosses the epithelial barrier intact, though we don't know exactly how yet. And while the amount of WGA that crosses the epithelial barrier is small, it's enough to have a huge impact on the immune system. In fact, even at these very low concentrations, WGA stimulates the secretion of pro-inflammatory cytokines.

As alluded to earlier, WGA is known to have a profound effect on both the innate and the adaptive immune systems. Some of the pro-inflammatory cytokines induced by WGA cause inflammation, including stimulating phagocytosis by neutrophils ("eating" of stuff by white blood cells) and stimulating the production of reactive oxygen species. Once again, this generalized inflammation can damage enterocytes, the innocent bystanders. WGA also induces cytokine production known to increase proliferation (cell division) of all helper T cells. However, WGA can also bind to cytokine receptors on T cells and thereby inhibit proliferation (which may actually contribute to overstimulation of one subset of T cells, as is often seen in autoimmune and immune-related disorders). WGA also stimulates the production of antibodies by B cells and binds to blood-derived immune cells, thereby increasing activation of inflammatory cells and increasing apoptosis of white blood cells.

WGA is so good at getting across the gut barrier that it is being investigated as a carrier for oral drugs, the idea being that WGA could be bound to a drug molecule and help facilitate its absorption into the body. Fortunately, a red flag has been raised about the possible toxic effects of WGA as a drug-delivery vehicle, with research suggesting that WGA may be the cause of various gastrointestinal disorders.

Of course, non-wheat lectins—both prolamins and agglutinins—can be harmful as well. While some agglutinins are largely deactivated by cooking (such as several of those in legumes; see page 290), others, including WGA, are not. Wheat germ agglutinin is so resistant to deactivation even through traditional food preparation methods that even when consumed as part of our food, it qualifies as a biologically active compound in our digestive tracts. (That is not a normal classification for a protein in food!) And while some other "blacklisted" foods are okay for occasional consumption (like dairy, beans, and rice), avoiding gluten and wheat altogether is wise even for people who do not have celiac disease.

A famous example of an agglutinin is ricin, which comes from castor bean casings. Ricin is so toxic that as little as 1 milligram, if inhaled or injected, is deadly. How much is 1 milligram of ricin? Roughly the size of a grain of sand. In fact, the Bulgarian dissident Georgi Markov was assassinated in London in 1978 with a pellet containing 0.2 milligram of ricin that was shot or injected into his thigh, allegedly with the tip of an umbrella.

Legumes are also particularly high in agglutinins, this being the primary reason legumes are excluded from the Paleo diet.

A toxic and immunogenic agglutinin called phytohaemagglutinin is found in high levels in kidney beans and to a lesser extent in broad beans, cannellini beans, fava beans, and common beans. As few as five raw kidney beans can cause extreme gastrointestinal distress, with symptoms similar to those of food poisoning (not that anyone would want to eat raw kidney beans!). Phytohaemagglutinin can cross the gut barrier, increase intestinal permeability, and stimulate the immune system. In fact, phytohaemagglutinin is easily detected in the bloodstream after consumption. It has also been shown to cause extensive overgrowth of *E. coli* in the small intestine; some *E. coli* is normal, but it is a common culprit in small intestinal bacterial overgrowth, or SIBO.

Other legume agglutinins, like peanut agglutinin (PNA, or peanut lectin), also enter the bloodstream quickly after being consumed, suggesting significant effects on intestinal permeability. Soybean agglutinin (or soybean lectin) and concanavalin (an agglutinin in jack beans, which are often used in animal feed) have been shown to increase epithelial permeability (that is, cause a leaky gut!) as much as wheat germ agglutinin does. Concanavalin stimulates the immune system and is being investigated as a drug for chemotherapy (because chemotherapy drugs are more toxic to cancer cells than they are to normal cells, which seems to be the case with concanavalin). Soybean agglutinin is also known to stimulate the immune system—so efficiently in fact, that it is being studied for use in vaccines to improve immunization.

Yes, legumes do have some compelling nutrition, but their agglutinin content puts many of them firmly in the no category when it comes to an optimal human diet. For more on traditionally prepared and fermented legumes as well as legumes with edible pods, such as snow peas and green beans, see Chapter 24.

Lectins in Context

When it comes to lectins, dose is another important factor. The vegetables and fruits that our prehistoric ancestors ate in large quantities (and that science validates are still excellent for us today) are generally very low in lectins and come with a friendlier defense strategy: we eat the delicious fruit encasing the seeds, and then the seeds pass through our digestive tracts intact. In our ancestors' time, those seeds would then be planted in rich manure. (That's much different than grains, whose lives depend on *not* getting eaten and crushed by our teeth!) And the lectins that fruits and vegetables do contain generally interact much less strongly with the gut barrier than the lectins found in grains. Grains (especially wheat) and legumes (especially soy) are high in prolamins and agglutinins, the two subclasses of lectins with the greatest negative impact on the barrier function of the gut. (That's where the gut is supposed to selectively allow digested nutrients from our foods into our bodies and keep everything else out.) And if damaging the gut lining and causing systemic inflammation isn't enough, lectins are also antinutrients, which means that they stop us from absorbing many of the vitamins and minerals in our food, like calcium!

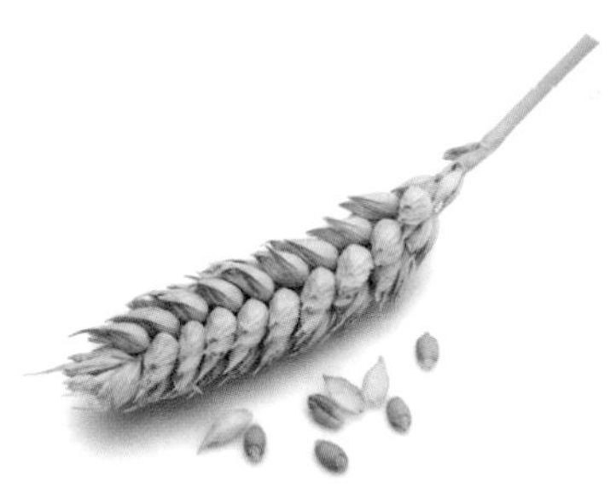

DIGESTIVE ENZYME INHIBITORS

Digestive enzyme inhibitors are compounds particularly concentrated in the seeds of plants that interfere with the enzymes our bodies secrete to help digest our food. There are different types of digestive enzyme inhibitors, each named for the type of digestive enzyme it inhibits. Grains, legumes, and pseudograins contain protease (protein-digesting enzymes) and amylase (starch-digesting enzymes) inhibitors. Grains are high in protease inhibitors, although soybeans are the most concentrated source of trypsin (a specific protein-digesting enzyme) inhibitors among commonly consumed foods. All legumes are high in amylase inhibitors, which is one reason they are called resistant starches—they are literally resistant to digestion. It is important to note that dairy products are also high in protease inhibitors.

Digestive enzyme inhibitors are considered antinutrients—substances that interfere with the absorption of nutrients in food. However, their effects are far more pervasive than simply decreasing the availability of micronutrients for your body. Consuming foods laden with digestive enzyme inhibitors stimulates the secretion of more digestive enzymes from the pancreas. Synthesizing digestive enzymes requires amino acids (typically sulfur-rich amino acids), so the hyperproduction of digestive enzymes by the pancreas, beyond causing undue stress on the organ itself, can cause a depletion of nutrients from the body. This idea is supported by animal studies in which pancreatic hypertrophy and hyperplasia (meaning that the cells of the pancreas increase in cell size and number, respectively, which is associated with disease) occur as a direct result of consuming potato- or soybean-derived inhibitors of the digestive enzyme trypsin.

As mentioned earlier, two main types of digestive enzyme inhibitors present in grains, legumes, and pseudograins that are known to be bad news for digestion and the gut barrier:

- **Protease inhibitors,** which block the digestive enzymes responsible for breaking apart proteins into individual amino acids from doing their job
- **Amylase inhibitors,** which block the digestive enzymes responsible for breaking apart starches into individual monosaccharides (simple sugars) from doing their job

There are many types of proteases and amylases, and the effects of inhibiting certain digestive enzymes is still being intensely studied (although, oddly enough, far more aggressively in regard to the health of farmed fish and poultry than of humans).

Whatever we cannot properly digest becomes food for gut microorganisms. In the presence of an overabundance of food, those microorganisms (or, worse, a subset of them) can become quite numerous, leading to bacterial overgrowth and gut dysbiosis. Recall that gut dysbiosis on its own can cause a leaky gut and interfere with the normal functioning of the immune system. In fact, studies in which rats were fed amylase inhibitors derived from kidney beans in doses suggested for the treatment of diabetes resulted in such severe bacterial overgrowth that the rats' cecums (the first part of the large intestine) ruptured; the rats then had to be euthanized. Other effects of amylase inhibitors include reduction in growth (owing to loss of nitrogen, lipids, and carbohydrates), hypertrophy of the intestines and pancreas, and atrophy of the liver and thymus gland (see page 81).

Perhaps most alarming is evidence that digestive enzyme inhibitors can cause inflammation directly. A recent paper showed that inhibitors of trypsin and α-amylase that were derived from wheat strongly activated the innate immune system and significantly increased production of pro-inflammatory chemical mediators (cytokines) both in the small intestine and in the blood. These digestive enzyme inhibitors also stimulated pro-inflammatory cytokine production in biopsy samples from celiac patients. The authors suggest that, while these findings are certainly relevant to celiac disease, the way that the immune system is activated (via Toll-like receptors) implies that the pro-inflammatory effects of these substances are widespread. This means the digestive enzyme inhibitors in grains, legumes, and pseudograins may play a critical role in both intestinal and nonintestinal inflammatory diseases. In fact, some scientists have suggested that non-celiac gluten sensitivity is a severe inflammatory reaction to amylase-trypsin inhibitors in wheat.

It's worthy to note that the amylase-trypsin inhibitor activity is highest in modern gluten-containing grains and is retained even after processing and cooking. A recent study compared the amylase-trypsin inhibitor activity of modern wheat varieties, ancient wheat varieties (emmer and einkorn), gluten-free grains, soy, and pseudograins, both processed and unprocessed, and discovered that gluten-containing cereals, especially modern varieties, have by far the highest concentrations of amylase-trypsin inhibitors that activate Toll-like receptor 4 (TLR4), causing intestinal inflammation. This may explain why some people do well with gluten-free diets even though they continue to consume gluten-free grains and legumes.

SAPONINS

Along with lectins, grains, legumes, and pseudograins (like quinoa and amaranth) are high in saponins, which are compounds with detergent-like properties. Saponins, typically concentrated in the bran or hull, are designed to protect plants from consumption by microbes and insects by dissolving the cell membranes of these potential predators. All plants contain saponins, but they're often concentrated in the seeds.

Saponins consist of a fat-soluble core (having either a steroid or a triterpenoid structure) with one or more side chains of water-soluble carbohydrates. This combination of a water-soluble and a fat-soluble component is what makes saponins act like a detergent—that is, something that can make oil and water mix. Because of their detergent-like structure, saponins can interact with the cholesterol molecules imbedded in cell surface membranes and create pores (holes) in the surface membrane of the cells that line the gut (enterocytes), allowing a variety of substances found in the gut to enter those cells.

A number of types of saponins exist, and some bind more easily and tightly to cholesterol molecules in cell membranes than others. As a result, different saponins can create larger or smaller pores, which may be more or less stable. The larger and more stable (and/or more numerous) the pores, the more difficult it is for the enterocyte to recover. Small doses of some dietary saponins (like those found in fruits and vegetables) might play a helpful role in the absorption of some minerals, and some food saponins have been shown to be anti-inflammatory or anti-cancerous. However, grains, legumes, and pseudograins contain *very* high doses of saponins (and, in general, contain types of saponins that interact more strongly with cholesterol). Saponins from these foods are known to increase gut permeability, which may be via either pore formation or killing enterocytes. Cells, in general, do not survive large, irreversible changes in membrane permeability. Oat, soy, and quinoa saponins in particular have been shown to markedly increase intestinal permeability.

Interestingly, even when a sub-lethal amount of saponin pores form in the enterocyte surface membrane, the cell loses its ability to transport nutrients, especially carbohydrates. While slowing sugar transport from the gut to the bloodstream may seem like a great thing (this is one reason why beans are so often recommended as a carbohydrate source for diabetics!), the potentially irreversible increase in gut permeability is just not worth it

KNOWLEDGE BOMB *Legumes tend to have a low glycemic load for three reasons. First, the carbohydrates in legumes are mainly polysaccharides, long starch molecules that take longer to digest before the monosaccharides can be absorbed into the body. Second, legumes are high in fiber, especially resistant starch, which slows carbohydrate absorption from the digestive tract. Those are both positives. Unfortunately, the third reason is the presence of saponins, which inhibit the ability of gut cells to actively transport carbohydrates into the body. This in and of itself wouldn't be a problem if saponins didn't damage gut cells.*

When large amounts of dietary saponins are consumed, especially in the presence of an already leaky gut, saponins can leak into the bloodstream. At sufficient concentrations, they cause hemolysis, or destruction of the cell membranes of red blood cells. Saponins also have adjuvant-like activity, which means that they are able to affect the immune system, leading to the production of pro-inflammatory cytokines (chemical messengers that tell white blood cells to attack) and can further contribute to inflammation in the body. Soyasaponin Ab (the major saponin in soy) strongly increases the release of the pro-inflammatory cytokines TNF-α and IL-1β as well as antibody production to an antigen. Quinoa saponins have also been shown to have adjuvant activity in addition to increasing epithelial barrier permeability (in both the intestine and the sinuses).

KNOWLEDGE BOMB *Grains, legumes, and pseudograins aren't the only foods that contain saponins. A particularly toxic class of saponins, called glycoalkaloids, are found in vegetables of the nightshade family and cause inflammation, have adjuvant properties, and increase intestinal permeability. Nightshade saponins are discussed further in Chapter 28.*

PHYTATES

Grains, legumes, and pseudograins contain high levels of antinutrients called phytates that can inhibit mineral absorption and damage the gut in additional ways. Phytates are the salts of phytic acid (that is, phytic acid bound to a mineral) and are present in the outer layer and bran of all plant seeds. Within the seed, the primary function of phytic acid is as a storage molecule for phosphorus, but it also serves as an energy store, a source of cations (positively charged ions) for various chemical reactions in the plant, and a source of a cell wall precursor called myoinositol. Our bodies cannot digest phytates.

Because phytates are formed when phytic acid binds to minerals (typically calcium, magnesium, iron, potassium, and zinc), these minerals are then unavailable to be absorbed by the gut—which is why phytates are considered antinutrients. As a result, the consumption of grains (as well as legumes) can cause mineral deficiencies, especially when these phytate-rich foods displace other mineral-rich foods in the diet.

Along with blocking mineral absorption, phytates limit the activity of a variety of digestive enzymes, including the proteases trypsin and pepsin, as well as amylase and glucosidase. This implies that phytates can be as devastating to the gut barrier and gut microbiota as digestive enzyme inhibitors, namely by causing intestinal inflammation and feeding bacterial overgrowth.

It's important to emphasize that *excessive* dietary phytates and phytic acid are the problem. Phytates are present in much lower concentrations in nonreproductive plant parts, like leaves and stems, as well as in nuts and seeds, the moderate consumption of which is endorsed within the Paleo template.

Consuming phytates in moderate quantities may actually provide an important antioxidant function and help reduce cardiovascular risk factors and cancer risk. Moderate consumption also means that a healthy amount and variety of gut bacteria will be able to liberate some minerals from the phytates to make them more absorbable. In that sense, the scientific literature reinforces the idea that vegetables (with their lower concentration of phytates) are extremely important in our diet, whereas grains deliver levels of phytates that surpass what benefits us.

KNOWLEDGE BOMB *Antinutrients in grains may lead to nutrient deficiencies. Epidemiological studies performed in the early 1980s showed that vitamin D deficiency and rickets (a disease characterized by soft bones caused by deficiencies in vitamin D, phosphorus, and calcium) were much higher in people who ate lots of unleavened whole-grain breads, despite adequate sun exposure. In an effort to understand why, a group of researchers compared the plasma vitamin D levels of volunteers eating a "normal" diet with those of volunteers whose diets were supplemented with 60 grams of wheat bran daily. After 30 days, the wheat-bran volunteers had significantly lower vitamin D levels. Although how wheat bran consumption influences vitamin D was not determined with certainty, the authors speculate that something in the bran interfered with enterohepatic circulation of vitamin D metabolites (that is, vitamin D recycling from gut to liver) and caused enhanced elimination of vitamin D in the intestines (so instead of being reabsorbed in the gut, vitamin D was excreted). Calcium deficiency may also increase inactivation of vitamin D in the liver.*

OMEGA-6 FATS

On top of all these problems, grains and legumes are very high in omega-6 polyunsaturated fatty acids (see page 158). Grains (including corn) and legumes are high in linoleic acid, the omega-6 fatty acid that seems to be at the root of many modern diseases.

Omega-6 fatty acids contribute to pro-inflammatory pathways in the body, and the huge increase in the proportion of dietary fat that comes from omega-6s (instead of omega-3s) is a major player in a wide range of health problems.

But it gets worse! These omega-6 fatty acids are concentrated in modern vegetable oils, which we've been encouraged to consume in place of natural animal fats due to unfounded fears surrounding saturated fat and cholesterol. Oils derived from grains and legumes (soybean oil, canola oil, safflower oil, peanut oil, corn oil, and so on) didn't exist until the process of mechanical extraction was invented. So we are consuming omega-6 fatty acids not only from grain-containing foods, but also from the vegetable oils in which they are cooked.

Another insidious way in which omega-6-rich grains have negatively impacted human health is through farmed meat. Cows, pigs, sheep, chickens, and even some farmed fish are fed grains instead of their more diverse, biologically appropriate diets. The meat from these animals no longer contains a balanced 1:1 ratio of omega-3 to omega-6 fatty acids, which it did prior to the advent of agriculture. Instead, the ratio is typically closer to 1:10! It's not enough to avoid grains; we need to be mindful of what we eat that eats grains, too. In a perfect world, we would eat grass-fed beef, pasture-raised poultry, wild-caught fish, and wild game while avoiding all grains, legumes, and vegetable oils. (For more information about vegetable oils, see Chapter 20.)

THE EMPTIEST OF CALORIES

A healthy diet doesn't need to be devoid of problematic compounds. In reality, just about every food has checks in both the pros and the cons categories. For example, a handful of phytochemicals in broccoli can actually increase cancer growth! Of course, these phytochemicals are balanced by hundreds of other phytochemicals that prevent cancer. The point is that avoiding compounds that undermine health is just part of the equation, and it's important to recognize that genetic susceptibility, as well as things like the overall nutrient quality of the diet, sleep, stress, and activity, all play a role in how damaging these compounds are. For some people, they're disastrous, and for others, they're relatively benign. But there's still another reason to avoid grains: poor nutrient value!

For a long time, grains (especially whole grains) have been promoted as nutritious foods, with the claim that they contain important vitamins and minerals and thus enhance the nutritional quality of our diets. This might be true if we compare grains to extremely refined products, like pure white sugar and industrially processed oils, but compared to the foods that make up a Paleo diet—vegetables, fruits, nuts, meat, eggs, and seafood—grains are nutritional weaklings! For example, half a cup of dry oats contains zero or minuscule amounts of vitamin A, vitamins B2, B3, B5, B6, B9, and B12, vitamin C, vitamin D, vitamin E, vitamin K, calcium, and potassium. In fact, oats contain only one vitamin in significant quantity: vitamin B1 (14 percent of the daily value). Meanwhile, cooked wild salmon is rich in not only vitamin B1, but also vitamins B2, B3, B5, B9, and B12, selenium, phosphorus, potassium, magnesium, and copper, and it even has some iron and zinc . . . need I go on?

And that's just one example. If we compare virtually any grain (even in whole form) side by side with any vegetable, fruit, nut, seed, or whole-food animal product in terms of vitamin and mineral content (see page 23), the grain will lose almost every time. Plus, vegetables and fruits contain just as much fiber for far less glycemic load and overall calories (see page 45), making them better choices every single time.

Removing grains from the menu and replacing them with nutrient-dense Paleo foods will automatically improve the nutritional quality of our diets. In turn, a higher intake of micronutrients will support numerous functions in our body and help safeguard us against disease. Even if specific harmful compounds in grains weren't an issue, they would still cause damage by displacing more nutrient-dense and nutrient-diverse foods.

So is there any reason to eat grains, legumes, and pseudograins when we have access to nutritious Paleo foods that are lower in lectins, digestive enzyme inhibitors, saponins, phytates, and omega-6 fats and higher in micronutrients? With a few exceptions (see Chapter 24), all signs point to no!

ARE PSEUDOGRAINS PSEUDOBAD?

Pseudograins are the starchy seeds or fruits of broadleaf plants—the most common of which are amaranth, buckwheat, chia, and quinoa—whereas cereal grains are the starchy seeds of grasses. Pseudograins definitely provide more nutrition than grains, having good amounts of vitamins B1, B2, B3, B6, and B9, magnesium, phosphorous, copper, and manganese as well as fiber and some iron. They also contain some antioxidant and anticancer phytochemicals. Chia is a rich source of omega-3 fats, albeit in the less-useful ALA form. Given that these starchy seeds are often touted as superfoods, why do they get lumped in with grains as a Paleo no-no?

As already referenced throughout this chapter, pseudograins contain many of the same problematic compounds found in grains and legumes—including prolamins, agglutinins, saponins, phytates, and digestive enzyme inhibitors—although the amounts tend to be lower. For example, quinoa contains about 7 percent prolamins as a percentage of total protein, compared to 65 percent in wheat. And while several studies have shown that quinoa does not aggravate celiac disease activity, one study that analyzed fifteen different cultivars of quinoa demonstrated that four contained gluten cross-reactive proteins and two (Ayacuchana and Pasankalla) stimulated T cells isolated from celiac disease patients comparably to gluten. Amaranth prolamins weakly bind with antibodies against gliadin, indicating some cross-reactivity, although studies generally conclude that amaranth is safe for celiac disease sufferers.

Quinoa is particularly high in saponins, which remain unchanged even after cooking (although they can be reduced somewhat by soaking and then rinsing quinoa). While quinoa saponins have been shown to reduce the production of some inflammatory cytokines in cell culture models, vaccine research has proven that quinoa saponins are powerful adjuvants, meaning that they're great at ramping up an immune response to an antigen. What's more, ingested quinoa saponins act as what's called a mucosal adjuvant, meaning that they both increase the amount of antigen that crosses from the gut into the blood (by increasing intestinal permeability) and exaggerate the antibody response to that antigen. They do the same thing for intranasal administration, so they can increase the permeability of other epithelial barriers, too. Quinoa saponins have also been shown to increase intestinal permeability in pigs (no human studies have been done).

Amaranth saponins have been shown to be toxic at very high doses in animal studies (it would be challenging for humans to consume anywhere near that level) and also to have some hemolytic activity (meaning that they can break blood cells apart), indicating that they could impact the health of the gut barrier. Amaranth also contains low levels of phytohemagglutinin (see page 249).

Buckwheat is often contaminated with wheat, making it difficult to determine whether issues caused are due to buckwheat itself or to gluten. However, the digestive enzyme inhibitors in buckwheat cause moderate activation of the innate immune system (about 20 percent of the bioactivity of gluten-containing grains). The digestive enzyme inhibitors in quinoa cause a low-level response (about 10 percent of the bioactivity of gluten-containing grains), and amaranth causes a very low-level response (about 2 percent).

What about chia? This pseudograin comes from a different family than quinoa, buckwheat, or amaranth, and it doesn't appear to contain the problematic compounds identified in other pseudograins. While chia doesn't get an automatic pass owing to its mucilaginous fiber content, which is discussed in more detail on page 308, chia is particularly high in calcium, phosphorus, potassium, and magnesium, with moderate amounts of sodium, iron, zinc, vitamin B3, and vitamin C. Chia contains between two and ten times more fiber than whole grains and a 3:1 ratio of omega-3s to omega-6s. Chia also contains antioxidant phytochemicals, including chlorogenic and caffeic acids, as well as the flavonols myricetin, quercetin, and kaempferol.

In summary, quinoa definitely deserves its place on the Paleo Foods to Avoid list, and compelling arguments can be made against buckwheat and amaranth, although more scientific studies are definitely needed. Chia is considered a middle-ground food.

BUSTING THE MYTH OF LEGUMES AS QUALITY PROTEIN

Plants are great sources of plenty of important nutrients . . . but protein isn't one of them! As discussed in Chapter 10, plant protein takes a back seat to animal protein in terms of quality, digestibility, and density.

Few plant foods provide complete protein, meaning all nine essential amino acids—the small number that do include quinoa, soybeans, chia seeds, hemp seeds, buckwheat, potatoes, pumpkin seeds, cashews, and a handful of others. Plus, even these top-performing plant foods contain protein that is hard for our bodies to digest and absorb, which is reflected by their low Digestible Indispensable Amino Acid Scores (DIAAS); see page 169. The nail in the coffin: plant foods are not dense sources of protein. While animal foods are predominantly protein (recall that chicken breast is 80 percent protein and light tuna is 94 percent protein), even those plant foods that we consider "high protein" contain only a fraction of those amounts: garbanzo beans are 19 percent protein, quinoa is 15 percent protein, and almonds are 13 percent protein; soybeans top the list at 30 percent. There's nothing wrong with the fiber and nutritive carbohydrates in whole plant foods—in fact, those things are pretty great—but when it comes to protein, plant foods aren't taking home any trophies!

SCIENCE SIMPLIFIED *It's a myth that plants can provide us with the same or better-quality protein than animal foods. Plant protein is harder for our bodies to digest and utilize, and plants are far less protein-dense than animal foods. Of course, vegetables and fruits abound with valuable nutrition (see page 62), which is why they make up two-thirds to three-quarters of the Paleo plate!*

Along with providing building blocks for protein synthesis, different sources of protein have different effects on our health. In numerous studies, vegan and vegetarian diets containing only or mostly plant protein have been associated with lower bone density and higher fracture rates. For athletes, animal protein (especially from meat) appears to support muscle growth and reduce the breakdown of lean mass more than vegetable protein. And one controlled trial showed that soy protein failed to raise participants' metabolic rates, diet-induced thermogenesis, and 24-hour spontaneous physical activity as much as pork protein.

It's a myth that legumes can provide our bodies with quality protein. But what if you're vegetarian for religious or ethical reasons? Although an omnivorous diet is optimal for supporting human health (see Chapter 3), people who choose vegetarian diets can still have an adequate protein intake by planning their diets wisely. No amino acids are exclusive to animal foods, and true protein deficiency is rarely seen outside of chronic starvation, crash diets, and medical conditions that result in malabsorption (including celiac disease and Crohn's disease)—so developing a true deficiency due to a plant-only diet is *really* unlikely.

The best ways for vegetarians to get a wide and sufficient intake of amino acids are to eat a diverse diet (including a variety of whole plant foods each day), consume adequate calories (or, in the case of weight-loss diets, a small calorie deficit that promotes slow but steady fat loss rather than a drastic reduction in energy intake), optimize digestion to avoid malabsorption (see page 77), and consume plenty of eggs and/or high-quality grass-fed dairy if tolerated. Although these diets will be missing out on other benefits of animal foods, including some important nutrients (supplementation will be required), they can still provide a spectrum of essential and nonessential amino acids. A great compromise is a pescetarian diet because seafood (see Chapter 9) can provide all the same nutrients found in red meat and poultry.

GRAINS, LEGUMES, AND PSEUDOGRAINS

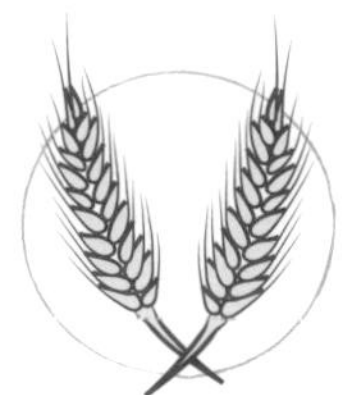

GRAINS are the starchy seeds of grasses and include:

- barley
- corn (aka maize)
- fonio
- job's tears
- kamut
- millet
- oat
- rice
- rye
- sorghum
- spelt
- teff
- triticale
- wheat (all varieties, including einkorn, durum, and semolina)
- wild rice

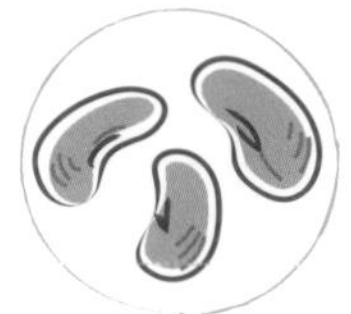

LEGUMES are members of the pea family. Often just the bean is consumed, but sometimes the pod is consumed as well, as in the case of snow peas or green beans. Legumes include:

- alfalfa
- carob
- chickpea
- clover
- common bean
- fava bean
- field pea or garden pea
- lentil
- lima bean
- lupin
- mesquite
- mung bean
- peanut
- pigeon pea
- rooibos
- runner bean
- soybean
- tamarind

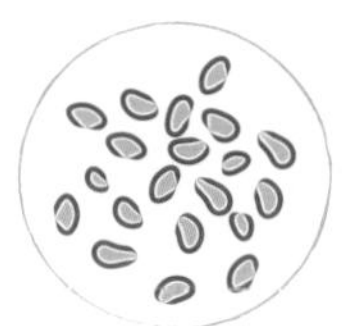

PSEUDOGRAINS are the starchy seeds of broad-leafed plants, including:

- amaranth
- buckwheat
- chia seeds
- quinoa

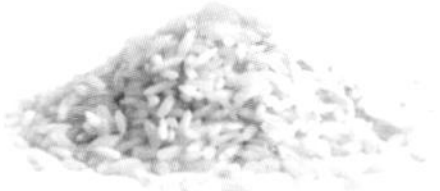

For more on rice, see page 302.

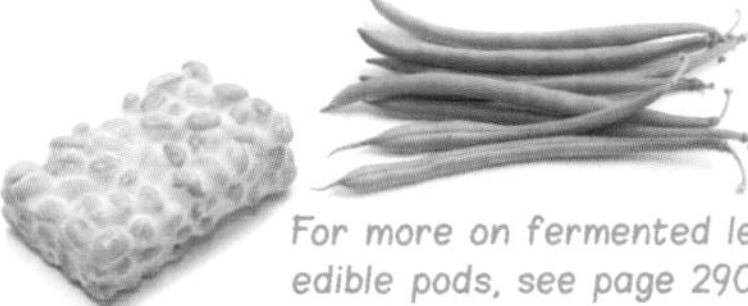

For more on fermented legumes and legumes with edible pods, see page 290.

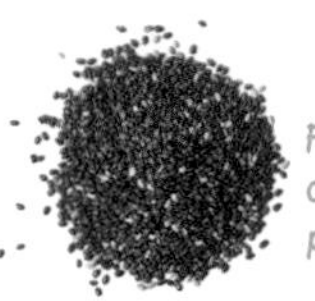

For more on chia seeds, see page 256.

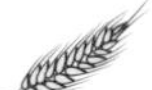

A variety of proteins in grains—including prolamins, such as gluten, and agglutinins, such as wheat germ agglutinin—cause increased intestinal permeability, feed bacterial overgrowth in the gut, and stimulate the immune system.

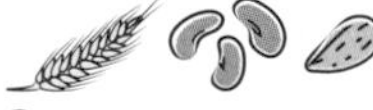

Digestive enzyme inhibitors in grains and legumes, as well as nuts, seeds, and dairy products, cause increased intestinal inflammation, feed bacterial overgrowth in the gut, and cause inflammation.

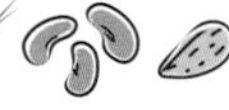

High dietary intake of phytates or phytic acid—found in grains and legumes, as well as nuts and seeds—causes increased intestinal permeability.

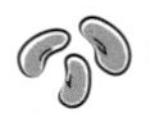
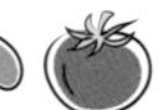

Saponins, found in legumes as well as vegetables of the nightshade family (see page 296), can cause increased intestinal permeability and significantly stimulate the immune system.

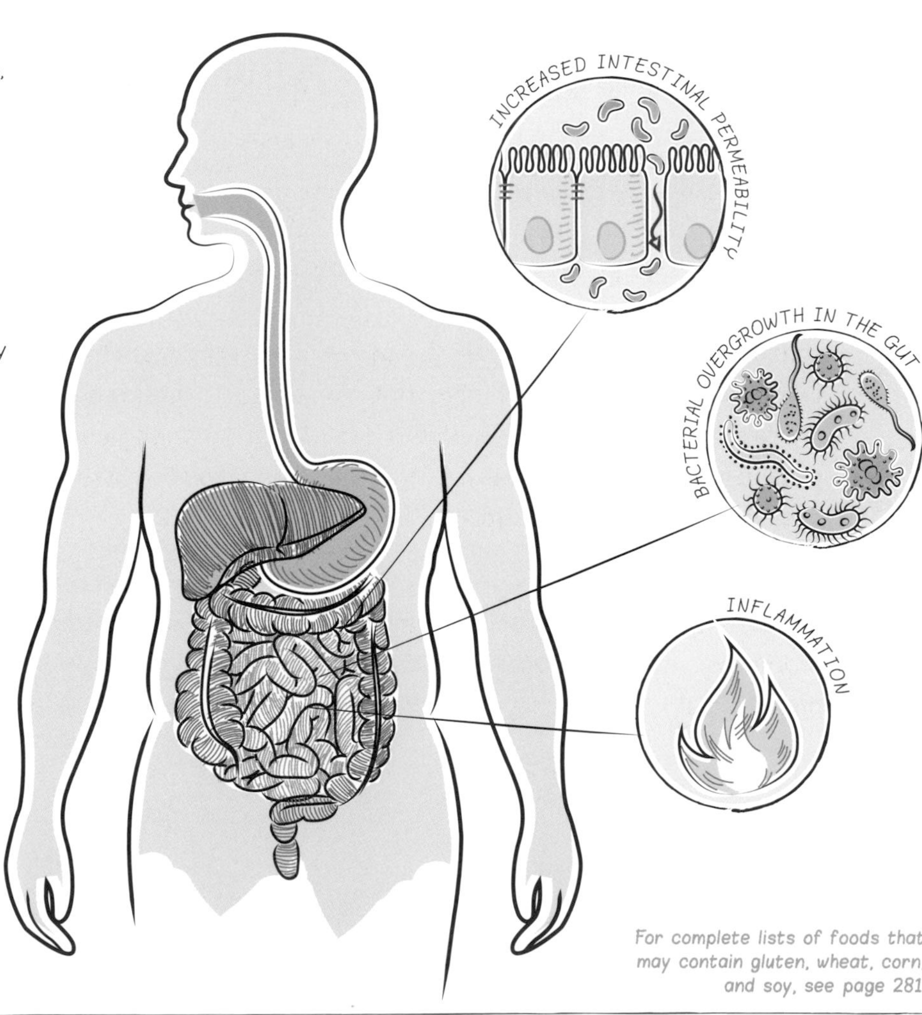

For complete lists of foods that may contain gluten, wheat, corn, and soy, see page 281.

Chapter 20: PROCESSED VEGETABLE OILS AND TRANS FATS

We've already looked at the evidence supporting the consumption of natural animal fats, omega-3 fatty acids, and cold-pressed plant oils rich in monounsaturated fat or medium-chain triglycerides. But what about the ubiquitous soybean, corn, canola, and other vegetable oils that seem to be in nearly every packaged food in the grocery store?

What comes as a surprise to many people is that these highly processed vegetable oils are among the worst fats we can put into our bodies. Unfortunately, plenty of high-profile institutions, including the American Heart Association, the USDA, and even Harvard Medical School, continue to promote processed vegetable oils based on the flawed logic that they tend to lower LDL ("bad") cholesterol and therefore must benefit cardiovascular health. In reality, the scientific evidence has a lot of bad news about these oils and what they do in our bodies.

So what exactly are processed vegetable oils? They are unsaturated oils extracted from seeds (including grains and legumes). Think soybean oil, corn oil, sunflower seed oil, cottonseed oil, and canola oil, to name a few. Vegetable oils require extensive processing because the types of plants that they come from don't give up their fat easily. (Imagine trying to extract fat from corn kernels!) That processing can include the use of mechanical extraction, high heat, industrial chemicals, deodorization, and toxic solvents. And because this type of mechanical and chemical extraction didn't exist until fairly recently, vegetable oils (and their unique fatty acid profile) are relative newcomers to our diet. In fact, there is a strong correlation between vegetable oil consumption and the rise in chronic disease seen over the last 70 years—and the mechanisms described in this chapter explain the link.

As Chapter 11 explains, some plant-based oils (like extra-virgin olive oil, avocado oil, macadamia nut oil, and coconut oil) are totally fine because they can be cold-pressed, require minimal processing, retain more micronutrients and antioxidants, and have a more beneficial fatty acid profile. On the flip side, processed vegetable oils are harmful for a few major reasons.

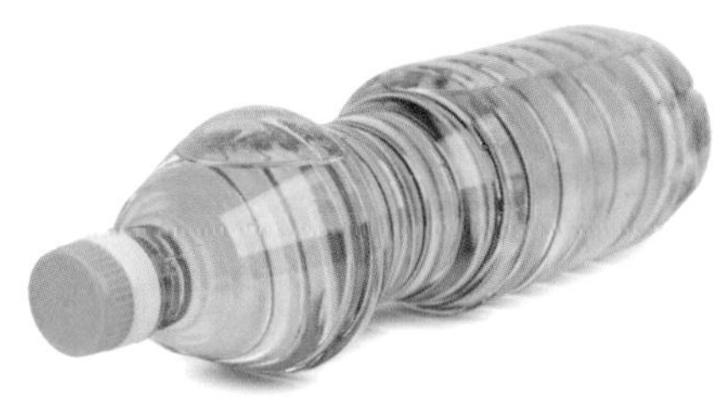

OMEGA-6 FATTY ACID CONTENT

The predominant fat in processed vegetable oils is omega-6 polyunsaturated fatty acids, mostly in the form of linoleic acid. Although small amounts of essential omega-6 fats are necessary for us to stay alive, most people eat *way* more than is required, especially relative to their omega-3 intake. (Recall that omega-3 and omega-6 compete for prostaglandin, thromboxane, and leukotriene formation, so balancing them is important; see page 158.) The ideal ratio between omega-3 and omega-6 fats is between 1:1 and 1:4, but the ratio in typical Western diets is closer to 1:16! And we owe a lot of that to a high intake of vegetable oils (along with grains and grain-fed animal products; see page 170). In fact, between 1909 and 1999, consumption of soybean oil alone increased one-thousand-fold in the U.S.! That led to a huge spike in the percentage of daily calories coming specifically from omega-6 fats.

SCIENCE SIMPLIFIED

Processed vegetable oils and products made with them (like many store-bought salad dressings) get the boot because they are very high in inflammatory omega-6 fatty acids.

While omega-3 fats contribute to anti-inflammatory processes, omega-6 fats contribute mainly to pro-inflammatory pathways. "Pro-inflammatory" sounds bad, but, in the balanced quantities that our ancestors consumed, it is critical for wound healing and fighting infections. There is a complex interplay between omega-3 and omega-6 fatty acids in our bodies, and both are essential for life. But when we combine excessive omega-6 fatty acid consumption with irritation to the gut lining caused by gluten and other lectins in grains and legumes as well as a host of modern lifestyle factors, our bodies have constant low-level inflammation. This sets the stage for many chronic diseases, a diminished ability to fight infection, and exaggerated allergies.

So when omega-6 fats are eaten in excess (or not balanced out with enough omega-3s), they can stir up tons of trouble. Studies have linked high intake of omega-6 (and a low ratio of omega-3 to omega-6) with a wide range of health problems, including certain cancers, cardiovascular disease, inflammatory diseases, osteoporosis, autoimmune disease, metabolic dysfunction, and obesity. Trials involving an increase in the omega-3 to omega-6 ratio have been shown to improve survival after the development of heart disease, reduce the proliferation of rectal cells in people with colorectal cancer, reduce asthma symptoms, and suppress inflammation in people with rheumatoid arthritis. Bottom line: the introduction of processed vegetable oils to our diet has pushed our omega-6 intake to unprecedented levels and may be at the root of many modern chronic diseases.

FAT COMPOSITION OF VEGETABLE OILS
Per 100-Gram Serving

	TOTAL FAT	SATURATED FAT	MONOUNSATURATED FAT	OMEGA-6 FATTY ACIDS	OMEGA-3 FATTY ACIDS	TRANS FAT
Canola oil	100 g	7.4 g	63.3 g	18.6 g	9.1 g	0.4 g
Corn oil	100 g	12.9 g	27.6 g	53.5 g	1.2 g	0.3 g
Cottonseed oil	100 g	25.9 g	17.8 g	51.5 g	0.2 g	0 g
Grapeseed oil	100 g	9.6 g	16.1 g	69.6 g	0.1 g	0 g
Margarine (stick, composite)	80.7 g	15.2 g	38.9 g	22.3 g	2.0 g	14.9 g
Margarine (tub, composite)	80.2 g	14.2 g	36.4 g	22.1 g	4.6 g	5.8 g
Margarine (Canola Harvest Brand)	80.3 g	21.3 g	45.3 g	15.1 g	6.1 g	0.3 g
Palm kernel oil (nonhydrogenated)	100 g	81.5 g	11.4 g	1.6 g	0 g	0 g
Palm kernel oil (hydrogenated)	100 g	88.2 g	5.7 g	0 g	0 g	4.7 g
Peanut oil	100 g	16.9 g	46.2 g	32.0 g	0 g	0 g
Safflower oil	100 g	6.2 g	14.4 g	74.6 g	0 g	0 g
Safflower oil (high oleic)	100 g	6.2 g	74.6 g	14.4 g	0 g	0 g
Vegetable shortening	100 g	25 g	41.2 g	26.2 g	1.8 g	13.2 g
Soybean oil	100 g	15.6 g	22.8 g	50.4 g	6.8 g	0.5 g
Sunflower oil	100 g	10.3 g	19.5 g	65.7 g	0 g	0 g
Sunflower oil (high oleic)	100 g	9.7 g	83.6 g	3.6 g	0.2 g	0 g

OXIDATION

One problem with highly unsaturated oils like processed vegetable oils is their susceptibility to oxidation. Because polyunsaturated fats (omega-3 and omega-6 fatty acids) contain multiple double bonds (compared to monounsaturated fats, which have only one double bond, and saturated fats, which have none), they're prone to reacting with oxygen. And worse, because processed vegetable oils contain very little in the way of vitamins and phytochemicals, there isn't much in these oils to prevent oxidation (as opposed to the polyphenol and vitamin E content of olive oil, for example; see page 184). When processed vegetable oils like sunflower and canola oil oxidize, they generate many degradation products, including aldehydes, ketones, epoxides, and hydroxy compounds. Many of these degradation products are considered toxic and potentially carcinogenic. And consumption of oxidized fats is conclusively linked to cardiovascular disease.

KNOWLEDGE BOMB

Did you just see the word ketones and think, "That doesn't sound bad!"? While you may have heard the term ketones used in conjunction with ketogenic diets (which I don't recommend for most people and discuss in detail in Chapters 2 and 33), ketones are not actually the energy molecule upon which ketogenic diets are based. What advocates are actually referring to are ketone bodies, which are any of three molecules (acetoacetate, β-hydroxybutyrate, and acetone) that are produced during fasting, starvation, prolonged intense exercise, and poorly treated type 1 diabetes. Ketone bodies can be converted to acetyl-CoA, which can then be oxidized in the mitochondria into the ubiquitous energy molecule ATP. Ketones, on the other hand, are simple chemical compounds that contain a carbonyl group (a carbon-oxygen double bond). They have uses as solvents, polymer precursors, and pharmaceuticals. Most are nontoxic, but they are still not something to be excited about when it comes to ingesting in oxidized vegetable oils.

Oxidation of vegetable oil can happen before the oil enters the body, such as during cooking or if the oil is improperly stored and becomes rancid. In fact, substantial oxidation and degradation of vegetable oil starts at about 210°F (99°C), a much lower temperature than most cooking applications and much lower than the smoke points of these oils, and the problem accelerates the longer and hotter the oil is heated. This is why commercial fried foods are such a problem; the vegetable oils in commercial deep fryers are typically heated to around 375°F (191°C) and kept at this temperature for long periods. In fact, some restaurants and fast-food joints change out their deep fryer oil only once per week (while filtering it up to several times a day).

Oxidation also can happen inside our bodies, when the fats we consume from vegetable oils get incorporated into our tissues. While consuming already-oxidized oil is bad, oxidation of fats inside the body is also highly problematic. One of the ways a high omega-6 intake may contribute to cancer is by increasing the proportion of omega-6 in our cell membranes, leading to lipid peroxidation (where oxidants react with lipids in the cell membrane and cause them to degrade, resulting in cell damage) and ultimately DNA damage. By contrast, saturated and monounsaturated fats are much less prone to oxidation as a result of their chemical structures.

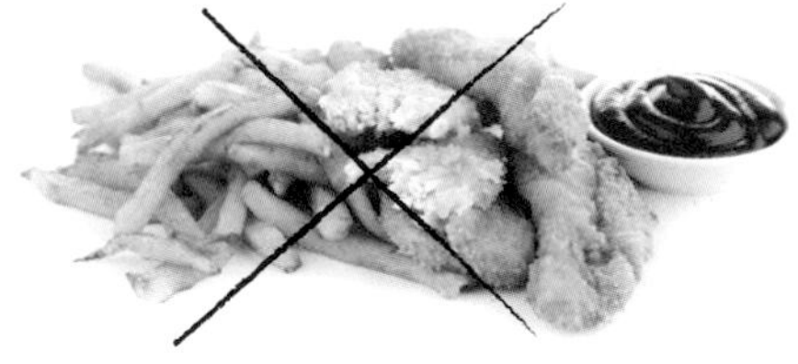

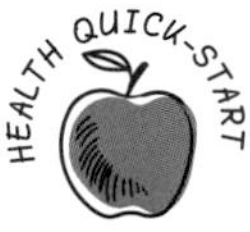

Beyond avoiding fast food, avoid the following:

- *canola oil*
- *corn oil*
- *cottonseed oil*
- *grapeseed oil*
- *margarine and other butter substitutes*
- *nonstick cooking spray*
- *palm kernel oil*
- *peanut oil*
- *safflower oil*
- *shortening*
- *soybean oil*
- *sunflower oil*
- *"vegetable" oil*
- *anything with the word hydrogenated*

TRANS FATS

Another harmful fat on the Paleo "avoid" list is man-made *trans* fats. For years, *trans* fats have been in the news as health hazards, with the potential to increase heart disease risk by lowering HDL ("good") cholesterol, raising LDL cholesterol, and increasing inflammation. In 2015, the FDA enforced a decision to phase out food companies' use of trans fat-rich oils. But even when we know they're bad, many people don't understand what exactly *trans* fats are and how they can harm us. What's really wrong with this type of fat?

Recall that a fatty acid is rendered monounsaturated or polyunsaturated by the presence of one or more double bonds in the hydrocarbon chain. The double bond can put a kink or bend in that chain, depending on where the hydrogen atoms are located in relation to the bond. This bend is called a "cis" configuration, and it is the most frequent configuration of double bonds found in monounsaturated and polyunsaturated fatty acids in nature. The other possible configuration is a "trans" configuration, in which the hydrocarbon chain is not bent at the location of the double bond and instead remains straight. There are some naturally occurring *trans* fats, but not many.

Commercially, *trans* fats are formed by taking a polyunsaturated oil (vegetable oil) and injecting it with hydrogen to make it more solid—a process called hydrogenation. This process converts some of the *cis* double bonds to trans double bonds, resulting in a partially hydrogenated oil that is high in *trans* fats. Because of their texture and long shelf life (saturating some of the double bonds makes these fats less susceptible to oxidation), hydrogenated oils were used extensively by food manufacturers to make cheap, shelf-stable products. The highest levels of *trans* fats are found in margarines, processed snack foods, frozen dinners, commercial baked goods, and fast food.

But what's good for the food industry isn't necessarily good for human health! In numerous studies, *trans* fats have been linked to higher LDL cholesterol, lower HDL cholesterol, and higher inflammation with a dose-dependent effect (that is, the more *trans* fat we eat, the more significant the changes in these risk factors). In mice, *trans* fats have been shown to reduce the responsiveness of a growth factor called TGF-β1 that helps control the growth, proliferation, differentiation, and apoptosis (programmed and controlled death) of cells. Population studies consistently link higher consumption of *trans* fats directly to heart disease. And some research shows a link between *trans* fats and diabetes, likely due to the effect on insulin sensitivity and glucose transport when these fats are integrated into cell membranes. Several studies have even suggested that *trans* fats could raise the risk of certain cancers.

Given the information above, the dangers of *trans* fats might seem like a case-closed issue. But there are other forms of *trans* fat that occur naturally in meat and dairy, and their health effects are much different from those of the *trans* fats in vegetable oils. Ruminants (like cows and sheep) have specific gut microbes that form *trans* fats through a process called biohydrogenation. These *trans* fats have a slightly different chemical structure than industrial *trans* fats and as a result behave differently in the human body. When scientists separate industrial *trans* fatty acids (iTFA) from ruminant *trans* fatty acids (rTFA) in studies, ruminant *trans* fats don't appear to raise cardiovascular risk factors at normal intake levels (and even up to over 4 percent of total energy intake, which is much more than most people would ever consume!). One type of ruminant *trans* fat, vaccenic acid, has been shown to suppress intestinal inflammation and reduce certain endocannabinoids in the liver and visceral fat. Another ruminant *trans* fat, the more widely studied conjugated linoleic acid (CLA), can help improve glucose tolerance, facilitate fat loss, and protect against certain cancers (by blocking the growth and spread of tumors), and in most studies has either a neutral or a protective effect against heart disease (see page 169).

Fortunately, if we stick to a Paleo diet based on whole, nutrient-dense foods and avoid commercially processed convenience foods and margarine, our intake of industrial *trans* fats will be zero (or close to it). And consuming grass-fed ruminant meat and dairy can supply us with the types of natural *trans* fats that can actually benefit our health.

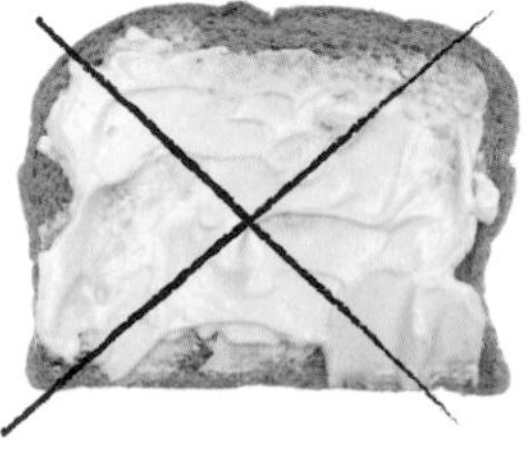

Chapter 21: INDUSTRIALLY PRODUCED DAIRY

When it comes to health benefits versus risks, dairy is a mixed bag. On the one hand, grass-fed dairy provides important fat-soluble vitamins, protein, and fatty acids like conjugated linoleic acid (CLA), and fermented dairy can be a good source of probiotic bacteria (see page 191). On the other hand, dairy products are insulinogenic (that is, they cause a release of insulin; see page 85), contain an array of hormones, and contain protease inhibitors, which may cause gut inflammation (see page 251), and the jury is still out on whether the fats in dairy prevent or cause cardiovascular disease and whether the proteins in dairy prevent or cause cancer. But when it comes to industrially produced dairy, the cons generally outweigh the pros.

"Industrially produced" dairy refers to non-organic, pasteurized, homogenized (in the case of milk) dairy products from cows eating grain in feedlots (instead of grazing on pasture). Compared to grass-fed dairy, industrially produced dairy has lower levels of vitamin A, selenium, vitamin E, CLA (five times less), and omega-3 fats (about 50 percent less alpha-linolenic acid), as well as a less-favorable omega-3 to omega-6 ratio. In fact, grass-fed dairy is an entirely different beast than industrially produced dairy, which is why it is discussed separately in Chapter 24.

Although the evidence is limited, concern also exists about a potential link between the artificial growth hormones used in conventional dairy farming (rbST and rbGH) and increased risk of cancer in humans via an effect on IGF-1 levels. These growth hormones can also cause problems in cows that require antibiotic treatment, such as a painful infection called mastitis. (In turn, antibiotic use can increase the spread of *Salmonella* bacteria among livestock.) In fact, rbST has been banned in Australia, Canada, Israel, Japan, New Zealand, and the European Union since the year 2000.

Similarly, industrially processed dairy is more likely to contain harmful additives such as carrageenan and xanthan gum (in the case of cream and cream cheese), high-fructose corn syrup, other refined sweeteners, and food dyes (in the case of yogurt and flavored milk beverages); see Chapters 18 and 22.

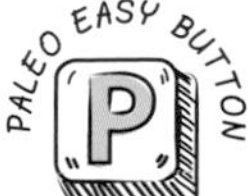

While most premade coconut and nut-based alternative dairy beverages contain emulsifiers (see page 235), making these drinks at home is actually quite straightforward. Recipes can be found on pages 480 and 481.

Industrially produced dairy offers few benefits to balance out its downsides, including potential issues involving lactose intolerance, dairy protein allergies, gluten cross-reactivity (see page 245), and the role of dairy in inducing leaky gut (all discussed in more detail in Chapter 24). For people who do tolerate dairy products, grass-fed sources are vastly superior. However, even grass-fed dairy comes with a number of ticks in the cons category, so it is not fully endorsed on the Paleo template.

BUT WHAT ABOUT BONE HEALTH?

Dairy products are not the only good source of calcium out there. In fact, fruits, vegetables, nuts, seeds, meat, and seafood all contain substantial quantities of calcium. Let's compare some Paleo foods to a glass of milk:

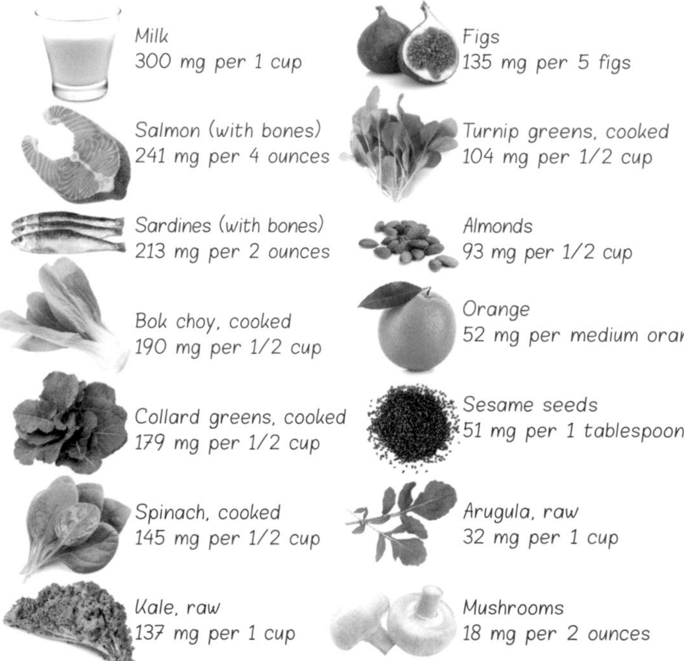
Milk
300 mg per 1 cup
Figs
135 mg per 5 figs
Salmon (with bones)
241 mg per 4 ounces
Turnip greens, cooked
104 mg per 1/2 cup
Sardines (with bones)
213 mg per 2 ounces
Almonds
93 mg per 1/2 cup
Bok choy, cooked
190 mg per 1/2 cup
Orange
52 mg per medium orange
Collard greens, cooked
179 mg per 1/2 cup
Sesame seeds
51 mg per 1 tablespoon
Spinach, cooked
145 mg per 1/2 cup
Arugula, raw
32 mg per 1 cup
Kale, raw
137 mg per 1 cup
Mushrooms
18 mg per 2 ounces

It's easy to see how a veggie-rich Paleo diet with an emphasis on seafood plus nuts and seeds in moderation can provide the Recommended Dietary Allowance of calcium every day. Another calcium-rich superstar is blackstrap molasses, discussed on page 304.

Not only do fruits, vegetables, nuts, seeds, and seafood contain substantial amounts of calcium, but there is scientific evidence that we absorb more calcium from cruciferous vegetables (like kale) than we do from dairy. Cruciferous vegetables (like kale, cabbage, broccoli, collard greens, and turnip greens) may be the best source of dietary calcium. In fact, several studies show that fruit and vegetable intake correlates much more strongly with bone health than dairy intake. In fact, the scientific evidence is mixed on dairy and bone health, with some studies indicating that higher dairy consumption may *increase* the risk of fractures and osteoporosis. Yes, to prevent osteoporosis and look after your bones, eat your veggies!

Other great sources of dietary calcium include green leafy vegetables, nuts (especially almonds), seeds (especially sesame seeds), figs, oranges, dried apricots, okra, bok choy, and seafood (especially when we eat the bones as you would with canned salmon or sardines).

Other fruits and vegetables also provide calcium, though to a lesser extent. Organ meat and long-cooked bone broth are sources of not only calcium, but also magnesium, phosphorous, and collagen, which are critical for bone health as well. The fact that minerals other than calcium are needed for healthy bones might be one of the reasons higher vegetable intake correlates with better bone health—vegetables also provide these other essential minerals, whereas dairy contains only a handful of nutrients.

Bone health is about much more than calcium. In fact, there are at least twenty micronutrients that are essential for bone health, either as constituents of bone, required for enzymatic activity involved in bone remodeling, or as regulators of bone formation. Bone is composed of a mixture of minerals (mainly calcium, phosphorous, magnesium, sodium, and potassium) deposited around a protein matrix that acts as a scaffold. It's the combination of inorganic (minerals) and organic (protein) materials that provide bone with both strength and flexibility. About 65 percent of bone tissue is minerals, chiefly calcium and phosphorous bound together in a molecule called hydroxyapatite. The remaining 35 percent is a protein matrix, 90 to 95 percent of which is type I collagen. Collagen fibers cross-link and twist around each other, forming the interior scaffolding upon which bone minerals are deposited.

Even after we're fully grown, our bones are constantly being remodeled—bone tissue is both resorbed (broken down), which is driven by a cell type called *osteoclasts*, and formed, which is driven by a cell type called *osteoblasts*. Osteoclasts erode the surface of bone by secreting enzymes that degrade the protein matrix and acids that solubilize bone minerals. Osteoblasts form new bone by secreting the protein matrix and then gradually mineralizing the matrix by secreting hydroxyapatite crystals. Osteoblasts then either die, become bone-lining cells, or become *osteocytes*, a cell type that regulates bone mass through signaling to osteoblasts and osteoclasts. The bone remodeling process loses equilibrium as we age: even by our mid-thirties, the rate of bone resorption can exceed that of bone formation (especially in the context of nutrient-deficient diets and sedentary lifestyles), leading to a loss of bone mass and higher rates of problems like osteoporosis and osteopenia (lower-than-normal bone density) as we age.

The major protein in bone is collagen, which we get richly from organ meat, seafood, and bone broth. The best sources of phosphorous are fish, shellfish, nuts, and seeds. We get magnesium from seafood, nuts, seeds, leafy dark green vegetables, and cruciferous vegetables. Potassium is found in leafy dark green vegetables, cruciferous vegetables, orange veggies, and some fruits (such as bananas and cantaloupe). In addition to protein and minerals as raw materials, fat-soluble vitamins (A, D, and K2 in particular) are essential regulators in bone mineralization. Where do we get these essential fat-soluble vitamins? Seafood, dairy fat from grass-fed cows (see page 288), and the fat from grass-fed and pasture-raised meats. Because the majority of people still don't buy meat and dairy from pasture-raised sources, for most people the dominant dietary source of these vitamins is seafood. No wonder high seafood intake also correlates with bone health!

Another major factor in bone health has nothing to do with food. Weight-bearing exercise-meaning exercise that involves moving your own body weight around, like walking-is excellent for our bones! Osteocytes are thought to be mechanosensor cells, meaning that they respond to mechanical stresses on bone, like the impact of walking, and signal to osteoblasts to produce more bone accordingly.

Basically, if you are eating plenty of fruits and vegetables (especially cruciferous vegetables) and seafood, sourcing the best-quality meat you can, maybe incorporating some bone broth into your diet, and getting some exercise (even if it's just walking), you are doing a great job of looking after your bones.

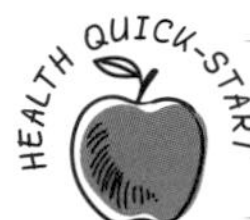

For a list of foods and ingredients that contain dairy, see page 284.

ESSENTIAL NUTRIENTS FOR BONE HEALTH

BORON (see page 28)
+ enhances calcium absorption
+ supports creation of bone-protecting hormones such as estrogen, testosterone, and DHEA

CALCIUM (see page 28)
+ a major component of bone
+ combines with phosphorous to form hydroxyapatite crystals
+ provides structure and microarchitecture

COLLAGEN (see page 179)
+ a major component of bone, making up 90–95% of the protein matrix of bone

COPPER (see page 28)
+ promotes bone mineralization and decreases bone loss
+ essential for cross-linking of collagen

FLUORIDE (see page 28)
+ component of mineralized bone, although too much makes bones brittle
+ stimulates new bone growth

INOSITOL (see page 27)
+ increases bone mineral density and improves bone strength

IRON (see page 28)
+ necessary for enzymes that form collagen bone matrix

L-ARGININE (see page 32)
+ increases bone mineral density and improves bone strength

MAGNESIUM (see page 28)
+ component of mineralized bone
+ important for bone mineralization
+ improves bone strength by controlling size of hydroxyapatite crystals

MANGANESE (see page 28)
+ necessary for creation of the connective-tissue components of bone

PHOSPHORUS (see page 29)
+ a major component of bone
+ combines with calcium to form hydroxyapatite crystals
+ provides structure and microarchitecture

POTASSIUM (see page 29)
+ preserves calcium in bones

SILICON (see page 29)
+ initiates the mineralization process
+ deficiency associated with bone abnormalities

VITAMIN A (see page 26)
+ regulates bone remodeling via osteoblast and osteoclast activity
+ both deficiency and excess linked to reduced bone mineral density

VITAMIN B6 (see page 26)
+ necessary for collagen synthesis

VITAMIN B12 (see page 27)
+ important for osteoblast function
+ low B12 is associated with reduced bone mineral density and higher fracture risk

VITAMIN C (see page 27)
+ necessary for collagen synthesis and cross-linking in bone

VITAMIN D (see page 92)
+ necessary for calcium and phosphorus absorption
+ promotes bone mineralization
+ osteoblasts have receptors for vitamin D

VITAMIN K (see page 27)
+ required for the creation of osteocalcin, a protein involved in the bone mineralization process

STRONTIUM (see page 29)
+ incorporated into bone to increase its strength
+ stimulates bone formation and inhibits bone resorption

ZINC (see page 29)
+ important for bone mineralization and collagen synthesis
+ decreases bone loss

Chapter 22: SUGARS

Over the past century, few foods have overtaken our food supply quite like sweeteners. Yet despite decades of research, the relationship between added sugar and human health is still a controversial topic. Around the globe, public health guidelines—including the World Health Organization, the Dietary Guidelines for Americans, the Nordic Nutrition Recommendations, and Public Health England—recommend limiting added (or "free") sugar intake to 10 percent of total calories or less, due to well-established effects on dental health, total caloric intake, obesity, inflammation, and related conditions. At the same time, some people question whether this upper limit is scientifically sound, leading to public confusion about how important it really is to avoid sugar.

Part of the confusion is due to aggressive action by the beverage industry (which relies on high-fructose corn syrup to sweeten drinks) to cast doubt on the validity of sugar research. For example, a systematic review published in December 2016 concluded that public health recommendations to reduce sugar intake were based on weak or inconclusive evidence, but this review was funded by the food and drink industry, which has a vested interest in neutralizing consumers' negative perception of sugar and sugary foods.

In reality, the evidence for greatly reducing or avoiding consumption of processed sweeteners is compelling. Beginning with sucrose (table sugar) and continuing with high-fructose corn syrup and artificial and noncaloric sweeteners (like sucralose, aspartame, and stevia), these ingredients can be large contributors to chronic disease. Even natural sweeteners like honey and maple syrup aren't off the hook, but since they have some redeeming nutritional features, they earn middle-ground status and are discussed separately in Chapter 24.

SUGAR AND INFLAMMATION

Carbohydrates are made up of sugar molecules, or *saccharides*. The most important and prevalent saccharide is glucose, the primary metabolic fuel for the human body and indeed most forms of life on Earth.

Carbohydrates are chemically classified based on the number of saccharides they contain: *monosaccharides* are made up of a single sugar molecule, *disaccharides* contain two sugar molecules, *oligosaccharides* are medium-length chains of three to ten sugar molecules, and *polysaccharides* are long chains that can be hundreds of sugar molecules long. From a dietary perspective, however, it's more relevant to classify carbohydrates based on how they're digested and absorbed:

- **Sugars,** also called *simple carbohydrates* or simple sugars, include monosaccharides like glucose, fructose, and galactose as well as disaccharides like sucrose (one fructose and one glucose), lactose (one glucose and one galactose), and maltose (two glucoses). Sugars give food a sweet taste and are naturally found in fruit, dairy products, and natural sweeteners like honey. They are digested and absorbed quickly, and the glucose they contain has a rapid effect on blood sugar levels and insulin secretion. (Note that the fiber present in whole fruit helps slow down the digestion of the sugars in the fruit.)

- **Starches** are *complex carbohydrates*, polysaccharides composed predominantly of glucose. Starch is produced by most plants as an energy storage molecule and is commonly found in grains, legumes, and root vegetables such as potatoes, sweet potatoes, and cassava. Starch takes longer to break down during digestion and has a more gradual impact on blood sugar levels than sugar.

- **Fiber** is also a complex carbohydrate, oligosaccharides and polysaccharides that don't get fully broken down by our digestive enzymes and instead are fermented by the bacteria and other microorganisms that live in our digestive tracts. Fiber is discussed in detail starting on page 39.

KNOWLEDGE BOMB *Whole-food carbohydrates, like fruits and vegetables, contain a mix of simple and complex carbohydrates, including fiber, which slows digestion and blunts the blood sugar response. Blood sugar regulation is further improved by consuming fruits and vegetables as part of a meal that also includes protein and fat.*

Refined carbohydrates refers to carbohydrates that have been processed. For example, when the bran and germ are milled away to make a refined grain product, most of the fiber is removed. The resultant starches are digested and absorbed rapidly, sometimes raising blood glucose levels as quickly as simple sugars do. See page 88 for more on glycemic index and glycemic load.

Simple sugars can also be refined. A prominent example of a processed sugar is high-fructose corn syrup. In this case, corn syrup is treated with enzymes to turn a portion of the syrup's glucose into fructose. High-fructose corn syrup is discussed further on page 275.

Most of the digestible carbohydrates that we consume are broken down into glucose, which is absorbed into the bloodstream and shuttled into cells by insulin (see page 85). Once in the cells, glucose is converted to adenosine triphosphate (ATP), the energy currency for all cells, in a series of chemical reactions collectively referred to as *cellular respiration* (since the process uses oxygen and produces carbon dioxide, much like our regular breathing does). Many ATP molecules can be formed from a single glucose molecule. Glucose molecules are first converted to pyruvate via glycolysis, which yields some ATP. Pyruvate then enters the mitochondria, where it is oxidized into acetyl-CoA, which can also yield some ATP. Acetyl-CoA is then converted to more ATP in what is called the *Krebs cycle* or *citric acid cycle,* an eight-step process involving eighteen different enzymes and co-enzymes. Other high-energy products of the Krebs cycle (NADH and FADH2) are converted to yet more ATP in the last step of cellular respiration, oxidative phosphorylation in the electron transport chain. This is complex biochemistry; the important takeaway here is that a whole lot of chemical reactions are required to turn sugar into a usable energy source for our cells!

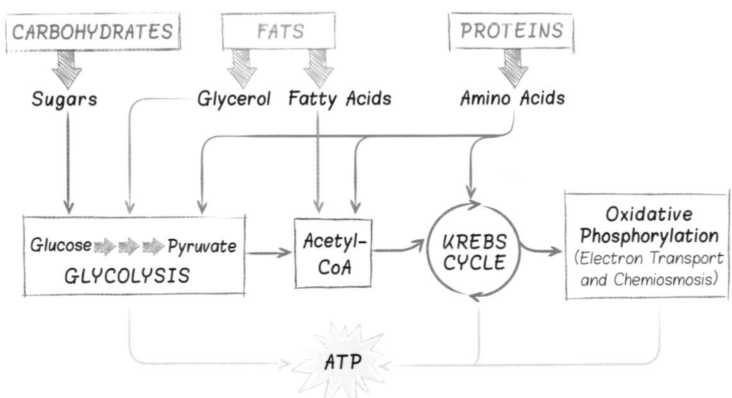

Glucose isn't the only molecule that can be converted to ATP via cellular respiration. Protein (amino acids), fats (fatty acids and glycerol), and other carbohydrates (like fructose) can be converted to various intermediates of the glycolysis, pyruvate oxidation, and Krebs cycle processes, allowing them to slip into the cellular respiration pathway at multiple points. However, glucose is the easiest to convert to ATP (it requires the least oxygen and can even produce some ATP anaerobically), so it is the preferred fuel for cells. Once the glucose that enters the bloodstream after a meal has been used up, cells metabolize stored fat and glycogen (stored carbohydrates) for energy.

A flexible metabolism is one that can easily switch between carbohydrates and fats, depending on what's available. Although protein is not a preferred source of energy, it can be used if needed—this is why people lose muscle mass in addition to fat when they are too severely calorically restricted, fasting, or starving.

Where does inflammation fit into this picture? A by-product of cellular respiration is the production of *reactive oxygen species* (ROS), also known as oxidants or free radicals. ROS are a group of chemically reactive molecules that contain oxygen. ROS have important roles in cell signaling (the complex communication between and within cells) and in homeostasis (the maintenance of a stable environment inside and outside the cell). But ROS are also potent signals for inflammation and can damage cells and tissue. In fact, they are produced and secreted by the cells of the immune system as one weapon in its arsenal to defend us from pathogens.

In general, the more energy (food) consumed, the more ROS produced. This production of ROS after meals is called postprandial oxidative stress or postprandial inflammation, and it continues to be a topic of intense study. In this sense, all foods are inflammatory—it is the price we pay for being aerobic organisms. Of course, our use of oxygen in metabolism is also what allows us to have such a wonderfully complex biological structure; anaerobic organisms are almost all single-celled. However, some eating patterns cause more oxidative stress and inflammation than others. Overeating in general is the biggest culprit, stimulating the production of ROS by flooding the body with energy, but so does high carbohydrate (especially refined carbohydrate) intake, even in the context of judicious caloric intake. High-carbohydrate diets cause more postprandial inflammation than low-carbohydrate diets, everything else being equal. Put simply, the more glucose we eat, the more inflammation we have!

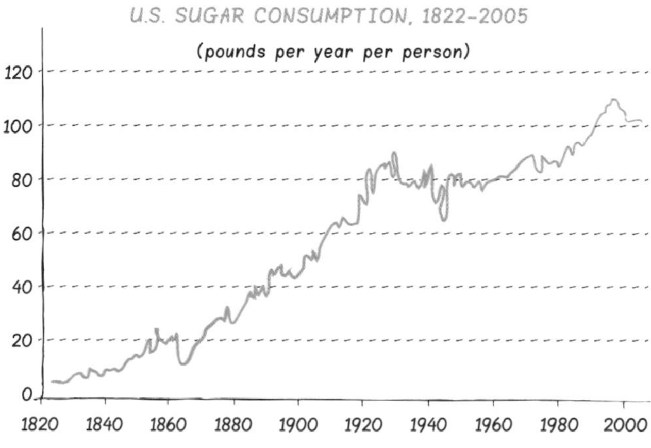

When it comes to sugar being inflammatory, dose matters. Today, the average American consumes almost 152 pounds of sugar each year, a staggering amount of refined simple carbohydrates equivalent to 6 cups of white sugar every week. This may be the single biggest dietary contributor to the rise in chronic disease. Consumption of glucose is associated with increased production of ROS and markers of inflammation, even in healthy people. However, it is exaggerated in those who are obese or have type 2 diabetes, high cholesterol, or metabolic syndrome. This is because postprandial inflammation is proportional to insulin sensitivity, or how effectively the body responds to insulin (see page 85): the less insulin sensitive (that is, the more insulin resistant) someone is, the more inflammation is created every time he or she eats. For this reason, simple sugars and refined carbohydrates that spike blood sugar levels cause more inflammation than whole-food sources of complex carbohydrates.

A healthy body has the ability to control both the amount of ROS and the damage they cause. In normal circumstances, the deleterious effects of these highly reactive molecules are balanced out by antioxidants: certain vitamins, minerals, and phytochemicals and the activity of some enzymes. However, when the production of ROS exceeds the availability of antioxidants, the resulting imbalance causes problems. Specifically, the overproduction of ROS stimulates inflammation and damages cells and tissue; this is called *oxidative stress.*

There is evidence that insulin itself is pro-inflammatory. A study of healthy subjects with controlled (and normal) blood glucose who were intravenously infused with insulin and glucose to achieve hyperinsulinemia (elevated blood insulin) showed that hyperinsulinemia caused an exaggerated inflammatory response to endotoxin (a toxin from the cell wall of Gram-negative bacteria; see page 186). An exaggerated stress response was also observed, meaning that hyperinsulinemia also contributes to increased cortisol (see page 85). Another study measured the levels of fasting insulin (the levels recorded first thing in the morning) in volunteers with normal blood sugar levels and found that those with higher fasting insulin levels also had more markers of inflammation, like C-reactive protein, or CRP. In a person who is insulin resistant, the pancreas secretes more and more insulin to handle elevated blood sugar, which contributes to inflammation and insulin resistance.

The takeaway here is that blood sugar regulation is essential for controlling inflammation. The Western diet is typified by the excessive consumption of calorie-dense, nutrient-poor foods that cause abnormal surges in blood glucose with little in the way of dietary antioxidants to balance things out. This doesn't mean that we should aim to eat a "low-carb diet" but that we should avoid eating a high-carb diet and instead focus on a variety of nutrient-dense whole foods (see Chapters 2 and 3). For more on how natural sweeteners like honey and maple syrup fit into the Paleo template, see Chapter 24.

SCIENCE SIMPLIFIED

Going low-carb isn't as important as simply making sure that blood sugar levels are well regulated by avoiding excessive carbohydrates, especially refined carbs and sugars. Most people can achieve healthy blood glucose levels by eating whole-food sources of slow-burning carbohydrates like those summarized on page 87 in the context of a nutrient-dense anti-inflammatory diet.

THE WORST OFFENDER: FRUCTOSE

A collection of recent research articles focuses on the effects of a simple sugar that could be causing a lot of trouble: fructose. In part because fructose makes up half of table sugar and in part because of the proliferation of high-fructose corn syrup, average fructose consumption is skyrocketing. Recent studies have shown that the average amount of fructose consumed daily is around 55 grams, which accounts for more than 10 percent of the total caloric intake of the American diet. Intake varies by gender and age group, of course; for example, young men consume an average of 75 grams of fructose per day! Compare this average to estimates of historic fructose consumption of between 15 and 20 grams daily, largely from fruit but also from vegetables. Today's average fructose intake is about three times higher, with our consumption having skyrocketed in the last 40 years.

U.S. PER CAPITA SWEETENER AVAILABILITY, 1966-2012

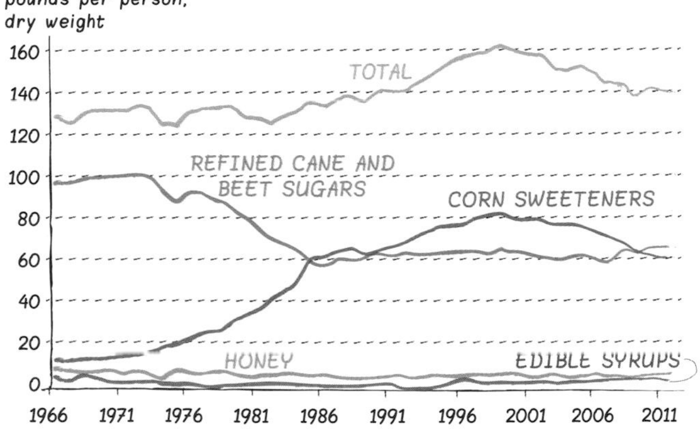

Source: USDA, Economic Research Service, Food Availability Data

Certainly, scientific studies support that a low to moderate fructose intake is healthful—it's only a high intake of fructose (like the typical intake of the Standard American Diet) that causes problems. While most of us following a Paleo diet automatically fall into the low to moderate range of fructose consumption, it's important to address the dangers of high fructose consumption, because this new science makes fructose look *really* bad, and because it's still possible to overdo fructose within a Paleo framework.

SCIENCE SIMPLIFIED

High fructose consumption—more than 50 grams per day—is linked to a huge variety of health problems, including all those that have grown to epidemic proportions over the last 50 years. And when you combine high fructose consumption with low vitamin D levels (approximately 75 percent of us are deficient in vitamin D; see page 92), you've got a perfect storm when it comes to bone health, liver health, and prostate health.

High fructose consumption has been linked to obesity, insulin resistance, hypertension, fatty liver disease, type 2 diabetes, cardiovascular disease, metabolic syndrome, and increased cancer risk. While the topic of fructose is still considered controversial within the scientific community, it won't be for much longer, thanks to the recent scientific studies elucidating the exact mechanisms of the negative health impacts of high fructose consumption. Correlation does not equal causation, at least until we have the mechanistic studies to explain how A causes B. And with fructose, we do!

Fructose consumption wasn't really a problem until high-fructose corn syrup was invented. Its use is so common due to its concentrated sweetness (meaning that companies can use less of it) and cheap manufacturing cost. There have been conspicuous parallels between the rise in obesity and fructose consumption. High-fructose corn syrup ranges from 42 to 60 percent fructose (the rest is mostly glucose), which is an incredibly high concentration relative to the amount found naturally in fruit. A mere 1½ tablespoons of high-fructose corn syrup—the amount in about half a can of Coke—has the same amount of fructose as a whole apple or 3 cups of strawberries. (See page 152 for the fructose content of common fruits.)

Here's where the problems begin! The difference between fructose and glucose is a small difference—just a couple of atoms—but that difference means a *lot* for metabolism. Glucose can be metabolized by virtually any cell in the body to create energy for all our cells, with extra glucose being stored as fat. Glucose is like fructose's overachieving sibling: it's able to do more with greater efficiency. When we consume glucose, it makes its way into the bloodstream through our intestinal walls and can be transported into cells using the receptor GLUT4, which is activated by insulin. When we consume glucose, the hormone leptin is released from fat cells, telling our brains that our stomachs are satiated and our bodies have enough energy to do their thing until our next meal.

Fructose, on the other hand, is more problematic both from an absorption standpoint (how effectively it is transported from the gut into the bloodstream) and from a metabolic standpoint (how it is used for energy and communicates with hormones). First, fructose consumed alone is more difficult for the gut to absorb than fructose consumed in combination with glucose and protein (such as enjoying a piece of fruit with a meal). Once fructose hits the bloodstream, it does *not* stimulate the release of insulin like glucose does. This lack of signaling is an issue because a large intake of fructose would not generate the appropriate response to sugar intake: the release of the hormone insulin, which is key for energy balance. This fact alone gives us a clearer understanding of how fructose could be contributing to the obesity epidemic.

Fructose cannot enter most cells to be metabolized; it requires transport via the GLUT5 receptor, which is found in a limited number of cell types, whereas GLUT4, which transports glucose, is found in almost every cell in the body (especially in fat cells and muscle cells, where energy is stored or used most). So while glucose is an easy-to-use energy source, fructose must find its way to where it is metabolized before it can be used for energy.

Here's where it starts to get really problematic: fructose is metabolized almost exclusively in the liver by the enzyme ketohexokinase-C (KHK-C). This process puts an additional load on our generally overstressed livers. And this enzymatic action is key for two reasons: overindulgence in high-fructose foods has recently been shown to upregulate GLUT5 transporters in the gut, and KHK is found only in the heart and liver. The latter point is really important because it translates to fructose being metabolized in the heart to create more heart cells—which can contribute to heart disease (more on this later).

When fructose is metabolized, the end products are triglycerides, uric acid, and free radicals, all of which are concerning. Triglycerides are long-chain fatty acids that can be stored immediately as fat or remain in the bloodstream, contributing to heart disease risk. Likewise, this production of triglycerides has been shown to contribute to the development and progression of nonalcoholic fatty liver disease. Uric acid has been directly linked with increased risk for metabolic syndrome and renal disease and is the cause of gout. Free radicals are highly reactive molecules that can damage DNA and have been directly linked with fructose-related issues with blood vessels in people who already have insulin resistance.

This is why high fructose consumption has been associated with a host of chronic health problems, including insulin resistance, dyslipidemia (high LDL ["bad"] cholesterol and triglycerides), hypertension, and obesity—all of which increase the risk of other health problems, like metabolic syndrome, diabetes, and cardiovascular disease. Even though the evidence on fructose is already damning, there is even more brand-new work demonstrating that fructose is a substance to worry about!

For example: heart failure. A recent study identified a previously unknown mechanism that specifically links high fructose consumption to increased risk of heart failure, alluded to earlier.

At this point, it is common knowledge that heart disease is a leading cause of death worldwide. Before heart disease develops, there is higher metabolic demand in the cells of the heart as the heart muscle grows to meet the increased need for oxygen in a straining, chronically stressed system. We might find this situation in someone with high blood pressure, for example. This increased growth puts more and more metabolic demand on the heart, so it triggers certain molecules that are present only in hypoxic states (when the body doesn't have enough oxygen to meet its

Consuming fructose results in the following concerning events:

- *Improper hormone responses to sugary foods*
- *Additional metabolic load on the liver*
- *Potential risk for undue growth of heart cells*
- *Elevated triglycerides*
- *Elevated uric acid*
- *Production of free radicals in the liver*

THE GOUT-FRUCTOSE CONNECTION

Gout is caused by *hyperuricemia*, or too much uric acid in the blood. Sharp needlelike crystals of urate (uric acid salts) form deposits in joints, especially in the cooler areas of the body, such as the metatarsophalangeal joint of the big toe. The symptoms include joint swelling, redness, and pain, especially in lower-body joints, and inflammatory arthritis (called gouty arthritis), which can affect any joint. Gout affects about 2 percent of people in Western countries at some point in their lives, with an estimated 3 million new cases annually in the U.S. Gout is associated with other chronic health problems and is frequently co-morbid with hyperlipidemia (high cholesterol), hypertension (high blood pressure), cardiovascular disease, kidney disease, diabetes, obesity, and metabolic syndrome.

Because purines are metabolized into uric acid (see page 231), gout is typically blamed on eating too much meat, which is high in purines. However, fructose seems to be a bigger player in the development of gout and the common denominator between gout and its co-morbidities. About one-third of Americans have hyperuricemia—no surprise when you look at our average fructose intake! Consuming fructose (or high-fructose corn syrup or sucrose) increases uric acid levels in the blood within 30 minutes, and with continued high fructose intake, uric acid in the blood can remain elevated. One study in men showed that those who consumed two soft drinks per day had an 85 percent higher chance of developing gout. And a recent meta-analysis showed that people who get 12 percent of their calories from fructose have a 62 percent higher risk of gout than those who get just 7 percent of their calories from fructose. To put this into perspective, eating meat increases the risk of gout by 41 percent compared to a meat-free (but not necessarily vegetarian) diet; drinking one alcoholic beverage per day increases the risk of gout by 10 percent but drinking two per day doubles the risk; and having a BMI over 27.5 increases the risk of gout by a whopping sixteen times!

Most studies show that eating more vegetables and fruit decreases the risk of gout as well as the risk of gout flares once diagnosed. Even eating high-purine vegetables reduces gout risk by 5 percent for each daily serving. This may be attributable to some important nutrients in vegetables and fruit. For example, getting more than 8 grams of fiber per day decreases the risk of gout by 62 percent compared to getting less than 6 grams per day—and 8 grams of fiber isn't very much (see page 45)! One study showed that consuming 62 milligrams or more of vitamin C per day decreased the risk of gout by 69 percent compared to consuming less than 51 milligrams. And consuming more than 63 micrograms of vitamin B9 daily decreased the risk of gout by 67 percent compared to consuming less than 52 micrograms.

Lifestyle is important, too; one study in men showed that the more active and fit they were, the lower their risk of gout.

So what can you do to decrease gout risk?

- Reduce sugar intake, especially fructose.
- Limit alcohol intake.
- Eat a veggie-rich diet.
- Maintain a healthy body weight.
- Live an active lifestyle.

Once gout has developed, a diet low in purine-rich animal foods is typically advised. While acutely high purine intake does increase the probability of a gout flare, the overall effectiveness of low-purine diets has not been proven. In addition, limiting fructose and alcohol intake, losing weight if needed (see page 400 for strategies), exercising, and eating tons of veggies are all prudent.

energy expenditure), called "hypoxia-induced factors," or HIFs. One such HIF was shown by the researchers of this recent study to turn on the genes that code for KHK-C, an enzyme that ramps up glycolysis and fuels the production of more heart cells.

KHK-C is found in the highest concentrations in the liver, where it has a high affinity for fructose. Because KHK-C is a driver for glycolysis, metabolizing fructose leads to an abundance of energy in the form of ATP, which can be used to create more molecules now or be stored for later (a large part of why excess fructose consumption leads to weight gain). For the first time, these scientists have shown that KHK-C can be found in the heart. Why is this scary? Because when we consume too much fructose, KHK-C can use it to fuel the growth of more and more heart cells; this cycle can exacerbate the progression of heart disease and even lead to heart failure. So consuming too much fructose, especially when cardiovascular problems are already present, is *really* bad—and it isn't the only recent study on fructose.

In addition to potentially exacerbating heart disease, a 2015 study published in the renowned scientific journal *Nature* has given us an additional clue as to whether fructose is making direct contributions to the obesity epidemic.

The current research does not directly demonstrate a cause-and-effect relationship between fructose and the health problems mentioned above that are related to obesity—in fact, there is some debate in the literature as to whether fructose is a cause of disease or a result of another issue; for example, some researchers argue that these effects would be seen from a high-calorie diet, regardless of fructose content. This recently released paper from Rendeiro and colleagues finally addresses this controversy and proves just how big a culprit fructose is.

The authors sought to examine how fructose consumption may be related to the above health concerns as well as to physical activity, cognition (learning and memory), and brain development. Scientists compared mice fed a diet of 18 percent fructose or 18 percent glucose for 11 weeks, which is considered a long-term diet for rodents. After the dietary intervention, the mice in the fructose condition had 11 percent higher body weight than their glucose-consuming counterparts. Additionally, the fructose mice seemed to consume more food (that is, calories) over time and had more fat mass at the end of the experiment.

How could this apply to human physiology? These findings suggest that a diet high in fructose could directly contribute to obesity. The researchers also found that the mice consuming fructose engaged in less physical activity, measured by the amount they moved around their cages. This result is of particular interest.

The notion that increased fructose consumption is directly related to inactivity is novel and certainly intriguing. Current thinking in the field suggests that poor diet and inadequate physical activity co-occur to contribute to obesity, yet this research seems to suggest a slightly different model: one in which fructose consumption directly leads to less activity, and these two effects additively cause weight gain.

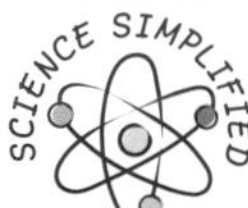

Current scientific research suggests that high fructose consumption both increases appetite and lowers motivation to be active. That's a bad combination when it comes to achieving and maintaining a healthy weight!

Fructose and Vitamin D Deficiency: The Perfect Storm

In case those problems aren't enough, fructose may also exacerbate vitamin D deficiency, as well as the *many* conditions that stem from this deficiency! It all starts when UVB radiation hits our skin and triggers the generation of vitamin D3 from cholesterol in our cells (or when we consume foods that contain vitamin D, like fatty fish or egg yolks). Vitamin D in the form of D3 or D2 doesn't have much biological activity in our bodies, so it gets passed on to the liver and kidneys to be hydroxylated into the most usable form of vitamin D, 1,25-dihydroxyvitamin D3 (also called calcitriol). From there, vitamin D goes on to work its magic—supporting skeletal health, working with parathyroid hormone, modulating inflammation, and performing other crazy-important functions.

True to its name, calcitriol plays a critical role in all things calcium: it regulates active calcium transport in the intestine, helping increase its absorption from food. (In fact, without enough vitamin D, we can absorb only 10 to 15 percent of the dietary calcium we eat!) When calcium levels in the blood get too low, vitamin

D increases tubular reabsorption in the kidneys so that less calcium is excreted in the urine.

So when we talk about vitamin D, the discussion isn't complete without bringing calcium into the picture. These two nutrients are inextricably linked, and getting sufficient amounts of both is vital for supporting a number of body functions. (It's not all about our bones!) Without enough vitamin D, calcium is excreted by the body instead of being incorporated into tissues, and without enough calcium, vitamin D must draw minerals from skeletal tissue in order to prevent blood levels of calcium from dipping dangerously low. So anything that threatens our levels of vitamin D or calcium is a major health concern. And that brings us back to . . . *fructose*.

Researchers have discovered that when we consume high levels of fructose (in quantities only possible from sweetened beverages and processed foods—I'm not talking about mangoes and apples here!), an enzyme called 24-hydroxylase (which is responsible for degrading vitamin D3) becomes more active, while another enzyme, 1α-hydroxylase (which helps synthesize vitamin D), becomes *less* active. The result is that our bodies start breaking down more vitamin D while creating less of it. That, in turn, causes calcium regulation to be thrown out of whack, with less calcium making it out of our food and into our bones, teeth, and blood. Our bodies must then release calcium from skeletal tissue to compensate. Sounds like a recipe for disaster, right? Yes, spending more of our lives indoors than at any time in human history is only part of the reason that 75 percent of Westerners are deficient in vitamin D! Let's look at some of the ways this chain of events can manifest.

Although the Standard American Diet and lifestyle contribute to poor bone health in many ways (insufficient vitamin A and K2 intake, sedentariness, lack of sunlight, and excessive alcohol consumption, to name just a few!), a high fructose intake may also play a role in osteoporosis through its effects on vitamin D and calcium. In fact, some researchers uphold that fructose is part of the reason soft drink consumption often correlates with fractures and bone density in population studies.

To maintain healthy nerve and muscle function (including the heart muscle), our bodies fight *really* hard to keep calcium levels in our blood within a specific range, drawing it from any place necessary—particularly skeletal tissue—if levels dip too low. (For the sake of immediate survival, it's more important to have a beating heart than it is to have strong bones!) When the body senses low levels of blood calcium, the parathyroid gland secretes calcium-regulating parathyroid hormone (PTH). Along with increasing the amount of calcium reabsorbed by the kidneys, parathyroid hormone stimulates osteoclasts, which are cells that break down bone tissue in order to release calcium into the blood and prompt the body to produce more calcitriol so that more dietary calcium can be absorbed.

This process works just fine as long as there's sufficient calcium in our diet. The increased dietary absorption facilitated by calcitriol makes it so that only limited amounts of skeletal tissue have to be broken down to release calcium (in other words, it's not a huge deal for our bones). But when fructose intake is at an unhealthy level, things stop working so smoothly. Because fructose triggers higher levels of vitamin D-degrading hormones (and lower levels of vitamin D-synthesizing hormones), our bodies have less vitamin D available and therefore have a harder time forming calcitriol. As a result, calcium absorption from food is curbed.

Because our bodies will do everything in their power to prevent calcium levels in our blood from tanking, the primary alternative is to start drawing more calcium from our bones to put back into the bloodstream. Boom: suddenly we enter a state of bone tissue breakdown because of a chain of events initiated by excess fructose. Over time, skeletal health becomes compromised, and the risk of osteopenia (lower-than-normal bone density), osteoporosis, and fractures may go up.

KNOWLEDGE BOMB *As counterintuitive as it seems, blood calcium levels have almost nothing to do with how much calcium we get from our diets. If those levels are too low or too high, it's generally a result of vitamin D status, parathyroid hormone disorders, or another health condition.*

Another scary consequence of a high-refined-fructose diet is its potential effects on prostate health. The prostate is full of vitamin D receptors, and hormonally active vitamin D (calcitriol) can help protect against prostate cancer through a number of mechanisms—for instance, contributing to cell cycle arrest, reducing inflammation, increasing cancer cell death, and inhibiting *nuclear factor-κB* signaling, which results in lower production of new blood vessels, an important factor in cancer progression. Basically, vitamin D is such a big player in prostate health that researchers are starting to test it as a therapy for people with early or precancerous prostate disease!

When high fructose consumption suppresses vitamin D levels, those protective mechanisms disappear, and the risk of prostate cancer has the potential to rise. It's important to keep in mind, though, that naturally occurring sources of fructose, like fruit, are packaged with tons of phytochemicals that exert strong anti-cancer effects. The foods we have to worry about here are heavily processed items like sodas, candy, and other items with abnormally high fructose but low nutrient density, like agave nectar and inulin fiber-based sweeteners.

In recent years, a number of studies have shown a link between vitamin D deficiency and nonalcoholic fatty liver disease (NAFLD), a condition in which extra fat builds up in the liver cells, in both children and adults. (Fatty liver disease has been found in alcoholics for a long time, but only in the last 35 years has it shown up in children and people who consume little alcohol.) Although fructose is believed to be directly involved in the progression of NAFLD by increasing the production of hepatic fat and inflammation, this is another instance where vitamin D may be mediating some of the detrimental effects of this sugar.

Here's how it works. Normally, vitamin D can help prevent liver fibrosis (a component of NAFLD) by reducing transforming growth factor-β (TGF-β) signaling. When excessive fructose intake suppresses levels of vitamin D in the body, the ability of vitamin D to interfere with that signaling decreases—leading to greater susceptibility to liver fibrosis and liver damage. And it doesn't end there! Low levels of vitamin D (whether caused by fructose intake or inadequate sun exposure) actually make the inflammatory effects of fructose more potent and, as a result, exacerbate its contribution to NAFLD. So a vicious cycle is created between fructose and vitamin D in the progression of this disease!

From the literature, we might conclude that the effects of fructose—at least when it comes to the mechanisms discussed here—can be offset by getting plenty of vitamin D. This is only part of the story, though! Vitamin D is a precious nutrient that most of us don't eat (or synthesize) enough of; at latitudes of 40 degrees north or higher, there isn't enough UVB radiation for people to produce much vitamin D for the entire winter season, and it's better to have a diet and lifestyle that support healthy vitamin D levels than to "make up" for excessive fructose intake by going crazy with vitamin D supplements. Plus, excessive fructose can exert detrimental effects through avenues completely separate from vitamin D and calcium, so a moderate intake is better than a high intake for other reasons as well.

When we consider the wide body of recent studies as well as the existing literature, fructose definitely seems to be a unique and significant contributor to many of the chronic diseases currently plaguing society.

There is good science showing the importance of consuming less than 10 percent of calories from added sugars. Following the Paleo template, your added sugar intake will be closer to zero, with only the occasional and moderate intake of unrefined natural sugar.

How to Moderate Fructose Intake

Of course, fructose isn't that commonly found in nature other than in fruit and honey, so following the Paleo principles naturally reduces our intake to levels far below those in the Standard American Diet. However, there are still ways to overdo fructose even within a Paleo framework. If we consume too much fruit (especially dried fruit) or use too much honey, agave (which can have a higher fructose content than high-fructose corn syrup), or other "natural" low-glycemic-index sweeteners in "Paleo treats," we can get just as much fructose as our SAD-eating counterparts (albeit from whole foods rather than processed foods).

That said, avoiding *all* dietary fructose is not necessary. In fact, moderate amounts of fructose are probably beneficial. For example, small quantities of fructose can actually reduce blood glucose levels in response to glucose consumption, as well as boost insulin sensitivity. Plus, unlike refined fructose sources, fruit and honey contain other beneficial nutrients and compounds that can offset some of the negative effects of fructose. It is the *over*consumption of fructose (especially from concentrated sources) that we need to worry about.

But how much exactly is overconsumption? Studies evaluating the health detriments of fructose consumption use 50 grams daily as the threshold for toxicity. That doesn't mean we want to be messing around with a daily intake just below toxic levels, of course. (Being only a little tipsy all the time isn't great for the liver, either!) Population studies show that obesity rates drop once fructose is lowered to the 25- to 40-gram range. Other scientists believe that returning to the pre-modern-food-era range of 10 to 20 grams per day is optimal (this makes sense as a daily goal with occasional or seasonally higher intake). This 10- to 20-gram range equates to two to five servings of fruit, depending on the fruit: one small apple (3 inches in diameter) has 10.7 grams of fructose, whereas a cup of sliced strawberries has 3.7 grams.

HEALTH QUICK-START

Aim for a daily fructose intake of no more than 40 grams—20 grams is even better! This means limiting fruit consumption to five servings and using honey and other natural sugars in moderation (see pages 152 and 303).

KNOWLEDGE BOMB

The lowest-fructose fruits are:

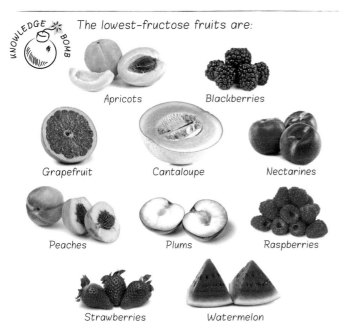

All of these fruits have less than 4 grams of total metabolic fructose (free fructose plus fructose bound in sucrose molecules) per 100-gram serving (see page 152). Five 100-gram servings per day from this list (plus abstention from sugars and sweeteners) will keep you in that optimal 10- to 20-gram range.

What About High-Fructose Corn Syrup?

A hotly debated topic (shrouded in plenty of unsubstantiated claims) is whether high-fructose corn syrup is even more harmful than table sugar. Some experts argue that because table sugar (sucrose) is metabolized into 50 percent fructose and 50 percent glucose in our bodies, there's not much difference between sugar and high-fructose corn syrup, which typically contains 55 percent fructose and 45 percent glucose. Other people point out that high-fructose corn syrup contains *free* (unbound) fructose and *free* glucose, whereas sucrose is composed of a glucose molecule and a fructose molecule that are chemically bonded together. Could that difference—the presence of free, rather than bound, fructose—cause HFCS to be more metabolically harmful?

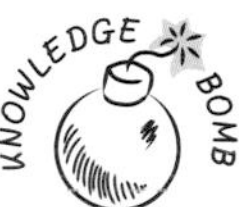

High-fructose corn syrup is not the only concentrated source of fructose to watch out for. The following sweeteners are composed largely of fructose:

- ***Agave nectar*** *contains an average of 70 percent fructose and as much as 90 percent. Yes, that's more than most HFCS!*
- ***Inulin fiber*** *is finding its way into many tabletop sweeteners. It is a high-fructose-content soluble fiber and thus is broken down into fructose in the digestive tract. It's also a FODMAP (see pages 434 and 435) and highly fermentable and thus can cause undesirable gastrointestinal symptoms, like bloating and gas.*
- ***Yacon syrup*** *is composed largely of inulin fiber.*
- ***Chicory root sugar*** *is another sweetener composed primarily of inulin fiber.*
- ***Coconut sugar/nectar*** *(or palm sugar/nectar) is purported to be largely inulin fiber as well. Note, however, that there are conflicting reports showing that the sugar composition of coconut sugar is not much different from cane sugar (that is, sucrose).*
- ***Sucrose*** *(table sugar, which can be derived from sugarcane or sugar beets but is also the dominant sugar in molasses and maple syrup) is a disaccharide composed of one glucose and one fructose molecule. Although it is a far preferable sweetener choice for occasional treats, sucrose in large quantities still provides excessive fructose.*

There aren't many studies that have looked at how free fructose differs from bound fructose after consumption, but the existing research doesn't give much weight to the "HFCS is worse!" theory. One study of type 2 diabetics found that 35 grams of sucrose or an equivalent amount of free fructose and free glucose produced similar blood sugar and insulin responses. Another study found that HFCS and sucrose resulted in the same satiety response (as well as the same energy intake at the next meal), refuting the idea that HFCS uniquely encourages excess calorie intake relative to other caloric sweeteners. While we definitely need more research to confirm whether the metabolism of HFCS differs from that of sucrose in important ways, especially when it comes to lipogenesis, fat accumulation in the liver, and inflammation, there currently isn't enough evidence to make the case that HFCS has different health effects than table sugar. Our best bet is to limit both!

ARTIFICIAL AND NONCALORIC SWEETENERS

The consumption of blood-sugar-spiking foods (both added sugars and refined carbohydrates) has been widely publicized as problematic, resulting in a surge in low-glycemic-index sweeteners heavily marketed to diabetics and those on low-carb diets. These products fall into three categories:

- Sugars that do not impact blood glucose levels as quickly or substantially as glucose or glucose-based starches, which are marketed as low-glycemic-index sugars (such as fructose and FODMAPs like inulin; see the previous page)
- Sugar alcohols (sorbitol, xylitol, and erythritol)
- Nonnutritive sweeteners, including acesulfame potassium, aspartame, neotame, saccharin, and sucralose, as well as the "natural" sugar substitute stevia

Our bodies are not designed to metabolize these sugars in the large quantities found in processed foods. Yes, even foods and tabletop sweeteners that are marketed as "natural," such as agave nectar and stevia, are not actually natural for our bodies. In most cases, consuming these glucose substitutes is more harmful than consuming glucose itself.

Bottom line? High fructose intake is clearly harmful, but consuming sugar alcohols or nonnutritive sweeteners in lieu of "regular" sugar or HFCS is like going from the frying pan into the fire. In Chapter 24, we'll take a look at some natural sweeteners that are less harmful and better suited to the Paleo framework. Now let's focus on the detrimental health effects of sugar alcohols and nonnutritive sweeteners.

Sugar Alcohols

Sugar alcohols (also called polyols) are hydrogenated forms of sugars, meaning that they contain a hydroxyl group, which is what makes them technically alcohols. They are naturally occurring sugars, typically found in small quantities in fruit. However, some sugar alcohols are refined and purified for use as sweeteners, including sorbitol, mannitol, xylitol, and erythritol. These sugar alcohols have gained popularity as sugar substitutes because, while they are relatively less sweet, they also have less of an impact on blood glucose levels.

Sugar alcohols are passively and, with the exception of erythritol, incompletely absorbed in the intestine. They are also fermentable, which means that they feed gut bacteria. In fact, the most common side effects of sugar alcohol consumption are severe gastrointestinal symptoms, such as watery stool, diarrhea, nausea, bloating, flatulence, and borborygmus (the rumbling noise produced by the movement of gas through the intestines). The dose required to produce these side effects varies depending on the specific sugar alcohol and the sensitivity of the individual.

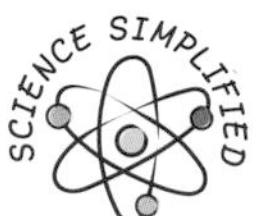

Sugar alcohols like sorbitol, mannitol, xylitol, and erythritol not only cause gastrointestinal symptoms like diarrhea, nausea, bloating, and flatulence but also can contribute to gut dysbiosis by preferentially feeding undesirable bacterial strains like E. coli *and can cause a leaky gut directly. They are a no-go on Paleo!*

There is evidence that sugar alcohols disproportionately feed Gram-negative bacteria and may contribute to gut dysbiosis (like alcoholic beverages, discussed in Chapters 15 and 24). Overgrowth of Gram-negative bacteria like *E. coli* has been shown to cause inflammation, may stimulate the immune system, and is linked to a variety of chronic diseases. This is also the most common form of small intestinal bacterial overgrowth (SIBO). Gut dysbiosis, such as SIBO, can also directly cause a leaky gut.

Furthermore, one study showed that the sugar alcohols xylitol and mannitol increase the permeability of epithelial cells (in a cell culture system) by directly opening up tight junctions. Tight junctions are the structures that hold epithelial cells together to create a solid barrier. When a substance causes the tight junctions to open, a leaky gut is the result.

Another study showed that erythritol has a similar effect on tight junctions and causes increased permeability of the epithelial barrier. Again, this means that erythritol, generally regarded as the safest sugar alcohol, can directly cause a leaky gut. To make matters worse, erythritol has also been shown to increase the virulence of bacteria from the *Brucella* genus, which includes pathogenic bacteria found in contaminated unpasteurized milk.

While the effect of sugar alcohols on intestinal permeability in humans has yet to be studied, this should be enough evidence for avoiding their refined forms.

Nonnutritive Sweeteners

Nonnutritive sweeteners are substances that taste sweet but don't provide a substantial number of calories. They include acesulfame potassium, aspartame, neotame, and sucralose, as well as the "natural" sugar substitute stevia, and have been linked to increased risk of obesity and metabolic syndrome. For example, studies have shown that the more diet soda we consume, the more likely we are to be overweight or obese and to develop metabolic syndrome; sugar-free soda, it turns out, has a greater impact on these conditions than any other dietary factor. In fact, in animal studies, the consumption of nonnutritive sweeteners causes a significant increase in body weight even with no change in food intake, which implies that these sweeteners affect metabolism or hormones.

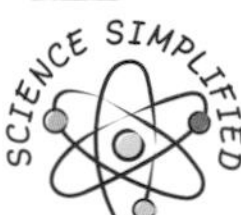

Nonnutritive sweeteners like aspartame and sucralose are linked to weight gain and obesity. This might be due to a direct effect on appetite, metabolism, and hormones.

In some people, the consumption of nonnutritive sweeteners causes the release of insulin in what is called *cephalic phase insulin release*. The body releases insulin upon tasting something sweet in anticipation of a blood sugar increase because the sweet-taste receptors on the tongue generate nerve impulses that are relayed to the brain. In the case of sugar consumption, this prerelease of insulin helps control blood sugar levels. However, in the case of nonnutritive sweeteners, it causes hyperinsulinemia (because of the absence of elevated blood sugar), which is inflammatory (see page 268). Cephalic phase insulin release seems to occur in some people and not others, and why is not clearly understood.

SCIENCE SIMPLIFIED

All low-calorie sweetener options, from aspartame to stevia, have the potential to stimulate the release of insulin in our bodies simply because they taste sweet and our brains tell our pancreas to release insulin in anticipation of higher blood sugar levels (which never come). High insulin without glucose to shuttle away into our cells can cause inflammation and increase appetite.

Recent studies show that nonnutritive sweeteners have physiological effects that alter appetite and glucose metabolism. There is evidence that these sweeteners bind to receptors on enteroendocrine cells (specialized cells in the gastrointestinal tract that interact with the endocrine system and secrete hormones) and pancreatic islet cells (cells in the pancreas that secrete the hormones insulin and glucagon). By interacting with these endocrine cells, nonnutritive sweeteners can either stimulate or inhibit hormone secretion. In particular, there is evidence that nonnutritive sweeteners cause an increase in the secretion of glucagon-like peptide-1 by enteroendocrine cells, which signals to the pancreas to increase the secretion of insulin and decrease the secretion of glucagon. Again, this results in hyperinsulinemia in the absence of elevated blood sugar.

There may be some direct effects of nonnutritive sweeteners on inflammation as well. For example, aspartame increases oxidative stress and inflammation in the brain, although how it does so remains unknown.

But Isn't Stevia Natural?

While many people in various "real food" communities agree that artificial sweeteners are a bad idea, stevia is often recommended as a natural sugar substitute because it comes from the leaf of a plant, *Stevia rebaudiana Bertoni*. It tastes sweet on the tongue, requires very small quantities to sweeten baked goods, and contains no sugar. While some experts advise caution against purified and manufactured forms of stevia, green leaf stevia is typically endorsed. On the surface, it sounds like a perfect solution.

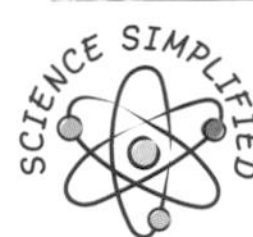

The jury is still out on whether stevia is truly safe for frequent consumption.

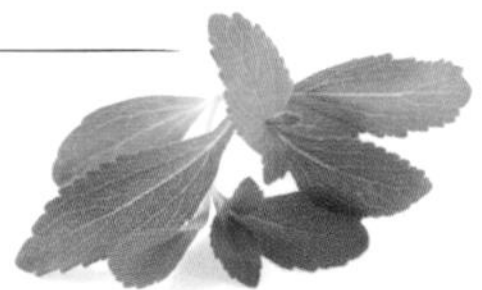

However, stevia requires major caution. The chemicals responsible for its sweet taste are called steviol glycosides, and there are at least ten different steviol glycosides present in the stevia plant. Purified/manufactured forms of stevia often isolate one or two of these steviol glycosides, whereas green leaf stevia (which is simply the dried and powdered leaves of the stevia plant) contains all ten.

Steviol glycosides are synthesized in the same pathway and end up being structurally very similar to the plant hormones gibberellin and kaurene. This means that steviol glycosides have a hormone structure. The majority of toxicological studies establish that stevia is safe, but some studies show that it can act as a mutagen and may increase the risk of cancer. (These studies are in the minority and tend to use quite high concentrations, so they are readily discarded in discussions of the overall safety of consuming stevia.) Whether or not stevia causes genetic mutations is not the only cause for concern, however, even if safety studies focus on this particular property.

There is evidence that steviol glycosides have contraceptive effects in both males and females. In particular, one specific steviol glycoside, called stevioside, has been shown to have potent contraceptive properties in female rats, implying that stevia may have an impact on estrogen, progesterone, or both. In another study, male rats fed stevia extracts showed decreased fertility, reduced testosterone levels, and testicular atrophy, potentially attributable to the binding of steviol glycosides with an androgen receptor. (Notably, other studies in male rats showed no such effects.) Although no studies have been conducted evaluating the impact of stevia on fertility in humans, the Guarani Indians in southern Brazil traditionally used the stevia plant to control fertility in women.

Occasional consumption of small amounts of stevia likely has little to no impact on general health. The World Health Organization has established 4 milligrams per kilogram (2.2 pounds) of body weight of steviol, in the form of steviol glycosides, as the safe upper limit for daily human consumption. For a 150-pound person, that equals approximately 40 packets of a stevia sweetener.

Unlike other nonnutritive sweeteners, studies show that stevia is pharmacologically active. Steviol and its conjugate (steviol glucuronide) can be measured in the blood after ingestion of feasible doses of either stevioside or rebaudioside. Unfortunately, there really is a shortage of human studies evaluating the full spectrum of possible negative effects of stevia (and no human studies exploring the potential effects on fertility!). In the case of stevia, caution is the better part of valor, especially for anyone struggling with fertility issues, hormone imbalances, high cancer risk, or chronic disease.

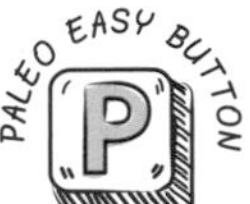

When it comes to sugars, our bodies know how to process sucrose, glucose, and fructose (the sugars found in fresh fruit) well, provided that the dose isn't too high and the consumption isn't too frequent. So when it comes to sweeteners, the safest options are natural sources of mainly sucrose that haven't been refined to remove valuable vitamins and minerals. The most nutrient-dense sugar is blackstrap molasses (see page 304), but unrefined cane sugar, maple syrup, and honey are all good options for occasional and moderate consumption. That bears repeating: sugars should not be part of an everyday diet but reserved for special infrequent treats. See Chapter 24 for details.

Chapter 23:
PALEO ELIMINATIONS

Well, here we are at Chapter 23, and we have finally come to the list of foods to avoid on the Paleo diet, what has classically been used to define this entire framework. I've included this chapter as a quick reference guide, which summarizes all the foods and ingredients discussed in Part 3.

Thanks to all the pages of science preceding this list of foodlike substances that are best eliminated from everyone's diets, you can understand the reasons for each item on this list. Hopefully, this list doesn't seem overwhelming—especially in comparison to all the nutrient-dense health-promoting foods summarized in Chapter 16. If it does, don't worry; making a gradual transition to eating a Paleo diet is discussed in Chapter 32.

Let's talk briefly about perfection versus balance, something that is discussed again in Chapters 25 and 31. The Paleo template is about using the scientific literature to inform a framework for the best dietary choices to achieve optimal health. However, individuals vary, lifestyle factors like sleep and stress influence how our bodies react to suboptimal foods, and our health histories and specific health goals need to guide our dietary choices. What does this mean? The complete list of verboten foods that follows may not apply to everyone all the time. Yes, you heard it here first, folks: Paleo is not a militant, black-or-white, perfection-or-bust approach to eating. While I encourage everyone to avoid all the following foods for at least several weeks (see Chapter 25 for more on elimination and reintroduction), if you find that your body tolerates some of these foods well, whether as an occasional indulgence or for more frequent consumption, you are allowed to call yourself a Paleo enthusiast while eating some foods that aren't strictly included in the Paleo diet. Just remember that none of the foods listed in this chapter are powerhouses of nutrition.

FOODS TO AVOID

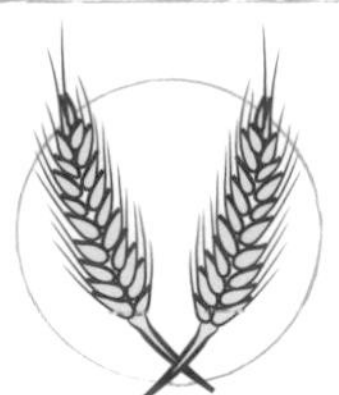

GRAINS:

barley
corn
durum
fonio
Job's tears
kamut
millet
oats
rice
rye
sorghum
spelt
teff
triticale
wheat (all varieties, including einkorn and semolina)
wild rice

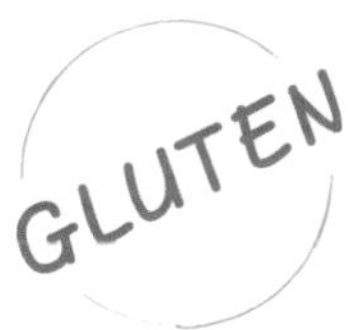

GLUTEN:

barley
rye
wheat
foods derived from these ingredients

(See page 281 for hidden sources of gluten and commonly contaminated foods.)

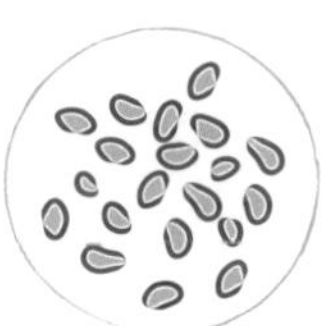

PSEUDOGRAINS AND GRAINLIKE SUBSTANCES:

amaranth
buckwheat
quinoa

(Chia seeds are a middle-ground food; see page 308.)

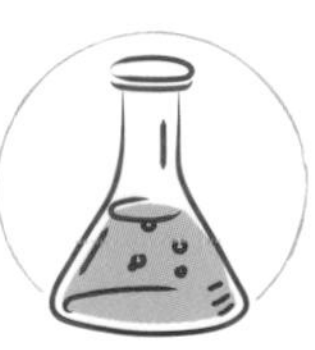

PROCESSED FOOD CHEMICALS AND INGREDIENTS:

acrylamides
artificial food color
artificial and natural flavors
autolyzed protein
brominated vegetable oil
emulsifiers (carrageenan, cellulose gum, guar gum, lecithin, xanthan gum)
hydrolyzed vegetable protein
monosodium glutamate
nitrates or nitrites (naturally occurring are okay)
olestra
phosphoric acid
propylene glycol
textured vegetable protein
trans fats (partially hydrogenated vegetable oil, hydrogenated oil)
yeast extract
any ingredient with a chemical name that you don't recognize (but see page 285 for some ingredients that sound unhealthy but actually aren't)

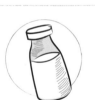

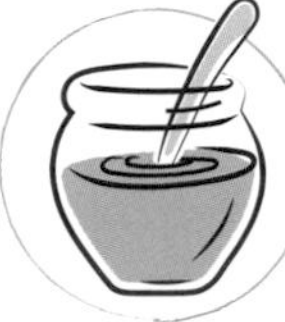

ADDED SUGARS:

agave
agave nectar
barley malt
barley malt syrup
beet sugar
brown rice syrup
brown sugar
cane crystals
cane juice
cane sugar
caramel
coconut sugar
corn sweetener
corn syrup
corn syrup solids
crystalline fructose
date sugar
dehydrated cane juice
demerara sugar
dextrin
dextrose
diastatic malt
evaporated cane juice
fructose
fruit juice
fruit juice concentrate
galactose
glucose
glucose solids
golden syrup
high-fructose corn syrup
honey
inulin
invert sugar
jaggery
lactose
malt syrup
maltodextrin
maltose
maple syrup
molasses
monk fruit (luo han guo)
muscovado sugar
palm sugar
panela
panocha
rapadura
raw cane sugar
raw sugar
refined sugar
rice bran syrup
rice syrup
saccharose
sorghum syrup
sucanat
sucrose
sugar
syrup
treacle
turbinado sugar
yacon syrup

(For a discussion on using natural sugars in moderation, see page 303.)

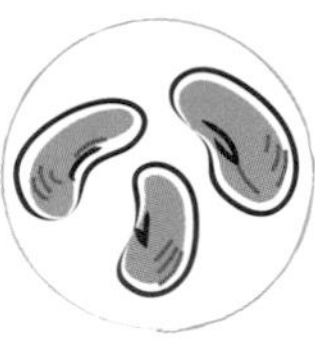

LEGUMES:

adzuki beans
black beans
black-eyed peas
butter beans
calico beans
cannellini beans
chickpeas (aka garbanzo beans)
fava beans (aka broad beans)
Great Northern beans
Italian beans
kidney beans
lentils
lima beans
mung beans
navy beans
pinto beans
peanuts
peas
runner beans
soybeans (including edamame, tofu, tempeh, other soy products, such as soy protein, and soy isolates, such as soy lecithin)
split peas
tamarind

(See Chapter 24 for more on legumes with edible pods and fermented and traditionally prepared legumes.)

DAIRY:

butter
buttermilk
butter oil
cheese
cottage cheese
cream
curds
dairy-protein isolates
ghee
heavy cream
ice cream
kefir
milk
sour cream
whey
whey-protein isolate
whipping cream
yogurt

(See Chapter 24 for more on grass-fed dairy.)

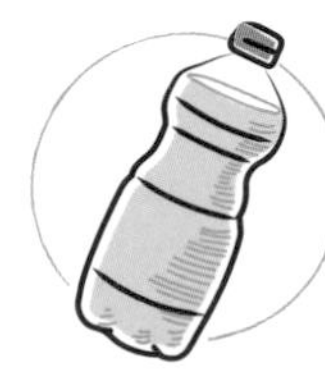

PROCESSED VEGETABLE OILS:

canola oil (rapeseed oil)
corn oil
cottonseed oil
palm kernel oil
peanut oil
safflower oil
sunflower oil
soybean oil

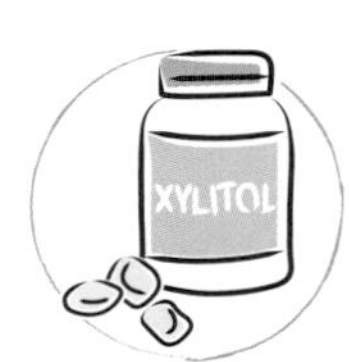

SUGAR ALCOHOLS:

erythritol
mannitol
sorbitol
xylitol

(Naturally occurring sugar alcohols found in whole foods like fruit are okay.)

NONNUTRITIVE SWEETENERS:

acesulfame potassium
aspartame
neotame
saccharin
stevia
sucralose

READING LABELS

Trying to figure out whether a product is Paleo-friendly?
It helps to know the many aliases that some pervasive foods go by.

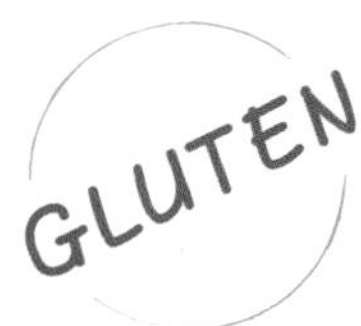

Gluten in Foods

Avoiding gluten takes some effort. Ingredients derived from wheat and other gluten-containing grains are found in a vast array of packaged and manufactured foods, but also in some foods not normally considered to be processed. The following list includes some of these hidden—and not-so-hidden—sources of gluten.

Asian rice paper
atta flour
bacon (check ingredients)
barley
barley grass
barley malt
beer (unless gluten-free)
bleached or unbleached flour
bran
bread flour
breading
brewer's yeast
bulgur
coating mixes
communion wafers
condiments
couscous
croutons
dinkle (spelt)
durum wheat
einkorn
emmer wheat
farina
farro (called emmer wheat except in Italy)
food starch
French fries
fu (a dried form of gluten)
gliadin
glues used on some envelopes, stamps, and labels
gluten peptides
glutenin
graham
gravies
hydrolyzed wheat gluten
hydrolyzed wheat protein
ice cream (may contain flour as an anticrystallizing agent)
imitation fish
kamut
lunch meats
maida (Indian wheat flour)
malt
malt vinegar
marinades
matzah (aka matso)
medications (prescription or over-the-counter)
mir (a wheat and rye cross)
nutritional and herbal supplements
oats
panko (bread crumbs)
pilafs (containing orzo)
prepared foods
processed cereals (often contain barley malt)
rye
salad dressings
sauces
seitan
self-basting poultry
semolina
soup bases and bouillon
soy or rice drinks (barley malt or malt enzymes may be used during manufacturing)
soy sauce (unless labeled wheat-free)
spelt
spice mixes (often contain wheat as an anticaking agent, filler, or thickening agent)
starch
stuffings
syrups
thickeners
triticale
wheat
wheat bran
wheat germ
wheat starch
wheatgrass

COMMON SOURCES OF GLUTEN/WHEAT CONTAMINATION:

- *art supplies: paint, clay, glue, and play dough (can be transferred to the mouth if hands aren't washed)*
- *flour dust*
- *foods sold in bulk (often contaminated by scoops used in other bins and by flour dust)*
- *grills, pans, cutting boards, utensils, toasters and other appliances, and oils that have been used for preparing foods containing gluten*
- *household products (may be transferred to the lips and ingested)*
- *knives (double-dipping knives into food spreads after spreading on bread can leave behind gluten-containing crumbs)*
- *millet, white rice flour, buckwheat flour, sorghum flour, and soy flour (commonly contaminated)*
- *personal care products, especially shampoos (may be transferred to the lips and ingested)*
- *powder coating inside rubber gloves (may be derived from wheat)*
- *waxes or resins on fruits and vegetables*

Gluten Cross-Reactors

Some foods have a higher likelihood of cross-reacting with gluten. The antibodies the body makes against gluten recognize similar proteins in these foods, so the body sees these foods and gluten as being one and the same. While having a gluten sensitivity doesn't automatically mean that you are sensitive to all or any of these foods, it's prudent to be cautious of them:

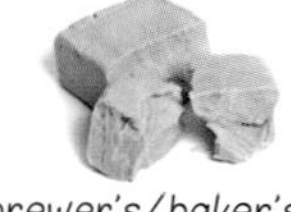
brewer's/baker's/ nutritional yeast

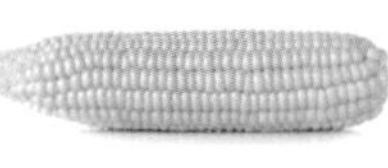
corn

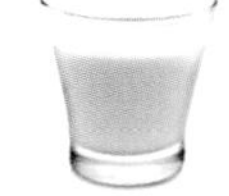
dairy proteins (casein, casomorphin, butyrophilin, whey)

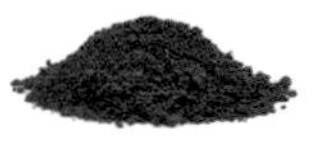
instant coffee

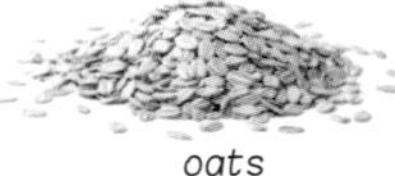
oats

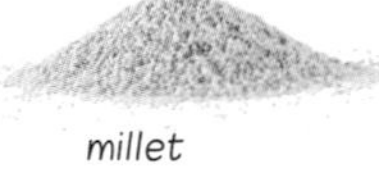
millet

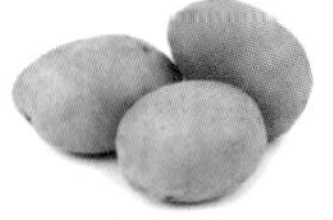
potatoes

rice

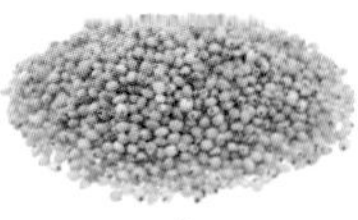
sorghum

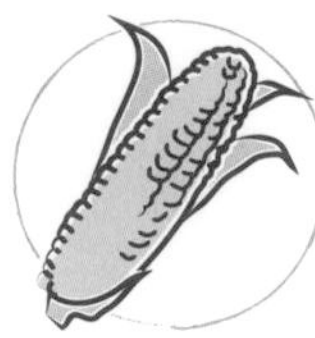

Corn in Foods

Ingredients derived from corn are found in the vast majority of packaged and manufactured foods. If you are very sensitive to corn-derived products, avoiding these pervasive ingredients can be overwhelming. However, avoiding processed foods in general will make a huge difference.

You may or may not need to go to the extent of avoiding all traces of corn-derived ingredients (in medications, for example); however, being aware of where corn exposure may be sneaking into your life will help you identify whether it is a problem. The following list includes some hidden—and not-so-hidden—sources of corn.

acetic acid
alcohol
alpha-tocopherol
artificial flavorings
artificial sweeteners
ascorbates
ascorbic acid
aspartame
astaxanthin
baking powder
barley malt
bleached flour
blended sugar
brown sugar
calcium citrate
calcium fumarate
calcium gluconate
calcium lactate
calcium magnesium acetate (CMA)
calcium stearate
calcium stearoyl lactylate
caramel and caramel color
carboxymethylcellulose sodium
cellulose, methyl
cellulose, microcrystalline
cellulose, powdered
cetearyl glucoside
choline chloride
citric acid
citrus cloud emulsion (CCS)
cocoglycerides
confectioners' sugar
corn oil
corn sugar
corn sweetener
corn syrup
corn syrup solids
cornmeal
cornstarch
croscarmellose sodium
crystalline dextrose
crystalline fructose
cyclodextrin
DATUM (a dough conditioner)
decyl glucoside
decyl polyglucose
dextrin
dextrose (such as monohydrate or anhydrous; also found in IV solutions)
D-gluconic acid
distilled white vinegar
drying agents
erythorbic acid
erythritol
ethanol
ethocel 20
ethyl acetate
ethyl alcohol
ethyl lactate
ethyl maltol
ethylcellulose
ethylene
Fibersol-2
flavorings
food starch
fructose
fruit juice concentrate
fumaric acid
germ/germ meal
gluconate
gluconic acid
glucono delta-lactone
gluconolactone
glucosamine
glucose
glucose syrup (also found in IV solutions)
glutamate
gluten
gluten feed/meal
glycerides
glycerin
glycerol
golden syrup
grits
hominy
honey
hydrolyzed corn
hydrolyzed corn protein
hydrolyzed vegetable protein
hydroxypropyl methylcellulose
hydroxypropyl methylcellulose phthalate (HPMCP)
inositol
invert syrup or sugar
iodized salt
lactate
lactic acid
lauryl glucoside
lecithin
linoleic acid
lysine
magnesium fumarate
maize
malic acid
malonic acid
malt
malt extract
malt syrup from corn
maltitol
maltodextrin
maltol
maltose
mannitol
margarine
methyl gluceth
methyl glucose
methyl glucoside
methylcellulose
microcrystalline cellulose
modified cellulose gum
modified cornstarch
modified food starch
molasses (corn syrup may be present)
mono- and diglycerides
monosodium glutamate (MSG)
natural flavorings
olestra/Olean
polenta
polydextrose
polylactic acid (PLA)
polysorbates (such as Polysorbate 80)
polyvinyl acetate
potassium citrate
potassium fumarate
potassium gluconate
powdered sugar
pregelatinized starch
propionic acid
propylene glycol
propylene glycol monostearate
saccharin
salt (iodized)
semolina (unless from wheat)
simethicone
sodium carboxymethylcellulose
sodium citrate
sodium erythorbate
sodium fumarate
sodium lactate
sodium starch glycolate
sodium stearyl fumarate
sorbate
sorbic acid
sorbitan
sorbitan monooleate
sorbitan trioleate
sorbitol
sorghum (syrup and/or grain may be mixed with corn)
Splenda (artificial sweetener)
starch
stearic acid
stearyls
sucralose (artificial sweetener)
sucrose
sugar
talc
threonine
tocopherol (vitamin E)
treacle
triethyl citrate
unmodified starch
vanilla, natural flavoring
vanilla, pure or extract
vanillin
vinegar, distilled white
vinyl acetate
vitamin C
vitamin E
vitamin supplements
xanthan gum
xylitol
yeast
zea mays
zein

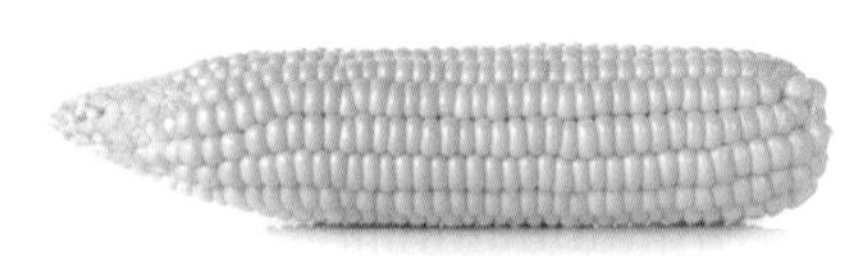

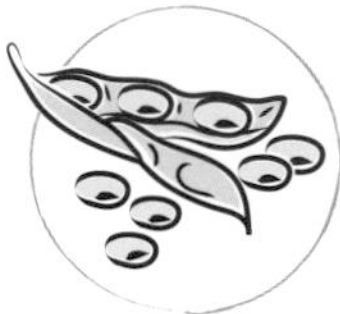

Soy in Foods

Soy is another ingredient that has permeated the food supply. Soy lecithin and soy protein are especially common ingredients in packaged foods. The following list includes foods and ingredients that are derived from soy:

POTENTIALLY CROSS-CONTAMINATED FOODS MUST BE LABELED:

- "MAY CONTAIN SOY"
- "produced on shared equipment with soy"
- "produced in a facility that also processes soy"

bean curd
bean sprouts
chocolate (soy lecithin may be used in manufacturing)
edamame (fresh soybeans)
hydrolyzed soy protein (HSP)
kinako
miso (fermented soybean paste)
mono- and diglycerides
monosodium glutamate (MSG)
natto
nimame
okara
shoyu
soy albumin
soy cheese
soy fiber
soy flour
soy grits
soy ice cream
soy lecithin
soy meal
soy nuts
soy pasta
soy protein (concentrate, hydrolyzed, isolate)
soy sauce
soy sprouts
soy yogurt
soya
soybean (curds, granules)
soybean oil
soymilk
tamari
tempeh
teriyaki sauce
textured vegetable protein (TVP)
tofu (dofu, kori-dofu)
yuba

PRODUCTS THAT COMMONLY CONTAIN SOY:

Asian cuisine (Chinese, Korean, Japanese, Thai)
baked goods
baking mixes
bouillon cubes
candy
cereal
chicken (raw or cooked) processed with chicken broth
chicken broth
deli meats
energy bars
imitation dairy foods, such as soymilk, vegan cheese, and vegan ice cream
infant formula
margarine
mayonnaise
meat products with fillers; for example, burgers and sausages
nutrition bars
nutrition supplements (vitamins)
peanut butter and peanut butter substitutes
protein powders
sauces, gravies, and soups
smoothies
vegetable broth
vegetarian meat substitutes (veggie burgers, imitation chicken patties, imitation lunch meats, imitation bacon bits)
waxes or horticultural oils on fruits

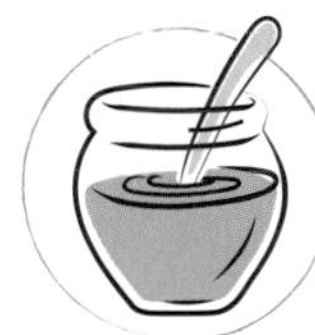

Sugar in Foods

When reading food labels, it is helpful to know how to decipher which ingredients are sugar. While most of them are refined, some are unrefined (which typically means that the sugar retains some minerals). Paleo is not a sugar-free diet, but added sugars should be kept to a minimum (less than 10 percent of total calories), and natural sugars should be reserved for occasional treats. It is common for manufactured products to contain more than one form of sugar. The following ingredients are all forms of sugar:

agave
agave nectar
barley malt
barley malt syrup
beet sugar
brown rice syrup
brown sugar
cane crystals
cane juice
cane sugar
caramel
coconut sugar
corn sweetener
corn syrup
corn syrup solids
crystalline fructose
date sugar
dehydrated cane juice
demerara sugar
dextrin
dextrose
diastatic malt
evaporated cane juice
fructose
fruit juice
fruit juice concentrate
galactose
glucose
glucose solids
golden syrup
high-fructose corn syrup
honey
inulin
invert sugar
jaggery
lactose
malt syrup
maltodextrin
maltose
maple syrup
molasses
monk fruit (luo han guo)
muscovado sugar
palm sugar
panela
panocha
rapadura
raw cane sugar
raw sugar
refined sugar
rice bran syrup
rice syrup
saccharose
sorghum
sorghum syrup
sucanat
sucrose
syrup
treacle
turbinado sugar
yacon syrup

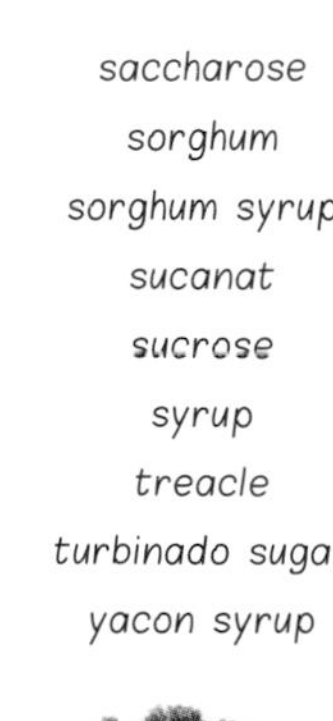

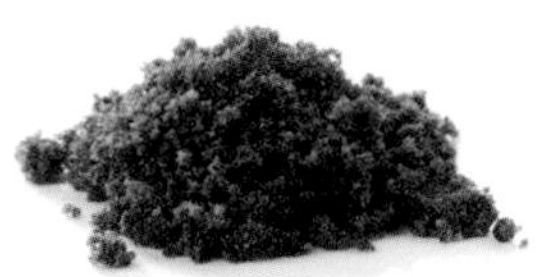

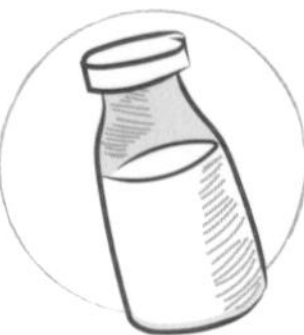

Dairy in Foods

Dairy ingredients are more and more commonly used in manufactured and packaged foods. The following ingredients indicate the presence of milk protein:

Milk: acidophilus milk, buttermilk, buttermilk blend, buttermilk solids, cultured milk, condensed milk, dried milk, dry milk solids (DMS), evaporated milk, fat-free milk, fully cream milk powder, goat's milk, Lactaid milk, lactose-free milk, low-fat milk, malted milk, milk derivative, milk powder, milk protein, milk solids, milk solid pastes, nonfat dry milk, nonfat milk, nonfat milk solids, pasteurized milk, powdered milk, sheep's milk, skim milk, skim milk powder, sour milk, sour milk solids, sweet cream buttermilk powder, sweetened condensed milk, sweetened condensed skim milk, whole milk, 1% milk, 2% milk

Butter: artificial butter, artificial butter flavor, butter extract, butter fat, butter flavored oil, butter solids, dairy butter, natural butter, natural butter flavor, whipped butter

Casein and caseinates: ammonium caseinate, calcium caseinate, hydrolyzed casein, iron caseinate, magnesium caseinate, potassium caseinate, sodium caseinate, zinc caseinate

Cheese: cheese flavor (artificial and natural), cheese food, cottage cheese, cream cheese, imitation cheese, vegetarian cheeses with casein

Cream, whipped cream

Curds

Custard

Dairy product solids

Galactose

Ghee (cultured ghee may be okay)

Half & half

Hydrolysates: casein hydrolysate, milk protein hydrolysate, protein hydrolysate, whey hydrolysate, whey protein hydrolysate

Ice cream, ice milk, sherbet

Lactalbumin, lactalbumin phosphate

Lactate solids

Lactic yeast

Lactitol monohydrate

Lactoglobulin

Lactose

Lactulose

Milk fat, anhydrous milk fat

Nisin preparation

Nougat

Pudding

Quark

Recaldent

Rennet, rennet casein

Simplesse (a fat replacer)

Sour cream, sour cream solids, imitation sour cream

Whey: acid whey, cured whey, delactosed whey, demineralized whey, hydrolyzed whey, powdered whey, reduced mineral whey, sweet dairy whey, whey powder, whey protein, whey protein concentrate, whey solids

Yogurt (regular or frozen), yogurt powder

MAY CONTAIN MILK:

Caramel flavoring

Flavoring

High-protein flour

Lactic acid

Lactic acid starter culture

Natural flavoring

> *"Nondairy" products may contain casein. Foods covered by the FDA labeling laws that contain milk must be labeled "contains milk"; however, prescription and over-the-counter medications are exempt.*

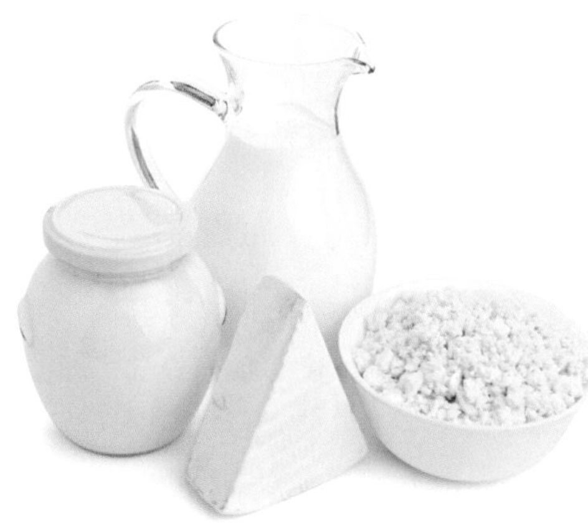

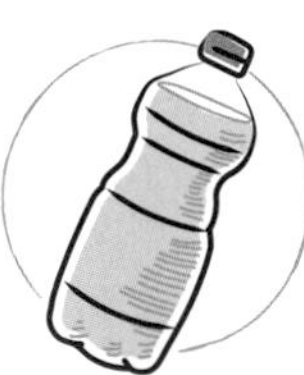

Processed and Refined Oils

Beyond avoiding fast food, do not use any of the following oils in home cooking, and avoid packaged foods with any of the following items on the label:

canola oil
corn oil
cottonseed oil
grapeseed oil
margarine
palm kernel oil
peanut oil
safflower oil
shortening
soybean oil
sunflower oil
"vegetable" oil
fake butter substitutes
butter flavor
nonstick cooking sprays
any oil labeled as refined
any oil labeled as hydrogenated
any oil labeled as partially hydrogenated

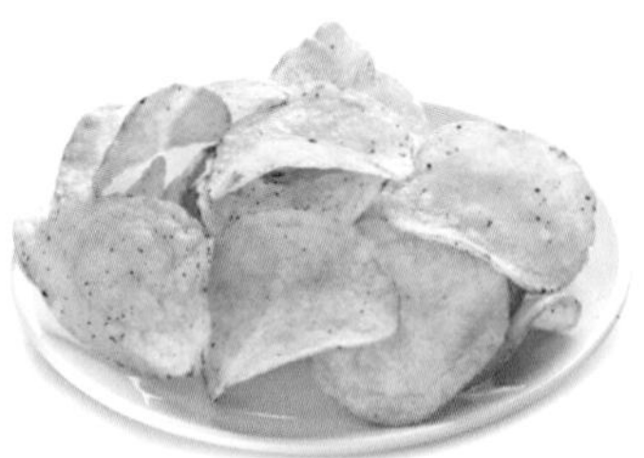

INGREDIENTS THAT SOUND SCARY BUT AREN'T

When reading food labels, it can be tempting to assume that any long, unpronounceable, or unfamiliar items in the ingredient list must be bad for us (and definitely aren't Paleo). But this isn't always the case! While some scary-sounding ingredients are worth watching out for, others are completely benign, and there's no reason to go out of our way to avoid them. Here's a rundown of some of the most common ingredients that sound harmful but aren't!

Vitamins added to food are sometimes listed under their less-familiar names and might not be recognizable at first glance. Some are used to enhance a food's nutritional value, but others (like ascorbic acid/vitamin C or mixed tocopherols/vitamin E) are used to prevent oxidation. If these ingredients appear on a food list, they're micronutrients, *not* toxic chemicals.

- α-tocopherol or mixed tocopherols (vitamin E)*
- Ascorbic acid (vitamin C)
- Ascorbyl palmitate (a fat-soluble form of vitamin C)*
- Biotin (vitamin B7)
- Calciferol (vitamin D)
- Choline
- Cobalamin or cyanocobalamin (vitamin B12)
- Folic acid, folate, folacin (vitamin B9)
- Niacin or nicotinic acid (vitamin B3)
- Pantothenic acid or calcium pantothenate (vitamin B5)
- Phylloquinone or menadione (vitamin K)
- Pyridoxal, pyridoxine, pyridoxamine (vitamin B6)
- Riboflavin (vitamin B2)
- Thiamin (vitamin B1)

**Some vitamins are derived from non-Paleo foods. For example, vitamin C is typically derived from corn, and vitamin E is typically derived from soy. When added to foods, there is no requirement to have "may contain corn/soy" on the label since these vitamins are purified. However, their presence may still be a problem for those with a severe allergy to corn or soy and a history of anaphylactic responses. Also note that synthetic forms of vitamins aren't always as bioavailable (easily absorbed and used) as the forms found in whole foods, so while we don't necessarily need to be worried about these vitamins being added to foods, we can't depend on them for nutrient sufficiency. For more on folic acid specifically, see page 422.*

Enzymes are sometimes added to meat tenderizers, cheeses, and other dairy products (as well as some supplements). The following ingredients are perfectly fine:

- Bromelain (an enzyme derived from pineapple)
- Papain (an enzyme derived from papaya)
- Ficin (an enzyme derived from figs)
- Rennet (commonly used in cheese)

Probiotic cultures. Certain foods (like yogurt, kefir, kombucha, kvass, and fermented veggies) contain health-promoting bacteria and yeasts that helped ferment the food. In some cases, these probiotics are listed in the ingredient list. Rest assured, they're beneficial (see page 191)!

- *Lactobacillus* species (including *L. acidophilus, L. johnsonii, L. casei, L. rhamnosus, L. gasseri, L. reuteri*)
- *Bifidobacterium* species (including *Bifidobacterium bifidum, Bifidobacterium longum, Bifidobacterium infantis*)
- *Saccharomyces boulardii*
- *Bacillus* species

Sodium chloride is just regular table salt. Even though it's always better to choose unrefined salt and moderate sodium consumption (see page 198), the presence of sodium chloride on a label isn't reason enough to turn tail.

Sodium bicarbonate is another word for baking soda.

Alginate (or sodium alginate or algin) is a harmless seaweed-derived salt found in some Paleo-friendly foods, like kelp noodles.

Acetic acid is the acid that gives vinegar its pungent smell.

Of course, some ingredients really *are* problematic. But there's no use eliminating foods just because we don't understand what some of the ingredients mean, unless there's actual evidence of harm.

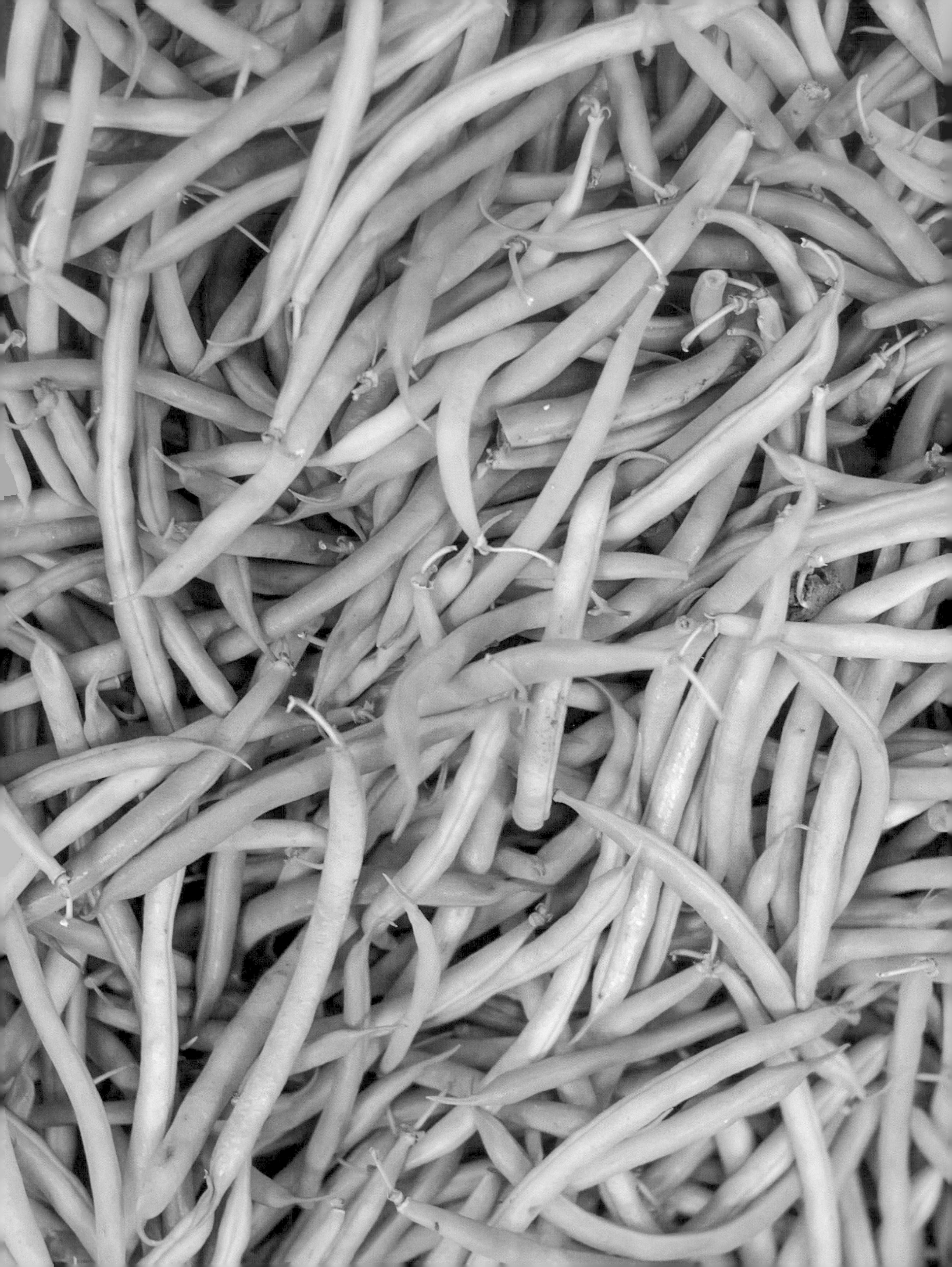

4.

THE MIDDLE GROUND: WHERE THE SCIENCE ISN'T CUT-AND-DRIED

The Paleo diet is often criticized because some of its tenets are not well supported by the scientific literature. This is absolutely true, and it's the motivation for separating certain foods into their own part in this book.

Yes, there are foods for which the science isn't cut-and-dried, or for which there are both pros and cons. At the end of the day, the labels "Paleo" and "not Paleo" are far less important than providing you with the tools to discern for yourself whether these foods work for you.

Let's revisit the idea of choosing foods based on how much Good Stuff (health-promoting nutrients) versus Bad Stuff (health-undermining compounds) they contain. Part 2 sanctions those "yes" foods that have tons of Good Stuff and little or no Bad Stuff, whereas Part 3 condemns the "no" foods that are best avoided. Now we will tackle the many foods that fall somewhere in the middle.

When it comes to identifying the role that these middle-ground foods should play in our diets, there are some important questions to ask. How much Bad Stuff can be tolerated for the sake of the Good Stuff in a food? And how much Good Stuff does a food need to contain to compensate for the presence of some Bad Stuff? How do our health histories affect where we draw the line? Is genetic makeup a significant factor? Might some foods be okay if we reserve them for special occasions? And how strict do we need to be if we are dealing with chronic health problems? Hard-and-fast answers to these questions are extremely difficult to pinpoint; each middle-ground food works for some people and not for others.

Many of the foods that fall into this middle-ground category feature heavily in other dietary recommendations that do have scientific backing, including red wine (which is said to lower Alzheimer's risk when consumed in moderation); grass-fed dairy products (which feature heavily in traditional diets like the Weston A. Price Foundation diet and the Primal diet); rice (a dietary staple of long-living Asian cultures and the Perfect Health Diet); lycopene-rich tomatoes; mineral-rich blackstrap molasses; and seeds and pseudograins (often labeled as superfoods).

Are these foods worth consuming? In this part of the book, I'll discuss the merits (or lack thereof) and nuances of each of these foods. And perhaps even more helpfully, Chapter 25 outlines a standard elimination-and-challenge protocol for identifying whether each of these foods (or even some of the foods discussed in Part 3) works for you.

Chapter 24:

FOOD FOR THOUGHT

It's important to recognize those foods for which there are potential arguments both for and against their inclusion in our diets. Rather than taking a dogmatic approach to the Paleo diet, let's discuss the merits and potential downfalls of these "middle-ground foods."

GRASS-FED DAIRY

The value (or lack thereof) of dairy products is one of the most fiercely debated topics within the Paleo community. Recommendations vary dramatically, from consuming no dairy whatsoever, to consuming only dairy fat (such as ghee, butter, and heavy cream), to consuming only raw grass-fed dairy, to consuming only fermented dairy or aged cheeses, to including any kind of dairy on a regular basis. All these positions are based on varying degrees of science and speculation, with no clear-cut (and evidence-based!) guideline that could apply across the board.

So should we include dairy in our diets or not? Let's start with the most legitimate arguments against dairy.

One of the biggest reasons many people must avoid or limit dairy products is lactose intolerance—the inability to fully digest lactose (the main sugar in milk). Rates of lactose intolerance vary widely based on ethnicity, ranging from 5 percent among northern Europeans to over 90 percent in some Asian and African populations. In fact, in the United States alone, somewhere between 30 and 50 million people are lactose intolerant!

Lactose intolerance results from a deficiency in an enzyme called lactase, which is secreted by cells in the upper part of the small intestine and is responsible for breaking down lactose into its simple sugar constituents, glucose and galactose. Lactose intolerance can be inherited (involving mutations in the LCT gene, which provides instructions for making lactase), or it can develop later in life due to certain health conditions (such as Crohn's disease, celiac disease, ulcerative colitis, gastroenteritis, or stomach infections) or as a result of chemotherapy. Regardless of how it forms, lactose intolerance is unpleasant: people experience symptoms like gas, bloating, stomach pain, nausea, and diarrhea after consuming dairy (all caused by undigested lactose in the gut).

Another issue that puts dairy on the "avoid" list for some people is dairy allergy. While lactose intolerance involves a reaction to milk *sugar*, a true dairy allergy involves reactions to various proteins in milk (including casein and whey). Epidemiological reports of cow's milk allergies (IgE antibody reactions to cow's milk proteins) range from between 1 and 17.5 percent in preschoolers, 1 and 13.5 percent in children ages 5 to 16 years, and 1 to 4 percent in adults in Western countries. The prevalence of cow's milk *sensitivities* (IgA and IgG antibody reactions to cow's milk proteins) is unknown, although one study of IBS patients showed that a whopping 84 percent of participants tested positive for IgG antibodies against milk proteins. That's an excellent rationale for eliminating dairy and then carefully reintroducing it to see how your body reacts (see Chapter 25).

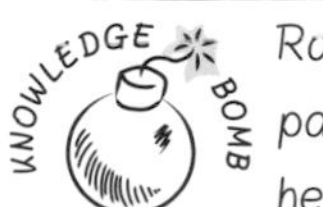

Raw milk is milk that has not been pasteurized—a process by which milk is heated to a high temperature to kill any potential pathogenic microbes. Carefully consider the risks and benefits before choosing to consume raw milk. One argument in favor of raw milk is the presence of active lactase, which aids in digestion even in those with lactose intolerance, and which is rendered inactive by the pasteurization process. However, it is important to recall that pasteurization was introduced in the late 1800s because serious infections—like tuberculosis, strep throat, scarlet fever, and typhoid fever—were transmitted via raw milk. In fact, the legal requirement that milk be pasteurized, introduced in 1908, is credited for preventing millions of cases of serious illness each year, nearly eradicating diseases like tuberculosis in the U.S., and is viewed as one of the greatest contributions to public safety in history. While many of the potential sources of milk contamination—such as zoonotic bacteria (bacteria that can infect more than one species, like tuberculosis) if milk comes from sick cows, or cow feces coming in contact with milk or processing equipment—can be mitigated, those opting for raw milk are strongly advised to thoroughly research the farming practices of their potential suppliers.

Cow's milk proteins are known gluten cross-reactors, which means that people with gluten intolerance may produce antibodies against gluten that also recognize dairy proteins (see page 245). For these people, eating dairy is essentially the same as eating gluten. Very importantly, for people with an allergy, an intolerance, or gluten cross-reactions to dairy proteins, even the trace proteins in dairy fats (like those found in butter and ghee) can be a problem.

Another issue with dairy involves gut health. Like grains and pseudograins (see Chapter 19), dairy contains protease inhibitors, which are molecules designed to neutralize the digestive enzymes that would normally degrade the proteins in food. (Milk specifically contains inhibitors of trypsin, chymotrypsin, and elastase.) When protease inhibitors are present in the digestive tract, the degradation of all proteins present at that time is affected. This can cause undue stress on the pancreas and may cause intestinal inflammation through activation of Toll-like receptors. (There's evidence that wheat-derived trypsin inhibitors cause intestinal inflammation, but this has not been confirmed in milk-derived protease inhibitors.)

Ultimately, dairy is designed to create a leaky gut. Scientists still don't understand all the mechanisms through which this occurs, but it seems to be an important aspect of what dairy is designed to do: feed babies (of the same species) optimal nutrition for rapid growth. In newborns, a leaky gut is essential so that components of mother's milk can get into the bloodstream, like hormones and all the antibodies a mother makes that help boost her child's immune system. When we're young and purely breastfed, a leaky gut is actually a good thing! But this becomes a problem in the adult digestive tract, where more things that we don't want leaking into the bloodstream are present. Drinking milk from a different species seems to exacerbate the problem, since the foreign proteins can trigger a stronger immune response.

Within the Paleo movement (as well as in other health communities), several more tenuous arguments are made against dairy consumption. Although they're worth considering, these arguments generally aren't sufficiently supported by enough real-world evidence to be considered reasons to avoid dairy. They include:

- **Insulin response.** Milk is highly insulinogenic, meaning that it causes a large spike in blood insulin, disproportionate to the amount of sugar and protein in milk. However, the available evidence suggests that dairy-induced insulin spikes don't lead to the development of chronic disease and obesity: as you'll see shortly, many dairy products (and specific components of dairy products) are associated with a *lower* risk of the chronic diseases linked with high insulin levels.
- **Hormones.** Milk contains active bovine (cow) hormones, which have the potential to alter our own hormone levels. For example, milk consumption tends to raise blood levels of insulin-like growth factor-1 (IGF-1), which has been linked to higher risk of breast, colorectal, and prostate cancer. However, other components of dairy have been shown to be cancer-protective and may negate the potential hormone-related risk increase.

So what about arguments *for* dairy? On the "pro" side, there are some compelling arguments for including dairy products in our diets. Studies have shown that consuming dairy, especially full-fat and fermented dairy products, can protect against metabolic syndrome, type 2 diabetes (fermented dairy only), and cardiovascular disease. In fact, one meta-analysis of 31 prospective cohort studies found that dairy consumption in general was associated with a 9 percent lower risk of stroke; calcium from dairy foods was associated with a 31 percent lower risk of stroke; and consumption of cheese was associated with an 18 percent lower risk of coronary heart disease and a 13 percent lower risk of stroke.

Grass-fed dairy (see page 170 for more on the benefits of grass-fed) is an excellent source of fat-soluble vitamins and conjugated linoleic acid (CLA), an anti-inflammatory fat that can potentially improve body composition and reduce cancer risk. Additional nutrients in dairy can be health-protective in a number of ways, such as calcium reducing vascular resistance and blood pressure; vitamin D improving insulin sensitivity and reducing cancer risk; and potassium, magnesium, and phosphorus playing a role in blood pressure management.

Fermented dairy (like yogurt and kefir) is an excellent source of probiotics, particularly *Lactobacillus* and *Bifidobacterium*. There are also some valuable proteins in dairy, such as glutathione (important for reducing inflammation and protecting against oxidative stress) and whey (which has been shown to have anti-tumor and immune-boosting properties in a wide variety of studies).

Finally, there is evidence that dairy proteins are beneficial for children due to their growth-promoting effects. Traditionally, children would have received some breast milk until approximately five years of age. In our modern society, however, most children are weaned by age one. The current scientific view is that cow's milk is a good substitute for human milk in terms of growth promotion, provided that it is not introduced too early in a child's life.

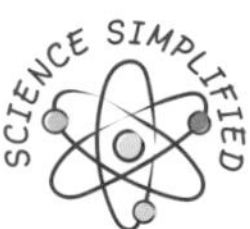

In the absence of allergy, lactose intolerance, or chronic health problems linked to leaky gut, grass-fed dairy has some compelling and beneficial nutrition!

So should we include dairy in our diets or not? The answer is entirely individual—hence the status of dairy as a middle-ground food. For a healthy person with no dairy intolerance or allergy, no autoimmune diseases, and no other conditions in which a leaky gut is a potential contributing factor, dairy may be perfectly fine and even beneficial (especially fermented dairy and full-fat, grass-fed dairy). For everyone else, it makes sense to omit dairy for at least one month and then experiment with reintroducing it to determine whether it causes symptoms (see page 315). In general, dairy fats that contain little to no sugar or protein (ghee and, to a lesser extent, butter and cream) tend to be less allergenic and more widely tolerated.

LEGUMES MIGHT NOT BE ALL BAD

One of the biggest sticking points for many Paleo diet critics is the fact that almost all legumes have historically been off the menu in the Paleo template. The current U.S. dietary guidelines recommend consuming 3 cups of legumes per week. Why? Legume consumption has been associated with lower cardiovascular disease risk, lower risk of colorectal cancer, and reduced markers of inflammation. These effects can be attributed to some compelling nutrient content. Analyses of total dietary nutrition reveal that consuming a mere half cup of cooked dried beans or peas daily results in higher intakes of fiber, protein, and an array of phytochemicals, as well as vitamin B9, magnesium, iron, and zinc. Plus, legume consumption tends to lower overall intake of saturated fat and total fat. In the context of the nutrient-deficient Standard American Diet, this is a good thing!

Legume consumption is also observed in some hunter-gatherer populations: the !Kung San diet relies heavily on the tsin bean, and Australian aborigines extensively harvest and eat acacia seeds. So how can we reconcile the purported benefits of legume consumption with our understanding of the health detriments of saponins (see page 253), excessive phytate consumption (see page 254), protease and other digestive enzyme inhibitors (see page 251), and agglutinins (see page 249)? It may be that lumping all legumes into one category and judging them based on their worst offenders is the wrong way to go about evaluating the merits of these foods.

The antinutrient content varies greatly from legume to legume, and these antinutrients are more or less stable during cooking and digestion. It's worthwhile parsing out the differences between legumes that clearly have more Bad Stuff than Good Stuff (such as soy and peanuts) and those that may be a worthwhile addition to a healthy diet if properly prepared (such as split peas, black beans, fava beans, and lentils).

In certain legumes (soy and peanuts being the biggest culprits, but also some types of dried beans, like kidney beans), the agglutinins are very resistant to deactivation and degradation. For example, peanut agglutinin is hardly affected even after cooking at 158°F (70°C) for several hours. (Incidentally, wheat germ agglutinin is also incredibly heat stable.) And it takes a whopping 40 minutes of cooking at 158°F (70°C) to deactivate only half of the total lectin in soybeans. In fact, there's nothing "middle ground" about soy, peanuts, or kidney beans: these foods should stay firmly on the "avoid" list, regardless of how they're prepared.

Soy does seem to be the worst offender when it comes to potential health detriments of legume consumption. It is linked to increased rates of some cancers, like bladder cancer, and worsening of hypothyroidism; studies are mixed on whether soy increases, decreases, or has no effect on cardiovascular disease.

It's harder to unilaterally recommend avoidance of all other legumes. Proper cooking of legumes can deactivate the vast majority, if not all, of the antinutrients, so the balance tips in favor of legumes due to their fiber and mineral content. This is supported by recent scientific studies that separate out non-soy legumes from soy in evaluating the effects of regular consumption on disease risk. And while there are still many unanswered questions, current data indicate that habitually eating non-soy legumes can reduce cardiovascular disease risk factors and markers of inflammation.

Until broadly designed studies that evaluate antinutrient deactivation in the full spectrum of commonly available legumes with a variety of different cooking techniques are performed, it's impossible to say with certainty which legumes are perfectly healthful foods under which cooking conditions. It is this lack of data that puts legumes other than soy, peanuts and kidney beans in the "middle ground" category. (Soy, peanuts, and kidney beans remain off the table.) What *can* be said is that many people might tolerate properly prepared lentils, black beans, chickpeas and other dried beans and that these legumes can make a positive contribution to a health-promoting diet. However, like all middle-ground foods, it's best to eliminate them initially and then methodically reintroduce to your diet using the protocol in Chapter 25.

Traditional Preparations Reduce Antinutrients

If you do choose to experiment with legume consumption, it's important to know that traditional preparations—soaking, fermenting, and prolonged cooking—greatly reduce the amount and activity of problematic antinutrients.

The biggest concerns cited in the scientific literature arising from the consumption of legumes is poor digestibility of proteins and poor absorption of minerals. As already discussed, legumes are naturally rich in a variety of antinutrients that adversely affect their nutritional properties and that, in high concentrations, can disrupt the gut barrier and cause inflammation. Yet many of these effects can be deactivated by traditional preparations, which typically involve prolonged soaking and extended cooking times.

The amount of deactivation of antinutrients in legumes depends both on the specific legume and on how it is prepared. For example, soaking pigeon peas for 6 to 18 hours reduces the lectin content by 38 to 50 percent, and soaking kidney beans for 12 hours reduces the lectin content by nearly 49 percent. Likewise, one study found that for white beans, broad beans, lentils, chickpeas, and soybeans, soaking for 12 hours at 78°F (26°C) reduced phytate levels by between 8 and 20 percent. Additional research shows that longer soak times in warmer water result in the greatest phytate decrease. (As an added bonus, soaking reduces the content of oligosaccharides, which are responsible for legumes' flatulence effects.) Lastly, fermentation—which occurs after extended periods of soaking—can reduce phytates and lectins even further. One study found that fermentation reduced phytates by 85 percent in kidney beans, 77 percent in soybeans, and 69 percent in mung beans, due in particular to the bacteria *Lactobacillus bulgaricus*. In fact, fermented legumes can be very nutrient-dense foods (see page 191).

Soaking and fermenting legumes is a fairly simple process: simply cover the legumes with warm water (approximately 140°F/60°C) and leave them in a warm place for 12 to 18 hours (the time varies depending on the type of legume), adding more water if needed to keep the legumes covered. Longer soaking times or the addition of bacterial cultures (especially the *Lactobacillus* species) begin the fermentation process. After soaking and/or fermenting, legumes should be thoroughly cooked to remove additional antinutrients.

The cooking method is also important. Studies have shown that microwave cooking is inadequate for destroying trypsin inhibitors and agglutinins in several commonly consumed legumes. But conventional cooking (boiling until the legumes are completely soft) can deactivate agglutinins and trypsin inhibitors in some legumes.

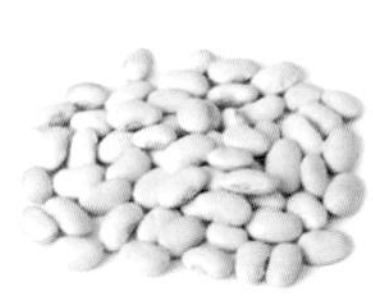

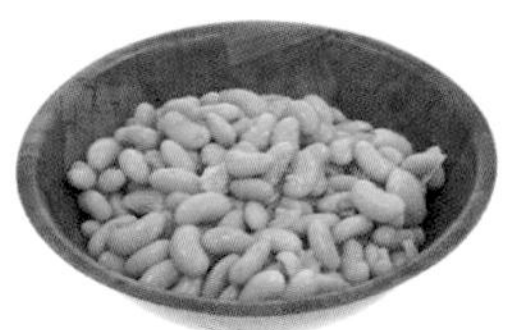

HEMAGGLUTININS AND TRYPSIN INHIBITORS IN LEGUMES BEFORE AND AFTER COOKING

	Agglutinins (extract minimum dilution causing agglutination of human erythrocytes)		Trypsin Inhibitors (trypsin inhibitor units per milligram)	
LEGUME	Raw	Conventional Cooking	Raw	Conventional Cooking
Black bean	12	3	31	2.6
White bean	12	0	31.3	1.4
Soybean	5	0	75.4	1.2
Green pea	0	0	2.5	1.6
Mature pea	3	2	3.5	2.5
Lentil	2	0	3.6	2.4
Fava bean	0	0	7.2	3.1
Chickpea	3	2	17.9	3.1

KNOWLEDGE BOMB

Because the problematic substances in legumes are concentrated in the seed, a few products that are made with other parts of the plant get a pass. These include tamarind paste (made from the fruit, separated from the seed and pod), carob powder (ground pod), sweet pea leaves, mung bean sprouts, mesquite wood or bark (often used in smoking), and some mesquite flour (when made with ground pod only).

If you read the table closely, you might think that soybeans aren't so bad when cooked. It's worthwhile to note that this data was derived from legumes that were cooked until completely soft, which is *not* the standard preparation for edamame (whole soybeans). Other studies show that only half of the lectins in soy are deactivated after 40 minutes of cooking at 158°F (70°C), which is still about four times longer than the more usual edamame cooking preparations. Many other soybean products, like soy milk and tofu, are not cooked as part of their manufacturing and are typically consumed raw or after a short cooking time.

Although most legumes are inferior to other plant foods in terms of nutrient density, they are a giant step above grains; legumes tend to be decent sources of iron, zinc, calcium, magnesium, and vitamin B9, contain modest levels of protein (about twice as much as most grains), and are rich sources of both soluble and insoluble fiber (including resistant starch). In epidemiological studies, consumption of legumes is frequently associated with greater longevity. It's worth noting that there is a much stronger correlation between fruit and vegetable consumption and disease risk. For example, not consuming fruits and vegetables daily may be responsible for up to 14 percent of heart attacks! So don't fret if legumes don't work for you. With a focus on consuming plenty of veggies, you won't miss out on anything.

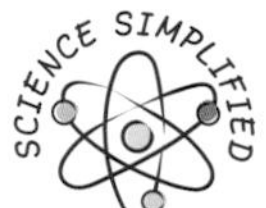

Soy, peanuts, and kidney beans are off the table (unless fermented like natto or tempeh), but other legumes, if properly prepared, might be okay. See Chapter 25 for how to challenge individual foods to determine how your body responds to them.

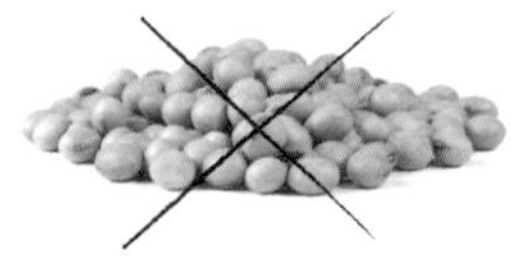

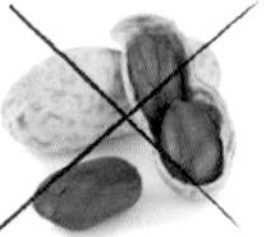

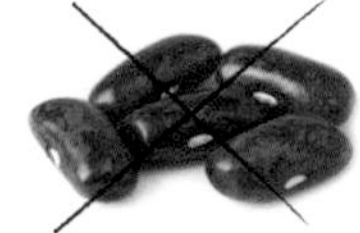

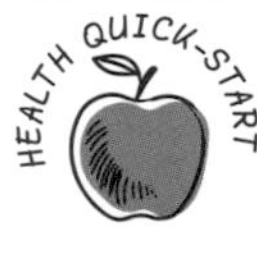

If you do choose to include non-soy and non-peanut legumes in your diet, it's important to cook them thoroughly. Proper preparation of dried beans requires five steps:

1. Clean. *Spread the beans in a single layer on a baking sheet. Discard any foreign objects (such as leaves, small stones, or twigs) and broken beans.*

2. Rinse. *Place the beans in a colander and rinse thoroughly under cold running water.*

3. Soak. *Put the beans in a bowl and pour warm water (approximately 140°F/60°C) over the beans to cover them. Leave them in a warm place for 12 to 18 hours (or up to 48 hours), topping up with water as needed to ensure that the beans remain completely submerged.*

4. Rinse again. *Discard the soaking water. Place the beans in a colander and rinse thoroughly under cold running water.*

5. Cook. *Place the beans in a large stockpot and cover with fresh cold water. Bring to a simmer and maintain a simmer over medium heat, stirring occasionally to prevent sticking. Add water periodically during cooking to keep the beans covered. Beans take 30 minutes to 3 hours, depending on the variety, to cook until soft.*

Legumes with Edible Pods Get a Pass!

Legumes are members of the pea family *(Fabaceae)* that produce long seed pods and include chickpeas, fava beans, lentils, mung beans, soybeans, peanuts, lima beans, alfalfa, Great Northern beans, broad beans, cannellini beans, black beans, common beans, kidney beans, red beans, snow peas, sugar snap peas, wax beans, and green beans . . . just to name a few!

In Chapter 19, I discussed legumes as foods to avoid due to their high lectin, saponin, and phytate content (including some lectins that are incredibly toxic). However, the playing field changes when it comes to edible-podded legumes like green beans (also called string beans or snap beans) and fresh peas (including sugar snap peas and snow peas). Unlike other legumes, which are harvested after their seeds (called pulses) have matured and dried, we eat green beans and fresh peas when they're still soft and immature.

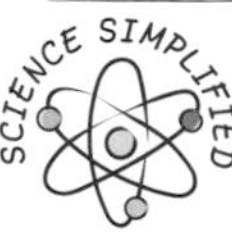

The arguments against legumes don't apply to those with edible pods, like green beans and fresh peas.

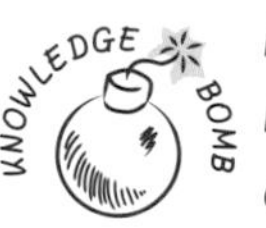

Not everything that grows in a pod is a legume. Vanilla, cocoa, coffee, and cashews are often misrepresented as belonging to the legume family. Vanilla actually comes from the orchid family, cocoa (chocolate) comes from the Malvaceae family, coffee is from the Rubiaceae family, and cashews are from the Anacardiaceae family.

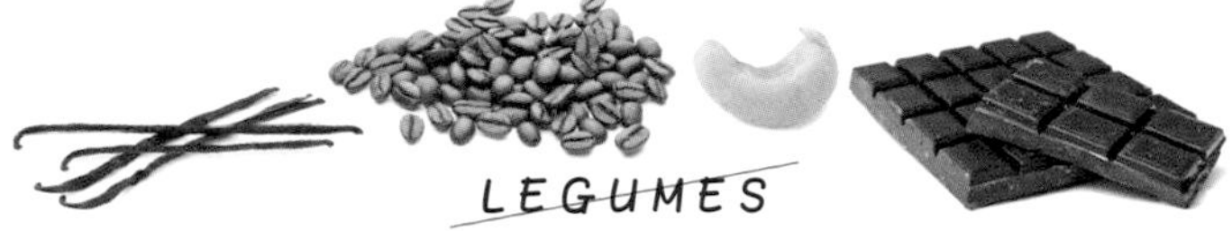

One benefit to eating soft, immature legumes is their lower phytate content. Phytates (the salts formed when phytic acid binds with minerals) are the main storage form of phosphorus in plants and tend to be high in grains, nuts, and legumes (see page 254). But studies of different legume varieties show that phytate levels increase as legumes get older and harder, so edible-podded legumes are naturally lower in phytates due to their earlier stage of maturity. And the data we have on actual phytate levels in legumes confirms that green beans and fresh peas are at the very bottom end of the spectrum. For example, one study found that fifteen Polish pea varieties had phytate levels ranging from 0.006 to 0.013 gram per 100 grams of dry weight, which is between 80 and 370 times less than the phytate content of soybeans.

GRAMS OF PHYTIC ACID PER 100 GRAMS OF LEGUME (DRY WEIGHT)

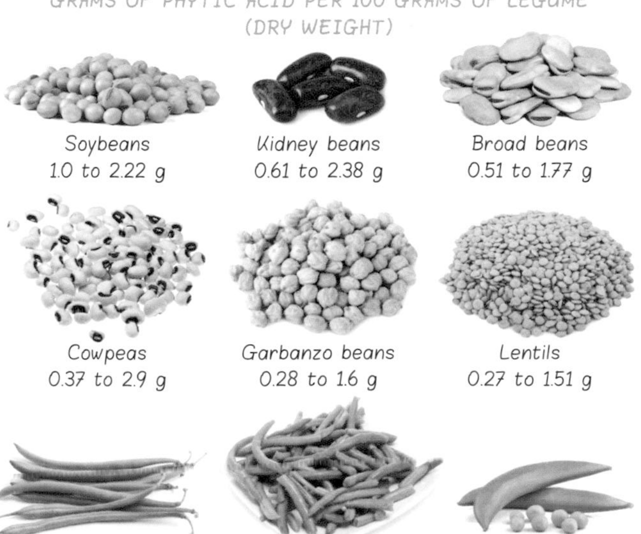

Soybeans 1.0 to 2.22 g

Kidney beans 0.61 to 2.38 g

Broad beans 0.51 to 1.77 g

Cowpeas 0.37 to 2.9 g

Garbanzo beans 0.28 to 1.6 g

Lentils 0.27 to 1.51 g

Green beans (raw) 0.15 g

Green beans (cooked) 0.05 g

Polish pea varieties 0.006 to 0.013 g

Likewise, compared to hard, dry legumes, fresh peas and green beans have lower levels of agglutinins, which are discussed in depth on page 249. It turns out that lectins are *not* a good reason to avoid green beans and fresh peas! Because of how they've been bred and their relatively early harvesting, edible-podded peas and green beans have low enough levels of phytohaemagglutin and other lectins to be safe to consume, even in their raw state. And the lectins they do contain are relatively instable, which means that they can easily be deactivated through cooking (see page 292).

On top of that, when we eat green beans or fresh peas, we're not just eating the seeds like we do with other legumes. We're also consuming the pod, which doesn't contain the same kinds of lectins (or the same high level of phytates) that legume seeds do. In fact, the nutritional profile of green beans and fresh peas is much more similar to nonstarchy vegetables than it is to other legumes (including a low calorie density and high content of vitamin C and vitamin A precursors).

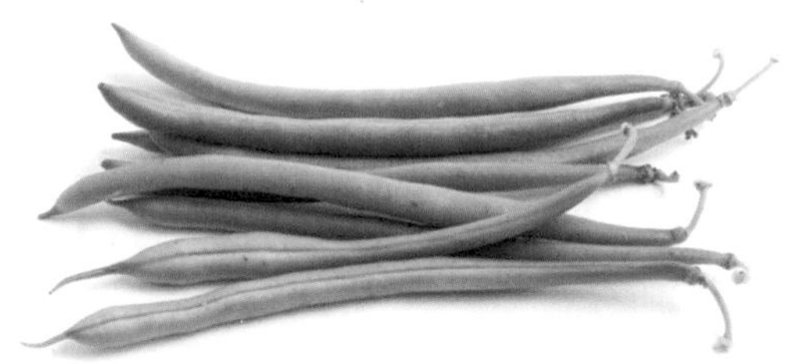

For example, if we compare edible-podded peas (which include both the pod and the peas inside) with mature split peas (which include only the seeds inside the pod), we can see that edible-podded peas have a higher concentration of micronutrients than mature peas per 120 calories of food (raw snap peas and snow peas versus cooked split peas):

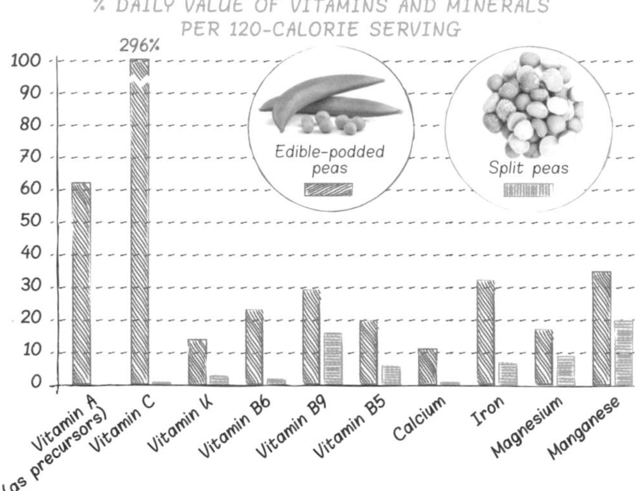

So what's the verdict? In terms of phytate levels, lectins, and overall nutrition, edible-podded legumes don't have much in common with the hard mature beans that typically come to mind when we hear the word *legume*. If you see green beans at the farmers market, are lucky enough to have sugar snap peas growing in the garden, or just want a tasty addition to your veggie menu, edible-podded legumes are a perfectly good choice!

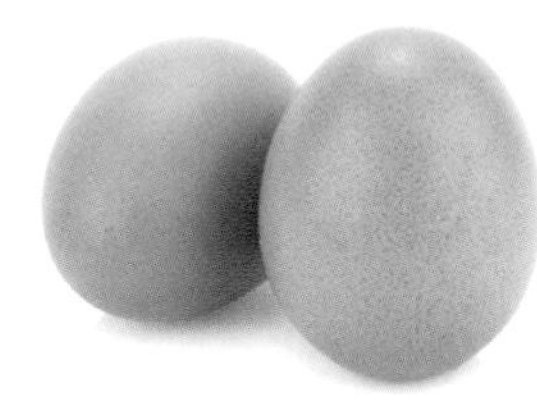

EGGS

Eggs are one of the most allergenic foods, affecting 2 to 3 percent of the entire population. Intolerance to eggs also appears to be fairly common; in one study of IBS patients, 57 percent of participants tested positive for IgG antibodies against eggs. (Recall that allergies are mediated by IgE antibodies and intolerances are mediated by any of the other four types of antibodies, IgG being the most common, but also IgA, IgM, and IgD; see page 246.) But for those without an allergy or an intolerance, what is it about eggs that lands them in the middle-ground category? To answer that question, we need to separate the whites from the yolks.

Egg Whites

One of the main functions of the egg white is to protect the yolk against microbial attack while the embryo grows. One way it achieves this worthy goal is through the activity of lysozyme. Lysozyme is an enzyme (a glycoside hydrolase) that is good at breaking down the cell membrane components of Gram-negative bacteria. In addition, lysozyme does a great job of transporting these bacterial protein fragments across the gut barrier.

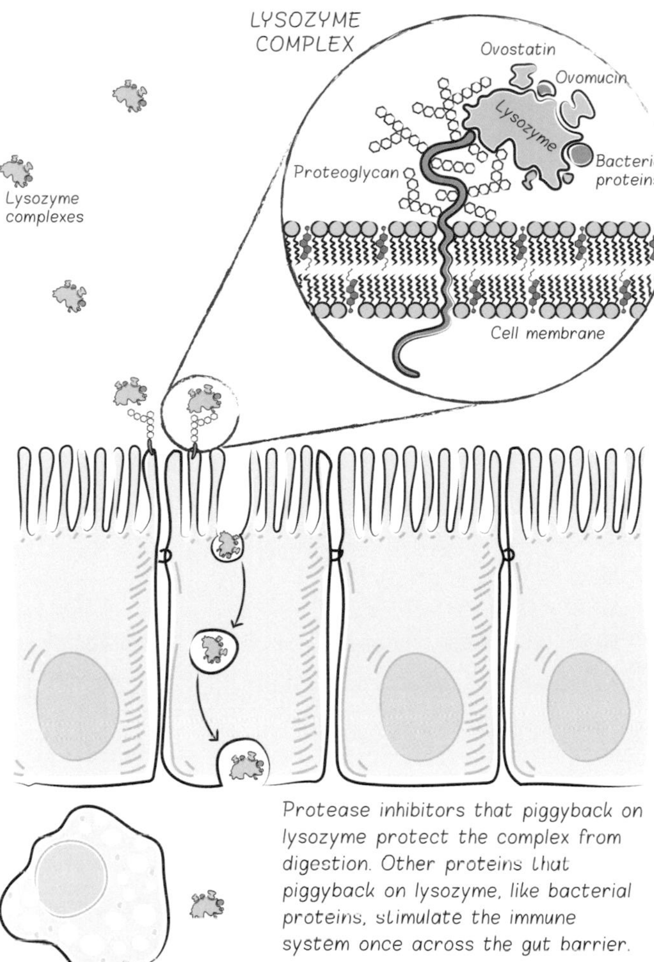

Protease inhibitors that piggyback on lysozyme protect the complex from digestion. Other proteins that piggyback on lysozyme, like bacterial proteins, stimulate the immune system once across the gut barrier.

Lysozyme works specifically and quickly to break apart peptidoglycans (a type of glycoprotein in bacterial membranes, especially Gram-negative bacteria); it is very resistant to heat and is stable in highly acidic environments. Humans also produce lysozyme as part of our normal defense against bacterial infections: it's found in our saliva, tears, and mucus (including the mucus layers in the intestines). So if we already make our own lysozyme, why is the lysozyme in egg whites a problem?

Lysozyme has the ability to form strong complexes with other proteins or protein fragments. This means lysozyme from egg whites typically passes through the digestive system in large complexes with other egg white proteins. Many of the other proteins in egg whites are protease inhibitors (see page 251), thus the lysozyme and egg white protein complexes become resistant to our digestive enzymes. The egg white protease inhibitors that are most likely to be bound to lysozyme are ovomucin and ovostatin, which are trypsin inhibitors (trypsin is one of our main digestive enzymes); cystatin, which is a cysteine protease inhibitor; and ovoinhibitor, which is a serine protease inhibitor. None of these protease inhibitors inhibits the activity of lysozyme. As the lysozyme complex travels, largely intact, through the gut, lysozyme can bind with bacterial proteins from the bacteria normally present in the digestive tract (such as endotoxin from the cell walls of Gram-negative bacteria like *E. coli*), adding it to the complex.

Lysozyme also maintains a positive charge, an unusual chemical property that allows it to cross through the enterocytes by electrostatic attraction to negatively charged glycoproteins (proteoglycans; an important part of the glycocalyx layer) embedded in the enterocyte cell surface.

Studies have confirmed that consumed lysozyme gets into the circulation (that is, circulates throughout the body via the bloodstream) even in healthy individuals, and even in conjunction with food intake (as opposed to isolated lysozyme taken as a drug or supplement, although the amount that enters the circulation is lower in that case). Absorption of pure egg white lysozyme into the circulation is probably not hazardous in itself (at least in the quantities that you would get from a plate of scrambled eggs; very high amounts do cause kidney damage). The problem is other proteins piggybacking on lysozyme across the gut barrier: the "leak" of other egg white proteins is the reason egg allergies are so common, and the high likelihood of bacterial proteins leaking out is why eggs (especially egg whites) cause difficulties for those with autoimmune disease.

SCIENCE SIMPLIFIED

A protein in egg whites can help bacterial proteins like endotoxin (see page 186) get into the body. The effect is pretty small, so this is really a concern only for people with unhealthy gut barriers or chronic disease. The other issue with eggs is that allergy and intolerance rates are quite high.

Egg Yolks

Egg yolk, on the other hand, is a rich source of vitamins A, B3, B6, B9, B12, and D (if free-range or pasture-raised), along with choline, phosphorous, and selenium; it also contains modest amounts of vitamin B1, vitamin E, calcium, iron, and zinc. The rich yellow or orange color comes from the presence of two antioxidant carotenoids—lutein and zeaxanthin (see page 38).

Contrary to decades of dogma, the cholesterol in egg yolks doesn't raise blood cholesterol; in fact, 47 percent of the fat in egg yolks is the ultra-heart-healthy oleic acid. Eggs also contain phospholipids, which are known to improve cholesterol (especially by supporting HDL), reduce blood pressure, improve vascular function, and reduce inflammation—all good things when it comes to cardiovascular disease!

It is generally accepted that egg whites are not an issue for those with a healthy gut, especially if eaten in moderate quantities. And egg yolks are a tremendous source of important nutrients. However, given the high rates of allergy and intolerance to eggs, it may be wise to eliminate eggs initially and then challenge (first yolks and then whites) using the protocol outlined in Chapter 25.

NIGHTSHADES

In general, "the more diversity, the better!" is a great motto when it comes to Paleo plant foods, but there's one potential exception to that rule: nightshades.

Nightshades are a botanical family of plants called *Solanaceae*. These plants have certain characteristics in common, like the shape of the flower and how the seeds are arranged within the fruit. There are more than 2,000 species in the nightshade family, the vast majority of which are inedible and many of which are highly poisonous (like deadly nightshade and jimsom weed). Tobacco is a nightshade that is known to cause heart, lung, and circulatory problems, as well as cancer and other health issues (although some of this clearly has to do with the other toxins found in tobacco products; see page 117).

The following are edible members of the nightshade family, a couple of which we might encounter only while on vacation in the tropics or in supplements:

Ashwagandha
Bell peppers (aka sweet peppers)
Bush tomatoes
Cape gooseberries (also known as ground cherries—not to be confused with regular cherries)
Cocona
Eggplant
Garden huckleberries (not to be confused with regular huckleberries)
Goji berries (aka wolfberries)
Hot peppers (such as chili peppers, jalapenos, habaneros, chili-based spices, red pepper, and cayenne pepper)
Kutjera
Naranjillas
Paprika
Pepinos
Pimentos
Potatoes (but not sweet potatoes)
Tamarillos
Tomatillos
Tomatoes

Note that many of the nightshades listed include dozens of varieties. There are many, *many* varieties of hot peppers, tomatoes, and eggplants, for example, and something like 200 varieties of potatoes. And the number of products that contain nightshades is enormous. In fact, if a label lists the vague ingredient "spices," that product almost always includes paprika. Many spice blends, like curry powder and steak seasoning, usually contain nightshades. You might see ingredients such as sambal, shichimi, or Tabasco listed and not immediately realize that those are sauces made with hot peppers. In fact, there are thousands of varieties of hot sauce, all of which contain nightshades.

You may recognize several "superfoods" in this list of nightshades. As a general rule, this family of vegetable-like fruits are packed with vitamins, minerals, fiber, and phytochemicals. Tomatoes, for instance, are high in phytochemicals and are one of the best food sources of lycopene. They also contain carotenoids (zeaxanthin, lutein, and β-carotene), flavonones (naringenin and chalconaringenin), flavonols (rutin, kaempferol, and quercetin), hydroxycinnamic acids (caffeic acid, ferulic acid, and coumaric acid), and glycosides (esculeoside A). This impressive list on top of being an excellent source of vitamin B7, vitamin C, molybdenum, and vitamin K, as well as containing moderate amounts of vitamins B3, B5, B6, and B9, choline, vitamin E, chromium, copper, iron, potassium, manganese, phosphorus, and zinc. Whew! So what's not to love?

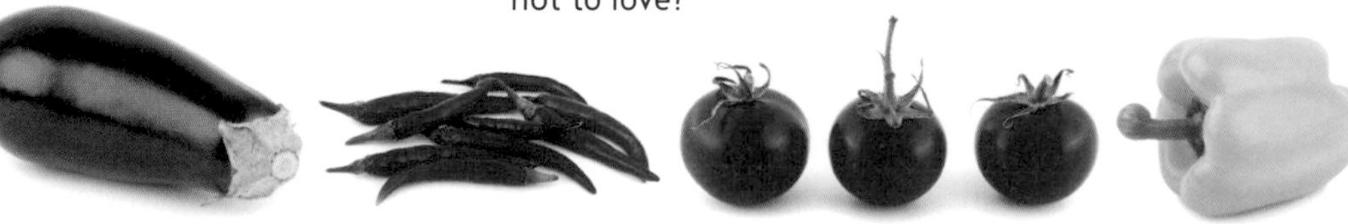

Of the edible species in the nightshade family, poisoning can actually occur with excessive consumption, and it is possible that the low-level toxic properties of the nightshade vegetables contribute to a variety of health issues as they progress over time. So let's talk about three key compounds in nightshades that make them such a common food sensitivity and potentially harmful for certain people: saponins, lectins, and capsaicin.

The "Bad Stuff" in Nightshades

Nightshades contain saponins (for a more detailed discussion on saponins, see page 253). More specifically, the flowers, fruit, and foliage of nightshade plants contain a type of saponin called glycoalkaloids (for example, α-solanine and α-chaconine in potato, α-solanine in eggplant, and α-tomatine in tomato).

Glycoalkaloids are natural toxins produced by nightshade plants. They help protect against insects, fungi, herbivores, and other predators. Unfortunately, they can also be harmful to humans. Solanum glycoalkaloids can disrupt cell membranes, induce developmental malformations, and inhibit cholinesterase (an enzyme needed for proper functioning of the central nervous system). The effects of glycoalkaloid toxicity include diarrhea, intestinal permeability, weight loss, and even death.

Very importantly for those with autoimmune conditions, some saponins, such as α-tomatine, have adjuvant activity. An *adjuvant* is a chemical that stimulates and exaggerates an immune response. In fact, the glycoalkaloid α-tomatine is such a potent adjuvant that it is used in vaccines to ensure that the recipient develops immunity against the virus against which they are being inoculated. In addition, glycoalkaloids inhibit a key enzyme, acetyl cholinesterase, which is required for nerve impulse conduction. There is also evidence that diets high in potatoes, in particular, result in increased markers of inflammation.

Based on reports of poisoning and death from high glycoalkaloid intake from potatoes (yep, there are quite a few of these!), an intake of 3 to 6 milligrams of glycoalkaloids per kilogram of body weight is considered a potentially lethal dose for humans, while 1 to 3 milligrams of glycoalkaloids per kilogram of body weight is considered toxic. And some researchers believe that the frequent consumption of potatoes and other nightshades may be a major contributor to the rise in chronic illness due to lower but more frequent intake of glycoalkaloids. According to researcher Yaroslav I. Korpan, PhD, "This discussion suggests that potato GAs [glycoalkaloids], particularly solanine and chaconine, are extremely toxic to humans and animals, and that this problem should no longer be ignored as it could turn into a serious health threat."

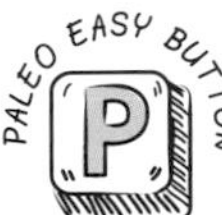

Tomatoes offer a great umami flavor to cooking, but you can add umami in other ways! Adding mushrooms, olives, or fish sauce to a dish is a great alternative.

However, certain people are much more sensitive to glycoalkaloids than others. In some individuals, for example, gastrointestinal symptoms have been documented after eating potatoes with a glycoalkaloid content of only 3 to 10 milligrams per 100 grams of potato. And people with autoimmune diseases (and certain other chronic conditions) can react to very low exposures that would be safe for the rest of the population. That's because glycoalkaloids are capable of decreasing the viability of intestinal cells (aka killing them) and increasing epithelial permeability (resulting in leaky gut). This increase in permeability is attributable not only to the effects on cell health, but also to an effect on cell-to-cell contact. The result is an exaggerated immune response when proteins enter the bloodstream, whether due to glycoalkaloids' direct influence on intestinal permeability or because of an already-leaky gut. That spells bad news for anyone with an autoimmune condition or other chronic disease involving compromised gut health.

Nightshades, like all plants, also contain lectins (see page 242), a class of sugar-binding proteins with many biological roles, including protecting plants (especially the seeds) against predation. Not all lectins are problematic; the lectins we want to avoid on a Paleo diet are the ones with the ability to increase intestinal permeability (which I hope is appearing as a common theme by this point!). These are lectins that resist digestion (typically due to high proline content), are relatively heat-stable (so there are still sufficient quantities to cause an issue after cooking), and have the ability to strongly interact with proteins in the membrane of the cells that line the intestine (and some can even bind to receptors in those membranes and be transported intact across the gut barrier).

So what do we know about nightshade lectins? Tomato lectin is known to enter the bloodstream relatively quickly in humans, which suggests that it can contribute to the development of a leaky gut. Based on this, most people should eat tomatoes in moderation. And because people with autoimmune disease are more likely have a leaky gut and have more challenges in healing a leaky gut once it has developed, these sensitive people should avoid tomato lectin entirely.

Another problematic substance in nightshades is capsaicin, a steroidal stimulant found in chili peppers. (It is one of the substances in peppers that give them heat.) While a variety of health benefits have been attributed to capsaicin, it is also a potent irritant to a variety of tissues, including skin, eyes, and mucous membranes. Very importantly, there is evidence that capsaicin can increase intestinal permeability.

SCIENCE SIMPLIFIED

Tomatoes, potatoes, peppers, and eggplant are full of great nutrients. Unfortunately, they're also pretty high in inflammatory compounds. Does the long list of pros outweigh the long list of cons? Since these foods work well for some people and not for others, they are included in this middle-ground category.

Overall, nightshades can certainly offer benefits (such as high micronutrient and phytochemical content), but their potentially harmful compounds put them squarely in the middle-ground category.

More on Potatoes

In Chapter 8, we looked at some of the benefits that potatoes offer—both for our cells (micronutrients) and for our gut microbiota (resistant starch). However, potatoes can be problematic for certain people.

As just highlighted, potatoes belong to the nightshade family of plants and thus contain glycoalkaloids. When determining whether the glycoalkaloid content is high enough to make potatoes harmful, it's important to understand that the effects of glycoalkaloids depend on two things: the amount we ingest and whether we have a chronic disease. Acute toxicity symptoms generally result from much higher doses of glycoalkaloids than we get from a moderate intake, or even a high intake, of potatoes. The upper limit of safety for glycoalkaloids is 20 milligrams per 100 grams of potato, and commercial varieties sold in the United States have been deliberately cultivated to remain well below this threshold. For example, the solanine content of some common cultivars are, per 100 grams (fresh weight):

- Washington russet potatoes: 0.58 mg
- White potatoes: 0.58 mg
- Idaho russet potatoes: 0.65 mg
- Red potatoes: 1.09 mg
- Benji potatoes: 2.8 mg
- Lenape potatoes: 21.6 mg

Compared to several cultivars from Pakistan that aren't sold commercially in the United States:

- SH-5 potatoes: 7.08 mg
- Diamant potatoes: 26.87 mg
- Cardinal potatoes: 30.83 mg
- FD 8-3 potatoes: 2,466.56 mg—whoa!

The most comprehensive experiment studying glycoalkaloid toxicity in humans found that symptoms of poisoning emerged at 2 milligrams of glycoalkaloids per kilogram of body weight (0.9 milligram per pound of body weight). Assuming that they're stored and prepared correctly (more on that in a moment!), it would take 20 kilograms (44 pounds) of russet potatoes to deliver that amount for a 150-pound adult! (Of course, variety matters. It would take only 10 ounces of Lenape potatoes to reach this threshold.)

So people with certain health conditions may need to eliminate potatoes to avoid triggering symptoms. But for everybody else, there are ways to store and prepare potatoes to minimize their glycoalkaloid content. Higher levels of glycoalkaloids result from exposure to light (as indicated by the greenish color that potatoes can develop), so storing potatoes in a dark area is important.

Between 30 and 80 percent of a potato's solanine content develops right under the skin; in some cases, the peel contains upwards of 98 percent of the total glycoalkaloid content! Peeling potatoes before cooking them reduces their glycoalkaloid content substantially.

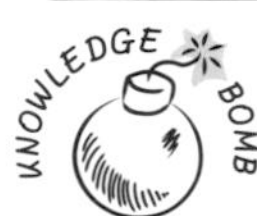

Choosing varieties like russet potatoes and peeling them before cooking is a great way to minimize glycoalkaloids.

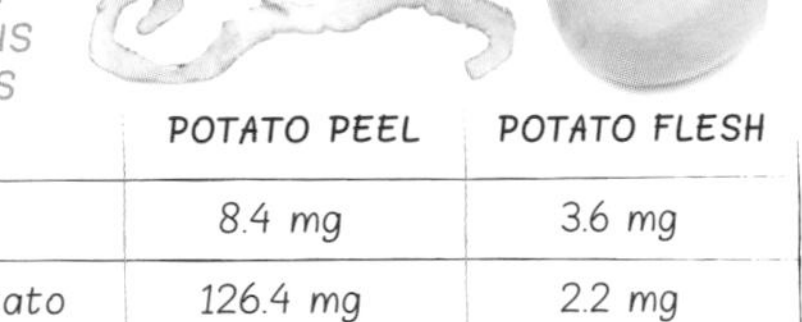

GLYCOALKALOIDS IN POTATO FLESH VERSUS SKIN PER 100 GRAMS (FRESH WEIGHT)	POTATO PEEL	POTATO FLESH
Atlantic potato	8.4 mg	3.6 mg
Dark Red Norland potato	126.4 mg	2.2 mg
Russet Norkotah potato	42.5 mg	6.4 mg
Snowden potato	325.6 mg	59.1 mg

Some research suggests that microwaving (more than boiling or other cooking methods) can reduce levels of these toxins by about 15 percent. Frying potatoes in oil at 410°F (210°C) or higher temperatures also reduces glycoalkaloid levels by about 40 percent, but only because the glycoalkaloids are retained in the oil—which makes it easy for these toxins to be reabsorbed by the potatoes if the oil isn't changed regularly, as is the case at some restaurants. Plus, this temperature is far above the smoke point for nearly all the healthy fat choices for deep-frying (see page 188).

GLYCOALKALOIDS IN POTATO PRODUCTS AND PREPARATIONS

POTATO PRODUCTS	GLYCOALKALOIDS (MILLIGRAMS PER 100 GRAMS OF PRODUCT)
French fries	0.04 to 0.8
Canned peeled potatoes	0.1 to 0.2
Frozen mashed potatoes	0.2 to 0.5
Frozen French fries	0.2 to 2.9
Frozen fried potatoes	0.4 to 3.1
Dehydrated potato flakes	1.5 to 2.3
Potato chips	2.3 to 18.0
Canned whole new potatoes	2.4 to 3.4
Boiled peeled potato	2.7 to 4.2
Baked potato with skin	9.9 to 11.3
Dehydrated potato flour	6.5 to 7.5
Frozen potato skins	6.5 to 12.1
Frozen baked potato	8.0 to 12.3
Potato chips with skin	9.5 to 72.0
Fried potato skins	56.7 to 145.0

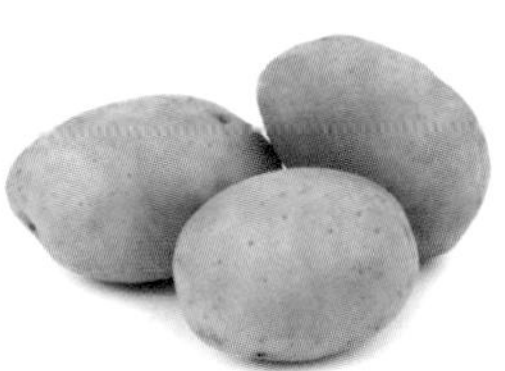

However, their nightshade status isn't the only reason potatoes can potentially be a problem. Another argument against these tubers is that they have a high glycemic index, meaning they cause a relatively high blood sugar response after consumption.

This is certainly true in some cases (a freshly baked potato has a glycemic index of 111, compared to a value of 100 for an equivalent amount of pure glucose), but the blood sugar response from potatoes is extremely context dependent. For example, cooling potatoes after cooking (or storing them in a cold environment, like the refrigerator) can reduce their glycemic response significantly, which may be due to the creation of retrograded resistant starch (see page 155). Glycemic index can also be lowered by adding an acidic food to the potato (like vinegar, citrus, or salsa), eating the potato with some fat (like olive oil or avocado), increasing the fiber content of the meal (such as by eating the potato with a leafy green salad), or boiling the potato instead of baking it. Simply storing a boiled potato in the fridge overnight and adding some vinegar can reduce its glycemic index by 43 percent!

Not only that, but analyses of different foods' satiety index, which measures hunger in the 2 hours following a meal, shows that potatoes are one of the most satiating foods out there, beating out fish, oatmeal, beef, beans, eggs, and cheese!

Plus, whether a food's glycemic index is really a concern is up for debate. Many studies show no link between foods' glycemic index values and whether those foods are associated with obesity and diabetes. In reality, the overall context of the meal (rather than an individual food in the meal, such as a potato) is what determines the body's glycemic response. And people can have significantly different glycemic responses to the same food depending on certain gene variations (such as AMY1 copy number and the level of amylase produced in the saliva).

Because choosing the right varieties, peeling the potatoes, preparation, and including them within a meal can have such a huge impact on the degree of problematic compounds in potatoes, they are included in the middle-ground category. The safest bet is to eliminate them initially and then use the protocol in Chapter 25 to reintroduce them to your diet and see how your body responds.

ALCOHOL

The conflicting claims surrounding alcohol can make it hard to know whether we should incorporate it into our diets. How does alcohol fit into a Paleo framework?

First, the good news: Moderate consumption of alcohol (and not just red wine) seems to provide diverse health benefits, including reduced risk of cardiovascular disease, reduced risk of type 2 diabetes, prevention of Alzheimer's disease, improved cognitive function and memory in people over 65, and potentially a reduced risk of some cancers. (Don't get too excited about the cancer prevention piece, though: moderate alcohol consumption also *increases* the risk of certain cancers, including breast cancer.) In small amounts, alcohol can help increase nitric oxide production (nitric oxide improves endothelial function by dilating blood vessels, controlling blood pressure, and facilitating the relaxation of vascular smooth muscles). It can also decrease iron absorption, which is bad in some cases (for people with higher iron requirements or iron deficiency anemia) but beneficial in other cases (for people with iron overload disorders like hemochromatosis). Some alcoholic beverages, particularly red wine, also contain high concentrations of the phenol resveratrol, which has potent antioxidant properties.

SCIENCE SIMPLIFIED *Unfortunately, alcohol can both damage the gut barrier and feed the wrong kinds of bacteria in the digestive tract. This allows toxins into the body that cause inflammation. For very healthy people, drinking in moderation may be fine. However, if you have a chronic disease and/or poor gut health, alcohol is probably not your friend.*

While the alcohol we consume today doesn't in any way resemble what our Paleolithic ancestors would have had access to, there is evidence that prehistoric man would consume fermented fruit and occasionally become intoxicated! Our gene to process alcohol goes back about 18 million years, long before humans were humans. Seeking out sweeter foods is thought to have given us an evolutionary advantage, and the same is thought about alcohol. Riper fruit has a higher alcohol content, so our ancestors' efforts to seek it out ensured that they got more vitamins and minerals, too. We are adapted to alcohol in small to moderate quantities (the bacteria in our guts also produce about 3 grams of ethanol per day), and we have the ability to effectively detoxify occasional and even semiregular higher consumption.

KNOWLEDGE BOMB *There are many examples of animals that get inebriated from fermented fruits: certain birds, bats, and tree shrews are known to get drunk off of wild fermented fruits. (Bats have been measured with a blood alcohol content as high as 0.3 percent! For reference, it's illegal to drive if your blood alcohol is above 0.08 percent.) There are even reports of larger animals like dogs and moose overindulging from time to time. Monkeys are known to enjoy the taste of alcohol; up to 20 percent of them even prefer alcohol to water and will drink to inebriation in lab environments. In the Caribbean, vervet monkeys are known to steal alcoholic beverages from beach bar customers, and as many as 5 percent of them are considered alcoholics!*

Yet despite all the research indicating that moderate consumption of alcohol (especially wine) is healthy, alcohol—even in moderation—can be a problem for people with certain health conditions, including autoimmune disease and other conditions related to leaky gut and gut dysbiosis (see page 73).

Moderate alcohol consumption is known to decrease the risk of some autoimmune diseases, including Hashimoto's thyroiditis, Graves' disease, celiac disease, type 1 diabetes, and systemic lupus erythematosus. However, it is linked to an *increased* risk of rheumatoid arthritis, psoriasis, and autoimmune liver diseases. An interesting study of the blood of patients who later developed rheumatoid arthritis found that alcohol consumption correlated with increased markers of inflammation, implying that alcohol may have contributed to their autoimmune disease. Another study of people with inactive inflammatory bowel disease showed that one week of moderate red wine consumption caused a significant increase in intestinal permeability (and a decrease is stool calprotectin, a marker of increased inflammatory bowel disease activity). So if you have inactive inflammatory bowel disease and drink red wine daily, you may be at increased long-term risk for a relapse.

Why? Alcohol consumption causes an increase in intestinal permeability (that is, a leaky gut). Alcohol unravels the tight junctions and adherens junctions (see page 67) that glue enterocytes together to form the barrier between the inside of the gut, where undigested food and bacteria live, and the inside of the body. Effectively, alcohol creates holes between the gut epithelial cells. Importantly, the "holes" that it makes in the gut epithelial barrier are known to be big enough to allow some very large molecules into the body, most notably endotoxin. Endotoxin is a toxic protein derived from the cell walls of Gram-negative bacteria, such as *E. coli*, which live in our guts. As these bacteria die (as part of their normal life cycle), endotoxin is released. If it gets into the bloodstream, it stimulates systemic inflammation, stimulates the immune system, and damages the liver.

Normally, the majority of bacteria that grow in our guts are Gram-positive bacteria (although some Gram-negative bacteria is normal). What do Gram-negative and Gram-positive mean? These terms refer to a staining technique that differentiates between these two major classes of bacteria. Basically, Gram-negative bacteria have more complex cell membranes/walls and tend to be pathogenic (that is, they cause disease). *E. coli* is an example of a Gram-negative bacteria. *Lactobacillus* (the probiotic found in yogurt, fermented vegetables, and supplements) is an example

PALEO BOOZE

If you do choose to drink alcohol, here are some important considerations!

HOW MUCH IS CONSIDERED MODERATE ALCOHOL CONSUMPTION?

- no more than four drinks for men or three drinks for women on any given day

AND

- a maximum of fourteen drinks for men and seven drinks for women throughout the week

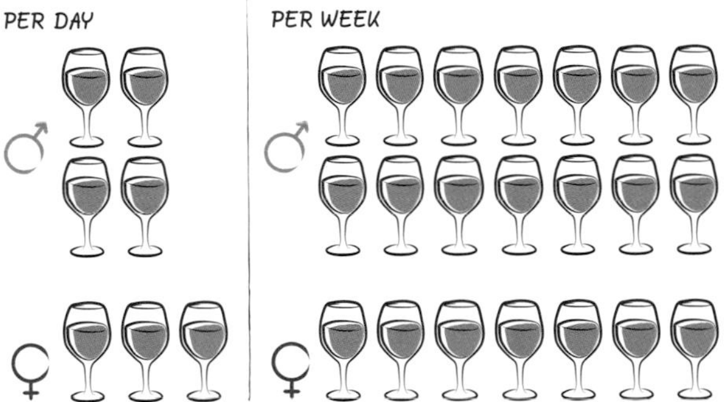

It's pretty unequivocal that once you're consuming two or three drinks most days, your risk of chronic disease and damage from alcohol consumption goes up dramatically.

WHAT ARE THE BEST CHOICES?

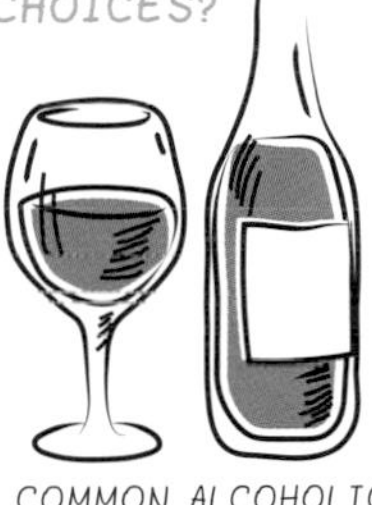
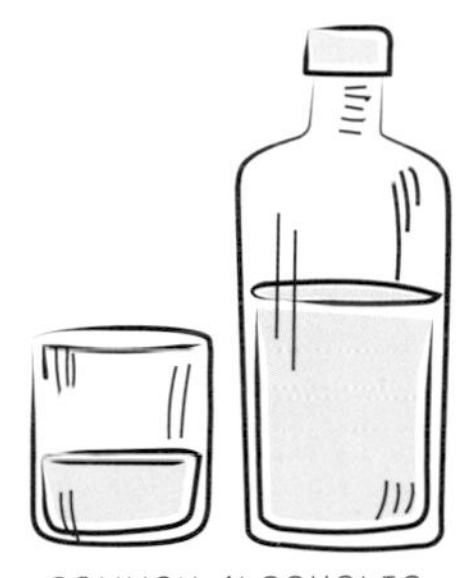

COMMON ALCOHOLIC BEVERAGES MADE FROM GLUTEN-FREE GRAINS:
- bourbon (corn)
- gluten-free beer (sorghum, millet, rice, and so on)
- sake (rice)

COMMON ALCOHOLIC BEVERAGES MADE FROM FRUIT:
- applejack (apples)
- brandy (grapes)
- champagne (grapes)
- cognac (grapes)
- vermouth (grapes)
- wine (grapes)
- apple cider (apples)
- kirsch (cherries)
- gin (juniper berries)
- grappa (pomace)

COMMON ALCOHOLIC BEVERAGES MADE FROM VEGETABLES:
- ginger beer (ginger root)
- rum (sugar cane)
- soju (sweet potato)
- tequila (agave juice)
- vodka (potatoes)

HOW MUCH IS ONE SERVING OF ALCOHOL?

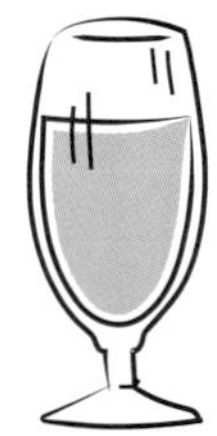
8 to 9 ounces of cider or gluten-free beer

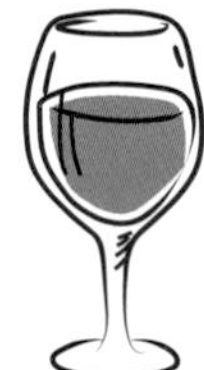
5 ounces of wine

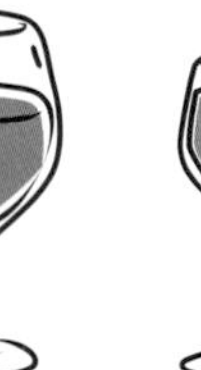
3 to 4 ounces of fortified wine (such as sherry, port, or Madeira)

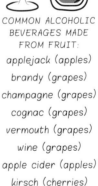

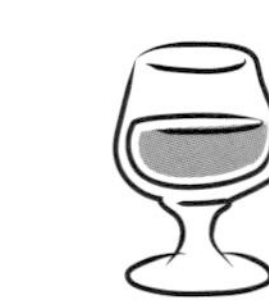
2 to 3 ounces of liqueur

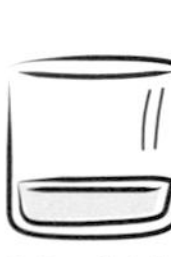
1 to 1 1/2 ounces of spirits

OTHER CONSIDERATIONS:

- Mixers can be full of refined sugars, nonnutritive sweeteners (in "light" versions), artificial flavors, and food dyes. It's better to stick with club soda and real fruit juice.
- Drinking within 2 to 3 hours of bedtime can wreak havoc on your sleep quality.
- Drinking alcohol makes us less inhibited with our food choices, meaning that it's harder to make good selections (in terms of both quality and quantity).

of a Gram-positive bacteria. So here's the kicker: alcohol consumption feeds Gram-negative bacteria such as *E. coli* to tip the microbial balance in the gut in favor of these more toxic bacteria and therefore excess endotoxin production in the gut. Excessive alcohol consumption is also correlated with Gram-negative bacteria growing very high up the digestive tract, in the duodenum and sometimes even the stomach.

So alcohol increases the production of endotoxin within the gut and increases intestinal permeability to endotoxin. Another toxin that is produced by both Gram-negative and Gram-positive bacteria is called peptidoglycan (another component of the cell wall that is released into the gut when the bacteria die). There is evidence that alcohol increases the permeability to peptidoglycan and that this toxin is very effective at stimulating the immune system and causing inflammation.

And that's not all. Even fairly small amounts of alcohol can damage the lining of the gut; specifically, alcohol damages the mucosa in the upper small intestine, induces epithelium loss at the tips of intestinal villi, and can cause hemorrhagic erosions and hemorrhage in the lamina propria. If that sounds bad, that's because it is. It's similar to the damage that gluten causes in celiac patients.

Most of the current understanding of the link between alcohol consumption and increased intestinal permeability comes from studies of chronic alcohol consumption. But there are studies showing that this damage occurs from even a single drink. Occasional drinkers don't damage their intestines as severely because they don't consume as much alcohol at once and thus their guts have more time to heal between drinks. This might lead to some adaptive mechanisms (hormesis), which could be part of the reason why low to moderate alcohol consumption can actually provide a health benefit.

In summary, alcohol is not good for anyone dealing with inflammation or gut issues: it's simply not conducive to healing an already leaky gut and remedying existing gut dysbiosis. However, for most of us, moderate alcohol consumption (especially wine) can be either health-neutral or somewhat health-protective. Cooking with alcohol is also generally okay, even for people who don't tolerate an actual drink, since the vast majority of the alcohol is cooked off. In other words, where alcohol falls within the Paleo framework is extremely individualized.

WHITE RICE

Rice is a gluten-free grain native to Asia. Brown rice is the whole grain with just the outermost layer (the hull or husk) removed. White rice is further polished to remove the bran and much of the germ, the next layer of the rice grain. While white rice has less fiber and lower levels of some nutrients than brown rice (noting that rice is not a particularly nutrient-rich food to begin with), it also has far fewer antinutrients (see page 230). That's because the antinutrients and toxins are concentrated in the bran, germ, and husk of the rice grain. When those are removed, as in the case of white rice, the result is a low-fructose source of complex carbohydrates. Yes, contrary to popular belief, white rice is a better choice than brown rice.

In Chapter 8, I mentioned that white rice can be less problematic than other grains; however, rice does not get an automatic green light for consumption.

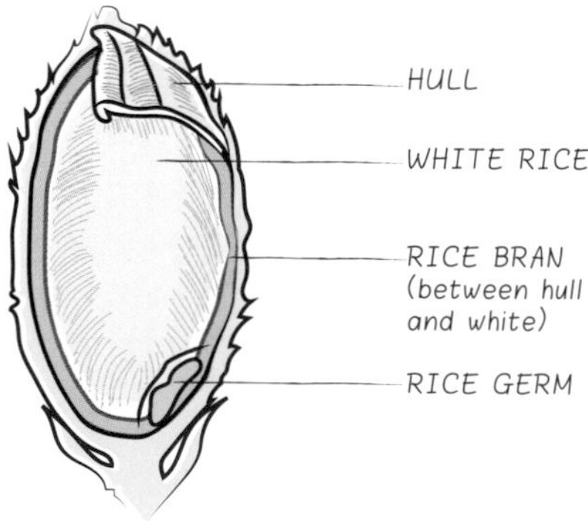

SCIENCE SIMPLIFIED *For those with suspected or confirmed celiac disease, gluten allergy, or gluten intolerance, it's much safer to avoid rice at least initially and then reintroduce it later using the protocol outlined in Chapter 25.*

First, rice can act as a gluten cross-reactor, meaning that people with celiac disease or gluten intolerance may potentially react to the proteins it contains (see page 245). So anyone on a gluten-free diet should also consider eliminating rice and later reintroducing it to see whether it triggers symptoms.

Second, rice is one of the riskiest crops as far as arsenic contamination goes. Arsenic is a toxic heavy metal that interferes with cellular energy production (blocking several key enzymes in the Krebs cycle; see page 267), causing cell death and oxidative damage. Chronic arsenic exposure can cause thickening and darkening of the skin, numbness, abdominal pain, and diarrhea and is linked to type 2 diabetes, heart disease, and cancer. Compared to other grains like barley and wheat, rice can absorb and accumulate very high levels of arsenic from the soil and water (which builds up in the land from motor vehicle traffic, waste incineration, industrial activities, mining operations, and fertilizer and pesticide use). The use of irrigation water in paddy fields can also increase arsenic levels in rice if the water contains heavy metals from nearby human activities. As a result, it's extremely important to eat only low-arsenic brands and varieties of rice.

The FDA monitors and publishes arsenic levels in rice, and other organizations perform independent testing as well. In general, most types of rice from Arkansas, Louisiana, and Texas tend to have the highest levels of arsenic, whereas white basmati rice from California, India, and Pakistan (as well as sushi rice from the United States in general) has lower levels. Likewise, because arsenic accumulates in the outer layers of the rice grain, brown rice (which retains that husk) tends to have much higher levels than white rice.

Rice can be an inexpensive source of important starchy carbs. When made with broth (see page 178), it can also be an easy way to increase our consumption of glycine and some minerals. However, given its potential health hazards, it's categorized as a middle-ground food.

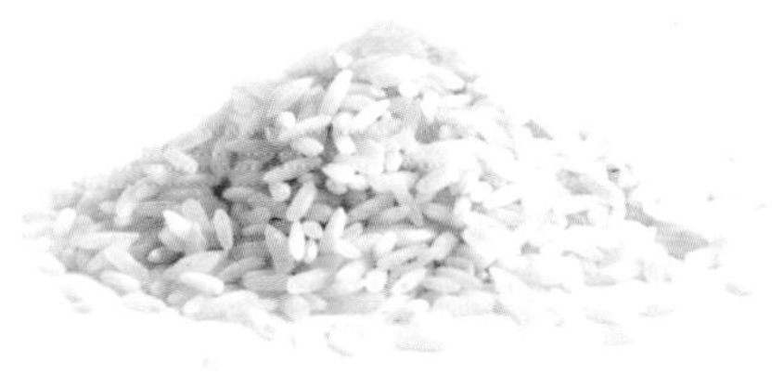

NATURAL SUGARS AND SWEETENERS

We've already looked at why high-fructose corn syrup and artificial sweeteners are worth eliminating completely. And the evidence clearly shows that sugar (in large quantities) should not be a staple in our diets. But what about natural sweeteners like honey, molasses, and maple syrup, or less-refined versions of cane sugar?

The good news is that small amounts of natural sweeteners are unlikely to be harmful and can even contribute some valuable micronutrients to our diets. The bad news is that it's still a case of "the dose makes the poison": these foods become harmful when they start displacing more-nutritious items from the menu or when they increase our energy intake beyond what we need. Therefore, they're *conditionally* allowed on a Paleo diet.

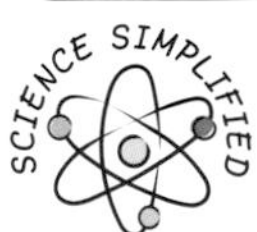

Our bodies can generally handle a little sugar now and then. The tricks are to keep treats minimally sweetened, to use a natural and preferably nutrient-dense sugar, and to indulge only occasionally.

How do natural sweeteners differ from refined table sugar and high-fructose corn syrup? In most cases, the ratio of glucose to fructose (after we've consumed and metabolized the sweetener) is actually very similar: about 50 percent glucose and 50 percent fructose (keeping in mind that sucrose is broken down into equal parts fructose and glucose in our bodies). The biggest exception is agave syrup, which is in the "avoid" list due to its extremely high fructose content (up to 85 percent or higher); see page 269.

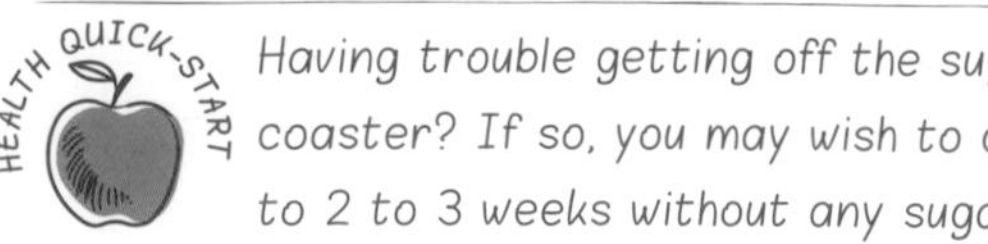

Having trouble getting off the sugar roller coaster? If so, you may wish to commit to 2 to 3 weeks without any sugars other than those naturally occurring in whole fruits to help your taste buds and metabolism adapt to a lower sugar intake. Making sure to get plenty of sleep and managing stress (see Chapters 26 and 27, respectively) will also go a long way toward minimizing sugar cravings.

The main reason natural sweeteners are considered superior to highly refined table sugar and high-fructose corn syrup has to do with micronutrients. Raw honey contains small amounts of vitamins A, B1, B6, B9, B12, C, D, and E, as well as calcium, sodium, phosphorus, magnesium, silicon, iron, manganese, and copper. Maple syrup contains small amounts of manganese and zinc. Unrefined cane sugar (sucanat, evaporated cane juice, muscovado/Barbados sugar, rapadura sugar, or jaggery) contains small amounts of vitamins A, B1, B2, B3, B5, and B6, along with calcium, iron, magnesium, zinc, copper, chromium, phosphorus, manganese, sodium, and potassium. By contrast, white sugar, brown sugar, and turbinado sugar ("raw sugar") contain close to zero micronutrients.

Among the natural sweeteners, though, molasses is king. Its nutritional content is exceptional, and while it should be used in moderation like any sweetener, it can make some truly beneficial contributions to our diets.

Molasses: King of Natural Sweeteners

Molasses is a brown, viscous by-product of sugar making, typically produced from sugarcane or sugar beets (although grapes, sorghum, dates, pomegranate, carob, and a number of other foods can also produce molasses-like products). After sugarcane is harvested and its juice is extracted (typically by cutting, crushing, or mashing), the juice undergoes multiple boilings to concentrate it and allow sugar crystals to form. The dark, thick syrup remaining after the sugar crystals are removed is what we call molasses.

Many of us have been led to believe that because molasses is associated with sugar, it must be a processed sweetener that's best avoided (or at least used very sparingly). This couldn't be further from the truth! Molasses is surprisingly nutrient dense and could even be considered a superfood based on its impressive vitamin and mineral content—not to mention that its robust flavor is an irreplaceable component of a number of recipes.

But, as with most foods, not all molasses is created equal. Three different types of molasses are available, distinguished by the number of times the cane or beet juice has been boiled. And each type differs not only in appearance and flavor but also in nutritional composition, since each subsequent boiling removes more sugar and further concentrates the remaining nutrients. It's important to know which molasses to look for to get the maximum nutritional benefit.

- **Light molasses** (also called Barbados molasses) is the result of the first round of boiling and sugar crystal extraction and is the sweetest and lightest in color. But it doesn't offer much in the way of micronutrients; it has only about 25 percent of the nutritional content of blackstrap (third boiling) molasses, and its sugar content is highest among all the molasses types (since less sugar has been crystalized and removed).

- **Dark molasses** (also called robust molasses) is the result of the second boiling and sugar crystal extraction. It's less sweet and slightly bitter compared to light molasses, with a relatively higher nutritional content. This is the type of molasses that is found in most grocery stores and is typically used for making gingerbread and other sweet baked goods.

- **Blackstrap molasses** is the residue remaining after the third and final boiling. As a result, it's thicker, darker, and more nutritious than any other molasses. It also has a much stronger flavor and a lower sugar content, since three rounds of sugar crystals have been removed (most of the remaining sugar is caramelized, contributing to the dark brown color of the syrup). Basically, as refined sugar is extracted, all the nutrients originally present are concentrated in this final product. This type of molasses is typically carried in specialty grocery stores and health food stores.

KNOWLEDGE BOMB

Blackstrap molasses has more than five times as much iron as steak and one and a half times as much calcium as cheese (per calorie). Not many foods can boast those kinds of micronutrient levels!

Let's take a look at just what blackstrap molasses has to offer. One tablespoon (20 grams) contains only 42 calories, but packs in:

27% OF THE RDA FOR **MANGANESE**

21% OF THE RDA FOR **COPPER**

20% OF THE RDA FOR **IRON**

17.6% OF THE RDA FOR **CALCIUM**

11% OF THE RDA FOR **MAGNESIUM**

9.7% OF THE RDA FOR **POTASSIUM**

7.5% OF THE RDA FOR **B vitamins, including B6, and smaller amounts of B2 and B3**

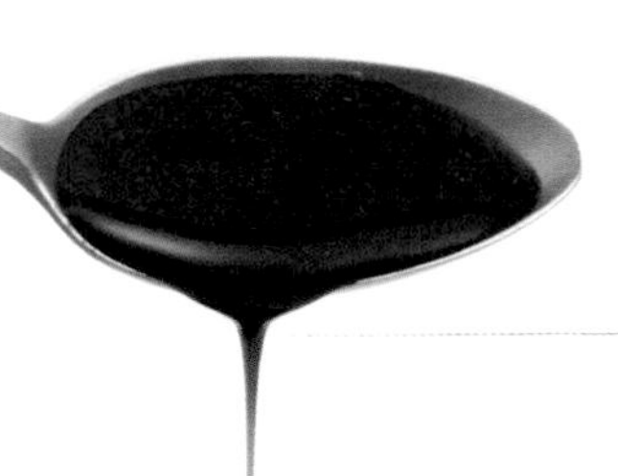

5.2% OF THE RDA FOR **SELENIUM**

Small amounts OF **SODIUM, ZINC, and PHOSPHORUS**

This qualifies blackstrap molasses as a nutrient-dense food. Yes, it does contain sugar (roughly 50 percent sucrose, 25 percent glucose, and 25 percent fructose), but the amount of nutrition per calorie is still impressive. Likewise, the glycemic index of blackstrap molasses is reported to be 55 (right on the border between low and moderate) compared to table sugar at 80 (high). That puts molasses in the same category as fruit and moderate glycemic load starchy veggies: it's a great choice in moderation.

Historically, blackstrap molasses has been used not only as a cooking ingredient, but also medicinally. It was traditionally given as a remedy for an upset stomach and used directly in the ear to treat earaches (although I don't recommend you try that!). Papers dating back to the 1930s and earlier discuss it as therapy for iron deficiency anemia due to its high iron content and ability to raise serum ferritin (an iron-storage protein that acts as an indirect measurement of the total amount of iron stored in the body). Even today, it's proposed as a treatment for anemia associated with inflammatory bowel disease and menorrhagia and can be an excellent supplement for vegetarians and anyone else who doesn't eat much iron-rich red meat or organ meat.

Thanks to its specific array of nutrients (at significant levels for human health), molasses helps support a number of body processes. It's a great food for enhancing oxygen transport and energy production (which involve iron); supporting healthy skeletal tissue, muscle and blood vessel contraction, and nervous system function (which involve calcium); producing red blood cells, forming collagen, and keeping nerve cells healthy (which involve copper); manufacturing sex hormones, supporting carbohydrate and fat metabolism, and forming clotting factors (which involve manganese); synthesizing protein, regulating blood glucose, and controlling blood pressure (which involve magnesium); aiding in nerve conduction and maintaining a normal water balance between cells and body fluids (which involve potassium); supporting cellular metabolism (which involves the B vitamins); and assisting with thyroid function, DNA production, and antioxidant defenses (which involve selenium).

Along with making sure the molasses is blackstrap instead of light or dark (to maximize the micronutrient content), there's another detail to watch out for. Look for *unsulfured* blackstrap molasses (typically spelled the British way, "unsulphured," on molasses bottles), which means that the molasses has been processed without sulfur dioxide (a bleaching and antimicrobial agent). Sulfur is sometimes used in molasses to extend its shelf life and kill bacteria and mold, and to assist in processing sugarcane that's been harvested at an early stage (as opposed to fully sun-ripened sugarcane). But it can be allergenic (especially to people who are sensitive to sulfites; see page 239) and gives the molasses a chemical flavor. Unsulfured molasses made from mature (rather than green) sugarcane is considered higher quality and better tasting.

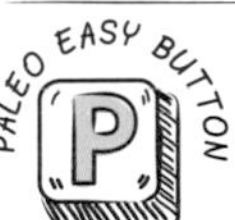

The recommendation to add some blackstrap molasses to your diet doesn't mean that you get a green light to eat dozens of gingerbread cookies! Molasses can be used as an ingredient in barbecue sauce (page 493) or meatloaf (page 543), or you can add a few tablespoons to stews (like on page 519) and pasta sauces for a savory, earthy flavor.

So how should we view natural sweeteners in the context of a Paleo framework? In general, micronutrient-containing sweeteners (molasses, honey, maple syrup or sugar, and unrefined cane sugar) are superior to nutrient-devoid sweeteners, and small amounts can be a perfectly acceptable addition to our diets. In the case of blackstrap molasses, the micronutrient benefit can be profound. But these foods are beneficial or neutral only to a point and should never crowd out more nutrient-dense items from our menus!

What's the Next Superfood Sweetener?

A few fruit-based sweeteners have found a niche within sugar-conscious communities. They include lucuma powder, made by grinding up the dried fruit of the subtropical South American *Pouteria lucuma* plant, and monk fruit extract, made by dehydrating the solvent-extracted and purified juice of the fruit from the East Asian *Siraitia grosvenorii* plant.

Lucuma tastes sweet owing to its sugar content, with 64 percent of its sugars coming from sucrose, 21 percent from glucose, and 15 percent from fructose. (A few other cultivars of lucuma have more glucose and fructose and much less sucrose.) However, the benefit of lucuma powder is that, because it's a dehydrated whole fruit, it also contains some fiber and some more complex carbohydrates. A 20-gram serving of lucuma powder has 80 calories and contains 16 grams of carbohydrates, 4 grams of which come from sugars and 8 grams of which come from fiber. This greatly reduces its impact on blood glucose levels, although the glycemic index of lucuma powder has not yet been established. Limited nutritional information is available for lucuma, although it is rich in several important phytochemicals, including phenolic compounds and carotenoids. No toxological studies on lucuma powder have been published in peer-reviewed journals, but given that lucuma fruit has been consumed in South America for centuries and that lucuma powder is a dehydrated whole food, it is likely a safe and nutrient-dense sugar choice.

Monk fruit contains sugars but also mogrosides, a glycoside that is about 300 times sweeter than sugar. Whole monk fruit is only about 1 percent mogrosides, which are concentrated to 80 percent in monk fruit extract using solvent extraction. The flavor is rendered more neutral through the use of deodorizing agents like sulfonated polystyrene-divinylbenzene copolymer or polyacrylic acid in conventional manufacturing and charcoal or bentonite in more chemical-conscious manufacturing. Very little nutritional information on monk fruit extract is available at this time; however, given that it is a processed and refined food, little nutritional value is expected.

While whole monk fruit has been consumed for centuries in Asia and is used as a cold and digestive aid in Eastern medicine, there is a scarcity of scientific studies evaluating the effects of regularly consuming high levels of mogrosides as a sugar substitute. On the pro side, mogrosides have anti-inflammatory, antioxidant, and anti-cancer properties. They have no effect on the gut microbiota and lower blood glucose levels in diabetics. On the con side, a thorough rat study evaluating possible toxicity of mogrosides over 4 weeks indicates some possible reasons for concern, at least for high consumption:

- Lower blood lymphocytes and leukocytes (two important types of white blood cells) indicate possible immune suppression.
- Increased liver weight, decreased bilirubin, and decreased prothrombin time indicate possible functional changes in the liver.
- Increased ovary and testes weights indicate a possible impact on reproductive systems.

Although no histopathological changes (changes in tissue structure that would indicate disease) accompanied the increased organ weights (adrenal gland weight also increased in male rats), increased organ weight is considered one of the most sensitive drug toxicity indicators, often preceding morphological changes to the organ (changes to the biological structure of the organs that distinctly indicate toxicity). Clearly, more data is needed before monk fruit extract, as opposed to the whole fruit, can be fully endorsed as a sugar substitute.

What about the next trendy superfood sugar? Contrary to all the hype you're likely to read, there really is no way to cheat sweet. The good news is that our bodies can generally handle moderate and occasional sugar consumption, so a treat now and then isn't out of the question. The best strategy is to avoid added sugars, even natural ones, on a daily basis, opting instead for whole fresh fruit (see page 151). As your taste buds adapt to a lower sugar intake, fruit and minimally sweetened treats will taste sweeter and more indulgent.

THE BEST SWEETENER CHOICES

The trick with all natural sugars and sweeteners is to keep your intake moderate and occasional. When you do want a treat, a natural sugar with some micronutrient content is the best choice.

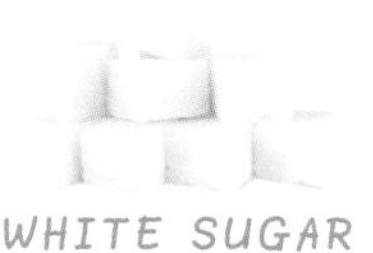

WHITE SUGAR

% Fructose	0	% Sucrose	100
% Glucose	0	% Other	0
Glycemic Index	65	Calories per 20 g	77

(about 1 tablespoon)

VITAMIN/MINERAL CONTENT:
none

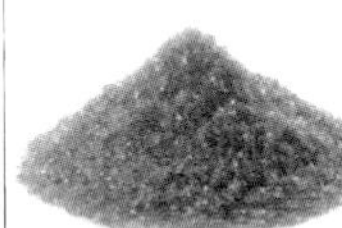

BROWN SUGAR (turbinado, sugar in the raw)

% Fructose	1	% Sucrose	97
% Glucose	1	% Other	1
Glycemic Index	65	Calories per 20 g	76

VITAMIN/MINERAL CONTENT:
Vitamin B6, calcium, iron, magnesium, potassium, copper, manganese

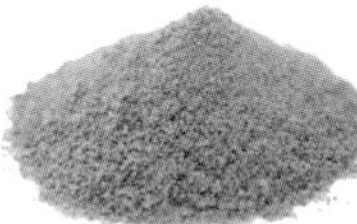

COCONUT SUGAR

% Fructose	3-9	% Sucrose	70-80
% Glucose	3-9	% Other	2-24
Glycemic Index	34-55°	Calories per 20 g	67

VITAMIN/MINERAL CONTENT:
Vitamins B1* and C*, calcium, copper*, sodium, phosphorous, potassium*, magnesium, manganese, sulfur, boron, iron*, zinc*

° Conflicting measurements.

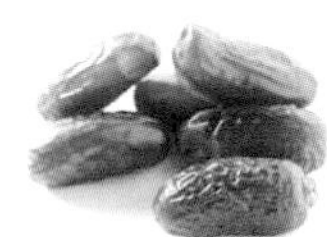

DATE SUGAR

% Fructose	31	% Sucrose	38
% Glucose	31	% Other	0
Glycemic Index	42	Calories per 20 g	67

VITAMIN/MINERAL CONTENT:
Vitamins B1, B2, B3, B6, and B9; calcium; iron; copper; magnesium; potassium*; phosphorous; zinc; manganese; selenium

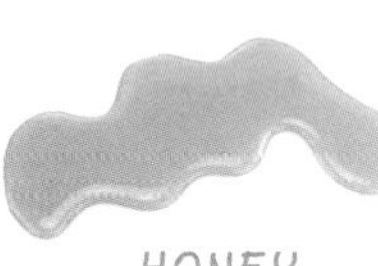

HONEY

% Fructose	28-56	% Sucrose	1-2
% Glucose	22-42	% Other	7-30
Glycemic Index	31-78°	Calories per 20 g	64

VITAMIN/MINERAL CONTENT:
Vitamins B3, B5, B9, and C; choline; calcium; sodium; phosphorus; magnesium; silicon; iron; manganese; potassium; selenium; fluoride

° Varies depending on exact sugar composition.

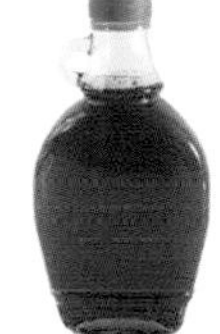

MAPLE SYRUP

% Fructose	1	% Sucrose	95
% Glucose	4	% Other	0
Glycemic Index	55	Calories per 20 g	52

VITAMIN/MINERAL CONTENT:
Vitamins B1, B2, B3, and B5; choline; potassium; phosphorous; calcium; manganese**; sulfur; iron; zinc*; copper; sodium; magnesium; selenium

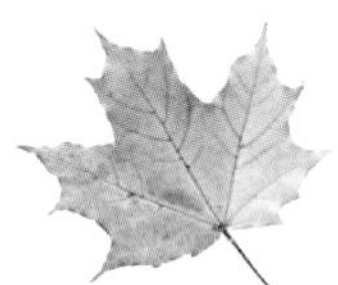

MAPLE SUGAR

% Fructose	1	% Sucrose	95
% Glucose	4	% Other	0
Glycemic Index	55	Calories per 20 g	70

VITAMIN/MINERAL CONTENT:
Vitamins B1, B2, B3, and B5; choline; potassium; phosphorous; calcium; manganese**; sulfur; iron; zinc**; copper; sodium; magnesium; selenium

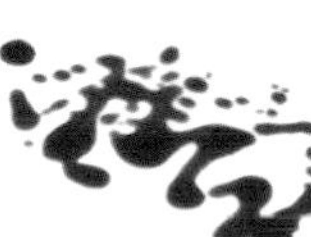

MOLASSES

% Fructose	23	% Sucrose	53
% Glucose	21	% Other	3
Glycemic Index	55	Calories per 20 g	58

VITAMIN/MINERAL CONTENT:
Vitamins B1, B3, B5, and B6*; choline; calcium; iron*; magnesium**; zinc; copper*; chromium; phosphorus; manganese**; sodium; potassium*; selenium*

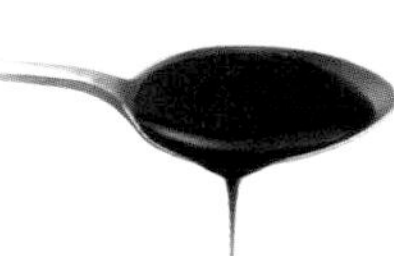

BLACKSTRAP MOLASSES

% Fructose	16	% Sucrose	54
% Glucose	13	% Other	17
Glycemic Index	55	Calories per 20 g	42

VITAMIN/MINERAL CONTENT:
Vitamins B1, B3, B5, and B6*; choline; calcium**; iron**; magnesium**; zinc; copper**; chromium; phosphorus; manganese**; sodium; potassium**; selenium*

UNREFINED CANE SUGAR (sucanat, evaporated cane juice, muscovado/ Barbados sugar, rapadura, jaggery)

% Fructose	2	% Sucrose	88
% Glucose	2	% Other	8
Glycemic Index	55	Calories per 20 g	76

VITAMIN/MINERAL CONTENT:
Vitamins B1, B2, B5, B6, calcium, iron**; magnesium*; zinc; copper; chromium; phosphorus; manganese*; sodium; potassium*

*Indicates greater than 5% of the RDA of that nutrient in 20 grams (about a tablespoon)

**Indicates greater than 10% of the RDA of that nutrient in 20 grams (about a tablespoon)

NOTE: Exact saccharide content can vary depending on exactly where and how these sugars are produced; the numbers in this table may not reflect the version you have purchased. Honey is especially variable in its glucose and fructose content. Also note that there is very limited and conflicting data on coconut sugar.

Now, don't get excited at the long list of vitamins and minerals in some of these natural sugars. With the exception of molasses, especially blackstrap molasses (see page 304), the amounts that you would need to eat in order for the micronutrient content to contribute meaningfully to your diet would far exceed what could be classified as moderate.

CHIA, FLAX, AND PSYLLIUM

As explained in Chapter 13, there's a benefit to moderate daily consumption of nuts and seeds, provided you don't have an allergy, intolerance, or sensitivity to them. But there's good reason to limit consumption of a few seeds typically labeled as superfoods, namely chia, flax, and psyllium.

Chia (technically a pseudograin; see page 256), flax, and psyllium, contain a type of viscous soluble fiber called *mucilage* that swells up and becomes gelatinous when it makes contact with water. For plants, mucilage comes in pretty handy: it can help barricade injuries from pathogens by forming a gelatinous layer on the wound site, helps plants develop a relationship with soil-dwelling life forms like fungus, serves as a barometer to check water loss, aids in germination, and helps facilitate seed dispersal. The unique properties of this fiber have led people to tout mucilaginous foods for their benefits to human health, especially when it comes to healing gut conditions. (In the case of flax seeds and chia seeds, their omega-3 and micronutrient contents have also painted them with a health halo.) However, in some situations mucilage may actually aggravate certain health problems and therefore is worth avoiding (at least temporarily).

First, the good: mucilage has long been praised for its role in human health, and in many cases, that praise is well earned. Plenty of research points to beneficial and therapeutic activity for this unique fiber. Mucilage-rich psyllium seed is often used to stimulate normal bowel function and absorb excess water (making it useful for both constipation and mild diarrhea). And the addition of mucilage to a calorie-reduced diet has been shown to lead to greater weight loss and greater reductions in triglyceride and total cholesterol levels than diet alone (possibly due to reduced intestinal absorption of bile acids).

However, mucilaginous foods also can operate as immune stimulators, which can be beneficial in some contexts but harmful in others. For instance, some types of mucilage specifically stimulate different subsets of the adaptive immune system: either the Th1 immune response (like flax seeds) or the Th2 immune response (like the mucilage in natto, or fermented soybeans). If someone has an autoimmune disease with one of these subsets already dominant (referred to as Th1 or Th2 dominance), stimulating the wrong pathway can aggravate the Th1/Th2 imbalance instead of helping to correct it, resulting in a worsening of autoimmune symptoms. Plus, regulating the immune system is far more complex than simply stimulating the suppressed pathway, as used to be standard in Th1/Th2 balancing protocols.

KNOWLEDGE BOMB

Recall that chia seeds and flax seeds are very high in phytoestrogens (see page 227). To review, flaxseed contains 305 milligrams of lignans per 100 grams, and chia seeds contain 114 milligrams per 100 grams. Yes, flax has a higher phytoestrogen content than soy! This is yet another reason to limit consumption of chia and flax.

If a person's immune system is not regulating itself well, as is the case with any chronic illness, since inflammation is a consequence of an immune system that isn't modulating itself properly, then stimulating inflammatory immune pathways is not likely to do that person any favors. When it comes to mucilage, individual responses vary greatly; the composition of the gut microbiota, exactly how the immune system is dysregulated, nutrient status, stress level, sleep debt, and the exact quantity (and food source) of mucilage are all inputs into the equation.

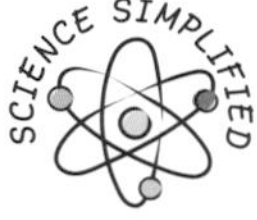

Those with chronic illness may wish to avoid chia, flax, and psyllium as well as other food sources of mucilage fiber due to their potential immune-stimulating effects.

Mucilage has the potential to cause harm in other ways as well. Although mucilage is only partially degraded by gut microbes, when it does become hydrolyzed in the intestines, its simple sugars get liberated and become potential food for bacteria—and not just the beneficial strains! A number of pathogenic microbes can chow down on the xylose, arabinose, rhamnose, galactose, glucose, mannose, and/or fucose contained in mucilage, especially if the gut is already compromised. Those bacteria species include:

- ***Clostridium difficile (C. difficile),*** which can eat the galactose, mannose, and glucose liberated from mucilage. When imbalanced, it can cause *C. difficile* colitis, a severe infection that can range from diarrhea to potentially deadly colon inflammation (and even the formation of a hole in the intestines!).
- ***Escherichia coli (E. coli),*** which can eat the glucose, arabinose, and xylose liberated from mucilage. Certain strains of *E. coli* are famous for causing foodborne illness due to producing the Shiga toxin, which can lead to vomiting, fever, severe stomach cramps, and bloody diarrhea. About 5 to 10 percent of people with this type of *E. coli* infection develop hemolytic uremic syndrome (HUS), which can be life-threatening.
- ***Staphylococcus aureus,*** which can eat the galactose liberated from mucilage. This major opportunistic pathogen produces a variety of toxins (both enterotoxins and cytotoxins) and can cause nausea, vomiting, diarrhea, cramps, fever, and loss of appetite. And it can alter the overall structure of the gut microbial community and reduce the production of beneficial short-chain fatty acids (SCFAs).

Basically, what this means is that for certain forms of gut dysbiosis, mucilage might feed the *wrong* bacteria and consequently worsen gut health instead of improving it. For example, someone with an overgrowth of *C. difficile* (and a shortage of beneficial resident bacteria to compete with it!) might find that mucilage encourages the *C. difficile* to flourish and cause infection. This could be an issue especially after a hospital visit or long-term antibiotic treatment that kills off intestinal bacteria that usually keep *C. difficile* in check.

Let me emphasize that there's no evidence that eating a diet rich in mucilage can cause gut dysbiosis if you're starting out with a healthy diverse gut microbiota. But this may explain why so many people report a worsening of gastrointestinal symptoms or symptoms of autoimmune disease when they eat foods like psyllium (whole or husks) and chia seeds.

Given the wide range of positive health effects from mucilaginous foods, mucilage isn't a definite no-no for a healthy, nutrient-dense diet. But it's worth noting that despite the glowing endorsements for this fiber, we may need to reduce or eliminate high-mucilage foods while building an optimal gut microbiota or addressing a dysfunctional and overstimulated immune system. And that may mean avoiding flax seeds, chia seeds, and psyllium (whole or husks) in the process.

The Dark Side of Psyllium Husk

Psyllium husks (also called ispaghula, isabgol, or just psyllium) are the protective sheaths around the seeds of the *Plantago ovata* plant, which grows across certain parts of Asia and Africa. Due to their high mucilage content, psyllium husks are hygroscopic, which means that they expand by attracting water and forming a slippery gel (which is part of what makes them a useful ingredient binder in recipes!). They're about 70 percent soluble fiber and 30 percent insoluble fiber, the majority of which isn't fermentable by the gut.

Psyllium husk has long been used to treat constipation and promote regularity (psyllium is the "magic" ingredient in Metamucil) due to its ability to increase stool bulk. It's also a common component of colon-cleanse programs promoted in some alternative health circles. And thanks to its texture and culinary chemistry properties, it's becoming a common ingredient in Paleo recipes that call for gluten-free (or low-carb) flour substitutes.

Most of what we hear about psyllium are its benefits. Not only does psyllium husk effectively soften stools (which makes it beneficial for people with constipation, hemorrhoids, anal fissures, and related conditions), it's also been shown in clinical trials to improve irritable bowel syndrome (IBS) symptoms, reduce cholesterol levels, reduce blood sugar levels in diabetics, and potentially assist with weight loss. In people with diarrhea, psyllium is sometimes prescribed to help soak up the excess fluid and improve bowel function. So, thanks to all those potential perks, psyllium husks are usually touted as being beneficial.

But we should keep in mind that none of these effects is unique to psyllium husk. Whole-food sources of soluble and insoluble fiber can exhibit these same health-promoting properties while also delivering fatty acids, amino acids, and micronutrients (all of which psyllium husks are practically devoid of, since they're merely the thin fiber layers around the more-nutritious seeds). And whole foods contain a mixture of fibers that feed beneficial gut flora, in contrast to the limited fiber composition of psyllium husk.

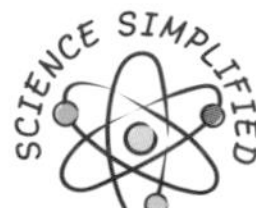

Whole psyllium seeds are probably okay for most people (but not those with gut dysbiosis or a dysfunctional immune system). However, psyllium husk comes with some legitimate risks and probably should not be consumed regularly, especially by those at a higher risk for colon cancer or bowel obstruction.

Despite some proven, albeit not unique, benefits, psyllium husks do pose risks as well, and yes, beyond psyllium's mucilage fiber content. Due to psyllium's ability to bind with water, mix with other substances, and dramatically expand in size, it can form what are called bezoars—and I'm not talking about the magical poison antidote in the Harry Potter universe. Bezoars are masses of material that obstruct the gastrointestinal tract and can cause serious damage. As early as 1938, reports were being published about psyllium causing intestinal obstruction and perforation, in some cases requiring surgery. Small bowel obstructions continue to occur even today in susceptible individuals taking this fiber. Psyllium husks (and psyllium-based products like the laxative Perdiem) have been shown to cause esophageal impactions as well, especially when consumed with insufficient amounts of water.

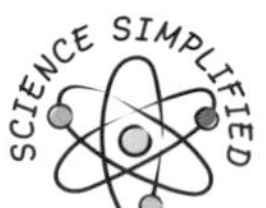

Psyllium husk has been linked with bowel obstructions and increased colorectal cancer growth.

Even more concerning is the possibility that psyllium husks can spur colon cancer progression in people who are already at risk. One trial gave a group of 665 patients with a history of colorectal adenomas (precursors to cancerous colon tumors) a daily calcium supplement, a daily psyllium husk supplement, or a placebo, for 3 years straight. By the end of the study, the people taking psyllium husk had a significantly higher rate of adenomas than everyone else. As revealed by colonoscopies, 29.3 percent of the psyllium group developed adenomas by the 3-year mark, compared to only 15.9 percent for the calcium group and 20.2 percent in the placebo group. That translates to an odds ratio of 1.67 for the study participants who took psyllium—or a 67 percent higher risk! Although other studies have produced contradictory results (some rodent studies show that psyllium should benefit intestinal cells), this news is concerning for anyone who has a history of colorectal adenomas or for whom colon cancer runs in the family.

And psyllium can interact with a number of medications. It can interfere with the effectiveness of antidepressants/tricyclics and reduce the absorption of the antiseizure medication carbamazepine and the heart medication digoxin. On top of that, allergic reactions have been reported, both from occupational exposure and from ingestion of psyllium.

So is it worth using psyllium (seed or husk) for the potential benefits (regularity, lower blood sugar, lower cholesterol, and maybe appetite suppression and weight loss)? The answer is probably no. Although eating psyllium occasionally (perhaps as an ingredient in a gluten-free baked good) probably won't cause harm except in certain people with autoimmune conditions or severe digestive sensitivity, the cons outweigh the pros. Psyllium husk doesn't have any special properties that make it better than other fiber sources, but it does carry some legitimate dangers and can displace far more nutritious items (like whole-food sources of fiber) from our diets.

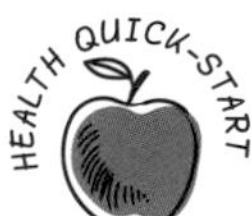

If treating constipation is a concern, it's a better idea to address any underlying gut dysbiosis issues, evaluate thyroid function, consume plenty of electrolytes (especially magnesium) to promote intestinal motility, eat a diverse array of plant foods, and invest in a Squatty Potty or Step and Go than to supplement with psyllium to put a bandage on the problem. And as far as Paleo cooking goes, there are other flour substitutes that can be used in recipes to support health!

Chapter 25:
EXPERIMENTING WITH FOODS

While many foods are clearly health-promoting or clearly harmful (when we look at the full scope of the scientific evidence), some are more ambiguous in terms of their effects on human health. Whether foods such as high-quality dairy, legumes, and natural sweeteners are damaging, neutral, or beneficial is far from case-closed and depends largely on individual tolerance and the overall context of our health.

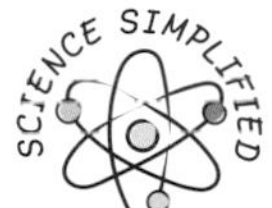

Yes, humans absolutely have adapted, at least somewhat, to the dietary changes that came with the advent of agriculture. But we're not fully adapted to our modern diets, as demonstrated by the links between diet and epidemics of chronic disease.

Which factors affect how our bodies react to specific foods? Major inputs to our health in general—including the nutrient density of our diet, sleep quantity and quality, stress, and physical activity—can affect how our bodies react to compounds in foods. A lot more is unknown than known in terms of specific mechanisms, but it's safe to generalize that our bodies are more tolerant of suboptimal foods when we're well rested, our stress levels are low, we live an active lifestyle, we have healthy gut microbiota, and we aren't deficient in any nutrients. Because these inputs can fluctuate even when we're trying to keep everything dialed in—stress levels may go up with an approaching deadline, or gut microbiota may be impacted by a course of antibiotics, for example—it can sometimes feel like identifying which foods work (or don't work) for us is a moving target. Layered underneath this variability are the more stable effects of genetics.

Genetic variation certainly accounts for some differences between individuals when it comes to which foods our bodies can tolerate. An oft-cited rationale for the Paleo diet is that the mere 10,000-ish years that have elapsed since the agricultural revolution is an insufficient amount of time for genetic adaptation to consuming grains, legumes, and dairy as dietary staples compared to the 4 million years of human evolution that preceded this massive dietary shift from foods that were hunted and gathered to foods that could be grown and harvested. However, this rationale doesn't hold up under scientific scrutiny.

While the human body has not adapted enough for us to thrive on the modern Western diet (if it had, we wouldn't be seeing chronic illness rising to epidemic proportions with such clear correlations and mechanistic links to various dietary factors), some genetic adaptations are apparent. A recent study sequenced the genomes of 230 ancient humans living in West Eurasia between 6500 BC, when farming first arrived in that area of the world, and 300 BC, analyzing for evidence of genetic adaptation driven by natural selection to the new environments, pathogens, diets, and social organizations that farming wrought.

The researchers found twelve areas of the genome where substantial genetic adaptations were apparent. While the function of some of these genes remains unknown, some relate to physical characteristics like height, skin pigmentation, and eye color. More relevant to this discussion, others relate to diet, metabolism, and immune function.

The most evident genetic adaptation is lactase persistence, spurred by the advent of animal husbandry, which allowed non-human milk to become an accessible food. Before this adaptation, humans produced only the enzyme lactase, which digests the milk sugar lactose, until weaning age (see page 423). However, starting around 4,000 years ago, a substantial proportion of Europeans continued to produce lactase into adulthood. Now, approximately 95 percent of people of northern European descent have lactase persistence, but only 10 percent of those of Asian or African descent continue to produce lactase into adulthood. Because this genetic adaptation has been driven by dairy consumption, variations in lactase persistence in different cultures is attributable both to how big a role dairy played in the traditional diets of these cultures and to how long ago dairy cows or goats were domesticated in these regions. Lactase persistence is an excellent example of genetic adaptation to new foods over a very short time, evolutionarily speaking.

Other genetic adaptations to the dietary shift that came with agriculture are also apparent, although the implications are not as well understood. Two adaptations relate to fatty acid metabolism, one affecting plasma lipid and fatty acid concentration and the other causing decreased serum triglyceride levels. Another adaptation relates to circulating vitamin D levels, likely relating to a variation in dietary or environmental sources of vitamin D.

Another relevant adaptation to agriculture is evident in the gene encoding the major histocompatibility complex, the HLA gene. Recall that even non-celiacs with either the HLA-DQ2 or the HLA-DQ8 gene variant secrete excess zonulin in response to gluten consumption, unraveling the tight junctions between enterocytes and causing increased intestinal permeability (see page 67). Well, these gene variants, associated with increased risk for ulcerative colitis, celiac disease, and irritable bowel syndrome, are believed to have hitchhiked onto an adaptation to protect against ergothioneine deficiency in agricultural diets. Ergothioneine is a naturally occurring antioxidant amino acid that our bodies can't produce, so we must get it from our diets, the highest food sources being edible fungi and organ meat. The full role of ergothioneine in human health remains unknown.

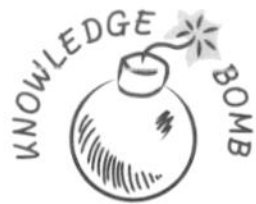

Some common gene variants of HLA are believed to come from Neanderthals breeding with Homo sapiens around 30,000 years ago. These Neanderthal variants are believed to have given modern humans an immune advantage in fighting off infections.

There are other heritable genes that influence how our bodies respond to individual foods representing genetic adaptation that has occurred over a much longer time. For example, AMY1 copy number affects how our bodies respond to starch-rich diets; the more copies of this gene we have, the more salivary α-amylase, a starch-digesting enzyme found in saliva, we produce. In fact, humans generally produce six to eight times more α-amylase than our chimpanzee cousins, who have only two copies of AMY1. If you are of Japanese or European descent, where starchy foods have long been dietary staples, you have a 70 percent chance of having six or more copies of AMY1. But if you harken from a culture with a traditionally low-starch diet, like the Inuit, you have only a 37 percent chance of having six or more copies of AMY1.

Yes, we have adapted, at least somewhat, to the dramatic dietary shift caused by the advent of agriculture. And in the face of this evidence, it would be ignorant to state that no one can thrive on a diet containing grains, legumes, and dairy or to state that everyone should avoid gluten for life. Of course, no gluten-containing or wheat-based food is a nutritional powerhouse (see page 23), but we see a spectrum in terms of the effects of consuming the inflammatory prolamins and agglutinins present in wheat. Individual sensitivity ranges from the severe and life-threatening damage caused in celiac disease sufferers, to the more subtle effects on intestinal permeability seen in non-celiacs with HLA-DQ2 or HLA-DQ8 gene variants, to examples of Blue Zone cultures (see page 137) in which homemade traditionally prepared whole-wheat bread is a dietary staple. This wide range of responses is partly attributable to genetics, but other aspects of our modern diet and lifestyles are also culprits. In fact, whether we are genetically adapted to eating wheat or dairy may be moot in the context of nutrient deficiency, poor gut health, high stress, and insufficient sleep—yeah, how most of us Westerners live our day-to-day lives.

Nutrient deficiency is definitely a contributor to how our bodies respond to specific foods. Not only are nutrient deficiencies themselves strongly linked to chronic diseases because the immune system requires so many nutrients to function well (see pages 24 and 82), but they are specifically linked to sensitivities and intolerances to various foods. Salicylate sensitivity, for example, may be purely a consequence of omega-3 fatty acid and zinc deficiency (see page 437). Zinc deficiency exaggerates the increase in activity of tissue transglutaminase in response to gluten consumption, thereby modulating the immune response to gluten as well as the likelihood of forming antibodies against tissue transglutaminase (see page 245).

Gut health is also a determinant of how the body responds to foods. This is, of course, most apparent when things go wrong. For example, histamine sensitivity, which is discussed further in Chapter 34, arises when there is a greater proportion of gut bacteria that convert the amino acid histadine into histamine and/or when the gut enterocytes do not produce sufficient deamine oxidase (DAO) to detoxify histamine (which may be due to poor enterocyte health, genetic mutations, or consumption of foods or drugs such as alcohol or antibiotics that interfere with DAO activity). When the gut barrier is leaky, the immune system is exposed to a greater amount of intact or only partially digested food proteins, increasing the likelihood of developing an allergic reaction (where IgE antibodies are formed against a food protein) or intolerance (where IgG, IgA, IgM, or IgD antibodies are formed against a food protein). And when our gut microbial community is out of balance, we can experience a variety of symptoms from eating specific foods, as in the painful bloating and other gastrointestinal symptoms that can occur in people with small intestinal bacterial overgrowth (SIBO; see page 70) after they consume foods rich in fermentable fibers and starches.

Both high stress and inadequate sleep increase insulin resistance, so the body is less able to handle spikes in blood glucose after eating a carbohydrate-rich meal or snack. Both high stress and inadequate sleep have direct detrimental effects on gut health and immune health, potentially magnifying immune reactions to foods or compounding issues like SIBO.

The Paleo framework is not about making unequivocal rules about which foods shall be included in or excluded from your diet. Instead, the Paleo framework respects our wide-ranging individual differences and remains flexible to further refinement as new scientific studies increase our understanding of the relationship between human health, diet, lifestyle, and our environment. Thus it is essential not just to provide you with a detailed education on the various health-promoting versus health-undermining compounds in different foods, but also to give you the tools to identify which foods work for you.

PALEO AS AN ELIMINATION DIET

So how do you go about determining whether a specific food works for you? The gold standard is a process called elimination and challenge. You cut that food out of your diet for a period of time (typically at least 2 to 4 weeks) and then consume it in a methodical way (that's the "challenge"), monitoring yourself for several days for signs of a negative reaction.

You can approach the Paleo diet as a sophisticated elimination diet, where you cut out those foods that scientific studies suggest have a higher likelihood of being problematic (like the foods discussed in Parts 3 and 4) while homing in on the most nutrient-dense foods available (like the ones discussed in Part 2), thereby addressing any health detriments arising from nutrient deficiency. When you think of the Paleo diet in these terms, challenging those eliminated foods becomes an integral aspect of the entire framework.

Identifying a link between specific foods and how we feel can be tough when we're chronically exposed to those foods, for a variety of reasons:

- We adjust to how bad we feel, making it difficult to realize that we don't feel our best.
- Our bodies can upregulate protective mechanisms, like producing more mucus in the gut, that can restrain reactions to a degree that makes them difficult to recognize.
- Symptoms can be amorphous—like feeling fatigued or moody—and we may not experience them immediately following consumption.

Elimination diets work by removing all these limitations.

Cutting out the foods that we may be reacting negatively to gives our bodies time to detoxify and recover from any negative health impacts. Many people express feeling renewed energy and well-being after adopting a Paleo diet, typically within a couple of weeks. When you're feeling great, it's easier to identify that you don't feel your best when a challenged food causes symptoms, even if those symptoms are fairly mild. The elimination phase also allows for the downregulation of any protective mechanisms, which means that reactions can be exaggerated and obvious when we consume foods that don't work for us. Finally, a methodical challenge protocol allows us to identify problematic foods even when our symptoms are vague and occur days after consuming those foods.

Let's take a moment to discuss exaggerated reactions to eliminated foods upon challenge. Exaggerated reactions typically occur in the case of food allergies and intolerances, and they can be very frustrating. It's common for people to misinterpret exaggerated reactions as Paleo "making them intolerant" to foods such as wheat. But that's not the case; in fact, the mechanisms behind these exaggerated reactions are exactly why elimination and challenge diets are the gold standard for identifying food sensitivities.

Even in a perfectly healthy gut, food-protein antigens are absorbed by a number of different cells, processed, and then presented to the immune system via a process called antigen presentation as part of the body's constant patrol for infectious agents. A type of sentinel immune cell in the gut called dendritic cells stick a long, armlike protrusion, called a dendrite, between enterocytes and into the lumen (inside) of the gut to "sample" the gut environment in search of infection. They then migrate to the gut-associated lymphoid tissues to present the antigens they've found (antigens from invading pathogens or food antigens) to other immune cells (naïve T cells and B cells). Other cells can do this same job, including a type of cell called an M cell in the Peyer's patches and even enterocytes themselves. It's a little like sticking your toe into a lake to see how cold the water is before you decide whether to jump in—the immune cells are constantly grabbing food proteins from the gut and showing them to the immune system so that the immune systems can decide whether to react.

That's right: the immune system doesn't react to all antigens all the time. It can "choose" not to react to an antigen through a process called immune tolerance.

Immune tolerance is mediated by regulatory cells of the adaptive immune system, called regulatory T cells. These cells can suppress the activity of those cells propelling an immune response to a food antigen (Th1, Th2, and memory cells) by producing anti-inflammatory cytokines (chemical messengers) that inhibit immune-cell activation, or they can actually cut the receptors off of immune cells so that they can't bind to the food antigen. But here's the kicker: these regulatory cells tend to have a shorter life span than the immune cells (there may be a genetic factor at play here since the life span of these cells can vary from a few days to months). If you have an immune reaction to a specific food, there is the period after eliminating it when the immune cells responsible for the reaction are still hanging around but the regulatory cells responsible for immune tolerance are too low in number to constrain the reaction. This is called loss of immune tolerance, and it is one cause of the exaggerated response to a challenged food.

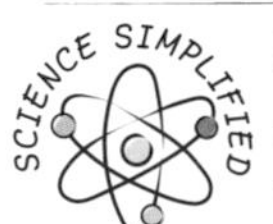

Perhaps you ate wheat your whole life, and then you cut it out for a while when you first "went Paleo." When you ate a dinner roll one evening as a treat, you became extremely ill. Did Paleo make you gluten intolerant? Nope. What actually happened is that eliminating wheat for a period of time unmasked a reaction that had been occurring all along. One of the cool, albeit frustrating, things about elimination diets is that they can magnify reactions to a food, making them easier to identify.

Immune tolerance is generally considered to be a good thing, but, of course, if you don't have an immune reaction to a food, you don't need to develop immune tolerance to it. The more a protein is broken down by healthy digestion (and compatibility with our digestive enzymes; see page 74), the less immunogenic (immune-stimulating) it is when it's "sampled." In fact, the mere act of restoring healthy digestion can make many food sensitivities disappear. Immune tolerance also relies on how much of an antigen crosses the gut barrier. In the case of a leaky gut, much more of a specific food antigen can cross into the body than when the gut barrier is intact. Once you have a healthy gut barrier, the "sampling" of antigens becomes a much more tightly controlled process.

KNOWLEDGE BOMB

Cruciferous veggies are rich sources of aryl hydrocarbon receptor (AHR) ligands, compounds that help modulate immune responses in the intestine. Studies have shown that supplementing with AHR ligands can help suppress allergic reactions to peanuts by improving immune tolerance. It's unknown whether dietary AHR ligands can do the same thing, but you can chalk this one up as yet another (albeit hypothetical) reason to eat your veggies!

Other factors may be at play in an exaggerated response to a food upon challenge. Perhaps the mucus layer of the gut was thickened as a protective mechanism before you eliminated the problematic food—basically, your body's way of minimizing your exposure to an antigen. Now that your body is healing, the mucus layer is thinner, so when you do eat a food to which you are allergic or have developed an intolerance, more of it can interact with your immune system.

If you react severely to a food, don't eat it. (If you are seriously allergic, talk to your doctor about getting a prescription for an epinephrine injector.) There are immune-sensitization protocols that can be performed under the guidance of an allergist to slowly introduce small amounts of the food antigen to stimulate the production of regulatory T cells, but this is something to consider only if you have a healthy immune system and the food in question is a nutrient-dense option that will contribute greatly to the quality of your overall diet.

For most people, these dramatic reactions will diminish over time, especially as gut barrier and immune health improve. Eventually, the number of immune cells responsible for the reaction decreases as well, so even if a food cannot be successfully reintroduced into your diet initially, it's worth trying again in a few months. In fact, a lack of serious reactions to foods is an excellent indicator of gut and immune health. By also addressing lifestyle factors (discussed in Part 5), you improve the chances of successfully reintroducing eliminated foods into your diet.

ELIMINATION AND CHALLENGE PROTOCOL

The Paleo diet can be thought of as a nutritional intervention for a diet gone badly awry, overabundant in calories and relatively lacking in vital nutrients. But how well an individual tolerates suboptimal foods depends on nutrient status, stress, sleep, activity level, genetics, and health history. As we improve as many of these as possible with diet and lifestyle changes, it's fairly common to see tolerance of certain foods increase.

At its core, the Paleo diet is an elimination diet, designed to cut out the most likely food culprits holding us back from achieving optimal health while flooding the body with nutrients. And the best part about an elimination diet is that eventually, you get to reintroduce foods that you've been avoiding.

How long is eventually? Ideally, you'd wait to reintroduce foods until you feel amazing, but as long as you're seeing improvements in your health thanks to your diet and lifestyle changes, you can try some reintroductions after 3 to 4 weeks.

In general, reintroduce only one food every 5 to 7 days and spend that time monitoring yourself for symptoms.

SYMPTOMS OF A REACTION AREN'T ALWAYS OBVIOUS, SO KEEP AN EYE OUT FOR ANY OF THE FOLLOWING:

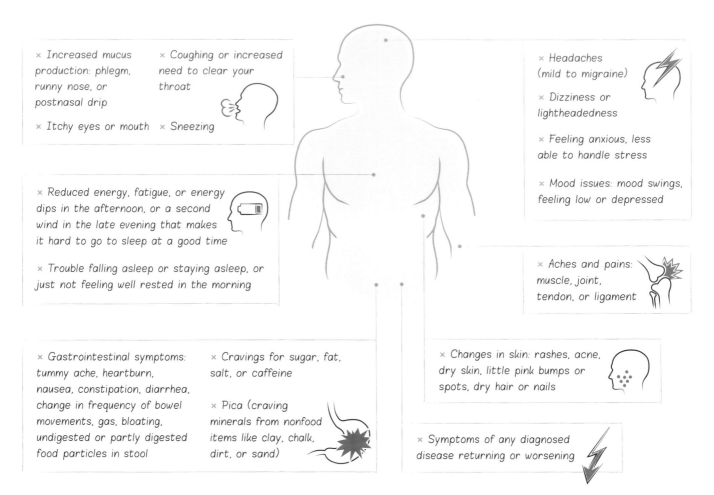

- × Increased mucus production: phlegm, runny nose, or postnasal drip
- × Coughing or increased need to clear your throat
- × Itchy eyes or mouth
- × Sneezing

- × Headaches (mild to migraine)
- × Dizziness or lightheadedness
- × Feeling anxious, less able to handle stress
- × Mood issues: mood swings, feeling low or depressed

- × Reduced energy, fatigue, or energy dips in the afternoon, or a second wind in the late evening that makes it hard to go to sleep at a good time
- × Trouble falling asleep or staying asleep, or just not feeling well rested in the morning

- × Aches and pains: muscle, joint, tendon, or ligament

- × Gastrointestinal symptoms: tummy ache, heartburn, nausea, constipation, diarrhea, change in frequency of bowel movements, gas, bloating, undigested or partly digested food particles in stool
- × Cravings for sugar, fat, salt, or caffeine
- × Pica (craving minerals from nonfood items like clay, chalk, dirt, or sand)

- × Changes in skin: rashes, acne, dry skin, little pink bumps or spots, dry hair or nails

- × Symptoms of any diagnosed disease returning or worsening

THE STANDARD PROCEDURE FOR FOOD CHALLENGE IS AS FOLLOWS:

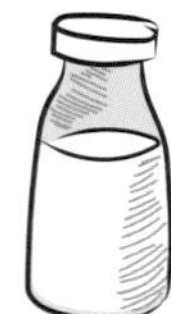

1. Select a food to challenge. Be prepared to eat it two or three times in a day, then avoid it completely for a few days.

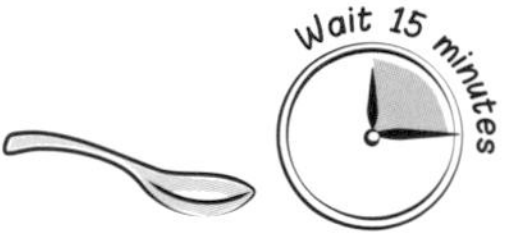

2. The first time you eat the food, eat 1/2 teaspoon or even less (one teensy little nibble). Wait 15 minutes.

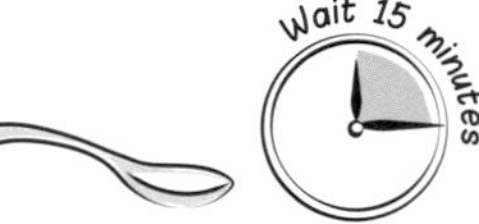

3. If you experience any symptoms, don't eat any more. If you don't, eat 1 teaspoon of the food (a small bite). Wait 15 minutes.

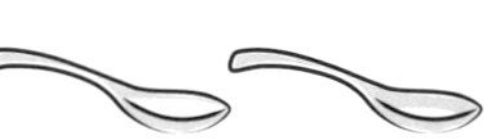

4. If you experience any symptoms, don't eat any more. If you don't, eat 1 1/2 teaspoons of the food (a slightly bigger bite).

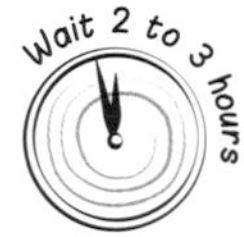

5. That's it for now. Wait 2 to 3 hours and monitor yourself for symptoms.

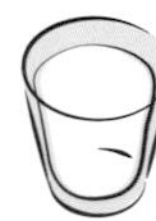

6. If you still haven't experienced any symptoms, eat a normal-sized portion of the food, either by itself or as part of a meal.

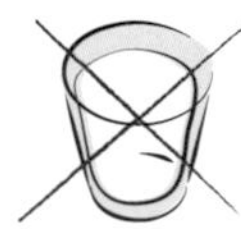

7. Do not eat that food again for 5 to 7 days, and don't reintroduce any other foods during that time. Monitor yourself for symptoms.

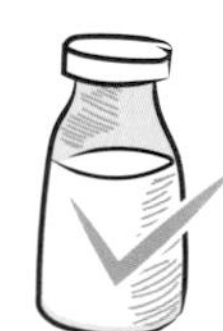

8. If you have no symptoms during the challenge day or at any time in the next 5 to 7 days, you may reincorporate this food into your diet.

It's best not to be in a hurry to challenge foods. Generally, the longer you wait, the more likely you are to be successful (thanks to improved gut and immune health). But when you reintroduce particular foods is ultimately your choice. How you feel is the best gauge, and only you will know whether you are ready. A word of caution, though: don't let cravings influence you. Your decision should be based on how good you feel and how much improvement you're seeing in your health.

WHICH FOODS SHOULD I EXPERIMENT WITH?

There is a compelling rationale for eliminating all the foods listed here when you first adopt a Paleo diet. Of course, there are no hard-and-fast rules about whether to eliminate all these foods or just some of them based on your health history and food intolerance suspicions. For more on transitioning to Paleo, see Chapter 32. Chapter 34 includes some additional eliminations to try if health troubleshooting is needed.

NIGHTSHADES (see page 206):

- ashwagandha
- bell peppers (aka sweet peppers)
- bush tomato
- cape gooseberries (also known as ground cherries—not to be confused with regular cherries)
- cocona
- eggplant
- garden huckleberries (not to be confused with regular huckleberries)
- goji berries (aka wolfberries)
- hot peppers (such as chili peppers, jalapeños, habaneros, chili-based spices, red pepper, and cayenne)
- kutjera
- naranjillas
- paprika
- pepinos
- pimentos
- potatoes (but not sweet potatoes)
- tamarillos
- tomatillos
- tomatoes

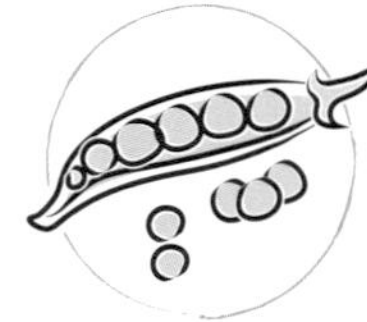

PROPERLY PREPARED SAFER LEGUMES (see page 290):

- black beans
- black-eyed peas
- butter beans
- calico beans
- cannellini beans
- chickpeas (aka garbanzo beans)
- fava beans (aka broad beans)
- Great Northern beans
- Italian beans
- legumes with edible pods (sweet peas, sugar snap peas, string beans, snap beans, wax beans, pole beans, runner beans)
- lentils
- lima beans
- mung beans
- navy beans
- pinto beans
- split peas
- tamarind

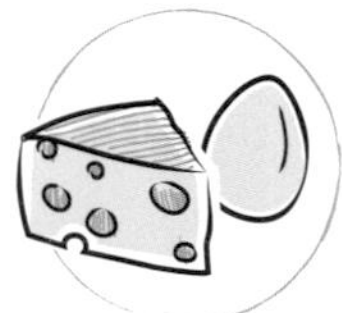

GRASS-FED DAIRY (see page 288) AND EGGS (see page 294):

- butter
- cheese
- ghee
- heavy cream
- kefir
- milk
- yogurt
- eggs

ALCOHOLIC BEVERAGES (see page 300):

- cider
- gluten-free beer
- gluten-free spirits
- wine

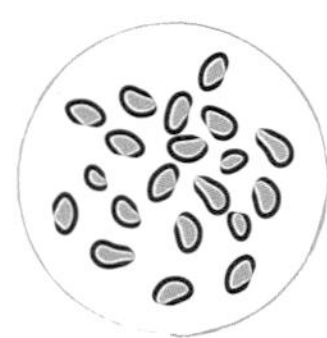

GLUTEN-FREE GRAINS, PSEUDOGRAINS (see page 256), AND SEEDS:

- buckwheat
- chia seeds (see page 308)
- flax seeds (see page 308)
- gluten-free oats
- millet
- non-GMO corn
- psyllium seed or husk (see page 308)
- sorghum
- white rice (see page 302)

ELIMINATIONS TO CONSIDER FOR TROUBLESHOOTING (see Chapter 34):

COMMON FOOD SENSITIVITIES:

- FODMAPs (see pages 434 and 435)
- high-histamine foods (see page 436)
- sulfites (see page 239)

TOP ALLERGENS:

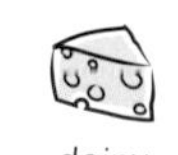
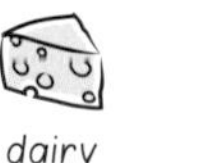
dairy (see page 288)

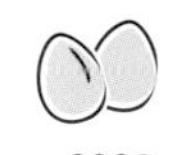
eggs (see page 294)

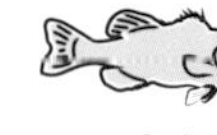
fish (see page 158)

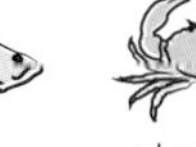
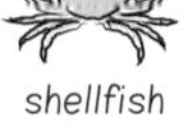
shellfish (see page 160)

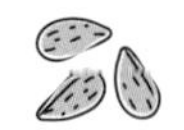
tree nuts (see page 194)

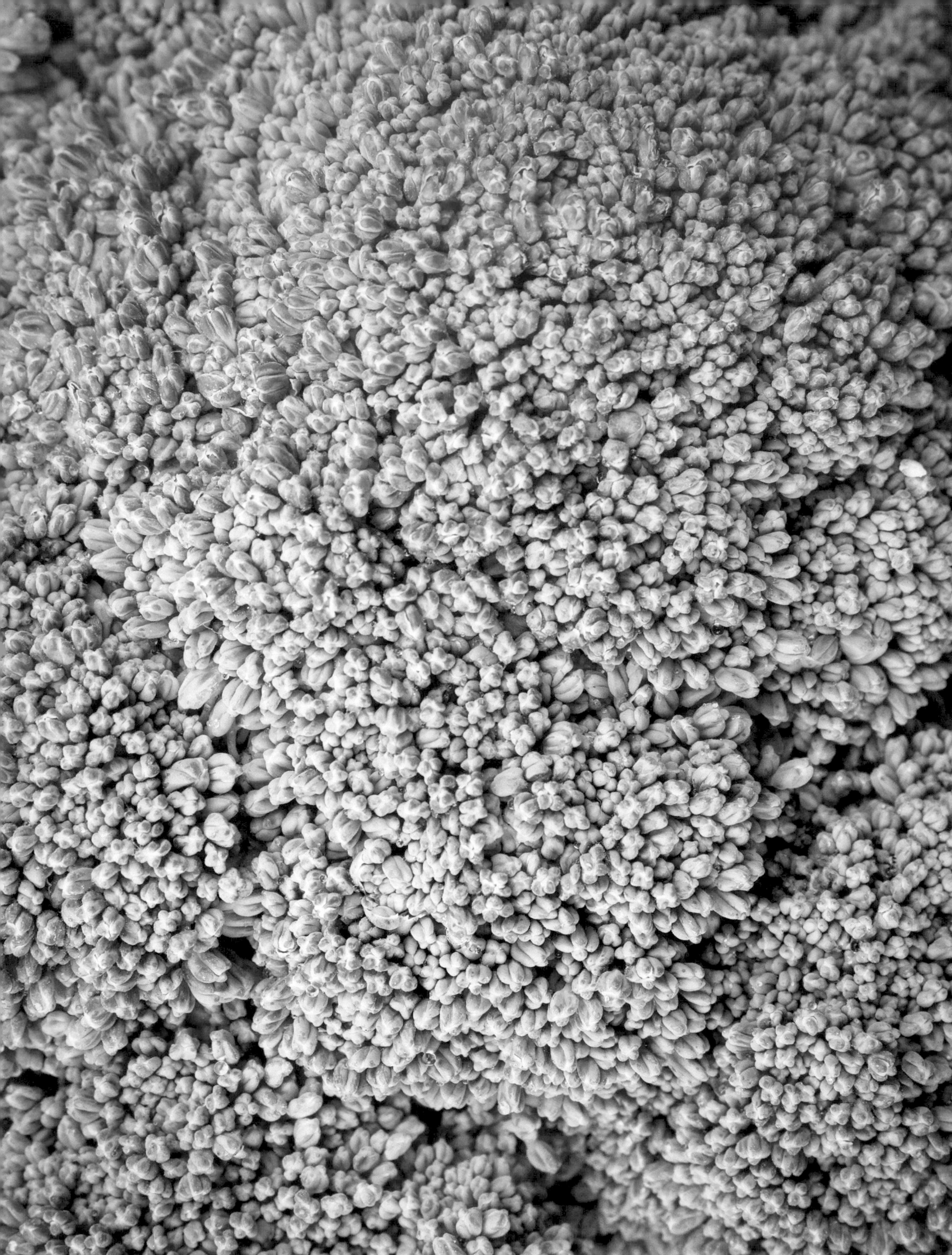

5.

PALEO LIFESTYLE

Although food plays a huge role in our health, diet is only one component of the Paleo framework—and only one aspect of the many elements that work together to support the numerous processes in our bodies. Various lifestyle components, including sleep, stress management, exercise and movement, nature, and social connection, play critical roles in thwarting disease, controlling hormone levels, stabilizing mood, regulating the immune system, and optimizing gut microbiota and overall gut health.

Not getting enough sleep increases the risk of all-cause mortality (your risk of dying, which is a pretty robust measure of overall health) comparably to being obese, living a sedentary lifestyle, and not eating many vegetables. There are strong causal links between inadequate sleep and cardiovascular disease, diabetes, obesity, autoimmune disease, cancer, inflammation, and susceptibility to infection. These links are due to the relationship between sleep (or lack thereof) and immune function as well as the effect that sleep has on many key hormones (such as immune modulators and hunger hormones) and neurotransmitter regulation (including our reward circuitry). In fact, getting sufficient quality sleep may be the single best thing you can do to improve your health.

Chronic stress increases the risk of depression and anxiety, cardiovascular disease, obesity, diabetes, autoimmune diseases, chronic headaches, memory problems, digestive problems, and infections and is linked with poor wound healing. These effects are believed to be mediated by the activation of the hypothalamic-pituitary-adrenal axis (HPA axis) and the impact that cortisol and other adrenal hormones have on immune function. Plus, chronic stress influences other behaviors, influencing our food choices (due to cravings for energy-dense foods and increased appetite) and making us more vulnerable to addiction.

Regular physical activity minimizes the risk of cardiovascular disease, obesity, diabetes, osteoporosis, and some cancers. These benefits are mediated by exercise's benefits to blood lipids, blood pressure, inflammation, insulin sensitivity, coronary blood flow, endothelial function, and oxidative stress. In fact, a sedentary lifestyle is one of the leading risk factors for chronic disease; for every hour of daily activity (even light) that replaces sedentary time, the risk of all-cause mortality drops by an impressive 16 percent! Simply walking briskly for 30 minutes five times per week can reduce the incidence of coronary artery disease by 30 to 40 percent in women and about 25 percent in men.

In fact, one could argue that lifestyle is an even more important contributor to long-term health than diet. For example, a recent study in dogs showed that a single night of sleep deprivation caused a greater increase in insulin resistance than 6 months of a high-fat Western-style diet. Insulin sensitivity declined by 33 percent after sleep deprivation but only 21 percent after 6 months of a poor diet.

Lifestyle factors also affect our food choices and behaviors. For example, getting sufficient sleep makes us much more likely to choose fruits and vegetables and less likely to choose fast food. A single night of insufficient sleep, on the other hand, leads to more snacking and an overall increase in caloric intake and makes us less inhibited with our food choices. Stress makes us crave energy-dense foods, like very fatty or sugary junk foods, which makes staying on any healthy eating plan more of a challenge.

As you work to adopt (and adapt) the Paleo dietary template, remember that paying attention to lifestyle factors will not only fast-track your health improvements but also help you succeed in maintaining your new dietary priorities.

Chapter 26:
SLEEP AND CIRCADIAN RHYTHM

Over the last 50 years, Americans' average sleep time has decreased by an average of 1½ to 2 hours per night. That's equivalent to a full month of sleep each year—and the effects of that loss have wide-ranging consequences for our health! In fact, adequate sleep is so important that it's considered a key Paleo principle.

First of all, what *is* sleep? That might seem like an easy question, but scientists have long struggled to come up with a definition—in part because sleep is a common experience for all animals and in part because we're still making frequent discoveries about the details and the "whys" of sleep. For now, scientists look at sleep in two ways: electrophysiologically and behaviorally.

In technical terms, the electrophysiological definition of sleep is a specific pattern of:

- Whole-brain activity
- Eye movement that includes patterns of both non-rapid eye movement (NREM) and rapid eye movement (REM)
- Muscle tone (the continuous and passive partial contraction of muscles)

The behavioral criteria of sleep are:

- Decreased behavioral activity
- Site preference (that is, a sleeping place, like a bed)
- Specific posture (such as lying down)
- Rapid reversibility (the ability to be woken up, unlike being in a coma)
- Increased arousal threshold (being unaware of our environment while asleep)
- Homeostatic control (the body rebounds and makes us sleep more after being deprived)

On a more detailed level, sleep involves a series of stages that cycle four or five times per night. In general, non-rapid eye movement (NREM) and rapid eye movement (REM) are the two main types of sleep. These types can be identified by examining brain activity. NREM is characterized by brain waves that are less frequent but stronger in amplitude and are more synchronized. REM brain waves, on the other hand, are more frequent and less synchronized. During NREM sleep, body position changes about once every 20 to 30 minutes, whereas the body is functionally paralyzed during REM sleep. As the name suggests, REM sleep is also characterized by observable rapid eye movement, whereas NREM involves no such eye movement.

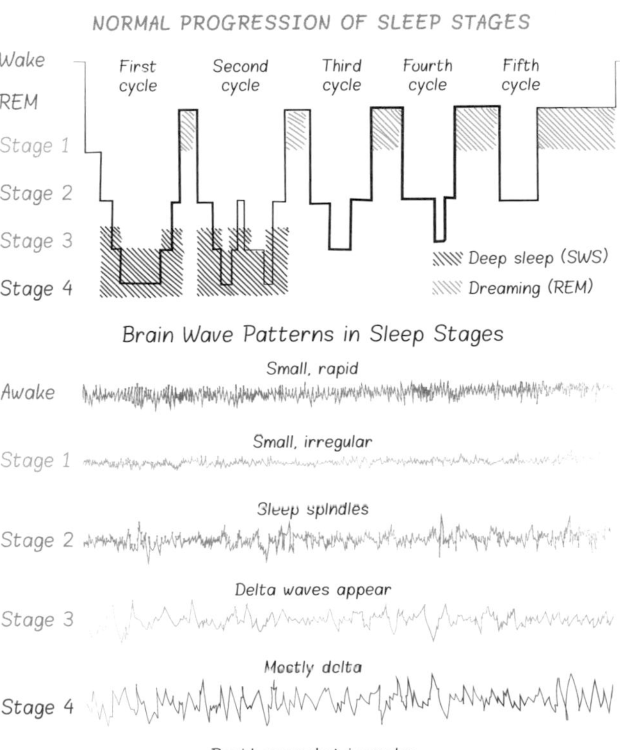

As noted earlier, one of the defining features of sleep is differences in brain activity, as measured by electroencephalogram (EEG). NREM sleep is sometimes called "quiet sleep" because the brain activity measured by EEG shows a much less active pattern than in REM ("active") sleep. These two types of sleep are separated into four stages that take place in cycles that repeat each time we sleep.

SCIENCE SIMPLIFIED *During deep sleep (stages 3 and 4), our bodies undergo the most physical repair, whereas REM sleep is psychologically restorative. Ideally, 20 to 25 percent of our sleep would be deep sleep, which we tend to get more of in the first half of the night, and 20 to 25 percent would be REM sleep, which we tend to get more of in the second half of the night. The rest of our sleep is light sleep, the phases between deep and REM sleep.*

Why do sleep stages exist? Each stage seems to allow for slightly different beneficial processes in the brain. Although the details remain a mystery, the sleep cycle stems from an interaction between the circadian clock (how our brains prioritize different processes depending on whether it's day or night; see Chapter 4) and a separate sleep-wake homeostatic process. There are four or five sleep stages, depending on how you count them, and healthy sleep has you pass through each stage sequentially in a cycle: stage 1, then stage 2, then stages 3 and 4 (which are sometimes combined into one "deep sleep" stage), and finally culminating in REM sleep. A complete sleep cycle takes an average of 70 to 100 minutes during the first part of the night and lengthens to 90 to 120 minutes later in the night, and the next cycle starts at the beginning with stage 1. The first sleep cycle of each night has a relatively short REM sleep and a long period of deep sleep (stages 3 and 4), but later in the night, the REM period lengthens and deep sleep time decreases (which is why we dream more frequently in the morning).

Stage 1 is a light sleep that begins the moment you drift off. Think of stage 1 as the transition from being awake to being asleep. From a brain wave perspective, this stage is the transition from waking-type brain waves when the body is resting, called "alpha waves," to sleeping-type brain waves, called "theta waves." During this stage, which lasts only about 5 to 10 minutes, your heart rate declines, your body temperature drops, and your eyes move in a pattern from side to side. This phase is usually dreamless and is easily disturbed. Have you ever woken with a start shortly after going to bed, thinking that you heard someone calling your name or that you were falling? These are relatively common phenomena during the early phase of sleep. Interestingly, stage 1 sleep varies per individual, so you might think you were just drowsy during this part of your sleep cycle, whereas your partner might consider it to be actual sleep.

After that, the body begins to transition into established sleep. In stage 2, which lasts between 10 and 25 minutes in the first sleep cycle (remember: each cycle lasts longer and longer), eye movement stops and brain waves become slower with only an occasional burst of rapid brain waves, called "sleep spindle," during which it is theorized that the brain is sorting through the information it picked up that day and synthesizing it with existing knowledge. As you might expect, memory consolidation occurs during stage 2 sleep. Along with sleep spindles, stage 2 sleep is characterized by sharp, short bursts of brain activity; these brain waves are called a "K-complex," and scientists believe that their purpose is to keep the brain prepared in the event that we need to be awakened.

Deep sleep begins when you enter stage 3 sleep, characterized by extremely slow brain waves called delta waves. During this stage, more of the brain's active centers shut down for the night, and the remaining active brain cells become more synchronized in their wave pattern. As the neurons emit brain waves in more synchronized patterns, their combined frequencies increase to create delta waves. The goal of stage 3 sleep is to get to this point. In stage 4 (which some scientists characterize as an extension of stage 3), the brain produces the slow delta waves almost exclusively. This is why stages 3 and 4 are referred to as slow-wave sleep, deep sleep, or delta sleep. In this stage, there is no eye movement or muscle activity, blood pressure is reduced by 20 to 30 percent, and the brain becomes much less responsive to external stimuli. It is difficult to wake someone from deep sleep—and if you happen to wake up during this stage, you will likely feel groggy and unrested. This is when some children experience bed-wetting, sleepwalking, or night terrors. Stages 3 and 4 combined typically comprise 20 to 40 minutes of each sleep cycle, although it is normal to not enter deep sleep at all in the last cycle or two of the night.

Deep sleep seems to be one of the most critical times for body repair. At the beginning of stage 3, the pituitary gland releases growth hormone, which stimulates the growth and repair of important tissues. The brain cools during this phase because less blood is directed to it (due in part the lowered blood pressure), which may help improve its function and allow for repair. Interestingly, levels of interleukins seem to increase (there are many types, all of which are released by white blood cells), indicating increased immune system activity during this phase of sleep—so immune function is related to deep sleep, too. Because slow-wave sleep is so important, our bodies designate a lot of time to it. At its peak importance, generally in young adulthood, deep sleep makes up 20 to 25 percent of total sleeping time, but then it declines in later adulthood, especially after the age of 65. And if you are sleep-deprived, you will pass more quickly through the earlier stages of sleep and spend more time in this stage.

After deep sleep, REM sleep begins. Brain waves during REM sleep increase to the levels experienced when awake, appearing more erratic in their pattern and with higher frequency. Unlike the restorative quality of NREM sleep, this dreaming, "active" sleep is just that: almost as active as if you were awake. In general, breathing becomes more rapid, irregular, and shallow; eyes jerk rapidly; and limb muscles are temporarily paralyzed (except in those who sleepwalk, acting out their dreams). Similarly, heart rate increases, blood pressure rises, sex organs become aroused, and the body loses some of the ability to regulate its temperature. Additionally, the sympathetic nervous system, which is responsible for the "fight or flight" response, is twice as active as when you're awake! However, despite all this activity, your body remains relatively still; all muscles except for those that control eye movement and breathing are paralyzed during this phase of sleep.

This is the time when most dreaming occurs. Scientists are still trying to understand how dreams contribute to our health and what they may mean, but dreaming sleep appears to be important for managing learning and memory. Studies have shown that repeated interruption of REM sleep (but not NREM sleep) decreases cognitive performance compared to a night with the standard three to five sleep cycles, each containing a REM stage.

Waking may occur after REM, when you cycle back to stage 1 sleep. If the waking period is long enough, you may remember the dreams from your most recent REM cycle. As the night progresses, REM sleep becomes longer and can last up to an hour depending on how long and how restfully you sleep. In total, REM sleep accounts for about 1 to 2 hours of total sleep each night.

Of course, how much time we spend in each sleep stage changes as we age. Infants spend almost half of their time in REM sleep. In contrast, adults spend nearly half of our sleep time in stage 2 and only 20 to 25 percent in REM sleep; the other 30 percent is divided between stages 1, 3, and 4. Older adults spend progressively less time in REM sleep. The differences in how much time is spent in each stage are called "sleep architecture," and scientists are still debating the best way to represent the transition between stages throughout the night.

Brand-new research is still coming out on this topic; there is so much that we still don't understand about REM and NREM sleep. A recent paper in the journal *Science*, which is considered to be one of the most prestigious scientific journals in the world, provided new insight on the cells that regulate the phases of sleep. Interestingly, they share a common developmental origin and work together to inhibit or promote the activity of the other. This mechanism is still being studied, but it's been shown that these cells are common among all mammals, so this is an ancient group of cells that we share with a vast number of other organisms. How cool is that?

THE IMPORTANCE OF SLEEP

With this broader understanding of sleep in mind, we can now ask: why is sleep important? The reason we need sleep is a question that evaded scientific researchers until very recently. One theory involves inactivity and energy conservation. Sleep is a process that mammals adapted over time in order to be inactive during the most dangerous time, nights. (Nocturnal predators sleep much more than their diurnal prey and hunt when their quarry are more vulnerable. Nocturnal prey animals utilize nighttime food sources, like night-blooming flowers, and evolved different defenses, like sleeping in trees.) Being inactive and in a safe resting space at night makes it easier to survive in the wild. Additionally, metabolism slows (by about 10 percent in humans), so sleep helps conserve energy.

Sleep also plays an important role in *synaptic plasticity*—the brain's ability to change. Although this concept sounds simple, scientists used to believe that we were hardwired from a young age and that the brain didn't change much until old age. However, our brains are flexible (like "plastic") and make new connections all the time. The brain is like a muscle in that the connections we use frequently are reinforced and strengthened, and the connections we rarely use tend to degrade or even disappear. These changes are related to memory and other brain functions, and brain plasticity depends on getting adequate sleep. So a newly discovered purpose of sleep is the formation of memories. Though learning happens while awake, sleeping improves our ability to encode and consolidate memories, and it looks like sleep is necessary for long-term memories.

Beyond this, we now know that the main purpose of sleep is to allow for detoxification processes in the brain. When our cells use energy, they produce waste. This waste is made up of a variety of chemicals, many of them toxic. Normally, this waste enters the bloodstream, and it's part of the liver's and kidneys' jobs to filter this waste to ensure that it's eliminated from the body via urine and stool.

A recent study of three different hunter-gatherer communities showed that these peoples tend to go "to bed" within a couple of hours of sunset and wake up just before sunrise. While their sleep duration ranges from 6.9 to 8.5 hours per night, their movement drops noticeably once the sun goes down, indicating that they are likely participating in quiet interaction before sleep and spending 8 to 10 hours per night in bed, depending on the season.

The brain uses 20 to 25 percent of the total calories we burn every day. Yes, the brain needs a lot of energy to perform all its wondrous functions! And this means a large accumulation of metabolic by-products concentrated in one comparatively small organ. To flush these waste products out of our brains, we need to sleep. During sleep, brain cells shrink by 60 percent, increasing the space between them so the toxins that built up during the day can be flushed away more effectively. Sleep is critical to remove these toxic compounds from the brain and draw them into the bloodstream (and then to the liver and kidneys so that they can do their filtering job).

Without sufficient sleep, these toxic metabolic by-products build up in the brain, which can negatively impact cellular health, neurotransmitter systems, hormone systems, and communication between neurons and stimulate inflammation in the brain. And anything that impacts the health of the brain affects every other system in the body. This is likely why inadequate sleep has been linked to so many health conditions and to broader issues like immune system dysfunction and hormone dysregulation.

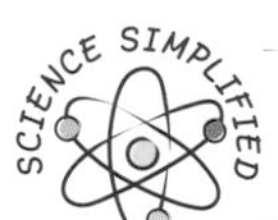

Sleep is necessary for the brain to flush out the toxins that build up during the day.

Indeed, the body of scientific literature linking inadequate sleep, more technically called "short sleep," with disease is vast—so vast that there are now huge meta-analyses combining data from multiple studies to establish a statistically powerful link. There's also a broad collection of studies exploring the cellular and molecular details of why we need sleep and all the bad things that can happen in our bodies when we don't get enough of it. The benefit for us is that quantifying the role that sleep plays in disease is pretty easy: we can pinpoint exactly how much our risk for diabetes, obesity, cardiovascular disease, cancer, and autoimmune disease goes up if we don't get enough sleep. This is also the body of scientific literature that the American Academy of Sleep Medicine and the Sleep Research Society used to establish its guidelines and consensus statement, published in 2015:

> *Adults should sleep 7 or more hours per night on a regular basis to promote optimal health. Sleeping less than 7 hours per night on a regular basis is associated with adverse health outcomes, including weight gain and obesity, diabetes, hypertension, heart disease and stroke, depression, and increased risk of death. Sleeping less than 7 hours per night is also associated with impaired immune function, increased pain, impaired performance, increased errors, and greater risk of accidents.*

The fact is, 35 percent of Americans never get 7 hours of sleep; 64 percent never get 8 hours of sleep. And however much sleep we think we're getting, we're likely getting less.

PERCENT OF ADULTS BY SELF-REPORTED SLEEP DURATION

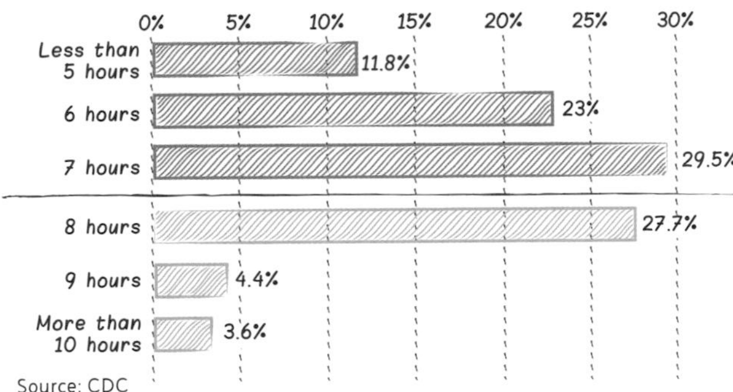

Source: CDC

Most of us overestimate how much sleep we get. We look at the clock when we turn out the light and think of that as the beginning of our sleep, and when we wake up in the morning, we check the time again to see how many hours have passed. But it's normal for it to take us 30 to 60 minutes to fall asleep. And it's normal to have at least a few brief wakings in the night.

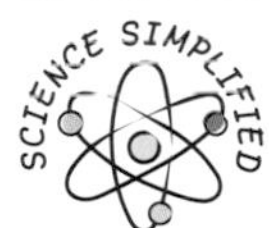

About two-thirds of Americans don't get enough sleep. This may be one of the single biggest contributors to the rise in chronic illness seen over the last 50 years.

Studies comparing how individuals report their sleep to how much they actually slept as measured by wrist actigraphy (like a Fitbit) have found that on average, subjects reported that they got 48 minutes more sleep than they actually did. But here's where things get interesting: the less people sleep, the more likely they are to overreport their sleep. So people who got 5 hours of sleep per night on average overreported by 1 hour and 20 minutes (so they said they got 6.3 hours instead of 5), whereas people who got 7 hours of sleep overreported by only 20 minutes. What does this mean? It means that if we get 6 hours or less, chances are good that our sleep situation is even worse than we think.

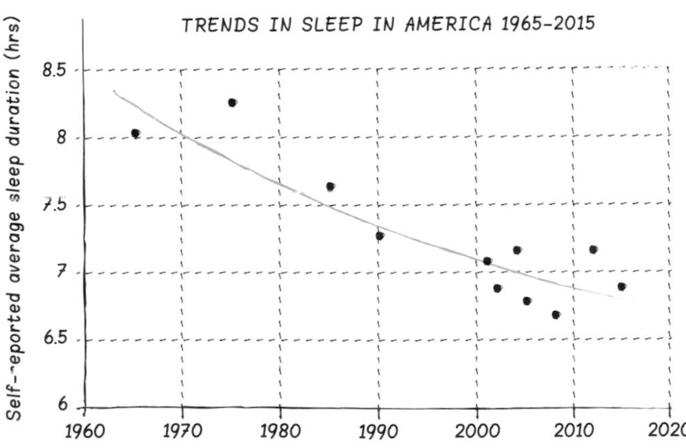

And self-reported sleep is used to estimate how much sleep Americans are getting! Compared to 50 years ago, when the average sleep duration was about 8 hours per night, we're averaging about 6.9 hours per night. In 50 years, we went from the Gold Standard of Sleep as our average to less than the minimum required to preserve health—and that 6.9 hours might be overestimated. This is a huge contributor to the rise in chronic health problems seen over that same time period. As tempting as it is to blame our high-PUFA, high-refined carbohydrate, processed food chemical-laden modern food supply, sleep is just as big, if not a bigger, factor . . . one that deserves much more airtime.

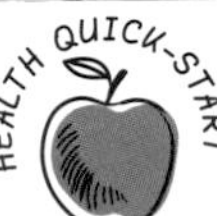

Aim to get at least 8 hours of sleep every night—remembering that you are almost certainly getting less sleep than you think. The number-one barrier that most people face to getting enough sleep is simply making sleep a priority.

Entrenching Circadian Rhythm

The term *circadian rhythm* refers to the fact that a huge array of biological processes within the human body cycle according to a 24-hour clock. Circadian rhythms are how your body knows what time it is so that it can prioritize functions based on the time of day and whether or not you are asleep—and properly regulated circadian rhythms are critical for health.

Your brain's circadian clock, located in the superchiasmatic nucleus of the hypothalamus, controls the ebb and flow of certain hormones (cortisol and melatonin being especially important) which act as signals of the circadian clock throughout the body. Using these signals, each cell aligns its own internal clock to the brain's circadian clock, allowing the body to synchronize its circadian rhythm.

The vast majority of our hormones cycle during the day (not just melatonin and cortisol), impacting the function of every system in our bodies. For example, the circadian clock drives metabolic pathways, bile acid synthesis, autophagy (destruction of damaged or redundant cellular components, like a spring cleaning in every cell), and immune and inflammatory processes. Additionally, how sensitive different types of cells are to different hormones can cycle. For example, in healthy people, insulin sensitivity is lower in the evening than in the morning, the effect of which is

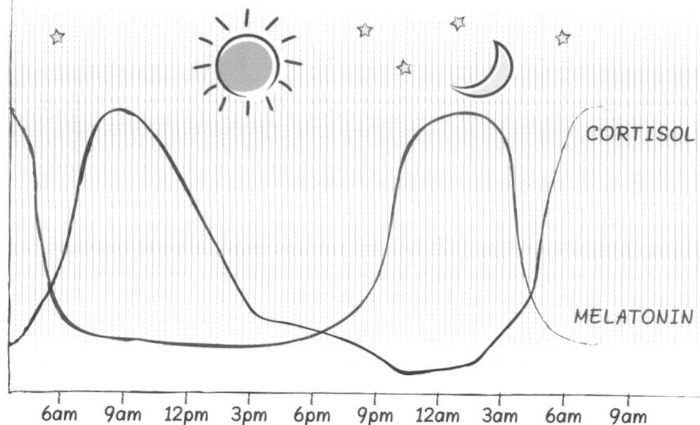

that blood glucose increases more after an evening meal than it does after a carb-matched breakfast. This natural cycling is why prioritizing circadian rhythm is so important: it not only helps regulate the levels of and sensitivity to different hormones, but even more importantly, it regulates the natural ups and downs that our hormones go through throughout the day and night. The effect of a well-regulated circadian rhythm is that biological processes are aligned with behavioral cycles; this reduces our risk of chronic disease.

To have healthy circadian rhythms, your circadian clock needs to be set to the right time. What can you do to set your circadian clock, protect your circadian rhythms, and therefore regulate so many important hormones? It's all about the zeitgebers! Zeitgebers are all the factors that influence our circadian clocks. And while the light-dark cycle is definitely the most important circadian rhythm signal, there are several other key zeitgebers worth discussing.

SCIENCE SIMPLIFIED *The best thing you can do to regulate your circadian clock is to live in tune with the sun. This means spending some time outside during the day every day, keeping your lights dim and red in the evening, and sleeping in a completely dark environment at night. Biohacks like light therapy boxes, light alarm clocks, amber-tinted glasses, and programmable light bulbs can all help simulate the day-night light cycle indoors.*

1. Get bright (blue) light exposure during the day.

The light-dark cycle mentioned above is the most important signal to our circadian clock. This means that one of the best ways to set your circadian clock is be exposed to bright light (ideally sunlight) during the day, but be in the dark at night. In fact, sunlight exposure during the day is probably the single most important thing we can do to support the normal production of melatonin in the evening.

The component of sunlight that tells your circadian clock that it's daytime is blue light. You have photoreceptors in your eyes and skin that are sensitive to blue light (the receptors in your eyes are much more sensitive than those in your skin) and convey that signal to the brain. How much time outside is enough? If it's a sunny day, as little as 15 minutes (without sunglasses!). If it's cloudy, 30 minutes to an hour is better. And of course, the more the better.

So what do you do if you're a shift worker or live in an ill-suited climate or have other barriers to being outside? There's a great biohack available for getting blue light exposure during the day: a light therapy box. There doesn't seem to be a difference between white light boxes and blue light boxes in terms of supporting melatonin production, so you can pick the least expensive option-but choose one that is bright, at least 10,000 lux. Use it for at least 15 minutes at roughly the same time every morning or midday. Another option is to make many small changes to brighten your environment during the day: use sunlight spectrum light bulbs in your house (but you'll want to avoid using these light bulbs in the evening), keep curtains open during the day, make sure your computer monitor and other screens are set to its brightest setting, drive with the windows down . . . all these things help, but they still aren't typically as bright as a light therapy box or just being outside, even on a cloudy day.

2. Avoid bright (and blue) light in the evening.

Just as it's important for your body to get the signal that it's daytime during the day (or your day, if you're a shift worker and using a light therapy box), it's important to tell your body it's nighttime once the sun goes down. This means avoiding blue light and sticking with red and yellow wavelengths of light as well as keeping the overall light level much dimmer.

You can achieve this important "darkness signal" to your circadian clock by keeping your indoor lighting as dim as possible in the evenings with dimmer switches, or just plain ol' turning on fewer lights, in conjunction with investing in red or yellow light bulbs for whatever lamps will be used in the evening. If you plan to use a computer monitor or watch TV, there are two options. The first is to install f.lux on your computer or Android devices, or use the Night Shift feature on Apple devices, and then set the screen brightness to the lowest setting. The second, and probably the best biohack for supporting evening melatonin production (more technically called dim-light melatonin production), is to wear amber-tinted glasses for the last 2 to 3 hours of your day. In fact, several scientific studies show that wearing amber-tinted glasses in the evening improves sleep quality and supports melatonin production. What are amber tinted glasses? Quite simple: glasses with yellow lenses. These could be driving glasses, glaucoma glasses, or safety glasses (my personal preference is for the larger lenses of safety glasses because they also block peripheral light and there are options that fit well over regular glasses . . . plus they're super cheap!). Amber-tinted glasses are also a great option for shift workers.

A more sophisticated option for getting both your bright blue light in the day and your dim red light in the evening is programmable light bulbs where you can set the color spectrum and the brightness for the time of day (and you can program them to automatically change at whatever time you want! how cool is that!). It's an investment, but then you can ditch the goofy safety glasses (although, you'll want to pull them out again if you're going to watch TV).

3. Reduce and manage stress.

You probably recognize cortisol as being the master stress hormone. It's also a very important circadian rhythm hormone. This means if you're under stress, not only do you have all the effects of elevated and dysregulated cortisol to deal with, but you also disrupt your circadian rhythms.

Reducing stress means removing stressors from your life. Whether it's saying no, asking for help, or making changes to the structure of your life, whatever you can do to reduce stress will make a difference. Oh, and coffee increases your body's response to psychological stressors, so you might want to cut down on coffee or give it up altogether.

Managing stress also means increasing activities that help regulate cortisol and make you more resilient to stressors. This might include meditating, doing yoga, going for a walk, taking a bath, or making time for a hobby. This is discussed further in Chapter 27.

4. Go to bed on time! (And get enough sleep!)

Just like being stressed can affect circadian rhythms, so can ignoring them. Your melatonin starts increasing about 2 hours before bedtime to prepare your body for sleep. If you're muscling through that with a sugary snack, a scary movie, or whatever else you do to keep yourself awake at night, you are affecting your circadian rhythms.

It's important to have a consistent bedtime and wake time. Allowing fluctuations in when we go to bed, when we get up in the morning, and how long we sleep not only negatively impacts sleep quality but also is a risk factor for obesity and diabetes.

Aim for 7 to 10 hours of sleep every night (most people need between 8 and 9). This means shifting your bedtime earlier so you aren't muscling through that fatigue to get a second wind (which, by the way, usually means you're increasing your cortisol right when it's supposed to be at its lowest). For more on optimizing sleep, see pages 335 to 338.

5. Sleep in a cool, dark room (and keep the indoor temperature warmer during the day).

Sleeping in a completely dark room is really important for protecting circadian rhythms. Cover up any LED lights on phones, toothbrushes, baby monitors, or whatever other gadgets you have plugged in in your room (masking tape works great for alarm clocks, and duct tape works great for little LED lights). And ditch the night-lights or switch to ones with red bulbs. Blackout curtains can be one of the greatest biohacks for getting a good night's sleep, as can white noise generators (especially if there are high-frequency/high-pitched noises inside or outside your home, as these are very stimulating for the brain).

While you're at it, ditch the alarm clock. Waking up to a jarring noise is very stressful. If you don't have the luxury of sleeping until your body naturally wants to wake every morning (which is the best option for protecting your circadian rhythms and overall health), a light alarm is a great investment.

The temperature of the room in which you sleep is also a cue to your circadian clock. Ideally, the indoor temperature at night should be 65°F or lower. And the converse is also true: being warmer during the day, typically above 75°F, supports circadian rhythms, but you can vary this range by season.

6. Get activity.

Getting some kind of activity during the day has been shown in clinical trials to support melatonin production. There are a few exceptions, though. For example, intense activity later in the day can delay melatonin production (basically keeping you revved up longer in the evening) unless it's routine (say, you always go to CrossFit in the evening and your body has adjusted). And working out in a really bright environment in the evening can be a problem; the combination of bright lights and activity suppresses melatonin. But, other than that, any kind of activity at any time of day (even better if it's outside!) will help support circadian rhythms.

7. Keep your blood sugar levels well managed.
Many hormones are sensitive to swings in blood sugar, including melatonin and cortisol. This doesn't mean eating low-carb (eating too low-carb can actually disrupt circadian rhythms by increasing cortisol and affecting insulin sensitivity, and high-starch meals about 5 hours before bedtime have been shown to improve sleep quality), but rather to avoid spikes in blood sugar from high-glycemic-load foods. If you're following a Paleo diet, chances are good that you're doing this already.

8. Be social during the day and intimate at night.
Social connection can influence our circadian clocks. To entrench circadian rhythms, limit big social gatherings (and even activities like watching TV shows with lots of characters) to the daytime, and keep things intimate (just your closest loved ones) in the evening.

9. Eat organ meat and seafood.
Melatonin is made from serotonin, which is made from tryptophan. Organ meat and seafood have more tryptophan and have less of the other amino acids that compete with tryptophan to cross the blood-brain barrier. So eating more organ meat and seafood is a great way to boost production of both serotonin and melatonin.

Eating seafood also contributes long-chain omega-3 fats (DHA and EPA) to your diet. Omega-3s help support circadian rhythms by improving neural health in the brain and by improving resilience to stressors (if you're getting high dietary omega-3s, you secrete less cortisol in response to stress).

10. Embrace seasonal variation.
It is natural, normal, and healthy to sleep more in the winter and less in the summer. But indoor lighting has robbed us of these natural seasonal variations in the amount of sleep we get, our activity levels, and even our appetites. Most of us live as though it's summer year-round. But you can embrace seasonal variation by adjusting things like bedtime (what time you dim the lights and put on your amber-tinted glasses) based on the time of year. Maybe aim for 9 or 10 hours of sleep in winter but only 7 or 8 in summer. Adjust your indoor temperature to more accurately reflect what's happening outside (this is also a great way to save on heating and cooling bills). Eat seasonally (which means your carbohydrate intake will likely vary by season, too, which will influence cortisol and melatonin through effects on insulin). All these things will help regulate your hormones in a healthy way, and you will feel the difference!

KNOWLEDGE BOMB *Could natural sleep patterns be different for those of us living at more extreme latitudes, where winter nights are longer and annual light exposure is different? The answer might be yes!*

Historical analyses have shown that until the Industrial Revolution (and scrolling way back through recorded history), something called "bimodal" or "segmented" sleep was dominant in Western civilization. Two distinct sleep periods occurred during the night: in general, 4 hours of sleep followed by 1 hour or more of wakefulness, followed by another 4 hours of sleep. Numerous ancient and medieval references talk about the "first sleep" and "second sleep," with the period between being used for writing, philosophizing, praying, reflecting, socializing, and other activities. (That period of wakefulness coincided with high levels of the pituitary hormone prolactin, possibly contributing to the sense of peace and creativity that people felt during their sleep intermission.)

So, while populations near the equator may naturally sleep uninterrupted, it could be normal for some people at extreme latitudes to rouse during the night (especially in the winter when periods of nighttime darkness are longer)—something we typically diagnose as maintenance insomnia. This is especially true for people with little or no exposure to artificial light and electronics after sundown (as was the case when bimodal sleep was the norm).

If your body naturally follows a bimodal sleep pattern, make sure not to turn on any lights when you wake in the night (this disrupts your circadian rhythm). Instead, use this time to listen to an audiobook, meditate, stretch in the dark, or, if you're lucky enough to have a partner with similar natural sleep habits, engage in quiet conversation, cuddling, or sexual activities. If you do need a light in the middle of the night, use a dim red light bulb in a lamp.

Inadequate Sleep and Disease Risk

One of the scientific strategies for quantifying how a factor impacts health is to look at something called *all-cause mortality.* Large cohorts of people are followed for years (sometimes decades), and every death is logged. Then scientists compare how many people died in each category of the factor being evaluated. These studies tend to define short sleep as less than 6 hours per night, normal sleep as 6 to 9 hours per night, and long sleep as more than 9 hours per night. Some studies look at narrower ranges—for example, less than 5 hours, 6 hours, 7 hours, 8 hours, 9 hours, and more than 10 hours. Comparing the number of deaths in each category gives us an indication of how sleep affects health. Yes, the number of deaths includes deaths that are the result of acute illness, chronic disease, old age, and accidents. However, looking at this number as a whole is a good way to measure overall health and longevity. More sophisticated statistics can account for other known health inputs, such as smoking, being overweight, and being active (or not), to home in on the effect of sleep independent of other risk factors.

A 2010 meta-analysis pooled data from twenty-seven different cohorts and found that sleeping less than 6 hours per night increased the risk of all-cause mortality by 12 percent. To compare, being obese increased the risk of all-cause mortality by 18 percent. Smoking about doubled the risk of all-cause mortality. For every hour of physical activity that replaced sedentary time, the risk of all-cause mortality dropped by 16 percent. And for every daily serving of vegetables (up to five servings), the risk of all-cause mortality dropped by 5 percent.

Using all-cause mortality as an indicator, the health impact of getting less than 6 hours of sleep per night is in the same ballpark as being obese, being sedentary, and not eating many vegetables. Getting less than 6 hours of sleep per night also increases a person's chances of being obese, being inactive, and not eating many vegetables. So, not only is not getting enough sleep an independent risk factor for disease, but then the probability of having additional risk factors goes up! Conversely, being well-rested improves our health both directly and indirectly by making it easier to make healthy food choices, increasing our motivation to move, and directly affecting hunger and metabolism—all major contributors to body weight.

We also have a huge variety of specific links between sleep and health problems. These are worth diving into to drive home just how essential sleep is for our health.

Sleep and Obesity

Sleeping less than 6 hours per night increases the risk of obesity by 55 percent in adults (and 90 percent in children!). But researchers have teased out some other fascinating links between how we sleep and obesity risk. During a week, variability in bedtimes of greater than 2 hours increases the risk of obesity by 14 percent. For example, if we normally go to bed at 10 p.m. on weeknights but stay up until midnight for a party on Saturday, our risk of obesity is higher. This is a normal pattern for students and working adults alike! Sleep duration variability increases the risk of obesity by 63 percent for every 1 hour of standard deviation. That means if some nights we get 6 hours and other nights we try to make up for it by sleeping 9 hours, that inconsistency is dramatically increasing our risk of obesity.

It's also important to sync our sleep time with the sun: following the night-owl patterns of late-to-bed, late-to-rise doubles the risk of obesity compared to early-to-bed, early-to-rise, even in people who get enough sleep.

How exactly does the sleep-obesity connection work? One mechanism by which inadequate sleep increases our risk of weight gain and obesity is its profound effects on hunger hormones and metabolism.

Not getting enough sleep increases appetite. When food intake is measured following sleep deprivation (5 consecutive days of 4 hours' sleep), people tend to eat substantially more than normal—20 percent more! However, it doesn't take 5 full days of inadequate sleep to see huge shifts in insulin, cortisol, leptin, and ghrelin, all of which impact appetite as well as metabolism. One study showed that even a single night of partial sleep (4 hours—something many of us experience more often than we'd like) causes insulin resistance (see page 86) in healthy people. Another study showed that a single night of partial sleep (3 hours in this case) caused a classic pattern of dysregulated cortisol, with lower morning cortisol levels (when cortisol should be at its highest), higher afternoon and evening cortisol levels (when cortisol should be waning), and high morning leptin levels (when leptin should be at its lowest). Yet another study showed that sleep restriction (4½ hours) caused not only an increase in leptin, but also an increase in ghrelin throughout the day and resulted in less of a drop in ghrelin in response to eating (see page 90 for more on the roles of these hunger hormones). The sleep-restricted healthy men consumed about 400 more calories per day, mostly in snacks rather than meals.

This means that a single night of 3 or 4 hours' sleep causes insulin resistance, dysregulated cortisol, increased leptin, increased ghrelin, and less of a drop in ghrelin after eating—all hormonal situations that lead to weight gain. That's *one night* of staying up past our bedtime to go to a late movie. One!

Through these hormonal effects, not getting enough sleep alters food preferences toward more energy-dense foods, increases hunger, decreases fat metabolism, and increases the stress response that affects basal metabolic rate.

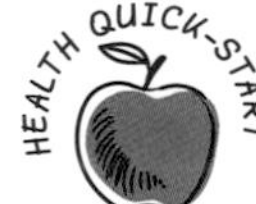

Trying to reduce caloric intake to meet weight-loss goals? Getting enough sleep is key!

However, there's a whole lot more to the link between sleep and obesity, and the dopamine link is perhaps even more impactful.

Dopamine is a neurotransmitter (and yes, also technically a hormone, but let's separate it from the other hormones because they aren't all neurotransmitters). It plays important roles in motor control, motivation, arousal, cognition, and reward as well as a number of lower-level functions, including lactation, sexual gratification, and nausea. But in order to perform its functions, dopamine must bind to a receptor, so its efficacy is only as good as both its levels and the levels of its receptors. In addition, receptors can be more or less sensitive to dopamine, adding another layer of complication to how this system impacts our health.

There's a huge body of scientific literature showing that people with obesity and/or binge-eating disorder (those are not the same thing and do not necessarily go together) have the same types of changes in dopamine receptors in their brains as drug addicts. In particular, the dopamine system in a region of the brain called the *striatum*—which is involved in reward, motivation, and food consumption—is altered. Food addiction is a real thing.

It's thought that food addiction arises from opportunistic overconsumption of highly palatable foods. Then the neuroadaptive response is triggered in the brain reward circuits (analogous to drug and alcohol addiction), which in turn drives the development of compulsive eating. This change in dopamine and its receptors increases the incentive to eat while counteracting satiety signals, which leads to overeating.

New research adds to our understanding of food addiction in an important way. Opportunistic eating behavior and body mass index (BMI) were both positively associated with something called dopamine D2-like receptor binding potential (how readily D2 dopamine receptors bind to dopamine), in a particular part of the striatum (an area of the brain essential for the reward system), but were negatively associated in the rest of the striatum (which is more important for motor systems). This pattern suggests that obese people have alterations in dopamine neurocircuitry that may increase their susceptibility to opportunistic overeating while making food intake less rewarding, less goal-directed, and more habitual.

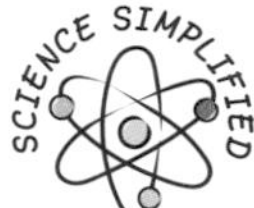

Not getting enough sleep causes the same changes in the brain as seen in addiction. No wonder inadequate sleep is linked to a higher likelihood of developing addiction or relapse!

It's believed that this change in dopamine receptors characteristic of food addiction and so common in those of us with a history of obesity and/or binge eating disorder is caused by opportunistic overeating. Well, it turns out that this altered dopamine receptor pattern in the brain may also be caused by a lack of sleep.

The study of how inadequate sleep affects the brain is an entirely different field, but one that is still very relevant to obesity research. A recent study measured the effects on dopamine receptors in the striatum region of the brain in healthy volunteers deprived of sleep. The authors of this study were interested in discovering the biological mechanism responsible for the decreased alertness that we experience after a night of lost sleep, so they looked at both dopamine levels and the levels of dopamine receptors. Sleep deprivation caused no change in dopamine levels but caused a major decrease in dopamine receptors in the same part of the striatum region of the brain (the ventral striatum) where dopamine receptors are decreased in those with obesity or binge eating disorder—the part that mediates the reward response to food and the motivation to eat.

What does this mean? From the perspective of understanding the effects of sleep on the brain, it means that sleep deprivation causes changes that make the brain less receptive to dopamine, so dopamine can't do all the things it's supposed to do. This likely explains common sleep deprivation behaviors, like increases in risk-taking behavior, impulsivity, and drug relapse (yes, addiction). The relevance to obesity is that these same changes in the brain are seen in people who are obese or who have binge eating disorder. Maybe it's not opportunistic overeating that leads us to food addiction, but chronically insufficient sleep—or both.

Genetics, too, may play a role in the sleep-obesity link. Several variants of the CLOCK (Circadian Locomotor Output Cycles Kaput) family of genes that control circadian rhythms (how our bodies know what time of day it is) may explain why inadequate sleep causes some people to gain significant weight but not others. People who have these particular CLOCK gene variants are much more susceptible to increased hunger and food cravings when they are sleep deprived.

The study that discovered this genetic link looked at appetite stimulation and the other hormonal effects of sleep deprivation. Because the dopamine receptor changes seen in the brains of sleep-deprived people was seen in all test subjects (who were healthy individuals), it's likely that the neurotransmitter link between lack of sleep and obesity does not require a genetic predisposition (or at least not the same genetic predisposition as the hormone link).

Most importantly, the simple act of routinely getting enough sleep turns off the effects on hunger and food preferences caused by a lack of sleep in people with these CLOCK gene variants. So, while genetics may make us more susceptible to gaining weight when we're not getting enough sleep, the environmental factor—inadequate sleep—is critical for the effect.

Sleep, Inflammation, and Infection

Not getting enough sleep causes inflammation—and with that inflammation comes increased risk of a wide assortment of diseases. A variety of studies evaluating the effects of acute sleep deprivation (typically by restricting sleep to 4 hours a night) for several consecutive days (typically 3 to 5) have shown increases in both markers of inflammation and white blood cells. Specifically, even three consecutive nights of not enough sleep can cause increased monocytes, neutrophils, and B cells in the blood, increased pro-inflammatory cytokines (including cytokines known to stimulate the maturation of naïve T cells into Th1, Th2, and Th17 cells; see page 79), increased C-reactive protein (a marker of inflammation), increased total cholesterol, and increased LDL ("bad") cholesterol.

Even one night of lost sleep (or 40 continuous hours without sleep) causes inflammation in young, healthy people. Pulling a single all-nighter dramatically increases markers of inflammation in the blood, including C-reactive protein and pro-inflammatory cytokines. Studies evaluating not just sleep deprivation but also recovery after sleep restriction—the idea being to simulate a typical workweek when someone might get inadequate sleep for four or five nights straight and then try to make up for it on the weekend—have also shown that the pro-inflammatory cytokine known to stimulate Th17 cell development persists for at least 2 days after increasing sleep to 9 hours a night, even though other measurements of inflammation have returned to normal. This means that even if we try to "catch up" on sleep over the weekend, the immune system doesn't fully recover from the overstimulation caused by the late nights and early mornings during the week. If we follow this typical pattern of not getting enough sleep during the week and sleeping in on the weekend, we run the risk of cumulatively wreaking havoc on our immune systems. We can recover from periods of undersleeping, but it takes persistence, consistency, and commitment—even during the week.

KNOWLEDGE BOMB *There is emerging evidence that sleep has a direct effect on the gut microbiota. A recent study evaluated the changes in the gut microbial composition after just two nights of partial sleep deprivation and showed an increase in the ratio of Firmicutes to Bacteroidetes and increased numbers of bacteria in the Coriobacteriaceae and Erysipelotrichaceae families with decreases in Tenericutes bacteria. These changes have all previously been associated with metabolic perturbations, like obesity and insulin resistance.*

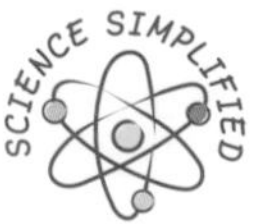

Not getting enough sleep is inflammatory. Even if you try to catch up on sleep on weekends, it's not enough for your immune system to return to normal.

Sleep deprivation is also associated with increased susceptibility to infections. The less sleep we get, the more likely we are to catch a cold. Conversely, getting adequate sleep can protect us from infections. One study even showed that the longer the duration of sleep, the lower the incidence of parasitic infections in mammals.

Sleep and Type 2 Diabetes

Considering the effects of sleep deprivation on insulin sensitivity (as it relates to obesity), the link between sleep and type 2 diabetes is hardly surprising. Sleeping less than 6 hours per night increases the risk of type 2 diabetes by 50 percent. If we pool diabetes and prediabetes (impaired glucose tolerance) together, that risk soars to a whopping 2.4 times!

Even a single night of restricted sleep (say 4 to 5 hours) causes measurable insulin resistance. This means that even in healthy adults, blood sugar responses to foods will be out of whack after a late night. Not only is this a good thing to keep in mind if you periodically don't get enough sleep (you may want to moderate your carbohydrate intake after a late night), but it's yet another compelling reason to prioritize sleep every single night.

Sleep restriction also increases the measurable free fatty acids in the blood, a contributor to insulin resistance that plays a central role in the development of metabolic diseases. A study found that getting 4½ hours of sleep per night compared to 8½ hours increased serum free fatty acids in healthy men by 15 to 30 percent.

What might be even more fascinating is that there's emerging evidence that sleep has an even greater impact on insulin sensitivity and glucose metabolism than diet does. Research presented at the 2016 Obesity Society's Annual Scientific Meeting shows that a single night of lost sleep was worse than 6 months of a high-fat Western diet in terms of insulin sensitivity and glucose metabolism.

Sleep and Autoimmune Disease

Research into risk factors for autoimmune disease is still in its infancy. There have yet to be large population studies looking at average sleep duration and autoimmune disease incidence. However, having a non-apnea sleep disorder (the most common is insomnia, which can be as mild as having a night or two a week where either we can't fall asleep or we wake up in the middle of the night and can't get back to sleep) increases the risk of autoimmune disease by an average of 50 percent. Some autoimmune disease incidence is more sensitive to non-apnea sleep disorders than others. For example, the risk of systemic lupus erythematosus goes up 81 percent, rheumatoid arthritis risk goes up 45 percent, ankylosing spondylitis risk goes up 53 percent, and Sjögren's syndrome risk goes up 51 percent. It's even worse if you suffer from obstructive sleep apnea, a condition that tends to go along with obesity and diabetes, which more than doubles your risk of autoimmune disease. Shift workers, known for having erratic sleep schedules and routinely getting inadequate sleep, have a 50 percent higher risk of autoimmune disease. It's also known that short sleep exacerbates symptoms of many autoimmune diseases.

In an animal model of psoriasis, sleep deprivation caused significant increases in pro-inflammatory cytokines, cortisol levels, and specific proteins in the skin associated with symptoms of psoriasis, like dry, flaking, scaly skin. Mice subjected to sleep deprivation developed multiple sclerosis earlier than mice allowed to sleep normally, and once they developed the disease, sleep deprivation increased its progress and the amount of pain the mice felt. Furthermore, sleep disturbances are commonly reported by people with chronic inflammatory conditions such as rheumatoid arthritis, systemic lupus erythematosus, inflammatory bowel disease, and asthma—in some cases, sleep disturbances are caused by pain or discomfort, and in other cases, sleep disturbances are caused by disruption of circadian rhythms, or both. Whether the sleep disturbances cause the disease or vice versa is not well understood (and might be different for different diseases), but sleep disturbances are known to worsen the course of the disease, aggravate disease symptoms such as pain and fatigue, and lower quality of life.

Sleep and Cardiovascular Disease

Routinely sleeping less than 6 hours per night doubles the risk of stroke, doubles the risk of myocardial infarction, increases the risk of congestive heart failure by 67 percent, and increases risk of coronary heart disease by 48 percent compared to getting between 6 and 8 hours of nightly sleep. Those are huge numbers! And while the dietary factors we've previously discussed absolutely influence disease risk, when we look at the body of literature explaining how inadequate sleep raises LDL cholesterol, raises blood pressure, increases heart rate variability, and causes inflammation, it's clear that diet is only part of the disease equation and that ignoring the role of sleep could have dire consequences.

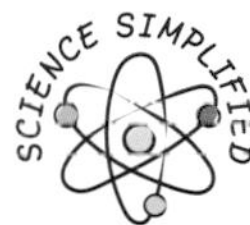

In terms of risk factors for cardiovascular disease, you get an even bigger bang for your buck out of sleep than exercise. Whoa!

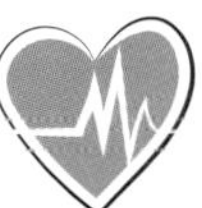

Sleep and Cancer

Finally, some less-bleak news: In the studies that have looked at prostate, breast, and lung cancer, there was no increased risk with short sleep, even when comparing people who get less than 5 hours of sleep per night to those who get 7 to 8 hours. The exception is studies of colorectal adenomas (precursors to cancerous colon tumors), in which the risk increases by 50 percent with less than 5 hours of sleep. However, how much sleep someone gets after a breast cancer diagnosis is a predictor of survival, and getting less than 6 hours of sleep increases the risk of death by 46 percent.

SLEEP REQUIREMENTS AND SLEEP DEBT

That brings us to the question: *how much sleep do we need?*

In addition to sleep specialists, the National Sleep Foundation recently convened experts from anatomy, physiology, pediatrics, neurology, gerontology, and gynecology to reach a consensus from a broad range of scientific disciplines. The panel revised the recommended sleep ranges and came up with the following guidelines:

AGE	SLEEP RECOMMENDATION
Newborns (0–3 months)	14–17 hours
Infants (4–11 months)	12–15 hours
Toddlers (1–2 years)	11–14 hours
Preschoolers (3–5)	10–13 hours
School-age children (6–13)	9–11 hours
Teenagers (14–17)	8–10 hours
Young adults (18–25)	7–9 hours
Adults (26–64)	7–9 hours
Older adults (65+)	7–8 hours

That being said, defining how much sleep we need within the normal range can be a challenge. Do you enjoy perfect health with 7 hours every night? Or do you need 9 hours on a regular basis? And what if you need even more sleep than the top end of the range, which happens during either chronic or acute illness? How do you know? While scientific researchers are working on a blood test to evaluate sleep debt (using serum levels of oxalic acid and diacylglycerol 36:3), being able to ask your doctor to run a test that will tell you whether you're getting enough sleep is probably at least a few years from being a reality.

In the absence of a definitive test, you can ask yourself the following questions:

- *Do I have to set an alarm in the morning? Would I sleep past my alarm time if didn't have one set?*
- *Do I drag myself out of bed? Do I need caffeine in the morning to get me going?*
- *Do I always sleep in on the weekends?*
- *Do I get less than 7 hours of sleep per night even once or twice per week?*

If your answer to any of these questions is "yes," you owe a sleep debt. And even if you're *almost* getting the right amount of sleep—that is, your sleep debt is very low—your health will suffer. A recent study showed that getting just 30 minutes less sleep per night than our bodies need on weekdays (while sleeping in on weekends) can have long-term consequences for body weight and metabolism.

Most research into the role of sleep uses "short sleep" as an investigatory tool. However, as researchers start to look at sleep debt instead of more dramatic situations, it's becoming clear just how sensitive the human body is to inadequate sleep.

In this case, the study participants kept sleep logs, and the researchers calculated how much less sleep they got than the recommended 8 hours a night over the workweek (not including sleeping in to "catch up" on the weekends). The participants were people newly diagnosed with type 2 diabetes. They were randomized into one of three groups: usual care, physical activity intervention, and diet and physical activity intervention. When the participants were recruited, those who typically didn't get enough sleep were 72 percent more likely to be obese. The researchers then followed the participants over a year to see what would change. Note that addressing sleep was not a part of any of the study interventions. The amount of sleep debt that individuals had didn't typically change during the study.

Sleep debt dramatically impacted the risk of obesity and insulin resistance, and the correlation between the two increased throughout the study—not surprising, considering the sleep-related disease risks we've already discussed. After 12 months, for every 30 minutes of weekday sleep debt, the risk of obesity was 17 percent higher and the risk of insulin resistance was 39 percent higher. Think about that for a second. If we get 30 minutes less sleep a night than we need just on weeknights, we have a 39 percent higher risk of insulin resistance. If we get an hour less sleep a night, we have a 78 percent higher risk. A separate study showed that Th17 cells, components of the immune system that become overactive during short sleep, do not return to normal after 2 days of sleeping in. Combined, these studies strongly reinforce the idea that we need to get adequate sleep every single night—and that when following a Paleo framework, sleep needs to be prioritized.

SLEEPING TOO MUCH?

The links between inadequate sleep and disease risk are pretty bad news for people who have difficulty carving out enough time for sleep in their lives. But the coin does have a flip side. A collection of studies show increased disease risk in long sleepers as well. A large meta-analysis looking at all-cause mortality showed a 25 percent higher risk for those who sleep more than 9 hours per night (compared to 7 to 8 hours) and a 54 percent higher risk for those who sleep more than 10 hours. However, there's a chicken-versus-egg discussion to engage in here. Are people sleeping more because they're sick, or are they sick because they're sleeping more? A 2014 study evaluated the effect of sleep on survival rate in groups with different levels of physical activity and found that long sleep (more than 9 hours) increased all-cause mortality only in physically inactive people.

And when the American Academy of Sleep Medicine and the Sleep Research Society reviewed the scientific literature on this topic, they came up with the following consensus statement:

> *Sleeping more than 9 hours per night on a regular basis may be appropriate for young adults, individuals recovering from sleep debt, and individuals with illnesses. For others, it is uncertain whether sleeping more than 9 hours per night is associated with health risk.*

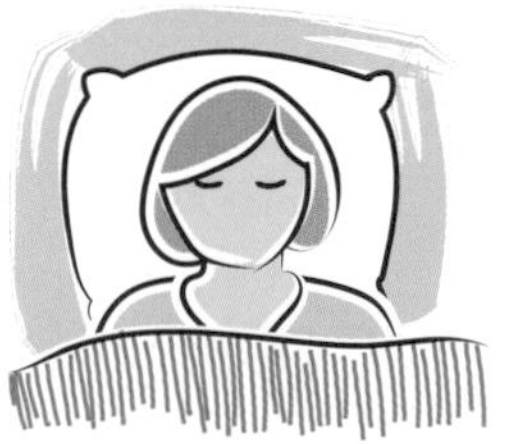

OPTIMIZING SLEEP

Unfortunately, learning about the many consequences of inadequate sleep is a lot easier than actually getting enough of it. Our modern lifestyles, overpacked schedules, work-centric culture, and early-morning obligations can make it difficult to avoid shortchanging ourselves on sleep. In fact, for many people, adequate sleep is the most difficult Paleo principle to implement. So how do we regulate our sleep-wake cycles and maximize our chance of getting a full night's rest—and reduce our disease risk in the process?

First, let's take a step back to look at some important neurophysiology. Our brains are made up of a network of many types of neurons. And neurons are fascinating cells. A typical neuron consists of a cell body, dendrites, and an axon. The purpose of dendrites is to receive signals from other neurons in order for the neuron to pass it on. Because one neuron can have many dendrites connecting to many other neurons, neural signaling can become amazingly complex. The axon extends from the cell body (by as much as a meter, or 3 feet!) and connects to other cells, acting as the primary transmission lines of the nervous system.

The most "basic" neurons communicate using a combination of electrical and chemical signals. When a neuron is activated (sometimes people say the neuron is "turned on" or "stimulated"), an electrical signal travels down the armlike axon of the cell, where the electrical impulse—called an action potential—triggers the release of chemical compounds called neurotransmitters from the axon terminus. The neurotransmitters travel a short distance and bind to the adjacent neuron at its dendrites, turning it on (starting another electrical signal) or off (preventing an electrical signal), depending on the neurotransmitters released, which type of neurotransmitter receptors are present on the receiving neuron, and something called membrane potential.

Because of the electrical component to neuron signaling, this process depends on the balance of ions (electrically charged atoms) between the cell and its surroundings. When the difference in ions between the inside and outside of the cell is greater, there is a stronger electrical signal, and the cell is more active and able to easily communicate with neighboring cells. A cell's membrane potential is when channels on the surface of the neuron's membranes determine which ions are allowed into and out of the cell, making it more or less active.

Why does this matter? It turns out that sleep is essentially regulated by this relatively simple mechanism. Researchers have identified that there is a small bundle of neurons that is connected to our circadian rhythm (see page 325), and the activity of these neurons is turned off and on by differences in membrane potential. These differences in membrane potential that allow a neuron to be turned on or off are determined by sodium and potassium pumps, which are regulated by time of day. During the day, more sodium ions are pumped into the cell and create more membrane potential, making the neurons more excitable and telling our bodies that it is time to be awake. At night, potassium pumps regulate the membrane potential such that the neurons are less excitable. When this happens, our brains are able to go into "sleep mode." Without this simple mechanism, our sleep-wake cycle could never be regulated.

What controls when these chemical changes occur is part of our physiology that has been understood for a while. Two major factors contribute to our sleep-wake cycle: circadian rhythm (our internal clock) and sleep homeostasis (our sleep debt).

The circadian rhythm was discussed in greater depth on page 325. A less-considered aspect of sleep-wake regulation is sleep homeostasis, which creates our drive for sleep. *Homeostasis* is a general biology term used to describe processes the body takes to stay in a stable and/or constant condition. We know much less about the details of sleep homeostasis than we do about circadian rhythm, but it appears to be controlled by the sleep-regulating substances that accumulate in the cerebrospinal fluid during waking hours. The best-understood sleep-regulating substance is the protein adenosine.

Adenosine is a protein that accumulates in the basal forebrain during wakefulness and is a natural by-product of using energy stores in the brain. Being the central protein for adenosine triphosphate (ATP, the basic energy molecule of the body that fuels biochemical reactions), free adenosine accumulation is a sign that the brain is using energy stores in the form of glycogen. During sleep, adenosine is cleared away and replaced by more glycogen; in fact, this was one of the examples of why we need sleep in the first place. Common stimulants like caffeine work as adenosine antagonists, preventing the effect of drowsiness. However, the details of this process and which other factors may be involved in regulating sleep homeostasis are still unknown.

The "sleep homeostat" is basically sleep debt. This is a term that refers to both the body's gauge of the amount of sleep we've experienced recently as well as its drive to return to balance—that is, to pay off any sleep debt. We can think of it as a sliding scale of how tired we feel based on how much sleep we've had in the last few nights. When our circadian clock tells our bodies that it's time to prepare for sleep and our sleep homeostat agrees that sleep is needed (and we actually listen and go to bed!), we have a good night's sleep. In combination, our natural circadian rhythm and sleep homeostat generate a drive for sleep each day that may be influenced by other factors. If we are looking to improve our sleep, regulating our sleep-wake cycles may be the key.

With all that said, what can we do to set our circadian clock, protect our circadian rhythms, and regulate so many important hormones?

The light-dark cycle is the most important signal to our circadian clock. One of the best ways to set our circadian clock is be exposed to bright light (ideally sunlight) during the day, but be in darkness at night. In fact, getting sunlight exposure during the day is probably the single most important thing we can do to support the normal production of melatonin in the evening.

You probably already know that our bodies make vitamin D in response to exposure to ultraviolet light. Recall that vitamin D is a steroid hormone that controls expression of more than 200 genes and the proteins that those genes regulate. In addition to its roles in mineral metabolism, bone health, and the immune system, vitamin D also activates areas of the brain responsible for biorhythms. However, that's hardly the only important aspect of sun exposure. Cells throughout the body, including the skin and eyes, are sensitive to blue light from the sun, which is strongest in the morning. When special cells in the retina of the eye are stimulated by sunlight, they directly affect the pituitary gland and the hypothalamus region of the brain. The hypothalamus is responsible for circadian rhythm, the regulation of hormones, and the nervous system. Proper regulation of circadian rhythm is crucial for quality sleep, stress management, and the cyclic pattern of expression of so many hormones in the body, which are independent of vitamin D production. So, while taking a vitamin D3 supplement is helpful when the sun is scarce in the winter months (or if you do shift work or face other challenges to getting outdoors into the sun), it can't replace the huge range of health benefits of plain old being outside. And while we're inside? Studies show that spending time by a bright window can be helpful. Another great alternative if you work in a dim room or are a shift worker is to invest in a light therapy box.

Just as it's important for our bodies to get the signal that it's daytime during the day, it's important to tell our bodies that it's nighttime once the sun goes down. Our bodies start releasing melatonin about 2 hours before we normally go to bed to start preparing us for sleep. This makes us feel sleepy and lowers our body temperature. But melatonin production can be inhibited by exposure to bright indoor lights. This means we need to avoid blue light and stick with red and yellow wavelengths as well as keep the overall light level much dimmer.

As discussed earlier, a useful biohack is to wear amber-tinted glasses—glasses with yellow lenses, also called melatonin glasses or blue-blocking glasses—for the last 2 to 3 hours of the day. Several scientific studies show that wearing amber-tinted glasses in the evening improves sleep quality and supports melatonin production. Sleeping in a completely dark room is also really important for protecting circadian rhythms.

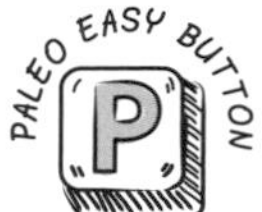

These three easy biohacks for great sleep will give you the biggest bang for your buck:

- *Use a light therapy box for at least an hour in the middle of the day if you can't spend time outside.*
- *Wear amber-tinted glasses (which can be as simple as a pair of yellow-lensed safety glasses) for the last 2 to 3 hours before bedtime every day.*
- *Have a consistent bedtime and sleep in a dark, cool, quiet room.*

SCIENCE SIMPLIFIED *The most important regulator of sleep is the light-dark cycle, meaning that you are in a bright environment during the day, a dim environment in the evening, and a dark environment at night. This is because sunlight (and the lack thereof at night) is an important signal to the brain's internal clock, telling the body which biological processes to prioritize, such as regulating the ups and downs of hormones that keep us energized during the day and help our bodies sleep restfully at night. The main problem with indoor lighting is that it's too dim to simulate sunlight's signals during the day and too bright to simulate nighttime signals in the evening.*

Avoiding eating for at least 2 hours before you go to bed can help protect circadian rhythms, too. Eating tryptophan-rich foods can also be particularly useful, and some herbal teas may assist the relaxing and unwinding process in the evening after a stressful day (chamomile is a classic, but any caffeine-free warm beverage can provide a soothing stimulus for sleep). But there are other ways to help optimize our sleep. They include the following:

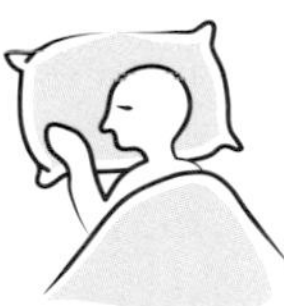

Make sleep a priority. This might sound like a no-brainer, but for most people it's the number-one barrier to getting enough sleep: simply making enough time for it! Truly, every one of us should have an established bedtime early enough that we can get at least 8 hours of sleep. And it's important to stick to that bedtime every single night. Consistency in bedtime not only lowers the risk of obesity, but it also pays off in terms of sleep latency (the time it takes to fall asleep) and overall sleep quality. Basically, our bodies better prepare for sleep when they know exactly what time to expect to be in bed.

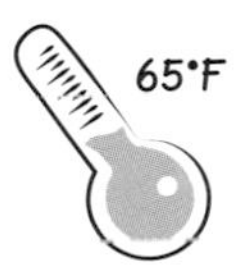

Regulate the temperature. The temperature in which we sleep is a cue to our circadian clock. There are a few contributing factors here. First, our core temperature is in sync with our circadian rhythm—they actually communicate! Our body temperature decreases during sleep, so when the bedroom temperature is lower, it is easier for the body to reach the correct sleep temperature. This makes sleep latency and sleep quality better. Ideally, the indoor temperature at night should be 65°F or lower. Being warmer during the day than we are at night—typically above 75°F—also supports circadian rhythms by saying, "it's time to be awake!"

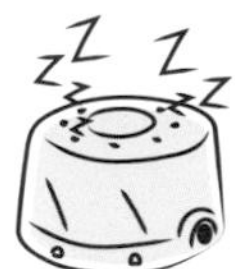

Make use of white noise. We've all been there: we've done all the right things to get ready for bed, but there's a noise outside that *will not stop*. Or maybe our ideal bedtime is an hour or two earlier than our family's. Since sticking our heads under a pillow isn't really conducive to restful sleep, a relatively inexpensive gadget can help solve the problem of environmental noise.

White noise generators (they sell for under $30) can be tremendously helpful, especially if we're looking to mask high-frequency or high-pitched noises inside or outside of our homes. Beyond the typical intrusive noise (cars driving by with music blaring, construction, teenage children watching TV downstairs), there are plenty of sounds in frequencies we can't hear that continue to stimulate our brains and block sleep. That makes it hard for our brains to get into sleep mode and keeps us in a very light phase of sleep. White noise generators can help drown out trains, traffic, barking dogs, and noisy neighbors by masking them with "radio static" that the brain can easily tune out.

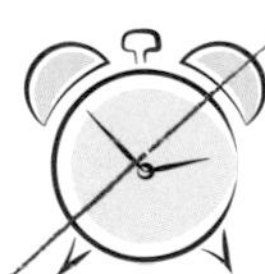

Ditch the alarm clock. Waking up to a jarring noise (even if it's your favorite radio station) is physiologically stressful and can impact the cortisol response that helps us wake up during the day—especially if we hit the snooze button multiple times. Think about it: if our bodies release a burst of cortisol upon our first alarm and we're sleeping through our body's "wake up" signals, then we're setting ourselves up to be tired for the rest of the day. Many of us live by that second or third alarm, but when we consider the effect on our cortisol, those extra 10 minutes probably aren't worth it.

The best option for protecting circadian rhythms and overall health is to sleep until our bodies naturally want to wake. Easier said than done, right? In a perfect world, we'd all be able to make that happen. But a light alarm clock—one that uses gradually brighter light rather than sound to rouse you from sleep—is a great investment that is considerably more soothing than a traditional alarm clock. Plus, it can help entrench our circadian rhythm even more effectively, especially during those darker winter months.

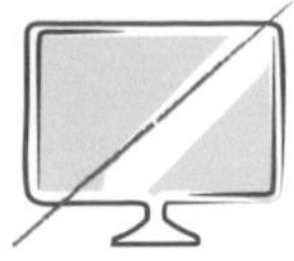

Be strict about what you do in bed. This one is tough for many of us to wrap our heads around. Even when we've ditched the TV before bed, we still want to be able to read in our own bedrooms. And while it's important that we cue our bodies for sleep by taking time to wind down before bed by reading, solving a crossword puzzle, cuddling with a loved one, or listening to relaxing music, ideally we wouldn't actually do these things in bed. If we frequently read, watch TV, surf the web, or eat in bed, our brains will begin to associate those activities with bedtime. That means when we lie down to sleep, our bodies will start revving up in anticipation of another episode of *Game of Thrones* or another chapter of *The Hunger Games*. And we all know what it's like to promise that we'll read only one chapter of a book and then get sucked into a particularly exciting part.

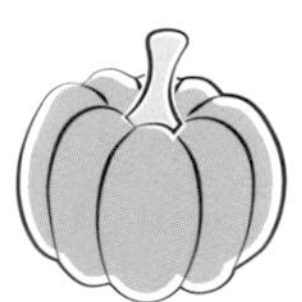

Eat starchy veggies with dinner. Keeping up with the news on carbs can be tricky these days, but there is evidence that monitoring the timing of carb intake could be just as important as the amount. Our bodies seem primed for slow-burn starchy carbohydrates in the evening. We produce more starch-digesting enzymes in the evening, and studies show that eating a decent quantity (say 30 grams) of starchy carbs from whole-food sources at dinner significantly improves sleep. Fiber intake also improves sleep quality and latency in addition to all the other good things fiber does. The great news is that we can kill two birds with one stone with a veggie-rich dinner that includes starchy veggies like sweet potatoes, plantains, cassava, taro, or acorn squash.

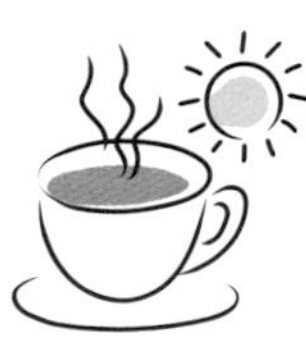

Drink caffeine in the morning *only* (if at all). Caffeine makes us feel more awake and energetic by blocking the sleep signal generated by adenosine, a protein waste product that accumulates over the course of the day. Unfortunately, when we consume caffeine, our levels of the stress hormone cortisol increase (dependent how well we manage stress and how much caffeine we consume), and they can stay elevated for up to 6 hours. In habitual consumers of caffeine (which is a huge majority of us!), cortisol increases much more dramatically in response to stress (like running late for an important meeting) than in someone who doesn't consume caffeine. With daily consumption, our bodies can adapt somewhat to not produce quite as much cortisol in response to caffeine, but complete tolerance never occurs. In addition, recent studies showed that caffeine intake disrupts circadian rhythm by pushing it back, so even if we're tired and want to go to bed early, consuming caffeine later than noon might make that goal impossible. (See page 214 for more on coffee.)

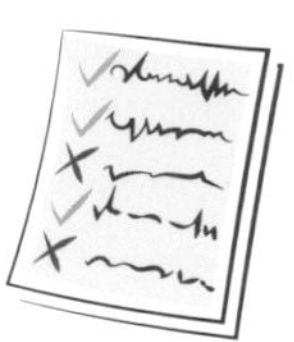

Fine-tune your schedule. It's important to evaluate how you are using your time and whether it would be smart to eliminate some activities to make more time for sleep. Perhaps you watch a couple of hours of TV after the kids go to bed. You might think about cutting back a little or not watching TV at all. Maybe you can limit how much time you spend on social media (which most of us know can be a big time drain). Maybe you're used to going out with your colleagues every day after work, in which case it may be a matter of going out only once or twice a week. Maybe you do all your household chores in the evenings, which might mean asking someone to help or restructuring the day or week to get those chores done at another time. Maybe your kids' after-school activities eat into your evenings, in which case asking a friend to help with transportation might mean that you can, say, get dinner on the table at a reasonable hour. Maybe freeing up time at night is as simple as planning ahead so you have a meal ready to go when you get home. Once again, asking for help and seriously evaluating what you can live without (Does the floor really need to be swept every day? Do you really need to work a 60-hour week?) are key aspects of looking after yourself.

Ultimately, getting enough sleep can be just as important (if not more so!) than the foods we eat. Yes, it plays *that* big a role in our health. It's imperative to avoid the temptation to skimp on sleep and mask the consequences with caffeine and other stimulants. The fact is, even those of us with incredibly busy lives can take measures to improve our sleep quality and maximize the amount of rest we get each night. Every bit of effort we put into optimizing our sleep will pay off exponentially.

Chapter 27:
STRESS AND RESILIENCE

The negative impact that chronic stress has on our health can't be stressed enough (pardon the pun). Stress contributes to the development and/or worsening of virtually every ailment, from the common cold to autoimmune disease. And stress is a bigger predictor of cardiovascular disease than any other factor.

However, lifestyle factors like stress can be far harder to prioritize than the foods we eat. And unlike sleep or physical activity, which are easy to quantify, it's sometimes difficult to know how we're doing in the stress arena. But let's be clear here: if we do not manage stress, it will undermine all the positive changes we make.

Chronic stress—that unrelenting kind of stress that never goes away—is known to affect health in a variety of ways. It can cause the development of metabolic syndrome (a nasty combination of obesity, insulin resistance, and high blood pressure), sleep disturbances, systemic inflammation, impaired immunity, and blood clots. It can even lead to increased appetite, cravings for energy-dense foods, uninhibited eating, and other poor health behaviors. No matter what spurs you on the path to going Paleo—whether it's losing a few pounds, increasing performance at the gym, or managing a chronic health problem—stress management is critical for success.

WHAT IS STRESS?

It may seem a bit facetious to explain what stress is. Chances are really good that most of us already know exactly what stresses we have in our lives. However, it's important to differentiate between acute stress and chronic stress.

Historically, almost all stress was acute. Acute stress includes situations such as being chased by a lion or slipping off the edge of a cliff. During this type of event, the fight-or-flight response is activated, and the hormones cortisol and adrenaline work together to ensure survival. At the end of the event, we are either dead (due to falling from the cliff onto craggy rocks 400 feet below) or alive and safe (due to grabbing onto a branch while falling and climbing back up to safety). After the event, there is no need for the body to continue producing adrenaline and excess cortisol (more on this momentarily). Levels return to normal—unless we're dead, of course—and we go on our merry way.

Chronic stress is a different story; it is *never over.* It can be mild: perhaps the everyday stresses from having a job, raising kids, and making ends meet. It can be moderate: perhaps from an impending deadline or exam, a kid getting into trouble at school, or ripping a favorite shirt. It can also be high: such as from illness, divorce, or a death in the family. What's different about chronic stress is that there's no big relief at the end where we can exhale and relax. It's always there, and its insidious effects build up over time. How quickly and severely we feel the effects of chronic stress depends on the severity of the stress and our individual resilience.

Interestingly, the occasional acute stressor may provide health benefits. Where we run into problems is with chronic stress, that low-grade stress that most of us face constantly.

HOW STRESS CONTRIBUTES TO DISEASE

The best-understood mechanism of stress is its impact on the immune system. Inflammation is a component of every disease and health condition. Worse, it's part of the pathogenesis (meaning how a disease develops) of every chronic health condition. Inflammation is controlled (or at least is supposed to be controlled) by the immune system. This doesn't mean inflammation is the sole cause of disease, but it is necessary for disease to develop. If the immune system is well regulated so that there is no inflammation, chronic disease will not develop.

The same is true of stress. It's not the sole cause of disease (at least there isn't any research to prove that it is). Rather, it contributes to the development of disease, so if we suffer from chronic stress, our risk of getting sick increases. To understand how being stuck in traffic or on a deadline at work can directly impact immune system function, it helps to describe what's happening inside our bodies.

The HPA Axis

The hypothalamic-pituitary-adrenal (HPA) axis is responsible for the fight-or-flight response—that is, how the body responds to stress. It is made up of the complex communication among three organs:

- **Hypothalamus:** The part of the brain located just above the brain stem that is responsible for a variety of activities of the autonomic nervous system, such as regulating body temperature, hunger, thirst, fatigue, sleep, and circadian rhythms
- **Pituitary gland:** A pea-shaped gland located below the hypothalamus that secretes a variety of important hormones, such as thyroid-stimulating hormone, human growth hormone, and adrenocorticotropic hormone
- **Adrenal glands:** Small, conical organs on top of the kidneys that secrete a variety of hormones, such as cortisol, epinephrine (also known as adrenaline), norepinephrine, and androgens

HYPOTHALAMUS
↓ ↓ ↓
PITUITARY GLAND
↓ ↓ ↓
ADRENAL GLANDS

The hypothalamus (which receives signals from the hippocampus, the region of the brain that analyzes information from all the senses and thus can perceive danger and make decisions) releases a hormone called corticotropin-releasing hormone (CRH), which signals to the pituitary gland to release a hormone called adrenocorticotropic hormone (ACTH), which signals to the adrenal glands to secrete cortisol as well as catecholamines (like adrenaline).

Cortisol has a huge range of effects in the body, including controlling metabolism, affecting insulin sensitivity and the immune system, and even controlling blood flow. If we're running away from a lion, all these effects (including the combined effects of catecholamines and some direct effects of CRH) come together to prioritize the most essential functions for survival—perception, decision-making, energy for our muscles so we can run away or fight, and preparation for wound healing—and inhibit nonessential functions, like digestion, kidney function, reproductive functions, growth, and collagen and bone formation.

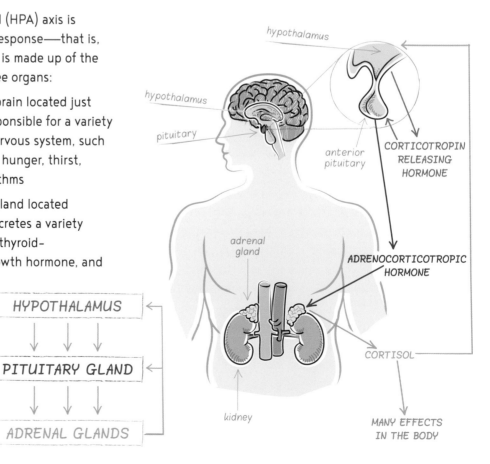

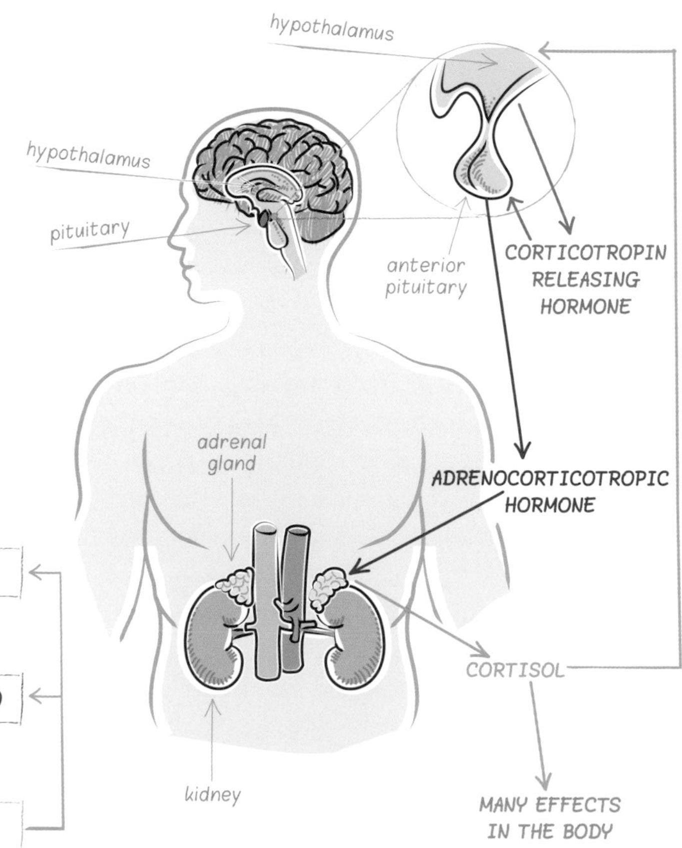

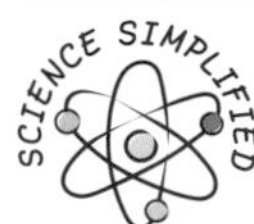

The HPA axis is the cross-talk between two areas of the brain and the adrenal glands responsible for the fight-or-flight response.

Cortisol also provides negative feedback to the pituitary and the hypothalamus. It's the body's way of saying, "Hey, we got the signal that we're supposed to be stressed now. Thanks, we're on it!" If the stressful event has ceased (the lion gave up and left), the HPA axis is deactivated. Of course, if a stressor is still being perceived (the lion is still there), the HPA axis remains activated. And this is why chronic stress (deadlines, traffic, sleep deprivation, teenagers, divorce, being sick, being inflamed, bills, and internet trolls) is such a problem. All those essential functions suppressed by high cortisol, catecholamines, and CRH never get a chance to be prioritized.

The HPG Axis

Another axis? Yes. This time, it's the hypothalamic-pituitary-gonadal (HPG) axis, the primary role of which is to control reproduction; it is also important for development (puberty and aging) and the immune system. Cross-talk between the HPA and HPG axes is one major way that chronic stress leads to health problems.

The hypothalamus releases gonadotropin-releasing hormone (GnRH), which signals to the pituitary gland to secrete two hormones: luteinizing hormone (LH) and follicle-stimulating hormone (FSH). LH and FSH signal to the gonads to produce estrogen and progesterone in women and testosterone in men (see Chapter 4).

Women's bodies are particularly susceptible to the effects of stress on sex hormone levels due to interaction between the HPA and HPG axes. Estrogen and progesterone also signal back to the pituitary gland and the hypothalamus. Generally, estrogen provides positive feedback, further stimulating the HPG axis (although there are some mechanisms for negative feedback as well). Progesterone provides negative feedback, inhibiting the HPG axis. In the menstrual cycle, the positive feedback from estrogen prepares the follicle in the ovary and the uterus for ovulation and implantation. When the egg is released, progesterone production inhibits the hypothalamus and pituitary gland, blocking the positive feedback from estrogen. If the egg is fertilized, the fetus takes over production of progesterone (which is why ovulation doesn't occur during pregnancy). If conception does not occur, progesterone production starts to decline, which allows the HPG axis to be stimulated, causing menses and the whole shebang to start over again.

This is an oversimplification because there are other hormones at play here. All these hormones control dozens of aspects of fertility and menstruation, as well as link back to thyroid function, bone formation, and immune health. And it's very important that these hormones cycle in rhythm with each other. When one of the players is out of tune, the whole symphony sounds wrong.

The Links Between the HPA and HPG Axes

The HPA and HPG axes are not isolated endocrine systems; there is plenty of cross-talk between them. For instance, progesterone activates the HPA axis. This is probably part of how the body shifts metabolism, immune function, and resource priorities during pregnancy. It may also be why women tend to have strong food cravings in the days before their periods.

But the links are more insidious than food cravings. Cortisol inhibits the HPG axis at every point. It reduces the production of GnRH by the hypothalamus. It reduces the production of FSH and LH by the pituitary gland. It suppresses ovary function, thereby reducing estrogen and progesterone secretion. This is because reproduction just isn't a priority if you are running away from a lion. The body takes those resources and channels them toward immediate survival.

But what if the lion never stops chasing you? Chronic stress—especially high levels of chronic stress (coupled with not spending time outside, not being active during the day, not getting enough sleep, and using caffeine and sugar to get through the day)—has the same basic physiological effect of running away from a lion all the time. Reproduction (as well as digestion, kidney function, growth, and collagen and bone formation) never gets prioritized.

SCIENCE SIMPLIFIED

Chronic stress can lead to hormone imbalances, such as progesterone or testosterone deficiency, because when we're stressed, our bodies use the precursor molecules for sex hormones to make more cortisol.

Let's examine how adrenal and sex hormone production is linked. This diagram shows how these essential hormones and their precursors and intermediaries are produced from cholesterol (yet again, the essential cholesterol!).

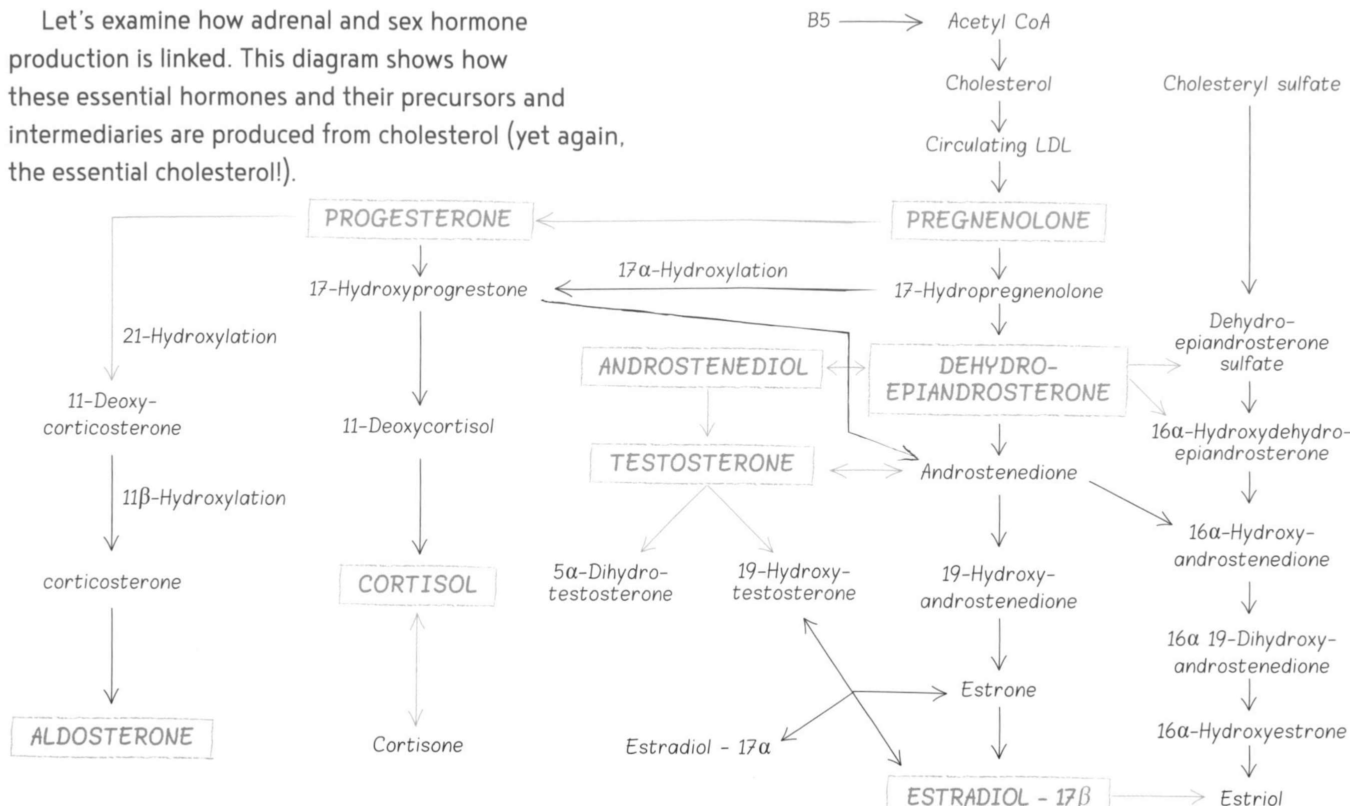

Yes, this is complex. Here's the important part: cholesterol (the backbone of all steroid hormones) is converted into pregnenolone. Pregnenolone is then converted into either dehydroepiandrosterone (DHEA) or progesterone. DHEA, produced by the adrenal glands and the most abundant steroid hormone in the human body, is converted to testosterone and estrogen. Progesterone is usually converted to cortisol but can also be converted to estrogen and testosterone.

When the body is stressed, it starts using up progesterone to make cortisol. It needs more progesterone, so it starts using more pregnenolone to make it. This process is called pregnenolone steal. The HPA axis is literally stealing the precursor for testosterone and estrogen (because pregnenolone is being used to make progesterone instead of DHEA) from the HPG axis. What's more, it's using up all that progesterone to make cortisol. This is how chronic stress causes hormone imbalances.

In women, this can lead to a deficiency in estrogen, progesterone, and/or testosterone. But there are some extra complications here. When DHEA is low, the body tends to convert testosterone and what little DHEA is being produced into estrogen. Environmental estrogens (like the phytoestrogens in soy, flax seeds, and walnuts and the xenoestrogens in some plastics; see page 112) further increase estrogen. Nutrient deficiencies and lifestyle factors like type and frequency of activity also influence exactly which hormones are produced and which aren't. This can result in an excess of one hormone (most commonly estrogen or testosterone) and a deficiency in the other(s). In the same way, chronic stress leads to low testosterone in men—one possible symptom of which is balding!

How do we know if chronic stress has negatively impacted our hormones? Symptoms of hormone imbalances caused by stress include depression, fatigue, anxiety, hair loss, facial and body hair growth, headaches, dizziness, brain fog, poor memory, low libido, vaginal dryness, breast swelling and tenderness, fibrocystic breasts, thyroid disorders, osteoporosis, PMS, dry or wrinkly skin, urinary tract infections, endometriosis, uterine fibroids, weight gain (or resistance to weight loss), water retention, bloating, sleep disturbances, mood changes, irregular periods, loss of periods (amenorrhea), heavy periods, and infertility. Although some of these symptoms can accompany normal hormone shifts like pregnancy and menopause, any one of them should otherwise be considered abnormal and worthy of intervention. If you suspect that a hormone imbalance is contributing to your health struggles, stress management and good sleep are extremely important, as is seeking out a functional or integrative medicine practitioner to properly diagnose you and identify your best options for hormone-balancing therapy (see Chapter 34).

CORTISOL AND THE IMMUNE SYSTEM

Cortisol has profound effects on the immune system and is required for healing wounds and fighting infections. Studies have shown that acute stressors (like running away from a lion) induce a redistribution of immune cells in the body, resulting in enhanced immune function in organs like the skin. White blood cells are released from bone marrow and travel to the skin during acute stress, most likely in preparation for wound healing. Other aspects of the immune system are activated in anticipation of being needed. In this situation, cortisol enhances the immune system response.

However, what is beneficial in acute stress becomes quite the troublemaker during chronic stress. The immune system responds to a high-cortisol environment in a range of ways, probably reflecting different effects at different cortisol levels and in the presence of other chemicals produced by the body and in the context of different levels of sensitivity to cortisol. The details are murky, but what is universally accepted is that chronic stress causes immune system dysfunction.

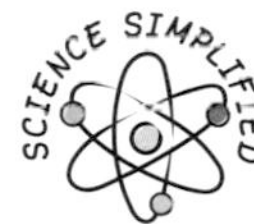

Inflammation is part of the pathology of every chronic disease. Chronic stress causes inflammation, which is why it's so strongly linked with disease risk.

Cortisol alters the chemical messengers of inflammation (called cytokines) secreted by cells in the immune system. This changes how the immune system communicates with itself, turning on some aspects (like the parts of the immune system that attack foreign invaders or produce generalized inflammation) while turning off others. A wealth of studies have shown that high cortisol causes inflammation.

The exact response of the immune system to chronic stress seems to depend on other physiological factors, such as hormones, cytokines, and neurotransmitters, as well as the state of activation of the immune system (if we're already fighting a cold virus, for example). Even genes might play a role in how the immune system responds to chronic stress. The immune system is complex and only just beginning to be understood by scientists, but the bottom line is that chronic stress greatly diminishes the immune system's effectiveness.

Chronic stress has been unequivocally shown to increase susceptibility to a variety of conditions, including autoimmune disease, cardiovascular disease, metabolic syndrome, osteoporosis, depression, infection, and cancer.

HUNGER HORMONES

Chronic stress also affects the hunger hormones leptin (which suppresses appetite) and ghrelin (which increases appetite), which themselves are immune modulators (see page 90). However, the effects of chronic stress extend to food preferences. Chronically stressed mice, for example, select high-fat diets over high-protein and high-carbohydrate diets and eat way more than normal. Interestingly, this desire for fat may help protect against anxiety and depression (while also stimulating weight gain). Appetite stimulation appears to be a result of decreased leptin levels and increased ghrelin, especially in the evening. Cortisol might also influence the reward value of food through interactions of leptin and insulin with neurotransmitters such as neuropeptide Y and dopamine, leading to more cravings for calorie-dense and highly palatable foods.

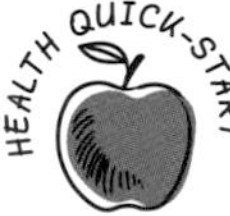

Do you battle intense food cravings? Stress might be to blame! Here are some easy things you can do to reduce stress:

- *Get enough sleep.*
- *Spend time outside, preferably in nature.*
- *Get some exercise. Even a simple walk can work wonders!*
- *Avoid excess caffeine (which magnifies stress responses).*
- *Learn to meditate (see pages 353 to 354).*

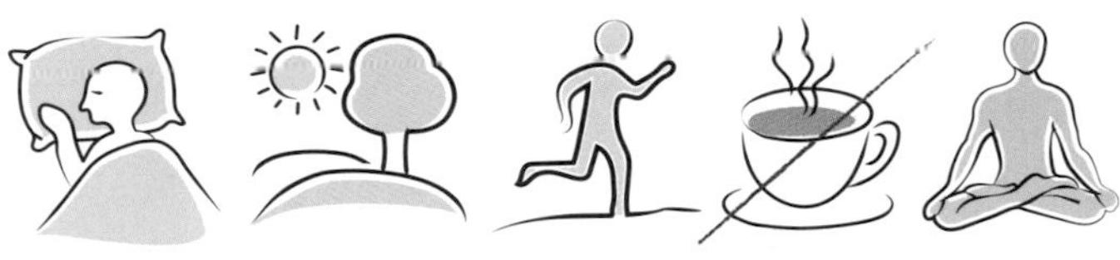

STRESS AND LEAKY GUT

We've looked at the issue of leaky gut and how it can affect so many aspects of our health (see page 67). To review, the gut is a barrier between the inside of the body and the outside world. Yes, as unintuitive as it may be, the stuff inside our digestive tracts is actually outside our bodies. However, the gut is a unique barrier. Its job is to let important nutrients into the body while keeping everything else out. This makes it a highly selective semipermeable barrier. Nutrients enter the body through a variety of tightly controlled mechanisms.

What forms this highly selective semipermeable barrier is a single layer of specialized cells called enterocytes. On the other side of that barrier is 80 percent of the body's immune system, acting as a sentinel, ready to attack anything that might try to cross the barrier.

When a person has a leaky gut, or, more technically, "increased intestinal permeability," things can get across the gut barrier that aren't supposed to. This happens when either the enterocytes or the complex structures that glue the enterocytes together are damaged. The things that leak into the body aren't big chunks of food, but a variety of small substances—like incompletely digested proteins, bacteria or bacterial fragments, infectious organisms, and waste products—all of which stimulate the immune system on the other side of the barrier. Some of these substances cause generalized body-wide inflammation; for example, bacterial fragments from those good bacteria that live and are supposed to stay in our digestive tracts can travel and stimulate inflammation throughout the body. Others stimulate targeted attacks by the immune system; for example, a food intolerance or allergy could result from incompletely digested proteins leaking into the body. The many symptoms and health conditions related to leaky gut are caused by this stimulation of the immune system.

Chronic stress is detrimental to our health in large part due to the direct effect of both cortisol and CRH on gut health. Chronic stress increases intestinal permeability, decreases gut motility (intestinal muscle contractions), decreases mucus production by goblet cells in the gut, decreases secretory IgA production, inhibits digestion (by inhibiting pancreatic enzyme secretion and gallbladder function), and decreases intestinal blood flow. Both a leaky gut and gut dysbiosis (see Chapter 4) are consequences of these actions.

Cortisol's actions on the gut epithelial tight junctions are complicated (see Chapter 4). Low cortisol causes tight junctions to open, whereas normal or high cortisol causes them to close (this implies that cortisol plays a normal role in digestion, which is supported by the fact that cortisol goes up every time we eat). But at very high levels of cortisol, there's a change in tight junction assembly that makes the gut barrier more permeable to small molecules and less permeable to large molecules.

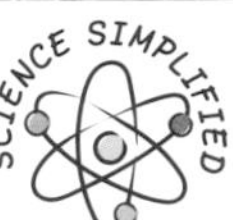

Stress wreaks havoc on gut health, in part because of the actions of cortisol, but even more importantly because of the actions of corticotropin-releasing hormone (CRH), which is released by the hypothalamus region of the brain when something stressful is first detected.

CRH is the stress hormone that does the biggest damage to our guts. It is known to increase epithelial permeability, not just in the gut, but also in other barrier tissues like the lungs, the skin, and the blood-brain barrier. This appears to be due to a direct effect of CRH on tight junction assembly; CRH increases the expression of a tight junction protein called claudin-2, which opens up tight junctions. CRH also stimulates the release of histamine, a blood thinner called heparin, and pro-inflammatory cytokines from mast cells (a type of innate immune cell characteristically found in connective and barrier tissues that is a major player in allergic reactions, including anaphylaxis), all of which contribute to inflammation.

CRH is perpetually produced by the hypothalamus if the perceived stress continues. This becomes an even bigger problem in the context of adrenal fatigue (discussed in the next section), where the adrenal glands can no longer keep up with demand and cortisol levels begin to fall in proportion to psychological stress. Since cortisol is an important negative feedback signal for CRH production (meaning that cortisol signals to the hypothalamus to produce less CRH), adrenal fatigue and chronic stress lead to even higher levels of CRH.

Given the growing list of health conditions linked to a leaky gut, including the further impact that a leaky gut has on the immune system, this is another check mark in the need-to-manage-stress column.

ADRENAL FATIGUE

Chronic stress can lead to a condition called HPA axis dysfunction, often called *adrenal fatigue*, which is caused by inadequate functioning of the adrenal glands and involves a collection of symptoms such as fatigue, poor sleep or insomnia, mood swings, unexplained weight gain or loss, inflammation, high cardiovascular disease risk factors, insulin resistance, decreased sex drive, joint pain, and frequent infections (like colds and flu). Although HPA axis dysfunction is not recognized by many conventional medical practitioners (unless you've pushed your adrenals to the level of chronic adrenal insufficiency or you suffer from Addison's disease), diagnosis rates are increasing dramatically within alternative health communities. When we pull together the clinical evidence, some concepts from evolutionary biology, and recent developments in laboratory testing, it's easy to see that our adrenal glands are being taxed as we deal with the relentless stress of modern life.

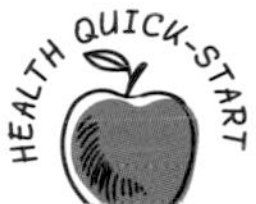

If you suspect that you have adrenal fatigue, it's important to get tested for it before taking any medications, supplements, or botanicals to treat it.

As we saw earlier, the adrenal glands are small, triangular glands located on top of the kidneys in the abdominal cavity. These glands are the major site of steroid hormone production and coordination, so when they're out of whack, a lot of processes—for example, blood sugar regulation—can go awry!

Adrenal fatigue occurs when chronic stress continues without relief (and "relief" means more than just a weekend getaway or an occasional day off; it means actual stress management on a daily basis) and the adrenal glands stop being able to function properly. In the naturopathic medical community, adrenal fatigue was originally referred to as the general adaptation symptom: that is, your adrenals are literally adapting to too much stress!

There are three phases to adrenal fatigue that, in some ways, mimic the release of cortisol. It's important to emphasize that this disorder occurs after a long period of chronic stress, and it presents in many different ways.

Phase 1: Alarm

Phase 1 of HPA axis dysfunction is often called the alarm phase because it involves the fight-or-flight response discussed earlier (see page 340). The alarm phase is a common phenomenon for those of us who've dealt with a lot of stress (basically everyone!). In this phase, we see the normal physiological response from cortisol but in greater amounts than what is considered to be normal:

- Blood sugar is elevated.
- Blood pressure is elevated.
- Heart rate and respiratory rate increase.
- Metabolism speeds up at the cellular level.

All these reactions are within normal limits, and after the stressor is removed, the body is able to recover normally. Importantly, most of us dip into and out of this phase as we experience the normal stresses of modern life. Because of how normal it feels, we can move in and out of this phase for years.

The symptoms during the alarm phase are easy to dismiss, but they generally include:

- Hypoglycemia (low blood sugar, which could manifest as feeling lightheaded or "hangry")
- Fatigue
- Insomnia
- Irritability
- Anxiety

These symptoms may be exaggerated or feel uncontrollable compared to other stressful times in your life. However, the longer you spend in Phase 1, the more likely it is that your levels of other hormones will be impacted as the pregnenolone steal occurs (see page 342)—and from there, you're on your way to Phase 2 as your body stops being able to bounce back from frequent, relatively normal-feeling alarm phase periods.

Phase 2: Resistance

Phase 2 of HPA axis dysfunction is referred to as the resistance phase. It begins when the focus shifts significantly from producing a balance of hormones to producing as much cortisol as possible. This phase is about "resistance" because the body has built up a tolerance to cortisol and has functionally adapted to chronic stress. The great irony here is that someone in Phase 2 might feel great; a lot of people describe this phase as feeling "wired" or "tired and wired."

Pregnenolone steal is in full force here, and people experience reduced sex hormones, which might manifest itself as fewer gains in the gym due to less testosterone, dysmenorrhea (problems with menses), or even a full loss of period due to low estrogen and progesterone levels. While we're excited to have the energy to be busy bees (or at least feel like we can be), our bodies are paying the price of chronically high cortisol levels. This can cause long-term changes to physiology and metabolism, such as:

- **Elevated blood lipids (that is, cholesterol and triglycerides).** This puts a significant stress on the liver because it requires that the lipids be repackaged and sent to cells to be stored.
- **Breakdown of skeletal muscle.** As discussed earlier, cortisol is catabolic—meaning it mobilizes the amino acids in skeletal muscle for use elsewhere—but in the case of adrenal fatigue, there is no need for those mobilized amino acids. So we end up with wasted muscle mass and a lot of difficultly making improvements in physical fitness and body composition.
- **Elevated blood sugar and hemoglobin A1C** (a measure of the saturation of heme with glucose in the past 3 months, which is used to diagnose type 2 diabetes). Along with burdening the liver, this creates problems for metabolism. Someone in this phase might have trouble losing weight or develop insulin resistance despite a healthy diet.
- **Water retention.** All this excretion madness is a huge burden on the liver and kidneys. One of the compensatory reactions is to retain water. As a result, people in this phase might have some swelling in their hands and feet and might get that "puffy" sensation in their faces.

So if all this subtle damage is being done, how is it that people in this phase feel fine? It's simple: cortisol activates the sympathetic nervous system and those catecholamines (also known as adrenaline or epinephrine and norepinephrine) that keep us running at warp speed. However, one of the signs of late Phase 2 HPA axis dysfunction is huge fluctuations in energy at inappropriate times of the day, like having a "second wind" at night without doing anything to instigate it.

At this point, most people start to self-medicate in some way, which might include increasing coffee intake, a drink at bedtime to wind down, or experimenting with adaptogenic herbs or stimulating vitamins. Here are some signs that you might need to ditch the crutches and visit a health-care practitioner instead:

- Changes in blood sugar regulation, like insulin resistance or hypoglycemia
- Dyslipidemia (elevated or abnormal triglycerides or cholesterol)
- Mood swings
- Unexplained weight loss or gain
- Decreased sex drive
- Fatigue with insomnia (especially feeling "tired and wired" in the evenings)

The bottom line is that Phase 2 of adrenal fatigue is much easier to treat than Phase 3, but most people don't seek help until Phase 3 hits.

Phase 3: Burnout

Phase 3 of HPA axis dysfunction is where the term "adrenal fatigue" comes from. Also called the exhaustion or burnout phase, it is where health starts to crash in a significant and scary way. Essentially, the pregnenolone steal has failed: we can't make cortisol at the rate our bodies demand, and the whole system crashes. Clinical intervention is often necessary at this point because leading a functional life can be incredibly challenging. The medical language around this issue can be dramatic: "collapse of vital systems" being an example.

The signs and symptoms of Phase 3 HPA axis dysfunction include:

- Severe fatigue that persists regardless of the amount of sleep you get
- Heart palpitations
- Hypoglycemia
- Low blood pressure
- Joint pain (likely due to very high systemic inflammation)
- Frequent infections, including colds and flus

This phase can involve a series of progressively worsening crashes, or it can culminate in an extended acute attack, which can result from even the smallest stressor. For most people, the symptoms are so severe that they must seek medical help. Depending on the type of practitioner, medications might be used to treat the symptoms rather than the adrenal problem itself (for example, antidepressants or sleeping pills might be prescribed). Unfortunately, there is no medication that can fix adrenal fatigue, but there *are* methods for measuring and then monitoring adrenal function that can reduce the recovery time. These methods can include a nutrient-dense anti-inflammatory diet (you've got that covered after reading this book!); a focus on stress management and resilience activities (discussed later in this chapter); a focus on sleep (see Chapter 26); avoidance of strenuous activity (see Chapter 28), stimulants, and depressants; and the use of carefully selected adaptogens. However, protocols to recover from adrenal fatigue need to be individualized, so it's imperative that you work with a health-care professional such as a functional or integrative medicine doctor (see page 439).

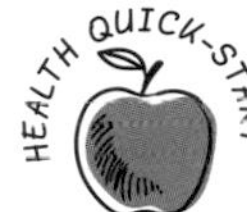

Getting plenty of sleep is essential for recovering from adrenal fatigue.

Diagnosis

When it comes to diagnosing HPA axis dysfunction, the gold standard is to utilize a series of salivary samples collected over the course of a day to complete an Adrenal Stress Index (ASI). Remember, cortisol is an essential part of our daily circadian rhythm: it helps us wake up in the morning with a spike that peaks at about 9 a.m. and gradually drops throughout the rest of the day (allowing melatonin to act and tell us that it's time to sleep).

The ASI measures cortisol throughout the day and then maps out how its variations compare to normal values. When someone is in Phase 2 or 3 adrenal fatigue, their daily cortisol pattern differs from the normal curve. In Phase 2, cortisol is chronically high. This pattern is what creates the "tired and wired" sensation that people in Phase 2 often experience; they might be trying to go to sleep but have a huge amount of energy in the evening due to excess cortisol (which also reduces the amount of melatonin they produce, making it hard for them to fall asleep). In Phase 3, cortisol production nosedives, and the ASI will indicate a very low curve throughout the day. There are also intermediary phases between Phases 2 and 3 where cortisol is too high at one point in the day but too low at another time.

To complete the test, you take four to five salivary samples throughout the day (depending on the company used), either by spitting into a tube or by allowing a cotton swab to absorb your saliva for a couple minutes and then placing it in a plastic tube. The samples need to be refrigerated, so it's important to keep that in mind when planning what day to complete the test. Likewise, the test needs to be completed on a day without caffeine or exercise, and women with menstrual cycles need to complete the test at a certain point in their cycle (typically between days 19 and 21) because of the intricate relationship between the HPA and HPG axes. Also, the samples are typically taken immediately before a meal and at least 2 hours after eating or drinking anything but water. Some practitioners allow the samples to be collected at any time during a woman's cycle and with normal caffeine use, but the reference ranges will be less valid with that method.

There are other ways to measure cortisol and identify adrenal fatigue:

Cortisol awakening response is a method of measuring chronic stress and adrenal function that is occasionally used in practice but is more generally seen in research. When we wake up in the morning, our cortisol spikes; this phenomenon is creatively called the cortisol awakening response and is an important part of our sleep-wake cycle. To measure this response, saliva samples are collected (in the same manner as the ASI) upon waking (while in bed!) and then 15 minutes later. There should be a measurable increase in cortisol between samples. A huge spike is a rough indicator that the individual has overactive adrenal glands. If the increase is minimal, then the person may have underactive adrenal glands.

Although this test can't be used as a diagnostic, it has been used in research studies that give us some insight on why adrenal function variation (and thus chronic stress) is so important.

Serum cortisol is sometimes measured as a part of standard bloodwork. Because cortisol fluctuates throughout the day, a single serum sample doesn't give us a lot of information about adrenal function (other than suggesting to physicians that they should order more tests). Fasting doesn't matter with this type of sample, but the time of collection is really important.

Even though it doesn't give a complete picture, one of the great benefits of blood samples is that they're collected so frequently that we have reference ranges that apply widely to adults and children. For a morning sample (8 a.m.), the range is 6 to 28 mg/dL for adults and 3 to 21 mg/dL for children. For a late-afternoon sample (4 p.m.), the range is 2 to 12 mg/dL for adults and 3 to 10 mg/dL for children. Anything outside of these ranges might indicate suboptimal or pathological adrenal function.

24-hour urine collection is based on similar logic to the ASI but does not map out cortisol patterns throughout the day. Cortisol that has been conjugated (modified by the liver) is excreted in urine, so urine is a good measure of the cortisol that has been used recently. This method is used less often simply because of the inconvenience: every single time you use the restroom, you have to go into a cup. As a result, the lab gets all the conjugated cortisol that is excreted in a day (as a total value rather than a series). A normal value is between 10 and 34 milligrams, although men can have higher levels. Since this method is an average, it might not be appropriate for someone who has a normal value but an abnormal pattern (like low cortisol in the morning and high cortisol at night).

Herbs and botanicals that affect adrenal function are called adaptogens, and they are commonly used to treat chronic stress and HPA axis dysfunction. In medical herbalist communities, adaptogenic herbs are used for their "normalizing" effect on our physiology to help make us more resistant to stressors; therefore, they are believed to lower cortisol output in Phase 2 and increase cortisol output in Phase 3. But within the spectrum of adaptogenic herbs, some are considered to be more stimulating (like ginseng), some are more relaxing (like ashwagandha), while others support adrenal health generally (so are neither stimulating nor relaxing). That's important because you would want to choose adaptogens based on what your cortisol is doing throughout the day (as determined by test results)—in other words, you want to suppress cortisol production when it's too high and stimulate it when it's too low. This can mean taking different adaptogens at different times of day. Many popular herbal formulas include both stimulating and relaxing adaptogenic and non-adaptogenic herbs, so pay careful attention to the ingredients in these products (usually in the form of a tea, tincture, tonic, or pill) and note which specific herbs they contain. The take-home message is that you don't want to self-diagnose or treat; instead, see a qualified health-care professional for proper testing and individualized treatment protocols.

OTHER ADRENAL DISORDERS TO CONSIDER

It's important to note that Phase 2 or 3 of adrenal fatigue might be confused with (or even overlap with) other adrenal disorders—namely hyperadrenalism (or Cushing's syndrome) or Addison's disease (also called primary or secondary adrenal insufficiency).

Cushing's syndrome is a medical condition in which the adrenal glands produce pathologically high amounts of glucocorticoid hormones (predominantly cortisol) all the time. Cushing's syndrome, specifically, refers to the clinical symptoms associated with too much cortisol. The syndrome may be the result of many different factors. Cushing's syndrome itself is most often a result of a tumor in the pituitary gland that produces ACTH. The increased serum cortisol has many effects:

- Hyperglycemia stimulates gluconeogenesis (buildup of glucose) and glycogenolysis (breakdown of liver glycogen) pathways
- Negative nitrogen balance
- Salt and water retention increases blood vessel volume and thus the potential to develop hypertension
- Reduced immune response increases susceptibility to infection by decreasing the activity of macrophages (resident immune cell sentinels present in nearly every tissue in the human body)

As a result of these big physiological changes, there can be other, secondary symptoms of Cushing's syndrome, including:

- Central obesity (a focus of adipose tissue around the stomach)
- Myopathy
- Bruising
- Hirsutism (inappropriate hair growth, like around the face in women)
- Acne
- Stretch marks
- Ankle swelling
- Easy fractures
- Missing or changing menstrual periods

If one or more of these symptoms sounds familiar, don't panic! But keeping them in mind as a complete picture of a disorder is important as we consider all the ways the adrenal glands can malfunction and manifest symptom patterns.

How does this compare to the main topic at hand, adrenal fatigue? In short, the symptoms are much worse. Rather than suboptimal function, the adrenal glands are hyperactive in a pathological way, and cortisol levels are likely to be much higher. This leads to severe symptoms like hypertension, osteoporosis, and muscle wasting (the result of tissue breakdown/weakness, because the cortisol keeps the body in the "breakdown" phase rather than in the "buildup" phase of metabolism).

Addison's disease is the result of the destruction of the adrenal glands by a variety of mechanisms, including autoimmunity, tuberculosis, tumor(s), or an infectious agent (for example, meningococcus). The consequence is that the hormones made exclusively in the adrenal glands, cortisol and aldosterone, are diminished (or become nonexistent if the disease progresses); other hormones, like sex hormones, are affected but are not eliminated due to their ability to be produced elsewhere. Addison's disease has an incredible number of possible symptoms:

- Fatigue
- Weakness
- Weight loss
- Poor appetite
- Mood changes (apathy, confusion)
- Abdominal pain
- Salt cravings
- Hyperpigmentation
- Hypotension (low blood pressure)
- Weak pulse
- Hair loss

Compared to adrenal fatigue and Cushing's syndrome, several of the symptoms associated with Addison's disease are unique. For example, hyperpigmentation is associated with an excess production of corticotropin, which increases melanocyte-stimulating hormone to produce more skin pigment. (Historical note: President John F. Kennedy always looked tan because of his Addison's disease.) So someone who is worried about adrenal fatigue may be less concerned about Addison's, but it's always good to know all the possible causes.

MANAGING CHRONIC STRESS

Chronic stress is epidemic in our society, and in truth, it is impossible to eliminate completely. Fortunately, living a stress-free life isn't the goal. Instead, we're looking to manage stress in such a way that our physiological responses to stress are proportional (meaning that our cortisol doesn't go through the roof just because we're stuck in a traffic jam), we recover quickly from stress (our stress hormone levels go back to baseline quickly after the stressful event is over), and there are breaks between stressors (meaning that chronic stress isn't so unrelentingly chronic after all). By managing stress, we can limit the negative health impact it can have.

Managing chronic stress is best handled from two sides: reducing stressors and increasing resilience. You can think of it this way: if you have too many apples to fit in your bucket, you can either get rid of some apples (that is, reduce stressors) or get a bigger bucket (increase your resilience)—or you can do both!

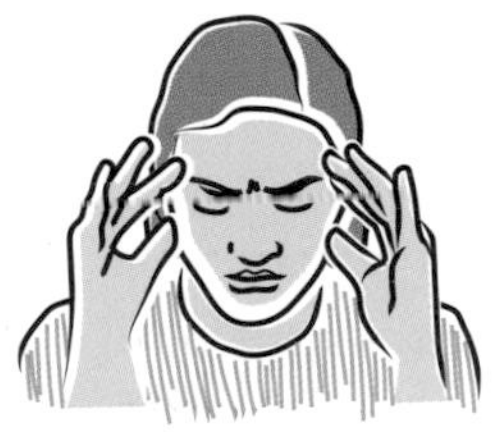

Reducing Stressors

A *stressor* is a chemical or biological agent, environmental condition, external stimulus, or event that activates the HPA axis, causing the release of stress hormones. Stressors can be categorized in the following ways:

- **Physical:** for example, injury, a vigorous workout, sitting for prolonged periods, not getting enough sleep, extreme environmental temperatures
- **Sensory:** for example, loud noises, too-bright lights, overcrowding
- **Chemical:** for example, tobacco, alcohol, drugs, allergens
- **Psychological:** for example, deadlines, traffic, bills, societal and family demands

Reducing stressors is a matter of setting boundaries to protect our mental and physical well-being, which can include:

- Reevaluating our goals and priorities to make sure we aren't taking on more commitments than we really need to
- Saying no to optional activities that would drain us more than benefit us
- Asking for help from our spouse, friends, family, coworkers, or others in our social support network when we're feeling overwhelmed
- Limiting the presence of negative, stressful people in our lives
- Making more time for sleep (which has the added benefit of increasing resilience)
- Reducing physical and mental stress at work (such as by taking time to stretch and breathe deeply throughout the day, discussing the possibility of a deadline extension or a more flexible schedule, leaving work *at work*, and finding ways to get up and move—for instance, taking the stairs instead of the elevator)

Increasing Resilience

Resilience is the ability to adapt in the face of adversity. Because we can never completely eliminate stress from our lives, actively making choices that help bolster our bodies against the effects of stress is an extremely important habit and skill. This doesn't mean stressful events won't affect us, but rather that we can handle them without the wheels falling off our cart.

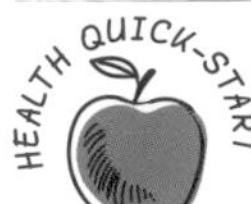

The healthy habits that increase our resilience to stress can easily be distilled as follows:

- *Sleep: Get enough of it and make choices during the day that improve sleep quality*
- *Move: Avoid being sedentary and make time for more moderately intense activity*
- *Meditate: Take up a daily mindfulness practice*
- *Play: Make time every day for fun, laughter, and other breaks from stressors like work*
- *Connect: With nature, family, friends, and even pets*

Resilience helps us deal with the unavoidable stressors we encounter throughout life—everything from bad traffic to a massive deadline at work to the death of a loved one. Without resilience, an unexpected or unavoidable stressor could take a serious toll on our health. The psychosocial characteristics of resilience include:

- Realistic optimism
- Active coping (using one's own resources to deal with a problem situation) and high coping self-efficacy (having high confidence in one's coping abilities)
- High cognitive functioning and autonomy (the ability to think things through independently)
- Planning, motivation, and positive risk-taking (taking risks only after weighing the potential benefits and harms)
- Strong cognitive reappraisal (adjusting an emotional response by reevaluating the emotional stimulus) and emotion regulation (the ability to effectively manage and respond to emotional experiences)
- Secure attachment and trust
- Strong social skills and social network

- Self-confidence and a positive identity
- Religious or spiritual belief that gives life meaning
- Humor and positive thinking
- Altruism and generosity

We don't need to be able to check off *every* item on this list in order to successfully navigate life's ups and downs. Being resilient is about more than personality traits; it's also about developing coping strategies, establishing healthful routines, and approaching life with a positive attitude. Here are some ways to develop these characteristics:

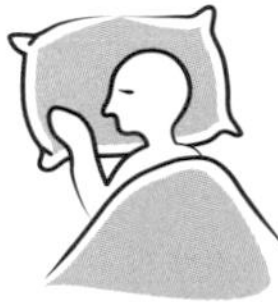

Get enough sleep. Getting adequate quality sleep is probably the single most important thing we can do for adrenal health. A growing number of studies show that poor-quality sleep or chronic inadequate sleep causes our physiological stress responses to be exaggerated in reaction to psychological stresses. That means that if we're not getting enough good sleep, our adrenal glands kick into high gear more easily in response to things like deadlines, psychotic bosses, and traffic jams. The combination of chronic stress and poor sleep is a recipe for HPA axis dysfunction.

A recent study showed that healthy men who were restricted to 4½ hours of sleep had a morning cortisol peak 2 hours earlier than men who were in bed for 8½ hours. Furthermore, cortisol levels in the evening hours were 23 percent higher in those who got 4½ hours sleep than in those who got a full 8½ hours. Noradrenaline levels were also about 30 percent higher in the sleep-restricted men during the early-night and early-morning hours. This adrenal activation caused extended evening wakefulness, implying a vicious cycle. High cortisol inhibits sleep, especially restorative deep sleep.

But increasingly, research indicates links between sleep and stress that highlight the potential for a vicious cycle. Poor sleep makes us less resilient to stress, and chronic stress wrecks our sleep quality. (Have you ever found yourself tossing and turning at night, worried about bills or thinking about your to-do list?) While it may seem like this link makes it doubly hard to claw our way back to healthy adrenals, it actually highlights the possibility of managing stress by managing sleep (and vice versa).

A few simple strategies can go a long way in terms of improving sleep quality. First and foremost is carving out enough time for sleep; on average, we need 7 to 9 hours' total sleep, which typically means being in bed for 7½ to 10 hours each night. Second, when stress is a confounding factor, it's even more important to make choices that entrench circadian rhythms. This means being mindful of important zeitgebers (see pages 326 to 328) like the light-dark cycle, meaning that we need exposure to bright (blue) light during the day, dim (red) light in the evening, and darkness while we're sleeping. Of course, there's a whole lot more we can do to improve sleep, mostly requiring only small adjustments to our choices; see Chapter 26 for details.

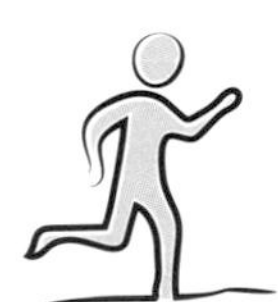

Engage in mild and moderate activity. Exercise is potent at reducing and normalizing cortisol levels, which can help reduce inflammation and promote healing. This makes it easier to burn stored energy (especially fat), improves your sleep, and makes you feel more relaxed and able to cope with life's surprises.

The key here is to move throughout the day, although more rigorous exercise sessions are beneficial, too. Our society tends to focus on going to the gym to "pay off" a caloric debt for all the "bad" foods we eat and the time we spend at desks. Elsewhere in the world, we see more realistic models of what the human body is adapted to in terms of daily movement (see Chapter 28).

To mimic this beneficial constant-movement model of hunter-gatherer lifestyles, set a timer to go off every 20 minutes and take a 2-minute movement break—walk around, stretch, and so on. Another strategy is to try being in a constant (or near-constant) state of gentle movement by using a nifty biohack like a treadmill desk, desk elliptical machine, or desk stationary bike.

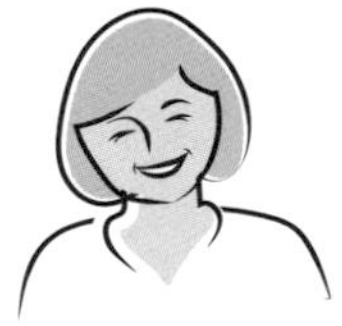

Have fun. Making time to have fun is a powerful way to reduce or cope with stress. So many of us get stuck in the daily grind of work, commuting, chores, looking after the kids or our parents, cooking, cleaning, and running errands that we forget to take time to do something we enjoy. Sometimes we're so busy and distracted that even when we're doing something we love, we don't appreciate it or have fun doing it.

It's important to carve out time every single day to do something that is fun for you: feeding the birds, listening to a podcast, watching a movie, listening to music, or even just being a little bit silly.

The simple acts of smiling and laughing can reduce stress and improve mood. Smiling and laughing activate the ventromedial prefrontal cortex, which produces endorphins (which are opioid peptides that function as neurotransmitters). They suppress pain through mechanisms similar to analgesics. Even more important, endorphins increase the release of dopamine, a neurotransmitter with many functions in the brain, including inhibiting negative emotions, boosting mood, improving sleep quality, and increasing motivation, cognition, and memory. Smiling and laughing also activate parts of the limbic system of the brain, specifically the amygdala and the hippocampus (see more on the HPA axis on page 340). The limbic system is a primitive part of the brain that is involved in emotions and helps us with basic functions necessary for survival. When the limbic system is activated, serotonin levels are increased, contributing to feelings of well-being and happiness. There are further effects on the autonomic nervous system, which balances blood pressure levels, heartbeat, and respiration. Smiling and laughing also lower blood sugar levels after a meal, help regulate the immune system, reduce muscle tension, and reduce cortisol, growth hormone (abnormally high growth hormone levels are associated with inflammatory conditions like rheumatoid arthritis), and catecholamines.

As you might expect, laughing and smiling work through the same pathways, but laughing is more powerful than smiling. Surprisingly, though, even a fake smile or laugh can have a positive effect on mood, stress levels, immune function, digestive health, vascular health, and blood sugar regulation. In fact, maintaining a fake smile through a stressful task decreases the body's stress response and improves your ability to recover from stress—although the effect is even greater when the smile is genuine. The converse is also true: frowning can exacerbate depression. Even if you don't feel like smiling, forcing your facial muscles into a smile causes the same, but less potent, body and brain chemistry changes as a real smile or laugh. That means forcing a smile will actually help you feel happier!

Enjoy and connect with nature. The importance of nature and spending time outdoors is discussed in more depth in Chapter 29. For the purposes of stress management and resiliency, virtually any contact with the sights, sounds, smells, and textures of the outdoors has positive effects on the body and brain. This includes both wilderness-type nature (such as going for a hike in the woods or sitting on the beach watching the waves) and tamed nature (like sitting in a tranquil garden or gazing at the mountains from a balcony). Even walking in the backyard with bare feet or listening to the birds sing while running errands can decrease stress and impart a feeling of peace. For city dwellers, visiting a rooftop garden or park or growing a few herbs on the windowsill can provide a connection with nature.

To get the most out of connecting with nature, it's helpful to stop and acknowledge the sensations of your surroundings. This means thinking about the feeling of the air on your skin, the scents in the air, the colors and organic shapes surrounding you, the sounds you hear, and the textures in your line of vision. If possible, take off your shoes and feel the ground beneath your feet, making note of whether it feels hard or soft, cool or warm, damp or dry. This is called "being present" and can be thought of as a form of mindful meditation.

Another way to connect with nature is to play in the dirt. Exposure to soil-based organisms, both topical (like digging your hands into rich, fertile soil) and ingested (through probiotic foods and beverages), can be extremely beneficial. This might mean simply growing some potted plants on the windowsill or balcony. It might mean taking up gardening. Or it might mean taking the opportunity to get dirty when you're out in the woods. Playing in good-quality organic dirt and not worrying about washing your hands (even before you eat) is good for you!

Spending time outside, even if it's not the great outdoors, can also help relieve stress by supporting circadian rhythms. The light-dark cycle (meaning it's light out during the day and dark at night) is a powerful signal to our circadian clocks, and spending time outside during the day is one of the best things we can do to protect our circadian rhythms, including evening melatonin production.

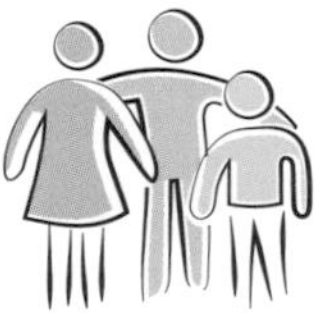

Connect with people. Physical and emotional connection—such as giving a family member a hug, cuddling with a loved one, or even cuddling with a pet—also has an important calming effect on the HPA axis. The importance of social connection is discussed in more detail in Chapter 30.

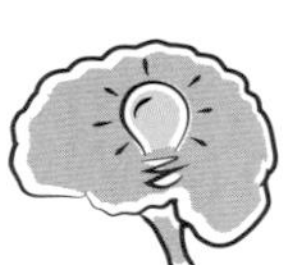

Use your brain. Using your brain for *fun* intellectual activities, whatever that might mean for you, can help increase blood flow to your brain, which is critical for resolving inflammation there. This is important for anyone dealing with gut-brain axis issues (see Chapter 4), because resolving inflammation in the brain can be a very slow process.

Intellectually stimulating activities come in many flavors: reading a challenging book (whether it's challenging due to the topic, the style of writing, or the language it's written in), learning to play a musical instrument, taking up a new craft (like knitting), solving a puzzle (crossword, Sudoku, Rubik's Cube, jigsaw), or getting down with some differential equations. Even if your job is intellectually demanding, taking 10 minutes a day to exercise your brain can be very healthful and can help bolster against the effects of stress.

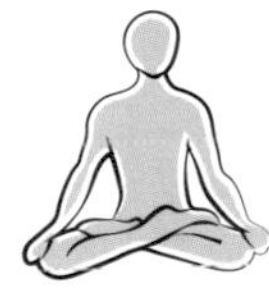

Engaging in active meditation. Active meditation, like yoga, tai chi, or more strenuous martial arts, helps manage stress. Beyond the benefits from the moderate intensity of these physical practices, their meditative quality is linked to decreased depression and anxiety, improved optimism, and reduced stress (and cortisol levels). If you are someone who has joined a gym only to have your membership card gather dust after the first couple months, try active meditation. Studies show that previously sedentary adults are more likely to stick with yoga classes than other physical activities, and yoga is generally more accessible for many people (and can be adapted to accommodate diverse physical challenges).

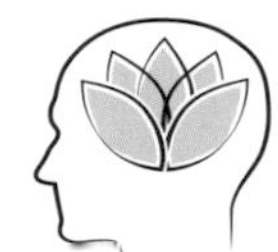

Develop a mindfulness practice. This aspect of increasing resilience to stress is so important, and so well founded in the scientific literature, that it deserves its own section for a more thorough discussion. So let's dive in!

Mindful Meditation

Meditation may not strike you as a likely subject of scientific investigation, but it's been thoroughly documented in the scientific literature that mindful meditation dramatically reduces stress and boosts cognitive abilities.

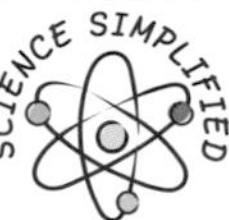

Even 10 minutes a day of meditation, whether you're doing a mindful breathing practice or listening to a guided meditation, can have tremendous benefits for your overall health. It sounds crunchy granola, but there's a ton of science to support it!

Mindful meditation—sometimes called mindful breathing practice or mindfulness—may be one of the most powerful stress management tools we have in our arsenal. We can reap huge benefits with a relatively short time commitment, and it can be practiced anywhere at any time by anybody. Mindfulness is a calm and self-aware mental state achieved by focusing on the present moment while acknowledging and accepting your feelings, thoughts, and physical sensations.

Mindful meditation is fairly simple. Choose a comfortable position—sitting, reclining, or lying down. Keep your attention on your breath. You might find it easier to maintain focus by doing a breathing technique that requires mental control, like equal breathing, diaphragmatic breathing, or alternate-nostril breathing; all of which are described next. Alternatively, you can simply breathe as deeply and slowly as possible or "watch" your breath while trying not to control it (which is harder than it sounds). As thoughts come to you and vie for your attention, acknowledge them ("Yes, I know I have to do the dishes when I'm done" or "Yes, yellow would be the perfect color for the kitchen walls") and then consciously let them go and bring your attention back to your breath. In many ways, mindful mediation is the practice of stopping repetitive or obsessive thoughts. It may help you become aware of which issues truly need your attention and which ones are less important. It may also help you become more in tune with your body.

You can practice mindful meditation in silence, outdoors with the sounds of nature, or with music playing in the background (typically a soothing instrumental track). While studies generally show that

10 to 15 minutes a day are beneficial, even 5 minutes will probably help you tremendously with stress management and your overall mood. You can either block off a time of day for meditation or do it as you feel the need throughout the day (or both).

Mindful meditation has even been evaluated as an adjunct therapy for a variety of chronic illnesses, including some autoimmune conditions. For example, clinical trials evaluating mindful practices in patients with cancer, fibromyalgia, chronic pain, rheumatoid arthritis, type 2 diabetes, chronic fatigue syndrome, multiple chemical sensitivity, and cardiovascular disease all showed benefits (albeit sometimes modest benefits). Meditative exercises have also been shown to decrease oxidative stress and increase levels of two important antioxidants, glutathione and superoxide. One of the best things about this stress management technique is that everyone can do it.

There are a wealth of guided meditations that can help you ease into mindfulness practice. Apps such as Insight Timer, Headspace, and Calm are all excellent sources of guided meditations to mitigate stress.

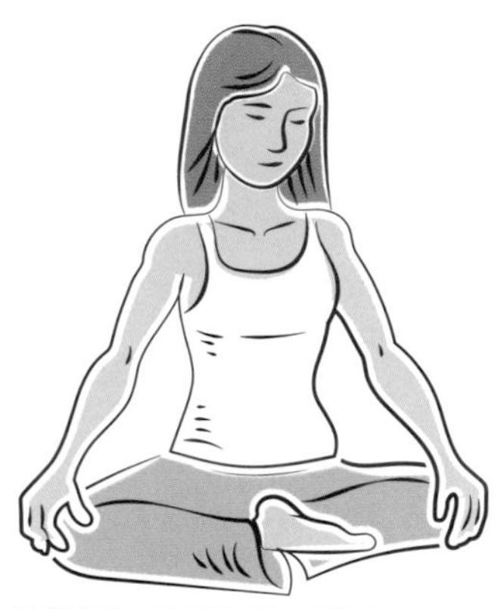

BREATHING TECHNIQUES FOR MINDFUL MEDITATION

These techniques can be done lying down on a flat surface (with your legs straight or your knees bent or even with a pillow under your knees to support your legs) or sitting up in a comfortable position, on the floor or in a chair.

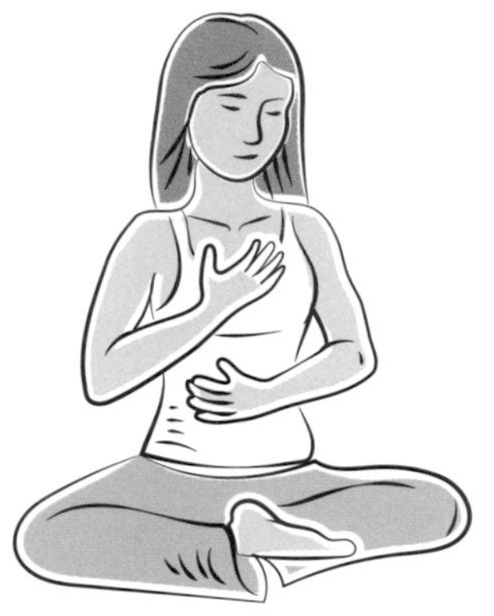

EQUAL BREATHING

1. *Inhale for a count of four.*
2. *Exhale for a count of four.*
3. *You can slow your breathing and inhale and exhale for a count of six or even eight as you settle into this technique (or just count to four more slowly). You can also try combining equal breathing with either diaphragmatic breathing or alternate-nostril breathing (see below).*

DIAPHRAGMATIC BREATHING

1. *Place one hand on your upper chest and the other on your abdomen—this will enable you to feel whether you are using your diaphragm instead of your chest muscles to breathe.*
2. *Breathe in slowly through your nose, letting your stomach expand against your hand as your lungs fill with air. The hand on your chest should remain as still as possible.*
3. *Let your stomach fall back inward as you exhale, and tighten your stomach muscles to help push all the air out of your lungs, exhaling through your nose or pursed lips. Again, the hand on your upper chest should remain as still as possible.*
4. *Make your breaths as deep and slow as possible.*

ALTERNATE-NOSTRIL BREATHING

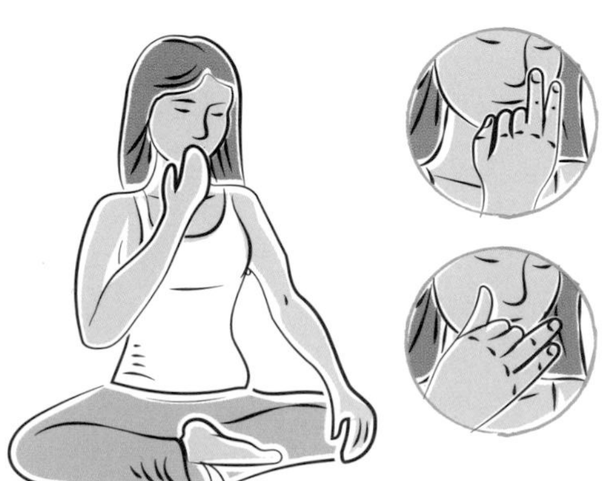

1. *Hold your right hand in front of your face, palm toward you. (Reverse these instructions if you're left-handed.)*
2. *Close your right nostril with your right thumb and inhale through your left nostril.*
3. *Immediately close your left nostril with your right ring finger or pinky finger, remove your thumb from your right nostril (this involves a simple rotation of your hand), and exhale through your right nostril.*
4. *Inhale through your right nostril and then close your right nostril with your right thumb, remove your ring or index finger from your left nostril, and exhale through your left nostril.*
5. *Continue like this, one round of breath starting with an inhale on the left side and finishing with an exhale on the left (it helps to remember to switch nostrils every time you inhale), keeping your breaths as deep and slow as possible.*

Chapter 28:
EXERCISE AND GENTLE MOVEMENT

The importance of exercise is ingrained in our minds, and for good reason: studies routinely show that physical activity is health-protective, and we've identified a wide range of mechanisms explaining why that's the case. Getting regular moderate exercise decreases the risk of cardiovascular disease, type 2 diabetes, depression, and some cancers. In fact, the World Health Organization has identified a lack of physical activity as the fourth leading risk factor for mortality, being responsible for an estimated 3.2 million deaths globally each year! With such strong science supporting its role in our lives, physical activity is a clear tenet of the Paleo framework.

First, let's get one thing straight: exercise is not just about "burning calories." The number of calories we burn when exercising compared to sitting and doing nothing is not really that significant. It certainly adds up slowly considering that 3,500 calories is equivalent to 1 pound of stored energy. If we want to lose weight, we should focus on dietary changes. But exercise still plays an important role in health (and weight) management. Instead of a calorie burner, we should think of exercise as a hormone manager.

Hormones are chemical messengers in contact with virtually every cell in the body, and they are sensitive to the demands of cells. When hormones sense changes in body chemistry, they respond rapidly to ensure that the cells get everything they need to stay healthy. Exercise has a profound effect on every hormone system in the body. Whether the exercise is aerobic or anaerobic, cardio intensive or strength training focused, low intensity or high intensity, and short duration or long duration, virtually every hormone system benefits. It also matters what time of day we exercise, whether we exercise in a fasted state, and what other stressors are present (mental stress, lack of sleep, poor-quality diet, and so on). However, what is uniformly true is that exercise improves hormone regulation.

Some of the advantages of exercise are obvious. Increasing muscle mass causes an increase in metabolism, making it easier to maintain a healthy weight. Of course, most people like the way they look when they have bigger, more defined muscles. In fact, there are no negative aspects to being stronger, faster, more flexible, and more agile.

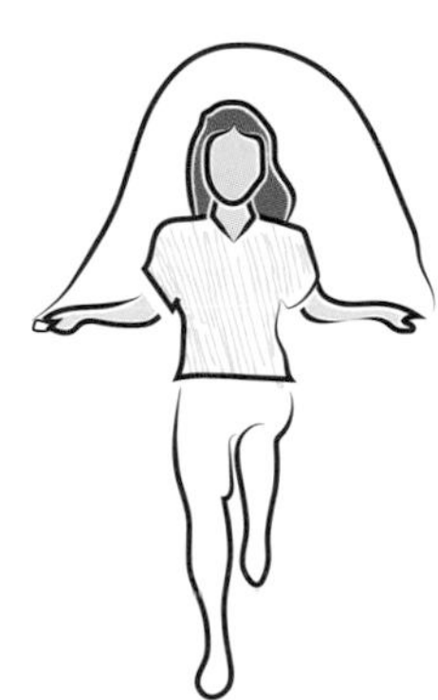

BENEFITS OF BEING ACTIVE

As you contemplate adding more or different types of activity to your life, there are some additional benefits that you might not immediately consider. For example:

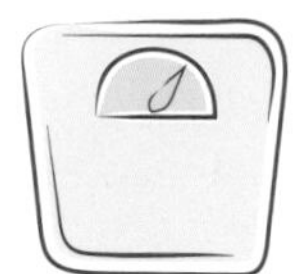

Appetite and weight control. Exercise is known to regulate key hunger hormones such as leptin and ghrelin and may promote healthier digestion through hormone regulation. It is not necessarily true that exercise makes us hungrier, although it may seem that way. In fact, for many people (and depending on the type of exercise), exercise makes it easier to consume fewer calories in an entire day, even if they eat a bigger meal right after working out—and as an added perk, exercise leads many people to crave healthier, more nutrient-dense foods. Exercise is also believed to help lower our body weight "set point," based on the controversial idea that there is a set weight at which the body "wants" to be, which is determined by hormones, which are, in turn, influenced by diet and lifestyle.

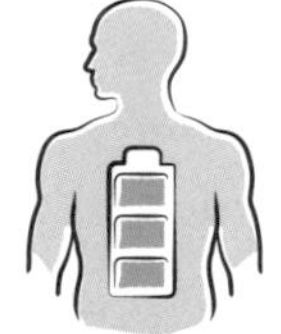

Metabolism and insulin sensitivity. Exercise helps improve insulin sensitivity through direct action on the glucose transport molecules in the individual cells of our muscles. It also affects the full range of hormones related to accessing stored energy and regulating how that energy is used. This "boost" in metabolism is one reason why exercising can make us feel more energetic throughout the day. It is also a major reason why exercise is linked with a reduced risk of diabetes and cardiovascular disease.

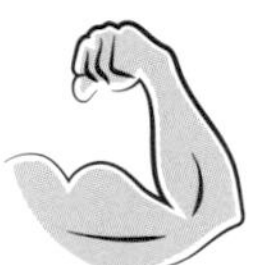

Body composition and bone health. When we exercise, our muscles get stronger (and sometimes bigger, depending on the type of exercise). This muscle gain is one contributor to increased metabolism. As an important part of long-term health, exercise—especially weight-bearing exercise—stimulates our bodies to make stronger and denser bones. Exercise (or lack thereof) is a bigger determinant of osteoporosis risk than diet!

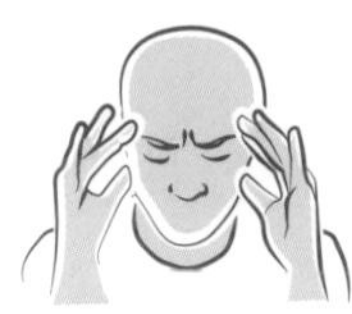

Stress management. Exercise is very effective at modulating levels of the stress hormone cortisol. This is a bit of a double-edged sword because exercising *too* intensely can raise cortisol levels too high and cause problems. However, if we keep exercise to an appropriate duration and intensity for our particular fitness level (and for how well we eat, sleep, and manage stress), exercise becomes potent at reducing and normalizing cortisol levels, which can also help reduce inflammation and promote healing. This makes it easier to burn stored energy (especially fat), in addition to improving sleep and making us feel more relaxed and able to cope with life's surprises.

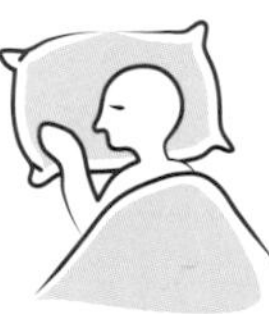

Sleep quality. Beyond its effect on cortisol, exercise regulates several key hormones related to circadian rhythm. Therefore, when we exercise during the day, we'll fall asleep easier, sleep more soundly, and experience more restorative sleep so that we wake up feeling more refreshed (provided that we allotted adequate time for sleep). As discussed in Chapter 26, sleeping better positively affects just about everything in our bodies, from cortisol levels to the ability to resolve inflammation. But be aware that exercising too intensely late in the evening can make it more difficult to fall asleep.

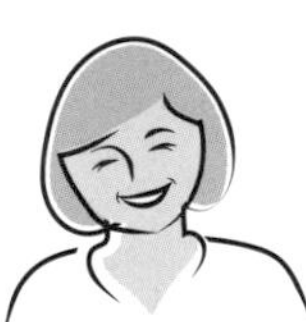

Mood. Beyond its effect on cortisol, exercise releases endorphins, which have a direct impact on several key neurotransmitters that are related to mood. Making time to exercise can help fight depression and anxiety and improve your general outlook on life. Exercising also increases blood flow to the brain and in turn helps reduce inflammation in the brain (which has the net effect of boosting mood). This is an important strategy for people with gut-brain axis problems (impaired signals between the brain and the digestive system; see page 96).

Gut health. While strenuous, exhaustive exercise is detrimental to gut health (we'll get to that on page 360), moderate-intensity exercise is a boon to the community of microorganisms in our gut. While more research is still needed, there is compelling evidence that exercise by itself increases gut microbial diversity and supports the growth of important probiotic strains like *Bifidobacterium* and *Lactobacillus* (see page 70). While most of the research to date has been performed in rodents, one human study comparing the gut microbiota of rugby players to those of healthy controls showed nearly double the number of microbial strains in the athletes.

How do you determine which exercise is best for you? There are different benefits of exercise, depending on the type, duration, and intensity, but with the exception of overtraining (exercising too intensely or for too long of a duration for your individual fitness level), all exercise is extremely beneficial. What activity is best for you depends on your goals and current health status. What matters most is that you do *something*—even if it's just a leisurely stroll. Even better, do something you really enjoy. If you enjoy the activity, you're far more likely to keep doing it!

HEALTH QUICK-START *Regular exercise doesn't have to mean pouring sweat and exhausting yourself at the gym for 2 hours every day. Simply going for a 30-minute walk most days, while also taking short movement breaks throughout the day, yields almost all the benefits of physical activity!*

GENTLE MOVEMENT VERSUS SITTING

Speaking of different forms of activity, one form in particular deserves the spotlight for a moment: frequent gentle movement. Many of us think we can cancel out an otherwise sedentary lifestyle (sitting at a desk job, commuting in the car, watching TV, and spending way too much time on Facebook) by going to the gym a few times per week and breaking a sweat. It's common to think of exercise as a sort of "payment" so we can veg out on the couch afterward (eating whatever food we want because we've "earned" it) and not feel guilty.

We've already seen the ways in which exercise can be tremendously beneficial, but isolated bouts of activity (like a workout at the gym) are *not* enough to make up for hours and hours of inactivity, especially sitting. In fact, a growing body of research is showing that it's not just the absence of exercise that makes sedentary behavior an issue: sitting itself, especially for long periods, is actually hazardous for our bodies.

SCIENCE SIMPLIFIED *Unfortunately, we can't make up for a day spent sitting at a desk with a rigorous workout in the evening. We need both gentle movement throughout the day and moderate or vigorous activity throughout the week.*

The scientific literature has been churning up data that should have all of us rethinking our sitting habits. A meta-analysis published in the *Annals of Internal Medicine* pooled the results of forty-seven studies on sedentary behavior, the largest study of its kind to date. Across the board, prolonged periods of sitting were linked to a higher risk of heart disease, cancer, type 2 diabetes, and death from all causes.

Just how big of a risk increase are we talking about? By some estimates, every extra hour we spend sitting in front of the TV each day is associated with an 18 percent increase in heart disease death and an 11 percent increase in death from all causes. Those are significant numbers! (Sitting in general almost certainly has the same detrimental effects, but TV time is a very accurate way for scientific studies to gauge sitting time.) And if we really want to scare ourselves, one study framed it this way: every hour of TV we watch after the age of 25 reduces our life expectancy—at least statistically—by almost 22 minutes.

Even more alarming, a recent meta-analysis showed that regular exercise did not wipe out the harmful effects of extended sitting. Although people who didn't exercise and also had sedentary lifestyles fared the worst overall, people who exercised on top of spending long periods sitting down still faced a higher risk of death and disease relative to those who were more active throughout the day. That means that no matter how many buckets of sweat we lose at the gym during the week, if we spend the rest of our time sitting and not moving, we're putting ourselves in danger.

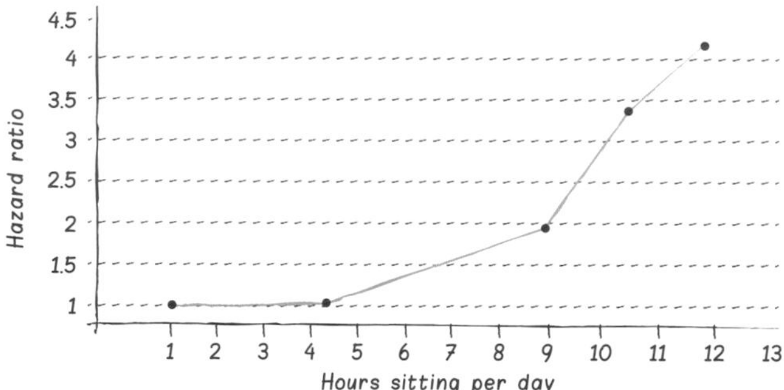

Associations of daily total sitting time with Hazard Ratio of all-cause mortality risk (with no adjustment for physical activity). Adapted from Koster, A., et al. "Association of sedentary time with mortality independent of moderate to vigorous physical activity." *PLoS One* 7, no. 6 (2012): e37696. doi: 10.1371/journal.pone.0037696. Epub 2012 Jun 13.

So how does sitting cause problems? Researchers are still trying to understand the exact mechanisms that make sitting such a hazard for our health. However, we have enough evidence from animal models and human experiments to start piecing the puzzle together.

The biggest issue is the effect of inactivity on certain metabolic processes in our bodies, especially in our muscles. Prolonged sitting can suppress the activity of lipoprotein lipase (LPL), an enzyme involved in lipid metabolism, and in turn contribute to high triglycerides and low HDL ("good") cholesterol. Likewise, the lack of muscle contraction that happens when we sit for a long time can reduce glucose uptake and contribute to elevated blood sugar. The cellular changes from sitting happen very quickly (and are improved as soon as we stand up), so even one day of extreme inactivity can be detrimental. All these problems start setting the stage for a variety of chronic diseases. (See also page 123.)

Here's where physical activity comes into play. "Frequent movement" doesn't mean we need to run a marathon every day. Even gentle movement like a slow amble has tremendous benefits. One of the major ways gentle movement can boost our health is through its impact on lymph flow. The lymphatic system, which transports lymph fluid through a network of tissues and organs—including the tonsils, spleen, adenoids, and lymph nodes—plays a huge role in immune function, fluid regulation, the absorption of lipids, and ridding the body of waste and other unwanted materials. Because it doesn't use pumping mechanisms to operate, the lymph system relies partially on the pressure and contractions from surrounding tissue, such as muscle. So one of the best ways to improve lymph flow is by—you guessed it—moving our bodies. Experiments using electrical stimulation show that muscle contractions can increase lymph flow to twice of what it is during rest, and voluntary muscle contractions (where we *don't* get zapped with electricity) have a similar effect. We can boost lymph flow by simply moving frequently in ways that gently engage our muscles.

There's more to the story, too. Gentle movement, when it also involves bearing weight, helps improve bone mineral density and protect against fractures—in men and women across all age groups. Mechanical loads from extra weight (from carrying dumbbells, grocery bags, a child, an overweight cat, or even our own bodies as we perform squats and similar exercises) stimulate cells called osteoblasts, which are responsible for synthesizing and mineralizing bone tissue. Engaging in gentle weight-bearing exercise throughout the day (hello, walking!) is a great investment for our skeletal health.

Traditional cultures offer us additional clues to the role and importance of gentle movement. The ability to be completely sedentary and still survive is brand-new in human history. Until just a few generations ago, most people had to move their bodies in order to find or grow food, travel from place to place, and communicate with friends and family. Now, virtually all of that can be taken care of with technology and gadgets (and social media), making our bodies somewhat useless for the tasks we once needed them for.

Elsewhere in the world, we can see more realistic models of what the human body is adapted to in terms of daily movement. Ethnographic accounts of hunter-gatherers show that both men and women participated in regular movement to keep their societies running smoothly. Men were often in charge of hunting large game, trekking long distances, and mixing periods of rest with spikes of brief, intense exertion. In many tribes, women were in charge of foraging for edible plants and small animals or eggs—with periods of rest interspersed with hours of walking, digging, stretching, and bending in order to collect food and bring it back to camp. Hunter-gatherer mothers also had to carry their children around through infancy and toddlerhood and by some estimates would walk nearly 3,000 miles with a child in their arms during the child's first four years of life. As anyone with children knows, that's no easy feat!

Despite what seems like an ultra-busy lifestyle, hunter-gatherer populations might not expend much more total energy than typical Westerners do. A recent study of the Hadza of Tanzania found that over the course of a day, the total energy expenditure of adult men and women carrying out their normal activities was about equal to that of industrialized Europeans and Americans. In 2013, a similar study of the Tsimane, forager-horticulturalists of the Amazon who are known for having extremely low rates of heart disease and diabetes, found that their 24-hour physical activity level was similar to that of developed populations. But they spent very little time being totally sedentary, and most of their movement was light to moderate rather than vigorous.

So how do traditional populations evade the chronic diseases and obesity plaguing the Western world? This evidence shows us that it's not the total quantity of activity that matters, but rather how it's dispersed throughout the day. Traditional populations don't go to the gym before work and then sit in a chair for the next 8 hours: they engage in frequent, lower-intensity activity pretty much from the time they get up to the time they go to sleep, with less-frequent bouts of intense movement. Frequency appears to be the protective factor as far as physical activity goes. That also means that contrary to what many of us envision, hunter-gatherers don't live like elite athletes and pack a ton of calorie-burning exercise into each day in order to stay lean and healthy, so we don't need to, either!

How often should we move, then? A growing body of scientific literature shows that moving around for just 2 minutes after every 20 minutes of being completely sedentary has tremendous health benefits. Repeatedly setting a 20-minute timer and then getting up and walking around for 2 minutes throughout the workday can negate the health detriments of prolonged sitting. Interestingly, one study showed that simply standing for 2 minutes didn't work, and that moving (a slow walk) is key.

PALEO EASY BUTTON *There are some great biohacks for incorporating movement into a desk job. Treadmill desks, desk elliptical machines, and desk cycles are available to help you move throughout a day when you might otherwise be sitting for extended periods. Typically, the intensity of this movement is low enough that you can work without being distracted or fatigued by your movement, so using one of these desk alternatives doesn't substitute for physical activity time. What it does do is remove sedentary time. There are also a variety of apps and fitness trackers that can remind you to get up and move on a regular schedule.*

That doesn't mean working at a standing desk is pointless, though. While a standing break isn't enough to avoid problems associated with too much sitting, working at a standing desk in lieu of a conventional desk has been shown to have great health benefits, one of which is that it tends to increase activity throughout the day. Maybe it's easier to scatter that gentle movement throughout the day if we're already standing? More research in this area is definitely needed.

It's also important to emphasize that the goal to incorporate gentle movement throughout the day is *in addition* to some form of moderately intense activity (see page 363) at least a few times a week.

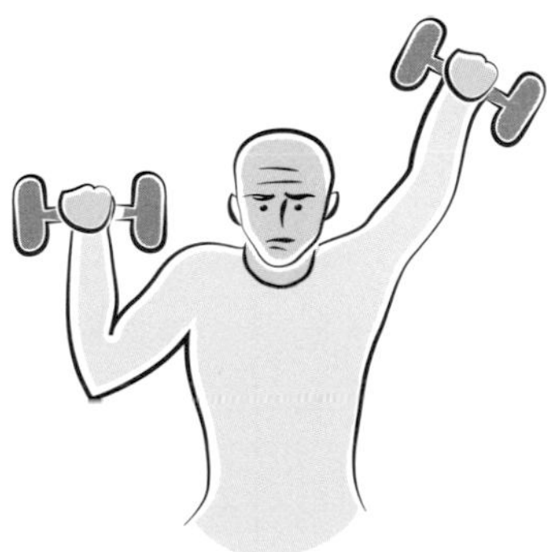

THE DOWNSIDE OF OVER-EXERCISING

When it comes to exercise, there's a happy medium that provides health benefits. Too little activity is associated with detrimental health effects, including a compromised immune system, decreased resistance to stress, and decreased resilience of circadian rhythms. However, as I touched on earlier, too much (too strenuous or intense) activity also negatively impacts health, such as by causing dysregulated cortisol, increased susceptibility to immune-related diseases and infection, and—here's the surprising one—a leaky gut.

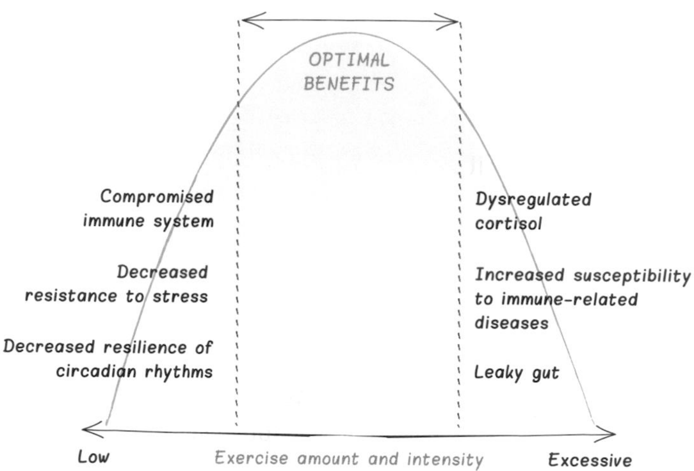

Yes, we can get too much of a good thing. This is called a U-shaped curve, where both too little and too much cause problems and there's a happy middle range. Let's discuss in more depth how strenuous activity directly affects the integrity of the gut barrier, ultimately causing a leaky gut.

Leaky Gut

It really shouldn't come as a surprise that strenuous activities cause gut problems. Up to half of all long-distance runners experience something called runner's diarrhea (colloquially referred to as "runner's runs," "runner's trots," or "the gingerbread man"). The symptoms include dizziness, nausea, stomach or intestinal cramps, vomiting, and diarrhea, which occur mainly while running. All symptoms point to something insidious happening in the gut (see Chapter 4).

While not all endurance athletes suffer overt symptoms, strenuous exercise does appear to increase intestinal permeability in everyone who indulges in it, albeit to varying degrees. A variety of studies have documented increased intestinal permeability in athletes who reported no gastrointestinal symptoms. And one study showed that well-trained athletes who suffered from exercise-induced gastrointestinal symptoms experienced significantly more intestinal permeability after exercise than asymptomatic athletes.

The way that exercise increases intestinal permeability is multifaceted. First, intense activity is a stress on the body and activates the hypothalamus-pituitary-adrenal (HPA) axis, otherwise known as the fight-or-flight response. It causes the release of two important hormones that directly affect gut health: cortisol and corticotropin-releasing hormone. In Chapter 27, I explained how these two hormones cause a leaky gut.

However, the stress response isn't the only way exercise causes a leaky gut. In order to prioritize blood flow to the heart and skeletal muscles during exercise, blood flow is diverted away from the gastrointestinal tract and other visceral organs, like the liver and spleen. This lack of sufficient blood flow results in what is called *ischemic injury* to the gut, which disrupts the intestinal barrier and thus increases intestinal permeability.

Participating in strenuous and exhaustive exercise further stimulates the production of a class of proteins called heat shock proteins (so called because the first of this family of proteins was discovered to be induced by fevers). Heat shock proteins have a direct effect on tight junctions by affecting the levels of two integral protein families called occludin and claudin, opening them up and causing a leaky gut.

Given all this, perhaps it's no surprise that vigorous exercise is also associated with a condition called food-dependent, exercise-induced anaphylaxis, in which the exercise-induced increase in intestinal permeability facilitates the absorption of allergens from the gastrointestinal tract.

A few conditions can aggravate the increased intestinal permeability caused by strenuous exercise. One study showed that the use of ibuprofen, a nonsteroidal anti-inflammatory drug (NSAID), significantly exacerbated both intestinal permeability

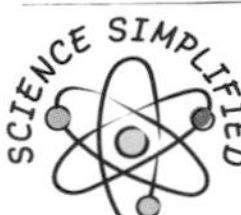

Unfortunately, intense and exhaustive exercise, especially endurance-type sports, causes health problems. The big issue is that this type of training causes a leaky gut and can dysregulate the immune system. That's why elite endurance athletes have much higher rates of some health problems, including lung infections and asthma.

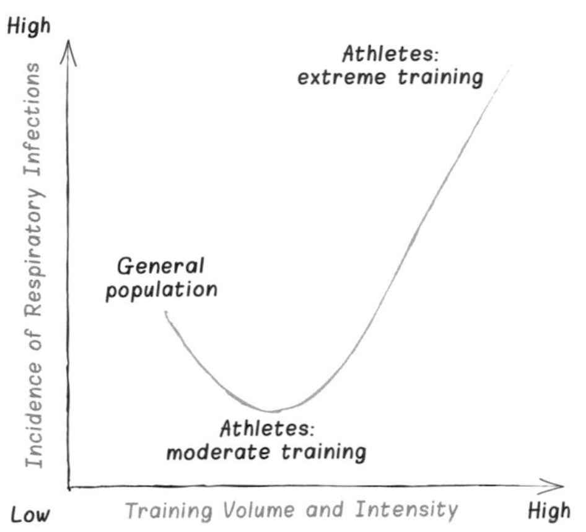

and intestinal damage caused by strenuous exercise in well-trained athletes. (Ironically, popping ibuprofen is a common practice for endurance athletes.) There is also a strong correlation between both food intake and the consumption of carbohydrate-dense, electrolyte-enhanced beverages and gastrointestinal symptoms in endurance athletes. Strenuous exercise inhibits gastric emptying (the movement of food from the stomach to the small intestine), which is then further inhibited as the concentration of carbohydrates and salt in the stomach increases, so sugary sports drinks can make the problem worse. Of course, dehydration also causes heightened symptoms. It remains unknown whether food and overly concentrated sports drinks actually increase intestinal permeability or simply magnify the symptoms felt by the athlete.

Environmental conditions also have an impact. One study showed that an hour-long run in either hot (91°F or 33°C) or mild (72°F or 22°C) conditions caused increased intestinal permeability, but the amount of endotoxin (bacterial protein from Gram-negative bacteria) detectable in the blood was much greater after strenuous exercise performed in hot conditions. This implies that strenuous exercise is more inflammatory if performed in the heat.

Probiotic treatment may help protect the gut from increased permeability caused by strenuous exercise. One study showed that probiotic supplementation reduced the amount of pro-inflammatory cytokines in the blood after strenuous exercise in male athletes and decreased the amount of zonulin detectable in the feces.

Runners, cyclists, and triathletes have been studied for exercise-induced intestinal barrier dysfunction. Although no definitive studies have been done on the connection between resistance training and intestinal permeability, it probably depends on the style of workout and the amount of rest time between sets. Certainly, high-intensity, short-rest workouts have been shown to increase cortisol secretion more than traditional resistance training. By contrast, regular exercise at a relatively low intensity may protect the gastrointestinal tract from becoming diseased. There is evidence that physical activity reduces the risk of colon cancer, gallstones, diverticulosis, and inflammatory bowel disease, which is yet another argument for increasing physical activity while avoiding strenuous exercise. Again, it's the happy medium phenomenon.

Effects on the Immune System

Along with leaky gut, physical activity has complicated effects on both the innate and adaptive immune systems (see page 78). This largely depends on whether the exercise is acute (meaning strenuous exercise that is not part of a regular training routine) or chronic (that is, regular). Acute exercise doesn't just refer to someone who is out of shape jumping into an intense cardio kickboxing class. Anyone working out at a level that is substantially more intense than what they're accustomed to, or for substantially longer than they're used to, is doing acute exercise. Therefore, depending on the exercise or sport and the intensity, some people may be unaware that they are doing acute exercise every time they work out.

Acute exercise, whether it is in the form of endurance or resistance training, stimulates inflammation. Both neutrophils and natural killer cells are mobilized, and their numbers in the blood increase dramatically following exercise, the magnitude of which is related to both the intensity and the duration of the exercise. Acute exercise also stimulates phagocytosis (eating of stuff by macrophages and monocytes) and increases the production of reactive oxygen species and pro-inflammatory cytokines. However, chronic exercise does not appear to appreciably increase neutrophils in the blood and may reduce both the number of blood monocytes and their reactivity to inflammatory stimuli. In fact, a few reports indicate that consistent training may provide anti-inflammatory benefits in those with chronic inflammatory conditions. By contrast, other studies show that even regular training increases natural killer cells and that this effect is probably exacerbated by intense training.

The effect of acute exercise on the adaptive immune system is only partly understood. During and immediately after acute exercise, helper T-cells and cytotoxic T-cell numbers in the blood increase but then rapidly return to normal. Furthermore, there is a differential effect on the helper T-cell subsets, in particular Th1 cells (which secrete cytokines that drive macrophage "eater" cell activity) versus Th2 cells (which secrete cytokines that drive antibody production by B cells). Specifically, acute exercise decreases the relative number of Th1 cells and increases the number of Th2 cells. Not surprisingly, given that Th2 cells are important modulators of B-cell activation, there is a concurrent increase in B cells in the blood. In the recovery period, the numbers of

MOVEMENT AND ACTIVITY GUIDELINES

WEEKLY ACTIVITY TARGETS

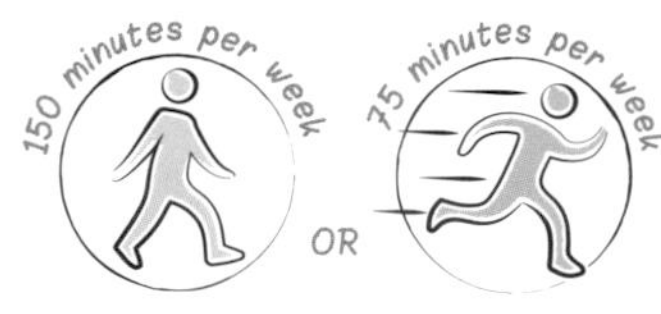

- Studies show major health benefits with at least 150 minutes (2 1/2 hours) of moderately intense activity or 75 minutes of vigorous activity each week.

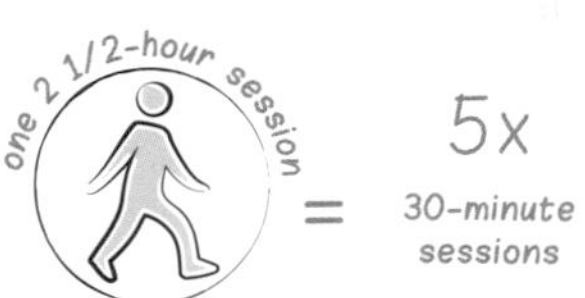

- Recent studies show that it doesn't make a difference whether you get your 150 minutes of moderate activity in one 2 1/2-hour session once per week or five 30-minute sessions spread throughout the week.

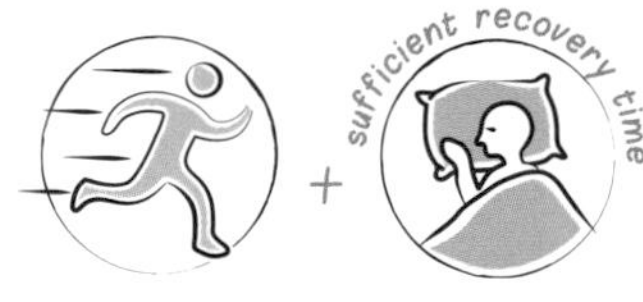

- The more active you are, the greater the health benefits, provided that you are giving your body sufficient recovery time between vigorous workouts.

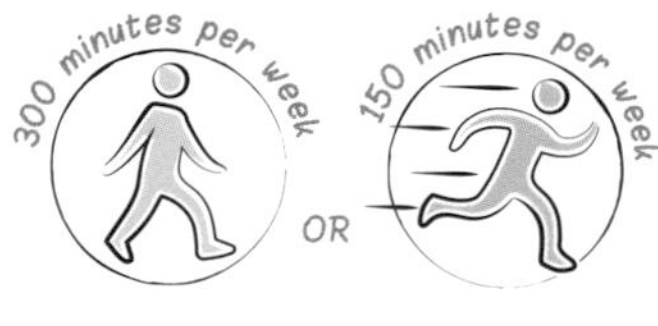

- For even greater health benefits, aim for 300 minutes (5 hours) of moderately intense activity or 150 minutes (2 1/2 hours) of vigorous activity each week.

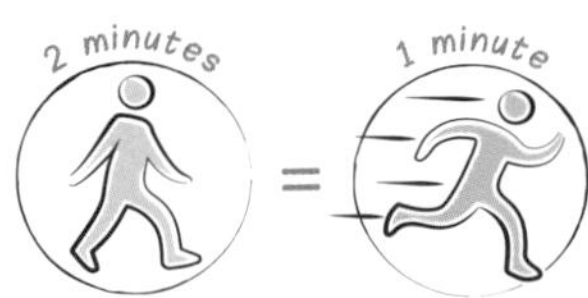

- You can absolutely mix it up with some moderate activity and some vigorous activity. As a general rule, 1 minute of vigorous activity is equivalent (in terms of health benefits) to about 2 minutes of moderate activity.

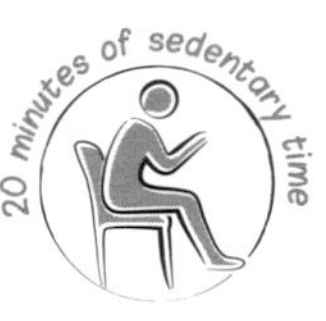

AVOID BEING SEDENTARY

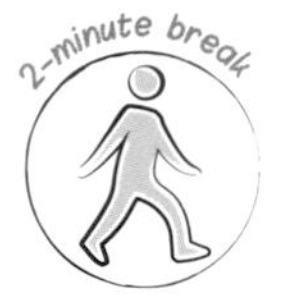

- Take a 2-minute movement break after every 20 minutes of sedentary (sitting) time.
- During your 2-minute breaks, walk around or move in some other way; research shows that it isn't enough to simply stand up.

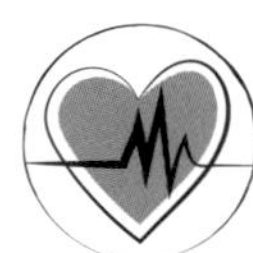

AEROBIC ACTIVITY

- Engage in aerobic activity (that is, elevate your heart and respiration rates due to exertion) for at least 10 minutes at a time.
- Spread aerobic activity throughout the week.

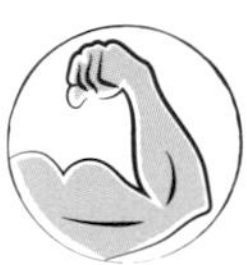

MUSCLE-STRENGTHENING ACTIVITIES

- Muscle-strengthening activities should be included two or more days a week.
- These activities should work all the major muscle groups (legs, hips, back, chest, abdomen, shoulders, and arms) within the week.

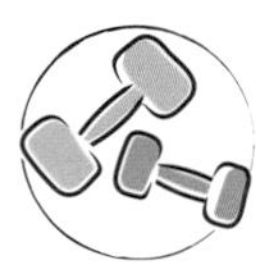

MAKE GRADUAL CHANGES

- Especially if you're starting out as an inactive person, add minutes of physical activity and increase the intensity of physical activity gradually.
- Some physical activity is better than none.
- You can gain health benefits from as little as 1 hour of moderately intense activity per week, so that's a great beginner's goal.

T cells and B cells drop below pre-workout levels, indicating a suppression of the adaptive immune system, before recovering to normal levels relatively quickly. Studies of elite athletes show that, in general, the numbers of T cells and B cells measured 24 hours after exercise are the same as in non-athletes, indicating that regular training probably does not cause persistent changes in the adaptive immune system. Problems arise, however, when there is insufficient recovery time between intense workouts, in which case immune suppression can result.

KNOWLEDGE BOMB

Regular, moderately intense activity improves immune function and lowers the risk of chronic disease and infections. One study showed measurable improvements in immune function (indicated by secretory IgA and defensin levels) immediately after a 90-minute yoga class. Another study determined that walking five times per week for 45 minutes gradually increased secretory IgA levels, reaching a maximum after 3 years. (Secretory IgA serves as the first line of defense in barrier tissues such as the gut, so unlike the other antibody types, having high levels of it is a good thing!) So not only do you get immediate immune benefits from moderately intense activity, but the benefits continue to build over years of commitment to an active lifestyle.

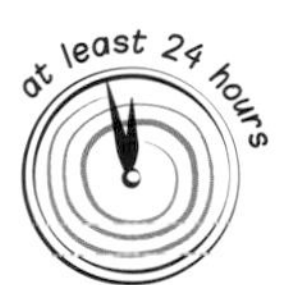

REST AND RECOVERY

- Make sure you are getting ample recovery time between training sessions (at least 24 hours).

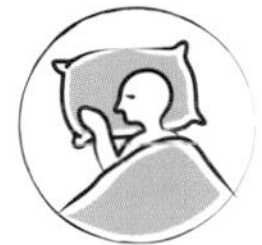

- Get enough sleep every night (see Chapter 26).
- Be sure to eat enough food to support recovery and repair between training sessions (see page 120).

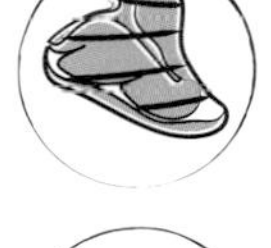

- During intense exercise, consume approximately 16 ounces per hour of a beverage that contains less than 10 percent carbohydrates but includes glucose, fructose, and electrolytes.

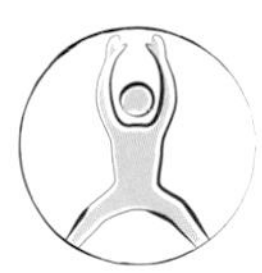

- Stretch before and after vigorous activity and any activity that might strain muscles. Self-myofascial massage ("rolling out" the muscles) is also very beneficial.

- Listen to your body and reduce the intensity of your workouts if you have very sore muscles, feel fatigued or sluggish, or feel like you may be getting sick.

DIALING IN INTENSITY

- The intensity of your activity is relative to your individual capacity. What is vigorous for one person might be moderate for another or impossible for someone else.
- During your workouts, use the rating of perceived exertion (RPE) scale to assign numbers to how you feel. Rate your perceived exertion on a scale from 1 to 20, with 1 being lying in bed and 20 being sprinting as fast as you can. Moderately intense activity usually corresponds to an RPE of 11 to 14. Vigorous activity usually corresponds to an RPE of 17 to 19.

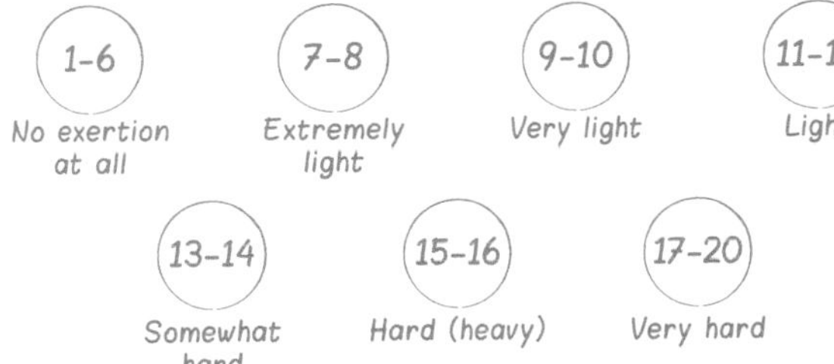

- You can also use the "talk test" to estimate the intensity of your workout. Most people are able to talk or hold a conversation during moderately intense activity. During vigorous activity, holding a conversation or saying more than a few words before running out of breath is challenging.

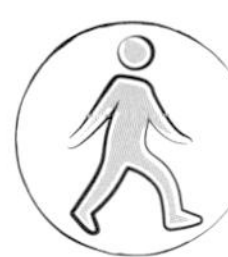

EXAMPLES OF MODERATE INTENSITY:

Walking briskly (generally 3 or more miles per hour, but not race-walking), water aerobics, bicycling slower than 10 miles per hour, tennis (doubles), ballroom dancing, general gardening

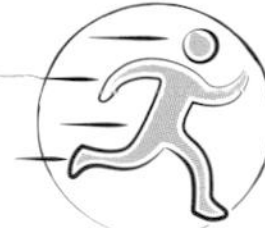

EXAMPLES OF VIGOROUS INTENSITY:

CrossFit, HIIT (high-intensity interval training) such as many boot-camp programs, race-walking, jogging or running, swimming laps, tennis (singles), aerobic dancing, bicycling 10 miles per hour or faster, jumping rope, heavy gardening (continuous digging or hoeing), hiking uphill or with a heavy backpack

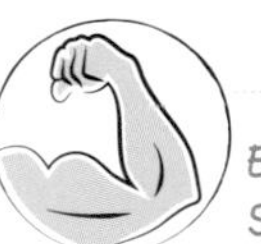

EXAMPLES OF MUSCLE-STRENGTHENING ACTIVITIES:

CrossFit, lifting weights, working with resistance bands, bodyweight movements such as sit-ups and push-ups, yoga, heavy gardening

Guidelines taken from American Heart Association and U.S. Department of Health and Human Services (HHS) 2008 Physical Activity Guidelines for Americans and updated to reflect current research.

LIVING AN ACTIVE LIFESTYLE

Ultimately, what all this means is that it's more important to be active than it is to exercise in ways that are too strenuous or acute. The best scenario for our health is to do light to moderate activity for as much of the day as possible. This includes gentle activities like going for walks, taking the stairs, parking in the farthest space instead of the closest, working at a treadmill desk, gardening, doing housework, playing actively with the kids or the dog, and maybe getting some moderately intense activity designed to build strength, like lifting weights or doing yoga. The key is to avoid being sedentary, especially sitting for prolonged periods, and to avoid doing overly strenuous or prolonged physical activities like endurance training and HIIT (high-intensity interval training) workouts.

It's important to understand that the meaning of "too strenuous" is different for different people. Clearly, how physically fit you are will determine what workout intensity is going to mean overdoing it. As previously discussed, other important lifestyle factors play into this as well: how long we give ourselves to recover after an intense workout (at least 24 hours, and preferably 48), how well we manage stress, whether we work out in the heat (which can increase leaky gut), and whether we're getting adequate sleep. The micronutrient density of our diet is almost certainly a player as well; our diet affects the health of our adrenal glands, neurotransmitter regulation, and the gut microbiome.

So what's the takeaway? There's no benefit to overexerting ourselves in the gym or on the pavement. Where to draw the "overexertion" line is an individual choice, and we have to listen to our bodies and experiment. While science can point us in the right direction, the details are up to each of us to dial in. For more guidance on dialing in intensity, see the previous page.

All that said, there are a few important things to keep in mind when implementing the "activity" tenet of Paleo:

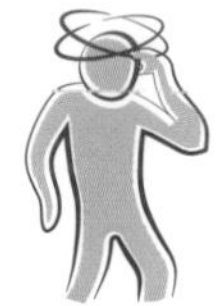

Don't overdo it. Pushing our bodies too hard can cause an increase in stress hormone production, harm gut health, compromise our immune systems, and lead to other problems. It's better to go for a long, slow stroll than to sprint for 20 minutes and induce feelings of imminent death. We can push our bodies to do more, but we should aim for gradual improvement.

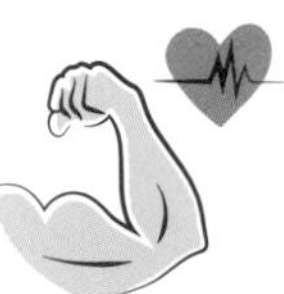

Diversify for more benefits. Find an activity that builds strength and an activity that provides some cardiovascular conditioning. Better yet, try something that does both. But remember that neither strength-building nor cardio activities should be strenuous.

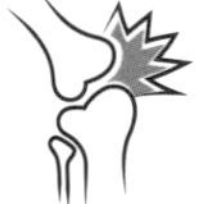

Protect your joints, back, and brain. Whatever activities you do, be aware of the injury risks involved and take precautions to protect your body. This means taking time for proper warm-ups and cool-downs, stretching, and practicing correct technique in addition to wearing the right gear and following safety protocols.

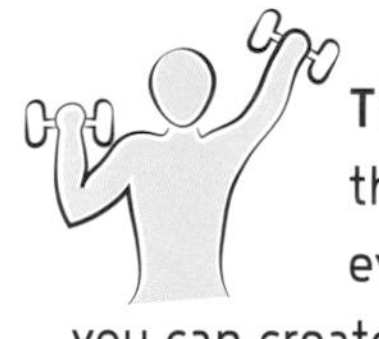

Think about the long term. Find activities that you can do for the rest of your life, even if the intensity decreases over time. If you can create a social aspect to your activities, all the better.

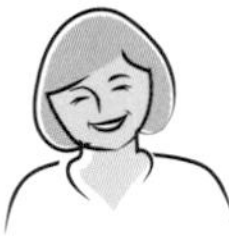

Do it for enjoyment. If you love doing a physical activity, chances are you'll want to do it more—to the point that it becomes more like a hobby than a chore. If you stop enjoying the activity, it's time to take a break and find something else to do. Having fun is key!

Chapter 29:
NATURE AND SUNLIGHT

Another critical component of a Paleo lifestyle is spending time outside. Unfortunately, many of us can go for days—if not weeks—with our only exposure to fresh air and sunlight happening while we walk to and from our cars. Modern living makes it easy to stay insulated indoors (at home, at school, at the office, at the gym, in our vehicles, in the grocery store . . . on and on), which is a far cry from the direct contact with nature that defined most of human existence. Today, science confirms that "nature time" remains extremely important for our well-being, in ways that no amount of healthy eating or exercise can compensate for.

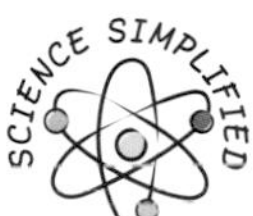

As a society, we are spending more time indoors than at any other point in human history. This deprives us of valuable sun exposure, fresh air, and connection with nature, all of which are likely impacting our health for the worse!

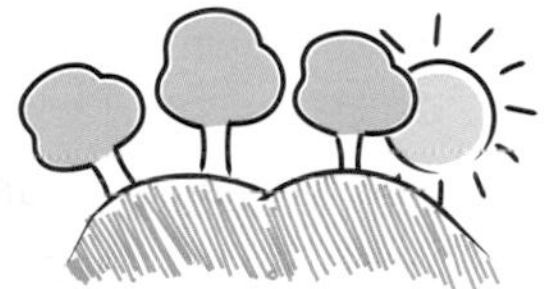

THE BENEFITS OF NATURE

The feelings of peace, relaxation, and tranquility that come from spending time in nature are so potent that they've been measured and confirmed by science. Everything from a short visit to a park to a long camping trip in the wilderness can benefit our physical and psychological health.

For example, spending several hours in a forest gives an impressive boost to the immune system, including increasing natural killer cell activity by 50 percent, which improves the immune system's capacity to detect and eliminate cancerous cells and cells infected with viruses and parasites. When that forest trip is increased to 3 days, research has shown that natural killer cell activity, the number of natural killer cells, and intracellular anti-cancer protein levels remain elevated for at least 7 days after the trip is over! That means an extended weekend of camping could continue benefiting us long after we're back at work.

What about those of us who only have time to sit amidst a tree grove on our lunch breaks? It turns out that nature has such a powerful effect on our health that spending as little as 30 minutes per *week* in a green space can reduce the rates of high blood pressure and depression by 7 percent and 9 percent, respectively. The more time spent in nature per week, the lower the risk—but even short visits to some greenery are worth it.

When we swap the green of the forest for the blue of the ocean, the benefits hold firm, especially for mental well-being. One study found that when people with psychological distress were exposed to either a natural park or an ocean beach for a period of 3½ hours, they experienced significant drops in their Total Mood Disturbance (TMD) scores, suggesting a major improvement in psychological health. When exposed to an urban environment, the participants' feelings of distress did *not* diminish.

Overall, a connection to nature—in its various forms—appears to boost memory and concentration, improve longevity, relieve stress, lower inflammation, enhance creativity, improve focus, support immune function, reduce risk of chronic disease (including cancer and cardiovascular disease), improve symptoms of mental illness, and help us sleep better. It sounds too good to be true, but this time, it's real!

HEALTH QUICK-START *It really is as simple as carving out a little bit of time to be outside every day. One easy way to do that is to move an activity that you normally do indoors to the outdoors. Perhaps you enjoy reading a book in the evenings; you could easily do so in your backyard. Maybe you usually eat your lunch at your desk, but you could just as easily take it outside. These little changes make a big difference!*

Nature Walks

For some of us, walking in nature is just another form of exercise—and maybe it's a little more interesting than walking in place on a treadmill. So it might come as a surprise that walking in nature is *much* more beneficial than walking indoors or in a city, and the benefits extend far beyond fitness.

Compared to a similar stroll in an urban setting, a 50-minute walk in nature has been shown to decrease anxiety, reduce rumination (repeated negative thoughts about ourselves or our experiences), lower negative affect (poor self-concept and emotions), improve positive affect (positive moods like joy and alertness), improve symptoms of major depressive disorder, and even offer cognitive benefits, such as boosting working memory performance. In other studies, a 90-minute walk in nature has been shown to reduce neural activity in brain areas linked with mental illness. (A 90-minute walk in an urban setting offered no such benefits.) Nature walks of 80 minutes also appear to lower blood pressure and adrenaline, increase mood test scores for vigor (defined in psychology as feeling energetic and lively, with a strong sense of well-being), and decrease mood test scores for depression, fatigue, confusion, and anxiety.

Strapped for time? Even short nature walks can boost our well-being. In one study, a 15-minute stroll through an urban park resulted in significantly lower heart rate, lower sympathetic nerve activity (the fight-or-flight response), and higher parasympathetic nerve activity (the "rest and digest" system) than a similar walk through the city. Likewise, participants reported feeling "comfortable," "relaxed," "natural," and "vigorous" after their nature walks and exhibited significantly lower levels of anxiety and negative emotions. These benefits occurred no matter what the season, even during the cold winter months.

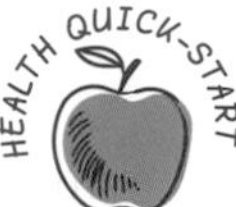

Making time for even a 15-minute walk through green space can have a measurable positive impact on your health. Aim for daily walks, but even two nature walks a week can reduce blood pressure and depression!

Sights, Sounds, Smells, and Earthing

So how does nature exert such profound effects on our well-being? The answer may lie in the sights, sounds, smells, and sensations that envelop us when we venture into the natural world.

Simply being surrounded by natural beauty could be enough to boost our physical health. One analysis found that people who live in scenic places—defined as having broad open areas unobstructed by buildings, roads, and other man-made objects—report significantly better health, regardless of their employment status, education level, income, access to services, exposure to air pollution, and proximity to crime and regardless of whether the location is rural or urban.

Even for people who don't live amidst natural beauty, simply viewing pleasant scenery can have similar benefits in the short term. In one experiment, participants spent 15 minutes sitting down while viewing either forest scenery or an urban area. When the participants viewed the forest, they exhibited a significantly lower heart rate, lower scores for anxiety, higher scores for "vigor" and "refreshed," and lower reports of fatigue than when they viewed the urban environment. Additional research shows that when surgery patients are placed in rooms that look out over natural scenes, they tend to have shorter postoperative hospital stays, receive better evaluations by nurses, and take less pain medication than matched control patients whose windows face the wall of a building.

Part of the reason that viewing natural scenery is so much more healing than viewing urban scenery has to do with the kind of attention each setting demands. According to attention restoration theory (ART), nature is restorative because it's filled with intriguing stimuli that only modestly grab our attention, without demanding much conscious action, decision-making, or focus. By contrast, urban settings tend to be more chaotic and stimulating, dramatically capturing our attention and sometimes requiring quick responses (such as moving out of the way of an oncoming vehicle!).

The sounds and smells of nature also have powerful effects on our health. Scientists have conducted indoor experiments in which participants experience various nonvisual elements of nature, including wood smells, tactile stimulation with wood, and forest sounds. As with studies that immerse participants in natural areas outdoors, these indoor experiments demonstrate that people's heart rate and blood pressure drop after they are exposed to nature sensations.

The reason natural sounds help soothe us may be due to their effects on our fight-or-flight response (associated with the sympathetic nervous system). In one study, participants worked on an attention-demanding activity while listening to a series of 5-minute recordings of either natural sounds or man-made sounds, while also receiving functional magnetic resonance imaging (fMRI) so that researchers could monitor changes in their brain activity. The natural sounds triggered brain patterns associated with externally focused attention (better concentration on the activity at hand), as well as a decrease in the body's sympathetic nervous response, indicating relaxation. Meanwhile, the man-made sounds were associated with internally focused attention (which includes worry and rumination and is associated with psychological distress) and more engagement of the sympathetic nervous system.

Smells, too, may play a part in nature's ability to boost our health. Phytoncides (the aromatic airborne chemicals that plants emit, and that give forests and other natural areas their scent) have the ability to decrease our stress hormone levels and boost several markers of immunity. Research shows that inhaling phytoncides such as α-pinene and β-pinene results in higher levels of natural killer cells as well as lower levels of cortisol, indicating less stress. Although being in a real forest is optimal for other reasons, the use of wood essential oils indoors can have a similar beneficial effect on immunity and stress.

And what about the textures of nature—the sensations of the natural world on our bodies? It turns out that bringing our bodies into contact with the earth offers many perks.

The concept of earthing (also called grounding) is sometimes dismissed right out the gate because of the unsubstantiated hype and "woo-woo" that often accompany it. Advocates of earthing claim that the practice works due to the transfer of free electrons from the earth's surface to our bodies, which in turn help neutralize free radicals and impact various biological processes, but studies assessing this claim have generally failed to confirm it. However, while this is a field that definitely needs more study, especially on a mechanistic level, there is legitimate evidence that the practice of earthing can benefit our health—whether or not we've correctly identified why.

Earthing involves making direct physical contact with the surface of the earth. This can involve walking barefoot outside, digging our feet into soft sand at the beach, or even doing a handstand or yoga in the backyard. (Various earthing products, such as grounding mats, are on the market, but until we have a better sense of why skin contact with the ground is beneficial, it's probably better to save your money and "earth" the old-fashioned way.) A number of pilot studies have suggested that earthing helps improve sleep quality, normalize circadian rhythms, reduce pain and stress, reduce blood viscosity, increase heart rate variability, and reduce signs of inflammation following injury (including heat, redness, pain, and swelling). Although these studies were small and need to be replicated before we can say that the evidence is solid, the findings so far are promising. And let's face it, who doesn't like walking around barefoot on fresh green grass?

Nature-Based Therapies

Nature-based therapies are emerging as promising ways to manage stress and boost both physical and psychological health. In Sweden, for example, nature-based rehabilitation programs are being used to help people with stress-related mental disorders recover from burnout, depression, and anxiety. And in Japan, "forest therapy" has been used for decades to combat the negative effects of urban life. This involves spending extended time—anywhere from several hours to several days—in a forest setting and engaging in specific timed activities such as walking, lying on the ground, and deep breathing.

A huge body of literature shows that for men and women across a wide range of ages, whether they are healthy or at risk of or experiencing chronic disease, forest therapy has wide-ranging benefits for health. Forest therapy reduces cortisol levels, lowers heart rate, increases positive feelings (both physical and emotional), lessens negative feelings, improves cognitive function, and measurably reduces oxidative stress and inflammation (as reflected by a decrease in the markers malondialdehyde, interleukin-6, and tumor necrosis factor). One study of 420 people found that after engaging in forest therapy, cortisol levels dropped by an average of 12.4 percent (see page 340), sympathetic nervous activity dropped by 7 percent, systolic blood pressure decreased by 1.4 percent, heart rate dropped by 5.8 percent, and parasympathetic nervous activity (indicating a relaxed state) increased by a whopping 55 percent.

For people with borderline hypertension, forest therapy helped restore blood pressure to the optimal range, potentially preventing the condition from progressing to clinical hypertension. And for elderly patients with confirmed high blood pressure, a 7-day forest therapy trip resulted in lower inflammation and the inhibition of the renin-angiotensin system (a hormone system involved in blood pressure regulation), thus reducing the risk of cardiovascular disease. Individuals with chronic widespread pain saw significant relief from their pain, as well as associated physical and psychological symptoms, following a 2-day forest therapy camp. And on top of all that, the physiological effects of forest therapy have included improved immune function and even a protective effect against cancer!

Other forms of nature-based therapy have had a positive effect on human health. Horticultural therapy, in which gardening is used to improve mental and/or physical well-being, shows potential as a mental health intervention as well as for the management and prevention of chronic diseases. Within the scientific literature, gardening consistently leads to benefits such as better life satisfaction, stronger sense of community, improved cognitive function, more vigor, reduced stress and anxiety, less fatigue, less anger, reduced depression symptoms, lower BMI, and greater overall happiness—just to name a few! A systematic review of horticultural therapy trials found that gardening may be an effective treatment for a variety of mental and behavioral disorders, including dementia, depression, and schizophrenia, and can have a positive effect on terminal cancer care.

Wilderness therapy (sometimes called adventure therapy or outdoor behavioral health care) is another form of nature-based therapy with impressive—and sometimes life-changing—benefits. Wilderness therapy involves excursions into the outdoors, typically with activity-based challenges and group or individual therapy, as a way to address mental, relational, and behavioral problems. This form of therapy has been used to help at-risk youth, victims of rape or abuse, and survivors of other forms of trauma, with documented success.

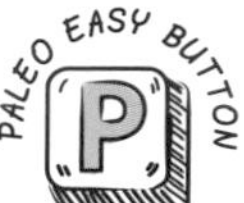

Here are some easy tricks for bringing nature into your life:

- *Make time for a nature walk, whether it's in the woods, on the beach, in an urban park, in your backyard, or in any other green space you can find.*
- *Grow a few plants in your backyard, on your balcony, or on your windowsill.*
- *Keep cut flowers or herbs in a vase.*
- *Listen to nature sounds while you work or commute.*
- *Look at scenic photos of nature.*
- *Use phytoncide-rich (wood) essential oils.*
- *Look for opportunities to spend time in nature when you go on vacation.*
- *Take up an active hobby that can be done in nature, like mountain biking, birdwatching, or mushroom hunting.*

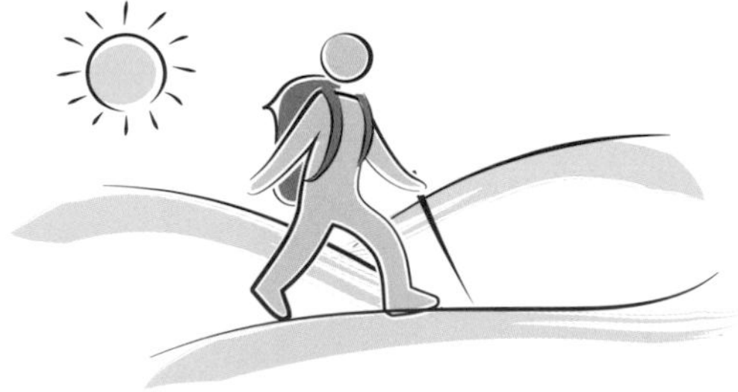

SUN EXPOSURE

Another important feature of being outside comes from the sun. Sun exposure plays a critical role in our health, both by helping us produce vitamin D and by regulating our circadian rhythm.

For decades, we've been told to limit sun exposure due to concerns about skin cancer. While it's true that too much exposure to intense ultraviolet light can cause DNA damage in our skin cells and increase our risk of skin cancer, it's also true that too *little* sun exposure creates a different set of health problems—including raising the risk of multiple forms of cancer (including, ironically, skin cancer!), cardiovascular disease, cognitive problems, eye diseases, multiple sclerosis, and diabetes. As long as we aren't getting sunburned, exposure to ultraviolet light is not only safe, it's essential for our health.

Vitamin D

In response to ultraviolet (UV) light exposure, our bodies produce vitamin D—a steroid hormone that controls the expression of more than 200 genes and the proteins that those genes regulate. When UVB radiation hits our skin, it triggers the generation of vitamin D3 (cholecalciferol) from its precursor (7-dehydrocholesterol), which is present in the outermost layer of the skin. From there, that cholecalciferol undergoes a series of metabolic steps (specifically, hydroxylation) in the liver and kidneys until it becomes the final—and biologically active—form of vitamin D3, called 1,25-dihydroxyvitamin D3 or calcitriol. That's a pretty impressive chain of events sparked by just a little sunlight!

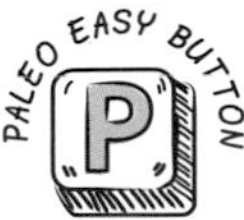

While getting a sunburn is definitely detrimental, vitamin D production is maximized when we're not blocking UV rays from penetrating our skin (by wearing sunscreen, UV-blocking clothing, and so on). Dim-light melatonin production is maximized when we're not wearing sunglasses. Clearly, the need for sun protection varies depending on the season, your location, and how long you plan to be outside; however, when it is possible and safe, go without.

To review, the roles that vitamin D plays in our bodies are vast:

- It is essential for mineral metabolism; it regulates the absorption and transport of calcium, phosphorous, and magnesium.
- It is crucial for bone mineralization and growth.
- It regulates several key components of the immune system, including the formation of important antioxidants.
- It has recently been shown to decrease inflammation and may be critical in controlling autoimmune and inflammatory diseases.
- It is involved in the biosynthesis of neurotrophic factors, regulating the release of such important hormones as serotonin, required not only for mental health but also for healthy digestion.
- It helps control cell growth, so it is essential for healing.
- It activates areas of the brain responsible for biorhythms.

Each year, scientists continue to discover new ways in which vitamin D is essential for human health!

Unfortunately, almost 50 percent of people worldwide (and up to 75 percent of Westerners) suffer from vitamin D insufficiency, putting billions at risk of earlier mortality and a long list of chronic diseases. Research shows that low vitamin D levels are associated with higher risk of colorectal cancer, breast cancer, bladder cancer, cardiovascular disease, metabolic syndrome, type 2 diabetes, Alzheimer's disease, cognitive decline, non-alcoholic fatty liver disease, dental cavities (in infants), macular degeneration, and myopia. Because most of our organs and cells have vitamin D receptors, it makes sense that inadequate vitamin D levels can have a negative effect on nearly every area of the body. By some estimates, almost 13 percent of all deaths in the United States could be attributable to low vitamin D levels!

Speaking of which: what vitamin D levels are considered healthy, exactly? This is a surprisingly controversial question! Many health authorities recommend levels of 25(OH)D (as measured by the 25-hydroxyvitamin D blood test) to be at least 30 ng/

ml, while other scientists and institutes, such as the Endocrine Society, recommend that levels be in the range of 40 to 60 ng/ml. At this point, we can say with confidence that levels significantly below 30 ng/ml (for men, women, and children alike) are unlikely to support optimal health, whether or not clinical symptoms of deficiency emerge.

In lieu of sun exposure, can we simply take a vitamin D supplement to stave off deficiency and decrease our risk of disease? While vitamin D supplementation can definitely be helpful (especially for people who can't get enough UVB exposure due to the time of year or the latitude of where they live), a surprising body of literature suggests that at least some of sunlight's protective effects are independent of vitamin D. In fact, in many studies, vitamin D levels may simply be a marker for UVB exposure rather than the active agent in disease risk reduction. For example, one experiment found that moderate UV radiation exposure could reduce the progression of malignant colon tumors but that vitamin D supplementation had no effect. Other studies have shown a negative relationship between sun exposure and multiple sclerosis, prostate cancer, and non-Hodgkin's lymphoma, but *not* between vitamin D levels (or intake) and those conditions.

How can sun exposure improve our health in ways other than boosting our vitamin D status? Hormones may be one piece of the puzzle!

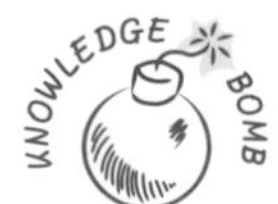

Ultraviolet is a higher-energy electromagnetic radiation than the light we can see, with wavelengths in the 10 to 400 nanometer range. (Visible light has wavelengths of between 400 and 700 nanometers.) About 10 percent of the total light output of the sun is in the form of UV light. It can classified into types based on its wavelength:

- *UVA is the longest-wavelength UV light and therefore has the least energy. Most of the UV light that reaches the Earth's surface (95 percent) is UVA. It causes the immediate tanning effect, contributes to skin aging and wrinkling, and increases the risk of skin cancer via indirect DNA damage.*
- *UVB is medium-wavelength UV light and has higher energy than UVA. Most of it is absorbed by the atmosphere, but about 5 percent of the UV light that reaches the Earth's surface is UVB. It is responsible for delayed tanning and burning and increases the risk of skin cancer via direct DNA damage. UVB is the type of UV light needed for vitamin D synthesis.*
- *UVC is short-wavelength UV light and would be the most damaging except that it is entirely absorbed by the atmosphere and does not reach the Earth's surface.*

Circadian Rhythm (Again!)

Cells throughout the body, including the skin and eyes, are sensitive to blue light from the sun, which is strongest in the morning (as opposed to the softer golden light that comes as sunset approaches). When special cells in the retina of the eye are stimulated by sunlight, they directly affect the pituitary gland and the hypothalamus region of the brain. The hypothalamus is responsible for circadian rhythm (the body's internal clock, discussed in Chapter 26) and regulation of hormones and the nervous system. Proper regulation of circadian rhythm is crucial for quality sleep, stress management, and the cyclic pattern of expression of many hormones in the body. The circadian clock also regulates certain components of cell survival and growth, making it a key player in protecting us from cancer.

The light-dark cycle (meaning that it's light out during the day and dark out at night) is a powerful signal to our circadian clock, and spending time outside during the day is one of the best things we can do to protect our circadian rhythm, including evening melatonin production. This is particularly true because our modern lives often flood us with the blue light of electronic screens at night, when our eyes should be receiving warm light in the yellow-orange range, which disrupts our bodies' clocks. This disruption can be so harmful that, according to multiple studies, exposure to unnatural light cycles is associated with higher risks of cancer and cardiovascular disease, sleep disturbances, mood disorders, and metabolic problems. Shift workers with an inverted schedule (who see little daylight but are exposed to long periods of nighttime illumination) are at a particularly high risk of obesity, diabetes, cardiovascular disease, and cancer.

One important circadian rhythm hormone, produced by the brain's pineal gland and regulated by sunlight, is melatonin. In addition to being critical for quality sleep, melatonin is a powerful antioxidant, is important for intestinal function, and can help prevent depression.

The hypothalamus and the pituitary gland influence the adrenal glands, which control cortisol production. Again, these important effects on brain activity, which increase alertness, improve cognition, and boost mood and vitality, are all independent of vitamin D production!

Of course, getting daily sun exposure is a piece of cake if you live in the tropics (and have a schedule that allows you to go outside during daylight hours), but what about those of us who do shift work, live in areas with gloomy climates, endure long, dark winters, or face other challenges to getting out in the sun?

Bright light therapy (sometimes called phototherapy) is one tool for helping us stay healthy when sunlight is out of reach. It involves exposing ourselves to full-spectrum light (resembling the composition of sunlight, but typically filtering out UV rays) early in the day, especially upon waking, with the use of special light boxes or lamps. Light therapy sessions typically last between 15 minutes and several hours. Although bright light therapy is most commonly used to treat seasonal affective disorder, a form of depression that strikes some people in late fall and winter, when days become shorter and sunlight becomes scarce, its ability to recalibrate our internal clock means it can benefit the many areas of our health affected by our circadian rhythm. Even so, bright light therapy is only a "plan B"; sun exposure is still our best bet!

Skin Cancer

What about skin cancer? For those of us who've spent years religiously lathering up with sunscreen—or avoiding the sun entirely—out of fear of developing skin cancer, it may seem counterintuitive that outdoor occupations and non-burning sun exposure are actually associated with a *lower* risk of skin cancers, particularly melanoma. In fact, some researchers believe that the rising rates of skin cancer over the past 80 years are due to the steady increase of indoor occupations and activities during that same time. Along with heightening global rates of vitamin D deficiency, these two lifestyle factors tend to make people more susceptible to burning when they finally do get outdoors.

From a mechanistic standpoint, we know that vitamin D (in its biologically active form) inhibits the growth of keratinocytes and melanocytes, the predominant cells in the skin, as well as promotes differentiation, which should in theory reduce the risk of skin cancer. But epidemiological studies haven't shown a clear connection between vitamin D levels and melanoma risk. So, while vitamin D certainly benefits our health in many ways, it's probably not the only reason non-burning sun exposure seems to protect against skin cancer.

Therefore, when it comes to the sun, there's a definite "Goldilocks" zone in which sun exposure is great enough to keep vitamin D levels high but not so intense that it causes burning. Where this sweet spot is depends on a few factors:

- **Where we live:** UVB radiation is more intense the closer we get to the equator.
- **How dark our skin is:** Darker skin contains more melanin, which reduces the risk of burns and increases the length of time we need to spend in the sun in order to produce vitamin D. Melanin is also the protein responsible for tanning: our skin cells produce it to absorb UV radiation and dissipate the energy as harmless heat, blocking the UV rays from damaging skin tissue.
- **What time of day we're outside:** The midday sun is the most intense.
- **A variety of hereditary factors:** Some people have genetically lower levels of vitamin D and may need more time in the sun to bring their levels up into the healthy range.

No matter which way we look at it, making time to get outdoors and enjoy nature's gifts—including sunshine, sights, smells, sounds, and sensations—is well worth it!

Chapter 30:
SOCIAL CONNECTION

Among the many lifestyle factors that influence our health (and serve as important Paleo principles), one in particular has been proven to greatly impact physical health yet is under-recognized in conventional medicine: *connection.* That is, our relationships with the individuals around us—our friends, family, neighbors, coworkers, and other members of our community (this can even include animals!).

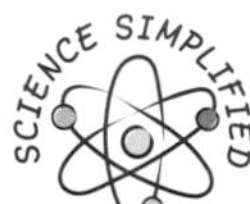

Connection is the subjective feeling of closeness to and belonging with others. It improves health through its impact on hormones (especially the stress hormone cortisol) and the immune system.

The benefits of having a strong social network go beyond the practical aspects of help and support in our day-to-day lives. Just knowing that we have people who are there for us and feeling connected to even a handful of people we trust and love can make a huge difference to our health. In fact, research shows that having an inner circle of eight to ten people we can depend on and confide in is optimal.

Researchers have examined the role that connection plays in our health by looking at the two "extremes" of connection:

- Social isolation and loneliness, which correspond with increased risk of morbidity and mortality
- A strong social support network, which corresponds with decreased risk of disease and increased longevity

Across the board, having strong social connections appears to protect us against disease and even extend our life span, while a lack of such a network significantly harms our health.

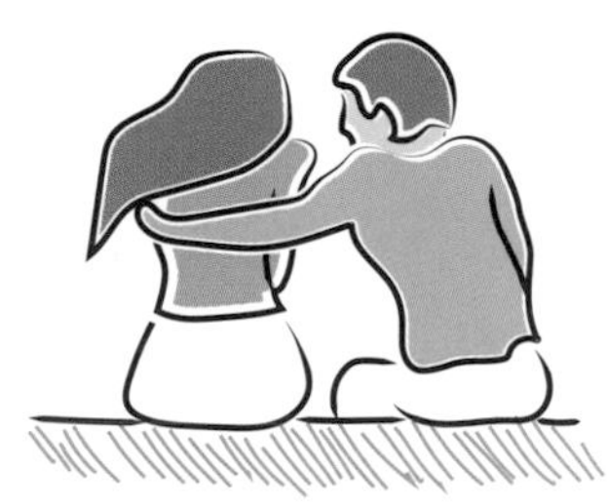

CONNECTION, DISEASE RISK, AND LONGEVITY

One meta-analysis of 148 different studies found that people with stronger social relationships had a 50 percent higher chance of survival than people with weaker social bonds, regardless of age, gender, cause of eventual death, length of follow-up period, or how healthy each person was at the beginning of the study. Another meta-analysis found that social isolation, loneliness, and solitary living raised the risk of death by 29 percent, 26 percent, and 32 percent, respectively. Additional research has shown that social isolation raises mortality risk independent of loneliness (and vice versa), meaning that even if we don't *feel* lonely, a lack of social support might still be harming our health. Conversely, if we feel lonely despite having plenty of social connections, we're still at risk of earlier death.

Among the elderly, loneliness is a major predictor of dementia; one study found a 64 percent higher risk among older patients who reported feeling lonely compared to those who didn't. In younger and middle-aged adults, having a greater variety of social ties—including with parents, partners, friends, coworkers, and other community members—is associated with a greater resistance to upper respiratory infections. In fact, the role of social connection on immunity has been confirmed in multiple studies: for example, one study evaluated how loneliness and a lack of social connection affected antibody production in response to a vaccine and showed that it was substantially inhibited, indicating a suppressed immune response. Among healthy adults, social isolation increases the risk of cardiovascular disease by dysregulating neuroendocrine, metabolic, and cardiovascular processes. And for adults already diagnosed with heart disease, a lack of perceived social support can worsen the progression and prognosis of the disease.

HEALTH QUICK-START *A feeling of social connection is subjective, meaning that what matters is whether you feel connected, not how many friends you have. A great place to start is by carving out time to nurture relationships, whether that's date night with your spouse or a weekly walk with your BFF.*

In short, virtually everyone is negatively affected by a lack of social connectedness and benefits from having strong ties to others! This quote sums up the profound impact of connection and community on our health:

> *Social relationships, or the relative lack thereof, constitute a major risk factor for health–rivaling the effect of well established health risk factors such as cigarette smoking, blood pressure, blood lipids, obesity and physical activity.*
>
> —House, J. S., K. R. Landis, and D. Umberson. "Social Relationships and Health." *Science* 241, no. 4865 (1988): 540–45.

How can social relationships affect our health so dramatically? In a basic sense, humans are hardwired to be social creatures. Positive social interactions stimulate changes in hormones that affect nearly every system in the body. People who feel more connected to others have lower levels of anxiety and depression. Connection also improves self-esteem and causes greater empathy for others. Those who feel connected to others are more trusting and cooperative, and therefore others are more open to trusting and cooperating with them. Social connectedness creates a positive feedback loop of social, emotional, and physical well-being.

This is all great news if you're close with your family, have an awesome group of friends, and live in a tight-knit community. But it's much less great if you're one of the growing number of people who live far from home, feel like you have friendly acquaintances rather than true friends, and generally have a sense that life would be better if you lived somewhere else. Sound familiar?

The bottom line is this: it's important to nurture relationships and feel connected to people (as well as the companion animals that share our homes!). This time investment is worth every minute when we think of not only the improvements in quality of life when that life is shared with wonderful people, but also the direct health benefits that we experience. There's a bit more scientific detail to go over, but if you're eager to take action on this key Paleo principle, feel free to jump to page 377 for tips on improving social connection.

CONNECTION AND CORTISOL

The benefits of connection go beyond knowing who to call at 3 a.m. when one of the kids needs to be taken to the ER on the same day your spouse is out of town on a business trip. A social network is important for hormone regulation. Research has shown that social interaction and connection reduce the body's secretion of cortisol.

As discussed in detail in Chapter 27, cortisol is the master stress hormone. It is synthesized from cholesterol by the adrenal glands and is involved in diverse essential functions in the body. As part of the fight-or-flight response, cortisol's primary action is to redirect fuel to the organs that need it most—basically, the brain and muscles for enhanced decision-making, reflexes, and speed. Cortisol does this by stimulating gluconeogenesis, the production of glucose from fatty acids and amino acids in the liver. Under normal conditions, this rapid rise in glucose would cause increased insulin secretion, which would shuttle the glucose into storage. However, cortisol also counteracts insulin, creating a state of hyperglycemia (high blood sugar). Cortisol takes over control of blood glucose concentration by simultaneously stimulating glycogen synthesis in the liver and glycogenolysis, the breaking down of glycogen to glucose (and glucose-1-phosphate) in the liver and muscles; this is achieved by increasing the activity of the hormone glucagon, which is basically the opposite of insulin. The increased glucose provides quick fuel for the body. By interacting with different receptors in different tissues, cortisol is also able to control which tissues can utilize this glucose and which tissues are low priority. Cortisol increases circulating ketone bodies (which the brain can use as energy) by stimulating lipolysis, the breakdown of triglycerides into free fatty acids. Cortisol also raises the level of free amino acids in the blood, probably in preparation for healing damaged tissues.

Cortisol shuts down nonessential processes to reserve resources for immediate survival needs. This means that increased cortisol suppresses the digestive system, the reproductive system, growth, the immune system, collagen formation, amino acid uptake by muscle, and protein synthesis, and it even decreases bone formation. Cortisol release also communicates with regions of the brain that control mood, motivation, and fear. In the context of surviving immediate danger, this has a negligible effect on overall health, but in the context of chronic stress, these "other" effects of cortisol become a very big problem.

While it is best known for its contribution to the fight-or-flight response, cortisol has many other essential roles in the body. Other functions of cortisol include regulating circadian rhythms, blood pressure, cardiovascular function, inflammation, and the immune system and controlling carbohydrate metabolism.

Chronic stress increases the risk of chronic disease through the actions of cortisol. Once we understand how cortisol interacts with so many different systems in the body, it's easy to understand just how detrimental chronic stress can be. In fact, chronic stress is thought to be the biggest contributor to cardiovascular disease (that's right, it's stress, not diet), but because chronic stress is itself inflammatory, it can contribute to every non-infectious disease.

The link to connection? Feeling socially connected lowers cortisol and makes us more resilient to psychological stressors, meaning that our bodies produce less cortisol when we're stuck in traffic. Positive social interactions reduce the effects of chronic stress, and that leads to improved health in the long term.

CONNECTION AND INFLAMMATION

One of the most intriguing ways in which social connection can benefit our health is by influencing the body's inflammatory responses. Inflammatory markers like C-reactive protein (CRP) and pro-inflammatory cytokines (such as interleukin-1, interleukin-6, and tumor necrosis factor-α) are reliable predictors for all-cause mortality, cardiovascular disease, arthritis, type 2 diabetes, Alzheimer's disease, and even periodontal disease, and inflammation is also believed to be a risk factor for most types of cancer. For each of these conditions, different mechanisms explain the link between inflammation and disease development; for example, pro-inflammatory cytokines contribute to diabetes by suppressing insulin signal transduction, and they increase cancer risk by influencing tumor cell survival, proliferation, and invasion; angiogenesis; and metastases.

The effect of social connection on inflammation (and, subsequently, inflammation-related diseases) is multifaceted. We now know that psychological and social stress can cause the body to produce pro-inflammatory cytokines in the same way that infection or injury can. For example, relationship conflict and inadequate social support have been shown to promote depression, which can influence the secretion of pro-inflammatory cytokines both directly (through changes in central nervous system, endocrine, immune, and neural pathways) and indirectly (by causing inflammation-promoting behavioral changes, such as disturbed sleep). In genomics studies, people who are socially isolated tend to under-express genes involved in anti-inflammatory responses while overexpressing genes involved in pro-inflammatory responses. In other words, being socially disconnected or stressed appears to promote inflammation in the body.

At the same time, higher degrees of social integration, which encompasses a person's ties to family, friends, and the larger community, are associated with lower levels of interleukin-6 and C-reactive protein. Pregnant women who are socially supported throughout their pregnancies have lower levels of CRP, and among older women, having trusting and satisfying relationships with other people is linked to lower levels of interleukin-6. Even in large observational and correlative studies, social connectedness, social integration, and lower interpersonal conflict are all associated with lower levels of interleukin-6 and CRP. Given how strongly biomarkers of inflammation predict disease and mortality risk, it makes sense that inflammation could be a major mediator in the link between social connectedness and human health.

CONNECTION AND OXYTOCIN

Physical touch is an important component of social connectedness and comes with its own set of health benefits. Research has shown that physical connection—hugging a family member, enjoying sexual relations with a partner, cuddling with a pet, or receiving therapeutic touch or massage—reduces cortisol. A variety of studies have shown that therapeutic touch, when added to hospital care, improves patient outcomes in a variety of ways.

Touch, love, and positive social interactions increase the hormone *oxytocin,* which is sometimes referred to as the "love hormone." Oxytocin is produced by specialized neurons in the thalamus and then stored and released by the posterior pituitary gland. Upon release, oxytocin is associated with feelings of contentment and calm, reductions in anxiety, and increases in human bonding and trust. It also inhibits fear and nervousness. We may recognize oxytocin as the hormone released during childbirth and breastfeeding. Like most hormones, it has many roles in the body.

Importantly, increased oxytocin levels lead to decreased activity in the hypothalamic-pituitary-adrenal axis (or HPA axis, which controls the production of cortisol) and enhanced immune function. Essentially, increasing oxytocin protects against stress. In fact, positive social interaction has been shown to have a direct impact on wound healing, attributable to increased levels of oxytocin. Oxytocin also modulates inflammation by decreasing some pro-inflammatory cytokines. Whether the effects of oxytocin are completely due to direct interactions with the immune system or to effects on cortisol and the HPA axis remains unknown. Either way, the feeling of connection is important for general health and well-being.

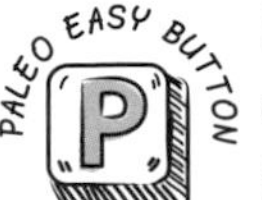

Many of the same activities that improve our resilience to stress also increase our feelings of social connection. Check out the tips for improving resilience on pages 350 to 353.

ONLINE CONNECTION

As our lives become increasingly "digitally connected," many of us find ourselves maintaining relationships through various social media platforms—sometimes at the expense of seeing each other in person. Do these online connections benefit us in the same way as face-to-face interactions?

The answer is: it's complicated! On one hand, research confirms that online relationships fail to deliver the same level of intimacy experienced when spending time with someone in person, that online interactions are less effective at delivering emotional support, and that social support contributes to overall life satisfaction only if it's delivered offline rather than on the internet. This is true even when internet users feel more connected on a very short-term basis—for example, right after posting or receiving a comment on Facebook. Worse, some studies suggest that spending significant time on social media is associated with greater feelings of social isolation, depression, and envy, although it's unclear whether time online *causes* these feelings or simply fails to relieve the loneliness of people who go online looking for a sense of community and support.

In support of the latter hypothesis, studies show that people with preexisting depression and anxiety are more vulnerable to the harmful effects of social media use, especially when exposed to negative social interactions like cyberbullying. In turn, these types of negative interactions are linked to lower self-esteem, decreased life satisfaction, and more rumination—or dwelling on adverse events and perceived self-shortcomings. People who score high on the "social comparison orientation" personality trait are at a particularly high risk of feeling lonely when broadcasting on social media; the same goes for people who have low perceived "communication competence" (a general evaluation of their communication behavior and skills)—suggesting that certain characteristics could mediate the link between social media use and negative psychological outcomes.

Social media use has also been linked to sleep disturbances. In one study, the young adults who spent the most time on social media each week had a 192 percent higher risk of sleep disturbances than those with the lowest usage. Instagram, specifically, is associated with lower psychological well-being, particularly among young adults, especially when it comes to orthorexia (an obsessive focus on eating only those foods perceived to be healthy) and other forms of disordered eating.

On the other hand, social media appears to be neutral or beneficial when used to keep in touch

A WORD ON PETS

Although human companions are absolutely important, owning a pet has also been associated with a variety of health benefits. The root of these benefits is probably the fact that owning a companion animal reduces stress and depression, resulting largely from the same oxytocin release that makes human touch so therapeutic. A number of fascinating research papers show that companion animals also reduce blood pressure, reduce blood cholesterol and triglycerides, improve outcomes in cardiovascular disease sufferers, lower risk of heart attack and stroke, alleviate allergies, reduce obesity, improve rheumatoid arthritis and osteoporosis, and benefit those with ADHD.

For example, among heart attack survivors, those who own dogs are significantly less likely to die within a year of the attack than those who don't own dogs. Spending 30 minutes interacting with a dog has been shown to boost dopamine and endorphin levels while also decreasing levels of cortisol; a similar effect was found in health-care workers after only 5 minutes of petting a dog. Even among children, sitting or reading near a dog results in lower blood pressure than performing the same activities with no animal nearby. Some research even suggests that being in the presence of a dog causes a more powerful reduction in cardiovascular stress than being in the presence of a friend or spouse. Dogs don't get all the credit, though: one recent study showed that owning a cat reduced the risk of dying from cardiovascular disease, especially stroke, much more than owning a dog. And of course, dozens of studies have looked at pet ownership in general and have shown health benefits across the board.

While pet ownership can never replace the social support we gain from our fellow humans, having a companion animal can be a boon to health (allergies notwithstanding!).

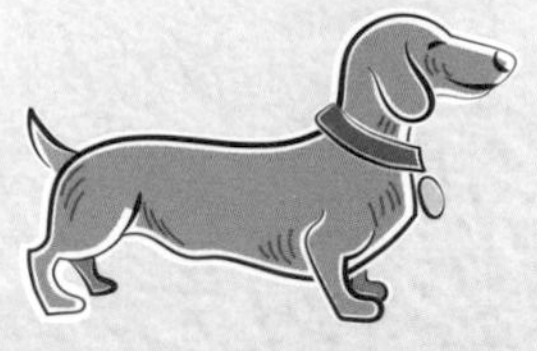

between in-person meetings with friends, family, colleagues, and significant others. People without depression or anxiety are more likely to experience benefits from communicating with others online, without the psychological harm documented in some studies. Likewise, individuals whose online social networks are made up primarily of people they know in real life (as opposed to strangers) are far less likely to experience depression or anxiety in association with social media use.

So what's the takeaway? When we use our online social connections to augment offline relationships rather than replace them, and when we're already psychologically healthy, social media can be a perfectly fine tool for helping us stay connected. This is particularly true for people who use social media to keep in touch with loved ones and for people who aren't prone to comparing themselves to others online. However, people who suffer from anxiety or depression, as well as people without strong real-life social networks, may experience more harm than good when they rely on the internet to meet their social needs. In other words, context is important!

SCIENCE SIMPLIFIED *Having hundreds of social media "friends" isn't doing you any favors if you aren't nurturing those relationships offline, meaning in person whenever possible but also in other one-on-one interactions, like phone calls.*

SIMPLE TIPS FOR IMPROVING SOCIAL CONNECTION

Spending meaningful time with others appears to be more difficult than ever before. So how can we gain the benefits of having a strong social network when our lives are busy, our friends and families live far away, and our communication is frequently online?

It's easier than it seems! Research shows that providing social support may be even more beneficial than receiving it. Research also shows that the subjective feeling of connection is much more important than the size of our support network; in other words, we don't need to be social butterflies to reap the health benefits of connection, as long as we have some close relationships that nourish our social needs. This is great news because it means that we have the power to create social connection simply by reaching out to others. There's no quota of friends or family members we need to have in our inner circle.

While there are many ways to improve social connection and shore up a support network, here are a few strategies to consider:

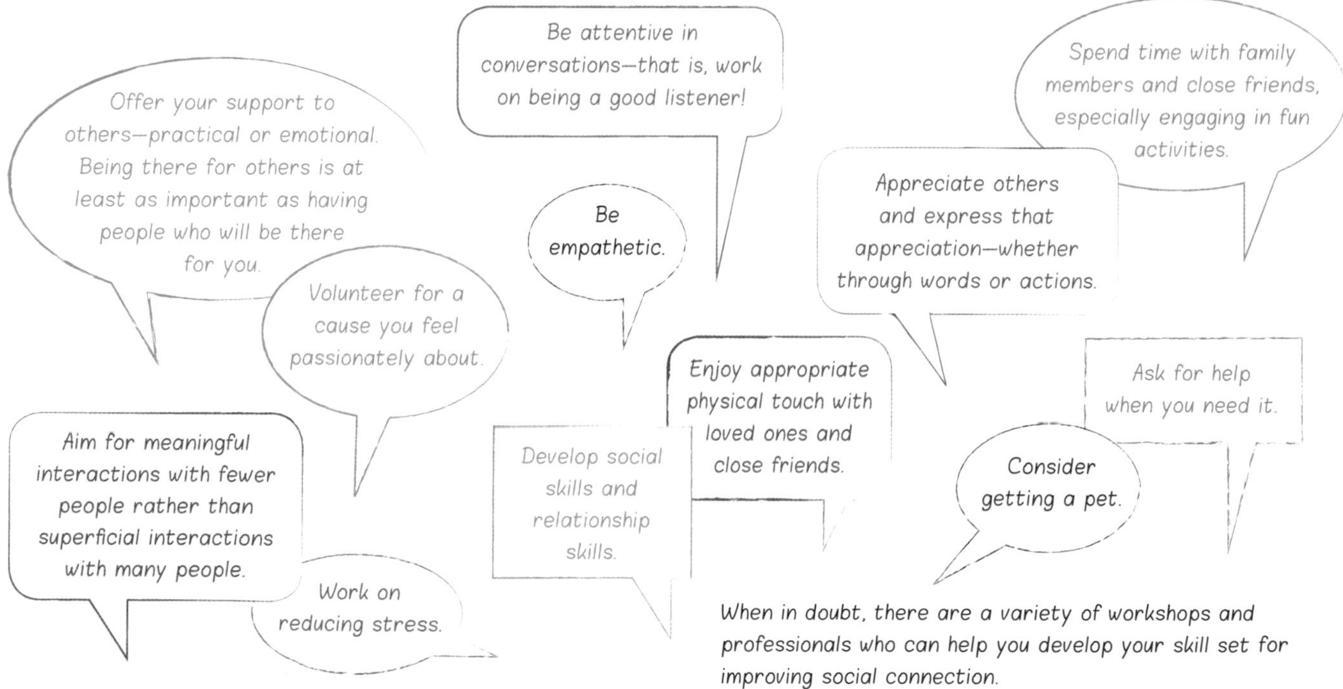

Offer your support to others—practical or emotional. Being there for others is at least as important as having people who will be there for you.
Be attentive in conversations—that is, work on being a good listener!
Be empathetic.
Spend time with family members and close friends, especially engaging in fun activities.
Appreciate others and express that appreciation—whether through words or actions.
Volunteer for a cause you feel passionately about.
Enjoy appropriate physical touch with loved ones and close friends.
Ask for help when you need it.
Aim for meaningful interactions with fewer people rather than superficial interactions with many people.
Develop social skills and relationship skills.
Consider getting a pet.
Work on reducing stress.

When in doubt, there are a variety of workshops and professionals who can help you develop your skill set for improving social connection.

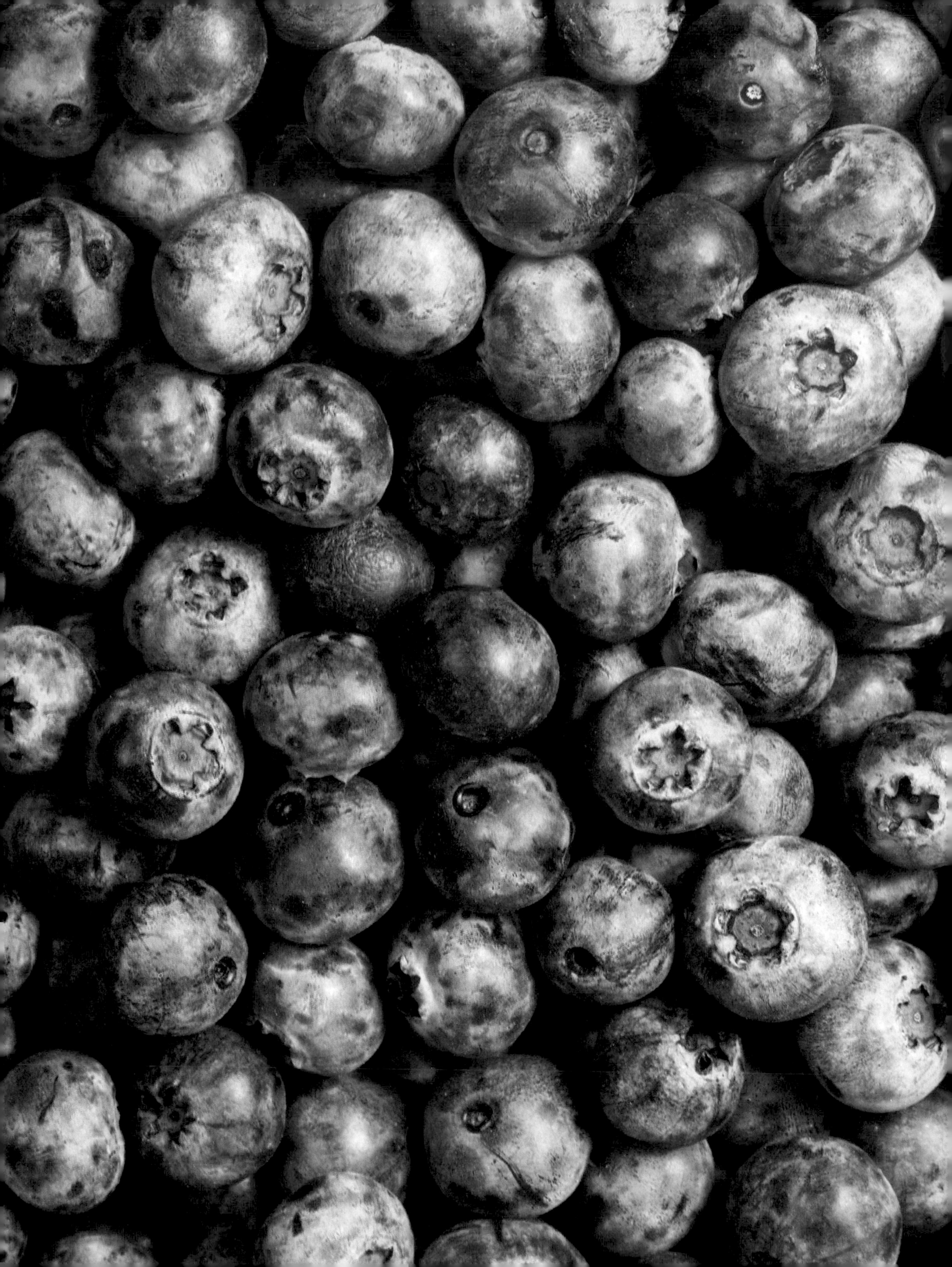

6.

PUTTING PALEO INTO PRACTICE

Congratulations! You have emerged from about three college courses' worth of nutritional science, physiology, anthropology, and cell biology. Now it's time to put all that knowledge into practice!

I fully expect that some readers will skip forward to this part of the book for a fast-track implementation of the Paleo principles while continuing to learn about the science behind them. That's totally fine! These chapters can be thought of as a review, distilling the tremendous amount of information in the Introduction and first thirty chapters of the book into actionable steps to help you regain your health and live your best life.

I am a person who needs to know the science behind my options in order to be consistently motivated to make the best choice. And I know I'm not alone in that regard. So as we move on to topics related to practical implementation, keep in mind that every recommendation is founded on scientific research and the big-picture implications of the current body of knowledge.

Also keep in mind that within the Paleo framework, there is a great deal of room for customization to meet your individual needs, preferences, and health goals. To help you identify the best choices for you, Chapter 32 outlines two different strategies for transitioning to a healthier diet, Chapter 33 summarizes many of the health goal/condition-specific information shared throughout this book, and Chapter 34 introduces some troubleshooting strategies to help you break through common barriers to success.

Chapter 31:
THE PALEO PRINCIPLES

When we think of Paleo, the *last* thing that should come to mind is a set of rigid restrictions that make our lives harder. We need to excel beyond a set of "healthy diet and living" rules by which we are expected to abide. I'll remind you of a statistic that I shared way back in the Introduction: at least 60 percent of people will choose to eat something unhealthy even though they know they "shouldn't." By understanding the detailed scientific rationale behind healthy eating and living guidelines, we can transcend the rules while improving the quality of our day-to-day choices.

Instead of a set of rules, the principles that Paleo is built upon are meant to liberate us, bringing us greater freedom from disease and closer to the health and wellness that we all deserve to experience. In that sense, these principles are more like stepping stones toward a better future.

To summarize what's been discussed in this book thus far, the guiding principles of the Paleo framework are:

Maximize nutrient density. Focusing on minimally processed whole plant foods (especially vegetables) and animal foods (including seafood and organ meat) while limiting energy-rich, nutrient-poor foods (like refined sugar, refined grains, and processed vegetable oils) helps us obtain the highest concentration of micronutrients per calorie of food we consume (see Chapter 1).

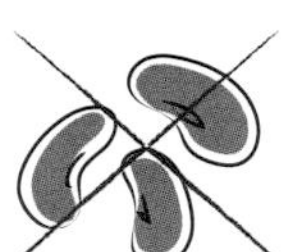

Avoid toxins. Grains, pseudograins, legumes, and even nuts and seeds, albeit in much smaller quantities, contain natural toxins that can harm the gut or inhibit mineral absorption, including prolamins (such as gluten), agglutinins (such as wheat germ agglutinin), and phytates (see page 228). Some vegetables also contain naturally occurring toxins that certain people are particularly sensitive to, such as the glycoalkaloids found in nightshades (see page 296).

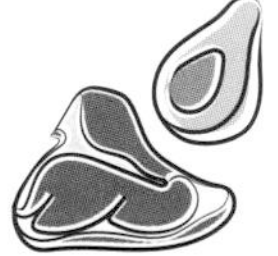

Embrace diverse omnivorism. Humans are omnivores, and our nutritional needs are best met with a diet that includes a variety of plant and animal foods. Neither veganism nor strict carnivorism is optimal for human health (see Chapter 3).

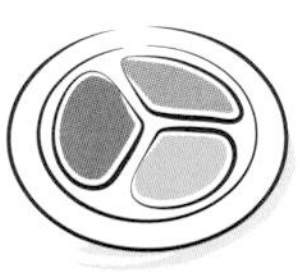

Eat balanced macronutrients. Fat, protein, and carbohydrate all play important roles in human health, but any one macronutrient in excess can be problematic; the same goes for eating too *little* of any macronutrient. Aim for a 30/30/40 ratio; it doesn't matter which one is the 40, and there's lots of wiggle room! (See Chapter 2.)

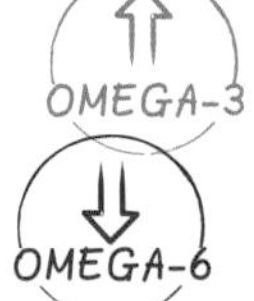

Balance omega-3 and omega-6 fats. The Standard American Diet is skewed heavily toward pro-inflammatory omega-6 fats, raising the risk of many chronic diseases. Eating more omega-3-rich foods, like seafood, while decreasing intake of omega-6 rich foods, like grains and vegetable oils, helps create a healthier balance (see page 183).

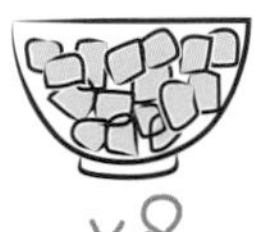

Eat eight (or more!) servings of vegetables per day. Along with being an incredible source of micronutrients, vegetables supply fiber and phytochemicals that can protect against numerous chronic diseases. Aim to eat the rainbow (red radishes, orange carrots, dark leafy greens, purple cabbage, white cauliflower, and so on) to ensure that you receive the full spectrum of what vegetables have to offer (see Chapter 8).

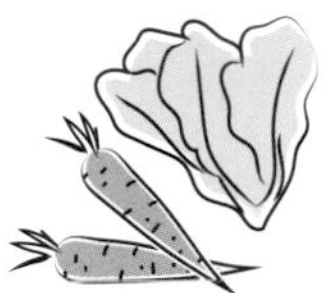

Eat plenty of fiber to support the gut microbiota. Fiber (including fiber from Paleo starches; see page 153) feeds the beneficial microbes in our guts, which in turn help neutralize toxins, produce certain vitamins and short-chain fatty acids, support digestion, protect against diseases, and assist in a number of metabolic processes. When our microbial colonies are healthy, our entire bodies benefit (see pages 39 and 70).

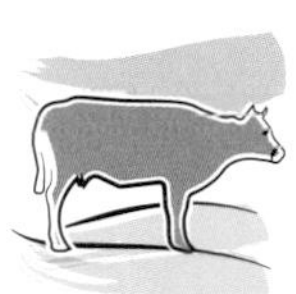

Focus on food quality. Whenever possible, buying food that's locally sourced, organic, fresh, and, in the case of animal foods, grass-fed, pasture-raised, or wild-caught helps ensure maximum nutrient density as well as promotes sustainability and lowers toxin exposure (see page 221).

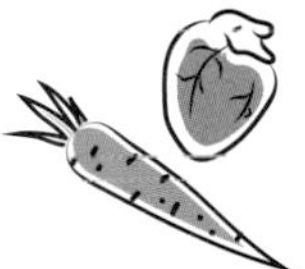

Focus on food variety. The more we can vary the foods on our plates day to day and season to season, the higher our chances of micronutrient sufficiency. Mix up the types of vegetables you eat, look for fun varieties of your staples (like purple carrots or heirloom lettuce), eat meats from different animals, and embrace snout-to-tail ideals (see page 220).

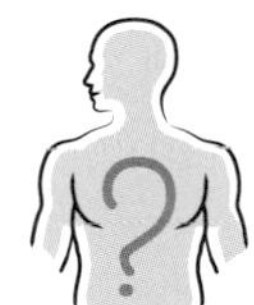

Understand your own body. Many foods have check marks in both the pros and cons categories; these foods may work well for some people but not for others. Methodically testing your individual tolerance to these foods while understanding whether these foods are likely to support your specific health goals is a prerequisite for determining whether to include them in your diet (see Chapter 25).

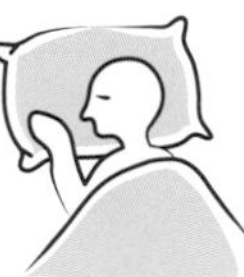

Sleep. Getting adequate sleep—7 to 9 hours for most adults—reduces the risk of a number of chronic diseases (including diabetes, heart disease, and stroke), improves vitality and mood, improves athletic performance and work performance, decreases inflammation, regulates the immune system, regulates hunger and metabolism, reduces stress, and gives us energy throughout the day. It can even help us live longer (see Chapter 26)!

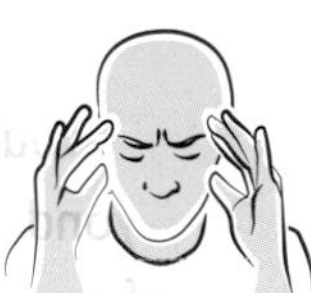

Manage stress. Reducing unnecessary stress in our lives (including saying "no" to optional activities that would drain us, asking for help when we're feeling overwhelmed, and reevaluating our goals and priorities), as well as taking measures to better handle the stress we can't avoid (such as through meditating, spending time in nature, walking, and stretching), helps support healthy hormone function, reduces inflammation, improves immunity and sleep quality, and reduces cravings and uninhibited eating behaviors (see Chapter 27).

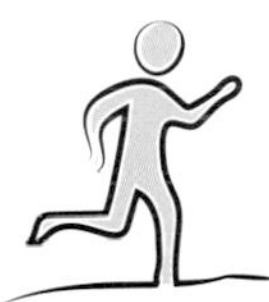

Be active. Frequent gentle movement (such as walking, yoga, or stretching), as well as moderate-intensity activity that you find enjoyable and that works with your particular health situation (such as hiking or lifting weights) can decrease your risk of cardiovascular disease, type 2 diabetes, depression, and some cancers, as well as improve your mood. At the same time, it's important to avoid *over*-exercising, which can create a new set of health problems. (See Chapter 28.)

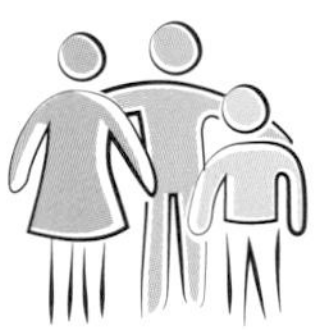

Seek community. Social connection provides profound health and longevity benefits. Even if you're not close to your family and don't have a spouse, making an effort to nurture existing relationships or form new ones can go a long way. Even owning a pet has been shown to reduce risk factors for chronic disease and obesity (see Chapter 30).

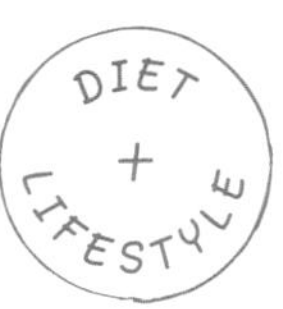

Focus on diet *plus* lifestyle. A great diet can only take us so far if healthy lifestyle factors aren't in place, and a healthy lifestyle won't keep us totally healthy if our diet is poor. Combining diet and lifestyle is the best way to see maximum benefit from the Paleo template.

PALEO CHEAT SHEET

EAT:

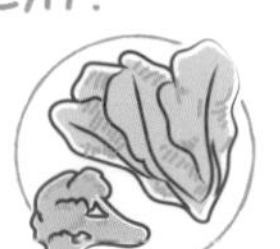
Vegetables of all kinds

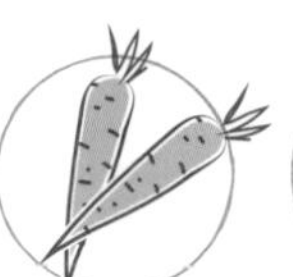
Roots and tubers

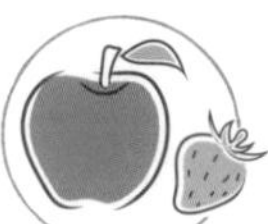
Fruit

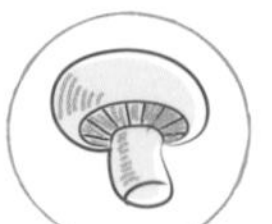
Mushrooms and other edible fungi

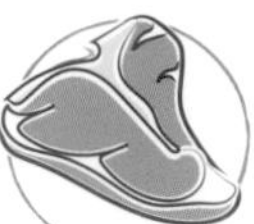
Red meat

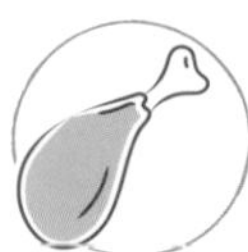
Poultry

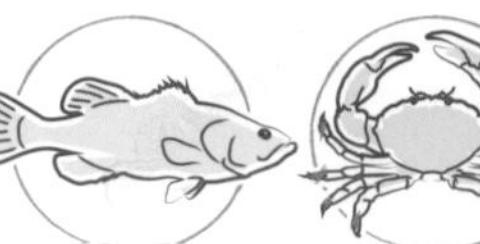
Fish

Shellfish

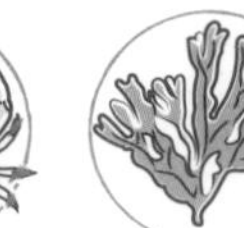
Sea vegetables

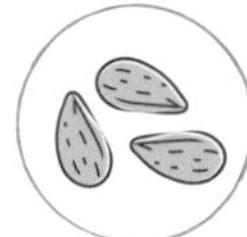
Nuts

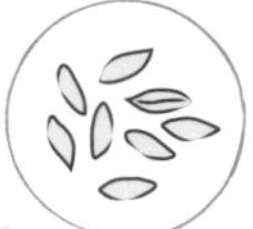
Seeds

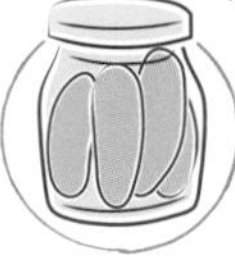
Fermented foods

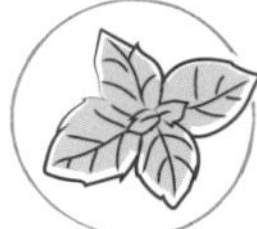
Herbs and spices

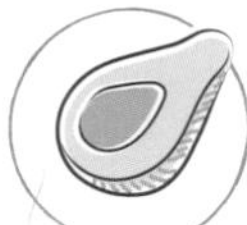
Healthy fats

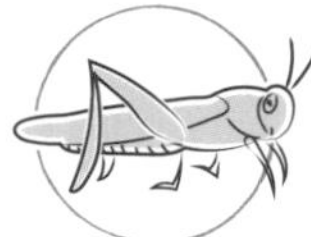
Edible insects

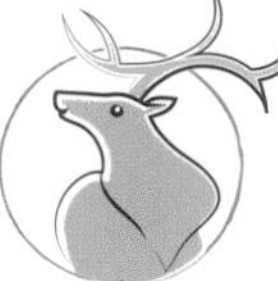
Wild game

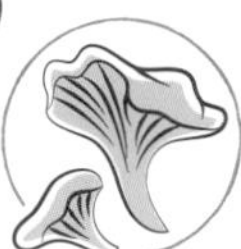
Wild edibles

AVOID:

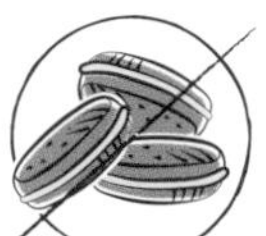
Processed and refined foods

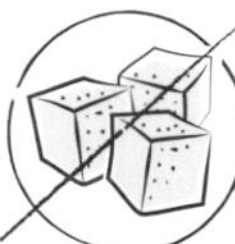
Refined sugars

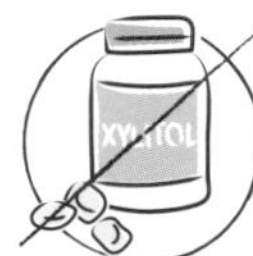

Sugar substitutes

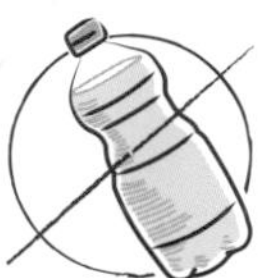
Refined vegetable oils

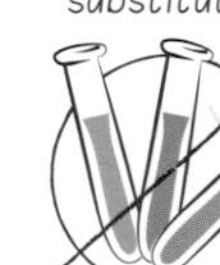
Trans fats

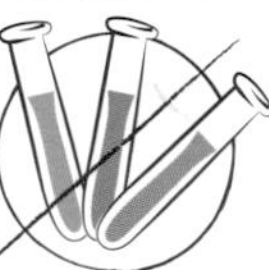
Chemical additives

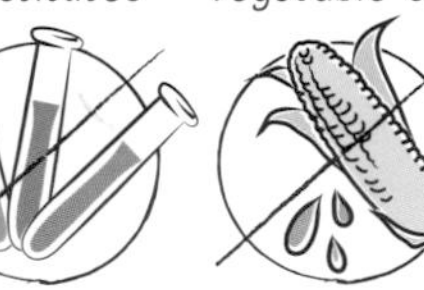
Artificial colors and flavorings

High-fructose corn syrup

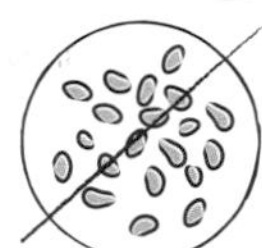
Grains (especially wheat, barley, and rye)

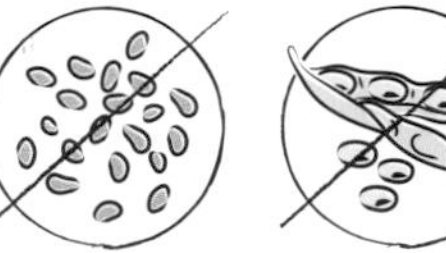
Pseudograins

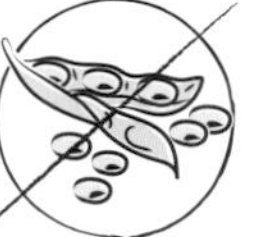
Legumes (especially soy, peanuts, and kidney beans)

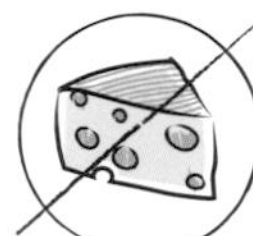
Conventional dairy products

IMPORTANT DIETARY FACTORS:

Nutrient density

Seasonal variation

High variety

Snout-to-tail (nothing wasted)

High fiber (lots of veggies!)

High phytochemicals (lots of veggies!)

Whole, unprocessed, unrefined foods

BALANCED MACRONUTRIENTS:

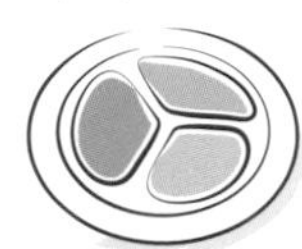

20% to 35% **PROTEIN**

20% to 40% **CARBOHYDRATE**

20% to 50% **FAT**

EXAMPLES OF PALEO FOODS:

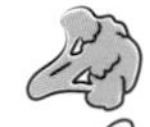
VEGETABLES: asparagus, broccoli, Brussels sprouts, cabbage, celery, kale, lettuce, spinach

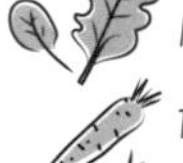
ROOTS AND TUBERS: beets, carrots, cassava, parsnips, sweet potatoes

FRUIT: berries, citrus, cucumbers, melons, squash

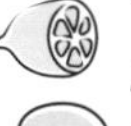
MUSHROOMS: button, cremini, oyster, portabella, shiitake

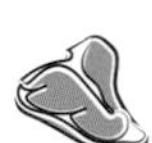
RED MEAT: beef, bison, lamb, pork, rabbit

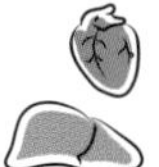
ORGAN MEAT: heart, kidney, liver, sweetbreads, bone broth

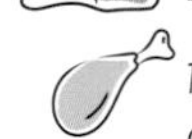
POULTRY: chicken, turkey, duck, goose, pheasant

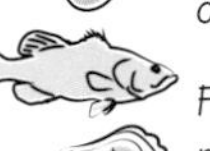
FISH: cod, halibut, mackerel, salmon, tuna

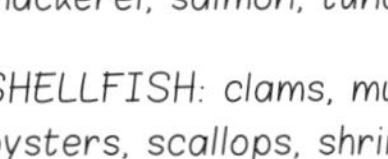
SHELLFISH: clams, mussels, oysters, scallops, shrimp

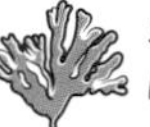
SEA VEGETABLES: arame, kelp, kombu, nori, wakame

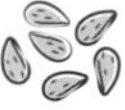
NUTS: almonds, Brazil nuts, macadamia nuts, pine nuts, coconut

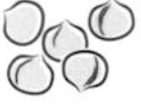
SEEDS: sunflower seeds, pumpkin seeds, sesame seeds

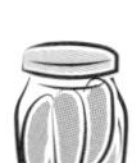
RAW FERMENTED FOODS: kimchi, pickles, sauerkraut, kombucha, water kefir

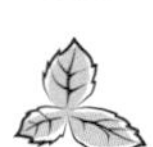
HERBS AND SPICES: basil, oregano, parsley, cinnamon, ginger

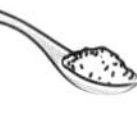
UNREFINED SEA SALT: Himalayan pink salt, Celtic sea salt, sea vegetable salt

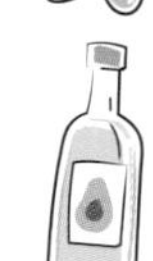
HEALTHY FATS: avocado oil, coconut oil, extra-virgin olive oil, grass-fed ghee, pasture-raised lard, grass-fed tallow

FIND YOUR INDIVIDUAL TOLERANCE TO THE FOLLOWING ITEMS (see Chapter 24):

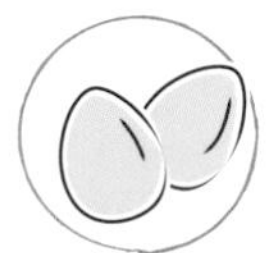
Eggs

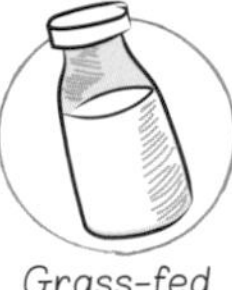
Grass-fed dairy

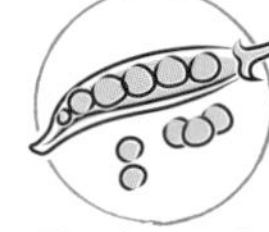
Traditionally prepared legumes

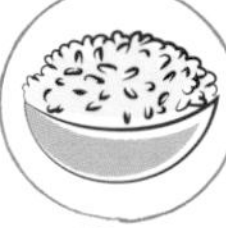
Rice

Nightshades (including white potatoes)

Alcohol

Coffee

Natural sweeteners like honey and maple syrup

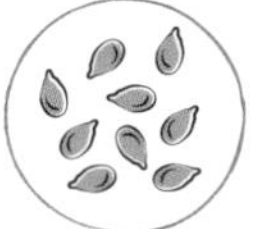
Chia seeds, flax seeds, and psyllium seed and husk

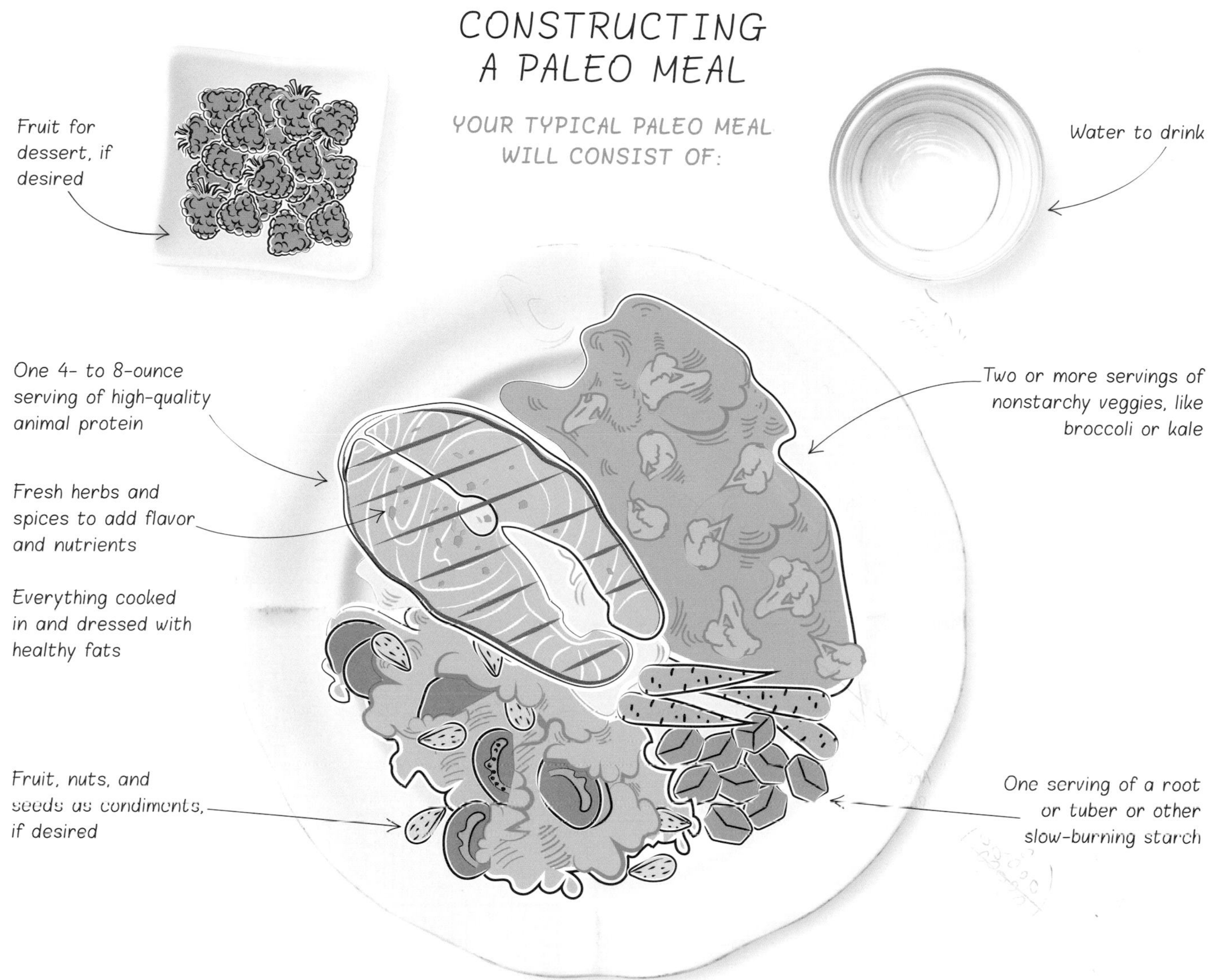
CONSTRUCTING
A PALEO MEAL
YOUR TYPICAL PALEO MEAL
WILL CONSIST OF:
Fruit for dessert, if desired
Water to drink
One 4- to 8-ounce serving of high-quality animal protein
Two or more servings of nonstarchy veggies, like broccoli or kale
Fresh herbs and spices to add flavor and nutrients
Everything cooked in and dressed with healthy fats
Fruit, nuts, and seeds as condiments, if desired
One serving of a root or tuber or other slow-burning starch

WHEN CONSTRUCTING A MEAL, THINK OF:

NUTRIENT-DENSE PROTEINS:
Choose fish, shellfish, and organ meat for proteins more often; seek the highest-quality meat you have access to and can afford (grass-fed or pasture-raised, organic).

TONS OF VEGGIES:
Aim for at least three servings per meal to hit your eight-a-day minimum.

EATING THE RAINBOW:
Choose vegetables of different colors.

MIXING UP RAW VERSUS COOKED:
Vary the way you prepare your vegetables.

SLOW-BURNING CARBS:
Choose starchy roots and tubers.

PHYTOCHEMICAL-RICH FRUITS:
Options like berries and citrus pack more antioxidant bang for your buck.

NUTS AND SEEDS AS CONDIMENTS:
Aim for up to 1 ounce of nuts and seeds per day.

CHOOSING HIGH-QUALITY FATS FOR COOKING AND DRESSING:
Use rendered fats from grass-fed or pasture-raised animals, high-quality cold-pressed extra-virgin olive oil, avocado oil, coconut oil, or grass-fed butter or ghee.

ADDING A PROBIOTIC FOOD:
Think of raw sauerkraut or pickles as a probiotic boost to your meal.

USING FRESH HERBS AND SPICES WHENEVER POSSIBLE:
Fresh herbs and spices not only provide tons of flavor and variety, but also are packed with vitamins, minerals, and phytochemicals.

COOKING AT HOME MOST OF THE TIME:
Take control of your food quality by committing to cooking your meals yourself; when eating out, choose healthier options like farm-to-table restaurants.

AVOIDING GETTING IN A RUT:
Aim for a wide variety of fruits, vegetables, cuts of meat, types of seafood, and so on.

LIFESTYLE CHANGES SUPPORT DIETARY CHANGES (AND VICE VERSA)

Although it's tempting to look at diet and lifestyle as separate topics, they're fundamentally linked in terms of how they impact our health.

Focusing on lifestyle can make a huge difference in terms of the ease of transition to a Paleo diet. For example, when we get adequate sleep and manage stress, we're less likely to crave sugar and overeat. Getting enough sleep not only makes us more likely to choose vegetables and fruit (and less likely to choose fast food and junk food), but it also regulates hunger so we snack less and consume fewer overall calories (without trying!). Getting enough sleep even helps us make better choices in the grocery store. Stress tends to make us crave energy-dense (high-sugar and/or high-fat) foods while depleting our bodies of important nutrients like vitamin C and magnesium.

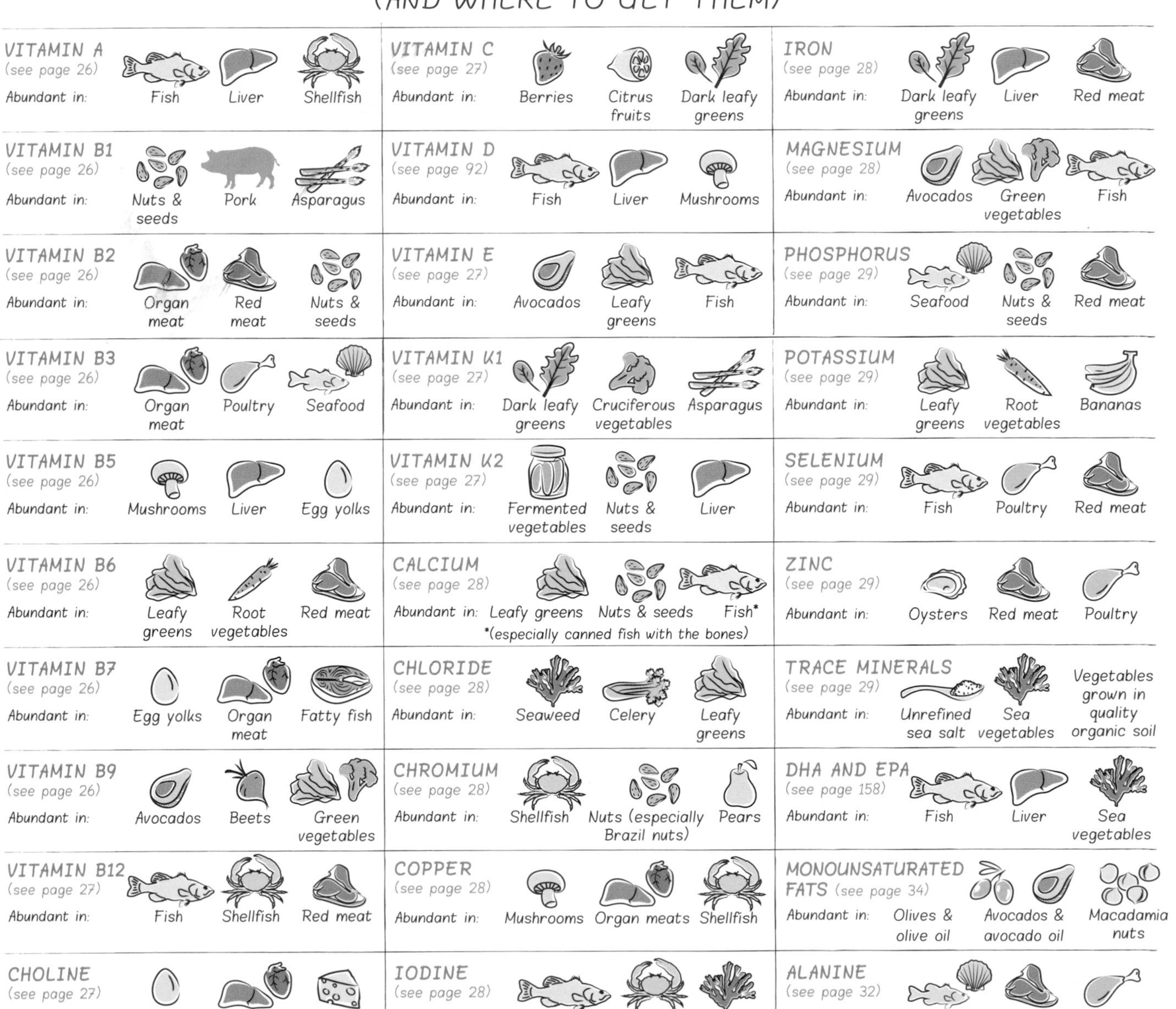

ESSENTIAL AND IMPORTANT NUTRIENTS (AND WHERE TO GET THEM)

		Abundant in
VITAMIN A	(see page 26)	Fish, Liver, Shellfish
VITAMIN B1	(see page 26)	Nuts & seeds, Pork, Asparagus
VITAMIN B2	(see page 26)	Organ meat, Red meat, Nuts & seeds
VITAMIN B3	(see page 26)	Organ meat, Poultry, Seafood
VITAMIN B5	(see page 26)	Mushrooms, Liver, Egg yolks
VITAMIN B6	(see page 26)	Leafy greens, Root vegetables, Red meat
VITAMIN B7	(see page 26)	Egg yolks, Organ meat, Fatty fish
VITAMIN B9	(see page 26)	Avocados, Beets, Green vegetables
VITAMIN B12	(see page 27)	Fish, Shellfish, Red meat
CHOLINE	(see page 27)	Egg yolks, Organ meat, Grass-fed dairy
VITAMIN C	(see page 27)	Berries, Citrus fruits, Dark leafy greens
VITAMIN D	(see page 92)	Fish, Liver, Mushrooms
VITAMIN E	(see page 27)	Avocados, Leafy greens, Fish
VITAMIN K1	(see page 27)	Dark leafy greens, Cruciferous vegetables, Asparagus
VITAMIN K2	(see page 27)	Fermented vegetables, Nuts & seeds, Liver
CALCIUM	(see page 28)	Leafy greens, Nuts & seeds, Fish*
CHLORIDE	(see page 28)	Seaweed, Celery, Leafy greens
CHROMIUM	(see page 28)	Shellfish, Nuts (especially Brazil nuts), Pears
COPPER	(see page 28)	Mushrooms, Organ meats, Shellfish
IODINE	(see page 28)	Fish, Shellfish, Sea vegetables
IRON	(see page 28)	Dark leafy greens, Liver, Red meat
MAGNESIUM	(see page 28)	Avocados, Green vegetables, Fish
PHOSPHORUS	(see page 29)	Seafood, Nuts & seeds, Red meat
POTASSIUM	(see page 29)	Leafy greens, Root vegetables, Bananas
SELENIUM	(see page 29)	Fish, Poultry, Red meat
ZINC	(see page 29)	Oysters, Red meat, Poultry
TRACE MINERALS	(see page 29)	Unrefined sea salt, Sea vegetables, Vegetables grown in quality organic soil
DHA AND EPA	(see page 158)	Fish, Liver, Sea vegetables
MONOUNSATURATED FATS	(see page 34)	Olives & olive oil, Avocados & avocado oil, Macadamia nuts
ALANINE	(see page 32)	Seafood, Red meat, Poultry

*(especially canned fish with the bones)

When we engage in gentle movement throughout the day, our insulin sensitivity improves and we can better handle Paleo-friendly carbohydrates. When we focus on lifestyle, it's much easier to make major or difficult changes to our diet.

The converse is also true: focusing on diet can help us dial in lifestyle factors. For example, habitually drinking too much coffee can magnify cortisol release in response to psychological stressors. Likewise, studies have shown that a deficiency in omega-3 fats exaggerates stress responses and that supplementing with fish oil reduces cortisol secretion in response to stress. Studies also show that consuming a serving of slow-burning carbohydrates with dinner can improve sleep quality, as can eating a high-fiber diet in general and moderating saturated fat intake. Consuming adequate amounts of quality protein aids in muscle recovery after workouts and helps preserve muscle mass while losing weight.

All this is to say that if you're struggling to implement some facet of the Paleo template, be it sticking with the dietary guidelines, getting enough sleep, managing stress, or getting enough activity, think about the challenge in a holistic way. You may find that improving another aspect of the Paleo template is the key to overcoming your challenge.

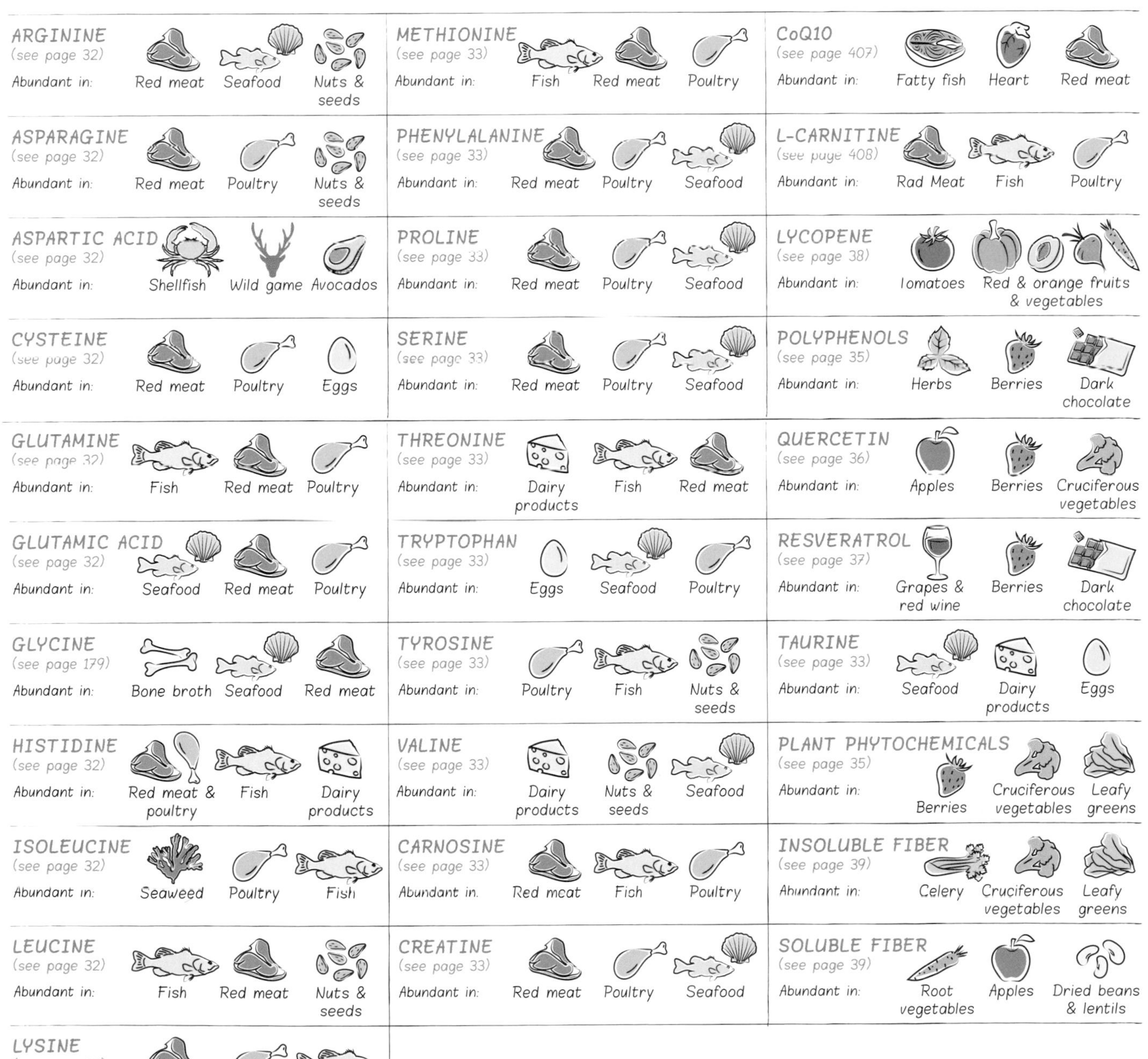

ARGININE (see page 32) Abundant in: Red meat, Seafood, Nuts & seeds
ASPARAGINE (see page 32) Abundant in: Red meat, Poultry, Nuts & seeds
ASPARTIC ACID (see page 32) Abundant in: Shellfish, Wild game, Avocados
CYSTEINE (see page 32) Abundant in: Red meat, Poultry, Eggs
GLUTAMINE (see page 32) Abundant in: Fish, Red meat, Poultry
GLUTAMIC ACID (see page 32) Abundant in: Seafood, Red meat, Poultry
GLYCINE (see page 179) Abundant in: Bone broth, Seafood, Red meat
HISTIDINE (see page 32) Abundant in: Red meat & poultry, Fish, Dairy products
ISOLEUCINE (see page 32) Abundant in: Seaweed, Poultry, Fish
LEUCINE (see page 32) Abundant in: Fish, Red meat, Nuts & seeds
LYSINE (see page 33) Abundant in: Red meat, Poultry, Fish
METHIONINE (see page 33) Abundant in: Fish, Red meat, Poultry
PHENYLALANINE (see page 33) Abundant in: Red meat, Poultry, Seafood
PROLINE (see page 33) Abundant in: Red meat, Poultry, Seafood
SERINE (see page 33) Abundant in: Red meat, Poultry, Seafood
THREONINE (see page 33) Abundant in: Dairy products, Fish, Red meat
TRYPTOPHAN (see page 33) Abundant in: Eggs, Seafood, Poultry
TYROSINE (see page 33) Abundant in: Poultry, Fish, Nuts & seeds
VALINE (see page 33) Abundant in: Dairy products, Nuts & seeds, Seafood
CARNOSINE (see page 33) Abundant in: Red meat, Fish, Poultry
CREATINE (see page 33) Abundant in: Red meat, Poultry, Seafood
CoQ10 (see page 407) Abundant in: Fatty fish, Heart, Red meat
L-CARNITINE (see page 408) Abundant in: Rad Meat, Fish, Poultry
LYCOPENE (see page 38) Abundant in: Tomatoes, Red & orange fruits & vegetables
POLYPHENOLS (see page 35) Abundant in: Herbs, Berries, Dark chocolate
QUERCETIN (see page 36) Abundant in: Apples, Berries, Cruciferous vegetables
RESVERATROL (see page 37) Abundant in: Grapes & red wine, Berries, Dark chocolate
TAURINE (see page 33) Abundant in: Seafood, Dairy products, Eggs
PLANT PHYTOCHEMICALS (see page 35) Abundant in: Berries, Cruciferous vegetables, Leafy greens
INSOLUBLE FIBER (see page 39) Abundant in: Celery, Cruciferous vegetables, Leafy greens
SOLUBLE FIBER (see page 39) Abundant in: Root vegetables, Apples, Dried beans & lentils

A DIET THAT'S NOT A *DIET*

Despite being called the "Paleo diet," we shouldn't think of Paleo in the same way we do the Atkins Diet, the South Beach Diet, or other programs designed as temporary ways to lose weight. Paleo isn't a quick fix (although many people do experience rapid results after adopting a Paleo lifestyle). Rather, it's a framework that informs our daily food choices and permeates other areas of our lives to become the "new normal" for how we think about food, sleep, stress, activity, and community. When we adopt this way of eating and living, the goal is to be in it for the long haul, not just to lose 10 pounds for an upcoming event.

Whereas fad diets are often scientifically unsound and hard to adhere to long-term, Paleo has abundant scientific support and is designed to provide everything we need in life. Unlike diets that have rigid rules about fat or carbohydrate grams, calories, "points," number of meals per day, or other metrics that take away the joy and spontaneity of eating, Paleo is simply a guide—a scientific foundation for understanding the optimal food choices that nourish our bodies.

When we refer to the Paleo diet, we're referring to the scientific definition of *diet*—that is, it describes the foods we habitually eat. Think of it this way: lifelong health requires a lifelong commitment to healthy habits. The Paleo principles inform those healthy habits and keep you motivated to make the best choices as often as possible.

BALANCE AND SUSTAINABILITY: THE 80/20 RULE

In a perfect world, we would all adhere to the Paleo principles at every meal (and in that same perfect world, we'd be able to get gluten-free, additive-free, organic, local, in-season grass-fed or pastured foods wherever we went). However, the goal of following a Paleo diet isn't to achieve perfection at the cost of making our lives harder! The 80/20 rule (also called the Pareto principle) states that 80 percent of the results of a situation are obtained by 20 percent of the causes. Applied to diet, this means we can obtain the majority of the benefits Paleo can bring by focusing on a handful of changes, rather than needing to adhere to the diet perfectly 100 percent of the time.

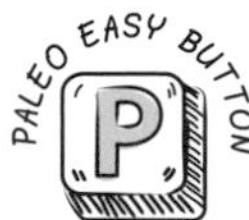

To help you stay on track for an entire week, consider allowing yourself one to three "cheat meals" per week. The caveat is to make sure that even your cheat meals avoid ingredients that you react to—like gluten, dairy, or soy—which you need to eliminate and challenge in order to identify (see Chapter 25 for the protocol).

What does this look like in practice? You do need to follow the guidelines more than 20 percent of the time! But what it *does* mean is that many people feel amazing when they home in on the most important Paleo principles (summarized on pages 380 and 381) without being fanatical about their execution. In terms of meals, this means:

- Swapping out empty calories (like pasta or bread) for vegetables
- Structuring most of your meals to include a quality animal protein, a few servings of veggies, and maybe some fruits or nuts
- Identifying and eliminating foods that are particularly problematic for you as an individual—gluten, dairy, and soy being the most common culprits
- Ditching junk food and fast food completely
- In terms of lifestyle, this means getting enough sleep, exercising on most days, and striving for work-life balance.

Some people opt to strictly follow the Paleo dietary guidelines most of the time but include one to three cheat meals during the week. Others opt for an entire cheat day once every 1 to 2 weeks. Yet others opt to include a few non-Paleo foods in their regular diets, knowing that any detriment from that food is counterbalanced by all their other good choices. On the other side of the spectrum, many people with chronic illnesses choose to eschew all non-Paleo foods all the time. Where you land on this spectrum is up to you, although it's worth emphasizing that it's much, much easier to make informed choices about which off-plan foods you eat and how often once you have done a period of elimination and challenge (see Chapter 25). Another word of caution: don't let missing an old favorite food cloud your judgment about how that food impacts your health.

In reality, most of us will be fine eating some non-Paleo foods occasionally, such as at business meetings, while traveling, or simply because we're craving something non-Paleo. During these off-plan moments, the biggest concern for most people is to remain gluten-free, since a large portion of the population carries the HLA-DQ2 or DQ8 genes associated with celiac disease and gluten sensitivity. (It's true that a minority of the population legitimately doesn't need to avoid gluten, but if you haven't done blood tests, genetic testing, and/or elimination and challenge to know for sure, it's best to steer clear.) However, any other foods that garner a reaction when you consume them should be considered off-limits for your cheat meals. Again, that's where methodically identifying your particular trigger foods comes in super-handy.

The trick to long-term health is to use the 80/20 rule as a way to strike a balance so that you can stick with the healthy habits defined by Paleo principles for the rest of your life. The 80/20 rule backfires when it is used as an excuse never to fully adopt the Paleo diet in the first place—or to derail, overindulge, and fall back down that slippery slope into old, unhealthy habits.

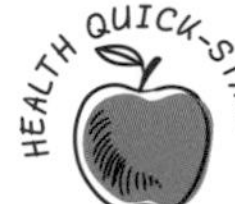

Those with autoimmune diseases or other chronic illnesses might not see substantial improvement in their conditions if they allow themselves cheat meals. For more on mitigating autoimmune and other chronic illnesses, read my book The Paleo Approach.

For a sustainable lifelong approach to Paleo, we need to understand which foods are optimal for our bodies and which foods our bodies merely tolerate (which we discover through an elimination and challenge protocol). This information forms the constraints for individual implementation and allows for the dietary flexibility that is necessary for continued success. For example, you will likely find that your body is happiest when you eat mostly organic local veggies, seafood, and grass-fed meat, but you might also discover that you feel fine when you consume some gluten-free grains, as long as they don't displace too many nutrient-dense foods. With this information, you might choose to eat some gluten-free products when traveling or eating out.

Ultimately, the 80/20 rule grants us more flexibility and enhances Paleo's long-term sustainability (and gives us permission *not* to beat ourselves up if we eat something non-Paleo on occasion!). It means that following the Paleo dietary guidelines most (but not all) of the time will still yield great results in terms of health for most people. The best part about the 80/20 rule is that it allows us to adapt the Paleo diet (in an informed way) to fit our lives rather than forcing our lives to conform to a rigid Paleo template.

IS PALEO TOO EXPENSIVE?

Grass-fed and pastured meats and wild-caught seafood, which are the pinnacle of quality and offer a better fat profile and more essential nutrients, can cost more than conventionally produced meat and seafood. Organic and locally grown vegetables and fruits, which can have double or more of the essential vitamins, minerals, and phytochemicals, are often more expensive than non-organic produce. And yes, that expensive estate olive oil *is* teeming with antioxidant polyphenols. But what if these options are too expensive for your budget? Or impossible to find near you?

From health and environmental perspectives, there are some compelling reasons to seek out the best-quality foods, but if they are not available to or affordable for you, that shouldn't be a nonstarter. The fact is, you can dramatically increase the nutrient density of your diet (while eliminating most problematic substances) and therefore improve your health simply by choosing foods that fall within the Paleo framework, even if you buy the conventionally grown versions at your local grocery or box store.

When a very tight budget puts even a diet based mostly on conventional meat and vegetables out of reach, using some of the inexpensive foods discussed in Chapter 24, such as white rice and traditionally prepared legumes, to stretch meals makes a ton of sense. Remember that there are no Paleo police. Use the information in this book to make the best choices you can within your means and let go of any guilt about not being "perfectly Paleo."

Likewise, you don't need an expensive gym membership to be active: walking is an incredible health-promoting activity. You can absolutely support your circadian rhythms and sleep quality without costly biohacks like light therapy boxes and amber-tinted glasses. Adopting the Paleo principles should not add to your stress but instead give you tools to improve your health, no matter where you start and no matter the individual challenges you face.

It's also worth noting that adopting a Paleo template often leads to savings in other areas. For example, you may find that as you cook more at home, you save a great deal of money that was being spent at restaurants and fast-food drive-thrus. You may be able to discontinue medications, saving on prescription drug costs and doctor's visit co-pays. You might find that by choosing to walk more, you save on gas. You may find a way to grow some vegetables in your backyard, saving you money at the grocery store or farmers market. As your health improves and your priorities shift, you may discover that you want to allot some of that saved money toward better-quality foods.

Of course, following the Paleo dietary guidelines does not automatically mean a larger grocery bill. Many families find that between shopping at local farms, farmers markets, and box stores; taking advantage of online discounts; discovering new inexpensive filler foods like sweet potatoes and cabbage; and avoiding expensive Paleo flour substitutes (these are used for Paleo adaptations of American favorites, but it's much better to stick with meals composed mainly of meat and veggies), they are absolutely able to stay on budget.

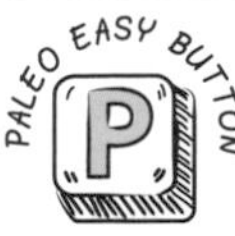

See page 390 for money-saving grocery shopping tips, as well as a list of priorities for those items worth an extra investment, if possible. Also see page 638 for a list of online vendors.

Nutritional Considerations for Conventional Foods

If you are restricted, by either budget or accessibility, to buying conventionally produced foods, what nutritional differences are there are to keep in mind?

Consideration #1: Omega-3 to Omega-6 Ratio

When buying conventionally produced meat and poultry, the biggest difference in terms of health is the ratio of omega-3 to omega-6 polyunsaturated fatty acids in those meats compared to their pasture-raised or wild equivalents. This is where the original recommendation to focus on lean meat, which is presented in the book *The Paleo Diet* by Loren Cordain, came from; that is, the assumption that most people will try to follow a Paleo diet using conventionally produced foods.

It may be tricky to achieve that optimal 1:1 to 1:4 omega-3 to omega-6 ratio, but it is possible with a little planning and careful choices. You will need to make an effort to both decrease your omega-6 intake and increase your omega-3 intake.

TO DECREASE OMEGA-6 INTAKE:

- **Limit consumption of nuts and seeds to 20 grams daily.** Most nuts and seeds are much (and sometimes much, *much*) higher in omega-6 fatty acids than omega-3 fatty acids. The exceptions are coconut, which is high in healthful medium-chain saturated fats; macadamia nuts, which have a very low polyunsaturated fatty acid content; and walnuts, which have a 1:3 ratio of omega-3 to omega-6.
- **Limit consumption of poultry.** Chicken and turkey have the highest omega-6 fatty acid content of any conventionally produced meat.
- **Stick with lean cuts of meat.** Fat is very healthful, so don't think this recommendation is about avoiding fat. The reason for this recommendation is that the fats in conventionally produced meat aren't the good fats that your body needs.
- **Really, *really* avoid refined vegetable oils.** See page 188 for a list of healthy fats for cooking and dressing food.

TO INCREASE OMEGA-3 INTAKE:

- **Eat more fish.** Even farmed fish has, at worst, a 1:2 omega-3 to omega-6 fatty acid ratio, and some fish have almost no omega-6 content whatsoever (and high omega-3!). Canned salmon, tuna, and sardines are inexpensive ways to include wild-caught seafood in your diet. You get the best omega-3 bang for your buck with oily coldwater fish like salmon and mackerel, but all types of seafood are good options.
- **Eat some sea vegetables.** Kelp noodles, seaweed snacks (avoid those cooked in canola oil), and nori are good options for boosting your omega-3s, especially DHA.
- **Buy omega-3 eggs.** If you can't afford or source completely pasture-raised eggs, which provide a great ratio of omega-3 to omega-6 fats along with a higher density of other nutrients, standard omega-3 eggs are a good option. (This higher quantity of omega-3 is typically achieved by feeding the chickens flax seed in addition to the other feed ingredients.) You will likely pay a bit more for omega-3 eggs than conventional eggs, but they are still a relatively cheap protein.

OMEGA-3

Consideration #2: Nutrient Density

Whether you're talking about meat or produce, conventionally produced foods have fewer vitamins, minerals, and antioxidants than their pasture-raised and locally grown equivalents, for a variety of reasons.

TO GET THE MOST NUTRIENTS YOU CAN FROM CONVENTIONAL MEAT AND PRODUCE, CONSIDER THESE GUIDELINES:

- **Eat vegetables as soon as possible after you buy them.** The longer vegetables are stored, the more the nutrients contained within them degrade.
- **Buy frozen veggies.** These are typically picked ripe (as opposed to ripening during storage and transport) and flash-frozen, which preserves many of their nutrients. They also tend to be cheaper—even organic!
- **Eat organ meat.** Organ meats have the advantage of being the most nutrient-dense foods available, and they are quite inexpensive. You can often find pasture-raised and grass-fed organ meat for cheaper than conventional ground beef! Even if you can't afford pasture-raised, conventional organ meat is a great choice.
- **Eat seafood.** Seafood is also extremely nutrient dense, even if it's farmed. While fresh seafood can be expensive, frozen and canned seafood is a much more affordable option.
- **Be picky about nuts.** If you're going to eat nuts and seeds, Brazil nuts, pumpkin seeds, sesame seeds, and sunflower seeds are the most nutrient dense. (See page 197.)
- **Mix up eating vegetables raw and cooked.** Some nutrients are enhanced by cooking, while others are degraded. (See page 143.)
- **Ferment your own fruits and vegetables.** Fermenting fruits and vegetables increases the digestibility, increases the bioavailability of nutrients, and makes these foods great sources of probiotics. It's also a great alternative to freezing when good-quality produce goes on sale.
- **Grow and gather your own!** Grow some of your own vegetables or gather wild edibles that grow around you (just make sure you are identifying wild berries and mushrooms accurately!).

Consideration #3: Variety

Variety is an important part of a healthy diet simply because different foods contain different nutrients. Eating a wide variety of foods is the easiest way to ensure that you aren't overdoing a particular nutrient or missing out on something your body needs to be healthy. What's the challenge when buying all your food at a typical grocery store? It's common for grocery stores to stock the same ol' standard fare, which limits the variety of meats, seafood, vegetables, and fruit available to you, especially as compared to what you can typically find at a good farmers market.

TO INCREASE THE VARIETY IN YOUR DIET:

- **Try shopping at different stores.** Even if you're limited to conventional grocery stores, one chain might carry some types of produce or meat that another chain does not. Ethnic and specialty markets are great places to find new foods that you can't get at your local grocery store.
- **Don't be afraid to buy things you've never tried.** Purchase that strange-looking root vegetable or that kind of fish you've never heard of. Try that cut of meat that you haven't eaten since you were a kid. The internet is a tremendous resource for recipes for those new foods.
- **Make an effort to cycle through the available foods at your local grocery store.** Even if you're stuck shopping at the same store every week, and even if the store doesn't have anything unusual to challenge your culinary skills, make sure to cycle through the variety to which you do have access; don't get stuck in a broccoli-and-carrots rut.
- **See if you can buy something different online.** If you've exhausted the variety available from your local stores, see what you can buy off the internet and have delivered to your door; this will help add a little "new" to your diet.
- **When you can't vary the ingredients, vary the cooking method.** Cooking foods in different ways can change their nutritional content and make some nutrients more available than others. Try cooking with different herbs, spices, and fats, too.

Getting the Best Bang for Your Buck

If you have a little extra cash to spend on just a few high-quality food items, it's helpful to know which ones will give you the most benefit for your dollar. Here are some great places to invest a little more money and see big returns in terms of nutrition:

- **Switch to unrefined sea salt or sea vegetable salt.** Yes, pink and gray salts are more expensive, but they offer a ton of trace minerals.
- **Buy grass-fed butter or ghee if you include dairy fat in your diet.** Butter and ghee are great sources of the fat-soluble vitamins A, D, and K2, in which many of us are deficient, and of the healthful fat conjugated linoleic acid (CLA). They also offer a good ratio of omega-3 to omega-6 fatty acids.
- **Buy lard from pasture-raised pigs and tallow from grass-fed cows.** Like grass-fed butter and ghee, these fats are great sources of vitamins A, D, and K2 and offer a good ratio of omega-3 to omega-6. Tallow is a good source of CLA. It's also very inexpensive to render your own lard and tallow; you'll find a recipe on page 485.
- **Eat some shellfish.** When it comes to nutrient density, shellfish is right up there with organ meat, although shellfish is definitely more expensive. The occasional serving of oysters can do wonders for the nutrient density of your diet.
- **Buy fatty cuts of grass-fed or pasture-raised meat.** Cuts like Boston Butt and 75 percent lean ground meat tend to be the cheapest cuts available. A growing number of companies ship meat nationwide, so ordering online is a great option if you don't have a nearby farmer to buy from. See page 638 for a list of online vendors.
- **Get familiar with the Dirty Dozen and Clean Fifteen lists from the Environmental Working Group.** Buy organic (or, better yet, locally grown and organic) produce on the Dirty Dozen list whenever possible. (See page 113.)
- **Check out produce stands, farmers markets, U-pick farms, co-ops, and CSAs (community-sponsored agriculture) for locally grown, in-season produce.** Depending on where you live, this can be a less-expensive option than you might think, plus some CSAs deliver, which may address accessibility options for some people. My favorite online directories for finding good produce near you are www.localharvest.org, www.eatwellguide.org, and www.pickyourown.org.

There's no question that the higher the quality of the foods you eat, the better. But don't let barriers to accessing and/or buying high-quality foods stop you from making positive changes to your diet.

IS PALEO TOO HARD?

The number-one criticism of the Paleo diet (apart from critiques that emphasize myths like Paleo being an all-meat or zero-carb diet) is that it's too hard to follow. One recent news article cited that Paleo is too hard because you have to get used to ordering your hamburger without the bun. Anyone who has been a member of the Paleo community for a while will roll their eyes at statements like this one—especially when vegetarian diets (where you'd have to get used to ordering your hamburger without the meat) and the low-sodium DASH diet (where you'd have to get used to ordering your hamburger without the seasoning) are ranked as being much easier to follow than Paleo. The millions of Americans who currently follow the Paleo diet are a testament to the fact that it's not hard. But instead of dismissing this criticism, let's discuss the challenges of following the Paleo diet in more detail.

The Paleo diet is classically presented as a list of eliminations. Many people look at the list of approved Paleo foods and see that all their favorites are off-limits. Viewing the Paleo diet this way makes it seem intimidating and elicits the idea that, by following it, we'll be constantly deprived. This is probably where much of the perception of Paleo as hard to follow comes from: an unwillingness to give up American comfort food staples like pizza and pasta. That perception is a major motivation for the structure of this book, which focuses first and foremost on the amazing wealth of delicious foods that are included on the Paleo diet, as well as the many foods that may be well tolerated even if not traditionally considered Paleo-compliant. It's also a major motivation for including recipes for Paleo adaptations of these "wheaty" staples in Part 8.

But even when it is viewed more positively and inclusively, the fact remains that adopting the Paleo diet entails a steep learning curve. Beyond simply familiarizing yourself with which foods to eat and which ones to avoid, there are the more practical challenges of finding more time to cook, developing a repertoire of quick meals for busy weeknights, finding new foods you like, restocking your pantry, learning what to pack for lunch, figuring out where to buy specialty ingredients, and discovering new portable snack foods and travel staples. Even after you have the day-to-day stuff mastered, new challenges can crop up, like navigating your first holiday season after adopting the Paleo diet or undertaking international travel. This book provides ample strategies for and solutions to all these hurdles, but you will need to gain some experience before it feels easy.

There's also the matter of physiological adaptation. For example, if you've been eating hyperpalatable junk foods regularly, whole fruits and vegetables will seem bland in comparison. The good news is that your taste buds turn over about every 2 weeks, so nutrient-dense whole foods should start tasting much more flavorful in a couple of weeks. Another common experience for people who transition to the Paleo diet cold-turkey is something called the "carb flu," where a dramatic reduction in carbohydrates (which will happen if you were eating a lot of grains before switching to Paleo) can temporarily cause you to feel pretty crummy (see page 395). Gastrointestinal symptoms can also occur as a result of a sudden substantial increase in vegetable intake. Giving up foods designed to be addictive while learning to cook new recipes *and* feeling crummy due to a drastic dietary shift—yep, that stuff is legitimately hard. So is quitting smoking or getting into the routine of going to the gym three times a week. Forming healthy habits takes persistence and dedication (see page 393), but it's worth it!

PALEO EASY BUTTON

The fact is, the more you do it, the easier it gets. So the best way to make Paleo easy is to stick with it!

Most people find that about a month into Paleo (right when you're ready to start challenging some eliminated foods; see Chapter 25), everything starts to fall into place. The human body rarely takes longer than a few weeks to adapt to a dietary shift, especially if you're getting ample sleep, and a few weeks of shopping and cooking while following the Paleo template is enough time for most people to feel like they're at least starting to get a good handle on it.

Following the Paleo template is not hard once you've adjusted and figured out how to fit Paleo into your life. But it can be tough at first. That's why this book is brimming with the reasons for each facet of Paleo. When we truly understand *why* a specific choice is the best one, we are much more motivated to choose that option, even if it's the toughest choice. And when we make that best choice regularly, it starts to become the easiest choice.

Navigating social situations like the office holiday party, a girls' night out, or your kid's birthday party is another challenge worth mentioning. Even after you've mastered the Paleo diet at home, at work, at school, and while traveling, there's always the issue of not fitting in. There are usually two sides to this coin: the feeling of having to rationalize our food choices to a deaf audience and the desire to communicate our newfound enthusiasm for our food choices, again to a deaf audience. While every person's social situation is different, it's worth making two statements in this regard:

- First, you do *not* need to rationalize your dietary and lifestyle choices to your friends and family. If they aren't ready to make health changes themselves, they may not understand why you're doing what you're doing. That's okay.
- Second, you can't force your diet and lifestyle priorities on others. Just as a person needs to find their own internal motivation to quit smoking in order to be successful, no amount of peer pressure can get someone to stick with healthy dietary choices long-term. What you *can* do is educate friends and family members who are curious (perhaps by giving them a copy of this book) and be a resource for them when they are ready to make changes themselves.

It's a fairly common experience to encounter people who don't (yet) understand how powerful nutrition can be in disease management. A conversation about why you eat the way you do is a great opportunity to share what you now know about the role that food (and sleep, and stress . . .) plays in health. Your willingness to share your experience may help someone else recover their health. Unfortunately, it's also fairly common to encounter people who just aren't ready to accept that giving up multigrain bread can make them healthier. Conversations with these people may leave you feeling frustrated or defensive as though you need to justify how you eat. But you don't need to explain your choices to anyone, especially if what you're doing is working! If you feel you have to say something, you can simply say, "This works for me." End of story. Or you might offer up something vague about allergies or food sensitivities to avoid a lengthy debate. If you do find yourself becoming engaged in philosophical debates about food that aren't likely to go anywhere, then share this book. That's one of the reasons I belabored the science—not just to help you understand why it's important to improve your diet and lifestyle, but also to enable you to talk knowledgeably about it with others.

MOVING BEYOND LABELS

I believe that scientific literacy is the key to improving public health. You can label the information in this book as Paleo (as I have done), or, just as legitimately, you can use the label Primal, ancestral, traditional, clean eating, real food, plant-based (although this differs from the trademarked Plant-Based Diet), or nutrient nerd. Or you can simply refer to it as a set of science-based nutrition guidelines. Whatever you want to call this way of eating (and it's fine if you prefer not to label your food choices with any of these terms), the takeaway messages from the scientific literature remain the same: a healthy diet is replete in nutrition and free from toxins and inflammatory compounds in order to support a healthy gut microbiome, regulate hormones, and aid in detoxification.

The Paleo movement has been growing exponentially since it was first popularized in 2002 with the publication of *The Paleo Diet* by Loren Cordain. As thought leaders and scientists have joined the discussion about the merits of individual foods and the importance of various lifestyle habits, Paleo has itself evolved from a restrictive set of dietary guidelines based predominantly on evolutionary biology and anthropology to the much more comprehensive yet flexible diet and lifestyle template described in this book, based in physiology, nutritional sciences, and cell and molecular biology.

One of the truly exciting things that we see happening today is the convergence of various dietary guidelines toward a consensus. For example, the 2015-2020 USDA dietary guidelines more accurately reflect current scientific research than perhaps ever before, with recommendations to eat a variety of nutrient-dense foods from all six food groups, a division of vegetables into five subgroups, and an emphasis on avoiding excess caloric intake and added sugar while eschewing refined and manufactured foods. Important concepts promoted by the Mediterranean diet and the Plant-Based Diet (like the importance of seafood, the benefits of olive oil, and the critical nature of eating lots of veggies) are being integrated into the USDA dietary guidelines, and they are also Paleo principles. Doctors around the world are recommending the Paleo diet, or some variation of it, to their patients. While it may be years down the road, this will culminate in a set of guidelines for a healthy diet and lifestyle that transcends labels.

For now, we call this lifestyle Paleo. In the future, we'll likely call it simply "making healthy choices."

Chapter 32: MAKING THE TRANSITION

When it comes to transitioning, there's no one-size-fits-all strategy that works for everybody. Some people do better embarking on a complete diet and lifestyle overhaul from day one. Others do best (both physically and psychologically) with a slower transition process. Neither strategy is better or worse than the other. The most important thing is finding what works best for *you* in terms of tackling change and sticking with it so that Paleo becomes your default lifestyle. Ultimately, this boils down to maximizing compliance and sustainability.

Compliance refers to how well you can adhere to a particular protocol as prescribed, whether it's a diet, a medication, an exercise program, or some other intervention. In the medical and pharmaceutical fields, compliance is seen as an indicator of not only how well a particular medication works, but also how severe (or tolerable) the side effects are. If a drug results in extreme side effects and doesn't work very well, fewer people end up taking the drug as directed, resulting in low compliance. On the other hand, if a drug works as promised and doesn't produce many side effects, more people will take the drug as prescribed, resulting in high compliance. When it comes to the Paleo framework, the concept is similar: compliance reflects how closely the way you eat follows the protocol. Certainly, there is some wiggle room with middle-ground foods (like high-quality dairy; see Chapter 24) and the exact assortment of Paleo-friendly foods you eat throughout the week (such as how often you eat fish or organ meat), but these choices don't fall under the banner of compliance. In this case, compliance refers to how often you eat something you know isn't good for you, will cause a negative reaction, or will interfere with your body's healing. For the purpose of transitioning, choosing the approach that maximizes your compliance is critical.

Sustainability refers to the ability to be maintained at a certain rate or level. Depending on which aspect of Paleo we're talking about, this could refer to environmental sustainability, economic sustainability, individual sustainability, or many other things. In the context of implementing dietary and lifestyle changes, though, the focus is on individual sustainability—your ability to stick with Paleo for the long haul. In that sense, it's important to choose a transition method that feels manageable and sets you up for long-term success.

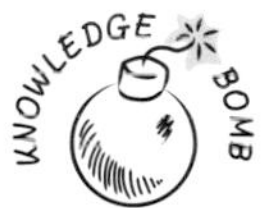

Transition is about making healthy choices a habit. Unfortunately, it's a myth that it takes only 21 days to make or break a habit. The vast majority of us must commit to repetitively performing a task for a much greater length of time before that task becomes automatic. Scientific research shows that the average length of time it takes to form a new habit is more like 66 days, but it can take up to 254 days before that new change we're working on feels completely natural and easy. Being prepared for a longer haul when it comes to creating new healthy habits is the first key to success.

Studies have identified these five simple steps for forming a habit:

1. *Decide on a goal that you would like to achieve.*
2. *Choose a simple action that will move you toward your goal and that you can do on a daily basis.*
3. *Plan when and where you will perform your chosen action. Be consistent: choose a time and place that you encounter every day of the week.*
4. *Every time you encounter that time and place, perform the action.*
5. *Within 10 weeks (or up to 8 months), you should find that you are performing that action habitually without even having to think about it.*

Congratulations, you've formed a healthy new habit!

THE 30-DAY CHALLENGE

The 30-day challenge is a tried-and-true transition method. You pick a day to start Paleo and then jump all-in, committing to staying strict for 30 days before you allow yourself "cheat meals" or try to challenge any non-Paleo foods. This strategy compresses both the physical and psychological adaptations along with the more practical learning curve into one short period. By the end of the 30 days, most people see substantial health improvements that help them stay motivated to continue, while also having dealt with the biggest practical challenges to long-term success.

Whom Does This Method Work For?

Think about your personality for a minute. Are you more likely to stick with something if you approach it as if you're breaking a bad habit, investing plenty of up-front effort to make a change until a new habit is solidified and the change feels effortless? Are you more likely to stick with a new dietary approach if you see quick results? Are you more likely to have an all-or-nothing attitude and throw in the towel if you aren't completely on board? If you answer "yes" to these types of questions, a 30-day challenge might be right up your alley. This approach fully immerses you in the Paleo lifestyle so that you can start forming new habits—and seeing results!—as quickly as possible.

How to Do It

Before diving in, it's important to take time to prepare. This often means setting up a meal plan, shopping for Paleo-friendly ingredients, cooking extra food to freeze for later, and organizing your support network. When it comes to jumping in with both feet, it's a good idea to clean out your pantry of foods you know you won't be eating anymore, which also helps you assess your food inventory. For example, you might already have olive oil, vinegar, spices, and other Paleo-friendly items on hand, so you won't need to buy them. Decide which meals you plan to cook over the first week (or use one of the meal plans in Part 9) and make a shopping list of all the ingredients you don't have. This strategy ensures that you'll be prepared during this cold-turkey approach and lets you stock your pantry slowly over the course of a few months, buying new items as you plan for the coming week.

What to Expect

Although a cold-turkey approach reduces the amount of time it takes to start feeling fantastic, it can be a little jarring. Fortunately, there's an advantage to forcing yourself to adjust quickly (and only once): this approach typically results in faster, more dramatic improvements. Be warned, though, that even when you "get the transition over with" this way, some people experience a lag while their bodies adjust to new foods and different macronutrient ratios before they start to see improvements. However, many others report phenomenal changes in long-standing symptoms, energy levels, mood, sleep quality, and overall well-being within the first few days of transitioning.

At the other end of the spectrum, rapid transitions can trigger symptoms resembling Jarisch-Herxheimer reactions (a reaction to the endotoxin-like products that are released when harmful microorganisms in the body die), though this isn't very common and certainly isn't permanent.

As a result of changes in gut microflora, increases in stool bulk (if your fiber intake goes up), increases in stomach acid requirements, increases in fat intake, and/or decreases in carbohydrate intake, certain symptoms are particularly likely in the first few days or weeks of a cold-turkey transition. Temporary gastrointestinal issues such as bloating, looser stools, constipation, and more or less frequent bowel movements can occur in response to gut microbiota shifts and higher fiber intake. As the stomach adjusts to producing more acid in response to high-protein foods, fiber-rich foods, and fat, symptoms such as heartburn, nausea, acid reflux, and belching can result.

When carbohydrate intake significantly decreases (which often happens when we stop consuming grains and processed sugars), the "carb flu" can occur; it is characterized by symptoms such as fatigue, headaches, muscle cramps, brain fog, and dizziness—many of which can be relieved by drinking more water; ensuring adequate intake of sodium, potassium, and magnesium; and upping carbohydrate intake by incorporating more tubers, root vegetables, and fruit.

That being said, transition symptoms should be temporary and mild enough not to cause serious alarm. If you experience symptoms that don't subside after the first several weeks of Paleo, that interfere with your ability to function throughout the day, or that indicate a worsening of a health condition (such as increased pain or stiffness), talk to your doctor. You could have introduced a particular food into your diet that isn't a good fit for your body; for example, you may have a sensitivity to a Paleo-friendly food that you weren't eating before.

TRANSITION GUIDE: GOING COLD TURKEY

The key to success with a 30-day challenge is to take some time in advance to prepare, using the following suggestions:

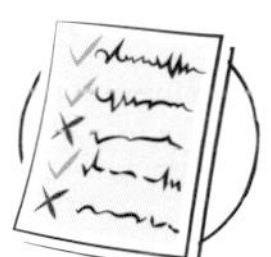

STUDY THE FOOD LISTS.
Know which foods are okay and which ones should be eliminated for the next 30 days by reviewing the food lists on pages 216 to 219. Decide ahead of time how you plan to handle middle-ground foods; most people choose to eliminate them for the first 30 days, but this is up to you.

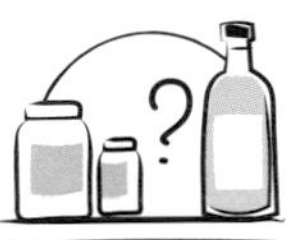

CLEAN OUT YOUR PANTRY.
Donate or dispose of any foods that might tempt you over the next 30 days.

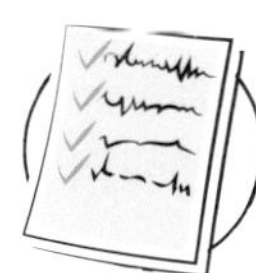

PLAN YOUR MEALS.
Whether you plan a week at a time or you simply make a list of a few new recipes you want to try, think about what your meals are going to look like. Check out the meal plans in Part 9!

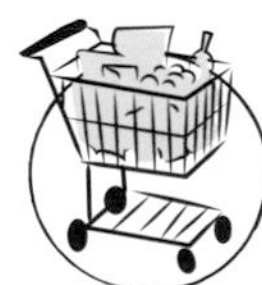

RESTOCK YOUR PANTRY.
Purchase healthy cooking fats, herbs, spices, and other flavoring ingredients you're going to need to cook tasty Paleo meals over the next month.

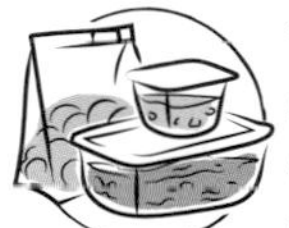

THINK ABOUT SNACKS, ON-THE-GO FOODS, AND QUICK AND EASY MEALS.
Consider how you're going to handle eating on the run or whipping up a quick meal when you get home super-tired from a long, busy day. Consider purchasing some portable Paleo foods (see page 456) or cooking some meals ahead of time to freeze for later.

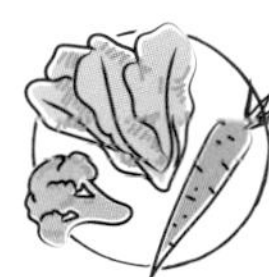

GO GROCERY SHOPPING FOR FRESH AND FROZEN INGREDIENTS.
Make sure to start your 30-day transition stocked with Paleo foods.

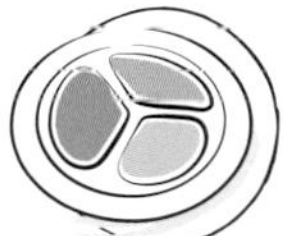

FOCUS ON YOUR MEAL COMPOSITION.
It's okay if nutrient density is an afterthought at first. Yes, eating organ meat, shellfish, and tons of veggies is important, but if you find it intimidating, don't worry about it just yet. Instead, your meals can be mostly veggies and a serving of meat. Just remember to come back around to this important Paleo principle once everything starts to seem a bit easier.

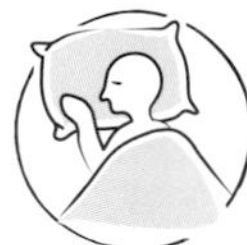

EVALUATE YOUR SLEEP.
The simplest first step to getting enough sleep is to establish a bedtime that's at least 8 hours before your alarm goes off in the morning. Commit to this bedtime for the next 30 days.

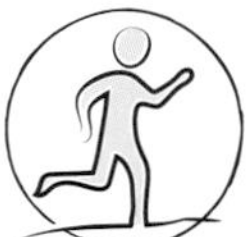

PLAN SOME ACTIVITY.
If you're starting the 30-day transition as a fairly sedentary person, don't go hog wild here. You're making a whole lot of changes at once, so keep it simple with activity. Aim for a 30-minute walk most days and take 2-minute movement breaks throughout your workday if you have a desk job.

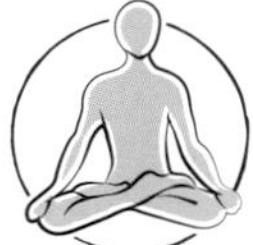

ASSESS YOUR STRESS LEVEL.
If you know that you're under a lot of stress, think about how you can simplify your life for the next month. Also consider adding 10 minutes of mindfulness or meditation (see pages 353 to 354), perhaps before bed to help improve your sleep quality.

THE STEP-BY-STEP APPROACH

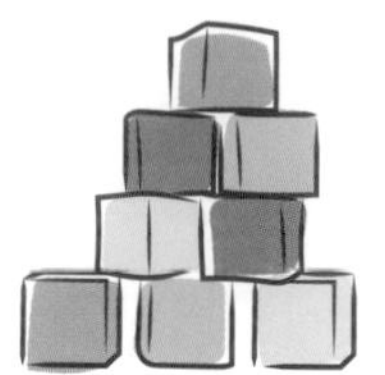

Another absolutely acceptable method of transition is to prioritize individual aspects of the Paleo diet and implement them iteratively. There's no prescribed length of time that each step should take, some people allot a week to each step while others simply move on once they feel like the previous step is mastered (which can take days or months). The key here is not to lose site of the end goal and keep progressing toward it.

Whom Does This Method Work For?

Are you more likely to stick with something if you ease into it and make one manageable change at a time? Can you be patient and optimistic if you don't see immediate results? Are you transitioning along with children or other family members who aren't ready for a sudden, complete overhaul of their current diet? Is Paleo your first foray into healthy eating, and is your current diet a long way off from your goal? These situations suggest that a step-by-step approach could be better for you. The results might not come as fast, but you're more likely to make lasting habits and avoid feeling overwhelmed, leading to better compliance and less risk of falling off the wagon.

How to Do It

The step-by-step approach involves implementing changes in phases and solidifying each new change before moving on to the next one. The best way to do so is by creating a game plan for which changes you want to make first, second, third, fourth, and so on. Different people will prioritize different changes for different reasons: If you suspect that you are gluten-intolerant, eliminating gluten may be your top priority. If you know that eating veggies is a particular challenge for you, adding a serving or two per meal might be where you start. If you're a junk food junkie, you might begin simply by finding healthier alternatives. And if you eat most of your meals out, simply getting into the routine of grocery shopping and cooking at home will be your first step.

As you adopt each new step in your plan, you'll know that you're ready to move on once you have adjusted to the absence of certain familiar foods (like bread and breakfast cereal) and have found a "new normal" in terms of what meals should look like—such as eggs and vegetables for breakfast instead of milk and toast. Some steps might seem easy, and you can move on to the next one in a few days. Others might be tough, and you might find that you aren't ready to tackle the next step for a few weeks or even months. The key with the step-by-step approach is never to lose sight of the end goal: even if you're making very gradual changes, make sure that you're still progressing toward full implementation of the Paleo template.

What to Expect

Although some people feel better and better with each step, many won't see major improvements—or, in some cases, even minor improvements—until they eliminate all problem foods from their diets. For example, if you're sensitive to gluten and dairy, you might not notice any big differences in how you feel until gluten and dairy are completely removed from your diet, regardless of the other changes you make. So when choosing the step-by-step approach, it's important to keep in mind that you can't expect to see substantial results until you've taken all the steps toward a fully Paleo diet.

Ultimately, how you transition is up to you. How you handle changing your diet and lifestyle will depend on a wide range of variables that are unique to your situation, including how you are eating now, what your personality is like, how strong your support network is, how motivated you are to heal from existing illnesses, how comfortable you are in the kitchen, and how accessible these changes are for you. As long as you end up reaching your goal, there's no right or wrong way to transition.

TRANSITION GUIDE: INCREMENTAL IMPLEMENTATION

There are about a million ways to implement a step-by-step approach to transitioning to a Paleo diet. The following are suggestions to prioritize dietary changes based on the health impact of each change:

1. ELIMINATE GUT-IRRITATING FOODS FROM YOUR DIET. This can be a multistep process while you work on other steps. Focus on eliminating gluten first. This means cutting out all foods that contain wheat, oats, and barley (as well as hidden gluten ingredients like malt; see page 281). But don't replace them with gluten-free alternatives like rice- or potato-based bread. Instead, try to get used to not eating bread or make your own (see Chapter 44). Also eliminate all junk food and fast food. Once you've got this step down, eliminate other problematic foods one by one or group by group, however it makes sense for you: legumes (especially soy and peanuts), conventional dairy, nightshades, and so on.

2. START COOKING ALL YOUR MEALS. Unfortunately, it's difficult to get healthy nutrient-dense Paleo meals from restaurants or prepackaged. This can be one of the biggest challenges to following a healthy diet because we are so used to convenience. Start collecting recipes for quick meals that can be prepared midweek. (For quick meals, try Shrimp Pad Thai on page 533, Taco Meat on page 544 served in lettuce wraps, Gremolata-Topped Fish Fillets on page 525, or Beef & Mushroom Risotto on page 526.) Cook large portions so you have enough food for a few days' worth of leftovers. And double or triple recipes so you can fill your freezer with meals that can be thawed and reheated when you're too busy or too tired to cook. (For your freezer, try Hamburger Stew on page 516, Pumpkin Chili on page 517, or Chicken or Beef Pot Pie on page 533, or make a bunch of Pizza Crusts on page 499 for pizza nights.) If you love to eat in restaurants, see the next page for tips.

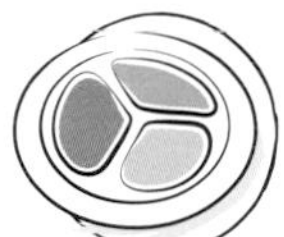

3. GET USED TO YOUR MEALS CONSISTING OF SOME KIND OF PROTEIN (MEAT, POULTRY, FISH, OR SHELLFISH), SOME VEGETABLES (IDEALLY OF A FEW DIFFERENT COLORS, INCLUDING AT LEAST ONE THAT IS GREEN), AND MAYBE SOME FRUIT, NUTS, OR SEEDS. Every meal should look like this—even breakfast! Focus on meals that were already part of your rotation that fit this criteria (or could easily fit with a simple swap or two, like cooking your favorite stir-fry with coconut aminos instead of soy sauce and serving it over cauliflower rice instead of white or brown rice) and expand from there. This would be a good time to try some unfamiliar vegetables or types of meat and fish and experiment with new ways to cook them.

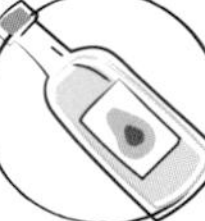

4. START THINKING ABOUT FATS. Switch to high-quality fats—such as lard, tallow, avocado oil, coconut oil, and olive oil—as your main cooking fats. Also start thinking about your omega-3 to omega-6 fatty acid intake ratio. This means sourcing quality meats and incorporating fish and shellfish into your diet as often as possible. This step also overlaps with the next step.

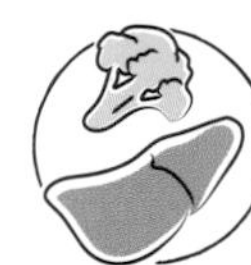

5. THINK ABOUT NUTRIENT DENSITY. It's time to work on eating some liver (even if you have to hide it from yourself; see page 177) and other organ meat, drinking or cooking with bone broth, making sure to eat at least eight servings of veggies a day, and getting seafood into your diet a few times a week. These nutrient superstars make a huge difference to the overall nutrient density of your diet and can accelerate health improvements substantially.

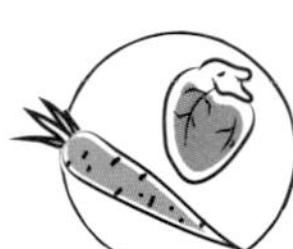

6. WORK ON EATING VARIETY AND MAYBE ADDING SOME NEW FOODS. If you find that you are eating the same foods day in and day out, it's time to broaden your horizons. Start trying new foods and increasing the variety in your diet. The more different foods you incorporate, the higher the likelihood of providing your body with all the nutrients it needs.

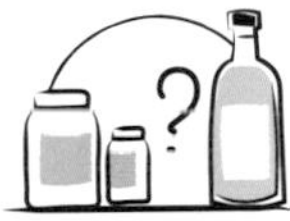

7. PURGE YOUR PANTRY. As you go through each step, throw out what you don't eat anymore (or compost it, feed it to some ducks, or give it to a food bank or a non-Paleo friend).

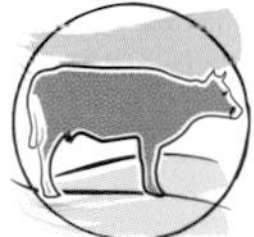

8. ADDRESS FOOD QUALITY. Start eating grass-fed and pasture-raised meat, wild-caught fish, and organic, locally grown, in-season fruits and vegetables, budget and access permitting.

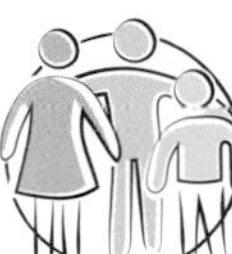

9. FIND SUPPORT. One of the toughest things about going Paleo can be the lack of understanding from friends and family. I suggest finding some blogs, podcasts, or forums where you can post questions and "meet" like-minded individuals who have limited diets (whether they're gluten-free or have food allergies), because they will be fairly sympathetic about your need to eat "off the grid." Having a sense of common cause will give you strength to cope with questions and judgments from the uninformed people around you.

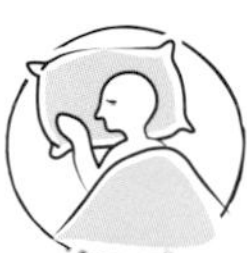

10. DON'T FORGET THE LIFESTYLE FACTORS! Make sure to address the lifestyle aspects of the Paleo template. You can work on increasing sleep, managing stress, protecting your circadian rhythms, and getting more mild- to moderate-intensity exercise while you improve your diet. In fact, making sure that sleep, physical activity, and stress management are priorities from the beginning will help make the dietary changes much easier. (See Part 7.)

RESTAURANTS AND TRAVEL

It can be tricky to stick with the Paleo principles when you eat out, but it is possible. It helps to know exactly which foods you fully tolerate, which ones you can tolerate in small, occasional amounts, and which are totally verboten for you (see Chapter 25).

If you are going out to eat, it's a good idea to call ahead and make sure that the restaurant can accommodate you. For most people, remaining gluten-free is the top priority, but you'll also want to avoid any other foods that elicit a reaction when you eat them, like soy, dairy, or tomatoes. Knowing what line you personally cannot cross is key to navigating restaurants. Fortunately, many restaurants are developing gluten-free menus and have gluten-free workspaces to cater to those with celiac disease or gluten sensitivities. There are also a growing number of Paleo-friendly restaurants, most of which can easily accommodate additional dietary restrictions. Farm-to-table restaurants are usually a good bet, as are burger chains that specialize in grass-fed beef.

It is important to have an open dialogue with your server. Explain which foods you cannot eat. (Even if they're not technically allergies, it can sometimes be helpful to express them as such to get the staff to take your needs seriously.) Ask specific questions: Is that meat dredged in flour before cooking? Is there any dairy in that salad dressing? What seasonings are used? Find out which dishes can be made to order: Can the fish be grilled instead of fried? Can you get a hamburger without the bun? And ask if the chef is amenable to making something off the menu for you. (That's a good question to ask before you arrive.)

Certain foods are more likely to be "safe" than others. Generally, grilled or roasted meats, grilled or poached seafood, salads (ask for the dressing on the side), and grilled or steamed vegetables can be ordered with a much greater certainty of being Paleo-friendly. They might not be cooked in the best-quality fats, but most people will tolerate these on occasion.

When it comes to eating at someone else's house, you should talk to your host beforehand. Explain what you can't eat—and also what you can! Make sure your host understands which foods might be hidden sources of gluten, like bottled sauces. It can also help to offer to bring something you can eat: maybe a protein if you know that item will be the hardest for your host to prepare, or a side dish or dessert to share.

Traveling can be a challenge as well. For a road trip, it's best to haul out and stock the cooler so you know you'll have good eats along the way. If you have to hit the grocery store to top off your supplies during a longer trip, look for rotisserie chickens (check the ingredients!), deli meats (again, check the ingredients!), canned fish or tuna in pouches, sweet potato chips, plantain chips, and raw vegetables and fruit. There are also slow cookers and microwaves that can plug into your car to reheat food.

Many of the same "convenience" foods work for air travel. If you are traveling internationally, check the regulations ahead of time to find out which food items you can bring with you. Generally, nonperishables such as jerky, protein bars (see page 457 for Paleo options), dried fruit, packaged plantain or sweet potato chips, and canned fish are okay. Depending on whether you technically cross the border before your flight or afterward, you might be able to bring perishable food on the plane but then be required to toss any leftovers before going through customs.

Eat a balanced meal before you leave home and have a plan for how to source good food once you arrive at your destination. If you're staying at someone's house, talk to your host ahead of time; if you're staying at a hotel, scope out the closest grocery store or specialty stores before you arrive. Spending a little extra for a hotel room with a mini-fridge or, better yet, a kitchenette will make your life much more pleasant. Then all you have to do is bring a paring or pocket knife (in your checked baggage!), a few utensils (camping utensils are very versatile), and maybe even a jar or two of your favorite fat or oil, seasoning mix, or good-quality salt, and you will have it made in the shade in terms of sticking with Paleo far from home.

The bottom line is that the best way to eat well away from home is similar to eating well at home: plan ahead! And do a little troubleshooting before you get in trouble: What will you do if your plane is delayed? If you arrive at your friend's house and discover that he marinated the pork in barbecue sauce that contains gluten? If the grocery store is closed by the time you get to your hotel? In some cases, not eating will be a better choice than eating a food that you know will cause an increase in symptoms. In other cases, eating a suboptimal food will be a better choice than enduring the stress of not eating. And you can avoid both of those contingencies by packing some emergency food (see page 638 for suggested prepackaged options).

Chapter 33: MODIFYING PALEO FOR SPECIFIC GOALS

The Paleo template is designed to improve the health of *any* human being by increasing the nutritional quality of the diet and eliminating foods that can contribute to chronic disease and obesity. However, for people who enter Paleo with existing health conditions or specific health goals, the diet can be modified even further to deliver maximum therapeutic value.

Scientific research into obesity, cardiovascular disease, diabetes, cancer, autoimmune disease, asthma and allergies, mental health, autism spectrum disorder, child development, and athletic performance has identified important dietary and lifestyle factors that should be considered if your health challenges and goals fall under any of these umbrellas. While none of the nutrition and lifestyle information we've covered so far is moot when it comes to these topics, a particular focus on specific nutrients or lifestyle factors can be immensely helpful in mitigating chronic health conditions or achieving specific health goals.

Of course, an entire book could be written to summarize the state of scientific research about each of these chronic health challenges and about athletic performance. (In fact, I've already written a book about autoimmune disease called *The Paleo Approach*.) However, given the huge amount of detail already provided about optimal diet and lifestyle choices, I'll be summarizing the most salient information in regard to disease prevention and mitigation.

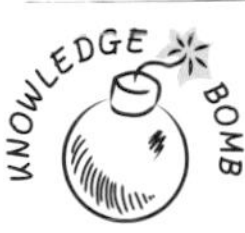

Dietary changes—specifically in the types and amounts of fiber and fat you eat—can be immensely corrective stimuli for the gut microbiota.

A diet rich in vegetables and fruit tends to promote a healthy diversity of microorganisms in the gut, with something like two-thirds to three-quarters of those species being Gram-positive bacteria (bacteria that don't have endotoxin in their cell membranes; see page 301), like the well-known Bifidobacterium and Lactobacillus. Low fiber intake or consumption of a lot of grain-based fiber, on the other hand, tends to skew the gut microbiota toward Gram-negative bacteria. The good news? Gut microbiota can undergo a monumental shift in as little as 3 to 4 days when you increase your vegetable and fruit intake. (Unfortunately, it also takes only a few days to start losing that great diversity of gut microorganisms, so consistently eating a diet rich in vegetables and fruit is very important!)

A high intake of omega-6 polyunsaturated fats is known to promote bacterial overgrowth in the small intestine (specifically the ileum) and deplete probiotic bacteria from the Firmicutes and Bacteroidetes phyla. A high saturated fat intake also skews gut microbiota unfavorably toward Bilophila, Turicibacter, and Bacteroides. This is one of the major rationales for moderating fat intake (see page 186). Studies show that fish oil supplementation can restore levels of probiotic bacteria in about 14 days.

HEALTHY WEIGHT LOSS

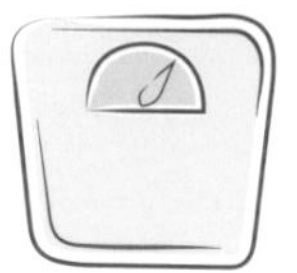

An estimated 213 million Americans (69 percent of the population) are overweight, with 111 million (36 percent) being obese. Because being overweight increases the risk of developing many other chronic health problems—including type 2 diabetes, heart disease, cancer, polycystic ovary syndrome (PCOS), infertility, pregnancy complications, gout, arthritis, erectile dysfunction, high blood pressure, and high cholesterol—achieving a healthy weight is one of the most important things we can do to improve our long-term health.

Thanks to the Paleo diet's focus on consuming nutrient-dense, satiating foods (along with removing many hunger-stimulating foods, like refined grains and sugars), many people lose weight when they first adopt the Paleo framework—even if they're not trying! The elimination of Standard American Diet (SAD) staples, along with an increase in bulky plant foods that are high in fiber and water, generally results in a spontaneous decreased caloric intake and a subsequent reduction in body fat.

However, when significant and sustained weight loss is the goal—or when the scale won't budge even after the adoption of a Paleo diet—there are some diet and lifestyle modifications that can help jump-start the process.

The Weight-Loss Magic Bullet: Portion Control

Portion control is the driving force behind every successful weight-loss diet, whether it be low-carb, Paleo, the Mediterranean diet, the DASH diet, Weight Watchers, or any number of short-lived fads. No matter what a diet's official rationale is, it induces weight loss chiefly by reducing the number of calories consumed. Different diets go about this in different ways, but energy intake is what ultimately ends up changing the number on the scale.

A large body of scientific literature confirms this concept. When calorie intake is held constant, different macronutrient ratios (such as low-carb/high-fat or high-carb/low-fat) don't have significantly different effects on the amount of body fat lost (or on overall energy needs). There's no substantial evidence to support that specific macronutrient ratios have a "metabolic advantage" when it comes to burning more fat or changing energy needs; the only thing that ends up influencing body mass is the calorie content of our diet. For example, a metabolic ward study from 1992 in which subjects were fed tightly controlled diets with equal calorie contents found no detectable difference in the amount of energy people burned when eating an extremely high-fat, low-carb diet (70 percent fat and 15 percent carbohydrate) versus an extremely low-fat, high-carb diet (0 percent fat and 85 percent carbohydrate). Another metabolic ward study found that when hypercaloric diets with different macronutrient ratios were compared, calories alone accounted for body fat gain.

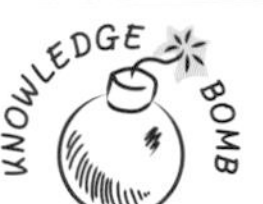

Metabolic ward studies are tightly controlled nutritional science studies that include rigorous and detailed measurements of metabolism, body composition, energy expenditure, and food intake. Participants live in a metabolic ward for the duration of the study, closely monitored and often spending days at a time in a metabolic chamber, which measures energy expenditure extremely accurately. These studies are extremely expensive to conduct but provide profound insight into how dietary factors impact metabolism and weight loss.

That being said, some studies *have* found an advantage to eating more protein when it comes to preserving lean mass (muscle) or burning a higher proportion of body fat relative to other tissue. But those findings aren't consistent across all studies and in some cases are gender-specific, with women having a greater advantage when it comes to lean mass preservation from high-protein diets. Ultimately, the research consistently shows that the most important component of weight loss is being in a negative energy balance (that is, consuming fewer calories than you burn).

However, just because weight loss boils down to calorie intake doesn't mean that all diets are created equal when it comes to portion control. Many processed foods (particularly those rich in refined carbohydrates, vegetable oils, salt, and sugar, as well as low in protein) are designed to induce overeating and override our bodies' satiety signals, especially when compared to whole foods closer to their natural state. For decades,

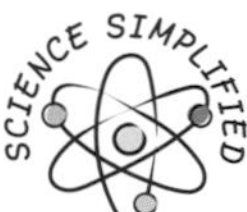

Many people purport that there are benefits to manipulating macronutrient ratios (including low-fat, low-carb, and even ketogenic diets), claiming that doing so will bolster weight-loss efforts. But this claim isn't supported by scientific research; in fact, studies attempting to confirm weight-loss improvements have debunked the concept.

rodent experiments have shown that energy-dense diets (those that are high in fat, refined carbohydrates, and total calories) result in overeating and obesity relative to lower-energy-density diets. In fact, an interesting study from 2014 found that energy-dense food (equivalent to potato chips) strongly activated the reward systems of rats' brains, leading to something called *hedonic hyperphagia:* eating for pleasure rather than to fulfill energy needs. This effect was *not* seen when the rats ate fat or carbohydrate separately! A similar phenomenon occurs in humans when we eat energy-dense processed foods.

This means one of the keys to losing weight without feeling deprived is avoiding hyperpalatable manufactured foods. Yes, portion control is yet another reason to avoid junk and fast food, but many foods purported to be healthy actually contain few nutrients and inadequate fiber and take advantage of that addictive combination of salt, sugar, and fat.

We can understand another key to weight loss by looking at studies of low-carb diets, in which a spontaneous caloric deficit is achieved via a focus on satiating foods like meat and leafy greens, which make you feel full after eating fewer calories. While low-carb diets have some limitations when it comes to supporting whole-body health (see Chapter 2), this advantageous quality of low-carb diets is shared by the Paleo diet.

A Paleo diet rich in fibrous plant foods (dark leafy greens, cruciferous veggies, seaweeds, tubers, fermented vegetables, berries, and so on) along with highly satiating high-quality meat and seafood (including organ meat, grass-fed beef, pasture-raised pork and poultry, and wild-caught fish and shellfish) puts us at an advantage for reducing energy density and increasing satiety. This concept is supported by scientific studies pitting the Paleo diet against other diets for weight-loss effects (see page 128). It's been demonstrated that transitioning to a Paleo diet results in a spontaneous reduction in calories of about 400 per day—that's almost a pound of weight loss per week, without any additional attention paid to weight-loss efforts! Furthermore, research has demonstrated that a Paleo diet improves the symptoms of metabolic syndrome, high blood lipids, and elevated fasting blood sugar, all of which may hinder weight-loss efforts due to the hormonal imbalances underlying these issues.

Generally, someone with weight to lose can expect to achieve a modest caloric deficit when adopting a Paleo diet—without feeling deprived, counting calories, or going hungry—as a result of replacing addictive empty calories with satiating, nutrient-dense whole foods. Unfortunately, that doesn't mean every overweight person following a Paleo diet will spontaneously achieve a caloric deficit and watch the pounds melt away. There are a few traps we can fall into that can stall or prevent weight loss:

- Tasty combinations of Paleo-friendly fat, carbohydrate, and salt encourage us to eat more than we might really need to. This includes Paleo breads and desserts, adaptations of SAD comfort foods, dehydrated foods, and chocolate. Even though the ingredients in these foods are acceptable components of a Paleo diet, when they're mixed together in hyperpalatable combinations, they can stall weight loss or even contribute to weight *gain*. (Just because the cookies are Paleo doesn't mean it's harmless to eat the entire batch at once!) Monitoring portion sizes with these foods can be helpful.
- A number of studies have shown that protein is the most satiating macronutrient, curbing appetite and potentially increasing thermogenesis (see page 52), so making lean sources of animal protein (like seafood and grass-fed beef) the centerpiece of our meals may assist with weight loss.
- Low-moisture foods like nuts, dried fruits, and Paleo-friendly chips tend to be easier to overeat than foods with greater volume and water content. Watch out for mindless munching! Fully hydrated foods (fresh fruit versus dried, a sweet potato versus sweet potato chips or fries, and so on) tend to be more difficult to overeat.
- Adding veggies to any meal will lower the energy density of that meal and provide more fiber and bulk, helping us reduce our calorie intake without even thinking about it.

By focusing on portion control and understanding the traps that can lead us to eat more than we need, we have a good shot at spontaneously reducing our energy intake and losing weight without the hassle of counting calories, weighing food, or stressing about every bite that goes into our mouths.

Eat Your Veggies!

I've covered the importance of a vegetable-rich diet ad nauseam already, but if healthy, sustained weight loss is your goal, there are some additional reasons to load up on veggies.

New research in the field of obesity is helping to explain the differences between normal-weight and overweight people. Successful weight loss is highly related to vegetable intake, which is no surprise. One difference is the way we approach vegetable (and fruit) intake. Overweight people are more likely to consume lots of vegetables and fruit when they have better planning—something we know is necessary when it comes to Paleo!—and inhibitory control (that is, the ability to resist hyperpalatable foods). And eating a veggie-rich diet improves our chances of maintaining weight loss. Choosing to incorporate more vegetables into our diet is one way to retrain our executive functioning, promote weight loss, and make it more sustainable in the long term.

KNOWLEDGE BOMB *Executive functioning refers to a collection of neurologically based skills related to cognitive control of behavior directed at achieving objectives. It includes skills such as organization and planning. Having good executive functioning means that we assess every choice and consider the benefits of each option in the context of both our short- and long-term goals. In the context of weight loss, this means we have more willpower and engage in healthier behaviors. Studies have linked obesity with poor executive functioning and show that improving executive functioning can help us successfully lose weight and keep it off.*

One of the most obvious reasons to eat vegetables is that they are relatively less calorically dense than other Paleo foods; this means we get more micronutrients and fewer calories from each bite. For example, 200 calories of a pure fat like ghee is just shy of 2 tablespoons, whereas 200 calories of kale is more than 6 cups!

Vegetables also supply plenty of fiber. This is important because a high fiber intake increases satiety by suppressing ghrelin (see page 90), meaning that we feel more satisfied more quickly. This significantly reduces the likelihood of overeating. Plus, fiber is essential for healthy gut microbiota, which is critical for optimal health (including weight loss and maintenance). Indeed, the types of gut bacteria have been found to be different in normal-weight people than in overweight people. Fiber (or lack thereof) is a likely reason why the microbes are different.

Phytochemicals are another compelling reason to eat tons of vegetables while pursuing weight loss. The process of liberating fat from adipocytes (fat storage cells) and then converting the stored fat to glucose creates oxidants (see page 267). While the production of reactive oxygen species (ROS) is a normal consequence of our metabolism, if we are losing weight and metabolizing a relatively large amount of stored fat, we can create too many ROS, causing an imbalance between oxidants and our bodies' ability to eliminate them using our natural antioxidant systems that may lead to cellular damage. This is one of the arguments against losing weight too quickly; it can increase our chances of some diseases, like cardiovascular disease, and may speed up cellular aging. However, eating phytochemicals helps balance the equation (see page 35).

Carbohydrate Confusion: Proceed Intelligently!

There are known setbacks to eating too many carbohydrates while trying to lose weight. Monitoring blood sugar regulation—knowing our levels of fasting blood glucose, fasting insulin, and HbA1c (a 3-month measure of how much glucose is stored in our red blood cells)—is essential. But even if your bloodwork is pristine, excess carbohydrate consumption can undermine weight-loss attempts. Here are the two main reasons to avoid a high-carb approach to weight loss:

- **Excess carbohydrates become stored fat.** When we do not maintain a caloric deficit, excess dietary carbohydrates are easily converted to fat (specifically triglycerides) and stored as fat in our cells. Eating too many carbs is like asking your body to store more energy for later—and it will happily comply!

· **Systemic inflammation is elevated.** Consuming too many carbohydrates, notably sugars, is a trigger for elevated systemic (or bodywide) inflammation. Sugar has been shown to increase the release of pro-inflammatory cytokines, immune system messengers that ramp up inflammation (see page 268). Systemic inflammation is associated with weight problems.

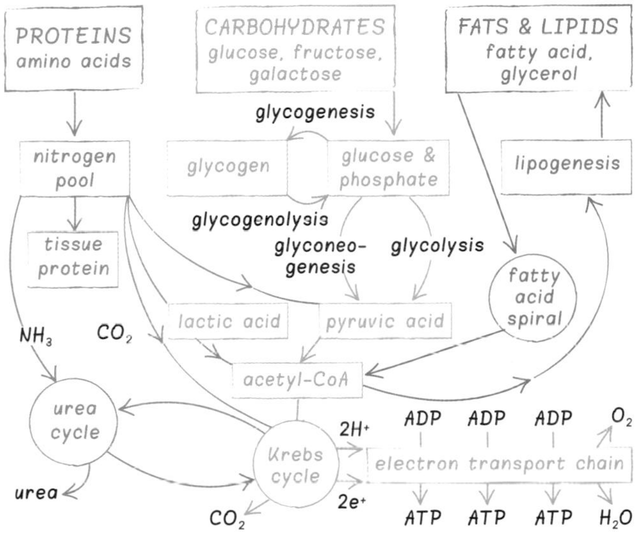

Conversely, low-carb eating is often touted as a tool for weight loss because it theoretically keeps insulin levels low, allowing for more stored fat to be released as fuel for the body (the insulin hypothesis of weight loss). But there is little to no scientific evidence supporting this theory, with the most recent data indicating that low-carb diets are simply a sneaky way to reduce calorie intake without actually counting calories. (Yes, that means portion control!) There are several reasons to avoid going too low-carb:

· **Hypothyroidism:** You may have heard the recommendation that we all need to eat enough carbs to support our thyroid gland and hormone production. It's true—you can induce hypothyroidism (insufficient thyroid hormone). Eating enough carbohydrate, specifically having enough available glucose, is essential for the production of functional thyroid hormone. This is why adding carbs to a chronically low-carb diet might jump-start weight loss: the additional thyroid hormone stimulates metabolism! See page 93.

· **Mood problems:** Serotonin, the "happy neurotransmitter," is produced largely in the gut, and this process depends on the presence of glucose. (That stereotypical low-carb crankiness is due in part to lower serotonin production.) If you have a propensity toward depression or anxiety, cutting off your serotonin supply might not be the best idea! Science also says that long-term low-carb diets might be problematic for cognitive function, so things like work performance might be sacrificed.

· **Insulin and hunger dysregulation:** Contrary to popular belief, some people experience insulin dysregulation when they go too low-carb. A recent study of the participants on the popular TV show *The Biggest Loser* demonstrated that there are long-term metabolic consequences to severe carbohydrate restriction that increase hunger and decrease a person's ability to lose weight and maintain weight loss. See page 85.

· **Gut health:** Dietary carbohydrates feed our microbiome. When we don't eat enough vegetables and fruit, we lose diversity in our gut bacteria. As previously discussed, this lack of diversity can have huge consequences for our health, including not just digestive upset but also issues with hormone regulation that undermine weight-loss efforts through effects on appetite and metabolism. See page 73.

· **Sleep:** Because of the role that carbohydrates, including fiber, play in hormone balance, they are essential for healthy sleep. In fact, research has demonstrated that less sugar and more fiber is the best formula for deep sleep. See page 338.

This is not to mention the importance of getting enough carbohydrates in certain states of being, like if you're an athlete (athletes' bodies need carbs to make glycogen and maximize athletic performance) or a pregnant woman (a growing fetus needs carbs for brain growth and other aspects of development). The notion that carbs are needed during pregnancy was corroborated by a recent study, which determined that a higher-carb diet is better for the metabolisms of pregnant women than a low-carb, high-fat diet.

So how many grams of carbohydrates should we aim for? An analysis of ethnographic data for 229 hunter-gatherer societies showed that the majority of these populations ate between 22 and 40 percent of their diets as carbohydrates. That translates to 110 to 200 grams of carbohydrates per day on a 2,000-calorie diet. A handful of societies fell outside that range; for example, some groups were eating as high as 50 percent carbohydrates. In general, hunter-gatherers living close to the equator had higher carbohydrate (and total plant food) intakes than populations living closer to polar regions, and virtually every group residing between 11 and 40 degrees north or south of the equator (equivalent to the range between the northern part of Colombia and New York City) ate between 30 to 35 percent carbohydrates as a percentage of total calories. On a 2,000-calorie diet, that comes out to 150 to 175 grams per day. Some critics of the data have pointed out that these levels could be underestimated due to a tendency for ethnographers to interact more with male hunters than with female gatherers and consequently under-document the contribution of gathered plant foods. But we can say with confidence that most hunter-gatherer groups eat about a third of their diet as carbohydrates.

Another way to frame the carbohydrate issue is to look at the bare minimum intake we'd need to get adequate daily fiber.

Current USDA fiber recommendations are 25 grams per day for women and 30 to 38 grams per day for men. This is definitely less than what most Paleolithic and modern hunter-gatherers consumed (Boyd Eaton and Melvin Konner estimate 45.7 grams per day for a typical hunter-gatherer diet of 65 percent plant foods, and Dr. Jeff Leach estimates that some hunter-gatherers eat as much as 200 grams of fiber per day), but I'll use the USDA numbers for the sake of illustration. If we look at nonstarchy vegetables with the highest ratio of fiber to non-fiber carbohydrates, spinach comes out near the top, with roughly half of its carbohydrates coming from fiber. In order to get 25 grams of fiber per day from spinach, our minimum carbohydrate intake would be 50 grams. (And for the record, we would need to eat about 45 cups of spinach—almost 3 pounds—to reach that level. That's pretty ambitious, even for those of us who love veggies!)

Using this logic, a carbohydrate intake of less than 50 grams per day is almost guaranteed to shortchange us on fiber. And that's assuming we eat nothing but the highest-fiber carbohydrates available. When our diet includes starchier or more sugary carbohydrate sources like tubers and fruit, which have a lower ratio of fiber to non-fiber carbs (while also being denser fiber sources), the minimum total carbohydrate we need to eat to meet our fiber needs rises even higher. For example, you'd need only about 3½ cups of baked sweet potato to get your 25 grams of fiber, but then you're looking at nearly 150 grams of total carbs—a similar amount to that consumed by hunter-gatherers.

SCIENCE SIMPLIFIED *Eating tons of veggies is key to losing weight and keeping it off, while supporting health in other ways. Instead of worrying about grams of carbohydrates, aim for one serving of a starchy root or tuber, like sweet potatoes, beets, or parsnips, with each meal in addition to two or more servings of nonstarchy veggies, like lettuce, broccoli, kale, cabbage, or celery.*

Provided that your carbohydrates are coming from whole fruits and vegetables, the 100- to 200-gram range is probably adequate from a fiber standpoint. Of course, emulating a hunter-gatherer fiber intake would be incredibly challenging without total carb intake creeping up toward 300 grams or more. When it comes to weight loss, we need to eat enough carbs to maintain health and support our metabolism. Planning to stay between 100 and 200 grams of total carbohydrates per day is a good "middle of the road" plan.

Lifestyle Adjustments for Weight Loss

While regular exercise is a fantastic tool for ensuring that we achieve a caloric deficit, research has demonstrated that exercise alone is not enough to induce spontaneous weight loss. So, while exercise contributes to weight loss, we can't spend endless hours at the gym without also altering other behaviors.

However, it's almost impossible to discuss exercise as a whole without addressing the different types of exercise individually. We know that the two different types of exercise (aerobic and anaerobic) have different effects on the body, and they have been studied separately in the scientific literature. Let's discuss how each type contributes to weight loss.

Aerobic exercise is essentially the scientific way of saying "cardio." From a scientific perspective, aerobic exercise involves cellular metabolism that utilizes oxygen. Really, this is normal human metabolism: aerobic exercise is just higher-intensity activity, so it involves the utilization of the stored glucose (as glycogen) in our muscles, and *that* is the enhanced caloric burn that we experience with this type of exercise. In a workout scenario, this translates to low to moderate activity that elevates heart rate and respiration rate and (almost always) involves sweating. Notably, extended periods of aerobic exercise utilize our available glycogen stores and promote the release of stored fatty acids. However, overexertion in the aerobic exercise realm can lead to muscular atrophy, so aim to keep this type of exercise to less than an hour per day.

SCIENCE SIMPLIFIED

In addition to contributing to a calorie deficit, exercise helps promote weight loss by increasing metabolism immediately afterward, increasing muscle mass, and increasing basal metabolic rate. Regular exercise is a key predictor of how successful someone will be at maintaining weight loss.

Apart from the obvious caloric-deficit aspect, there are other benefits to engaging in this type of exercise. Countless studies have demonstrated the metabolic benefits of aerobic activity specifically during weight-loss efforts, including increased insulin sensitivity and improved liver function. Why does this matter for weight loss? Because insulin acts on fat cells, it's critical for someone attempting to lose weight to be as insulin sensitive as possible. Aerobic exercise improves the functionality of fat cells and the liver, so we know that the fat being released from storage is going to be properly processed and used as energy.

Anaerobic exercise is the other main type of exercise. *Anaerobic* means that cellular metabolism is taking place without oxygen. Like aerobic metabolism, anaerobic cellular metabolism is totally normal; it is just used by different tissues and under specific conditions. In particular, type IIX fast-twitch muscle, which is used for sprinting and resistance training, utilizes this type of metabolism (see page 102). Why? It allows for faster movements and provides energy more quickly. The downside is that the by-product, lactic acid, is created by anaerobic metabolism and can build up in tissues (this is what causes the classic "burn" that we experience during intense exercise). Because anaerobic metabolism is a limited system, the limit of true anaerobic activity is only about 4 minutes. And because anaerobic metabolism does not utilize glucose in the same way that aerobic metabolism does, we don't understand how this type of activity specifically contributes to calories burned.

Still, there are compelling reasons to engage in high-intensity, anaerobic activity. Specific to weight loss, we see an increase in the release of stored fat immediately after anaerobic exercise. Plus, resistance training increases lean muscle mass. Relative to fat cells, muscle cells burn much more energy, so when we gain muscle mass, our metabolic rate goes up, even if we haven't lost any fat. For that reason alone, adding weight training focused on building muscle is essential for long-term weight-loss success and especially maintenance.

Although we typically think of weight loss as a matter of diet and exercise, a number of other lifestyle components can stand in the way.

Sleep is critical for keeping hormones in balance. Through changes in hormone signaling throughout the body (both our sensitivity to those signals and the amounts of hormones we produce), a lack of sleep alters our food preferences toward more energy-dense, hyperpalatable foods, as well as increases hunger, decreases fat metabolism, and increases the stress response, which affects basal metabolic rate. See Chapter 26.

Inadequate sleep has profound effects on hunger hormones and metabolism—up-regulating ghrelin (making us hungrier) and down-regulating insulin and leptin (making us insulin resistant), which makes us more prone to hormone resistance (such as insulin resistance, leptin resistance, and cortisol resistance, in which the body is less responsive to the actions of those hormones) that can easily complicate, delay, or even prevent weight loss. In studies, when food intake is measured following sleep deprivation, people tend to eat substantially (20 percent!) more than normal.

It's also critical to manage stress in order to lose weight. The net effect of cortisol is catabolic, meaning that it prepares the body for action without giving it an opportunity to rebuild. Plus, because cortisol increases blood glucose levels, chronically high cortisol can lead to increased storage of fat and makes it very difficult for us to use the fat we already have.

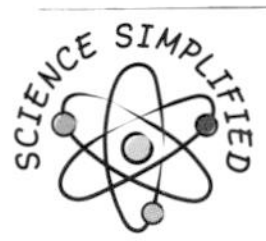

Getting enough sleep on a regular basis is key to successful weight loss and maintenance. See Chapter 26.

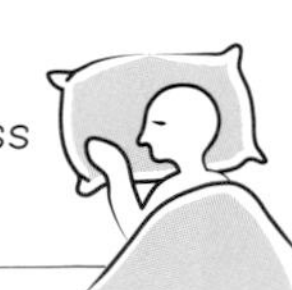

Nutrients to Metabolize Stored Energy

Just to be clear: there are no "magic bullet" nutrients (or foods, for that matter!) that will turn us into fat-burning machines. However, certain nutrients play important roles in mobilizing and metabolizing stored fat, and being deficient in any one of them could stand in the way of weight loss. To see how this works, let's first look at what goes on inside our bodies when we lose fat.

We all have energy stored in the form of fat in adipose tissue (fat cells) throughout our bodies and in the form of glycogen in our muscles and livers. When we lose weight, we want to lose weight in the form of fat (rather than just lose water from depleting glycogen stores—a common side effect of crash diets and low-carb/ketogenic diets). From a biochemical perspective, the fat molecules must be liberated from storage so that they can be converted to cellular energy, or adenosine triphosphate (ATP), in the energy-production organelles called mitochondria (see Chapter 22)—this is called lipid metabolism. This process includes help from assorted micronutrients, which act as cofactors (meaning their presence is necessary for a biological activity to take place) for the various enzymes involved in pyruvate oxidation and the Krebs cycle or as antioxidants. In fact, micronutrient sufficiency (especially of the micronutrients below) is necessary to "burn" fat, regardless of how many calories we consume. The following nutrients act as key players in this process.

Vitamin A

Vitamin A is one of the least obvious vitamins that promote fat burning, but it has one of the clearest mechanisms! Vitamin A is a fat-soluble vitamin known to play key roles in vision, neurological function, healthy skin, and antioxidant function. There are several forms, including active forms such as retinal and retinoic acid and vitamin A precursors called *carotenoids*.

One of the active forms of vitamin A is retinal. This molecule is best known for its role in vision, but it has also been implicated as a regulator of lipid metabolism. Vitamin A can burn fat in several ways. An enzyme called retinaldehyde dehydrogenase 1 (RALDH1), which converts retinal to retinoic acid, is dense in white adipose tissue. Down-regulating this enzyme (that is, turning it off) by taking in large doses of vitamin A makes it possible for white adipose tissue to start thermogenesis, a characteristic normally isolated to brown adipose tissue.

Let me clarify this a little bit: there are different kinds of adipose tissue. White adipose tissue (WAT) is what we commonly think of when we think of fat; it is simply a type of cell that stores fat. Brown adipose tissue (BAT), which is rich in mitochondria, is another story. While some lipids are stored here, BAT cells undergo thermogenesis, which occurs when mitochondria use fat molecules to produce heat rather than energy. This process is useful for maintaining basal body temperature. So, to restate the above: it looks like high doses of vitamin A (specifically retinal) is a potential "biohack" to increase metabolism by making WAT act like BAT. Retinal also seems to be involved in the regulation of how fats are stored and used in our bones—yet another reason to focus on getting plenty of vitamin A in our diet.

So vitamin A is capable of some awesome biochemical magic! Where do we get it? The richest dietary source of vitamin A is liver. Bonus: liver is rich not just in vitamin A precursors but also in retinal, the active form specifically implicated for lipid metabolism. There are other Paleo sources of vitamin A, though the amount and form depends on the food; vegetables like sweet potatoes are more likely to feature precursors (like β-carotene) rather than active forms.

Vitamin B1

Vitamin B1 (thiamin) is one of the many B complex vitamins, all of which are involved in metabolism (and thus are super-helpful when we want to burn fat!). Vitamin B1 is necessary for the normal metabolism of several molecules, including carbohydrates, lipids, and branched-chain amino acids. Thus this water-soluble vitamin is essential for the "end stage" process of using previously stored fat—the lipids have already been liberated from fat cells and transported to the liver, where they've been converted to acetyl-CoA to be broken down for energy. Thiamin acts as an enzyme cofactor in two parts of cellular metabolism: glycolysis and the Krebs cycle. Plus, it is a cofactor for the endogenous production of simple carbohydrates (this process maintains blood sugar levels overnight and when all the carbohydrate stores in the liver have been used up). So vitamin B1 is necessary for life (our cells need energy to live!) but is particularly necessary for someone who is hoping to metabolize stored fat.

The best sources of vitamin B1 are organ meat, pork, seeds, squash, and fish like mackerel, salmon, trout, and tuna.

Vitamin B3

Vitamin B3 (niacin) is another water-soluble B complex vitamin that is used in cellular metabolism within the mitochondria. Much like B1, this vitamin is part of our primary metabolic system, meaning that we need it to produce energy from any macronutrient (fat, protein, or carbohydrate—it all ends with glycolysis!). Specifically, vitamin B3 is necessary for oxidation-reduction reactions, which involves the transfer of electrons (an essential part of converting glucose to ATP). Plus, it is used in the production of many molecules important for health, like cholesterol, and L-carnitine, which is essential for lipid metabolism.

Vitamin B3 is found in dairy, poultry, fish, meat, eggs, and some plant sources (including vegetables, nuts, and seeds). While deficiency is pretty rare, focusing on getting enough vitamin B3 definitely makes it easier for our bodies to metabolize fats.

Vitamin B5

Vitamin B5 (pantothenic acid) is yet another B complex vitamin involved in cellular metabolism, making it essential for life. The main reason vitamin B5 is so necessary is that it is a precursor to coenzyme A (CoA), which cells use to make energy, steroid molecules (which are hormone precursors), or ketone bodies (which the brain can use for energy if it runs out of glucose). So we need vitamin B5 to burn fat *and* for all the hormones that regulate our metabolism! Beyond that, vitamin B5 is used to make a fatty acid carrier molecule that is necessary for the storage of fatty acids.

Like vitamin B3 deficiency, vitamin B5 deficiency is extremely rare because this vitamin is found in so many plant and animal foods. However, emphasizing foods that are particularly rich in B5 (especially shiitake mushrooms) makes a lot of sense for weight loss.

Vitamin B6

Vitamin B6 refers to a group of six forms of a water-soluble vitamin that cannot be synthesized in our bodies, so we must get it from our diet. Vitamin B6 is a cofactor for more than a hundred enzymes that catalyze essential chemical reactions. One of the many roles it plays is in fatty acid metabolism, including synthesizing essential fatty acids (which help control inflammation, making it easier to lose weight!).

Many foods in the Paleo diet are high in vitamin B6, including organ meat, fish, summer squash, banana, pistachios, and blackstrap molasses.

Vitamin B7

Vitamin B7 (biotin) is also essential for metabolism, and we need exogenous sources, as we can't synthesize vitamin B7 on our own. Its main role is as an enzyme cofactor within biochemical pathways, including cellular metabolic pathways such as glycolysis, fatty acid oxidation (fat burning), and fatty acid synthesis.

Studies have shown that vitamin B7 deficiency is related to issues with glucose metabolism, and we know that impaired glucose metabolism is associated with weight gain (that is, fat gain). Plus, a higher intake of vitamin B7 is associated with reduced plasma triglycerides, further demonstrating how vitamin B7 can be used to alter metabolism in our favor.

Vitamin B7 is easy to acquire from a Paleo diet. The foods highest in vitamin B7 include egg yolks, liver, and yeast. Since we need to get vitamin B7 from food, there is a chance of deficiency. Ensuring that we get enough vitamin B7 is absolutely necessary if we have some fat to burn!

CoQ10

CoQ10 (coenzyme Q10) is a non-vitamin micronutrient that is part of the ubiquinone family of compounds. Our livers make the majority of the CoQ10 that we need, but there is some benefit to consuming additional CoQ10 either in supplement form or in food (especially for people on statin medications, which are known to lower blood levels of CoQ10).

CoQ10 is found in the cell membranes of virtually all cells. Its main function is as an electron acceptor—a key part of cellular metabolism. In fact, CoQ10 is known to act within the mitochondrial electron transport chain (see page 267), facilitating the conversion of glucose and fatty acids to cellular energy. CoQ10 is also a fat-soluble antioxidant. Given that fatty acid oxidation (read: weight loss, fat loss, and so on) can generate free radicals that can damage our DNA (progressing aging and potentially increasing our chances for disease, like cancer and cardiovascular disease), having some CoQ10 and vitamin E (another fat-soluble antioxidant) around to absorb extra electrons is important. While we don't know much about clinical levels of deficiency in this cofactor, we do know that impaired energy metabolism is associated with lower serum (a component of blood) levels of CoQ10. Organ meat (especially heart) and sardines are high in CoQ10.

Iron

Iron is a well-known dietary mineral that is rich in any Paleo diet that includes red meat. (Iron is also present in some vegetables, though it is not as bioavailable as the iron in animal foods.) Iron is perhaps best known for its role in oxygen transport and storage; this metal ion is featured in heme-containing proteins like hemoglobin, which is responsible for transporting oxygen through our blood, and myoglobin, which is responsible for storing oxygen. We need oxygen to complete the process of cellular metabolism, in which oxygen acts as an electron acceptor (similar to CoQ10, but at the end of the chain).

Beyond its role in oxygen transport, iron has an even more direct role in cellular metabolism: it is featured in the proteins of the electron transport chain itself. These proteins are called *cytochromes*, and they facilitate the movement of electrons through the chain. Finally, iron is a cofactor in an incredibly important family of enzymes called the cytochrome P450 family, which are proteins in the liver responsible for the metabolism of many molecules, including fatty acids. Basically, having enough iron is super-important for metabolism on multiple levels, so it should be on everyone's list of pro-fat metabolizers. Consuming vitamin C-rich foods at the same time as iron-rich foods can help increase iron absorption.

L-Carnitine

L-carnitine is perhaps the best-known "fat burner" there is, which is why many people take it in supplement form (though we know that we need it along with other vitamins and minerals, so taking it on its own is less effective than getting it from food). This molecule is another non-vitamin micronutrient (it's actually a derivative of the amino acid lysine) that we know to be involved in the metabolism of fatty acids.

L-carnitine is specifically involved in the oxidation of long-chain fatty acids, so it's directly involved in fat-burning. This amino acid derivative is most concentrated in areas that use fatty acids as their primary fuel, such as skeletal and cardiac (heart) muscle, though it is found in all cells. L-carnitine binds a long-chain fatty acid (which is bound to CoA, a derivative of vitamin B5, as discussed earlier) so it can bring it across the outer mitochondrial membrane into the mitochondria. From there, it passes the inner membrane to the mitochondrial matrix, where it is oxidized before entering the other biochemical pathways of cellular metabolism (the Krebs cycle and electron transport chain, specifically). Plus, the addition of L-carnitine is considered the rate-limiting step, meaning that metabolism proceeds at the rate at which L-carnitine is available. Without L-carnitine, we cannot utilize stored fat for energy!

Healthy people without metabolic diseases seem to be able to generate enough L-carnitine to meet the cellular demands of everyday life. However, someone hoping to promote the use of fat for fuel may want to ensure that they have more than enough L-carnitine to meet the demands of a lot of fatty acid oxidation. L-carnitine is particularly abundant in red meat.

Creatine

Creatine is a nutrient touted by bodybuilders for its ability to aid in muscle building. But what about fat loss? This connection is a little less direct because there is no specific mechanism for fat metabolism. However, dietary intake of creatine is known to promote muscle building, which increases the metabolic needs of our bodies. Basically, muscles need more energy to function (fat cells are super energy-efficient because their one goal is to store energy), so building and maintaining muscle increases our basal and active metabolic rates.

Creatine is found in meat (including organ meat) and fish, so most people following a Paleo diet will be sufficient in this micronutrient. This muscle booster can also be made from the amino acids glycine and arginine. One of the richest sources of these is collagen, which is abundant in bone broth and can also be taken in supplement form.

Vitamin D

Vitamin D is a fat-soluble vitamin that is synthesized in the skin upon exposure to sunlight and then metabolized and activated by the liver and kidneys. This amazing vitamin, which also has some hormonal properties, carries out an incredible variety of functions in the body, including regulation of the metabolism. While scientists are still trying to determine the exact mechanisms, we know that people with excess fat tend to be deficient in vitamin D, and at least one study has shown that supplementing with vitamin D decreased body fat. Foods rich in vitamin D include fatty fish, liver, and egg yolks—but my favorite way to get vitamin D is with some sunshine!

About 75 percent of Westerners are deficient in vitamin D. Optimal serum vitamin D levels are between 40 and 60 ng/ml; ask a health-care provider to test your levels. If you're deficient, it can be tough to get enough vitamin D from foods (natural sources include grass-fed and pasture-raised meat and seafood), so consider supplementing with vitamin D3 and recheck your levels every 3 months to make sure you don't overshoot the mark. Serum vitamin D levels in excess of 100 ng/ml can also cause health problems.

These nutrients are just a sample of the incredible breadth of micronutrients that our bodies use to go through the vast number of chemical reactions that allow us to function every minute of every day. While nutrient density is a fantastic goal within a Paleo template, we know that focusing on these particular micronutrients will make it easier for us to burn fat.

WEIGHT-LOSS TIPS

A caloric deficit is essential for weight loss. That means you must eat fewer calories than you burn. Increasing activity is clearly helpful here, but the biggest factor is how many calories you take in.

Slow and steady wins the race. Thanks to leptin's dual response to overeating and undereating (see page 90), aiming for a modest caloric deficit (say, 10 to 20 percent) typically leads to more easily maintainable weight loss. That's a common spontaneous caloric deficit achieved simply by following a standard Paleo diet.

Nutrient deficiencies can increase appetite and cravings, as well as inhibit the body's ability to access and burn stored fat. Thus a nutrient-dense diet is key.

The best strategy for spontaneously achieving a caloric deficit is to eat tons of veggies. Aim for eight to ten servings and at least 30 grams of fiber from veggies and some fruit daily.

Low carbohydrate or low fat won't help you lose weight. Instead, aim for balanced macronutrients (say, 30-30-40; it doesn't really matter which one is the 40 percent) and make sure to get enough protein to support muscle mass and metabolism.

Eating a protein-packed breakfast sets you up for better food choices during the day. Eating within a couple of hours of bedtime increases metabolism and suppresses the release of growth hormones, which makes it difficult to lose weight. And eating right before bed can negatively affect your sleep quality.

Yes, there are some hyperpalatable foods within the Paleo framework! Natural sugars (such as honey), Paleo treats, nut-based baked goods, and the like should be avoided when weight loss is your goal.

Getting enough sleep and managing stress help regulate appetite and reduce cravings, as well as improve metabolism, reduce inflammation, and restore insulin and leptin sensitivity.

Getting plenty of moderately intense physical activity helps boost metabolism and contributes to a caloric deficit. Also engage in some anaerobic activity, like sprinting or resistance training, to build lean muscle mass.

Generally, your basic Paleo plate will contain a 5- to 8-ounce serving of not-too-fatty, not-too-lean meat or seafood and three or more servings of veggies. Think of nuts and seeds as condiments. Limit fruit to three to five servings per day. Eating less frequently (two or three meals a day) is better for insulin and leptin sensitivity.

Counting calories isn't a great long-term solution, but when in doubt, you can use it as a tool to educate yourself on what your plate should look like and use this information to improve your food choices.

REDUCING CARDIOVASCULAR DISEASE RISK

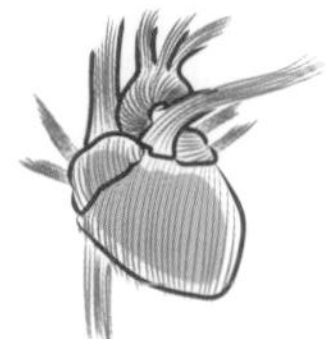

Cardiovascular disease, including coronary heart disease, hypertensive heart disease, and stroke, is the number-one global killer and is unequivocally rooted in diet and lifestyle. Approximately 84 million Americans suffer from cardiovascular disease, with approximately 610,000 deaths annually from heart disease alone. The good news is that multiple clinical trials have demonstrated that a Paleo-style diet can reduce virtually every risk factor for cardiovascular disease, including high triglycerides, high LDL ("bad") cholesterol and low HDL ("good") cholesterol, high blood pressure, high insulin, high blood sugar, high C-reactive protein, and other markers of inflammation.

That being said, what can we do to fine-tune the Paleo template to offer the best possible protection against cardiovascular disease? This question is particularly relevant for people who have a family history of heart disease or stroke (which can indicate a genetic component that raises disease risk, such as carrying the ApoE4 phenotype; see page 187) or who have already been diagnosed with cardiovascular disease. Luckily, Paleo can easily be modified to offer even more support for the cardiovascular system.

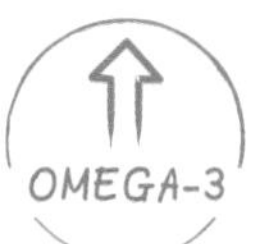

- **Eat plenty of omega-3-rich seafood.** Across numerous studies, omega-3 fats are consistently associated with a reduced risk of cardiovascular disease, as well as reduced mortality from sudden cardiac death. These fats promote cardiovascular health in a variety of ways, including by lowering triglycerides and reducing inflammation. Seafood is also a good food source of vitamin D, which is important because deficiency is linked to increased cardiovascular disease risk.

- **If you smoke, quit!** Smoking is a powerful risk factor for cardiovascular disease. If you're a smoker, embarking on even the most nutritious Paleo diet won't be enough to offset the damage and disease risk created by smoking.

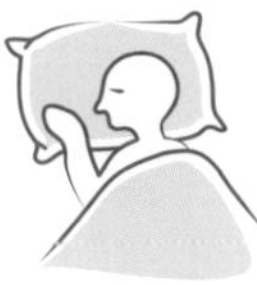

- **Get plenty of sleep.** Sleep deprivation is a major contributor to cardiovascular disease risk and is associated with higher blood pressure, weight gain, obesity, and higher rates of heart disease and stroke. In fact, routinely sleeping less than 6 hours per night (compared to getting between 6 and 8 hours) doubles the risk of stroke, heart attack, and coronary heart disease while also raising the risk of congestive heart failure. (See Chapter 26.)

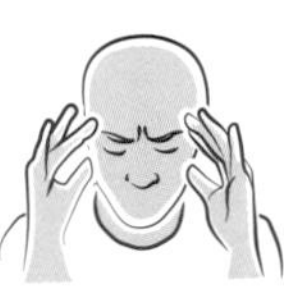

- **Manage stress.** Stress is a bigger predictor of cardiovascular disease than any other diet or lifestyle factor. Every effort to reduce avoidable stressors or to manage existing chronic stress translates to increased protection against cardiovascular disease. (See Chapter 27.)

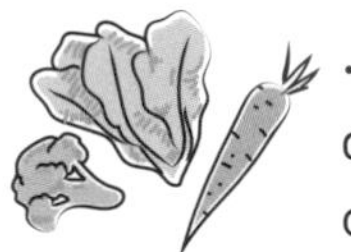

- **Focus on fiber.** The fiber in nutrient-dense vegetables, fruits, nuts, and seeds can go a long way toward protecting the cardiovascular system. Fiber consumption is associated with a lower risk of stroke and heart disease, and some types of fiber can reduce LDL cholesterol, lower blood pressure, and promote a healthy body weight. (See page 39.)

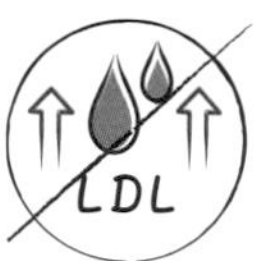

- **Eat saturated fat in reasonable, not excessive, quantities.** Although the idea that high-saturated fat animal foods cause heart disease has been discredited, eating excessive quantities of saturated fat (such as by going hog wild on butter, ghee, and coconut oil) is a question mark in terms of long-term effects on human health. Certain genetic factors, such as being an ApoE4 carrier (see page 187), may make some people more sensitive to the LDL-raising properties of some forms of saturated fat.

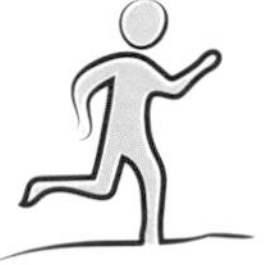

- **Engage in gentle movement throughout the day.** Although chronic overtraining can actually harm the cardiovascular system by raising cortisol and inflammatory markers, frequent gentle movement helps improve insulin sensitivity and circulation.

MANAGING DIABETES

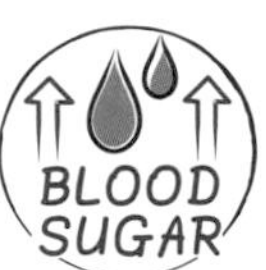

Diabetes affects more than just the 29 million Americans who have been diagnosed with it—an estimated 8 million Americans have undiagnosed diabetes, and an estimated 87 million Americans are prediabetic, meaning that they have insulin resistance.

Trials of Paleo-style diets on type 2 diabetics (and others with poor glycemic control) consistently show that Paleo can be a powerful tool for reducing both the risk factors and the symptoms of diabetes. Compared to conventional low-fat diabetes diets, Paleo leads to greater improvements in blood sugar, triglycerides, blood pressure, body weight, waist circumference, and body mass index. Logically, this makes sense: Paleo carbohydrates tend to be low glycemic, Paleo fats and proteins contribute to steady blood sugar levels, and the Paleo template overall encourages weight loss in people carrying extra body fat (the accumulation of fat in the pancreas contributes to insulin resistance and eventually diabetes).

Although Paleo can help many people manage diabetes without any special modifications, diabetics should be cautious of the handful of higher-glycemic foods that are technically Paleo-friendly—including dried fruits (raisins, dried figs, dried apricots, and so on), watermelon, pineapple, mangoes, white potatoes (although their glycemic index is reduced after they are cooked and cooled—see page 298), and unrefined sweeteners like maple syrup, honey, sucanat, muscovado (Barbados) sugar, and molasses. Likewise, emphasizing fiber-rich foods, protein, and nutrient-dense sources of fat can help prevent insulin spikes and keep blood sugar levels on an even keel throughout the day. It's also important to focus on other components of the Paleo framework that help improve insulin sensitivity, such as getting adequate sleep, managing stress, and engaging in gentle movement throughout the day (see Part 5).

If you are a diabetic adopting the Paleo template, it's still important to monitor your blood sugar levels after meals and adjust your insulin doses accordingly, if taking. If you have type 1 diabetes, it's valuable to learn more about mitigating autoimmune disease with the Autoimmune Protocol; see pages 412 to 414.

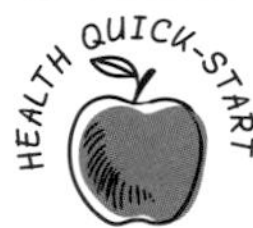

Each of the following independently reduces the risk of diabetes. That means the more items you check off this list, the lower your risk:

- *Getting at least 8 hours of sleep every single night (see Chapter 26).*
- *Managing stress by reducing stressors and increasing resilience (see Chapter 27).*
- *Living an active lifestyle and avoiding prolonged periods of inactivity during the day (see Chapter 28).*
- *Moderating fructose intake to 10 to 40 grams daily and avoiding eating too many calories (see Chapter 22).*
- *Eating tons of veggies and fruits; berries, leafy greens, yellow veggies, and cruciferous veggies all independently reduce diabetes risk (see Chapter 8).*
- *Consuming plenty of the nutrients important for insulin sensitivity, including vitamins B3, B6, B9, B12, and D, as well as chromium, calcium, magnesium, zinc, inositol, alpha-lipoic acid, omega-3 fatty acids, carnitine, and fiber (see Chapter 1).*

REDUCING CANCER RISK

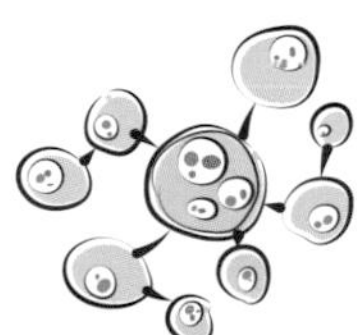

Cancer is the number-two global killer, with 15 million Americans affected and an estimated 595,000 annual deaths in the United States alone.

No diet or lifestyle protocol has ever been proven to cure cancer. (Despite claims made about Gerson therapy, the Gonzalez protocol, and other regimens, there is no peer-reviewed evidence demonstrating that these programs can treat existing cancer.) Likewise, the Paleo diet has not been evaluated for treating cancer patients and should not be viewed as a cure for this disease.

However, there *is* ample evidence that Paleo can help reduce cancer risk (keeping in mind that reducing cancer risk is different from *treating* cancer). Whole, fresh plant foods are rich in a massive spectrum of phytochemicals with proven anti-cancer properties, such as cyanidins and resveratrol in grapes, curcumin in turmeric, crocetin in saffron, apigenin in parsley, lycopene in tomatoes, fisetin in strawberries and apples, gingerol in ginger, kaempferol in broccoli and grapefruit, and indole-3-carbinol, isothiocyanates, and sulforaphanes in cruciferous vegetables. Maintaining sufficient levels of vitamin D (through sun exposure, supplementation, and/or food sources like salmon) helps protect against a wide range of cancers. Likewise, some types of fiber appear to protect against colorectal cancer.

If you have a family history of cancer or know via genetic testing that you have cancer genes like specific mutations in the BRCA1 or BRCA2 gene, your best bet is an even greater focus on vegetables and high-antioxidant fruits in addition to tracking micronutrients to ensure nutrient sufficiency. There is emerging evidence that deficiency in important immune system nutrients like zinc, omega-3 fatty acids, and vitamin D may increase cancer risk.

Additional lifestyle practices embraced by the Paleo framework, such as getting enough sleep and managing stress, are also associated with reduced cancer risk.

MITIGATING AUTOIMMUNE DISEASE

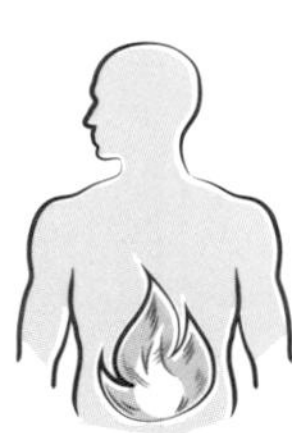

Autoimmune disease is an epidemic in our society, affecting an estimated 50 million Americans. There are more than a hundred confirmed autoimmune diseases—some of the most common being Graves' disease, Hashimoto's thyroiditis, lupus, rheumatoid arthritis, multiple sclerosis, Sjögren's syndrome, alopecia, psoriasis, ulcerative colitis, Crohn's disease, and type 1 diabetes—and many more diseases that are suspected of having autoimmune origins. Although each condition brings unique symptoms, the root cause of all autoimmune diseases is the same: our immune system, which is supposed to protect us from invading microorganisms, turns against us and attacks our own proteins, cells, and tissues instead. Which proteins, cells, and tissues are attacked determines the specific autoimmune disease and its symptoms. For example, in Hashimoto's thyroiditis, the thyroid gland is attacked. In rheumatoid arthritis, the tissues of the joints are attacked. In psoriasis, proteins within the layers of skin cells are attacked.

Although genetic predisposition accounts for approximately a third of the risk of developing an autoimmune disease, the other two-thirds comes from diet, lifestyle, and environmental factors. In fact, experts are increasingly recognizing that certain dietary factors are key contributors to autoimmune disease, placing these autoimmune conditions in the same class of diet- and lifestyle-related diseases as type 2 diabetes, cardiovascular disease, and obesity. That means that in many cases, managing autoimmune disease and preventing (or at least minimizing) flares is within our power.

Because the Paleo diet naturally eliminates a number of autoimmune triggers (including foods that cause or aggravate a leaky gut) while including key nutrients that support healthy immune and hormone function, simply adopting a Paleo diet may lead to noticeable improvements in symptoms. However, a modified form of Paleo called the *Paleo Autoimmune Protocol* (typically abbreviated AIP) takes the therapeutic effects of Paleo even further. The AIP is a powerful strategy that uses diet and lifestyle to regulate the immune system, putting an end to the attacks and giving the body the opportunity to heal.

The Autoimmune Protocol is a specialized version of the Paleo diet with an even greater focus on nutrient density and even stricter guidelines for which foods should be eliminated. The elimination list includes some foods typically allowed on the Paleo diet that have compounds that may stimulate the immune system or harm the gut environment, including nightshades (like tomatoes and peppers), eggs, nuts, seeds, and alcohol. The goal of the AIP is to flood the body with nutrients while avoiding any food that might be contributing to disease (or at the very least interfering with efforts to heal). It is an elimination diet strategy, cutting out those foods that are most likely to hold back our health. After a time, many of the excluded foods, especially those that have nutritional merit despite also containing some (but not significant quantities of) potentially detrimental compounds, can be reintroduced by using the protocol outlined in Chapter 25.

The key focuses of the Autoimmune Protocol are:

• **Nutrient density.** The immune system (and indeed every system in the body) requires an array of vitamins, minerals, antioxidants, essential fatty acids, and amino acids to function normally. Micronutrient deficiencies and imbalances are key players in the development and progression of autoimmune disease. Focusing on consuming the most nutrient-dense foods available enables a synergistic surplus of micronutrients to correct both deficiencies and imbalances, thus supporting regulation of the immune system, hormone system, and detoxification system and the production of neurotransmitters. A nutrient-dense diet further provides the building blocks that the body needs to heal damaged tissues.

• **Gut health.** Gut dysbiosis and leaky gut are key facilitators in the development of autoimmune disease. The foods recommended on the AIP support the growth of both healthy levels and a healthy variety of gut microorganisms. Foods that irritate or damage the lining of the gut are avoided, while foods that help restore gut barrier function and promote healing are endorsed.

A PRIMER ON THE AUTOIMMUNE PROTOCOL

The Autoimmune Protocol (AIP) is the most nutrient-focused and anti-inflammatory version of the Paleo diet. In addition to eliminating all the foods listed in Part 3, it omits middle-ground foods and foods with a high likelihood of intolerance and allergy, as described in Chapter 24.

"YES" FOODS

Here are some examples of foods from each of the major Paleo Autoimmune Protocol food groups.

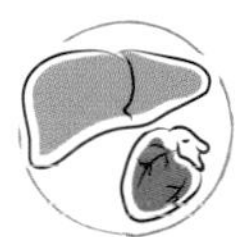

ORGAN MEAT

bone broth
heart
kidney
liver
tongue

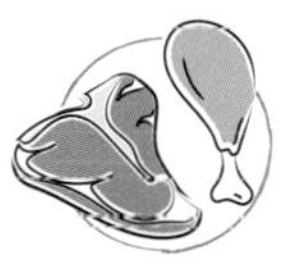

RED MEAT AND POULTRY

beef
bison
chicken
lamb
mutton
pork
turkey
wild game

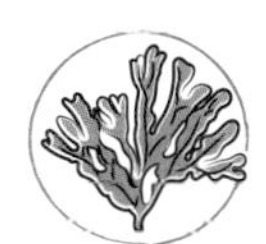

SEA VEGETABLES

arame
dulse
kombu
nori
wakame

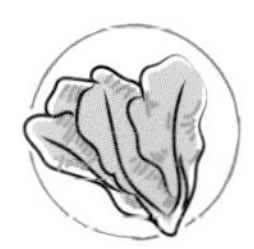

LEAFY GREENS

beet greens
bok choy
carrot tops
dandelion greens
endive
herbs
kale
lettuce
spinach
Swiss chard
turnip greens
watercress

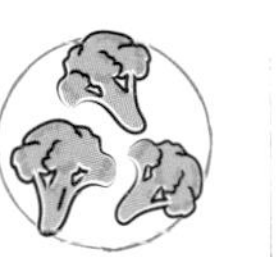

CRUCIFEROUS VEGETABLES

arugula
broccoli
Brussels sprouts
cabbage
cauliflower
collard greens
kohlrabi
mustard greens
napa cabbage
radishes
radicchio
turnips

ROOT VEGETABLES AND WINTER SQUASH

arrowroot
beets
carrots
cassava (aka tapioca, yuca)
jicama
pumpkin
rutabaga
squash
sweet potatoes
taro
yams

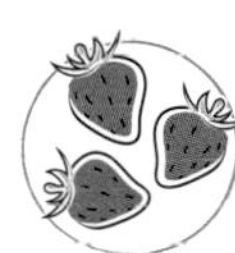

BERRIES

blackberries
blueberries
cranberries
currants
grapes
raspberries
strawberries

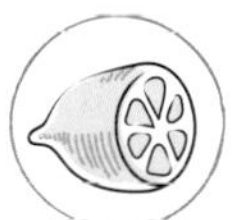

CITRUS FRUITS

clementines
grapefruit
lemons
limes
mandarin oranges
navel oranges

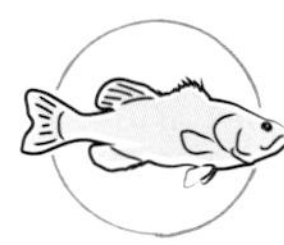

FISH

anchovies
catfish
cod
halibut
herring
mackerel
mahi mahi
salmon
sardines
snapper
tilapia
trout
tuna

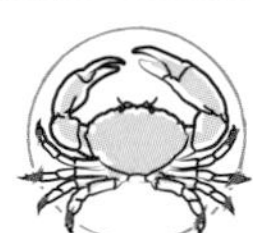

SHELLFISH

clams
crab
crawfish
lobster
mussels
octopus
oysters
prawns
scallops
shrimp
squid

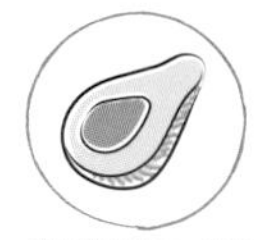

OLIVES AND OTHER HIGH-FAT FRUITS

avocados
coconut
olives (black and green)

ONIONS, GARLIC, AND OTHER ALLIUMS

chives
garlic
leeks
onions
scallions
shallots
spring onions

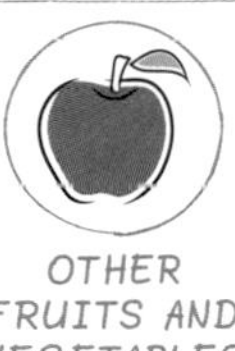

OTHER FRUITS AND VEGETABLES

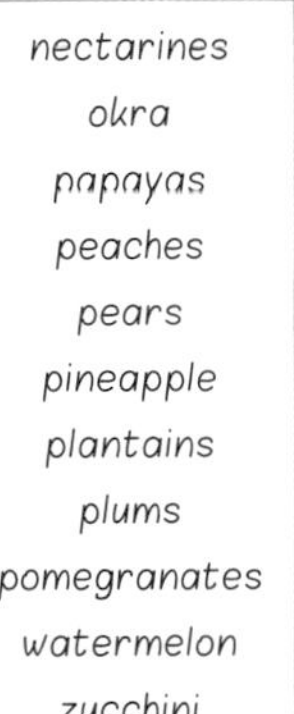

apples
apricots
artichokes
asparagus
bananas
cantaloupe
capers
celery
cherries
cucumbers
dates
figs
honeydew melon
kiwis
mangoes
mushrooms
nectarines
okra
papayas
peaches
pears
pineapple
plantains
plums
pomegranates
watermelon
zucchini

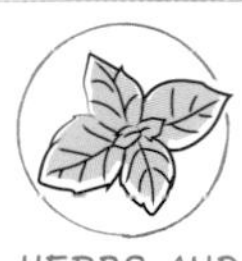

HERBS AND SPICES

basil
chives
cilantro
cinnamon
ginger
mint
oregano
parsley
rosemary
sage
sea salt (unrefined)
thyme
turmeric

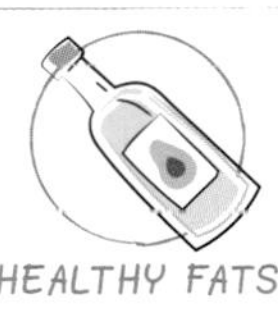

HEALTHY FATS

avocado oil
coconut oil
olive oil
lard (preferably pastured)
tallow (preferably grass-fed)

· **Hormone regulation.** What, when, and how much we eat affect a variety of hormones that interact with the immune system. When dietary factors (like eating too much sugar or grazing rather than eating larger meals spaced farther apart) dysregulate these hormones, the immune system is directly affected—typically stimulated. The AIP is designed to promote regulation of these hormones, thereby regulating the immune system. These and other essential hormones that impact the immune system are also profoundly affected by how much sleep we get, how much time we spend outside, how much and what kinds of activity we get, and how well we reduce and manage stress.

· **Immune system regulation.** Immune system regulation is achieved by restoring a healthy diversity and healthy number of gut microorganisms, restoring gut barrier function, providing sufficient amounts of micronutrients, and regulating the key hormones that regulate the immune system.

A PRIMER ON THE AUTOIMMUNE PROTOCOL

"NO" FOODS

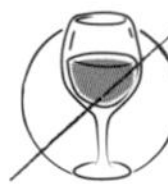

ALCOHOL: beer, wine (okay for cooking), spirits

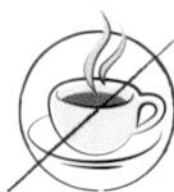

COFFEE: except for perhaps an occasional cup

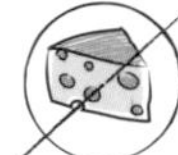

DAIRY: butter, buttermilk, butter oil, cheese, cottage cheese, cream, curds, dairy protein isolates, ghee, heavy cream, ice cream, kefir, milk, sour cream, whey, whey protein isolate, whipping cream, yogurt

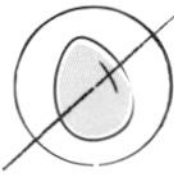

EGGS

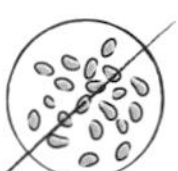

PSEUDOGRAINS: amaranth, buckwheat, chia, quinoa

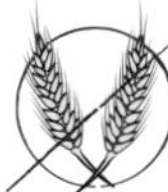

GRAINS: barley, corn, durum, fonio, Job's tears, kamut, millet, oats, rice, rye, sorghum, spelt, teff, triticale, wheat (all varieties, including einkorn and semolina), wild rice

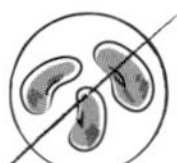

LEGUMES: adzuki beans, black beans, black-eyed peas, butter beans, calico beans, cannellini beans, chickpeas (garbanzo beans), fava beans (broad beans), Great Northern beans, green beans, Italian beans, kidney beans, lentils, lima beans, mung beans, navy beans, peanuts, peas, pinto beans, runner beans, soybeans (including edamame, tofu, tempeh, other soy products, soy isolates [such as soy lecithin]), split peas

NIGHTSHADES AND SPICES DERIVED FROM NIGHTSHADES:

ashwagandha, bell peppers (sweet peppers), cape gooseberries (ground cherries, not to be confused with regular cherries, which are okay), cayenne pepper, eggplant, garden huckleberries (not to be confused with regular huckleberries, which are okay), goji berries (wolfberries), hot peppers (chili peppers and chili-based spices), naranjillas, paprika, pepinos, pimentos, potatoes (sweet potatoes are okay), tamarillos, tomatillos, tomatoes (Note: Some curry powders contain nightshade ingredients.)

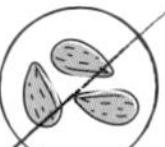

NUTS AND SEEDS: almonds, Brazil nuts, cashews, chestnuts, flax seeds, hazelnuts, hemp seeds, macadamia nuts, pecans, pine nuts, pistachios, poppy seeds, pumpkin seeds, sesame seeds, sunflower seeds, walnuts, any flours, butters, oils, or other products derived from nuts or seeds

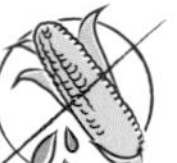

PROBLEMATIC SUGARS AND SWEETENERS: agave, agave nectar, barley malt, barley malt syrup, brown rice syrup, brown sugar, cane crystals, cane sugar (refined), caramel, corn sweetener, corn syrup, corn syrup solids, crystalline fructose, dehydrated cane juice, demerara sugar, dextrin, dextrose, diastatic malt, evaporated cane juice, fructose, fruit juice, fruit juice concentrate, galactose, glucose, glucose solids, golden syrup, high-fructose corn syrup, inulin, invert sugar, lactose, malt syrup, maltodextrin, maltose, monk fruit (luo han guo), panela, panocha, refined sugar, rice bran syrup, rice syrup, sorghum syrup, sucrose (saccharose), syrup, treacle, turbinado sugar, yacon syrup

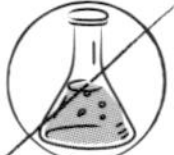

PROCESSED FOOD CHEMICALS AND INGREDIENTS: acrylamides, artificial food color, artificial and natural flavors, autolyzed protein, brominated vegetable oil, emulsifiers (carrageenan, cellulose gum, guar gum, lecithin, xanthan gum), hydrolyzed vegetable protein, monosodium glutamate, nitrates or nitrites (naturally occurring are okay), olestra, phosphoric acid, propylene glycol, textured vegetable protein, trans fats (partially hydrogenated vegetable oil, hydrogenated oil), yeast extract, any ingredient with a chemical name that you don't recognize

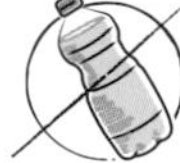

PROCESSED VEGETABLE OILS: canola oil (rapeseed oil), corn oil, cottonseed oil, palm kernel oil, peanut oil, safflower oil, soybean oil, sunflower oil

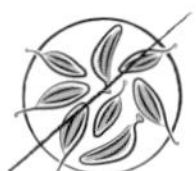

SPICES DERIVED FROM SEEDS: anise, annatto, black caraway (Russian caraway, black cumin), celery seed, coriander, cumin, dill, fennel, fenugreek, mustard, nutmeg

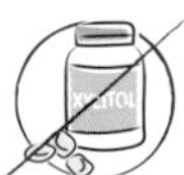

SUGAR SUBSTITUTES: acesulfame potassium (acesulfame K), aspartame, erythritol, mannitol, neotame, saccharin, sorbitol, stevia, sucralose, xylitol

Although scientific research on Paleo and autoimmune disease is still in its infancy, studies of multiple sclerosis patients have already shown that the AIP has therapeutic potential for the debilitating autoimmune disease secondary progressing multiple sclerosis, and studies of inflammatory bowel disease have shown that full remission occurs in a matter of weeks in the majority of patients. And while anecdotal stories cannot be used to validate any dietary approach, the tens of thousands (and counting!) of people who have successfully used variations of the Paleo diet, including the AIP, to mitigate and even completely reverse their diseases is compelling. For a comprehensive guide to the Autoimmune Protocol, read my book *The Paleo Approach.*

ALLEVIATING ASTHMA AND ALLERGIES

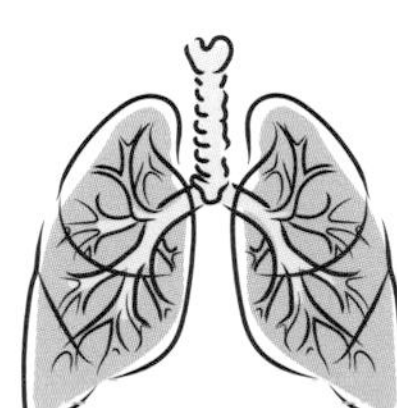

Asthma and allergies affect huge portions of the population: about 8 percent of Americans have asthma, and allergies affect as many as 30 percent of adults and 40 percent of children! Although we don't have any studies looking specifically at the effects of a Paleo diet on these conditions, plenty of evidence suggests dietary changes that reduce inflammation and regulate the body's immune response can improve asthma and allergies—without the harmful side effects that many medications bring. Three nutrients, in particular, have been shown in clinical trials to improve asthma and allergy symptoms.

Dietary Fermentable Fiber

In case we need yet another reason to embrace fiber, here it is! The short-chain fatty acids produced when our gut microbes metabolize fiber may suppress airway inflammation, leading to improvements in asthma symptoms. One study in mice found that a high-fiber diet increased the production of acetate (a short-chain fatty acid) in the gut, in turn enhancing the number and function of regulatory T-cells (see page 79) and suppressing the animals' allergic airway disease (the equivalent of human asthma). Another rodent study found that increasing the fermentable fiber content of the diet altered gut and lung microbiota, leading to higher levels of circulating short-chain fatty acids and in turn protecting against allergic inflammation in the lungs (in contrast to a low-fiber diet, which increased allergic lung inflammation). Likewise, the immune-regulating effects of short-chain fatty acids appear to benefit both food allergies and environmental allergies. Although we're just beginning to understand the role of our bodies' resident microbes in asthma and allergies, the evidence so far is compelling!

So what does this mean for our food choices? Although a well-designed Paleo diet is naturally loaded with fiber, regular consumption of fermentable fiber (the type of fiber that our gut microbes can metabolize into short-chain fatty acids) is the best bet for battling asthma and allergies. Rich sources include alliums (garlic, onions, leeks, scallions, and shallots), bananas (especially green or under-ripe bananas), Jerusalem artichokes, potatoes (especially potatoes that have been cooked and then cooled to room temperature), nuts, berries, plantains, and cassava.

Vitamin D

Low vitamin D levels have been convincingly linked to an increased risk of asthma attacks in both children and adults (and, although the evidence is much less clear, might impact allergy risk due to vitamin D's role in immune function). One study found that Canadians with vitamin D levels lower than 20 ng/ml were 50 percent more likely to have asthma than people with levels between 20 ng/ml and 30 ng/ml. A 2016 Cochrane Review found that vitamin D supplementation significantly reduced the number of asthma attacks requiring a hospital visit and reduced the number of asthma attacks that needed to be treated with steroids. In addition, vitamin D may indirectly benefit asthmatics by helping to protect against colds and flu, both of which can trigger or worsen asthma.

So how much vitamin D should we be taking? There's no clear answer. The optimal dose varies depending on a person's starting vitamin D level, latitude, sun exposure, age, and other factors. In general, whatever intake is needed to boost vitamin D levels out of the deficiency range will likely have a positive effect on asthma (and potentially allergies). Although small amounts of vitamin D are present in some foods, such as fatty fish and liver, the levels are generally too low to meet our daily needs, especially for people living at high latitudes. See page 328.

Omega-3 Fats

Due to their role in regulating inflammation, omega-3 fats (and the overall ratio of omega-3 to omega-6 of the diet) may influence the occurrence and severity of asthma and allergies. In fact, some researchers speculate that a sky-high intake of omega-6 fats relative to omega-3 fats is one reason why the United States and other Western nations have such high rates of asthma. Several trials have confirmed that omega-3 supplements (in the form of fish oil) can reduce exercise-induced bronchoconstriction in asthma, and research shows that an omega-3 to omega-6 ratio of 1:5 has a beneficial effect on patients with asthma, whereas a ratio of 1:10 becomes detrimental. Likewise, omega-3 fats express an anti-allergic effect through their conversion to certain metabolites (particularly 17,18-epoxyeicosatetraenoic acid) in the gut, helping to explain the role of omega-3 in reducing allergy risk.

Although a number of studies on omega-3 fats, asthma, and allergies have used supplements such as fish oil to boost omega-3 intake, consuming these fats in whole-food form may offer even greater benefits by providing additional nutrients that can boost immunity and suppress inflammation, such as vitamin E in omega-3-rich walnuts. For combating asthma and allergies, fatty fish (including salmon, mackerel, tuna, and sardines) can be helpful dietary additions.

REDUCING KIDNEY DISEASE RISK

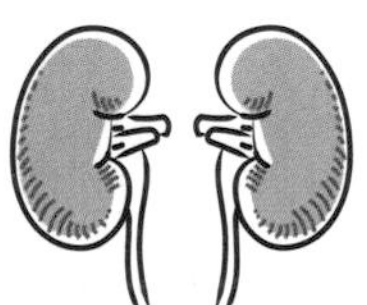

Chronic kidney disease is a condition in which a gradual and progressive loss of kidney function occurs. It affects about 10 percent of the American population, with older people at a much greater risk—for example, prevalence is only about 4 percent for people in their thirties compared to 47 percent for people over 70. The two main causes of chronic kidney disease are diabetes and high blood pressure, which are responsible for up to two-thirds of the cases. Choices that mitigate diabetes and normalize blood pressure will also help reduce the risk of chronic kidney disease. High-fiber diets (see page 39), high vegetable and fruit consumption (see page 138), a daily serving of nuts (see page 194), and proper hydration (see page 106) have all been shown to decrease the risk of kidney disease. As discussed in detail on page 201, avoiding excess sodium consumption is also important for kidney health. Vitamin D deficiency increases the risk of chronic kidney disease as well as all-cause mortality in chronic kidney disease sufferers.

A veggie-rich diet may also help treat chronic kidney disease once diagnosed. Recent studies have shown that simply adding more fresh vegetables and fruits to the diets of people with chronic kidney disease caused by hypertension could not only protect the kidneys from further deterioration but even improve kidney function. The less advanced the disease, the better the results. Fish oil supplementation has been shown to reduce markers of inflammation and cardiovascular disease risk factors in patients with chronic kidney disease—this is important because cardiovascular disease is the principal cause of death in chronic kidney disease sufferers.

Chronic kidney disease can also cause gout, which is discussed in detail on page 271.

Kidney stones are another potential cause of chronic kidney disease, especially if they are recurrent. They can impact any part of the urinary tract, from the kidneys to the bladder. There are several types of kidney stones, the three most common of which are the following:

- **Calcium oxalate stones** are the most common type, accounting for about 80 percent of all kidney stones. While oxalate is naturally occurring in some vegetables, there doesn't seem to be a direct relationship between the oxalate you eat and the formation of calcium oxalate stones—oxalate is also produced by the liver. High dietary sodium, calcium deficiency, excessive calcium intake via supplementation (but not diet), high fructose intake, and insufficient fluid intake all increase the risk of calcium oxalate stones.

- **Struvite stones** account for 10 to 15 percent of all kidney stones. They form in response to an infection, such as a urinary tract infection. While these stones are not directly linked to diet, people with gout as well as those with underlying metabolic disorders (like hyperparathyroidism) are at greater risk.

- **Uric acid stones** account for 5 to 10 percent of all kidney stones. They form in people who don't drink enough fluids and get dehydrated; those who eat a high-meat, low-veggie diet; those who consume too much fructose; and those who have gout. Certain genetic factors also may increase your risk of uric acid stones.

High vegetable and fruit consumption is the most important dietary factor in preventing kidney stones (except for stones related to infection or hereditary disorders). Maintaining a healthy weight also lowers kidney stone risk.

Gallstones are different in composition than kidney stones. While calcium is a common constituent of gallstones, they are composed predominantly of cholesterol or bilirubin (a product of heme breakdown that is normally excreted in the bile). Constipation, nutritional deficiency (especially in vitamin B9, vitamin C, calcium, and magnesium), insufficient fluid intake, high fructose intake, low fiber intake, consumption of fast food, and hypercaloric, high-carbohydrate diets all increase the risk of gallstones. Consuming plenty of vegetables and fruit, high fiber intake, high intake of monounsaturated fats and omega-3 fatty acids, and vitamin C supplementation reduce the risk of gallstones.

SUPPORTING MENTAL HEALTH

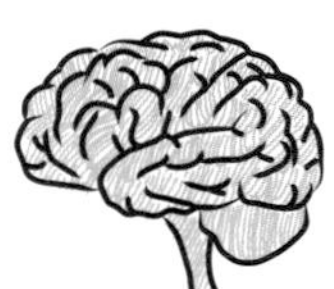

Although there isn't much research (yet!) examining how a Paleo diet impacts mental health (including conditions like anxiety, depression, attention deficit disorder [ADD], attention deficit and hyperactivity disorder [ADHD], autism spectrum disorder, schizophrenia, and bipolar disorder, along with general cognition), we have plenty of evidence showing the effects of different micronutrients and lifestyle practices on these conditions. With that in mind, we can modify the Paleo template to offer maximum support for mental health.

Omega-3 Fats

Due to their role in serotonin and dopamine transmission, gene expression, membrane fluidity, neurite growth, neuronal survival, transcription, and other elements of neural activity, omega-3 fatty acids (especially in the form of EPA and DHA) are important for brain health, and deficiencies may contribute to mental illness. Numerous studies show an association between low omega-3 intake and depression, and clinical trials have shown that omega-3 supplementation can improve symptoms of depression, schizophrenia, bipolar disorder, and possibly borderline personality disorder and ADHD. On the whole, an omega-3 intake of 1 to 2 grams per day appears to have benefited depression and bipolar disorder across multiple studies, and intake of 1 gram per day of EPA and DHA combined is recommended to support cognitive function. The best sources of omega-3s are seafood (especially fatty fish like salmon and mackerel) and some nuts and seeds, particularly walnuts and sacha inchi seeds.

KNOWLEDGE BOMB

Generally, ALA, the plant form of omega-3s, must be converted to the longer, active forms DHA and EPA to be used by our bodies (although there are processes that use ALA). Unfortunately, conversion is typically inefficient, approximately 6 percent for EPA and 3.8 percent for DHA, which is why it's important to get most of our omega-3s from animal sources like fish. Study after study has shown that increasing consumption of DHA and EPA reduces disease severity and symptoms—for instance, it improves the symptoms of rheumatoid arthritis—and lowers the risk of developing certain diseases, such as cardiovascular disease.

Here's where unusually rich sources of ALA like sacha inchi seeds stand out. There is scientific evidence that, thanks to the synergistic presence of other nutrients and the unusually high concentration of ALA, consuming sacha inchi seeds increases bioavailable ALA in all tissues, with a subsequent increase in DHA in the liver and brain and an increase in EPA in red blood cells, liver, kidney, small intestine, and heart.

Vitamin D

Along with its many roles in bone health, cardiovascular health, cancer prevention, and immune function (just to name a few!), vitamin D may be an important player in mental health. Many studies have linked low vitamin D levels with depression, and others have demonstrated a reduction in depressive symptoms following vitamin D supplementation (although due to differences in dosage, duration of supplementation, populations being studied, ways of measuring depression, and other elements of study design, the research is sometimes conflicting). Links have also emerged between low vitamin D levels and schizophrenia.

Apart from direct sun exposure, the best sources of vitamin D are fatty fish, liver, full-fat dairy, and egg yolks, but for many people (especially those in extreme latitudes or overcast climates), supplementation may be necessary to obtain enough vitamin D to impact mental health.

Although researchers are still exploring the mechanisms linking vitamin D with mental health, a likely possibility has to do with the presence of vitamin D receptors in the hypothalamus, which may give vitamin D a role in regulating neuroendocrine function.

B Vitamins

Deficiencies in vitamin B6, vitamin B9, and vitamin B12 may raise blood levels of homocysteine (due to their involvement in homocysteine metabolism), which is associated with impaired mental health, possibly due to the effect of homocysteine on neurotransmitters, oxidative stress, and neurotoxicity. Vitamin B9 deficiency in particular may worsen depression through its effect on central monoamine metabolism, and when compared to healthy controls, people with depression have vitamin B9 levels that are 25 percent lower on average.

B vitamins are abundant in liver, beef, leafy green vegetables, broccoli, and beets; animal foods are the exclusive source of B12. It's also useful to test for MTHFR gene variants that impact methylation because of MTHFR's role in creating the active form of vitamin B9 (methylfolate), because of the role that methylation plays in neurotransmitter regulation, and because elevated homocysteine is more common in people with certain MTHFR gene variants; see page 108.

Zinc

Zinc plays a critical role in neurotransmitter metabolism and in maintaining brain structure and function, and deficiency in this mineral may influence mental health status. In children, zinc deficiency has been strongly linked to ADHD, and double-blind, placebo-controlled studies have shown that zinc supplementation (compared to a placebo) can significantly reduce hyperactivity, impulsivity, and impaired socialization. Similarly, zinc deficiency has been linked with higher rates of clinical depression. Good sources of zinc include liver, pumpkin seeds, beef, oysters, and shrimp.

Amino Acids

Specific amino acids may help support mental health and reduce symptoms of certain mental illnesses. Depression has long been linked to low levels of neurotransmitters (namely dopamine, serotonin, noradrenaline, and GABA), all of which require certain amino acids as precursors. In particular, tryptophan (found in nuts, seeds, red meat, poultry, eggs, and fish) serves as a precursor to serotonin and can reduce symptoms of depression and obsessive-compulsive disorder, as well as improve sleep and increase feelings of tranquility. The amino acids tyrosine (found in beef, lamb, chicken, fish, pork, nuts, seeds, eggs, avocados, and bananas) and phenylalanine (found in liver, eggs, chicken, pork, fish, and beef) are converted to the neurotransmitters dopamine and norepinephrine and can improve mental alertness and well-being. When combined with ATP, the amino acid methionine (rich in most muscle meats, shellfish, eggs, and nuts) produces S-adenosylmethionine (SAMe), which helps facilitate neurotransmitter production in the brain and can likewise alleviate symptoms of depression. Glycine (high in bone broth, tendons, and meat with cartilage and connective tissue still attached) has been shown to reduce some symptoms of schizophrenia, including emotional flatness, apathy, and social withdrawal. Taurine (found in most animal products, including beef, dark chicken meat, eggs, lamb, and fish) may play a role in reducing manic episodes in bipolar disorder.

In general, a diet rich in high-quality protein from animal foods will provide a wide array of neurotransmitter precursors. Researchers are still studying the effects of amino acid supplementation (including what doses are needed) on depression and other measures of mental health.

Exercise

Exercise is a well-known mood booster; studies confirm that it can reduce anxiety, negative moods, and depression while boosting cognitive function—most likely through an impact on endorphins, monamines, and blood circulation to the brain.

Exercising outdoors with exposure to natural sunlight may be even more beneficial for mental health than exercising inside. Trials combining exercise (a brisk 20-minute walk outside, 5 days per week) with increased light exposure show that for people with mild to moderate depression, this regimen can improve mood, overall well-being, happiness, and self-esteem. Other less rigorous studies have shown that compared to walking at an indoor shopping center, walking outside (referred to as "ecotherapy") can lead to greater improvements in depression, self-esteem, and tension.

AUTISM SPECTRUM DISORDER

A great deal of research has been conducted on the use of gluten-free, casein-free (GFCF) diets in people with autism spectrum disorders. Although researchers are still trying to understand what causes autism, one theory suggests that the peptides in gluten and casein could produce opioid-type effects that lead to behavioral symptoms.

Despite the biologically plausible connection between diet and autism, GFCF diets have had mixed results in the scientific literature. A subset of individuals react to the diet with a decrease in autism symptoms (responders), whereas others don't see any behavioral benefit (non-responders).

Why is this the case? One, a GFCF diet isn't necessarily healthier than a diet containing these proteins: it all depends on which foods replace gluten and casein. Swapping out gluten-containing foods for gluten-free pasta, gluten-free pastries, gluten-free cookies, and other heavily processed grain-based items won't improve the nutritional quality of the diet, and the diet will still contain grain-based lectins that may aggravate a leaky gut (ditto for swapping out casein-containing dairy products for soy-based cheese, soy milk, and other processed dairy substitutes). A diet that replaces gluten and casein with higher-quality carbohydrate and protein sources (think fresh fruit, tubers, seafood, and meat) will have a higher nutrient density and fewer problematic proteins and may stand a better chance of benefiting autistic individuals.

Two, any link between gluten and casein and autism is likely mediated by the state of the gut. Some studies have found physiological abnormalities in the guts of people with autism spectrum disorders, including greater intestinal permeability (leaky gut)—something also found at higher frequency in first-degree relatives of people with autism spectrum disorders, suggesting a hereditary component. Individuals with these abnormalities may be more likely to respond to GFCF diets.

The length of time spent eating a GFCF diet, the age at which the diet is first started, the strictness of adherence, and possible food sensitivities and allergies might also dictate who ends up responding positively to a diet that omits gluten and casein. Overall, there's a shortage of well-controlled, randomized trials testing the effects of GFCF diets on autism spectrum disorders, and more research is needed to clarify why certain people respond dramatically to GFCF diets and others don't.

SUPPORTING ATHLETIC PERFORMANCE

Can the Paleo diet work for athletes? This is a common question among fitness enthusiasts, and the answer is a resounding yes! The sports and fitness industry tends to be flooded with foods that are heavily processed, low in micronutrients, and high in ingredients that disturb gut health—for example, artificially sweetened protein powders, meal replacement bars, carbohydrate gels, and energy drinks. Although many of these products can boost performance and recovery in the short-term, those benefits may come at the expense of longer-term health, especially if these processed foods start forming the bulk of the diet. Fortunately, Paleo supplies all the raw materials needed to support performance and help the body recover from physically demanding activities while also improving micronutrient status and removing dietary components that can undermine health over time. This can benefit virtually anyone interested in performance, from amateur CrossFitters to professional athletes!

A performance-supporting version of Paleo includes an emphasis on nutrients necessary for muscle growth and contraction—particularly protein, but also the electrolytes calcium (found in leafy greens and small bone-in fish, like sardines), magnesium (rich in many plant foods, like dark green leafy vegetables, avocados, bananas, nuts, and seeds, as well as some animal foods, like fish), potassium (abundant in tomatoes, bananas, sweet potatoes, squash, avocados, and coconut water), and sodium (found in any salted food, as well as in shellfish, beets, celery, and some other vegetables). These electrolytes are vital for controlling contraction and relaxation in all muscles, including both skeletal muscles and the heart. Iron (especially the more absorbable heme form found in red meat and shellfish, but also non-heme iron found in some leafy greens) is used for producing red blood cells, which carry oxygenated blood to the muscles (and the rest of the body). In addition, vitamin D plays a role in maintaining muscular health by helping the body absorb calcium and zinc (found in shellfish, organ meats, and pumpkin seeds), which helps the body utilize protein and facilitates muscle growth.

Consuming adequate carbohydrate also is important for fueling muscles during workouts and replenishing muscle glycogen after exercise, so Paleo carbohydrate sources like tubers and fruit should be emphasized (see page 87). In lieu of electrolyte replacement drinks that often contain high-fructose corn syrup or artificial sweeteners, coconut water delivers significant levels of electrolytes, as well as other micronutrients. And of course, the many high-quality protein sources available on a Paleo diet—eggs, fish, poultry, and other meats—take center stage for supplying extra protein (protein requirements may increase for some athletes, especially those involved in muscle-building activities). Combined with adequate sleep (critical for tissue repair) and an exercise routine that avoids overtraining and incorporates adequate recovery time, Paleo foods can easily support performance in any sport.

COCONUT WATER AS NATURE'S SPORTS DRINK

	COCONUT GROOVE Coconut water per 100 ml	STAMINADE ADVANCED Lemon/Lime Fusion per 100 ml	POWERADE ISOTONIC Gold Flush per 100 ml	GATORADE PERFORM Lemon-Lime per 100 ml
Calories	23.5	24	31	24.5
Protein	0	0	0	0
Fat - total	0	0	0	0
- saturated	0	0	0	0
Carbohydrate	5.8 g	5.8 g	7.3 g	6.0 g
Sugar Total	5.8 g	5.1 g	5.7 g	6.0 g
as Glucose	2.9g	--	--	0.5 g
as Sucrose	2.03 g	5.1 g	5.7 g	5.5 g
as Fructose	0.87 g	--	--	--
Maltodextrin	--	0.7 g	1.6 g	--
Dietary Fiber	0	0	0	0
Sodium	26.9 mg	42.4 mg	2.7 mg	51.0 mg
Potassium	133.0 mg	20.52 mg	14.1 mg	22.5 mg
Calcium	10.5 mg	4.2 mg	--	--
Magnesium	6.6 mcg	1.5 mg	--	--
Phosphorus	5.99 mg	--	--	--
Manganese	0.30 mg	--	--	--
Zinc	0.25 mg	--	--	--

PALEO FOR PREGNANT AND LACTATING MOTHERS

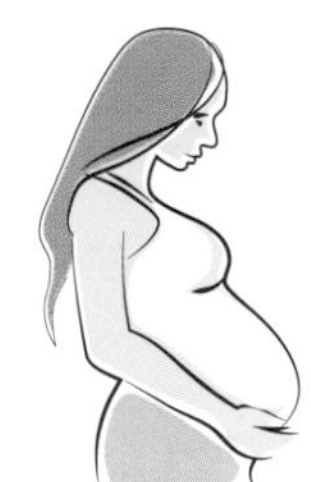

Eating a nutrient-dense diet is vital for every stage of human life, but it takes on an even greater importance during pregnancy and lactation. Not only do nutrient requirements increase for expecting and breastfeeding mothers, but the mother's diet directly influences fetal brain development, birth weight, the risk of birth defects, and even the baby's immune function. That makes the Paleo diet, with its focus on nutrient-dense foods, a great framework for ensuring that pregnant and lactating women receive the nutrition they need to support a healthy pregnancy and child.

That being said, the Paleo framework can be adjusted to emphasize the nutrients that are in particularly high demand during pregnancy and lactation. These include:

- **Vitamin A:** Vitamin A is vital for embryonic development, including the growth of the eyes, heart, lungs, kidneys, central nervous system, respiratory system, and circulatory system. Although vitamin A precursors (particularly β-carotene) are found in many plant foods, including carrots and sweet potatoes, some people have difficulty converting these precursors to "true" vitamin A, so it's best to get some retinol from animal foods such as liver, eggs, and grass-fed dairy. The recommended intake of retinol activity equivalents (RAE) is 770 mcg daily for pregnant women and 1,300 mcg daily for breastfeeding women. Although higher amounts can be safe, note that vitamin A overdose from retinol is a possibility, especially in the context of inadequate vitamin D and supplemental (non-food) vitamin A.

- **Vitamin B9 (folate):** Folate is needed from very early on in pregnancy to support healthy neural tube development in a fetus's brain and spinal cord. In fact, folate deficiency is strongly linked to a form of birth defect called *neural tube defects*, including spina bifida and anencephaly, which occur in the first month of pregnancy. The recommended intake for pregnant women (as well as women planning to conceive) is 600 to 800 mcg daily, and the best sources are leafy green vegetables, asparagus, broccoli, avocados, nuts, seeds, beets, cauliflower, and squash.

- **Vitamin D:** Along with facilitating calcium absorption and metabolism, vitamin D plays a critical role in immune function and, according to some research, can potentially help prevent pregnancy complications such as gestational diabetes, preeclampsia, low birth weight, and preterm birth. Vitamin D intake during pregnancy can also reduce the risk of wheezing and asthma developing in early childhood. Although the recommended daily intake for pregnant women is 600 IU, one study found that women taking 4,000 IU of vitamin D per day saw the most benefit in terms of preventing infections and preterm birth without any evidence of harm. The best way to get vitamin D is from skin exposure to the sun (and in lieu of that, supplementation), but the highest dietary sources are egg yolks, fatty fish (like salmon, herring, and mackerel), and cod liver oil.

- **Calcium:** Calcium is needed for skeletal development, blood pressure regulation, and proper muscle and nerve functioning, and it becomes particularly important for the fetus during third-trimester bone development. Pregnant or lactating women need 1,000 to 1,300 milligrams per day. The best Paleo-friendly sources are leafy green vegetables, broccoli, small bone-in fish like sardines, and grass-fed dairy.

- **Choline:** Choline is important for the development of the fetal nervous system, neural tube, and brain. Pregnant women should consume at least 450 milligrams per day. The richest sources are egg yolks, liver, shrimp, and beef.

- **Iron:** Iron is needed for a fetus's rapidly developing blood supply and for the expanding blood supply of the mother. For pregnant women, 27 milligrams daily is recommended. The best sources are red meat, organ meat, and leafy green vegetables.

- **Zinc:** Zinc is used for fetal cell growth, as well as supporting immunity, enzyme production, and insulin production in the mother. Pregnant women should aim for 11 milligrams per day from rich sources like beef, pork, poultry, seafood (especially oysters), nuts, and seeds.

- **Omega-3 fats, especially DHA and EPA:** DHA has been consistently shown to support fetal brain, eye, and central nervous system development (it's a major structural fat in the retina and brain), while EPA plays a role in transporting DHA across the placenta, as well as supporting DHA intracellular absorption. Inadequate omega-3 intake can negatively affect pregnancy outcomes and increase the risk of preterm labor and preeclampsia. Although there aren't clearly established omega-3 requirements for pregnant women, essential fatty acids are recommended, with the best sources being low-mercury fatty fish and other seafood, walnuts, and omega-3-enriched eggs.

FOLIC ACID VERSUS FOLATE

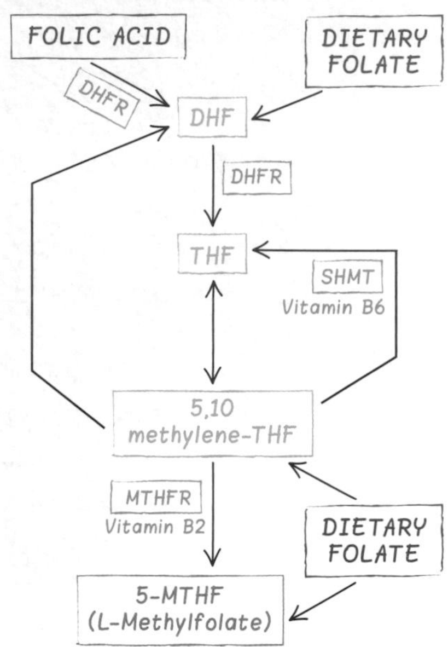

It's typically recommended that pregnant women and women who may become pregnant take a folic acid supplement because it can prevent neural tube defects and other congenital malformations linked to folate deficiency. But it's important to differentiate between these two different forms of vitamin B9, folic acid and folate.

Folic acid, also known as pteroylmonoglutamic acid, is a synthetic form of vitamin B9 used to fortify foods and used in supplements. *Folate* is naturally occurring in many foods. Folic acid is better absorbed than folate—folate from vegetables, fruits, and liver is absorbed into our bodies at about 80 percent of the rate of folic acid—so folic acid has traditionally been considered more bioavailable. But even though we can absorb folic acid more easily, in order for our bodies to use it, it must be converted to the active form of folate, L-methylfolate (also known as 5-methyltetrahydrofolate, so it's abbreviated as 5-MTHF), via a multistep process. We now know that this conversion is slow and inefficient (and even more so in people with MTHFR gene variants because the MTHFR enzyme is responsible for the last step of the conversion; see page 108).

While the body is working on converting folic acid to L-methylfolate, the absorbed folic acid circulates in the blood. Why is this an issue? High blood levels of folic acid are associated with increased cancer risk and can mask vitamin B12 deficiency. And if your body isn't very good at converting folic acid to folate (due to gene variants in MTHFR or vitamin B2 deficiency, for example), you can be folate deficient even though you have plenty of folic acid in your blood.

In contrast, folate from food occurs in many chemical forms, including L-methylfolate. So while some food folate will need to go through the same series of chemical reactions as folic acid to be converted to the active form of folate, some can be converted in fewer steps, and some does not require conversion at all. For this reason, it's preferable to get folate from natural food sources like leafy greens and liver rather than from fortified foods or supplements.

The most important thing during pregnancy is to avoid folate deficiency. The recommended daily allowance (RDA) of folate for pregnant women is 600 micrograms. The following foods are good sources of folate:

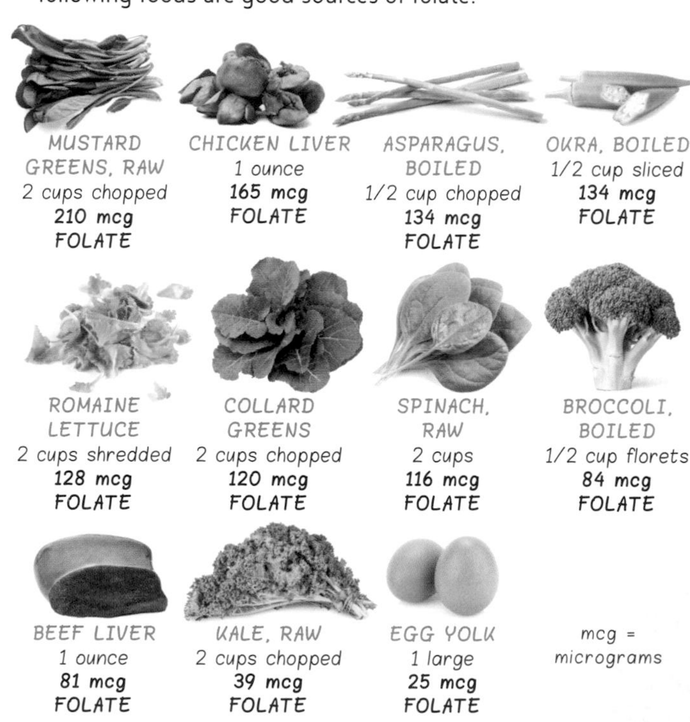
MUSTARD GREENS, RAW
2 cups chopped
210 mcg FOLATE
CHICKEN LIVER
1 ounce
165 mcg FOLATE
ASPARAGUS, BOILED
1/2 cup chopped
134 mcg FOLATE
OKRA, BOILED
1/2 cup sliced
134 mcg FOLATE
ROMAINE LETTUCE
2 cups shredded
128 mcg FOLATE
COLLARD GREENS
2 cups chopped
120 mcg FOLATE
SPINACH, RAW
2 cups
116 mcg FOLATE
BROCCOLI, BOILED
1/2 cup florets
84 mcg FOLATE
BEEF LIVER
1 ounce
81 mcg FOLATE
KALE, RAW
2 cups chopped
39 mcg FOLATE
EGG YOLK
1 large
25 mcg FOLATE
mcg = micrograms

Supplementation may still be advisable, depending on your risk factors, so it's important to discuss this with your doctor. Studies also show that supplementing with L-methylfolate (sometimes labeled 5-MTHF) is effective at increasing blood levels of folate and may be a safer option than folic acid.

Pregnancy increases a woman's energy requirements by 200 to 300 calories a day, depending on how much weight gain is advised for the woman's particular situation. Breastfeeding also burns significant energy—up to 500 calories a day or more—and inadequate calorie intake during lactation can reduce the mother's milk supply. These extra calories should come from a mixture of protein (which all fetal body systems use to develop and grow), carbohydrates (which provide energy), and fats (which assist with nutrient absorption and help the fetal nervous system develop properly).

Fluid requirements also increase during pregnancy and lactation, making it extremely important to stay hydrated by drinking plenty of water, too.

Breast Is Best

It's worth taking a quick moment to emphasize that the perfect baby food is human breast milk. Beyond meeting the baby's nutritional needs, breast milk provides important probiotics to help colonize the baby's digestive tract and support a healthy gut microbial community and provides important immunoactive compounds to complement the baby's immune system and protect against infection. Studies show that breastfed babies have lower risks of serious infections, including gastroenteritis and pneumonia, and sudden infant death syndrome (SIDS). Breastfed babies also have a lower risk of chronic disease later in life, including asthma, allergies, eczema, childhood obesity, diabetes, and leukemia.

Breastfeeding is health-promoting for the mother, too. Declining to breastfeed increases a woman's risk of premenopausal breast cancer, ovarian cancer, type 2 diabetes, and metabolic syndrome. It also increases her chances of retaining weight gained during pregnancy.

The World Health Organization (WHO) recommends breastfeeding children for at least their first 2 years of life, breastfeeding exclusively (meaning no supplementing with formula or baby foods) for the first 6 months. In hunter-gatherer societies, babies are typically weaned gradually during their fourth year, usually during the mother's next pregnancy. When the mother doesn't get pregnant again, children are generally breastfed longer, until age 5 or even older.

Unfortunately, in the United States, only about a third of babies are breastfed exclusively at 3 months, and a mere 11 percent of babies are breastfed exclusively at 6 months. These statistics reflect many cultural barriers to breastfeeding, such as short maternity leaves, lack of social support, and insufficient troubleshooting resources. Mothers can greatly improve their chances of successfully breastfeeding their babies by seeking knowledgeable support, such as a lactation consultant or a local La Leche League chapter (www.llli.org).

PALEO FOR FAMILIES

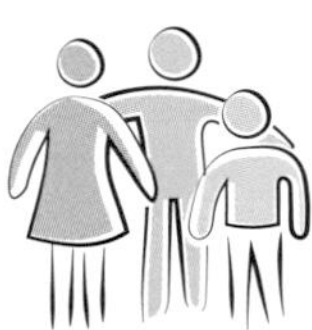

Is Paleo safe for kids? Absolutely! In fact, children might benefit from Paleo even more than adults because their food habits and associations are just starting to form, and the nutrient density of the Paleo diet readily supports the demands of growth and development. A diet rich in colorful fruits and vegetables provides a wide spectrum of vitamins and minerals for a healthy body and immune system, and a diet rich in omega-3 fatty acids is crucial for brain development. Plus, gluten and the other lectins in grains and legumes can be even more damaging to a child's immature digestive tract than to an adult's mature one, so minimizing their presence in a child's diet can go a long way toward supporting gut health from an early age.

That being said, making sure children get all the nutrients they need is important with any dietary framework, and Paleo is no exception.

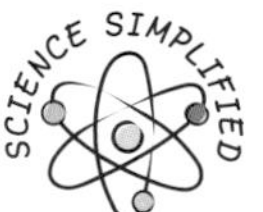

Your kids won't miss out on any nutrients by adopting a Paleo diet. In fact, they'll almost certainly beat out their peers in terms of essential vitamins, minerals, fiber, antioxidant phytochemicals, essential amino acids, and essential fatty acids.

Micronutrient Requirements for Children

Due to their faster rate of growth and higher metabolism, children have greater micronutrient needs relative to their total body weight than adults do. This makes it very important to emphasize the most nutrient-dense foods, like organ meats, seafood, healthy fat sources, and vegetables, and limit "empty calories," which take up volume in a child's stomach without contributing to daily nutritional needs. A few micronutrients are particularly critical due to the specific developmental processes that children are going through, including the following:

- **Vitamin A** is important for healthy vision, immunity, and gene expression (vitamin A deficiency is the leading cause of childhood blindness in developing nations and puts children at significantly increased risk of infection). The best sources of vitamin A in the form of retinol are liver, eggs, and full-fat dairy, and the best sources of vitamin A precursors are sweet potatoes, leafy green vegetables, squash, carrots, and many other orange and green fruits and vegetables.

- **Vitamin B12** is used in many metabolic processes and is important for neurological health. It plays a role in myelination from early fetal development all the way through early adulthood. The best sources are animal products like red meat, fish, shellfish, poultry, and eggs.

- **Vitamin C** plays a role in synthesizing collagen and neurotransmitters during childhood and beyond. It's also critical for proper immune function, helping children fight off infections as they're exposed to new pathogens. The best sources of vitamin C are citrus fruits, melons, berries, kiwis, papayas, mangoes, and pineapple.

- **Vitamin D** supports growing bones and teeth through its role in facilitating calcium metabolism (vitamin D deficiency is a major cause of rickets, which occurs when bones fail to mineralize and results in bowed legs and arms). The best sources of naturally occurring vitamin D (apart from what the body produces during sun exposure) are fatty fish, liver, eggs, and full-fat dairy.

- **Calcium** is used to build bones and teeth. An adequate intake during childhood and adolescence is necessary to attain strong peak bone mass and reduce the risk of osteoporosis later in life. See page 87 for the best Paleo calcium sources.

- **Iodine** is needed for brain development in infancy, is used to synthesize thyroid hormones, and helps control a number of bodily processes, such as growth, metabolism, and development. Because some Paleo diets omit iodized salt and processed foods made with iodized salt—the most common sources of iodine in the modern diet—dietary sources of iodine are extremely important for young children: sea vegetables, fish, eggs, and dairy.

- **Zinc** plays a role in growth, development, neurological function, immune function, and cell metabolism. Zinc deficiency can impair a child's physical growth and increase the susceptibility to infection, so adequate intake is important for preventing "failure to thrive." The best sources of zinc are organ meat, shellfish, nuts, and seeds.

- **Omega-3 fats** are critical for healthy brain development, vision, gene expression, nervous system function, and building cell membranes. The best sources are fatty fish such as salmon, mackerel, tuna, and sardines, as well as walnuts and sacha inchi seeds.

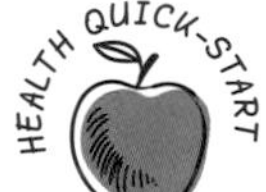

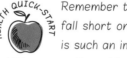

Remember that many standard Paleo diets fall short on calcium intake. Because calcium is such an important nutrient for growing children, use the table on page 264 to choose calcium-rich foods to include in your children's diet.

Essential Vitamin and Mineral Requirements for Children

Recommended Dietary Allowances (RDAs) are established for a variety of demographic groups by the Food and Nutrition Board of the Institute of Medicine (see page 30). Remember that an RDA is the dietary intake level of a specific nutrient considered sufficient to meet the needs of 97.5 percent of healthy individuals, implying that this intake would be harmfully inadequate for just 2.5 percent of the healthy population. RDAs are calculated based on the estimated average requirement for each nutrient, something that some specialists believe is an underestimation of our true biological need, as these levels are generally determined based on symptoms of deficiency rather than amounts needed for optimal health.

The following are the established RDAs for essential vitamins and minerals for babies and toddlers.

	RDA FOR AGES 0–6 MONTHS	RDA FOR AGES 7–12 MONTHS	RDA FOR AGES 1–3 YEARS
Vitamin A	375 mcg RE	375 mcg RE	300 mcg RE
Vitamin B1 (thiamin)	0.3 mg	0.4 mg	0.5 mg
Vitamin B2 (riboflavin)	0.4 mg	0.5 mg	0.5 mg
Vitamin B3 (niacin)	5 mg	6 mg	6 mg
Vitamin B5 (pantothenic acid)	2 mg	3 mg	2 mg
Vitamin B6 (pyridoxine)	0.3 mg	0.6 mg	0.5 mg
Vitamin B9 (folate)	25 mcg	35 mcg	150 mcg
Vitamin B12 (cobalamin)	0.3 mcg	0.5 mcg	0.9 mcg
Vitamin C	30 mg	35 mg	15 mg
Vitamin D	7.5 mcg	10 mcg	15 mcg
Vitamin E	3 mg TE	4 mg TE	6 mg TE
Vitamin K	5 mcg	10 mcg	30 mcg
Calcium	400 mg	600 mg	700 mg
Copper	600 mcg	700 mcg	340 mcg
Iodine	40 mcg	50 mcg	90 mcg
Iron	6 mg	10 mg	7 mg
Magnesium	40 mg	60 mg	80 mg
Manganese	0.6 mg	1 mg	1.2 mg
Phosphorus	300 mg	500 mg	460 mg
Selenium	10 mcg	15 mcg	20 mcg
Zinc	5 mg	5 mg	3 mg

mg = milligrams, mcg = micrograms, RE = Retinol Equivalents, TE = Tocopherol Equivalents

The following are micronutrient requirements for fully weaned children:

	RDA FOR AGES 4–8 YEARS	RDA FOR AGES 9–13 YEARS
Vitamin A	1,333 IU	2,000 IU
Vitamin B1 (thiamin)	0.6 mg	0.9 mg
Vitamin B2 (riboflavin)	0.6 mg	0.9 mg
Vitamin B3 (niacin)	8 mg	12 mg
Vitamin B5 (pantothenic acid)	3 mg	4 mg
Vitamin B6 (pyridoxine)	0.6 mg	1 mg
Vitamin B9 (folate)	200 mcg	300 mcg
Vitamin B12 (cobalamin)	1.2 mcg	1.8 mcg
Vitamin C	25 mg	45 mg
Vitamin D	600 IU	600 IU
Vitamin E	7 mg TE	11 mg TE
Vitamin K	55 mcg	60 mcg
Calcium	1,000 mg	1,300 mg
Copper	440 mcg	700 mcg
Iodine	90 mcg	120 mcg
Iron	10 mg	8 mg
Magnesium	130 mg	240 mg
Manganese	1.5 mg	1.9 mg
Phosphorus	500 mg	1,250 mg
Selenium	30 mcg	40 mcg
Zinc	5 mg	8 mg

Macronutrient Requirements for Children

When it comes to macronutrient ratios for kids, we can get a clear idea of how they should eat by looking at the composition of human breast milk. In prehistoric cultures, children likely received at least some breast milk until age 4 or 5, so it's a pretty safe bet that the macronutrient ratio of breast milk is a good guide for kids up to that age. Mother's milk is considered the perfect food for a growing young child, and we can continue to use the macronutrient ratio of breast milk as a general guide for children's diets for as long as they are growing; after all, the macronutrient ratio of breast milk is often used as a guide for carbohydrate consumption for adults!

The macronutrient ratio of human breast milk is quite variable, depending on the diet of the mother, the frequency with which the baby nurses, and the age of the baby. It is likely that much of this variability reflects the baby's specific dietary needs at the time. The carbohydrate content of breast milk varies from 57 to 70 percent of total milk solids. Fat makes up 28 to 39 percent of total milk solids, and protein makes up 7 to 10 percent of total milk solids. Translating each of these numbers to a percentage of caloric intake—a far more familiar number to most of us—the carbohydrate content of breast milk is 40 to 55 percent, the fat content is 40 to 55 percent, and the protein content is about 10 percent.

Human breast milk is high in fat, with approximately 40 to 55 percent of its calories coming from fat. On average, 43 percent of that fat is saturated, 37 percent is monounsaturated (including up to 7 percent of total fat being natural trans fatty acids like conjugated linoleic acid), and 20 percent is polyunsaturated. Fat is necessary for brain development, hormone regulation, and immune system development. Fat is also needed for the baby's digestive system to absorb fat-soluble vitamins like A, D, E, and K.

Children's carbohydrate needs vary with growth spurts, developmental spurts, and age. On average, their carbohydrate needs tend to go down as they get older (protein, in particular, begins to take the place of carbs). Caloric intake also varies dramatically with growth spurts, developmental spurts, and age, so it's tough to convert this to a number of grams of carbohydrates a child should be eating. Instead, think of it this way: to achieve 40 percent of calories from carbohydrates, something like half to three-quarters of a child's plate should be fruit and vegetables (including plenty of starchy vegetables; see page 153 for details on Paleo-friendly starches). The reason 40 percent of calories from carbohydrates doesn't translate to 40 percent of the plate being fruits and vegetables is that non-starchy vegetables are not very carbohydrate/calorie dense (especially compared to whatever fat might be on the plate).

The point isn't to suggest that we count the grams of each macronutrient that a child is eating, but rather to point out that eating a lot of fruit and vegetables is just fine for a growing child. As long as they are eating some meat and healthy fats as well and are presented with a variety of healthy options—think meat, fish, organ meat, healthy fats (such as avocados, olives, and coconut oil), green veggies, other colorful veggies, cruciferous veggies, starchy veggies, all kinds of fruit, and probiotic foods like sauerkraut—it's generally not worth worrying about.

First Foods FAQ

When it comes time to start feeding their babies solid foods, parents tend to have a lot of questions. Here are answers to some of the most common ones.

When should solid foods be introduced? The general rule is that you can introduce solids once your baby is *at least* 5 months old (6 months old is better since the gastrointestinal tract is more mature by then), is sitting up well, and is interested in your food; *and* you have the go-ahead from your pediatrician. Watch closely for signs of choking, and never leave a baby or toddler unattended while eating. You can help prepare your baby's digestive tract for solids by breastfeeding exclusively (which helps provide probiotics and hormones and enzymes that help mature the digestive tract). You can also give your baby a small amount of *Acidophilus bifidus* (buy a capsule that you can break open and rub a small pinch in the baby's mouth before nursing or offering a bottle) once or twice a day, starting at about 3 months old (again, with the approval of your pediatrician). Many people prefer a baby-led weaning strategy, whereby you wait until the baby is able to self-feed soft finger foods; some babies are able to do this as early as 5 or 6 months, but 8 to 10 months is more typical.

What consistency should baby food be? First foods for younger babies should be thinned with breast milk, bone broth, or formula and be very runny; it should pour off a spoon and be only slightly thicker than breast milk. Over the first few months, gradually increase the thickness of the baby food. By 8 months of age, most babies can start to handle a little texture in their food (think oatmeal consistency). By 10 months, most babies can handle soft food mashed with a fork. Sometime between 8 and 10 months, your baby will probably show interest in finger foods, such as small pieces of soft fruit or cooked veggies. Watch your baby's cues and don't rush it.

What time of day should a baby be fed? Start with just one feeding a day, usually in the middle of the day, when your baby is not tired. Stop feeding as soon as your baby loses interest. Your baby may eat only a few mouthfuls for the first few meals (or even few weeks of meals). You can also introduce sips of water as you are introducing foods, from either a cup (regular, sippy, or straw) or a spoon. Over the first few months, you can gradually increase the number of times a day that your baby eats. By 9 or 10 months of age, most babies will happily eat three solid meals a day and maybe even a snack or two.

How do I watch for allergies? It can take several days for an allergic reaction to a food to present itself. Introduce only one new food every 4 to 7 days (on the longer end of this range if food allergies run in your family). You do not need to give that new food every day for those 4 to 7 days; one or two exposures is sufficient. Watch for symptoms such as:

- hives or welts
- flushed skin or rash
- swelling of face, tongue, or lips
- vomiting and/or diarrhea
- inconsolable crying
- coughing or wheezing
- difficulty breathing
- loss of consciousness

When it comes to introducing high-allergy foods like berries, citrus, egg whites, nuts, shellfish, and tomatoes, it's best to wait until your baby is at least a year old (but see page 428).

Is it easy to make your own baby food? Not only is it quite easy, but it yields much more nutritious and tastier food. To save time, make a fairly big batch of individual ingredient purees and freeze (before thinning so that you can control the thickness as your baby gets older) in ice cube trays; once the food is frozen, you can pop the cubes into a bag and label the bag for easy defrosting later.

Can foods be mixed together? Absolutely! Play with different combinations. Something that might seem odd to you might taste delicious to your baby. And most babies prefer one taste at one meal, so mixing foods together is a great way to increase variety and balance nutrition—for example, most babies would rather their meal of sweet potato, avocado, broccoli, and chicken be mixed together into a single puree. Just make sure to use only ingredients that you've introduced before (or add only one new food at a time).

What are the best first foods? The best first foods for most babies are mashed ripe avocado, mashed ripe banana, mashed cooked sweet potato, mashed cooked winter squash, pureed liver (preferably pastured or grass-fed), and mashed or crumbled pastured egg yolk. For babies who are at least 6 months old, well-cooked meats very well pureed with broth or breast milk and grass-fed whole milk yogurt are excellent early foods. Babies can usually start digesting well-cooked pureed green veggies at around 6 months, too.

What goes into a balanced baby meal? Once you have introduced single foods to rule out allergies, your little one will be ready for balanced meals. A meal should consist of mostly fat and carbohydrates (something like 40 to 50 percent of calories each) with a moderate amount of protein (ballpark 10 percent of calories). Choose whole, preferably organic vegetables, fatty fruits like avocados, and quality meats. Making a puree with a mixture of cooked vegetables (including a sweeter starchy veggie like sweet potato and a green veggie like kale or broccoli) and meat is an easy way to achieve this balance as well as cater to a baby's typical preference to eat only one flavor at any given meal. There's no need to count carb and fat grams, though; this simple rubric will get you into the right ballpark for a balanced baby meal:

Children's Nutrition Hot Topics

Calories and Energy Density

While adults can benefit from eating an abundance of high-volume, low-calorie Paleo foods (like fibrous vegetables), children under the age of 5 may struggle to obtain enough calories from a high-volume diet due to their smaller stomach size. (This is also why snacking is appropriate for children.) For this age bracket, denser (but still micronutrient-rich) foods should be emphasized. Compared to adults, who generally require 25 to 30 calories per kilogram of body weight (11 to 14 calories per pound), infants require more than 100 calories per kilogram (45 calories per pound), and children 4 months to 3 years old require about 83 calories per kilogram (38 calories per pound). After that, relative calorie needs decline (but remain higher than in adults) based on height, weight, and physical activity levels.

Dairy Products

The inclusion (or exclusion) of dairy from a child's diet is a tricky topic. While dairy—especially cow's milk—can be allergenic or poorly tolerated by many adults and some children, there is evidence that children need milk proteins until at least the age of 5. This makes sense from an evolutionary point of view because prehistorically (and indeed until only the last 100 years or so), children were breastfed until at least age 3 or 4. Today, this is rare. So supplementing a child's diet with dairy seems like a good idea. But how can we avoid the gut irritants found in commercially pasteurized cow's milk? The best options are cultured dairy, like yogurt and kefir (especially full fat) and high-quality cheese from grass-fed cows. Some children (and adults, too) tolerate goat's milk better than cow's milk. Sheep and camel milk are also great less-allergenic alternatives to cow's milk.

BALANCED MEAL PUREE

Puree the ingredients in a food processor or blender until smooth and thin with breast milk, broth, cooking liquid, or formula. Store extra baby food in small freezer-safe containers in the freezer for up to 3 months.

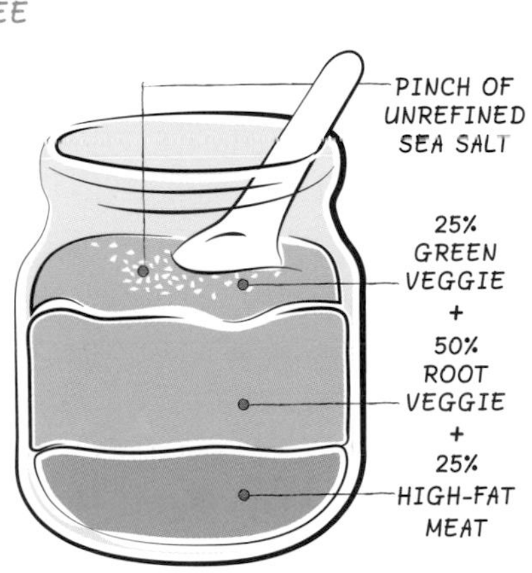

Going Gluten-Free

Occasionally, the internet becomes filled with dire warnings about gluten-free diets being unsafe for kids and putting them at risk of dangerous deficiencies. Critics are all over the media warning people that gluten-free diets are less nutritious and that there is no reason to avoid gluten unless you have a diagnosed allergy or celiac disease. However, this is an absolute myth.

In contrast, more and more parents are discovering that gluten-free (or gluten-free, casein-free, grain-free, or full-blown Paleo) diets lead to improvements in a variety of nebulous health issues in their kids, such as sleep disturbances, digestive symptoms, and behavioral problems. But is it safe to put a kid on a gluten-free diet if that child doesn't have a diagnosed health problem that is improved by going gluten-free? If one member of a family needs to be gluten-free, is it safe for the entire family to eat the same way? Will depriving a child of grains really deprive the child's developing brain of essential nutrients?

As discussed in detail on page 255, gluten is not a nutrient. Grains are not unique sources of any nutrients. And when you replace grain-based foods with vegetables and fruit, you get way more vitamins, minerals, and phytochemicals for the same amount of fiber and less sugar. A child who eats a diverse array of quality meats, seafood, vegetables, fruits, nuts, seeds, healthy fats, herbs, and spices will not be deficient in any vital nutrient—in fact, in terms of nutrient consumption, that child will far outperform peers consuming even fortified and enriched grain-based foods.

Immune Tolerance

You may hear from medical professionals that it's important to feed your baby grains and dairy. The erroneous belief that avoiding these foods will result in nutrient deficiencies has already been thoroughly debunked in this book. But another oft-cited reason why babies and toddlers should be exposed to allergenic foods, including the top-eight allergens (wheat, fish, shellfish, peanuts, tree nuts, dairy, eggs, and soy), has some interesting science to support this idea that's worthy of discussion here. The idea is that early introduction of these foods increases the chance of developing an immune tolerance to those foods.

Immune tolerance is a situation in which the immune system "tolerates" an antigen, meaning that it does not mount an immune response against something that normally would elicit one. Encompassing a range of physiological mechanisms, immune tolerance is why a mother's body doesn't attack a fetus, why we can suffer chronic infections, and why we can grow out of allergies. When it comes to allergenic foods, immune tolerance means that we have no symptoms of a reaction when we consume those foods.

A recent study called the LEAP study (LEAP stands for Learning Early About Peanut allergy) evaluated whether regularly consuming peanuts starting at an early age (4 to 11 months old) in high-risk babies (those with severe eczema and/or egg allergy) could affect the rate of peanut allergy in those kids at 5 years old. Babies were tested for peanut allergy at the beginning of the study and then randomly assigned to either a peanut avoidance group or a peanut consumption group, where they were given at least 6 grams of peanut protein per week—the equivalent of about 7½ dry-roasted peanuts—distributed in three or more meals throughout the week.

The results were dramatic: in those babies who did not test positive for peanut allergy at the beginning of the study, regular peanut consumption was associated with an 86 percent reduction in peanut allergy at age 5; and in those who did test positive, regular peanut consumption led to a 70 percent reduction in peanut allergy at age 5. This means that early and regular consumption of peanuts increased the probability of developing immune tolerance to peanuts substantially. In fact, these results and supportive data from other studies have led to a major shift in recommendations for when to introduce allergenic foods to babies, even in those with a high risk of food allergies.

It's important to note that breastfeeding is a major factor here. By shifting the introduction of these allergenic foods to a much earlier age, a much higher percentage of kids are being exposed to these foods while still breastfeeding. And the increased rates of immune tolerance may be attributable to the effects of breast milk on the gut microbiota. Studies show that breastfeeding is important for the establishment and growth of normal gut microorganisms, and these are important regulators of the immune system (see pages 70 and 78). In particular, breast milk contains probiotics, and for the duration of breastfeeding, the guts of babies are being constantly inoculated with these beneficial bacteria.

Another study looked at two cohorts of Swedish 12-year-olds. The first was a group born in 1993 during an epidemic of celiac disease (believed to be attributable to changes in government recommendations for the age of gluten introduction to 6 months old, combined with a concurrent increase in the gluten content of baby foods), and the second was a group born in 1997 after the epidemic (after the government revised the guidelines to lower the age of gluten introduction to 4 months and the amount of gluten in baby foods was reduced). The study sought to determine the impact of breastfeeding in relation to gluten introduction on the future development of celiac disease.

More than 13,000 children were enrolled in the study. The incidence of celiac disease was 2.8 in 100 in the 1993 cohort versus 2.2 in 100 in the 1997 cohort. The median age of gluten introduction was the same (5 months old) in both cohorts. But the infants in the 1997 cohort were breastfed an average of 2 months longer than the 1993 cohort (the age of weaning increased from an average of 7 months to an average of 9 months between 1993 and 1997). What this means is that the number of babies who were breastfed during and beyond gluten introduction was significantly larger in the 1997 cohort (the number of babies breastfed beyond gluten introduction was 70 percent in the 1993 cohort versus 78 percent in the 1997 cohort). From this, the authors conclude that introducing gluten before weaning reduces the risk of celiac disease.

This study supports others indicating that breastfeeding during and beyond the introduction of first foods reduces the incidence of food allergies. But is it immunoactive compounds in breast milk or breast milk's beneficial effects on the gut microbiota that mediate the development of immune tolerance? If breastfeeding is protective because of its probiotic effects, then it could be that it doesn't matter when allergenic foods are introduced (if ever), as long as the gut is healthy when the introduction occurs.

Another compelling result from the LEAP study is that once established, immune tolerance to peanuts persisted even after subsequent avoidance of peanuts for a year. That's good news because it means that once established, immune tolerance is not dependent on regular consumption.

Unfortunately, there are still many unanswered questions with regard to promoting immune tolerance to allergenic foods in children. It could be argued that immune tolerance isn't even desirable if the food in question is empty calories replete with problematic compounds. It could also be argued that the promotion of a healthy gut trumps the introduction of foods that may undermine gut barrier or microbiota health. And if one did wish to promote immune tolerance to the top-eight allergen foods, a definitive protocol has not yet been established.

However, it's worth considering introducing foods that would otherwise be eliminated on the Paleo diet to babies while they are still breastfeeding and in the context of an otherwise nutrient-dense and anti-inflammatory diet, with a few very small servings per week of those foods with high rates of allergy and sensitivity. Developing immune tolerance to common foods could be beneficial to protect against accidental or occasional exposure later in life. Because this is an area of active research and few definitive answers, this decision must be an individual one.

Flexibility

While even a strict Paleo diet is absolutely adequate for a growing child from a nutritional standpoint, life often gets in the way of perfect adherence—and that's *totally* fine. In an ideal world, children would eat a 100 percent Paleo diet at home, allowing all the gray-area foods (apart from alcohol and caffeine, and staying conscious of any known food sensitivities or allergies) and limiting refined sugars, while not worrying about carbohydrates, especially from fruit and starchy vegetables. But what happens when a child goes to a birthday party? Birthday cake, cookies, and ice cream are rites of passage for a child, and depriving children of those experiences won't (in most cases) have any true benefit for their health. What happens if a child goes to a school with a mandatory lunch program? Hopefully there will at least be a gluten-free option available. Do you worry about your child eating pizza at a playdate?

It's important to do whatever we can to raise our children with optimal nutrition, but with a healthy, not obsessive, attitude toward food. Let's not make a big deal out of occasional treats like pizza at a playdate, but strive for a tasty, healthy variety of Paleo foods at home. Of course, do be aware of whether your child is extra-sensitive to occasional exposures to off-plan foods. Most kids will be okay, but trust your instincts and observe their reactions.

Chapter 34:
TROUBLESHOOTING

If you are motivated to make dietary and lifestyle changes because you are sick or very overweight, you might find yourself in the position of needing to adjust a certain aspect of your diet or lifestyle to reflect your specific health challenges, or you might need to add adjunct medications, supplements, or therapies. This book has focused on defining what the best diet and lifestyle choices are and explaining why. While the previous chapter included some additional considerations for common chronic health problems and goals, one thing I have yet to discuss is how to troubleshoot when the diet and lifestyle changes you are implementing are insufficient for regaining your health and meeting your particular goals.

A common roadblock is continuing to consume foods to which you have an allergy, intolerance, or sensitivity. For that reason, I'll summarize the most common food sensitivities in this chapter. But what this chapter really boils down to is the recommendation that you seek guidance from a qualified health-care professional. While healthy diet and lifestyle choices can lead to amazing reversals of chronic disease and help us achieve the best health of our lives, these recommendations aren't intended to replace a doctor's care.

FIRST, ASK YOURSELF THESE QUESTIONS

The internet is teeming with the testimonials of people who have experienced rapid and dramatic results after switching to the Paleo template. These stories are inspiring, and the rapid growth of the Paleo community over the last decade is at least partially attributable to them. But what do you do if you aren't seeing impressive results right away? Don't be discouraged: often a few tweaks here and there can make all the difference.

Before you jump into additional food eliminations, try fad versions of Paleo, or fork over hundreds of dollars for the services of an alternative healthcare provider, ask yourself the following few key questions. The answers will help you identify where you may be able to improve your implementation of the Paleo template in addition to providing some guidance for troubleshooting.

How differently did you eat before committing to a Paleo diet? Generally, the more differently you are eating now compared to before you began eating Paleo, the harder and longer your adjustment period will be—especially if you were eating a lot of carbohydrates and very little fiber. It can take up to a month for your body to switch to a flexible and efficient metabolism that runs on whichever fuel (fat or carbohydrates) happens to be available; in the meantime, you may feel tired or lethargic, have headaches, and generally feel pretty terrible. It also takes a while to build up sufficient nutrient stores to promote optimal health. (However, this isn't true for everyone; the opposite can also be true. Some people were made so sick by the foods they were eating before that they notice a near-instant improvement in their health when they switch to Paleo.)

What health issues are you challenged with? Most gut health issues will improve dramatically in the first couple of weeks following a relatively strict Paleo diet and then continue to improve more slowly over the next 6 months as the gut continues to heal. During this period of healing, it's extremely important to avoid gluten while focusing on vegetables, omega-3 fats, fermented foods, and healing foods like bone broth. Issues relating to inflammation typically take longer to show significant improvement, depending on how well you are sleeping and managing your stress and how effectively you're addressing nutrient deficiencies. For many chronic health issues, you really need to dial in all the Paleo principles (diet plus lifestyle) to experience dramatic improvements. You might also benefit from implementing the Autoimmune Protocol (see page 412).

Are you truly complying with the Paleo template? It's true that many people experience tremendous health benefits from being "almost Paleo." But if you are asking, "When will I feel fabulous?" without following the Paleo guidelines as strictly as you can, then you might be a person who just can't cheat or tolerate even occasional gluten exposure. You might also be a person who can't tolerate many or any of the middle-ground foods discussed in Chapter 24. Another common stumbling block is to be super-strict about diet while not managing stress or prioritizing sleep. Make sure to consider the lifestyle aspects of the Paleo template equally to the dietary aspects.

Are you skimping on nutrient-dense foods? There's the old stereotype of a Paleo meal consisting of a chicken breast and steamed broccoli. But the truth is that if you don't actively try to include organ meat, fish, shellfish, sea vegetables, fermented foods, and a diverse array of vegetables, you're going to fall short on essential nutrients (see page 47). If you're following a narrower version of the Paleo diet that adheres to the basic template of meat and vegetables but doesn't include these nutrient superstars, nutrient deficiencies might be keeping you from your best health.

Are you in food sensitivity denial? Some people don't react overtly to specific foods, making it tough to identify triggers even after methodically eliminating and challenging them. If you had mild or delayed symptoms upon challenging a food, you might not have recognized that continuing to eat that food is holding you back. Try eating only the foods outlined in Part 2 and see if you experience more rapid improvements. If not, you may have developed an intolerance or allergy to one or more of those healthy foods, the possibilities of which include FODMAP sensitivity, salicylate sensitivity, histamine sensitivity, and allergies to latex, citrus, fish and shellfish, tree nuts, eggs, and/or dairy, all of which are discussed later in this chapter.

How is your digestion? You might need to add some digestive support supplements for a little while so that you can better absorb the nutrients from the healthy foods you're eating. These include digestive enzymes, ox bile, and stomach acid supplements (which are contraindicated for those with ulcers or blood clotting disorders or those who are taking NSAIDs). See page 77 for details.

Did you inappropriately discontinue a medication? When organs are damaged as the result of disease, they need to be supported. This might mean taking insulin for a type 1 diabetic or thyroid replacement hormone for someone with Hashimoto's thyroiditis. Generally, in these conditions, going medication-free is counterproductive to health. For example, thyroid hormones control a vast array of functions in the human body, from metabolism to immune function. Without adequate thyroid hormones, the body is less responsive to diet and lifestyle changes. In this case, it's in your best interest to properly support the damaged organ through pharmaceuticals—don't consider this a failure! Taking a medication, even for the rest of your life, does not make you a failure. But it doesn't mean that you don't have everything to gain from making diet and lifestyle changes, too. These meds can help prevent further damage to your organ and prevent the development of additional chronic health problems, so going medication-free should not be the goal.

Did you go too low-carb? While blood sugar regulation is extremely important, going too low-carb can be tough on your thyroid and can decrease leptin sensitivity (see page 402). Eating adequate carbohydrate, especially insoluble fiber, is critical for the proper regulation of ghrelin levels (see page 90). We need a minimum amount of carbohydrate just to meet our fiber requirements for a healthy gut microbial community. If you found yourself cutting out fruit or starchy carbs to spur weight loss or because you heard some dogmatic proclamations about the benefits of low-carb diets, try gradually increasing your starchy carbohydrate intake. The reason for a gradual increase (say, one-quarter serving every couple of days) is that prolonged periods of low-carb dieting can actually cause insulin and leptin resistance (see page 402). In addition, the bacteria that thrive on these fiber sources tend to be slow-growing, so allowing your gut microbiota to adjust gradually can prevent gastrointestinal symptoms.

Are you inappropriately "IFing"? IF stands for intermittent fasting, and there are many enthusiastic supporters of this strategy to lower overall caloric intake and spur autophagy (see page 92). But it's important to understand that fasting is appropriate only for very healthy people and perhaps only healthy men. If your sleep is not great, your stress in not managed, you are substantially overweight, or you have any kind of chronic disease, skipping breakfast (or breakfast and lunch) can cause dysregulated cortisol and undermine your other efforts. Fasting is not something to experiment with early on in your Paleo journey.

What are your weight-loss goals, and how far from those goals are you? If you have a lot of weight to lose, you will probably notice a big drop fairly quickly. This will be mostly water weight, but don't worry; fat is also being burned, and you should eventually settle into a nice, steady weight loss. (Slow and steady wins the race, so there is no reason to be frustrated with weight loss if you are losing "only" a half pound per week—that's actually very healthy!) If your body seems resistant to weight loss, try addressing sleep quality and stress levels, but also be aware of the impact of female hormones and hunger hormones (levels and sensitivity). See page 400.

Are you working on lifestyle factors? While most of this book focuses on explaining dietary factors, that doesn't mean we shouldn't make lifestyle improvements, too. Sleep and circadian rhythms, stress management, physical activity, sunlight exposure, and social connection all profoundly impact our health and well-being. If you're not experiencing the health improvements you were hoping for, critically evaluate your adherence to the lifestyle aspects of the Paleo template.

Do you have an undiagnosed underlying health challenge? Gut dysbiosis (see page 73), methylation defects (see page 108), hormone imbalance (see page 341), cortisol dysregulation and adrenal fatigue (see page 345), hypothyroidism (see page 93), autoimmune disease (see page 412), persistent infections (like Epstein-Barr, Lyme disease, *H. pylori*, or parasites), neurotransmitter imbalances, heavy metal exposure, and chronic nutrient deficiencies (see Chapter 1) are all examples of health challenges that you may not know about but can hold back your progress. Working with a functional or integrative medicine practitioner is your best bet for diagnosis and effective treatment.

As you reflect on your answers to these questions, chances are high that you've realized there's a Paleo principle that you're not fully implementing (sleep, stress management, and nutrient density being the three most common culprits). In the event that you've got the Paleo diet and lifestyle dialed in and you still aren't seeing results, it's time to dig deeper. Let's start with the possibility of reactions to healthy foods.

REACTIONS TO HEALTHY FOODS

Another obstacle to healing is continuing to eat foods (or be environmentally exposed to substances) to which you have developed an allergy, intolerance, or sensitivity. It's possible to have a reaction to one or a few of the healthy foods discussed in Part 2; those foods are great for optimal human health in general, but they may not work for you as an individual. Identifying the problematic food(s) and eliminating it from your diet will help you reach your health goals. Figuring out which foods (or substances, like chemicals) might be an issue for you can be tricky, though, so it's worth summarizing the most common culprits.

Food Allergies

An *allergy* is an immune reaction in which IgE antibodies (see page 246) are produced against a food or a specific substance in your environment, like pollen. This triggers histamine release from two types of immune cells, mast cells and basophils, which causes the symptoms normally associated with allergies, including hives, rashes, swelling (of the lips, nasal tissues, eyes, ears, face, tongue, and/or throat), a flushing or burning sensation in the skin, abdominal pain, bloating, vomiting, diarrhea, ear pain, sneezing, coughing, wheezing, shortness of breath, red or itchy eyes, runny nose, and increased heart rate. These symptoms may be dramatic, as in the case of anaphylaxis (a life-threatening severe allergic reaction typified by hives, severe swelling, trouble breathing, and shock), or subtle, as in the case of mild seasonal allergies.

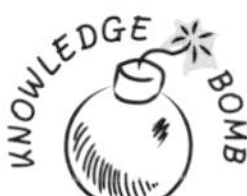

It is possible for allergies to diminish and even completely disappear over time. For example, in children with food allergies, about 20 percent outgrow peanut allergy by age 8, 75 percent outgrow dairy allergy by age 3, and half outgrow egg allergy by age 5. While it's generally accepted that if an allergy starts in adulthood, the chances of it going away are much lower, there are currently no studies to tell us how likely (or unlikely) that is.

Many common food allergens are eliminated on a Paleo diet, including peanuts, wheat, and soybeans, but of those that remain, the most common are fish, shellfish, dairy, tree nuts, and eggs. These are the top-eight food allergies that account for more than 90 percent of all food allergies; the FDA mandates that they be included on all food labels if the possibility of contamination is present.

Other common allergies include:

- **Latex-allergy foods:** apples, avocados, bananas, carrots, cassava, celery, kiwi, melons, papaya (and to a lesser extent apricots, cherries, citrus fruit, coconut, figs, grapes, lychee, mangoes, nectarines, passion fruit, peaches, pears, plums, persimmons, pineapple, strawberries, shellfish, dill, oregano, sage, and zucchini)
- **Birch-pollen-allergy fruits and vegetables:** apples, carrots, celery, cherries, peaches, pears, plums
- **Ragweed-pollen-allergy fruits and vegetables:** bananas, melons
- **Mugwort-pollen-allergy fruits and vegetables:** apples, carrots, celery, kiwi, parsley
- **Poison ivy family:** mangoes, pistachios
- **Citrus fruits**
- **Yeast:** all fermented foods, wine, cider, vinegar, some fruits (especially grapes and plums), many dried fruits, Marmite, Vegemite, processed meat and fish, many canned foods, B vitamin supplements (unless explicitly labeled), some other supplements
- **Beef**
- **Garlic**
- **Kiwi**

Note that not all latex allergy *foods* are an issue for those with an allergy to latex, and similarly for birch, ragweed, mugwort pollen, and poison ivy. However, if you have previously been diagnosed with an allergy to latex or poison ivy or if you have bad seasonal allergies that may be attributable to birch, ragweed, or mugwort pollens, eliminating the foods on the appropriate list above may be very helpful.

Food-allergy testing can be done by blood test or skin test. Blood tests are fairly straightforward. The most common test, called a RAST, measures the presence of IgE antibodies in the blood against up to 160 different foods. In skin tests, which are considered more accurate, small amounts of allergens are placed on the skin of the arms or back in a grid pattern, and the skin is then pricked where the allergens were placed. (Alternatively, allergens can be injected just under the skin.) After a set amount of time, the skin is evaluated for severity of reaction (usually redness, puffiness, or hives).

If you have a diagnosed or suspected allergy to any food, you should avoid that food completely. Severe food allergies are not likely to disappear entirely with the adoption of a Paleo diet, although the severity of your reaction may diminish.

Food Intolerances

You may also have *intolerances*—that is, immune responses other than IgE reactions (typically IgG, IgA, or IgM antibodies; see page 246). If you have a severely leaky gut, proteins from anything you eat can cross the gut barrier and interact with your immune system. And the more damaged your gut barrier and the more activated your immune system, the more likely you are to develop food intolerances. While these foods don't irritate the gut or activate the immune system in most people, because of your food intolerance they perpetuate inflammation in your body.

KNOWLEDGE BOMB *Unlike a food allergy, a food intolerance tends to be much more dynamic. With careful avoidance, IgG antibodies against food disappear within 3 months to 2 years, depending on how high they were initially.*

You may be able to figure out which food(s) you are intolerant of by eliminating the suspect(s) for 2 to 3 weeks and seeing if it makes a difference. This is a simple process if you notice symptoms when you eat one specific food. However, if there are multiple culprits, it might be a good idea to ask your health-care practitioner to order an IgG food sensitivity test (even better if it includes IgA and IgM as well) and help you interpret the results. In the case of a severely leaky gut, many foods may test positive, and your health-care practitioner can help you determine which you should exclude from your diet (those with the strongest reactions) and which you can continue to eat in moderation or on a rotation (so when you do eat a food to which you have a mild intolerance, you don't eat it again for several days).

Among the foods that are generally included on the Paleo diet, the most common intolerances are dairy, eggs, and tree nuts.

Legumes and cereal grain intolerances are also common and worth investigating if you're including some of these middle-ground foods in your diet. Other food intolerances that occur with higher frequency include:

Apples	Chicken	Pork	Wine
Apple cider vinegar	Fish	Shellfish	Yeast
Beef	Lamb	Tapioca (aka cassava, yuca, manioc)	
Celery	Nuts		

Unlike food allergies, food intolerances tend to be transient. After removing those foods from your diet for an extended period (at least 6 months for most people) and restoring gut barrier function, you may be able to reintroduce them without problems by following the protocol outlined in Chapter 25.

Food Sensitivities

Food *sensitivities* are distinct from allergies and intolerances in that they do not involve antibody production. Instead, sensitivities may arise through a variety of other mechanisms, including from the effects of severe gut dysbiosis (production of bacterial metabolites, for example may be the cause of your sensitivity) or from an inability to process or metabolize a substance (which can cause inflammation, damage to the gut, strain on the liver, or damage to other tissues).

There are no specific tests for food sensitivities; the only way to figure out whether you are sensitive to certain foods is the elimination and challenge protocol in Chapter 25. The following are the most common food sensitivities that might be hindering your ability to heal:

- FODMAP sensitivity
- Histamine sensitivity
- Salicylate sensitivity
- Sulfite sensitivity (discussed on page 239)

FODMAP Sensitivity

For people who have gastrointestinal symptoms, FODMAP sensitivity (sometimes called fructose malabsorption or FODMAP intolerance) is a distinct possibility. FODMAP is an acronym for "fermentable oligosaccharides, disaccharides, monosaccharides, and polyols," which are basically a group of highly fermentable, short- and medium-chain carbohydrates (typically high in fructose or lactose) and sugar alcohols. These carbohydrates are inefficiently absorbed in the small intestine, even in very healthy people, and the gut bacteria love them (which is what makes them highly fermentable).

When too many fermentable sugars enter the large intestine, which has the highest concentration of gut microorganisms, they feed the bacteria, producing excess gas and, in more extreme cases, an overgrowth of bacteria. This is exactly what happens in FODMAP sensitivity. The presence of these carbohydrates in the large intestine can also decrease water absorption (one of the large intestine's main jobs). This overfeeding of the gut microbiota causes a variety of digestive symptoms, most typically bloating, gas, cramps, diarrhea, constipation, indigestion, and sometimes excessive belching.

Almost everyone who eats FODMAP-dense foods experiences some degree of gastrointestinal symptoms (the source of "Beans, beans, the musical fruit . . .").

In fact, eating a lot of inulin fiber (a FODMAP that is often added to foods and included in supplements as a prebiotic) has been shown to significantly alter the composition of the gut microflora—although whether for the better or worse and whether a healthy body is well adapted to large amounts of inulin is in dispute. In the case of FODMAP sensitivity, these symptoms are magnified for a few reasons. FODMAP sensitivity simply means that the body is less able to digest these types of carbohydrates. This may be due to a lack of digestive enzymes to break down these particular molecules (see page 77) or to an insufficient amount of GLUT5 transporters in the cell membranes of the enterocytes to transport fructose across the gut barrier (see page 270). In most cases, both of these mechanisms are probably at work, the end result being that a far greater portion of these sugars enter the large intestine unabsorbed, causing magnified symptoms and an overgrowth of bacteria in the large intestine.

A large number of clinical trials have shown that removing FODMAPs from the diet is beneficial for sufferers of irritable bowel syndrome (IBS) and other functional gastrointestinal disorders. However, this should be seen as a short-term intervention. Whole-food FODMAPs feed some very beneficial strains of bacteria in the gut and are an important source of fermentable substrate for a healthy gut microbiota.

SCIENCE SIMPLIFIED

FODMAPs are types of carbohydrates that can cause gastrointestinal symptoms in those who have a sensitivity to them, however, they also feed some of the most desirable strains of probiotic bacteria in our guts. For this reason, a low-FODMAP diet should be followed for only 2 to 4 weeks before gradually adding them back in. If you can't reintroduce FODMAP-rich foods without severe symptoms, it's time to see a doctor.

For that reason, if you suspect that you have a FODMAP sensitivity, it's best to eliminate FODMAPs for 2 to 4 weeks. Then you'll want to reintroduce FODMAP-rich foods, especially alliums and cruciferous veggies, increasing the amount you eat very, *very* gradually. Try to stay just below symptomatic levels as you increase the amount of high-FODMAP foods you eat; you can be as conservative as increasing by a teaspoon a day. Fortunately, FODMAP sensitivity will likely disappear for most people as their guts heal and their gut microbiota levels and diversity normalize.

If severe symptoms return with the reintroduction of FODMAPs, it's likely that you have severe gut dysbiosis, such as small intestinal bacterial overgrowth (SIBO; see page 70). The current consensus among experts is that diet alone is insufficient to reverse SIBO. Your best bet is to see a qualified health-care provider for thorough testing in order to find an antimicrobial protocol specific to the type of bacteria overgrowth you have.

When it comes to modifying your diet to address a suspected FODMAP sensitivity, how much FODMAP-rich food you eat is the key. The standard recommendation for people with suspected FODMAP sensitivity is to avoid eating foods that contain:

- More than 0.5 gram of free fructose in excess of free glucose per 100-gram serving
- More than 3 grams of free fructose in an average serving regardless of glucose content
- More than 0.2 gram of fructans per serving

Most of the foods with the greatest amounts of FODMAPs are excluded from a Paleo diet, including wheat, barley, rye, legumes, high-fructose corn syrup, agave nectar, and sugar alcohols. Dairy products and some fruits and vegetables are also high in FODMAPs. Other high-FODMAP foods include:

All canned fruit
All dried fruit
All fruit juices
Apples
Apricots
Artichokes, globe
*Artichokes, Jerusalem**
Asparagus~
Avocados
Bananas (ripe only)
Beets
Blackberries
Blueberries
Broccoli~
Brussels sprouts
*Bulb onions**
Buttermilk
Butternut squash~
Cabbage~
Cashews
Cauliflower
Celery
Cheese
Cherries
Chicory root
Coconut (except coconut oil)
Cream
Cream cheese
Custard
Dandelion greens
Dates
Evaporated milk
Fennel bulb~
Figs
*Garlic**
Gelato
Grapefruit
Grapes
Green onions (white part only)
Guava
Honeydew melon
Ice cream
Kefir
Kiwi
Large servings of any fruit
*Leeks (white part only)**
Longans
Lychees
Mangoes
Milk
Mushrooms
Nashi pears
Nectarines
Okra
Onions
Peaches
Pears
Persimmons
Pistachios
Plums
Prunes
Rambutan
*Shallots**
Snow peas
Sour cream
Sweet potatoes
Watermelon
Yogurt
Zucchini

FODMAP

** Denotes very high fructan content*
~ Conflicting measurements; some sources found no FODMAPs

However, there are still no exhaustive studies measuring the FODMAP content of all foods, so this list should be considered incomplete.

Histamine Sensitivity

Histamine sensitivity results when there is more histamine in the body than the body can handle. Histamine (which you will recognize as the key chemical produced by the body during an allergic reaction; see page 433) is a type of molecule called a *biogenic amine*, which is created when the carboxyl group is removed from an amino acid (see page 30). In the case of histamine, the amino acid that is "decarboxylated" is histidine. Histamine is a normal part of the diet (at least in small amounts) and a normal product of the bacteria in our guts. In healthy people, histamine is rapidly detoxified by gut enzymes. In the case of histamine sensitivity, however, either production of histamine is unusually high or activity of these detoxification enzymes is unusually low (or both). Histamine sensitivity may be more likely if you have a thyroid condition or are taking thyroid hormone replacement drugs, especially if your dose of thyroid hormone is too high.

Some other factors contribute to histamine sensitivity. If basophils and mast cells (the two major cell types responsible for histamine release during immune and allergic reactions) are activated as part of health conditions you have, your sensitivity to histamine from foods may increase simply because your basal level of histamine production is higher. A variety of drugs inhibit the activity of the main enzyme that detoxifies histamine, deamine oxidase (DAO), including some commonly prescribed muscle relaxants, narcotics, analgesics, local anesthetics, antihypertensives, diuretics, antibiotics, H2 blockers, and antidepressants. And not only does alcohol inhibit DAO activity, but wine (especially red wine) and beer contain a lot of histamine.

Symptoms of histamine sensitivity resemble those of allergies and may include diarrhea, headache, sinus symptoms (congestion, runny nose, post-nasal drip, sinus pressure and/or pain, sneezing, or problems with sense of smell), itchy or watery eyes, asthma, low blood pressure, arrhythmia (rapid, slow, or irregular heart rate), hives, rashes, and flushing. Typically, a response is felt relatively quickly after consuming high-histamine foods. A food and symptom journal is the most common way to diagnose histamine sensitivity, but blood tests can measure both histamine and DAO and may help confirm diagnosis (although there is some debate over whether serum DAO is truly indicative of gut DAO). It is estimated that 1 percent of the population has histamine sensitivity, and most of these people are middle-aged. However, many researchers believe that this is a gross underestimation because histamine sensitivity has only very recently been recognized as a pathology.

The typical recommendation for those with histamine sensitivity is to follow a histamine-free diet. Doing so can be challenging because the histamine content of foods can vary significantly depending on handling and processing as well as on the specific bacteria used in fermentation. Furthermore, histamine content is not usually indicated on food labels and is measured only to ensure food safety (since high levels cause food poisoning). Antihistamines are recommended only when high amounts of histamine are accidentally consumed, and not for long-term therapy. Although DAO supplements are available (generally pig kidney enzymes), clinical trials have not been performed to test their efficacy. Also note that medium-chain triglycerides (MCTs), the healthy fats in coconut and palm oil, increase DAO activity and may be beneficial for those with histamine sensitivity.

Foods that are likely to contain significant amounts of histamine include:

- *Alcoholic beverages*
  - Beer
  - Champagne
  - Sherry
  - Wine
- *Chocolate and cocoa*
- *Coffee*
- *Eggplant*
- *Fermented dairy products*
  - Yogurt
  - Sour cream
  - Cheeses (Gouda, Camembert, Cheddar, Swiss, Harzer, Tilsit, Parmesan)
- *Fermented cured meats*
  - Dry-cured sausages (like salami and pepperoni)
  - Fermented ham
  - Fermented sausages
- *Fish*
  - Anchovies
  - Bonito
  - Butterfly kingfish
  - Dried milkfish
  - Fish paste (such as anchovy paste)
  - Fish sauce
  - Herring
  - Mackerel
  - Marlin
  - Pilchard
  - Sardines (amount varies; some contain no histamine)
  - Saury
  - Scad
  - Shrimp paste
  - Smooth-tailed trevally
  - Tuna (amount varies; some contain no histamine)
- *Any fish if stored too long or handled improperly*
- *Fruit*
  - Bananas
  - Grapes
  - Oranges
  - Pineapples
  - Strawberries
  - Tangerines
- *Green tea*
- *Pork*
- *Sauerkraut (and potentially other lacto-fermented fruits and vegetables)*
- *Spinach*
- *Tomatoes and tomato-based products like ketchup*

HISTAMINE

Some foods are more susceptible to histamine formation than others. Of the foods listed above, the average histamine content ranges from 2 to 4,000 milligrams per kilogram, with pineapples, strawberries, grapes, tangerines, and bananas on the low end of the scale and sausage, herring, mackerel, pork, and spinach at the high end.

Other foods have histamine-releasing capacities, meaning that although they do not necessarily contain histamine, once they are ingested they can stimulate the release of histamine from mast cells. These include:

Citrus fruits	*Nuts*	*Tomatoes*
Chocolate and cocoa	*Papaya*	*A variety of food additives*
Crustaceans	*Pineapples*	
Egg whites	*Pork*	
Fish	*Some spices*	
Licorice root	*Spinach*	
	Strawberries	

HISTAMINE-RELEASING CAPACITIES

Salicylate Sensitivity

Salicylates are the salts and esters of salicylic acid, an organic acid that is a key ingredient in aspirin and other pain medications, is frequently found in cosmetics and beauty products, and naturally occurs in varying concentrations in plants. In plants, salicylates act as an immune hormone and preservative, protecting the plants against diseases, insects, fungi, and bacterial infection.

Salicylates are converted to salicylic acid in the body. Salicylic acid is toxic in high doses and is one of the leading causes of death from accidental poisoning. In high doses, its effects include:

- **Respiratory alkalosis:** Salicylic acid stimulates the respiratory center in the brain stem. This causes hyperventilation, which increases the pH of the blood (making it less acidic and more alkaline).
- **Metabolic acidosis and hyperthermia:** Salicylic acid interferes with mitochondrial metabolism (the Krebs cycle; see page 267), which limits ATP production and causes a shift from aerobic to anaerobic metabolism. This results in a buildup of pyruvic and lactic acid and an increase in heat production, thus lowering the pH of the blood and body tissues (making them more acidic and less alkaline) and raising body temperature.

In the initial phases of acute salicylic acid poisoning, respiratory alkalosis produces alkaline urine because potassium and sodium bicarbonate are being excreted. Symptoms typically include nausea, vomiting, excessive sweating, tinnitus (ringing in the ears), vertigo, hyperventilation, rapid heart rate, and hyperactivity. As poisoning progresses, the urine becomes acidic despite respiratory alkalosis because pyruvic and lactic acid build up and potassium levels fall. Additional symptoms that may occur include fever, agitation, delirium, hallucinations, convulsions, lethargy, and stupor. The final stages of salicylic acid poisoning are characterized by dehydration, hypokalemia (low potassium levels), and progressive metabolic acidosis. Severe salicylate poisoning is fatal if not treated.

In the case of salicylate sensitivity, it takes much smaller doses than normal to produce symptoms of toxicity. Salicylate sensitivity was initially described in terms of adverse drug reactions, and to date most of the studies regarding it are performed in the context of medications that contain salicylates or salicylic acid. Although more research is needed, the definition has expanded to include sensitivity to foods and to cleaning and beauty products that contain high levels of salicylates. The typical reactions are gastrointestinal, asthma-related, or pseudo-anaphylactic (the symptoms of anaphylaxis through a non-IgE-antibody-mediated pathway). Symptoms of salicylate sensitivity include:

- Asthma and other breathing difficulties, such as persistent cough
- Changes in skin color
- Depression and anxiety
- Fatigue
- Headaches
- Itchy skin, hives, or rashes
- Memory loss and poor concentration (linked to ADHD)
- Nasal congestion or sinusitis
- Sore, itchy, puffy, or burning eyes
- Stomach pain, nausea, or diarrhea
- Swelling of hands, feet, eyelids, face, or lips (angioedema)
- Tinnitus

There is no diagnostic test for salicylate sensitivity. The only way to determine whether you are sensitive to salicylates is to significantly reduce your exposure to them and see if you improve. This involves avoiding oral, topical, and inhaled exposure since salicylic acid is readily absorbed through the skin and lungs. The following items usually contain substantial amounts of salicylates or salicylic acid:

Acne treatment products	Hairsprays, gels, and mousse	Skin cleansers and exfoliants
Air fresheners	Lotions	Soaps
Antacids	Lozenges	Sunscreen
Breath mints	Medications (including aspirin and other NSAIDs)	Toothpaste
Bubble baths	Mouthwash	Topical creams
Cleaning products	Muscle-pain creams	Wart and callus removers
Cosmetics	Shampoos and conditioners	
Detergents	Shaving cream	
Fragrances and perfumes		
Gum		

SALICYLATE

It is extremely important to emphasize that salicylic acid is believed to be an essential micronutrient, potentially even qualifying as a vitamin. It appears to have critical anti-inflammatory, anti-atherogenic and antineoplastic roles, meaning that it may prevent cardiovascular disease and cancer. In fact, some researchers believe that diets rich in fruits and vegetables decrease the rates of cardiovascular disease and cancer because of the benefits of dietary salicylic acid—giving salicylic acid a greater role than fiber, vitamins, and minerals! Even in the case of salicylate sensitivity, whether or not food sources of salicylates should be avoided in addition to medications and environmental sources (which are by far the bigger contributors to salicylate exposure) is a hot topic of debate.

Salicylate sensitivity may really be a consequence of omega-3 fatty acid or zinc deficiency. One of salicylic acid's jobs is to inhibit production of pro-inflammatory prostaglandins as a result of the COX-2-mediated metabolism of arachidonic acid (see page 115). However, salicylic acid might not be able to do so if there is insufficient DHA and EPA in the cell membranes (see page 159). Studies evaluating supplementation with high doses of omega-3 fatty acids (in the form of fish oil) in people with salicylate sensitivity show enormous reductions in symptoms. Animal studies also show that supplementation with zinc (concurrent with toxic doses of salicylic acid) completely prevent the symptoms of salicylate poisoning.

Studies evaluating the levels of salicylates (and the related compounds acetylsalicylates) show that dietary intake is typically very low, especially compared to other types of exposure. What this most likely means for those with salicylate sensitivity is that avoiding salicylate-containing foods is probably not necessary—especially if your diet is rich in omega-3 fatty acids and zinc. However, for reference, the following foods are the biggest Paleo sources of salicylates:

Alcoholic beverages	Nightshades (tomatoes, peppers, eggplant, and so on; see page 296)	Most berries
Asparagus	Many herbs and spices (cinnamon, rosemary, thyme, oregano, turmeric, and mint)	Oranges
Black tea		Pineapples
Dried fruits		Tangerines
Green apples		
Fruit juices		
Nectarines		

SALICYLATE

Cross-Contamination

If you have a food allergy, intolerance, or sensitivity, even a trace amount of that food can be a problem, the operative word being *can:* for example, gluten can elicit violent reactions even in very small quantities in some individuals, but a FODMAP sensitivity may produce symptoms only if a threshold quantity is consumed. But if you react strongly to a certain food, it's important to be very conscious of the possibility of cross-contamination.

For example, if you have an issue with gluten and you live in a home in which others eat gluten-containing foods, you will need to take precautions to ensure that even trace amounts of those foods do not contaminate your plate. For example, have one cutting board designated for gluten-containing foods and another designated for gluten-free foods (not stored nested together, either). Keep gluten-containing foods in separate cupboards or areas of the fridge and freezer. Wear gloves when you handle foods that contain gluten—or, better yet, have someone else handle them for you. Best option: Have all household members commit to eating gluten only outside the home. Wash everything very well if you are going to use the same utensils for both gluten-containing and gluten-free foods.

These precautions may be excessive for your particular sensitivity, and certainly not everyone needs to go to such extremes. But if you are reading through this chapter for ideas on what could be holding back your progress, cross-contamination might be the culprit. It's also worth re-examining ingredient labels (see pages 280 to 285).

WORKING WITH YOUR DOCTOR

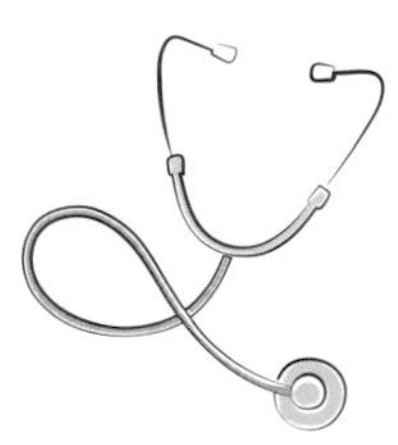

Now it's time to call in the reinforcements. When it comes to underlying health challenges that can't be addressed with diet and lifestyle modifications alone, it's important to take advantage of your health-care providers' expertise. Just as a prescription medication can't replace the benefits of eating healthy food, even the best diet and lifestyle can't replace a doctor's care—although I hope you'll need to see her less frequently.

When it comes to medical expertise, you have a lot of choices, and you can work with several practitioners. Depending on your particular situation, you may avail yourself of a variety of conventional and alternative health-care providers, including your primary care physician, a medical specialist, naturopathic doctor, chiropractor, acupuncturist, therapist, physical therapist, massage therapist, nurse practitioner, registered dietitian, nutritionist, nutritional therapy practitioner, or certified health coach, among others! These experts are part of your team, and each of you has the same goal: for you to be as healthy as you can be.

It's important to be an informed patient (but don't self-diagnose with Dr. Google before you even enter the exam room!), to be your own patient advocate, and to use medical interventions judiciously. For example, as discussed on page 116, antibiotics can be a lifesaving medication, but their overuse has led to antibiotic-resistant strains of bacteria, like MRSA. The goal is to take advantage of modern medicine when it's truly needed and practice preventative medicine the rest of the time.

HEALTH QUICK-START *You get the best of both worlds. You now know the optimal diet and lifestyle choices for your best health and you get to utilize the miracle that is modern medicine when needed.*

Preventative Medicine

The goal of preventative medicine, as the name implies, is to prevent the development of disease and disability through promotion of a healthy diet, lifestyle, behaviors, environment, and community. Effective preventative medicine requires active collaboration between patient and health-care provider. Thorough medical evaluation allows practitioners to identify underlying health challenges so that they can be addressed, boosting the efficacy of the patient's healthy living efforts. The patient's end of the deal is to be self-motivated to make healthy day-to-day choices.

However, preventative medicine is not what's typically practiced in the current health-care system. It may be a cliché, but I agree with the many others who say that it's sick care, not health care. I know how difficult it can be to find a doctor who wants to treat the whole person rather than throw pills at a problem. I know how much harder it is to dig deep into the root causes of a person's health conditions and devise a multifactorial approach to fixing it rather than prescribe a regimen that merely alleviates symptoms. But if we want to turn the tide of chronic disease in our society, we need to change the way care is provided. We need a shift toward preventative medicine, holistic approaches, integrative and functional medicine, and a routine of providing robust health science education to the general public. It's impossible to make the right choices to get healthy if you don't know what the right choices are!

Of course, this entire book is about providing that scientific education to help you understand the best diet and lifestyle choices for optimal health. And while discussing the merits and drawbacks of various supplements, medications, surgeries, therapies, and other treatments goes way beyond the scope of this book, it's worthwhile to elaborate on the types of health-care professionals who best align with the Paleo principles. So let's take a moment to discuss functional and integrative medicine.

According to the Institute for Functional Medicine, functional medicine practitioners (MDs, DCs, NDs, physical therapists, and even nutritionists) "address the underlying causes of disease using a systems-oriented approach" and seek to engage "both patient and practitioner in a therapeutic partnership."

The Academy of Integrative Health & Medicine has a similar definition of integrative medicine: "The field of integrative health and medicine reaffirms the importance of the relationship between practitioner and patient, focuses on the whole person, is informed by evidence, and makes use of all appropriate therapeutic approaches, health-care professionals and professions to achieve optimal health and healing."

Both integrative and functional medicine practitioners look for the root causes of disease (like food sensitivities, nutrient deficiencies, gut dysbiosis, hormone dysregulation, persistent infection, and organ dysfunction) and use multifaceted approaches (that encompass diet, lifestyle, supplements, botanicals, medications, and so on) to promote health.

So why doesn't everyone move to a functional or integrative medicine model? For one thing, this model of disease treatment simply isn't taught in a majority of medical programs, which focus on treatment instead of prevention. Thanks to the constrictions of our health-care system, it's also difficult for functional and integrative medicine practitioners to receive reimbursement from insurance companies; this means treatment is often prohibitively expensive. Despite these limitations, functional and integrative medicine are hugely important to the future of medicine and to the successful reversal of the current epidemics of chronic disease.

Finding a Practitioner

Functional and integrative medicine practitioners are doctors or alternative health-care providers with supplemental training who specialize in diagnosing and treating the root causes of disease. The recommendations presented in this book, such as the importance of gut health and nutrient density, are generally compatible with the philosophies of functional and integrative medicine specialists. Beyond ordering a wider range of tests than many other health-care professionals would, functional and integrative medicine specialists often use supplements, botanicals, and herbal remedies instead of, or in conjunction with, pharmaceuticals for a more diverse approach to disease management and prevention.

A few online directories can help you find a like-minded health-care provider near you. Try:

- www.a4m.com
- www.functionalmedicine.org
- www.paleophysiciansnetwork.com
- www.re-findhealth.com

Here are some questions you might wish to ask a potential provider:

- How would you describe your practice and general approach?
- Do you have experience treating my condition or diagnosing others with similar symptoms?
- What are the costs of office visits and your most commonly recommended tests? Do you take insurance? Will my insurance cover at least part of the cost of treatment?
- What are your first-line treatment options upon diagnosis? Do you predominantly recommend dietary changes, herbals or botanicals, chiropractic adjustment, nutritional supplementation, hormone replacement, and/or prescription medications?
- Do you use laboratory studies (urine, stool, saliva, and/or blood tests) to aid your diagnoses, or do you rely on other assessment tools? What other diagnostic tools do you use, and what is the science that supports those diagnostic tools?
- How long are your standard office consultations and follow-ups? Is there someone in your practice who is available for after-hours phone calls?

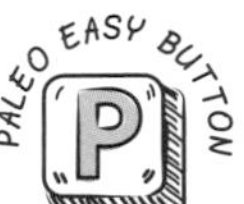

If you're working with a practitioner who does not accept your health insurance, it's worth asking your primary care physician to order some tests. While different doctors have different preferences for annual checkup bloodwork, many doctors will order the following:

- *Complete blood count with differential*
- *Lipid panel*
- *Diabetes panel*
- *Thyroid panel (usually partial)*
- *Serum ferritin test*
- *Kidney panel*
- *Vitamin D test*

You can take a copy of your results to an alternative health-care provider and thus save some money on testing.

Functional Intake Exams

When you start working with a functional or integrative medicine practitioner, you can expect to undergo a wide range of tests that will provide your doctor with a complete picture of your health status. You can expect the tests to fall under a variety of categories and to include a collection of the following (chosen based on your history and symptoms), among others.

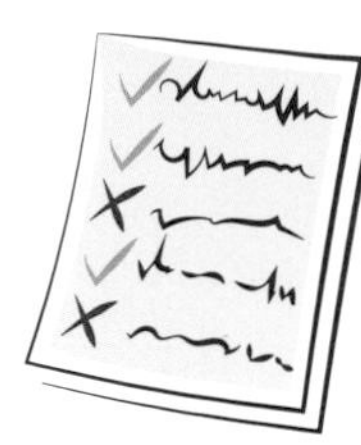

MEDICAL HISTORY:

Complete review of medical history, including the use of questionnaires

Immunization status and updating, if needed

Medication review and screening for drug interactions

Preventive screening review and planning (for example, colonoscopy or mammogram)

Risk factor analysis (for example, looking at lifestyle habits, cholesterol levels, and blood pressure to establish cardiovascular disease risk)

PHYSICAL EXAMINATION:

Standard physical examination (for example, vital signs)

Nutrition-focused physical assessment

Body composition analysis

Dermatologic screening exam

Electrocardiogram

Glaucoma and vision screening

Pap smear (for women)

Screening audiometry

Spirometry—FEV1 and FVC

COMMERCIAL LABORATORY TESTING:

Advanced lipid profiling

Antibody testing for autoimmune conditions

Complete blood count with differential

Comprehensive metabolic profile

Glucose tolerance testing

Gluten antibodies and gluten enteropathy

Heavy metal testing

Hormone levels

Inflammation/oxidation markers

Kidney function

Liver function

Metabolic markers

Mineral/electrolyte analysis

Thyroid function

Vitamin D levels

Other testing as indicated by your medical history or unique risk factors

IMAGING:

ABI index for peripheral vascular disease

Bone density testing

Carotid and abdominal aortic aneurysm screening

Colonoscopy

Coronary calcium scoring

Echocardiogram

Mammogram or thermography (for women)

Thyroid ultrasound

FUNCTIONAL TESTING:

Autonomic nervous system testing

Comprehensive stool analysis

Food sensitivity and allergy testing

Functional nutritional testing

Genetic testing for risk genes (for example, ApoE and MTHFR variants)

Grip strength test

Hormone profiling (looking at how levels change or cycle over time)

Hydrogen/methane breath testing for digestive problems

Red blood cell membrane fatty acid analysis

Salivary cortisol analysis

Urine organic acid analysis

SELF-ADMINISTERED TESTS:

Basal body temperature

Colon transit time

Resting heart rate or heart rate variability

ADVANCED BIOMARKER TESTING PANELS:

Autoimmune disease

Cancer

Hormonal imbalances

Metabolic disorders

Yes, that list may seem overwhelming, and it's true that some doctors are a little test-happy—which is especially frustrating if you're paying out of pocket. Have a conversation with your health-care provider about the reasoning behind any particular test and ask if any tests can wait until the results are available from the first round of testing.

Depending on the test results, your functional or integrative medicine practitioner may recommend specific dietary or lifestyle changes. You might be prescribed medication, but you might also be recommended a regimen of nutritional supplements, herbal remedies, or botanicals to address your health challenges. Treatments like chelation therapy, IV nutrition therapy, or detoxification regimens may be recommended. But chances are high that your practitioner will be pleased to know that you're implementing the recommendations laid out in this book.

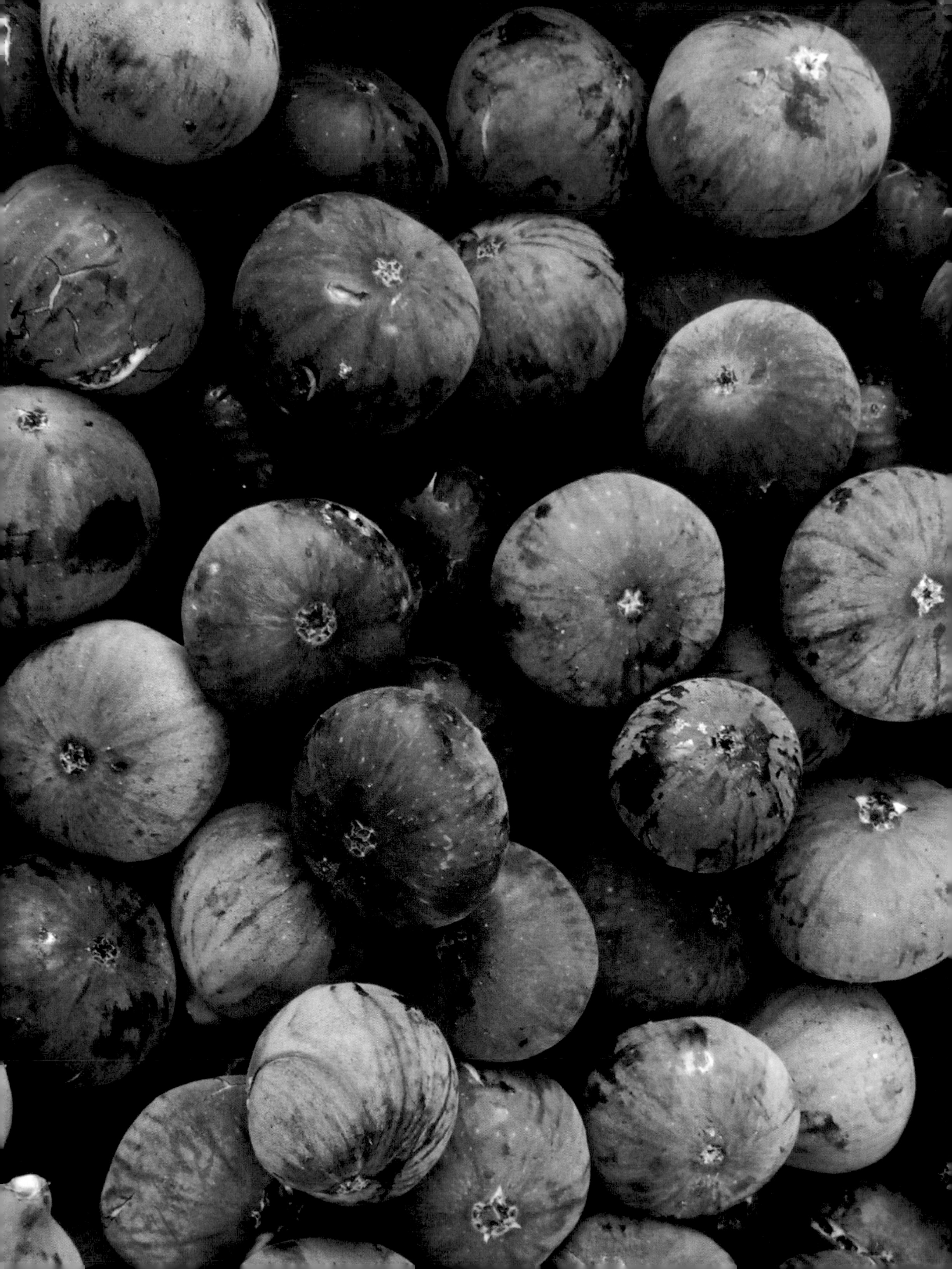

7.

PALEO COOKING BASICS

One effect of dramatically changing the way you eat that many people find difficult at first is that convenience foods are mostly a thing of the past. No longer are you able to pick something up from a drive-through or dial a number to have a meal delivered to your door (with a few exceptions, depending on where you live).

Over the last few decades, we've gotten used to eating more and more meals outside the home. About half of Americans eat two or more meals prepared outside the home each week, with 16 percent of us eating five or more weekly meals away from home. And the more you eat out, the more likely you are to be overweight or obese and to eat few fruits and vegetables. On average, we spend about half of our food budget on home-cooked meals and half on takeout, fast-food, and restaurant meals.

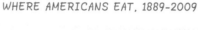

WHERE AMERICANS EAT, 1889-2009

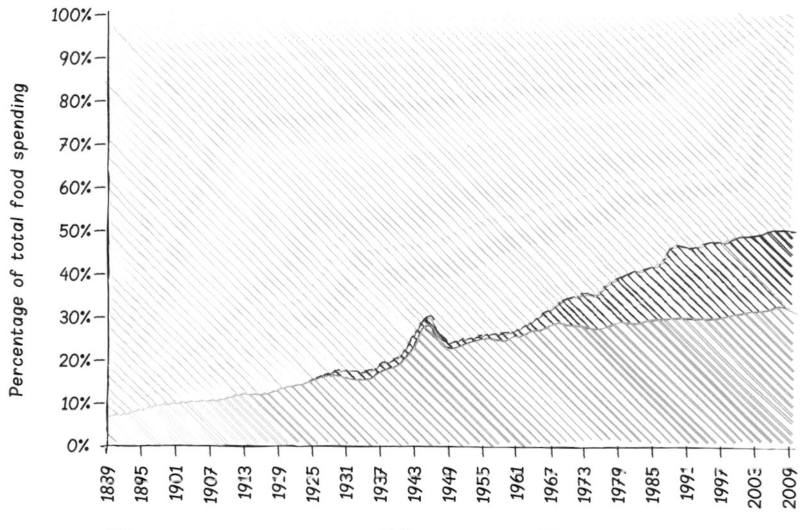

Data from ers.usda.gov. Fast food expenditures were not tracked before 1929.

The good news is that meals you make yourself from whole-food ingredients are almost always cheaper than packaged, prepared, or restaurant options. And while you may be operating within a tight budget, saving money on prepared foods, fast food, and takeout can more than offset the cost of higher-quality meat and fresh vegetables.

Cooking at home isn't the time sink you may think it is. The Environmental Working Group compared the time it took to prepare organic meals at home with the average time it took to pick up a fast-food meal or order and be served a restaurant meal and found that cooking at home can actually *save* a few minutes every day!

Even grabbing fast food isn't necessarily that fast: by the time you add up how long it takes to drive, order, and wait for your meal, you're looking at an average of about 14 minutes. And if you make the healthier choice of eating at a casual dining restaurant, you're looking at an average of 44 minutes. Committing that time to preparing food at home instead is one of the most important steps toward improving your health!

WAITING AND COOKING TIMES CLOCKED BY EWG

	EATING OUT		ORGANIC COOKING	
MEAL	MINUTES	RESTAURANT MEAL	MINUTES	RECIPE
breakfast	4	McDonald's Egg McMuffin	4	Breakfast sandwich
lunch	8	Baja Fresh's Baja Ensalada	10	Fiesta salad with chicken
dinner	30	Applebee's Savory Cedar Salmon	19	Salmon, asparagus, and potatoes
	42	TOTAL MINUTES	33	TOTAL MINUTES

adapted from www.ewg.com

Preparing your own food is one of the most important aspects of changing your diet. When you shop for and cook your food yourself, you have complete control over which ingredients are used and the quality of those ingredients. You also have the opportunity to cater to your own tastes! You can think of your food choices in terms of the nutrition your body needs and plan your meals to ensure that you're getting the full complement of nutrients throughout the week.

But what if you don't know how to cook from scratch? This is definitely part of the Paleo learning curve for many people. For that reason, most of the recipes in Part 8 of this book are straightforward, requiring either very little hands-on time and/or requiring very little time to whip together, while still being delicious!

Whether you're learning how to cook or simply learning how to translate your current kitchen skills to the Paleo diet, it's worth covering a few kitchen basics. So, before we dive into recipes, let's discuss shopping for and storing foods, budget concerns, time management strategies, important kitchen tools easy ingredient swaps, and cooking and ingredient basics!

Chapter 35:
SHOPPING FOR QUALITY FOODS

Making delicious, healthy meals at home starts with shopping for fresh, quality ingredients. The good news is that it's so much easier to find affordable and healthy Paleo options now than even 5 years ago. Grass-fed and pasture-raised meat, wild-caught fish (perhaps frozen), and organic produce can be found in most grocery stores and even discount superstores. With the local-foods movement taking hold, farmstands, farmers markets, and community-supported agriculture are more accessible than ever before. And the array of online vendors offering discounted quality ingredients delivered to your door easily fill in all the gaps.

Of course, if you aren't familiar with all the quality staples in a Paleo kitchen, figuring out where to find them and how to fit them into your budget can seem a bit overwhelming. So let's talk about where to shop and how to save money while doing so.

HOW AND WHERE TO SHOP

If you're intrigued by the extra health benefits that come from the best-quality foods, you may be wondering where you can find them.

Local farmers (farmers markets, farmstands, pick-your-own farms, farm shares, community-supported agriculture, and co-ops): Sourcing food from local farmers is one of the best ways to maximize quality and can be a vital tool for getting high-quality food on a tight budget. It's also a great way to get organ meat, buy a half or whole butchered animal, and find less-common vegetables and fruits.

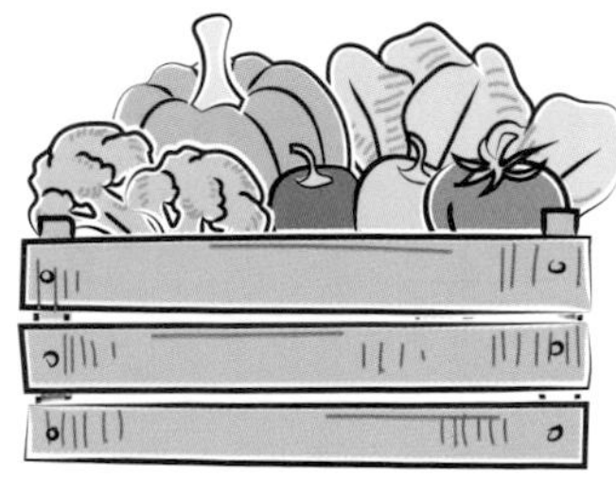

Specialty stores (health-food stores, natural-food stores, supplement stores, cultural food markets, and co-ops): From big-chain natural-food stores to mom-and-pop cultural food markets, these stores can be a boon to seekers of unusual ingredients and high-quality foods. Even supplement stores and small health-food stores often stock local produce. Cultural markets are a great place to find unusual fruits and vegetables, although the produce is typically imported unless there's a large ethnic community to cater to, in which case the produce may be locally grown.

Online: Frozen high-quality meat and seafood, farm-fresh produce, and the full range of pantry ingredients used in this and other Paleo cookbooks are all available online. In fact, these foods are often cheaper online than in stores (though not always, so make sure to compare prices!). And there's something about the convenience of having foods delivered to your door that can't be beat. Some of my favorite online vendors are:

Amazon.com

Barefoot Provisions

ButcherBox

Farmbox Direct

Grass-Fed Traditions

One Stop Paleo Shop

Thrive Market

US Wellness Meats

Check out the Appendixes for even more online shopping options!

Regular ol' grocery stores: Never fear if the kinds of food vendors listed above are beyond your reach either geographically or budgetwise. More and more grocery stores are stocking grass-fed and pasture-raised meat, wild-caught fish and shellfish, and organic produce. Most of the pantry ingredients used in this cookbook can be found in most grocery stores. And if your grocery store has an organic foods aisle, a gluten-free aisle, and/or a vegan/vegetarian aisle (these are often combined into one space) and/or a cultural/international foods aisle, these can be great places to find some of the more unusual pantry ingredients. When in doubt, ask a store employee. Not all grocery stores are willing to special-order foods, but if a store perceives a market for an ingredient that it doesn't usually carry, it may hop on the bandwagon.

But don't worry if your local grocery store doesn't carry anything more than the industrially produced basics or if higher-quality options are simply beyond your budget. You can still see substantial improvements in your health (see page 387)! Simply choose fresh or frozen plain meats, seafood, vegetables, and fruits—that's really all there is to it. For additional strategies for revamping your diet without expanding your budget, see page 390.

SHOPPING ON A BUDGET

Following a specific diet on a budget requires the same tools as doing anything else on a budget, namely knowing your prices, comparison shopping, taking advantage of sales and coupons, buying in bulk, and knowing how to get the best bang for your buck.

Knowing your prices doesn't require a photographic memory for numbers or an uncanny ability to convert the per-banana price at one store to the per-pound price at another store (although that skill would come in handy!). You can use a simple notebook to list your most commonly purchased items at each store you frequent, or you can use an app like Out of Milk to keep track for you. While you're getting used to eating this way, shop around, not only at different grocery stores and specialty markets (you'd be surprised how often the specialty markets with a reputation of being more expensive are actually cheaper for the specialty items you'll be looking for) but also online (factor in the cost of shipping, of course!). Before long, you'll have your regular stops for different types of foods: perhaps your local warehouse club for seafood, a local farmstand for certain produce and grass-fed meat, a regular grocery store for the rest of your produce and meat, and online sources for cooking fats and flavoring ingredients.

Almost everything goes on sale. Even online retailers have sales and coupons. Subscribing to a retailer's newsletter is typically the best way to find out about discounts. Having ample freezer space is useful when it comes to taking advantage of sales, but even if your freezer space is limited, you can benefit.

Buying in bulk is a great way to save money. The price per pound often decreases as you buy more. Many local farmers will give you a deal when you buy a quarter, half, or whole cow or pig. For example, you might pay $7 per pound for grass-fed ground beef, but if you buy a quarter or half a cow, you'll get a variety of cuts, from ground beef to prime rib, for $4 or $5 per pound (or less!). If you don't have the freezer space for half a cow, find some friends or family members to share a quarter cow with you.

It's helpful to know what you can get for heavily discounted prices. For example, organ meat can be

NAVIGATING YOUR GROCERY STORE

One of the biggest changes you might see in your shopping is how you navigate your grocery store. You'll likely never go down many of the interior aisles that used to be your go-to aisles.

Grocery stores are all laid out slightly differently, but here's the general path you'll likely take through your store and what you'll find where.

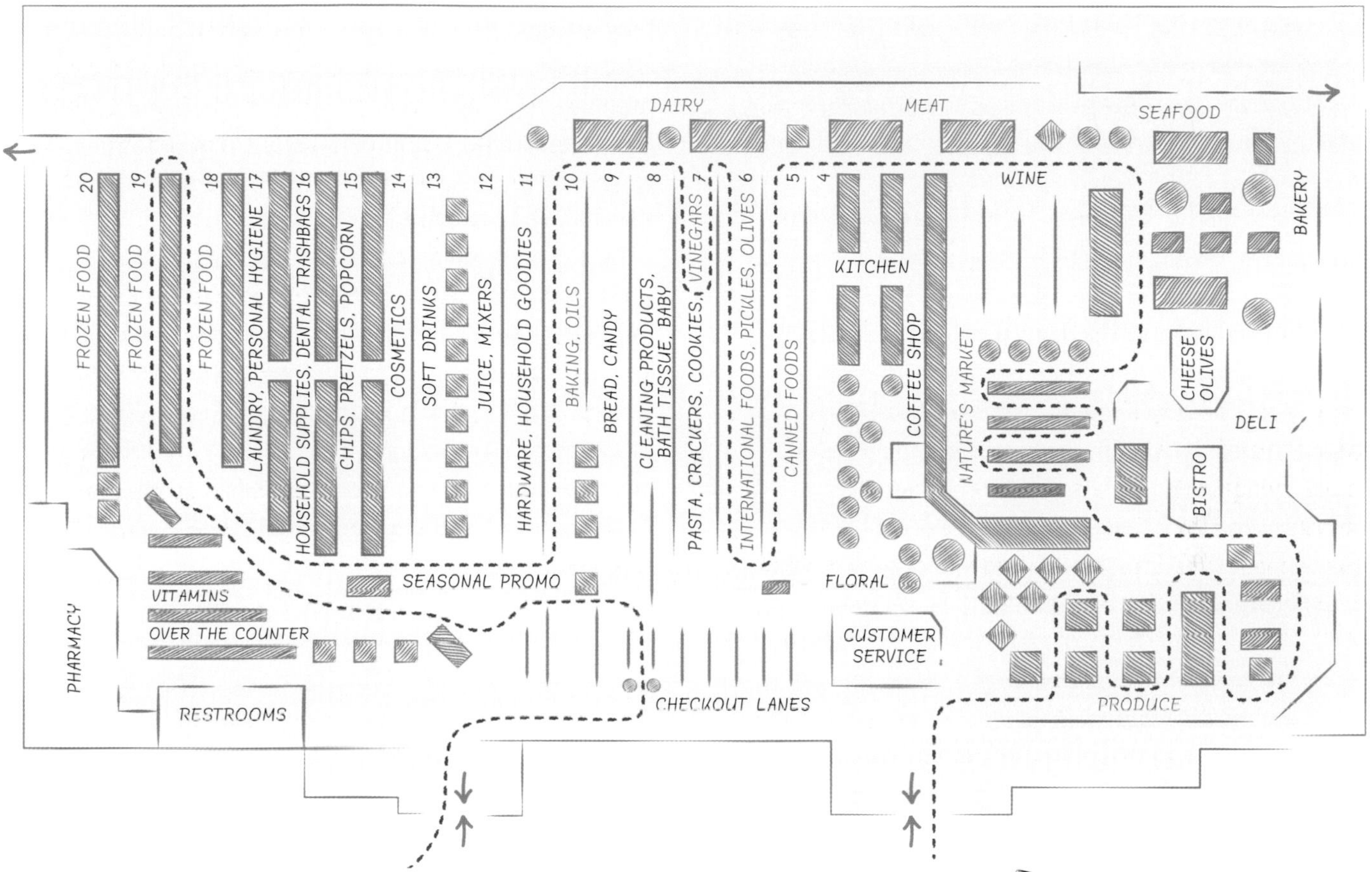

DAIRY
MEAT
SEAFOOD
WINE
BAKERY
20 FROZEN FOOD
19 FROZEN FOOD
18 FROZEN FOOD
17 LAUNDRY, PERSONAL HYGIENE
16 HOUSEHOLD SUPPLIES, DENTAL, TRASHBAGS
15 CHIPS, PRETZELS, POPCORN
14 COSMETICS
13 SOFT DRINKS
12 JUICE, MIXERS
11 HARDWARE, HOUSEHOLD GOODIES
10 BAKING, OILS
9 BREAD, CANDY
8 CLEANING PRODUCTS, BATH TISSUE, BABY
7 PASTA, CRACKERS, COOKIES, VINEGARS
6 INTERNATIONAL FOODS, PICKLES, OLIVES
5 CANNED FOODS
4
KITCHEN
COFFEE SHOP
NATURE'S MARKET
CHEESE OLIVES
DELI
BISTRO
PHARMACY
VITAMINS
OVER THE COUNTER
SEASONAL PROMO
FLORAL
CUSTOMER SERVICE
RESTROOMS
CHECKOUT LANES
PRODUCE

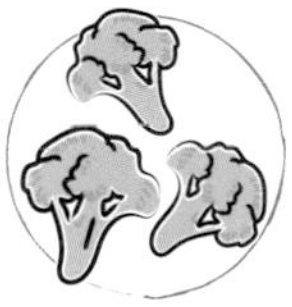

PRODUCE SECTION

Fresh vegetables

Fresh fruits

Fresh herbs

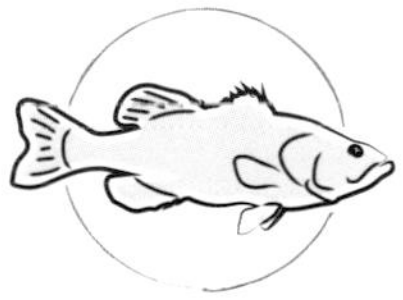

SEAFOOD COUNTER

Fresh fish

Fresh shellfish

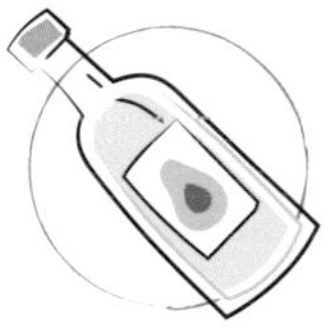

BAKING AISLE

Avocado oil

Coconut oil

Dried fruits

Dried herbs

Nuts and seeds

Olive oil

Sea salt

Spices

Vinegar (apple cider, white wine, red wine)

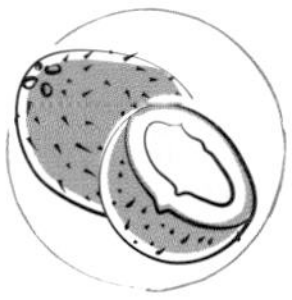

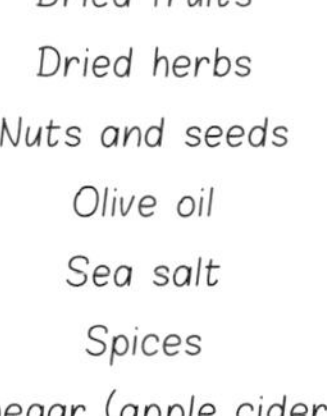

INTERNATIONAL FOODS AISLE

Coconut aminos

Coconut milk

Dried seaweed

Fish sauce

Nori wraps

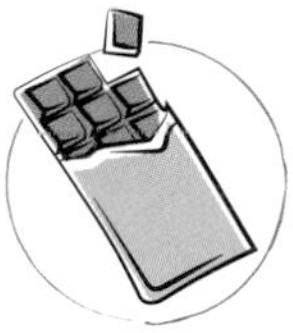

NATURE'S MARKET (ORGANIC/ GLUTEN-FREE AISLE)

Almond meal/flour

Arrowroot powder

Coconut flour

Dark chocolate

Palm shortening

Plantain chips

Sweet potato chips

Tapioca starch

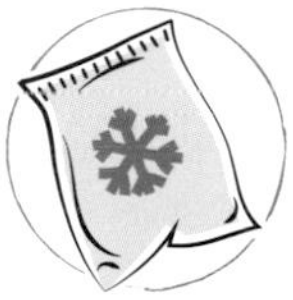

FROZEN FOODS AISLES

Frozen 100% beef burger patties

Frozen chicken breast

Frozen ground beef

Frozen seafood

Frozen vegetables

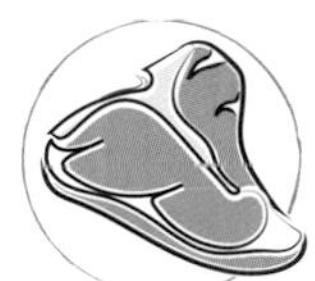

MEAT SECTION

Fresh meats

Bacon

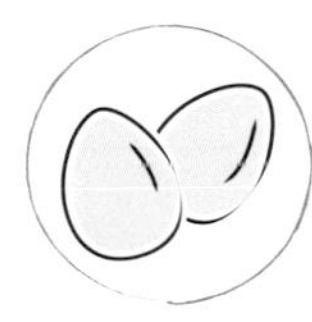

DAIRY AISLE

Eggs

Grass-fed butter

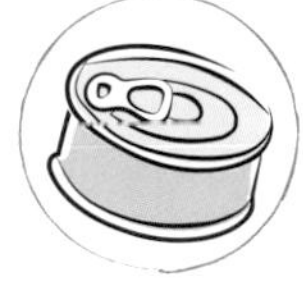

CANNED FOODS AISLE

Canned fish

Canned pumpkin

Coconut milk

Olives

some of the cheapest meat available simply because there isn't a huge market for it. Sometimes local farmers will give it to you for free (or at a steep discount) because they can't find anyone to buy it. It also helps to know what is typically thrown away. If you ask, a butcher will set aside grass-fed beef trimmings for you so that you can render your own tallow (and typically will give it to you for free or at a significant discount). Fish heads might normally be thrown away, but the fishmonger may give them to you for free if you ask; you can use them to make soup or cook them in other ways.

It's also helpful to know which meats tend to be cheaper per pound and which vegetables and fruits will stretch a meal further. Depending on where you live, chicken might be cheaper than pork, which is cheaper than beef. And when buying high-quality meat, it's helpful to know that grass-fed beef is typically cheaper than pasture-raised pork, which is cheaper than pasture-raised chicken. Tougher cuts of meat, like chuck roast, stew meat, pork shoulder, shanks, and short ribs, are usually less expensive (and very flavorful). Certain vegetables give you great bang for your buck, too. Cabbage, for example, is typically extremely inexpensive as compared to baby greens. In fact, cruciferous vegetables in general, except perhaps for the most common cauliflower and broccoli, tend to be very reasonably priced. Using root vegetables and plantains is a fantastic way to stretch a meal. Bananas tend to be much cheaper than apples, which tend to be cheaper than grapes or berries. And when you can buy vegetables in bulk, you'll save even more. Freezing (see page 456) or canning your own vegetables and fruit is a useful strategy to capitalize on a great deal.

Food that requires you to put in more time also tends to be cheaper. For example, a whole chicken is typically cheaper per pound than a chicken cut into parts. A beef roast is cheaper per pound than steaks, and a pork roast is cheaper per pound than chops. Vegetables that require peeling and chopping tend to be cheaper than those that can be thrown straight into a pot or onto a plate, which are cheaper than prepared or prewashed vegetables in plastic containers or microwave-safe bags.

Canned and frozen foods are often cheaper than fresh. While you probably won't want to buy canned vegetables because of the additives they usually contain, canned fish and shellfish are fantastic inexpensive options for increasing your seafood intake. (Look for BPA-free cans!) Canned seafood is typically cheaper than frozen, which is typically cheaper than fresh. However, when fish and shellfish are in season, the fresh and frozen offerings tend to go on sale, so knowing when your favorite types are in peak season can be a great way to save money. Frozen vegetables are a fantastic way to increase nutrient density since they are typically picked at their peak and frozen soon after. In fact, frozen vegetables tend to have more nutrients than fresh vegetables from the grocery store because the ones in the produce section tend to be picked before they are ripe and lose nutrients during shipping and storage.

When foods do go on sale or are offered in bulk, you can save money by freezing your own. You can freeze the raw food right in the package in which you bought it, prepare the food before freezing so that it saves you time when you're ready to use it (like chopping or blanching veggies), or cook and freeze meals for convenience on busy weeknights. For tips on freezing fresh meat, seafood, vegetables, and fruit, see Chapter 37. You can also ferment fruits and vegetables as an alternative to freezing them. For example, when cabbage is in season, you can make a large batch of sauerkraut (see page 491) to take advantage of both peak-season produce and the typically cheaper peak-season prices. Buying what's on sale is also a great way to buy in-season produce, since spikes in supply are a major reason for drops in price.

It's really helpful to know the people who grow your food. If you arrive at the farmers market or your local farmstand at closing time, you will often be rewarded with good deals on whatever didn't sell. Bruisies (or seconds), the produce that has some flaws like bruises or bird beak holes, can often be purchased heavily discounted; the trade-off is that they tend not to keep for long, so plan on eating or freezing them as soon as you get home. Joining a farm share or CSA is typically a great way to save on farm-fresh produce. Doing some of the work for your vegetables and fruits is another way to save money. In addition to pick-your-own farms, some farmers will trade your labor on the farm (weeding, harvesting, and so on) for produce if you ask. Do you have something else to trade? Don't be afraid to barter! Your local farmers are also a helpful resource for knowledge on what you can most easily grow in your backyard in your climate.

Also, check the food quality guide on page 221 to help you prioritize which foods are worth the extra bucks.

MONEY-SAVING STRATEGIES

SAVINGS STRATEGIES:

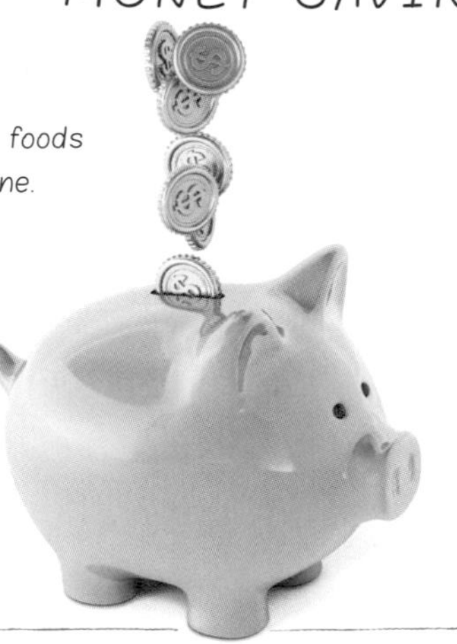

- Know the average prices for foods and shop around, including online.
- Clip coupons.
- Shop sales.
- Buy in bulk.
- Haggle or barter.
- Grow your own.

"LONGCUTS" TO SAVE MONEY (NOT SHORTCUTS, BUT WORTH THE EFFORT):

- Buy bigger cuts of meat, which are typically cheaper per pound, and butcher them yourself or roast whole and freeze leftovers.
- Buy tough cuts of meat that take longer to cook.
- Buy veggies in bulk rather than washed and chopped in packages.
- Buy meat, seafood, veggies, and fruits when heavily discounted and freeze them yourself.

SURPRISING WAYS HEALTHY FOOD AND LIFESTYLE CHOICES WILL SAVE YOU MONEY:

- You'll no longer eat at fast food joints or restaurants or grab prepared foods.
- You'll cut out completely or cut down on expensive beverages like soda, fancy coffee drinks, beer, wine, and spirits.
- Walking or cycling more will save you money on gas.
- You may reduce the need for medications, supplements, and doctor visits.

CHEAP VEGGIES THAT STRETCH A MEAL:

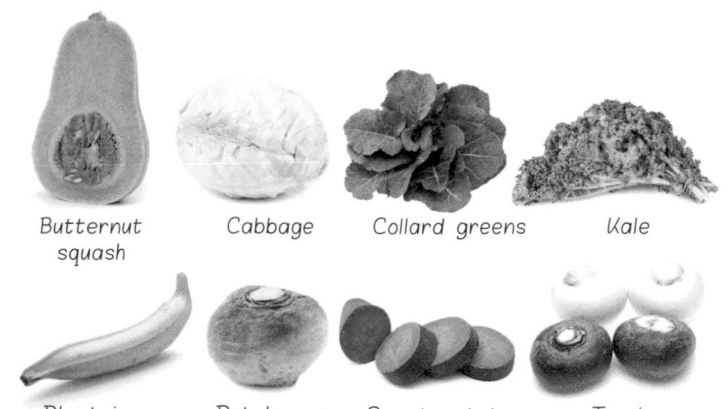

Butternut squash · Cabbage · Collard greens · Kale

Plantains · Rutabagas · Sweet potatoes · Turnips

THE CHEAPEST OPTIONS:

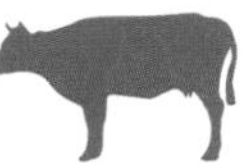
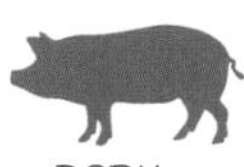
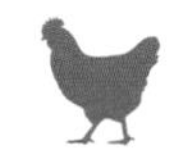

BEEF:	PORK:	CHICKEN:	SEAFOOD:
chuck roast	Boston butt	whole chicken	canned seafood
ground beef	picnic	chicken thighs	frozen seafood
sirloin	shoulder	ground chicken	cod
tri-tip	ground pork	liver	farmed salmon
liver	belly	heart	tilapia
heart	loin		
kidney			
bones			

VEGETABLES:

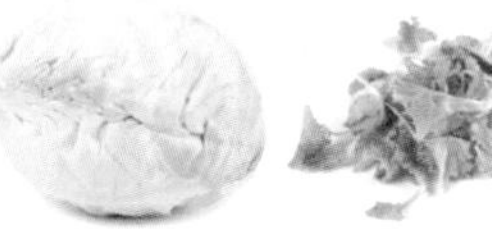

Cabbage

Lettuce

Carrots

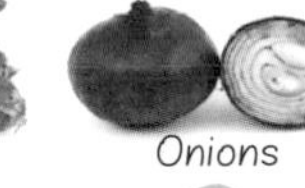

Onions

Celery

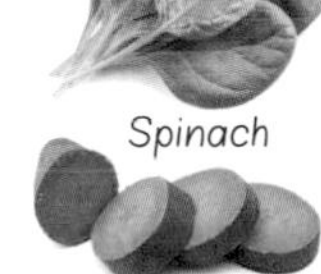

Spinach

Sweet potatoes

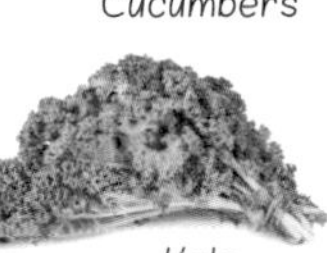

Cucumbers

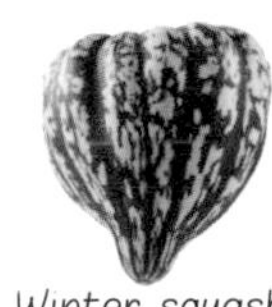

Kale

Winter squash

FRUITS:

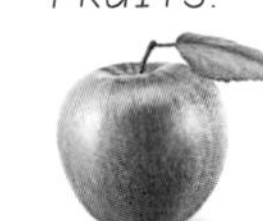

Apples

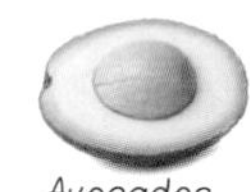

Avocados

Bananas

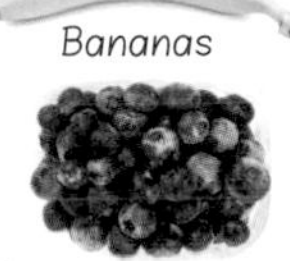

Frozen berries

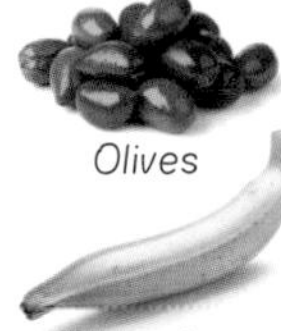

Olives

Plantains

Frozen is usually much cheaper than fresh!

FROZEN FOODS:

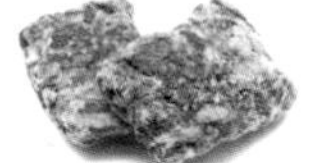

Veggies

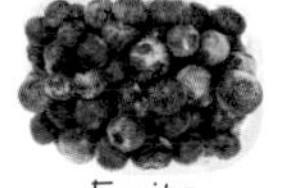

Fruits

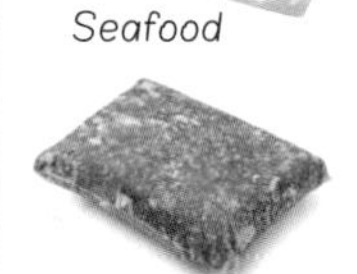

Seafood

Meats

FOODS THAT GIVE YOU A GOOD BANG FOR YOUR BUCK (AND YOUR HEALTH):

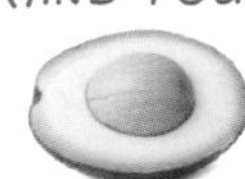

Avocados

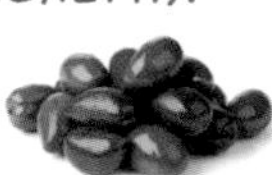
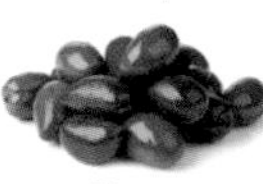

Olives

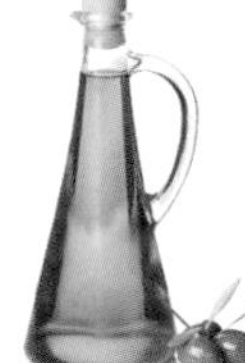

High-quality olive oil or coconut oil

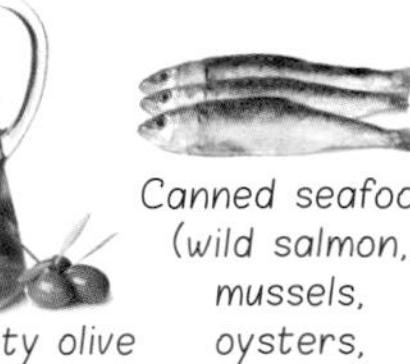

Canned seafood (wild salmon, mussels, oysters, sardines)

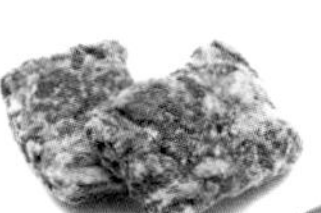

Chicken livers (and any other organ meat)

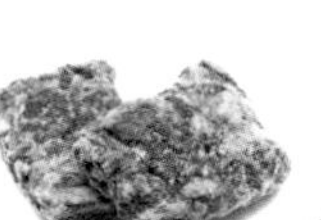

Frozen organic berries

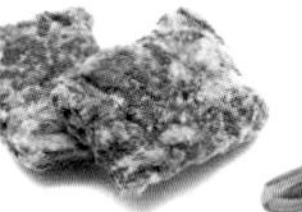

Frozen organic spinach

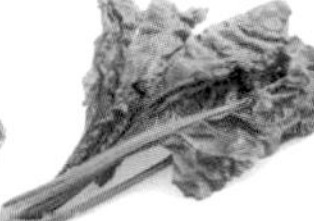

Leafy greens (kale, Swiss chard, spinach, dandelion greens)

Cruciferous veggies (arugula, Brussels sprouts, cabbage, kale)

Sweet potatoes

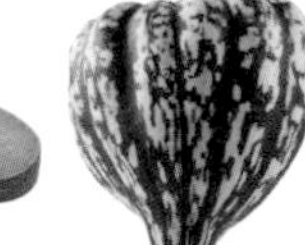

Winter squash

Sea salt

Chapter 36:
STOCKING YOUR KITCHEN

It really is true that a well-stocked kitchen is your best tool for creating flavorful and healthful meals in the shortest time and with the least stress. You have so many options for quick meals if you have broth in your freezer, a selection of healthy cooking fats in your pantry, an abundance of fresh vegetables in the crisper drawer of your fridge, and fresh herbs growing in pots on your kitchen windowsill.

The essential Paleo foods may be fairly different from what you're used to, although the general categories are the same: common base ingredients (mainly vegetables, meats, and seafood), cooking fats, oils for dressing foods, herbs and spices, and other flavoring ingredients. Having at least some of these foods on hand before you adopt the Paleo diet will definitely make the transition easier. Of course, there's a lot of room to expand on the basics so that you have a wide variety of ingredients handy for your cooking adventures.

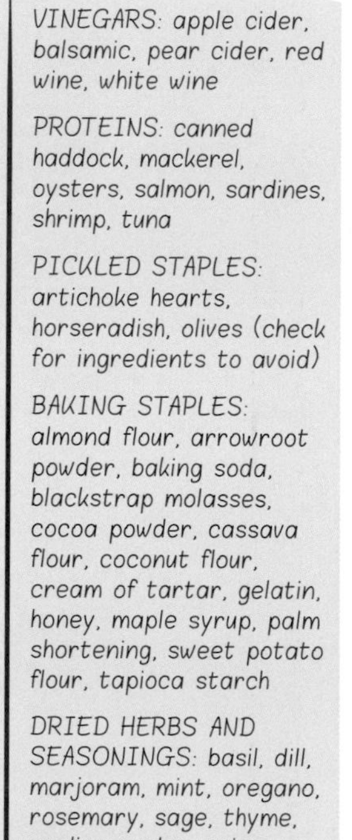

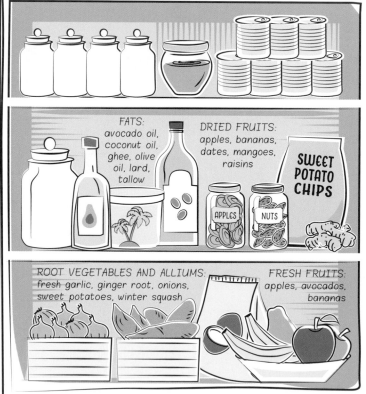

FLAVORINGS: anchovies, coconut aminos, fish sauce (check for ingredients to avoid), wasabi (check for ingredients to avoid)

CONDIMENTS: avocado oil mayonnaise, horseradish, ketchup (check for ingredients to avoid), mustard, salad dressing made with olive oil or avocado oil

EXTRAS: coconut wraps, nori wraps, apple chips, banana chips, cassava chips, plantain chips, sweet potato chips, coconut flakes, coconut milk or cream

NUTS AND SEEDS: almonds, Brazil nuts, cashews, coconut flakes, pine nuts, pumpkin seeds, sunflower seeds

Now that you have the right information about how to eat healthy, the next big hurdle is actually doing it! This means throwing out (or donating to a food bank or composting) all the food in your home that you don't plan to eat anymore and then restocking your freezer, fridge, and pantry with nutrient-dense choices.

When it comes to restocking your pantry, you don't need to go out and buy everything listed here in one enormous (and expensive!) shopping trip. Instead, add a few items to your pantry each week, prioritizing those ingredients that you'll need for the meals you plan to make that week. Stocking a few emergency proteins and grab-and-go snacks also makes life easier!

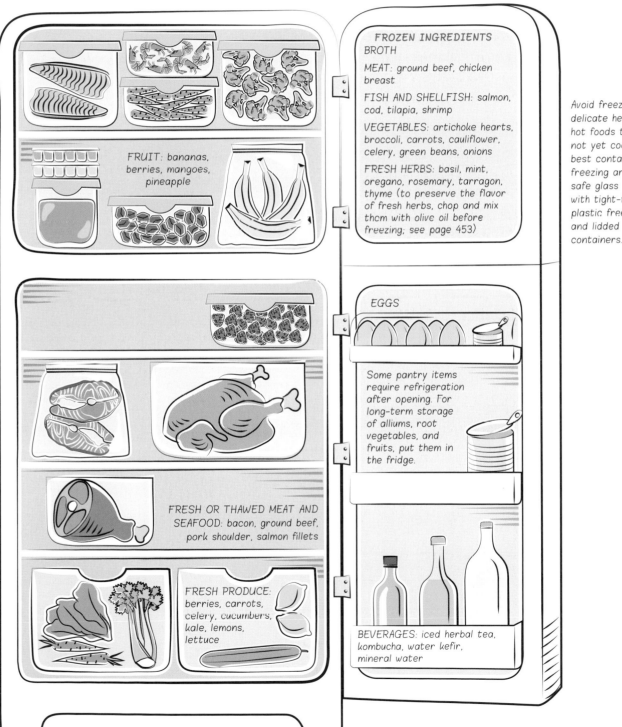

Avoid freezing salads, delicate herbs, and hot foods that have not yet cooled. The best containers for freezing are freezer-safe glass containers with tight-fitting lids, plastic freezer bags, and lidded plastic containers.

FOOD STORAGE

As a general rule, any product that you purchase from a refrigerated display case or that is shipped with ice packs should be stored in the fridge at home. For products that you buy off store shelves or that are shipped in regular packaging, check the labels. If a product needs to go directly into the fridge, the label will say so. Other products may be fine in your cupboard until you open them, after which time refrigeration is required. If a label does not list storage instructions, the product is typically fine at room temperature. If you're buying products from local manufacturers, ask how to store them when you purchase them.

Fats and oils deteriorate with exposure to light, heat, and air. To increase the longevity of your cooking fats, store them in tightly closed containers in the refrigerator or freezer. Rendered tallow and poultry fat will keep for about 6 weeks in the refrigerator and for a year in the freezer. Lard has a longer shelf life; it will keep for a year in the refrigerator or for 2 years in the freezer. Solid plant oils like coconut oil and palm shortening should be stored in a cool, dry place. An opened jar or can will keep for about a year, and an unopened jar or can will keep for up to 2 years. Olive oil and avocado oil should be stored at room temperature in a dark cupboard. They will retain their flavor and quality for up to a year after being opened.

When you buy an item for your freezer or pantry that does not have a date on it (manufactured on, best by, expiration, etc.), it's a good idea to label it with the date you purchased it. When in doubt, use the item within 3 months and examine it closely for signs of spoilage before consuming it.

Storing Meat and Seafood

When it comes to meat and seafood, you'll probably find that you buy it frozen more often than fresh because farmers and online grass-fed meat producers typically sell their meat frozen. Store frozen meat in the original packaging for up to 6 months for best quality (but pretty much indefinitely in terms of safety).

When buying fresh meat, keep it in the original packaging and store it in the coolest part of your refrigerator (typically at the back on the bottom shelf). Most fresh meat will keep for 2 to 3 days in the fridge before being cooked; ground meat and meat cut into small pieces, like stewing beef, will keep for 2 days, while larger cuts like steaks, chops, and roasts will typically keep for 3 days. I like to store meat on a rimmed baking sheet or plate to prevent the juices from leaking onto other foods. When buying fresh seafood, keep it in its original packaging if possible and store it in a bowl of ice in the refrigerator. However, live shellfish (like clams) should not be put on ice; instead, open or poke holes in the packaging and store on a rimmed baking sheet or plate in the fridge.

If you want to freeze meat or seafood that you bought fresh, place the entire package in a resealable freezer bag. Better yet, use a home vacuum sealer if you have one. If you plan to store meat or seafood that didn't come in a vacuum-sealed package in the freezer for several months, unpack it and wrap the pieces individually in plastic wrap before placing them in a resealable freezer bag to help prevent freezer burn. (If your meat is vacuum-sealed, there's no need to do so.) Make sure to label the bag with what's in it and the date you froze it!

The bigger challenge with freezing meat and seafood is thawing it safely. There are three safe ways to thaw frozen food:

- **In the refrigerator:** The best and safest way to thaw frozen food is in the refrigerator. A small package of meat typically defrosts overnight, but most foods require a day or two, so plan ahead. Large roasts and whole turkeys will take even longer—approximately 1 day for every 5 pounds of weight.

- **In cold water:** For faster thawing, place the package of frozen food in a leak-proof plastic bag and immerse it in cold water. Check the water frequently to be sure that it stays cold, and change the water every 30 minutes. Small packages of food can thaw in as little as 1 hour with this method, and larger items will thaw in 4 to 6 hours. (Thawing a turkey or very large roast may take 24 hours using this method, which usually means that the several-days-in-the-fridge plan is the more practical way to go.) Once it's thawed, cook the meat or seafood immediately.

· **In the microwave:** Thawing meat or seafood in the microwave is perfectly safe, although it's difficult to achieve even thawing without starting to cook the edges, which sometimes leads to overcooking those edges when you prepare your meat or seafood. Follow your microwave's directions for thawing meat (because the optimal time and power setting will depend on your microwave). If you thaw meat or seafood in the microwave, cook it immediately.

· **Cooking without thawing:** Cooking frozen meat or seafood is perfectly safe to do; however, the cooking time will increase by approximately 50 percent. Always check the internal temperature with a meat thermometer to make sure that your meat or seafood is thoroughly cooked.

FRESH VERSUS DRIED HERBS

Without exception, the flavor of fresh herbs is better than dried, but you can't beat the convenience of having an assortment of dried herbs in your pantry. Some herbs—like oregano, rosemary, sage, and thyme—retain their flavor well when dried. Others, including basil, cilantro, mint, and parsley, taste better fresh.

You can freeze fresh herbs when they're in season so you preserve the flavor and enjoy the convenience of having them on hand without having to buy them every week. To freeze fresh herbs:

- For every 2 cups of packed fresh herb leaves, add ⅓ cup of olive oil, avocado oil, or melted and cooled coconut oil.
- Pulse the herbs and oil in a food processor, scraping down the sides of the bowl from time to time, until you have a chunky paste and all the leaves are chopped.
- Spoon by the tablespoon into ice cube trays.
- Cover the ice cube tray with plastic wrap or aluminum foil and store in the freezer. These frozen herb cubes can be added directly to a pot or quickly thawed to season meat before cooking; each cube is equivalent to 1 tablespoon of chopped fresh herbs.
- Freeze fresh herbs individually (an ice cube tray full of cilantro, another one of mint, and so on) or freeze your favorite combinations (rosemary and thyme, basil and oregano, and so on).

Storing Vegetables and Fruits

Farm-fresh organic vegetables and fruits often don't keep as well as their grocery store counterparts, so knowing the optimal way to store different types of produce is even more important!

Do not store fruits and vegetables together. Fruits that give off high levels of ethylene (a ripening agent), like apples, can prematurely ripen and spoil the surrounding vegetables. (You can take advantage of this property to speed up the ripening of other fruits, like avocados, bananas, and peaches.)

As a general rule for vegetables, remove any ties or rubber bands and store the veggies in the refrigerator in plastic bags punctured with holes to allow for good airflow or in open containers covered with a damp towel. Root vegetables, winter squash, and alliums can be stored in a cool, dry, dark place that has good airflow, meaning you'll want to store them in a basket in the pantry and not in a plastic bag. Some veggies, like leafy greens, can be soaked in a sink full of cool water before being stored, while others, like mushrooms and herbs, should not be washed until just prior to use. See the list below for storage information for specific vegetables.

Most fruits will continue to ripen if left sitting out on the countertop. Once perfectly ripe, these fruits can typically be refrigerated for at least a few days; even bananas can be refrigerated once ripened to your liking, although the peels will darken in the fridge. The exceptions are berries, citrus fruits, and grapes, which will only deteriorate on the counter and should be refrigerated. The list below provides storage information for specific fruits. All fruits and vegetables stored at room temperature should be stored out of direct sunlight.

If you find yourself with a surplus of produce, nearly all fruits and vegetables can be stored in the freezer. Fruits will keep in the freezer for about a year; vegetables will keep for about 18 months. They are best used in recipes in which they are cooked or in smoothies because they will have a mushier texture when thawed compared to fresh. Vegetables and fruits can be used directly from frozen in your favorite recipes. Partially thawed frozen berries make a wonderful topping for Coconut Milk Yogurt (page 481) or Vanilla Ice Cream (page 585).

STORING COMMON VEGETABLES

ARTICHOKES: Store in the fridge in an airtight container with a piece of damp paper towel inside.

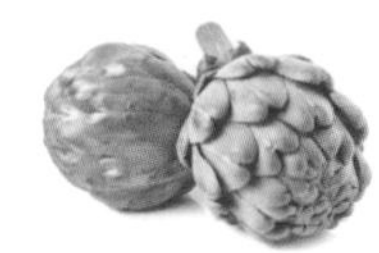

ASPARAGUS: Store upright in a glass or bowl filled with water at room temperature for up to a week, or store in the fridge.

BASIL: Store on the counter loosely packed in a jar with a damp piece of paper towel inside.

BEETS: Wash and store in an open container with a wet towel on top. Cut off any tops and store them separately.

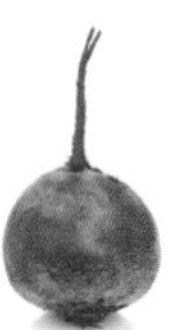

BROCCOLI: Wrap in a damp towel and place in an open container in the fridge. Use as soon as possible.

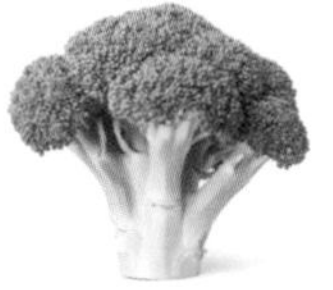

BRUSSELS SPROUTS: If on the stalk, store the entire stalk in the fridge. If loose, store in an open container with a damp towel on top.

CABBAGE: Store on the counter for up to a week, or in the crisper drawer of the fridge. Peel off the outer leaves if they start to wilt.

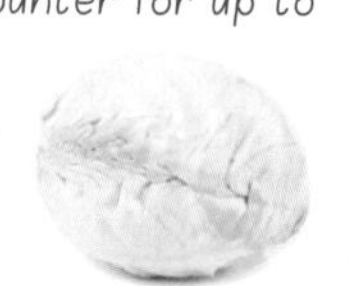

CARROTS: Wrap in a damp towel and store in a closed container in the fridge. Cut off the tops and store them separately.

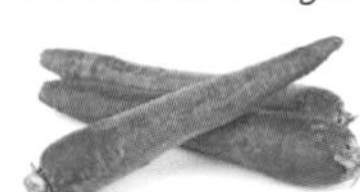

CAULIFLOWER: Store in a closed container in the fridge. Use as soon as possible.

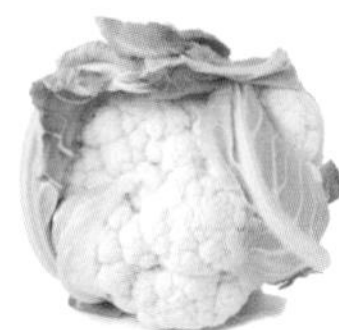

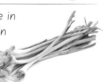

CELERY: Store in a cup or bowl of shallow water on the counter for up to a week. For longer-term storage, wrap in aluminum foil and place in the fridge.

CELERY ROOT: Wrap in a damp towel and place in the crisper drawer of the fridge.

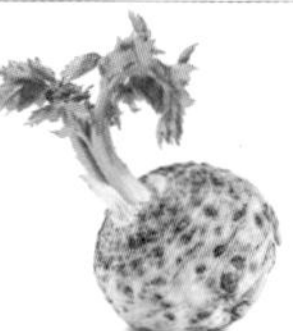

FENNEL: Store in a cup or bowl of shallow water on the counter for up to several days. For longer-term storage, place in the fridge in a closed container with a little water.

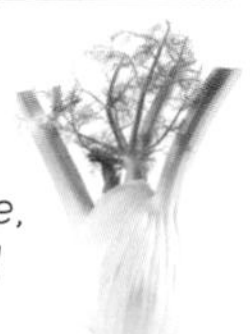

GARLIC: Store in a cool, dark, dry place.

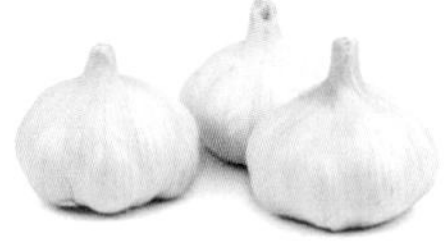

GINGER: Store unpeeled in a plastic bag in the crisper drawer of the fridge. Ginger roots can also be frozen and Microplaned directly from frozen.

GREEN GARLIC: Store in an airtight container in the fridge.

HERBS: Store in a glass or vase full of water in the fridge.

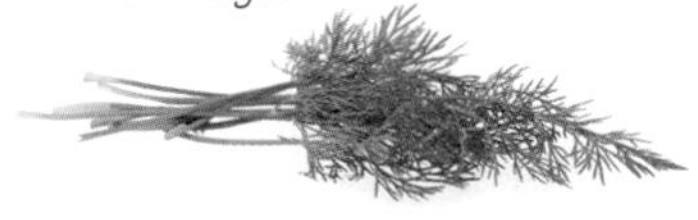

LEAFY GREENS: Remove any bands or twist ties and store in an airtight container with a damp cloth.

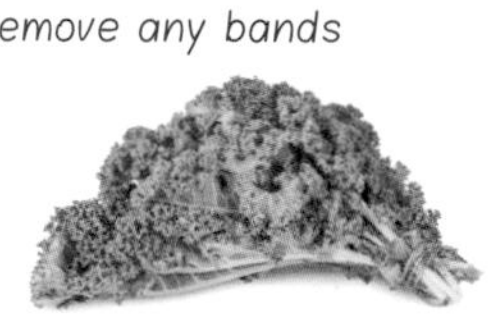

LEEKS: Store in a shallow cup of water on the counter (so that only the very bottoms of the stems are in water) or wrapped in a damp towel in the crisper drawer of the fridge.

MUSHROOMS: Keep in the fridge in their original packaging or in a paper bag.

OKRA: Store with a dry towel in an airtight container in the fridge. Use as soon as possible.

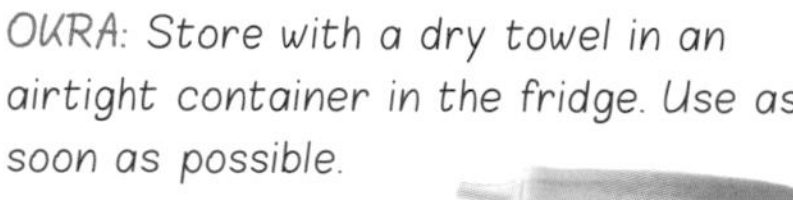

ONIONS: Store in a cool, dark, dry place.

PARSNIPS: Wrap in a damp cloth and store in an open container in the crisper drawer of the fridge.

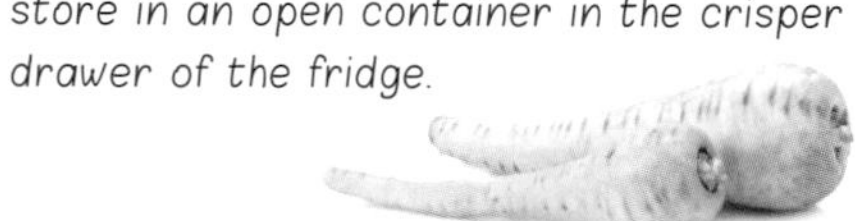

POTATOES: Store in a cool, dark, well-ventilated place.

RADISHES: Store in an open container in the fridge with a wet towel placed on top. Remove the greens and store them separately.

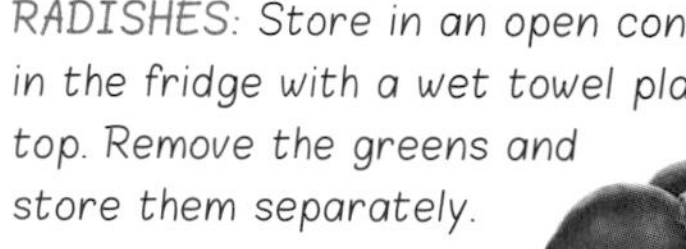

RHUBARB: Wrap in a damp towel and place in an open container in the fridge.

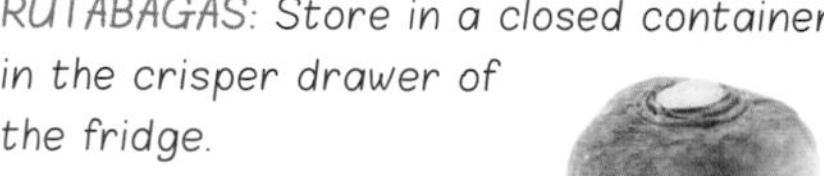

RUTABAGAS: Store in a closed container in the crisper drawer of the fridge.

SPINACH: Store loose in an open container in the crisper drawer, and refrigerate as soon as possible. Spinach loves to stay cold.

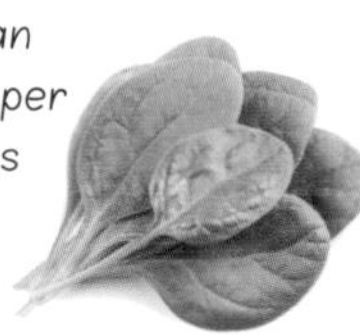

SPRING ONIONS: Remove any bands or twist ties and store in the crisper drawer of the fridge.

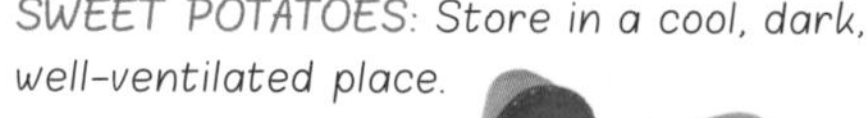

SWEET POTATOES: Store in a cool, dark, well-ventilated place.

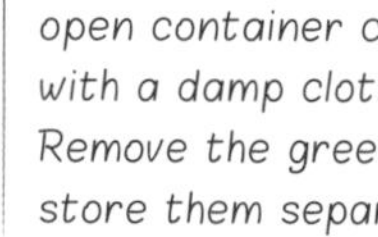

TURNIPS: Store in an open container covered with a damp cloth. Remove the greens and store them separately.

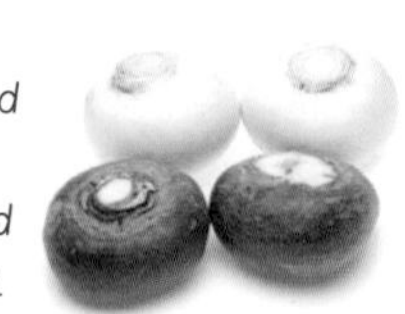

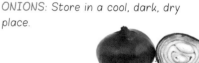

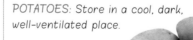

STORING COMMON FRUITS

APPLES: Store in a bowl or basket with good airflow at room temperature. For longer storage, keep in a cardboard box in the fridge.

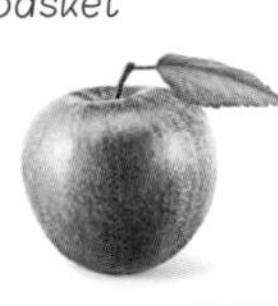

APRICOTS: Store in a bowl or basket with good airflow at room temperature. Store in the fridge when fully ripe.

AVOCADOS: Store in a bowl or paper bag at room temperature. To speed up ripening, place in a paper bag with an apple.

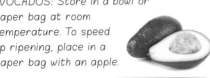

BANANAS: Store in a basket with good airflow or hang on a banana holder at room temperature. To slow down ripening, pull them apart and store them spaced apart.

BERRIES: Store in the refrigerator and wash right before you eat them.

CHERRIES: Store in an airtight container in the fridge and wash right before you eat them.

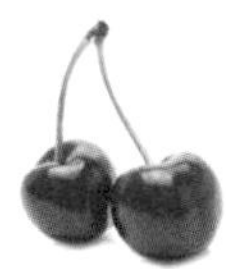

CUCUMBERS: Store wrapped in a moist towel in the fridge.

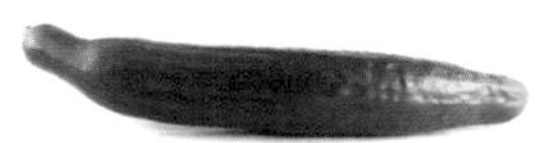

DATES: Drier dates (like Deglet Noor) can be stored in the original packaging in the cupboard. Moist dates (like Medjool) should be refrigerated in a container that allows for airflow.

EGGPLANT: Store in a container with a moist towel in the fridge.

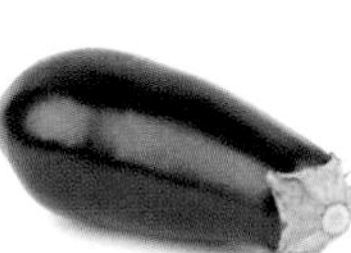

FIGS: Store in a paper bag or a container that allows airflow in the fridge.

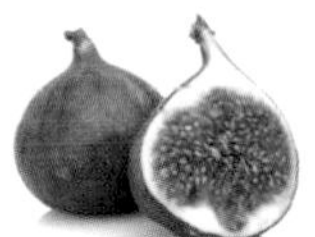

GRAPES: Store in a bag or a container that allows airflow in the crisper drawer of the fridge and wash right before you eat them.

KIWIS: Keep at room temperature until ripe, then refrigerate.

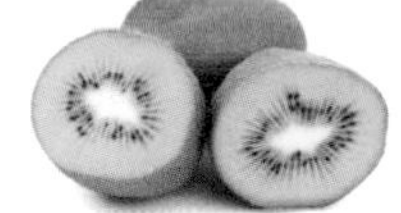

LEMONS AND LIMES: Store in a bowl that allows airflow on the counter. For longer storage, keep in the refrigerator (but note that they can absorb odors from foods stored beside them).

MANGOES: Store on the counter until ripe, then move to the refrigerator.

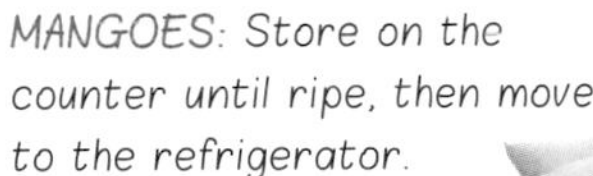

MELONS: Store uncut in a cool, dry place, out of the sun, for up to a couple of weeks. Softer melons like cantaloupe should be moved to the fridge when ripe. Keep cut melon in the fridge with the cut side covered with plastic wrap or cut side down on a plate.

NECTARINES: Store in a bowl that allows airflow on the counter and refrigerate only when fully ripe. To hasten ripening, place in a paper bag with an apple.

ORANGES AND OTHER CITRUS: Store at room temperature in a bowl or basket that allows airflow. For longer-term storage, move to the refrigerator.

PEACHES: Store in a bowl that allows airflow on the counter and refrigerate only when fully ripe. To hasten ripening, place in a paper bag with an apple.

PEARS: Store in a bowl or basket that allows for airflow or in a paper bag. To hasten ripening, store in a paper bag with an apple.

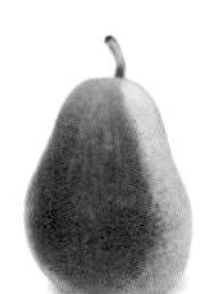

PEPPERS: Store in a container with a moist towel in the fridge.

PERSIMMONS: Store at room temperature until fully ripe, then move to the refrigerator. To hasten ripening, place in a paper bag with an apple.

PLUMS: Store at room temperature until fully ripe, then move to the refrigerator.

POMEGRANATES: Store in a cool, dry place.

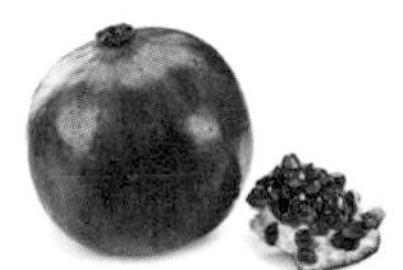

PINEAPPLES: Whole pineapples can be stored on the counter until ripe. Once ripe, store whole or peeled and cut in an airtight container in the fridge.

RASPBERRIES: Wash in a solution of 1 part vinegar to 3 parts water and drain well. Place the berries in a bowl lined with a dry paper towel, replacing the paper towel when it gets damp.

STRAWBERRIES: Store in a paper bag in the fridge and wash right before you eat them.

TOMATOES: Store in a bowl that allows airflow on the counter. Use immediately when ripe or freeze for cooking.

WATERMELON: Keep uncut on the counter at room temperature. Store in the fridge after cutting.

WINTER SQUASH: Store in a cool, dark, well-ventilated place.

ZUCCHINI AND OTHER SUMMER SQUASH: Wrap in a damp cloth and store in the fridge.

TO FREEZE FRUIT:

- Wash and sort for spoiled fruit before freezing. Damaged areas of larger fruit (like a bruise on an apple) can be cut out and the rest of the fruit can be prepared for freezing.
- Slice, peel, and remove pits, stones, seeds, and cores as you would if serving fresh.
- For fruits that tend to brown, like apples, peaches, and nectarines, toss with lemon juice before freezing. (You can dilute 1 tablespoon of lemon juice into up to 1 cup of water.)
- Drain the fruit on a kitchen towel or paper towels to remove as much water as possible before freezing.
- Arrange the fruit in a single layer on a baking sheet.
- Place the baking sheet in the freezer. The colder the freezer, the better, because the faster the fruit freezes, the more of its original texture it will retain once thawed.
- Once frozen, transfer the fruit to a plastic freezer bag or other container. Fill the container to the top or remove as much air as possible from the freezer bag. One cool trick is to place a straw in the opening and close the bag around the straw; suck out as much air as possible and then quickly seal the bag as you remove the straw.

TO FREEZE VEGETABLES:

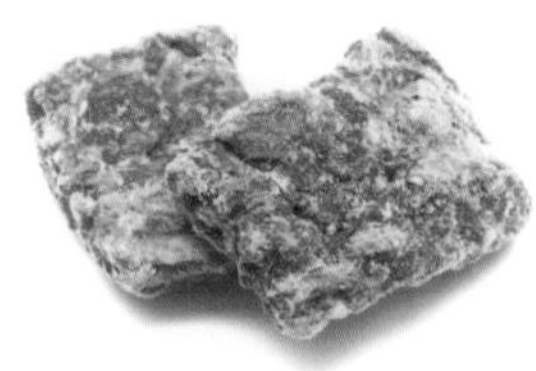

- Peel, trim, and slice vegetables as you would if serving fresh.
- It's best to blanch and shock the vegetables first. (While this step is optional, it improves the texture once thawed and prolongs freezer life.) To do so, prepare a pot of boiling water and a bowl full of heavily iced water. Working in batches, place your vegetables in the boiling water, being careful not to overcrowd the pot. Boil for 1 to 2 minutes (the veggies should remain crisp and be only partially cooked), then transfer to the ice water. Remove from the ice water once the vegetables have cooled completely.
- Drain the veggies on a kitchen towel or paper towels to remove as much water as possible before freezing.
- Arrange the prepared vegetables in a single layer on a baking sheet.
- Place the baking sheet in the freezer. Again, the colder the freezer, the better.
- Once frozen, transfer the veggies to a plastic freezer bag (using the same tip as at left to remove as much air as possible) or other container.

SNACK OPTIONS STRAIGHT FROM THE STORE

It is generally healthier to eat large meals spaced 5 to 6 hours apart and avoid snacking, but this approach isn't necessarily the best choice for everyone. For example, if you have a history of metabolic syndrome or adrenal insufficiency (adrenal fatigue), if you have difficulty managing chronic stress, or if your schedule forces you to go more than 6 hours between meals, you may find yourself in need of a snack.

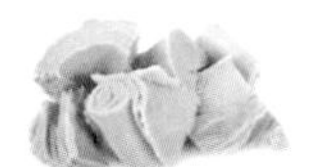
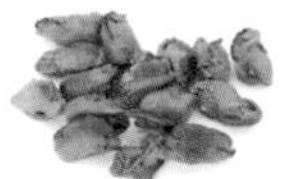
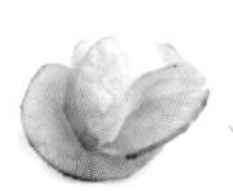
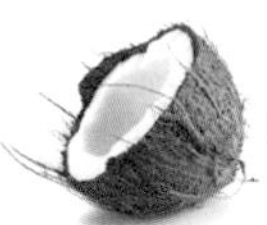
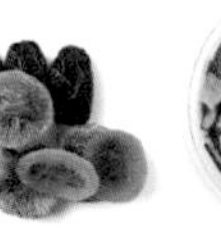
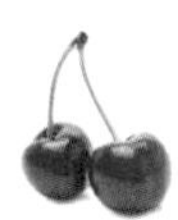
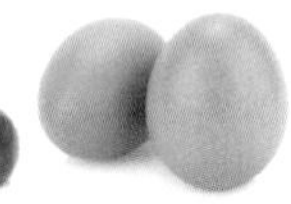
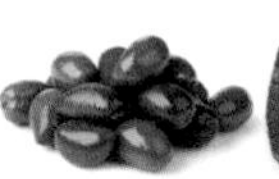
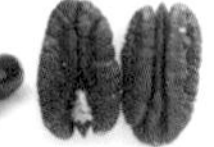

Canned or pouched fish (salmon, tuna, sardines, herring, kippers)

Canned shellfish (shrimp, crab, oysters, clams, mussels)

Cassava chips

Coconut flakes

Dried fruits (dehydrated or freeze-dried; in moderation)

Dried vegetables (dehydrated or freeze-dried)

Fresh fruit

Hard-boiled eggs

Olives

Nuts

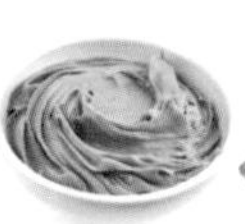
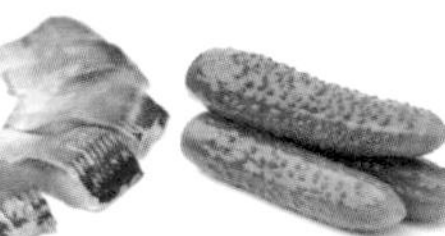
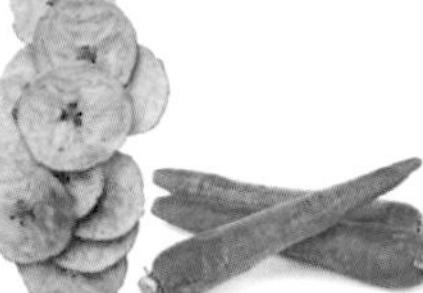
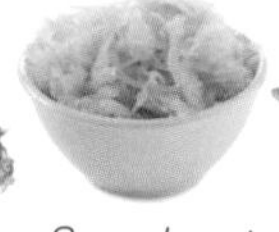
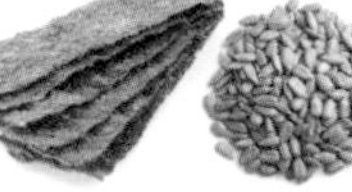
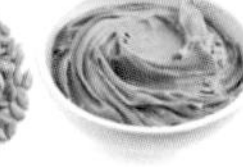
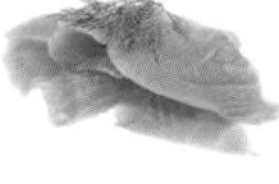
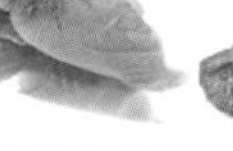
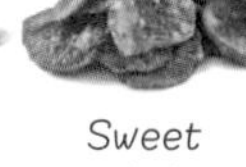

Nut butters

Pickled herring and mackerel

Pickles (preferably raw)

Plantain chips

Raw vegetables

Sauerkraut (preferably raw)

Seaweed snacks

Seeds

Seed butters

Smoked fish (such as salmon, trout, kippers; can be hot-smoked or cold-smoked)

Sweet potato chips

For more prepackaged snack options, see page 638.

SWAPPING OUT STANDARD AMERICAN DIET INGREDIENTS

Trying to figure out how to replace a component of a favorite meal or snack? Here are some simple swaps for old favorites:

NOODLES

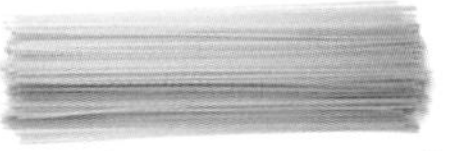

Spaghetti → spaghetti squash, zucchini noodles ("zoodles"), sweet potato noodles (dangmyeon), kelp noodles, wakame noodles, broccoli slaw, Cappello's grain-free noodles

Lasagna noodles → thinly sliced zucchini, yellow squash, butternut squash, eggplant, plantain, or sweet potato; Cappello's grain-free lasagna sheets

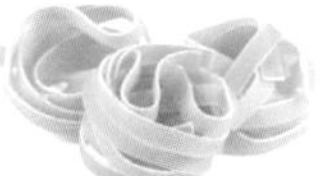

Linguine → spiral-sliced, shredded, or julienned peeled carrots, celery root, parsnips, sweet potatoes, turnips, kohlrabi, sweet potato, yellow squash, or zucchini; Cappello's grain-free noodles

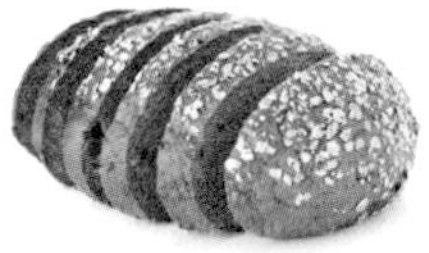

BREAD → homemade bread made with Paleo ingredients, sliced apple, sliced cucumber, sliced and baked sweet potato, sliced zucchini; blanched collard, kale, and Swiss chard leaves; iceberg and Bibb lettuce leaves; coconut wraps; nori wraps

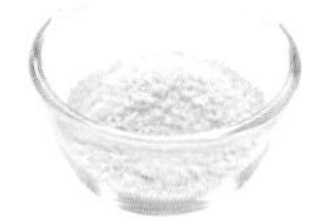

BREADCRUMBS FOR BREADING OR TOPPING → almond meal, crushed plantain chips or sweet potato chips, crushed plantain crackers, shredded coconut

FLOUR FOR BAKING → cassava flour (can substitute 1:1 for wheat-based flour in most recipes) or a mix of almond flour, coconut flour, arrowroot powder, tapioca powder, chestnut flour, plantain flour, sweet potato flour, and/or tiger nut flour

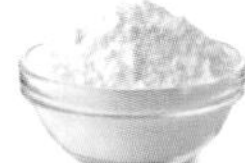

CORNSTARCH → arrowroot powder, kuzu starch, water chestnut powder, sweet potato starch

BAKING POWDER → baking soda mixed with cream of tartar (see page 473)

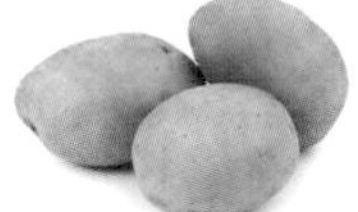

POTATOES → cauliflower, green plantains, sweet potatoes, root vegetables

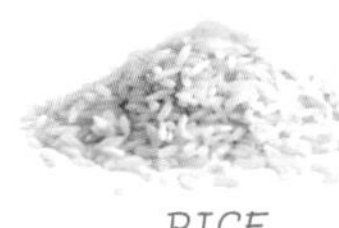

RICE → cauliflower or broccoli pulsed in a food processor or blender; finely shredded or chopped butternut squash, carrots, parsnips, plantains, or sweet potatoes

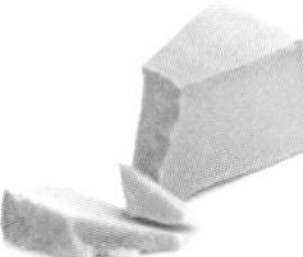

CHEESE FLAVOR → nutritional yeast

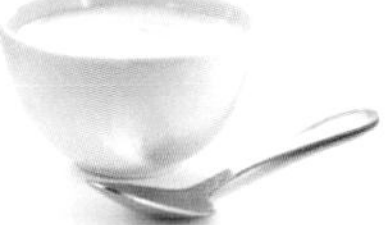

YOGURT OR SOUR CREAM → plain coconut milk yogurt or kefir

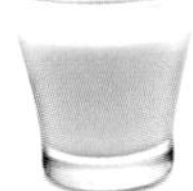

MILK → almond milk, cashew milk, coconut milk, pecan milk, sunflower seed milk, walnut milk

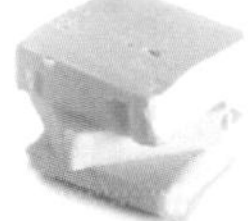

BUTTER → ghee, lard, tallow, palm shortening

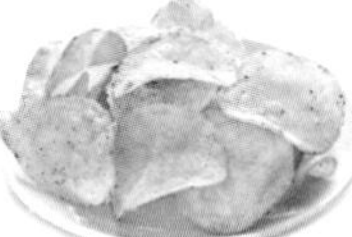

CHIPS AND CRACKERS → cassava chips, plantain chips, seaweed chips, sweet potato chips cooked in coconut oil, homemade Paleo crackers or chips, pork rinds

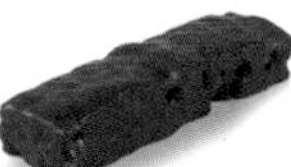

PROTEIN BARS → jerky (store-bought or homemade), Rx bars, Epic bars, Exo bars

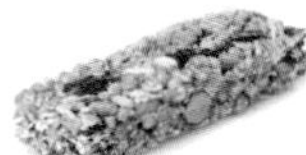

GRANOLA BARS → homemade Paleo granola bars, Larabars

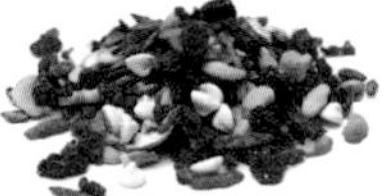

TRAIL MIX → homemade mix of dried fruit, nuts, seeds, and coconut flakes

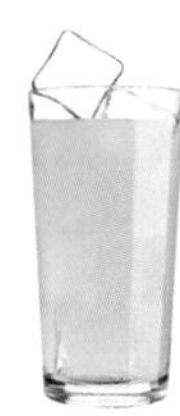

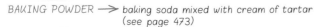

SODA → sparkling water flavored with citrus slices or chopped fruit, kombucha, water kefir

Chapter 37:

TIME MANAGEMENT IN THE KITCHEN

The amount of time we spend cooking has decreased dramatically over the last 50 years, correlating with the rise in chronic disease. Cooking more often means choosing more fresh foods, which naturally have way more nutrition than anything prepackaged or manufactured. Simply embracing home cooking is the smartest way to make better food choices!

Surveys have consistently shown that we are unwilling to dedicate more than an hour a day to cooking, or about 20 minutes per meal. The good news is, that's ample time to cook delicious, healthy Paleo meals at home! To help you make the most out of your kitchen time investment, this chapter outlines my favorite time-saving strategies.

BATCH COOKING

You can approach batch cooking as "cooking for the freezer," as "cooking for leftovers," or both. Batch cooking simply means that you are cooking a larger quantity of food than you would make for a single meal. Even though it may take a little longer to make a double or triple batch of a recipe, the time you save over cooking that recipe on two or three separate occasions can be enormous.

Freezing and Thawing Foods

Having a freezer full of already-cooked meals, ready to be reheated in a flash, can be a lifesaver. On those busy weeknights when you arrive home starving, you can simply pull a meal out of the freezer and throw it directly into the microwave. Think of your freezer as your own fast-food restaurant. Having a variety of ready-made meals in your freezer means that there's always more than one thing on the menu!

When freezing foods, let them cool prior to placing them in freezer-safe containers—unless you're using mason jars, in which case placing hot foods in the jars and loosely securing the lids allows you to get a seal prior to freezing and extends the freezer storage life. Foods such as muffins and sausage patties and ingredients such as berries are best frozen on a baking sheet, separated so they aren't touching, and then placed in a freezer bag or other freezer-safe container once frozen; this prevents them from sticking to each other and makes it easier to grab what you need out of a large batch. When choosing a freezer container, think about how many servings you want to freeze in each container. A large container is great for freezing a family meal's worth of food, whereas smaller containers are handy for individual portions or items that you will use as ingredients in smaller quantities, like broth.

Contrary to popular belief, refreezing previously frozen foods is safe to do most of the time. If you thawed an item in the refrigerator, it is safe to refreeze it without cooking it, although there may be a loss of quality due to the moisture lost through thawing. After cooking raw foods that were previously frozen, it is safe to freeze the cooked foods. If previously cooked and then frozen foods are thawed in the refrigerator, you may refreeze the unused portion. If you purchased frozen meat or seafood, you can refreeze it if it has been handled properly (meaning that it's been kept cold). Do not refreeze any foods that are left outside the refrigerator for longer than 2 hours or that have spent more than an hour in temperatures above 90°F. Do not refreeze meat that was thawed in a microwave without cooking it first. Always freeze leftovers within 3 to 4 days of cooking.

Thawing food in the fridge is the safest method and preserves food quality the best. You can also use the water bath method described on page 461, even for soups, stews, broth, and other frozen prepared-ahead-of-time meals, provided that they are in sealed containers or bags. However, if you use the water bath method to thaw a food, don't refreeze the leftovers. If you're reheating cooked foods, you can typically skip thawing, especially if you are reheating them in the microwave or oven. (Frozen foods can burn on the stovetop, so if you choose this method, use low heat and watch the food carefully.)

When it comes to reheating leftovers or thawed frozen foods, you can use the microwave, the oven, or the stovetop, depending on the type of food you are reheating. Cooked food can be reheated from frozen—while it takes longer than reheating thawed food, it takes less time than thawing and then reheating. Reheating from frozen can affect texture, so it's not always the best choice in terms of food quality, but sometimes it is the only choice in terms of getting food into your mouth when you're ravenous!

You can prepare several ready-made freezer meals by using any of the following strategies:

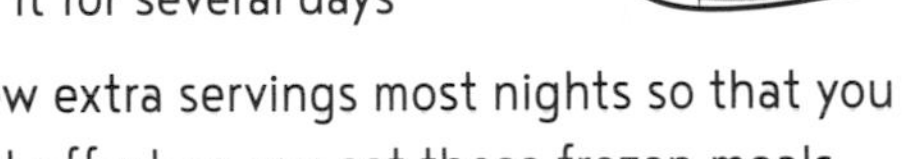

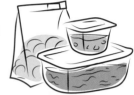

- cooking all the food that you will eat for the week in one big weekend session
- doubling or tripling a recipe so you can eat it for several days
- making a few extra servings most nights so that you have a night off when you eat those frozen meals
- preparing another recipe, specifically for the freezer, while you're cooking dinner—like making a batch of waffles for the next week's breakfasts

Cooking for Leftovers

If you are cooking for leftovers, think about what will save you time when you reheat your meal. Will it help if you slice the entire roast tonight so that it's presliced and ready to serve tomorrow? Will it help if you refrigerate your leftovers as full dinner plates as opposed to putting the chicken in one container and the veggies in another?

I recommend investing in good containers for storing your leftovers, whether in the fridge or the freezer. Glass is a great option because it can go straight from the freezer or fridge to the microwave. (Some glass containers are ovenproof, but you'll need to shop around if that's a necessity.) Look for round or square glass containers that are stackable—a feature that should not be underestimated in terms of handiness. Wide-mouthed mason jars are great for storing leftovers, and some sizes are freezer safe. These also have some stacking ability and seal tightly enough that they can go from freezer to water bath to microwave (after the metal lid is removed!)—and that means fewer dishes. Mason jars can even be packed in an insulated lunch box for an easy meal at work or school.

Batch Food Prep

Another way to save time without going to all the trouble of a massive cooking session on the weekend is to dedicate an hour to wash, peel, and chop veggies for the week. This might mean making veggie sticks for easy lunches and snacks, chopping vegetables for stir-fries or roasting, processing cauliflower for cauli-rice, or making a huge salad (minus the dressing, which is added right before eating).

Sauces and dressings can also be prepared ahead. Having your favorite salad dressing on hand can make a huge difference in terms of veggie servings during the week, plus it can be used on steamed vegetables or as a meat marinade. Making a batch of a favorite stir-fry sauce, pasta sauce, or dip can also save you tons of time during the week.

You might also choose to precook a few handy recipes that aren't meals by themselves but can make throwing together a quick meal super-easy. This could include anything from baking a batch of breakfast egg muffins or crackers to roasting a whole chicken to use the leftover meat in soups, salads, and stir-fries.

PLANNING AHEAD

The best tool you have for making the transition to Paleo is planning ahead. It's important to know in advance what you're going to eat on a rushed weeknight, how you're going to handle getting out the door in a hurry in the morning, and what you'll do when the rest of your (non-Paleo) family is enjoying a tempting treat.

Batch cooking is a way of planning ahead, but it's not the only way. You can put ingredients in a slow cooker in the morning so that dinner will be ready when you get home. Or you can take some meat out of the freezer to thaw the night before you cook it. Planning ahead might mean ordering some ingredients online. Or it can be as simple as making a shopping list and sticking to it!

This technique doesn't just encompass the mental planning of what you're going to make/eat and when; it also encompasses food prep that can be done ahead of time. Beyond the more obvious example of slow-cooking, planning ahead might mean chopping some vegetables when you have a few spare minutes. Or it might mean combining the ingredients for a sauce or dressing or putting a meat into a marinade in the fridge before you leave for work. Every minute you invest ahead of time is a minute less that it will take you to get dinner on the table when you're in a rush.

Do you normally hurry to get out the door in the morning? Having some leftovers or precooked sausage or breakfast egg muffins on hand can make a huge difference in terms of actually eating breakfast before leaving the house. If you know that you're going to be tempted by a treat, having a special indulgence premade in your freezer can mean the difference between feeling a sense of deprivation that drives you to fall off the wagon and feeling pampered and content.

USING THE RIGHT TOOLS

As simple as it sounds, having the right tools can make all the difference in the world when it comes to saving time in the kitchen. Whether it means having sharp knives as opposed to dull ones, or using an immersion blender instead of a wire potato masher, or having a pair of tongs to flip slippery foods instead of struggling with a spatula, the right tools can have a significant impact on the amount of time it takes you to accomplish any kitchen task. Consider splurging on higher-end tools, gadgets, utensils, and small appliances if you can. You typically (but not always) get what you pay for; a more expensive kitchen tool often does the job better and faster and is easier to clean. See Chapter 39 for a list of essentials and my favorite tools.

PULLING TOGETHER QUICK MEALS

Having a solid repertoire of quick meals that you can pull together in a pinch is an absolute must. Quick meals come in several flavors (pardon the pun):

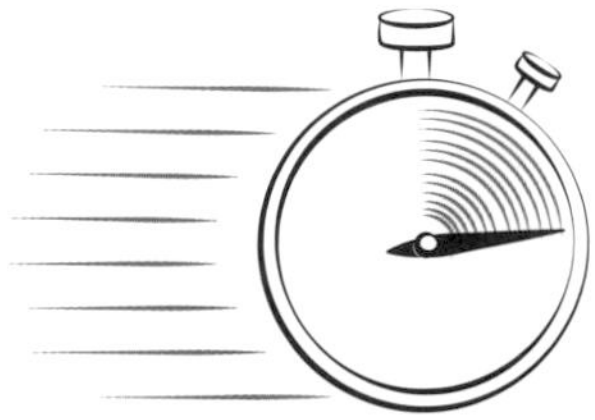

1. "Oops, I forgot to pull some meat out of the freezer, so I'll make ________." Fill in the blank with a meal from your big-batch cooking day, or some poached fish (which can be done from frozen), or some frozen precooked shrimp that can be force-thawed under cold water, or even smaller packages of pork chops or steaks that will thaw in less than an hour in a sink full of water and broil in about 8 minutes. It could even be a rotisserie chicken from the hot bar at your local natural-foods store (check the ingredients).

2. "I have the benefit of planning ahead, but I'm going to have only 15 minutes to cook." This is one of those cases where using a slow cooker or programmable pressure cooker is super-handy. But that's not the only way to tackle this scenario. If you're going to have more time in the morning for food prep, you can chop or even precook vegetables, season meat, assemble sauces and dressings, and make a salad. Then it might just be a matter of throwing everything into a frying pan or under the broiler at dinnertime. Many recipes in this cookbook have very short cook times if you've done the food prep in advance.

3. "I don't have time to prepare AND I don't have time to cook." While there are premade foods that will work in a pinch, like the aforementioned rotisserie chicken, canned fish, and raw veggies, if you find that you just can't ever make time to cook, it's time to reevaluate your schedule and your priorities. Maybe you can do some batch cooking on the weekends so that meals during the week are composed of leftovers and frozen favorites.

Leftovers, Leftover, Leftovers!

I've already covered cooking for leftovers, but I want to reiterate just how useful—and versatile!—leftovers can be. Eating leftovers doesn't have to mean that you eat the same meal night after night (although it can if you enjoy it). There are lots of ways to use leftovers and not feel bored by repetition in your meals.

One simple way is to cook a large batch of meat—for example, a sizable roast, a leg of lamb, or a whole chicken or two—while switching up your side dishes every night. One night you might make braised greens and roasted sweet potatoes, the next night you might have steamed broccoli and wild mushrooms with tarragon, and the next night you might have leftover sweet potatoes but change it up with a salad and some cauliflower gravy. Even leftover vegetables can be changed up by adding a dressing (page 484), tossing them with some chopped fresh herbs, or simply mixing together two different dishes of leftover veggies.

You can also completely reinvent your leftovers. Cooked meat can be added to stir-fries, salads, and soups to radically change their flavor, texture, and appearance. Try mixing cooked meat or seafood with some veggies and wrap the mixture in coconut or nori wraps. And when in doubt, freeze a meal of leftovers. Even though you'll be eating the same meal when you do reheat it, you can enjoy several days, weeks, or months of different meals before you get to it.

Using Convenience Foods

If you're struggling to make everything from scratch, there is no shame in taking advantage of some convenience foods. Precut veggies in microwavable steamer bags, prewashed salad greens, precut fruits and raw veggies that don't require any preparation, packaged sweet potato chips and plantain chips, and frozen vegetables ready to be added to a pot are all great time-savers. Meat that your butcher has already sliced (usually for no extra fee), fish that your fishmonger has already filleted (sometimes for a higher price per pound), rotisserie chicken, precooked shrimp, canned or smoked fish, and high-quality deli meats can save you a ton of time when it comes to getting quality protein on your plate. Canned coconut milk or cream, specialty flours, and other specialty foods like coconut wraps, nori wraps, and seaweed snacks all save you time and can help you pull together a meal when your schedule is packed. There are also a variety of Paleo baking mixes available, including pancakes, muffins, cakes, pizza crust, bagels, and dinner rolls, all of which add a comfort food component to a meal while requiring little time investment.

The caveat, of course, is that items that save you time tend to cost more money; conversely, items that are less expensive tend to require more time. If these two qualities are a trade-off for you, take a week to clock the time you spend doing various food-prep activities to home in on which time-saving items are worth the extra investment.

KNOWLEDGE BOMB

Great news! Microwaves are completely safe to use for cooking and heating your food. In fact, some studies even show that microwave cooking can better preserve the nutrients in your food compared to other cooking techniques. For an in-depth discussion of the safety of microwaves, see thepaleomom.com/are-microwaves-safe-to-use/

Chapter 38: COOKING TECHNIQUES AND TOOLS

In many ways, Paleo cooking bridges modern favorites with old traditions. When grain had to be milled by hand and yeast cultures had to be continuously grown in the kitchen to make leavened bread, meals tended to be centered around meat and in-season, local vegetables. Soups and stews were staples among many traditional cultures because they made use of the whole animal and even the whole vegetable. Slow-roasted wild game or tough meats like mutton would be paired with simply boiled root vegetables. Everything that was edible was used somehow—turnip greens in addition to the turnips, organ meat and bones in addition to the muscle meat, fish heads to make soup—and you can see this waste-not-want-not approach to meals reflected in traditional recipes.

Today, we have access to so many more flavoring ingredients, a huge range of fruits and vegetables throughout the year, and ingredients grown in other regions of the world, like olive oil and macadamia nuts, and we can cook them quickly in our own homes using our modern kitchen tools. We're spoiled compared to our ancestors, but just because we're adopting many of the same strategies when it comes to our food choices doesn't mean that we need to eschew modern conveniences like slow cookers and microwave ovens or ditch all but those seasonings we can grow in our backyards. The recipes in this book are about taking the best of both worlds: enjoying the full range of delicious, nutrient-dense whole foods available to us; embracing nutrient density principles like eating organ meat and lots of veggies; and appreciating the wealth of kitchen tools, gadgets, and cooking methods at our disposal.

Whether you're completely new to cooking or simply cooking beyond your current comfort zone, this chapter has a lot of useful information about basic cooking techniques and essential cooking tools.

COOKING TECHNIQUES

There are many cooking techniques out there, and it's not my intention to wrap up hundreds of pages of detailed science with a community college cooking course. But for those of you coupling your venture into healthier eating with learning how to cook, it makes sense to summarize some of the most common and useful cooking techniques, tools, and safety considerations.

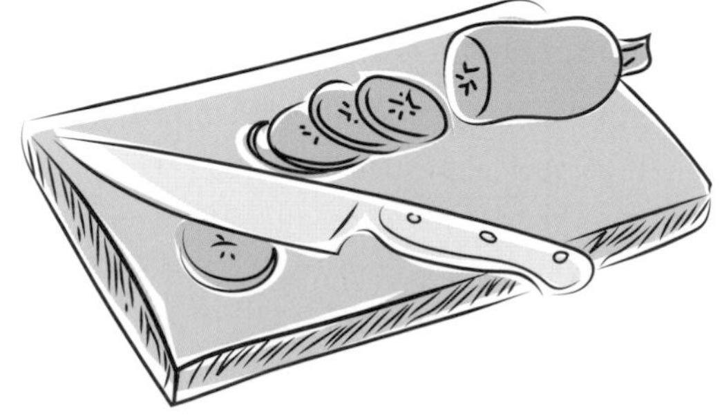

Roasting and Broiling Basics

Roasting meat and vegetables is probably the quickest cooking method in terms of hands-on time. Roasting typically requires simply seasoning meat or tossing veggies in a tasty fat and some seasoning and placing the food in a relatively hot oven for a period of time. Some foods will need to be flipped or tossed during cooking, but in most cases, once the dish is in the oven, it's "set it and forget it."

Broiling is also accomplished in the oven, but the broil function heats just the top element of the oven to a very high temperature, typically around 500°F. Food is then cooked 6 to 8 inches away from the top element—consult your oven's manual to find out whether to leave the door closed or slightly open.

You can think of broiling as upside-down grilling; most recipes that you would cook on a barbecue or grill can be broiled instead and cooked for the same amount of time. Broiling is particularly useful for quickly cooking tender cuts of meat, like rib-eye steak or pork loin chops, and also for browning foods that were cooked at a lower temperature, like some casseroles.

Steaming Basics

Steaming is a great way to cook vegetables and fish quickly. This is sometimes accomplished by adding only a tiny amount of water to a pot full of vegetables, but more typically a steamer rack or insert is placed in a pot, Dutch oven, or wok.

Steamer inserts and racks can be made of perforated metal (similar to a colander), wire, or bamboo. When using a wire steamer rack, make sure the food you are steaming is cut large enough that it will not slip through the openings in the rack. If the openings are too large, cover the rack with aluminum foil and punch small holes in it before putting the food on the rack. Bamboo steamers typically sit on a wire rack inside a wok.

It's common for sets of pots and pans to include a perforated metal steamer insert that fits perfectly into the same pot that might be used as a double boiler or into the stockpot. Woks also typically come with a wire steamer rack. If you don't own a steamer insert or rack, consider investing in one; they are inexpensive and quite versatile. Beyond steaming veggies and seafood, they can be used to cook soft- or hard-boiled eggs and even to sterilize small canning jars and lids.

TIPS FOR ROASTING:

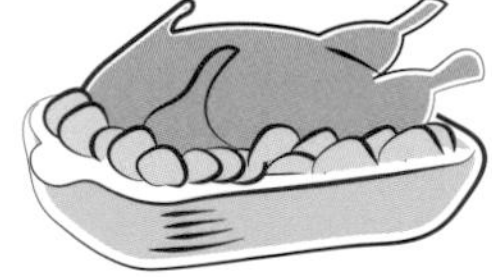

- Use a heavy pan or rimmed baking sheet. These pans absorb and distribute heat evenly, allowing meat and veggies to cook more evenly.
- Using a high-rimmed pan or casserole dish helps retain moisture. You can make use of this property if you want a juicy roast, or choose a pan with a low rim if you want a roast chicken with crispy skin.
- Avoid roasting pans with handles that fold down since they're difficult to remove from a hot oven with oven mitts.
- If you're not planning on making a pan gravy, line the bottom of your roasting pan with aluminum foil. You can save yourself a whole lot of cleanup time by preventing the drippings from crusting on the bottom of your pan.
- Don't overcrowd the pan. The best way to get browning and develop flavors is to have enough separation between meat pieces or vegetables so that the heat circulates evenly. Crowding causes the food to steam rather than roast.
- Use an instant-read thermometer for meats. To gauge doneness, insert the thermometer into the center of the piece of meat, being careful not to allow the tip of the thermometer to touch bone or go through to the bottom of the pan. It's especially important to check doneness early on when roasting grass-fed and pasture-raised meats since they tend to cook substantially faster than conventional meats.
- Let meat (as well as casseroles) rest. Meat will continue to cook after it is removed from the oven, heating up an additional 5°F to 10°F. As meat rests, the fibers relax and retain more juices (rather than releasing onto your plate when you slice into the meat), so wait at least 5 minutes before carving for juicier meat.

TIPS FOR STEAMING:

- Whatever equipment you are using, add enough water to have 1 inch of space between the bottom of the steamer rack or insert and the water.
- Bring the water to a boil over high heat. Once the water is boiling, arrange the food on the steamer rack or insert and place the rack in the pot.
- Secure the lid, making sure it fits tightly so that very little steam escapes. A dome-shaped lid is best because the water can't condense and drip on the food.
- Check the water level occasionally to make sure that it hasn't boiled away. Add more boiling water as needed.
- Anytime you remove the lid, tilt it away from you to avoid burning yourself.

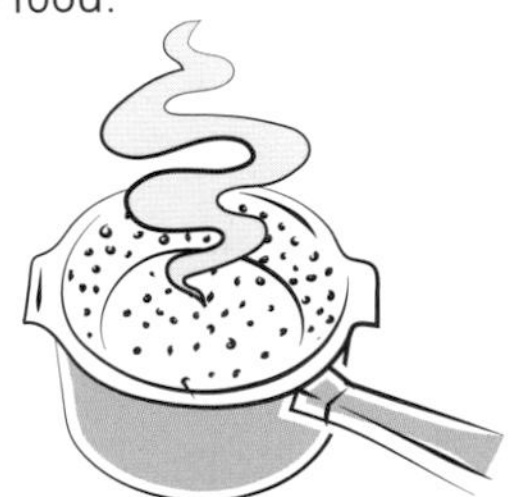

Sautéing and Pan-Searing

Sauté is a cooking term that means to cook a food quickly over relatively high heat using a small amount of fat in a shallow, uncovered pan. You can use a frying pan or a sauté pan, which has slightly higher sides than most frying pans.

Because food cooks quickly when sautéing, you'll want to either shake the pan or stir the food frequently. The traditional shaking technique makes the food jump, which is where the word *sauté* comes from—the French word for "jump" is *sauter*.

You can sauté just about anything: meat, fish, vegetables, and even some fruits, like apples, pineapples, peaches, and pears. One important trick is to cut the food into pieces that are uniform in size and thickness so they cook evenly.

It's always useful to have a pan that is much bigger than you think you need. As with roasting, you want some space between the pieces of food so that they brown instead of steam.

GENERALLY, TO SAUTÉ, YOU DO THE FOLLOWING:

- Preheat the pan over medium to high heat, depending on the fat being used, the ingredients being sautéed, the material the pan is made of, and the heat setting the recipe calls for.
- Add 2 to 3 tablespoons of a high-smoke-point oil or fat to the hot pan. You can mix fats, too—for example, you can use butter in conjunction with a higher-smoke-point fat like a quality olive oil to protect the butter from burning.
- Immediately spread the oil or fat by gently tipping the pan or with a spatula.
- Carefully add the food to the pan. At this point, the heat is often reduced somewhat. Do not add liquid unless it is called for in your recipe. (When a recipe uses both fat and liquid to cook a food, it's called *braising*, not sautéing.)
- Stir the food relatively frequently with a spatula or wooden spoon. Alternatively, you can use the pan's handle to shake the pan in a back-and-forth motion. Stirring or shaking the food frequently ensures that the food cooks evenly without scorching.
- Cook the food until done and then immediately remove it from the pan. If you sautéed meat, let it rest as you would if you had roasted it (see page 463).

Pan-searing is a related technique that is worth mentioning. To *pan-sear* is to sauté/fry a piece of meat or fish without disturbing it as frequently to brown one or both sides. In this case, you simply flip the piece of meat or fish after 3 to 5 minutes. The pan-seared meat or fish may be finished in the same pan in the oven or over lower heat on the stovetop, but it may cook quickly enough that by the time the second side is done searing, it's ready to serve!

Making a pan sauce is a great way to make use of the wonderful flavor achieved by sautéing and pan-searing. After cooking pieces of meat, transfer them to a serving dish and cover to keep warm. Add a cup or two of liquid, such as wine or broth, to the pan, along with some herbs or spices if you like. As the liquid comes to a boil, stir to scrape up the browned bits from the bottom of the pan. Continue cooking until the liquid has reduced to the desired consistency. To thicken a sauce, you can add a tablespoon of arrowroot powder (this makes it more of a gravy) or add a couple tablespoons of coconut cream, butter, ghee, or lard, 1 tablespoon at a time, stirring after each addition. Serve the sauce immediately.

Stir-Fry Basics

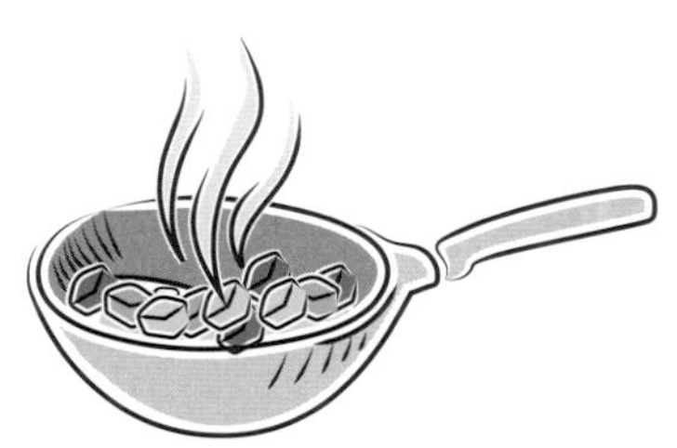

Stir-frying is similar to sautéing, but it is done in a wok, typically with a little more fat or oil and at a higher temperature. Most often, meat is cooked in oil with aromatics like ginger and garlic, then removed from the pan while vegetables are cooked (sometimes requiring more fat to be added to the pan). Sometimes the wok lid is used to help the vegetables cook, and liquid may be added to help cook vegetables that take a bit longer to soften, like carrots and broccoli. A sauce is created or added after the vegetables are cooked, when the meat is added back to the wok.

Stir-frying is a great way to reinvent leftovers or to prepare a quick meal with prechopped meat and veggies. The sauce can be as simple as a tiny bit of vinegar, a quarter cup or so of broth or water, and a tablespoon of arrowroot powder or kuzu starch. Or you can use a variety of more flavorful sauces, such as hoisin or teriyaki sauce (see Chapter 39 for recipes!).

Low-and-Slow Cooking

The slow cooker may be the king of the low-and-slow cooking method, but you can also use a Dutch oven (a special heavy-duty pot designed for this type of cooking) or other oven-safe lidded pot in a low- to medium-hot oven or over low heat on the stovetop.

In most slow cookers, the low setting is 200°F and the high setting is 300°F. You can usually make a slow cooker recipe just as easily in the oven in a covered oven-safe pot with the oven set to the equivalent temperature. You can often cook the same recipe on the stovetop over low or medium-low heat (at a gentle simmer), as long as the recipe calls for some kind of liquid. The caveat for making a slow cooker recipe on the stovetop is that you need to check the food every so often and give it a stir.

Whatever tool you choose, the advantage of low-and-slow cooking is that you can throw your ingredients in a pot in the morning (sometimes after searing the meat) and have a fully cooked meal at dinnertime. Not only is slow-cooking a great strategy for those short on time, but it's also budget-friendly. It's a great cooking method for tougher, typically cheaper cuts of meat like chuck roast and pork shoulder.

Every slow cooker recipe can also be cooked in a pressure cooker. There are no hard-and-fast rules for converting cooking times from slow cooker to pressure cooker, but for every 2 hours in a slow cooker, you're generally looking at 30 to 40 minutes on high pressure in a pressure cooker. This can be a real time-saver! There are lots of safety concerns with pressure cookers, so make sure to read the instruction manual before using it. If possible, opt for a countertop model with added safety features, like the Instant Pot (which does more than just pressure cook).

Low-and-slow techniques don't always involve wet heat, where liquid is added to the pot (think pot roasts, braised meats, and stews). Dry heat is also an option, where tough cuts of meat are cooked in a fairly cool oven (typically 200°F to 275°F) for a prolonged period. Leaner cuts of meat (like brisket) can be wrapped in aluminum foil to keep them moist during cooking, whereas fattier cuts (like pork shoulder) stay moist thanks to the constantly dripping fat.

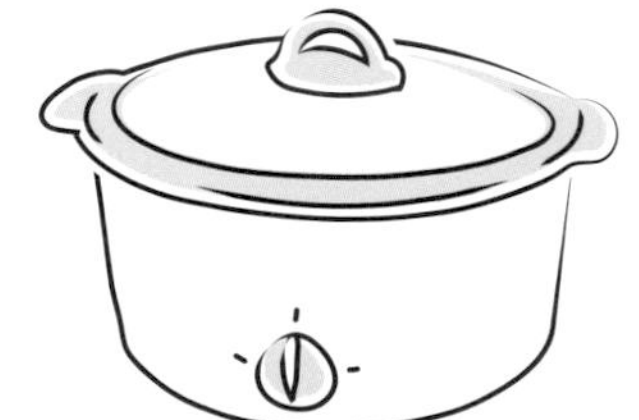

WHAT SALT DO I USE?

French sel gris, Himalayan pink salt, or Celtic gray unrefined sea salt are always preferred over other choices because they are an important source of essential minerals, typically containing in excess of eighty different trace minerals. The recipes in this cookbook assume that you are using finely ground salt (table salt). If using coarsely ground salt instead, you may want to adjust the seasoning, since 1 teaspoon of finely ground salt is equivalent to approximately 1¼ teaspoons of coarsely ground salt. If you purchase pink or gray salt in rock form, you can easily grind it yourself in a spice grinder, mortar and pestle, food processor, or blender.

Truffle salt can always be used as a substitute in savory dishes; look for a truffle salt with unrefined sea salt as its base. Sea vegetable blends (in which sea salt may or may not be one of the ingredients) are also nutrient-dense finishing salt substitutes.

Grilling Basics

Grilling is as much an art as it is a science. While there are general rules to follow, grilling requires intuition, which is generally gleaned from experience, and the ability to improvise. I fully admit to being merely a competent griller myself; but the good news is that grilling is a very forgiving cooking technique—you don't need to be an expert to make great food on a grill.

Grilling—or, more technically, *direct-heat grilling*—involves cooking food directly over a hot flame, whether from a campfire, a charcoal barbecue, or a gas grill. The exact procedure depends on the equipment you're using, and it's always best to follow the manufacturer's recommendations for lighting your grill and adjusting the temperature.

Gas grills generally need to preheat for 10 to 15 minutes with the burners on high and the cover closed before you adjust the temperature and put your food on the grates. For charcoal grills, light the coals and let it preheat with the cover off 30 to 45 minutes before you start cooking. How hot you want your grill depends on what you plan to cook. In general, larger pieces of meat that need to cook longer require a lower temperature, or else the outside will burn before the inside cooks through.

A grill thermometer is the most foolproof way to gauge the heat of your grill, but if you don't have one, you can always use the hand test. Carefully hold your hand (making sure you aren't wearing flammable clothing and you don't have jewelry or a sleeve hanging down over your hand), palm side down, about 4 inches above the grate. Count the number of seconds you can hold your hand in that position before the heat forces you to pull it away. Then use this guide to determine the approximate temperature:

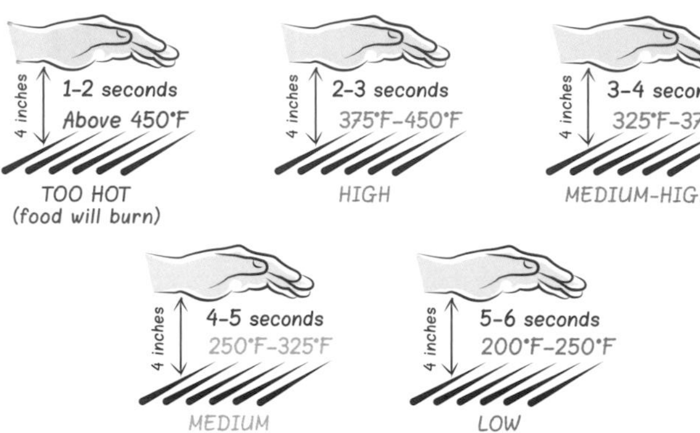

Controlling the temperature on a gas grill is a simple matter of using the knobs to adjust the settings. When cooking with charcoal, you lower the temperature by spreading the coals farther apart or by raising the cooking grate. To raise the temperature in a charcoal grill, you lower the grate or move the coals closer together and tap off the ash. To change the temperature quickly using either type of grill, open or close the lid.

Curious about *indirect-heat* grilling? This is a way of turning your charcoal barbecue into an oven—perfect for larger cuts of meat and fish—cooking food slowly and evenly but still imparting all that smoky flavor. With this method, you push all the coals to the edges of the barbecue and place a foil drip pan in the middle. Use the hand test to make sure that the grill is at medium heat in the middle, above the drip pan. Place your food in the center of the grill and cook it with the lid closed; there's no need to flip your food with this grilling method. Cooking times are similar to oven baking times (see the Appendixes), although, because cooking with charcoal can yield more variable temperatures, exact cooking times do vary.

HERE ARE SOME GENERAL GRILLING TIPS:

- Have the proper tools for the job. These include long-handled tongs (if using charcoal, one pair for food and one for coals), a long-handled basting brush, a long-handled metal spatula, a meat thermometer, a grill thermometer, heavy-duty oven mitts, metal or disposable foil drip pans, and a wire brush to clean the grates. There are lots of additional accessories for specific grilling applications, but these basics will get you started.
- Keep your grill a safe distance from anything flammable, like lighter fluid, fences, trees, and your house. A good general rule is at least 10 feet.
- Always keep your grill grates clean to prevent sticking and for better taste and general safety. Scrub the grates with a wire brush while the grill is still warm but not hot.
- Oil the food, not the grates. Avocado oil has a very high smoke point and, because it's liquid at room temperature, is very handy for coating food in preparation for grilling.
- Always keep an eye on what you're grilling. Besides the fact that you have an open flame probably not too far from your house, food can burn quickly, so check it frequently.
- It's easier to fix undercooked food than overcooked food. When you think it might be ready, remove the food from the grill, test it for doneness (either by thermometer or by taste test), and return it to the grill if it needs to cook longer.
- If making kabobs on bamboo skewers, soak the skewers in water for at least 20 minutes before grilling to prevent the skewers from burning. Soak cedar planks for at least an hour before placing them on the hot grill.
- Season your food at least an hour prior to grilling. It's generally best not to apply sauces prior to grilling since they can burn before the meat is fully cooked. Most recipes suggest basting with sauces for only the last 5 minutes of cooking.
- Cook vegetables and fruits at the outer, cooler edges of the grill since they tend to burn more quickly than meat.
- Do not use a spray bottle of water to control flare-ups. Flare-ups are caused by too much fat (or sugar from a sauce) and too much heat. If you have a fatty cut of meat, trim the excess fat before grilling or use a drip pan so that any fat dripping off doesn't land directly on the hot coals or flame.
- Turning food is essential for even cooking and to prevent burning. It's okay to turn your food more than once, but typically, the less often the food is turned, the better it tastes (in other words, don't get flip happy!).
- Place the food on a clean plate after grilling.

Deep-Frying Basics

Deep-frying can be done in fat that is anywhere between 320°F and 400°F, but the ideal temperature for most foods is 350°F to 375°F. Deep-frying in this temperature range allows less absorption of fat into the food while searing the outside to lock in moisture and create that wonderfully crispy outer layer. However, it's important to keep your fat below its smoke point—at least 5°F lower to be safe. If you're deep-frying in coconut oil, keep the temperature at 345°F. If you're using lard, keep the temperature at 360°F. This is most easily accomplished with a countertop deep-fryer, an inexpensive appliance that regulates the temperature for you. You can also use a large heavy-bottomed pot and an oil thermometer. Controlling the fat temperature can be tricky when using this setup, however, so you will want to aim to keep the fat at least 20°F below its smoke point, even though this is less than ideal from a cooking chemistry standpoint.

The best fats for deep-frying are those with higher smoke points, such as palm shortening, tallow, and lard (or a combination; see page 189). Each fat gives its own flavor, which may influence your choice. Palm shortening has very little flavor, whereas beef tallow and lard are just plain tasty! Also, when you mix fats, you average their smoke points. So if you want to use lard for flavor when higher-temperature deep-frying, try mixing it with an equal amount of palm shortening, which has a higher smoke point.

HERE ARE A FEW RULES FOR DEEP-FRYING:

- Never drop food into the hot fat, which could cause a dangerous splatter of hot fat. Instead, bring the food right to the surface and let it slide into the hot fat.
- Make sure to drain the food or pat it dry before frying. Excess moisture will cause the hot fat to bubble and splatter.
- Don't overcrowd the fryer. Making sure that there's plenty of space between items in your deep-fryer will ensure that they cook evenly.
- Always use a deep-fryer basket or strainer to remove food from the fat—don't be tempted to use a fork or chopsticks!

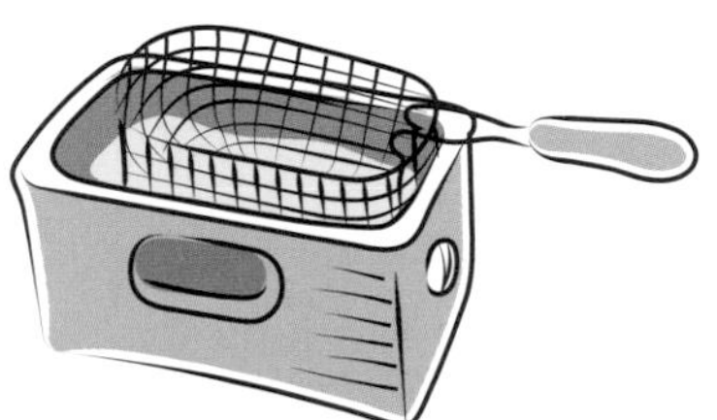

You can reuse the same fat many times as long as it never goes above its smoke point. When you're done frying, let the fat cool slightly and then pour it through a very fine mesh sieve or paper towel-lined sieve to filter out any food crumbs. Store the fat in a cool, dark place. The next time you deep-fry, top it up with some fresh fat. Change your fat when it doesn't taste good anymore or has darkened in color considerably.

BAKING BASICS

Baking with Paleo-compliant ingredients can be a bit tricky. This is because most of the flour substitutes don't bind as well as wheat flour. There are plenty of tried-and-true recipes for baked goods in this book, but if you're looking to experiment or to adapt some old family favorites, it's worth taking a brief tour of Paleo flour substitutes and binding ingredients.

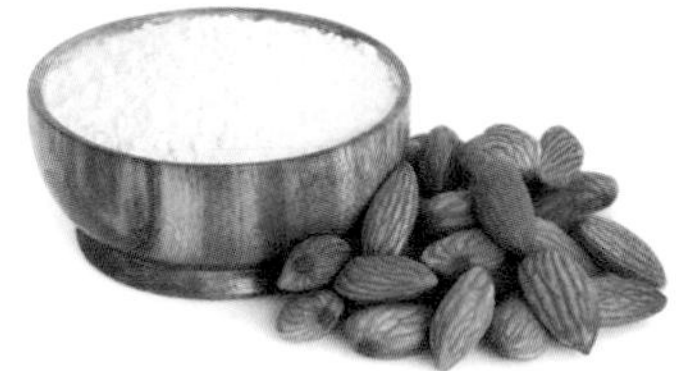

A Tour of Paleo Flours and Starches

Almond flour: The most common Paleo flour substitute. A high-quality blanched almond flour is very finely milled and can be quite light compared to other nut and seed flours or even a less finely milled almond flour. Generally, it can be substituted 1:1 for wheat flour. It works well when you want a denser crumb, as in muffins, coffee cakes, and chewy cookies. In recipes that call for a fairly large amount of wet ingredients, adding a starch or coconut flour can be helpful.

Almond meal: A less finely ground version of blanched almond flour. Almond meal typically uses the whole almond, but some products are made from blanched almonds. It is best for breading meat but can also be used for dense baking, like fruitcakes, some cookies, and pie crusts. If you are using almond meal in place of almond flour in a recipe, use slightly less, as it tends to be denser.

Arrowroot powder: The dehydrated and ground arrowroot tuber (not the cassava root). It is mostly a starch and is great for adding lightness to a recipe. It is also lovely for thickening sauces, gravy, and stews. Arrowroot powder can replace cornstarch in a recipe 1:1. You can also mix arrowroot powder with very finely ground granulated sugar to make an acceptable substitute for confectioner's sugar. If you are replacing wheat flour with arrowroot powder to add lightness to a recipe, replace up to one-fourth of your flour with arrowroot powder. I love using arrowroot powder in conjunction with coconut flour for cake recipes. It doesn't add much hold to baked goods that don't have a lot of binding ingredients, though.

Cassava flour: The newest flour available to Paleo bakers and definitely the easiest and tastiest to work with. It is the dehydrated and ground entire cassava root (as opposed to tapioca starch, which is the isolated starch of the cassava root) and because of its fiber content, it subs 1:1 for wheat flour in almost every circumstance. If you're looking to adapt a family favorite recipe, cassava flour is the best place to start.

Chestnut flour: This flour can be used interchangeably with almond flour but often yields a lighter texture owing to its higher starch content. It has more hold than almond flour and is quite a bit sweeter, so it's a useful flour substitute for coffee cakes, muffins, and other desserts.

Coconut flour: This flour has a high fiber content and absorbs liquid very efficiently, so it is used only in recipes that call for large amounts of wet ingredients. Because it makes for a finer crumb than nut flours, I like to use coconut flour for cake and cupcake recipes. It is also good for shortbread-style cookies. This is a very tricky flour to work with; often, 1 teaspoon can make the difference between the texture you are going for and something completely different. Sift coconut flour before adding it to a recipe unless you are blending your batter in a blender or food processor. When you add coconut flour to wet ingredients, the batter will thicken as it sits for the first few minutes. It's always a good idea to give your batter time to thicken before baking. The general rule is to replace wheat flour with one-fourth the amount of coconut flour. This quantity will be sufficient for some recipes, but you can add some nut or seed flour if you need to bring up the volume of the dry ingredients a little (try starting with the same volume you are using of coconut flour). Different brands of coconut flour behave slightly differently depending on how finely ground they are.

THE VERSATILE PLANTAIN

Plantains are an incredibly handy ingredient for Paleo recipes, acting as a flour substitute in recipes for pancakes and waffles (see pages 500 and 503), as lasagna noodles (see page 537), as a potato substitute (see page 554), and as a thickener for clam chowder and pot pie (see pages 512 and 532).

The plantain is a member of the banana family, and it's sometimes called a cooking plantain or raw banana. While plantains technically can be eaten raw, they are typically cooked (this is the dominant differentiator between plantains and bananas).

Green plantains should be dark to light green and firm. The peel can be challenging to remove; it helps to quarter the plantain first and then pry the peel off. Green plantains have a high starch content and a neutral flavor and can be used as a substitute for potatoes or for flour in grain-free baking. You can store them in the crisper drawer of your fridge for up to 2 weeks or peel and freeze them (either cut into large pieces or puréed). Keeping plantains in the fridge slows the ripening process, but note that the peel will continue to yellow in the crisper drawer even though the inside is still green.

Ripe plantains have less starch and more sugar than green plantains and have a lovely apple-meets-banana flavor. They should be nearly all black. They can be prepared in a variety of ways, and their natural sweetness lends itself well to desserts. Plantains take a long time to ripen from green to ripe, typically 3 to 4 weeks. Ripe plantains can be stored in the crisper drawer of your fridge for up to 5 days or be peeled and then frozen.

Finely shredded coconut: Coconut is a good bulking ingredient, similar to ground nuts and seeds but with a slightly different texture and flavor. Because of the fiber content, it will absorb a little liquid (although not nearly as much as coconut flour), so it behaves slightly differently than other nuts and seeds.

Ground nuts and seeds: Ground nuts and seeds are a wonderful way to add texture and bulk to baked goods. Many of them can act as binders as well. You'll likely be grinding your own in a food processor or blender. A finer grind will act more like a nut flour, but more coarsely ground nuts or seeds can replicate the texture of oatmeal or other whole-grain ingredients very well.

Hazelnut flour: This can be used interchangeably with almond flour but yields a different flavor.

Kuzu starch: Kuzu starch is ground dehydrated kuzu root and is often used in Asian cooking. It's great for thickening sauces and can substitute for arrowroot powder or sweet potato starch in most recipes.

Plantain flour (aka green banana flour): Plantain flour is simply ground dehydrated plantains. It has a distinct plantain taste, so it doesn't work in all baking. It has a lovely ability to bind (similar to tapioca starch, but with a texture and crumb more like wheat flour) and generally can be substituted 1:1 for wheat flour. It seems to work well in soft, cakey, and/or chewy recipes but not as well if you want some crunch or crispness. A word of caution: Some flours labeled as plantain flour actually contain a mix of different tubers, often including potato starch. If you are buying plantain flour from a store, make sure to check the ingredient list. I buy Barry Farm brand plantain flour from Amazon.

Pumpkin seed flour: Another seed-based alternative to almond flour. It has a distinct flavor and a slightly green color and is easier to make at home than most other nut flours. Simply place raw pepitas in a high-speed blender and blend on high for a minute or so.

Pureed green plantains: Green plantains are very starchy, have a fairly neutral flavor, and can act as a binder and give bulk to a recipe. A number of recipes in this book use fresh green plantains in place of flour.

Pureed root vegetables: Don't underestimate the versatility of canned or pureed root vegetables in your baking. You aren't limited to canned pumpkin, either. Sweet potato, yuca, taro, parsnip, carrot, and winter squash are all good options. When cooked and pureed, they can both act as a binder *and* add bulk to a recipe. They also add some sweetness without the use of sugars, and their flavors are often well camouflaged by other ingredients.

Sunflower seed flour: For those who are allergic to nuts, sunflower seed flour can be used interchangeably with almond flour. It has the fun property of turning green when used in baked goods that also contain baking soda (it's totally safe to eat the resulting baked good!).

Sweet potato powder: This is sometimes labeled as sweet potato flour, which can be very confusing. Sweet potato powder is ground dried whole sweet potatoes and retains its orange color. Sweet potato powder is an interesting flour because it has some fiber and can absorb liquid, so it has more ability to hold baked goods together.

Sweet potato starch: This is also sometimes labeled as sweet potato flour, but this fine white powder is actually a processed starch. It substitutes well for arrowroot powder but has almost no ability to hold baked goods together. You can use it as a substitute for cornstarch or in combination with other flours as a flour substitute.

Tapioca starch: This starch is extracted from ground cassava (aka yuca, manioc, tapioca) root, but it is not the same as arrowroot powder or cassava flour. Even though many people use tapioca starch and arrowroot powder interchangeably, they actually have fairly different properties in baking. Tapioca adds elasticity to baked goods, helping bind as well as giving more bounce (the cassava root is a naturally slimy starch). Tapioca is nice to use in Paleo breads and can be useful in cake recipes as well. You can replace up to about half of the wheat flour called for in a recipe with tapioca starch. Tapioca isn't a good substitute for cornstarch.

Vegetable powders: Along with the aforementioned sweet potato powder, pumpkin, carrot, spinach, winter squash, red cabbage, and beet powders are available. These powders are a great way to add natural color to recipes and can pack a serious nutrient punch even when used in moderation in conjunction with other flour substitutes.

Egg Substitutes

Agar powder: To replace one whole egg, dissolve 1 tablespoon of agar powder into 3 tablespoons of water. You can also use agar powder as an egg white substitute. For each egg white, dissolve 1 tablespoon of agar powder into 1 tablespoon of water; whip, chill, and then whip again before adding it to your recipe.

Applesauce: Apples are high in pectin, a fiber that has a fair bit of thickening and binding ability (pectin is added to jams to make them gel). Pears can also work, although they don't have quite as much binding ability. Applesauce also adds moisture, so it's a great binder for cakes, muffins, brownies, coffee breads, and so on. It also has a fairly mild flavor that can be hidden by other ingredients. Chunky applesauce (applesauce that is fork mashed as opposed to blended) can add a nice texture to muffins and coffee breads, while blended applesauce gives baked goods a smoother texture. Substitute ⅓ cup of applesauce for each egg.

Coconut oil (and other fats): Adding some extra fat to your recipe will help it hold together. Coconut oil is probably the best at holding baked goods together and gives them a bit more chew (great for cookies, brownies, and so on). Palm shortening, butter, ghee, or lard will give your baked goods a bit more lightness and still help them hold together, generally with a cakier texture. As a general rule, ¼ cup of coconut oil is equivalent to one egg.

Gelatin: This works brilliantly as an egg substitute for custards, cakes, and muffins. Dissolve 1 tablespoon of gelatin into 3 tablespoons of warm water and substitute this for one egg. If you replace too many eggs with gelatin, however, you will get an overly spongy, chewy texture, so if your recipe calls for several eggs, you can replace half with gelatin and half with one of the other egg substitutes listed here.

Mashed bananas: You know how bananas feel slimy when you mash them? That's what makes bananas such a great binder. It's because of their starch and fiber content (this is true for plantains, yuca, and taro, too). The only downside is that bananas have a habit of overwhelming any other flavors in a recipe, so this really only works if you want a distinct banana flavor in your baked good. Substitute ¼ cup of mashed banana (about half of an average-sized banana) for each egg.

Nut and seed butters: You can use a variety of nut and seed butters as egg substitutes, such as almond butter, sunflower seed butter, tahini, hazelnut butter, macadamia nut butter, cashew butter, sprouted macadamia nut butter, walnut butter, and pecan butter. Adding nut butters to replace or add to the fat ingredients in a recipe can help a recipe hold together quite well due to the fiber and fats in nut butters. This is a great strategy for cookies and bars since nut butter doesn't add much moisture. I wouldn't recommend replacing all of the eggs in a recipe with nut or seed butter, but you could replace one or even two eggs. Substitute ¼ to ⅓ cup of nut butter for each egg.

Plantain puree (ripe or green): Both green and ripe plantain puree can add substantial hold to a recipe (yep, because of the fiber). Green plantains add more starch and a little less hold than ripe plantains, but have a neutral flavor. Ripe plantains are fantastic binders and add a little sweetness, but similar to bananas, they add a distinctive flavor. To substitute for one egg, add ¼ cup of mashed ripe plantain or ⅓ cup of mashed green plantain (one average-sized plantain typically yields ¾ cup of puree).

Pumpkin puree: Pumpkin puree can act as a binder (because of its starch and fiber), although it is not as effective as mashed bananas or applesauce. It also has a flavor that is easy to mask. Use ⅓ cup of pumpkin puree in place of one egg.

Pureed root vegetables: Yuca (aka cassava, tapioca, or manioc) is brilliant at holding baked goods together. Peel and cube it (removing the tough string that runs down the middle) and boil it in salted water as you would potatoes until the pieces slide off a knife when poked (typically 20 to 30 minutes, depending on the size of your cubes). Drain and mash by hand with a potato masher or strong fork. Yuca is incredibly slimy and will do bad things to a blender or immersion blender; taro is similar. To use taro, steam whole (unpeeled) taro roots for 10 to 20 minutes depending on size, until they are soft enough to pierce with a sharp knife but are still a little firm. Let cool, peel, and mash by hand. Taro and yuca are a little sweet, which can be very helpful in some recipes. Other pureed vegetables can help hold baked goods together, too, including sweet potatoes, parsnips, winter squash, zucchini, and carrots. Typically, the starchier the vegetables are, the better.

A Primer on Chocolate

Chocolate is made from cacao beans. First, the beans are fermented, dried, cleaned, roasted (except for use in raw cacao products), and shelled to make *cacao nibs*. These nibs are ground to make *cocoa mass*, which is either liquefied by heating to make *chocolate liquor* or cold-pressed to make raw *cacao powder* and *cacao butter*. Chocolate liquor may be cooled and processed into its two components: *cocoa solids* (also called cocoa powder) and *cocoa butter*. Note the vocabulary here: *cacao* refers to raw, unheated ingredients from cacao beans, whereas *cocoa* refers to roasted, heated ingredients.

Chocolate can be made with any of these ingredients, typically in combination with sugar; most inexpensive chocolate also contains added fat (typically dairy) and emulsifiers like soy lecithin. The various terms used to describe chocolate are not tightly regulated, so a product containing as little as 10 percent chocolate liquor or cocoa mass can be called chocolate. At 35 percent, a product can be called dark chocolate, although most manufacturers use this label only when the cacao percentage is over 55 percent. It's important to read labels and know what to look for because there's a world of difference between high-quality high-cacao chocolate and all the other stuff.

Cacao is rich in antioxidant phytochemicals, flavonoids and polyphenols in particular, which is why very dark (over 70 percent cacao) chocolate is linked with diverse health benefits, like lowering cardiovascular disease risk factors, fighting depression, preventing diabetes, and even lowering the risk of some types of cancer. Cacao is also rich in several important minerals, including magnesium, zinc, iron, copper, manganese, potassium, and chromium (see Chapter 1). It's the other ingredients in chocolate that dilute and possibly negate these benefits: sugar is discussed in Chapter 22; dairy is discussed in Chapter 21 (plus, note that milk may bind to the flavonoids in chocolate, making them harder to absorb); and soy lecithin is discussed on page 236.

So high-quality dark chocolate is definitely on the menu: look for a high cacao content (at least 70 percent) and no dairy ingredients. (You may want to seek out chocolate that does not contain soy lecithin as well. Recall that soy lecithin, though not a gut irritant, is metabolized into TMAO in the gut, which can increase cardiovascular disease and cancer risk.) Good options include the following:

Cocoa or cacao powder: Look for natural, non-alkalized, unsweetened cocoa or cacao powder. Avoid Dutch-processed cocoa, which is additionally processed with alkali to neutralize its natural acidity, lowering the antioxidant content substantially. (The flavanol content of Dutch-processed cocoa can be as much as 90 percent lower!)

Dark chocolate with a high cacao content, generally 70 to 99 percent: The higher the percentage, the healthier the chocolate. You may see dark chocolate labeled as *semisweet* (typically 55 to 70 percent cacao, but this term isn't regulated) or *bittersweet* (typically 70 percent or darker), but it's still a good idea to read the label to find the exact cacao percentage. Look for chocolate sweetened with natural sugars like cane sugar, coconut sugar, maple syrup or sugar, or honey. Many brands contain unhealthy ingredients, so make sure to read the ingredient list. You can find high-quality dark chocolate in mini chip, regular chip, chunk, and bar forms. This type is great to use in recipes or for a sweet treat.

Unsweetened baking chocolate: Look for a product that lists only chocolate, cocoa mass, cocoa butter, and/or chocolate liquor as ingredients. The packaging should also say "100% cacao." This type is best used in recipes.

See the Appendixes for my favorite vendors of dark chocolate and other pantry items.

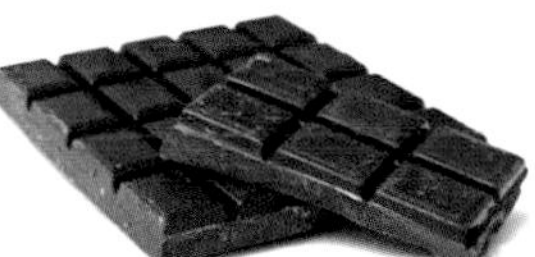

Everything Coconut

A dizzying array of products are made from the sap or the fruit of the coconut palm tree, and most of them find their way into Paleo recipes! The fruit of the coconut palm has several layers, including the husk, the shell, the meat, and the water. (When you buy a mature coconut from the grocery store, the husk typically has been removed.) Most coconut products are made from the meat of mature coconuts. These include:

- **Virgin or extra-virgin coconut oil** is the edible oil extracted from coconut meat, typically fresh, although it can be cold-pressed from dried coconut meat as well. Virgin or extra-virgin coconut oil retains the aroma and taste of coconut. The health benefits of coconut oil are discussed on page 184.

- **Refined coconut oil** is processed to remove the coconut flavor, which may or may not involve bleaching and chemical extraction using solvents. Refined coconut oil can also be made using a natural physical extraction process, so read labels carefully.
- **Coconut butter** (also called creamed coconut, coconut manna, or coconut cream concentrate) is a peanut butter-like paste formed when coconut oil and coconut meat are ground together.
- **Shredded coconut** (sometimes referred to as "desiccated coconut") is dried and grated coconut meat found in a range of sizes; it can be toasted or untoasted. Look for unsweetened shredded coconut.
- **Coconut flakes or chips** are also made from dried and grated coconut meat, but the pieces are much larger than shredded coconut. Again, look for unsweetened. There are many options of snacking chips made with coconut flakes.
- **Coconut milk** is the flavorful fatty liquid extracted from grated fresh coconut meat. (It is not the liquid found in the middle of the coconut; that's coconut water.) Full-fat coconut milk is made from the first press of the coconut meat. Light coconut milk is typically made from the second press, so it has a much lower fat content; this type is rarely used in Paleo cooking. Look for canned or boxed coconut milk that does not contain emulsifiers like guar gum.
- **Coconut cream** (not to be confused with creamed coconut) is the concentrated milk extracted from fresh grated coconut meat. It has an even higher fat content that full-fat coconut milk and a thick, creamy texture. Again, look for canned or boxed coconut cream that does not contain emulsifiers.
- **Coconut milk beverage or coffee creamers** are boxed cow's milk substitutes that are typically teeming with additives like sugars, emulsifiers, and titanium oxide. These are best avoided.
- **Coconut milk powder** is prepared by dehydrating coconut milk under controlled conditions. Look for varieties with better anticaking agents like tapioca maltodextrin.
- **Coconut flour** is made by grinding the dried coconut meat or pulp left over from making coconut milk. See page 468 for tips on baking with coconut flour.

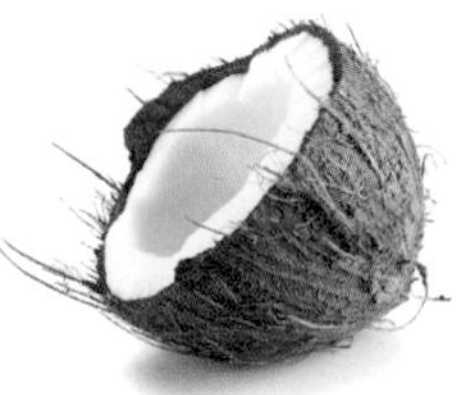

While mature coconuts do contain some coconut water in their centers, the coconut water that you buy is typically extracted from young, or green, coconuts because they contain a lot more of it. Young coconuts are the immature fruits of the coconut palm and have soft, gel-like meat.

- **Coconut water beverages** contain the electrolyte-rich, slightly sweet, clear liquid found inside a young coconut. Look for coconut water beverages that don't contain added sugars or artificial flavors.
- **Coconut water vinegar** (sometimes called coconut vinegar) is vinegar made from fermenting coconut water with the same *Acetobacter* bacterial cultures that are used to make other kinds of vinegar. It has a flavor similar to rice wine vinegar.

There are also products made from the coconut sap, obtained by tapping the thick flowering stems of the coconut blossom. These include:

- **Coconut aminos** are made from aged coconut sap blended with sea salt. It has a flavor similar to soy sauce while being entirely soy- and gluten-free and containing substantially less sodium.
- **Coconut nectar** (also called coconut palm nectar) is made by concentrating coconut sap via low-temperature evaporation. It can be used in place of honey or maple syrup in most recipes.
- **Coconut sugar** (also known as coconut palm sugar) is made by boiling and dehydrating coconut sap until it forms a granular sweetener similar to cane sugar. See page 307 for more on coconut sugar.

Other Baking Essentials

Other ingredients commonly found in Paleo baked goods recipes include natural sugars like maple syrup, maple sugar, unrefined cane sugar (evaporated cane juice or muscovado sugar), blackstrap molasses, and honey. Sometimes dates or other fruits are used as a source of nutrient-rich sweetness as well. Leavening agents are also typically used.

Baking soda is sodium bicarbonate. It comes from a natural mineral that was originally mined but is now made industrially using the awesomeness of chemistry. Sodium bicarbonate is an alkali, so when it mixes with acid, it undergoes a chemical reaction and CO_2 bubbles are released. Depending on how much acid it is mixed with, it reacts slowly or very quickly (think homemade volcano science projects). If your recipe calls for baking soda, then no substitution is necessary.

Baking powder is not Paleo compliant due to its cornstarch content (although corn-free versions using potato starch or arrowroot powder are available). However, the active ingredients in baking powder, baking soda and potassium hydrogen tartrate (aka tartaric acid or cream of tartar), *are* Paleo. Tartaric acid, which is naturally found in grapes, is a byproduct of winemaking. You can buy cream of tartar in the spice or baking section of just about any grocery store. This acidifying agent provides the necessary acid for baking soda to react with to make its little CO_2 bubbles.

If a recipe calls for baking powder, here are some simple Paleo-friendly substitutions:

1 tsp BAKING POWDER = 1/4 tsp BAKING SODA + 1/2 tsp CREAM OF TARTAR

1 tsp BAKING POWDER = 1/4 tsp BAKING SODA + 1/2 tsp VINEGAR or LEMON JUICE

Baker's yeast is a perfectly acceptable ingredient to use in Paleo baking, provided that it's gluten-free. There are several recipes that use yeast as a leavening agent in this book.

Coconut milk and almond milk are often used as cow's milk substitutes. You can almost always substitute another nut or seed milk for coconut milk or almond milk in a recipe. Sometimes you can use water or water mixed with a little fat in place of nut milks or dairy, too.

Most flavoring ingredients used in traditional baking, like sweet spices (cinnamon, cloves, and nutmeg) are perfectly Paleo. Vanilla extract is not necessarily gluten-free, however (the alcohol used to make it is typically grain-based), so check the label or use fresh or ground vanilla beans instead. Use half as much ground whole vanilla bean as vanilla extract. Alternatively, you can scrape the seeds from whole vanilla beans; the seeds scraped from one vanilla bean are equivalent to about 1 teaspoon of vanilla extract.

COOKING TOOLS

Cooking tools can be divided into two categories: essential and nonessential but awesome. The essentials list contains basic implements—a few pots and pans, a few good knives, a cutting board, various spatulas and stirring spoons, and a can opener—basically higher-quality versions of what probably graced the shared kitchen in your college dorm. The nonessentials list includes a variety of gadgets and small appliances that, while not absolute necessities, can save you an amazing amount of time and energy in the kitchen.

Essential Tools

If you're starting from scratch, here are the barest essentials:

Baking pan: A large metal, glass, or ceramic pan, either 9 inches square or 13 by 9 inches, with 2-inch-high sides. This versatile pan can be used for a variety of dishes.

Can opener: Even though you won't be eating many canned foods, a can opener is still a necessity. Look for a safe-cut or smooth-edge model that cuts around the outside of the can rather than the lid; this type will produce smooth edges and won't lower the lid into your food.

Casserole dish: A glass, ceramic, or enameled metal baking dish, sometimes with higher sides. Casserole dishes come in a variety of shapes and sizes and often come with lids. They are typically more aesthetically pleasing than baking pans, so they can be used for both baking and serving.

Dutch oven: This versatile pot can be used on the stovetop or in the oven. A heavy enameled pot is best, but a small stockpot with ovenproof handles and a tight-fitting lid will do the job. A 7-quart or 8-quart Dutch oven is the most useful size.

Garlic press: Whenever a recipe calls for crushed garlic, a garlic press is a required tool. Look for one that includes a reverse-side matching grid of blunt pins to clean out the holes of the press.

Grater: A flat or box-shaped tool that typically can be used to zest (or finely grate), coarsely grate, shred, or slice many different foods. The easiest type to use is a box grater, which also gives you the most versatility.

Ladle: Look for a large bowl that makes it easy to serve soups. A bent handle at the top enables you to hook the ladle on the side of a pot to keep it from falling in.

Knives: I emphasize the importance of having high-quality sharp knives. Sharp knives are much safer than dull ones—not only are you less likely to cut yourself, but should you accidentally slice a finger, a wound from a sharp blade heals much faster than one from a dull blade. Rather than buy an expensive knife set, you can purchase high-quality knives individually to get you through prep to serving.

- **Chef's knife:** A knife with a large triangular blade, typically 6 to 9 inches long, used for chopping, slicing, dicing, and mincing.
- **Paring knife:** A knife with a small triangular blade, typically 3 inches long, used for paring and cutting fruits and vegetables.
- **Utility knife:** A knife with a medium triangular blade, typically 4 to 6 inches long and thinner than a chef's knife blade, used for a variety of tasks in the kitchen.
- **Serrated knife:** A knife with a saw-like edge, typically at least 6 inches long, useful for slicing fruits and vegetables with waxy surfaces, such as tomatoes, watermelons, citrus fruits, and peppers.

Measuring cups and spoons: Having a way to measure your ingredients is an essential part of following any recipe. You will need a variety of sizes, from ¼ teaspoon to 1 tablespoon for measuring spoons, from ¼ cup to 1 cup for dry measuring cups, and from 1 cup to 8 cups for liquid measuring cups.

Meat thermometer: Using a meat thermometer ensures that you won't overcook your meat. Look for an oven-safe meat thermometer so you can stick the probe into your meat at the beginning of cooking and monitor the internal temperature throughout the cooking process. Digital thermometers (with an oven-safe probe and a display that remains outside the oven) often have alarms that you can set to go off when your meat reaches the desired temperature. Note that grass-fed and pasture-raised meats tend to cook faster than conventionally raised meats, and the time it takes the meat to reach the target internal temperature can vary by farm and by season.

Metal spatula: Often called a flipper, a metal spatula is a necessity for turning foods. An offset, thin blade allows you to get under delicate items like pancakes. A medium-length blade keeps you from picking up foods at an awkward angle.

Rimmed baking sheet: Also known as a jellyroll pan, a rimmed baking sheet has a low lip on all four sides to keep juices from dripping into your oven.

Roasting pan: A large, deep pan typically made of stainless steel, enameled steel, or aluminum. A low, open roasting pan with a rack is the most versatile type.

Rubber spatula: Useful for mixing and folding batters and scraping the sides of a bowl or pot to ensure that all the contents get poured into the target container. Silicone spatulas are heat resistant and can be used in hot pots.

Saucepan: A small pot ranging from 1 quart to 4 quarts in size (it's nice to have a couple of different sizes) and typically about 4 inches deep, with a tight-fitting lid. Look for ovenproof saucepans for the most versatility.

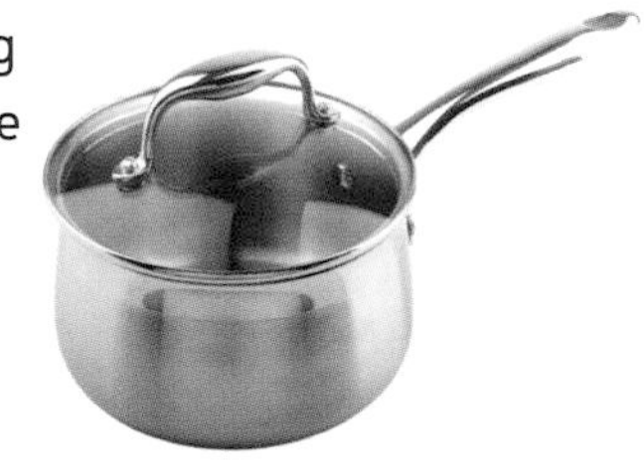

Saucepot: A deep, wide, and fairly light pot used for making soups and stews. A pot between 5 quarts and 8 quarts with a tight-fitting lid will be the most useful.

Scissors and shears: A good pair of kitchen scissors comes in handy for opening food packages, cutting strings, snipping fresh herbs, cutting bacon, and trimming artichoke leaves—to name just a few uses. Shears, which are larger and spring-loaded, make sectioning poultry and cutting pork skins much simpler. Look for sturdy models that are easy to clean.

Sharpening or honing steel: A rod of coated steel used to maintain sharp knife blades.

Sieve or strainer: This tool can be used to sift dry ingredients (like coconut flour) and to strain liquids (like broth). It's handy to have a few different sizes.

Skillet: A 10-inch or 12-inch cast-iron skillet is a wonderful investment. Enamel-lined skillets are more expensive but have the benefit of not requiring seasoning. It's also useful to have a 10-inch or 12-inch stainless-steel skillet, which is great for browning meat and then deglazing.

Slotted spoon: A large spoon with holes in the bowl that is used for scooping solid foods out of a liquid. Pick a sturdy spoon with a stainless-steel handle that won't get too hot.

Steamer basket or insert: While you can "steam" veggies in a regular pot with just a little bit of water, a steamer basket or insert does a much better job of retaining nutrients and preserving taste and texture. A collapsible-style metal steamer basket can fit into pots and pans of various sizes. A two-tier steamer pan looks like a double boiler (in which you boil water in the bottom pan to heat the top pan, which fits inside it) but with holes in the bottom and sides to let steam through. A bamboo steamer fits into a wok or over a pot of simmering liquid.

Stir spoons: Having a variety of sturdy spoons for stirring soups, stews, batters, sautéed vegetables, and other similar items is a must.

Stockpot: A tall, narrow, and very large pot used for cooking soups and stocks as well as bulky foods like lobster. Look for at least a 10-quart size; 12 quarts or 16 quarts is even better.

Tongs: Useful for picking up slippery, hot, or messy foods to flip, move, or serve them without piercing them (especially useful for flipping and serving meat). Select a style with nonslip handles and scalloped tips for a firm grip.

Vegetable peeler: While you can use a paring knife to peel vegetables, a vegetable peeler is an inexpensive tool that saves so much time in the kitchen that it makes the essentials list. A swivel blade removes less peel than a fixed blade since it conforms to the shape of the vegetable; however, a fixed blade gives you more control.

Whisk: A tool that has thick wire loops attached to a handle, a whisk can be used to mix sauces, batters, gravies, salad dressings, and dips. Different sizes are suited to different tasks, but a medium to large whisk will get most of these jobs done.

Zester (or Microplane grater): If your box grater doesn't have a side for very fine grating (or zesting), then a zester is a must. When pulled across citrus fruit, it removes only the peel, leaving the bitter pith underneath. A Microplane grater can also be used to grate garlic, ginger, and whole spices like nutmeg.

Nonessential (But Awesome to Have) Tools

You can cook glorious meals with very simple tools. There are, however, a variety of additional gadgets and small appliances that will save you time and energy in the kitchen. And when you are embarking on a diet and lifestyle change that requires you to prepare your own food, any time-saver is hugely appreciated.

Barbecue or indoor grill: Let's be honest: food cooked on a barbecue is just plain delicious. Whether you opt for a gas grill or a charcoal grill is a matter of personal choice. An electric indoor grill does all the same jobs, typically with less hassle, but the flavor it imparts is not quite the same.

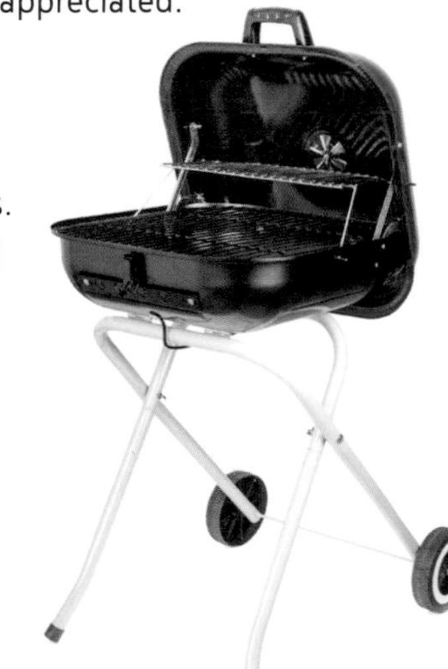

Blender: A high-powered, high-quality blender can do so much more than a standard blender. It is definitely an investment, but one that pays off in time saved in the kitchen.

Citrus juicer: Whether you choose a simple glass mold on which to smash citrus halves or a sophisticated electric model, a citrus juicer is much more efficient at extracting juice, especially from lemons and limes, than simply crushing the fruit with your fingers. Tip: Roll the whole fruit on the countertop while applying some pressure with your palm before slicing it in half to juice. This breaks up the fibers of the fruit and makes juicing easier, faster, and more efficient.

Countertop deep-fryer: If you plan to deep-fry foods, you have two options: a large, heavy-bottomed stovetop pot with an oil thermometer or a countertop deep-fryer that controls the temperature for you. Countertop deep-fryers tend to make less of a mess than a pot on the stove due to their built-in vented lids, and the temperature control feature ensures that the fat comes back up to temperature as quickly as possible after you add your food without heating it above its smoke point. There are many options in terms of size and amount of fat required. Models with the heating element under the fat compartment (as opposed to submerged in the fat) tend to require less fat. See page 467 for deep-frying basics.

Dehydrator: Dehydrators range from simple, low-powered, super-inexpensive versions to sophisticated programmable models. They open up a whole new range of cooking options, from drying your own fruits and vegetables (for snacking or for use in soups and stews) to making homemade vegetable flours and jerky.

Food processor: A food processor with a few different blades, especially for grating and slicing in addition to processing, is a tremendous time-saver. Certain jobs, like pureeing plantains, shredding cabbage for coleslaw, or slicing root vegetables extra-thin to make potato chips, go so much faster with a good food processor. Look for one that comes with different-sized bowls for versatility.

Freezer: A freezer isn't really a cooking tool, but it's such a handy appliance when you're making your own food from scratch, buying meat by the quarter or half animal, and batch cooking for quick meals that it deserves a spot on the list. Look for one that isn't frost-free. While you'll have to sacrifice some time to thaw your freezer to defrost it every year or two, the food you store in your freezer will have double or triple the storage life (the temperature swings of a frost-free freezer can cause freezer burn). Bonus: A freezer without the frost-free feature is typically much cheaper. Chest freezers tend to be the least expensive options, whereas upright freezers are easier to keep organized.

Grill pan: An alternative to using a barbecue or an electric indoor grill, this combination griddle/grill provides a versatile way to cook foods with less cooking fat than frying to better replicate the dry heat of a barbecue. The bottom surface is ridged, allowing fat to drip away. Use a grill pan over high heat for the best results.

Ice cream maker: One of the simplest and healthiest Paleo treats you can make is homemade ice cream or sorbet. Ice cream makers range from hand-crank options that use ice and rock salt in an outer compartment to freeze your mixture to electric models with a chamber that is stored in your freezer until ready to use to fully automated and programmable models with a self-refrigerating compressor.

Juicer: While I hope you are eating whole vegetables rather than juicing to get your greens, an inexpensive home juicer can be a useful tool. It can replace a citrus juicer in addition to being used for smoothies or added to soups, stews, and desserts in place of water or broth. You probably won't use a juicer often, so look for a cheap one that will get the job done.

Mandoline: This gadget speeds things up in my kitchen like no other tool. It slices, minces, and juliennes, and for small to medium-sized jobs it is often much faster to clean than a food processor (which can't slice long slices or julienne like a mandoline can). Look for a mandoline with several different blades for versatility. And always use the finger guard!

Meat grinder: You will likely find yourself grinding meat at home when adopting the Paleo template, mainly as a strategy to camouflage organ meat. While you can grind meat in a food processor, a meat grinder yields a better texture. You can find manual and electric countertop models or attachments for a stand mixer.

Pressure cooker: Stovetop pressure cookers are less expensive, but I recommend a digital countertop model. A programmable pressure cooker gives you the flexibility of setting a timer and has many built-in safety features. There are also all-in-one multi-cookers that enable you to sear meat and steam vegetables and even have slow-cooking and yogurt-making functions.

Salad spinner: While a colander and paper towel can do a great job of removing excess water from washed leafy greens, a salad spinner does a better job, and does it more quickly. Look for one with a solid bowl for both swishing greens clean and serving them.

Sausage stuffer: Typically an attachment for a meat grinder (although standalone models exist), a sausage stuffer is a must-have if you intend to stuff sausage mix into casings.

Silicone bakeware: If you plan to bake from this cookbook, having silicone muffin and cake pans is tremendously useful. Gluten-free baked goods can be hard to remove even from greased and "floured" (with arrowroot powder) pans, but silicone bakeware makes it a snap!

Silicone baking pan liners: Lining a baking pan with parchment paper or aluminum foil can make a huge difference in terms of cleanup. Silicone liners serve the same purpose and have the added benefit of being reusable and very versatile.

Smoker: While smoking your food isn't the healthiest method for everyday cooking, it's a fantastic treat; you just can't beat the taste of some foods cooked in a smoker! Look for one with a built-in thermometer and a mechanism for controlling the temperature. There are also smoker-barbecue hybrids, which give you two great cooking tools in one.

Spice grinder or mortar and pestle: The fresher your spices, the better their flavor. Freshly grinding whole spices like mace arils, cloves, cinnamon sticks, and pink rock salt in an electric or manual spice grinder (or mashing them with a mortar and pestle) can have a huge positive impact. You can also use an electric spice grinder to make your own coconut flour, pumpkin flour, and plantain flour. A mortar and pestle can be used to crush fresh herbs to make a paste for seasoning meat.

Spiral slicer: Spiral-cut vegetables are a fun and nutrient-dense replacement for pasta. Look for a spiral slicer with several different-sized blades for flexibility in the shape of your finished product.

Stand mixer: A stand mixer probably won't see as much action in your kitchen while you follow the Paleo diet, but for some tasks a stand mixer is very useful. Some mixers come with a slot for attachments like meat grinders, sausage stuffers, and ice cream makers. It's always handy to have a tool that can do more than one thing.

Wok: A wok is a pan with a rounded bottom that is used for frying and steaming in Asian cooking. Woks are available in different materials and sizes, are relatively simple to use, and have advantages over flat-bottomed frying pans or skillets, namely a large cooking surface area and the ability to take advantage of both the hot area at the bottom of the pan to sear food and the lower temperature at the sides of the pan for slower cooking.

Yogurt maker: This inexpensive gadget is a must-have if you intend to make homemade coconut milk yogurt. Simple models have an on/off switch, whereas more sophisticated models include a timer.

Certainly, there are lots more fun time-saving gadgets that you may find useful. If you're anything like me, visiting a kitchen supply store is even better than shoe shopping! This list represents those tools that are suggested in this book's recipes. Feel free to expand on your current supply of kitchen gadgets with anything you think will save you time or make a task easier and/or safer.

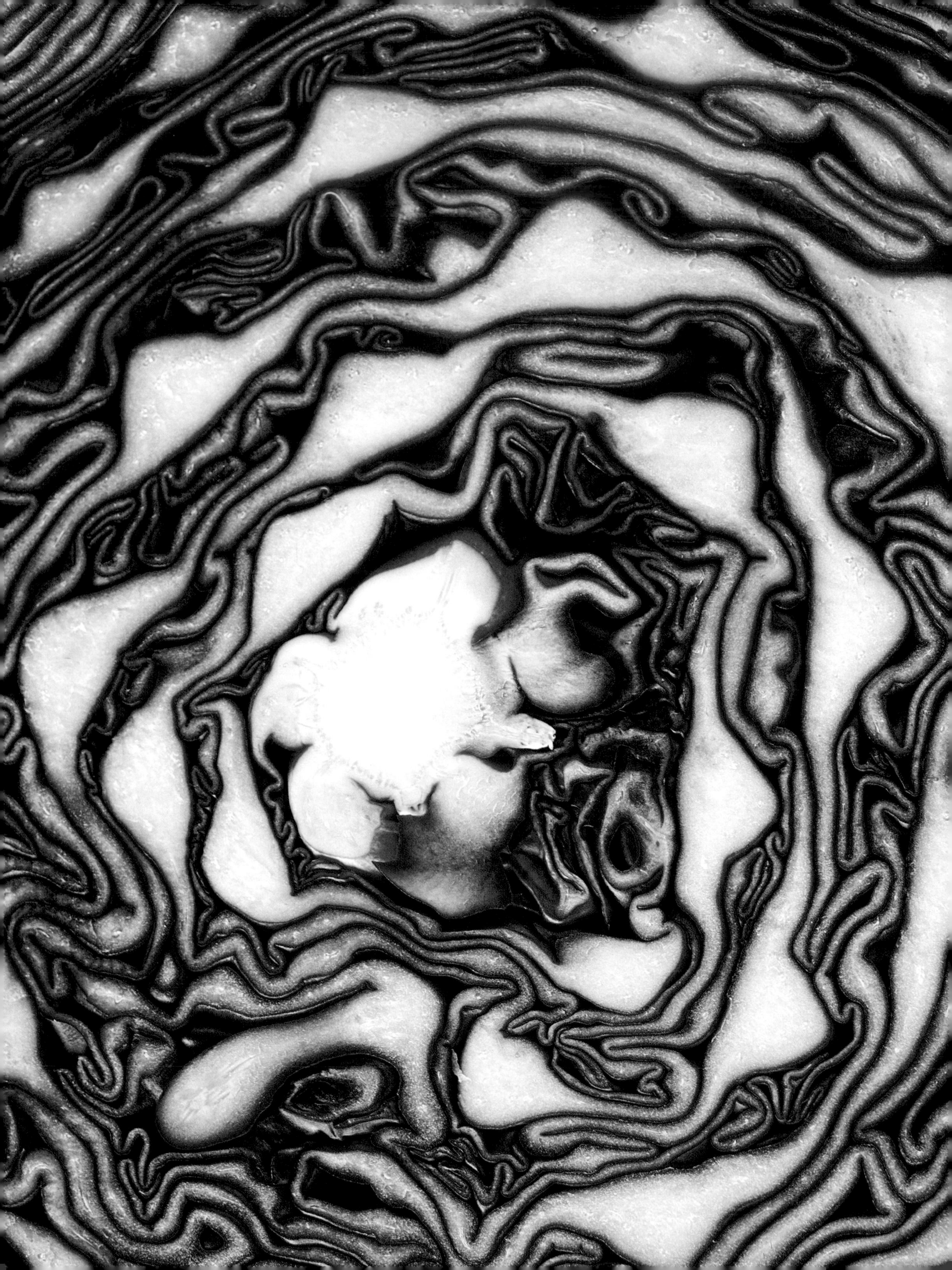

8.

RECIPES

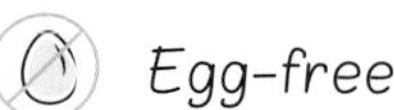
Egg-free

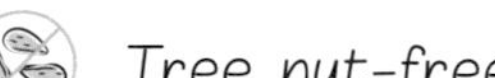
Tree nut-free

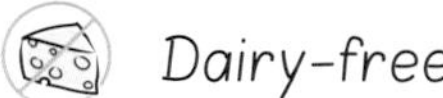
Dairy-free

Fish-free

Shellfish-free

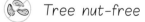

Coconut-free

Low-FODMAP

Nightshade-free

AIP Autoimmune Protocol compliant (see page 413)

★ Look for modifications below the recipe

Chapter 39:
KITCHEN BASICS

COCONUT MILK & CREAM

  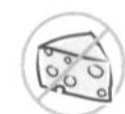 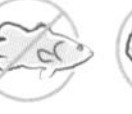 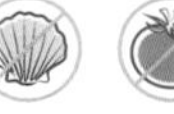 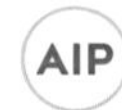 AIP

PREP TIME: 5 minutes

COOK TIME: 1 hour (hands-on time is about 5 minutes)

YIELD: 1 2/3 cups milk (equivalent to 1 [13 1/2-ounce] can) or 2/3 cup cream

2 cups finely shredded unsweetened dried coconut

2¾ cups water

1. To make coconut milk, combine the coconut and water in a saucepan and bring to a boil over high heat. Turn off the heat, cover, and let sit for 1 hour.

2. Pour the coconut and water into a blender. Blend on high for 2 to 5 minutes (less time for a high-powered blender, more time for other blenders), until the texture is thick and only slightly granular. Place a tea towel or other cloth over the lid of the blender and keep your hand over the top while the blender is running.

3. Pour the pulp into a nut milk bag, yogurt cheese bag, paint-straining bag, or fine-mesh strainer set over a glass bowl, mason jar, or measuring cup. Either let the coconut milk strain out by gravity or squeeze the pulp through the bag.

4. If not using immediately, store the coconut milk in a jar in the refrigerator for up to 2 weeks or in the freezer for up to 1 year. Shake well, blend, or gently warm before using.

5. To make coconut cream, complete Steps 1 through 4 and place the coconut milk in the refrigerator to chill thoroughly until the cream separates, at least 6 hours or overnight. Spoon the separated cream off the top. You can also do this with a can of coconut milk!

TIPS: You can make large batches of coconut milk and freeze it in freezer-safe mason jars so that you always have some handy. Make sure to leave an inch of space between the milk and the lid to allow for expansion.

Because there are no emulsifiers in this homemade coconut milk, it will naturally separate and be a little clumpy when chilled. If you want to drink the milk, blend it in a blender just before drinking.

It should go without saying, but never use a paint-straining bag for paint and then for food!

COCONUT WHIPPED TOPPING

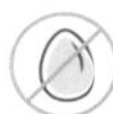 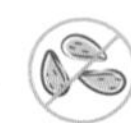 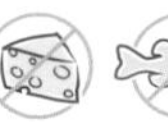 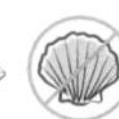 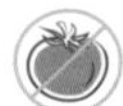 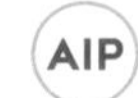 AIP

PREP TIME: 5 minutes, plus time to chill

YIELD: 2/3 to 3/4 cup

1 batch Coconut Milk (at left), 1 (13½-ounce) can full-fat coconut milk, or ⅔ cup chilled coconut cream (at left)

1. If using coconut cream, skip to Step 3. If using homemade or canned coconut milk, place the milk in the refrigerator to chill thoroughly, until the cream separates, at least 6 hours or overnight.

2. Spoon the separated cream off the top of the chilled coconut milk. Discard the watery liquid at the bottom or reserve it for smoothies.

3. Place the cream in a blender and blend on high for 1 minute. Then transfer the whipped topping to a jar and place in the refrigerator to chill for at least 1 hour. Coconut whipped topping will retain its texture for a day or two in the fridge, after which time you can repeat this step and chill the whipped topping again.

4. Serve over berries, sliced peaches, Waffles (page 503), or Crepes (page 505), or enjoy with your favorite dessert! Use within a week.

TIP: Anytime a recipe calls for coconut cream, you can use the separated cream off the top of a batch or can of chilled coconut milk.

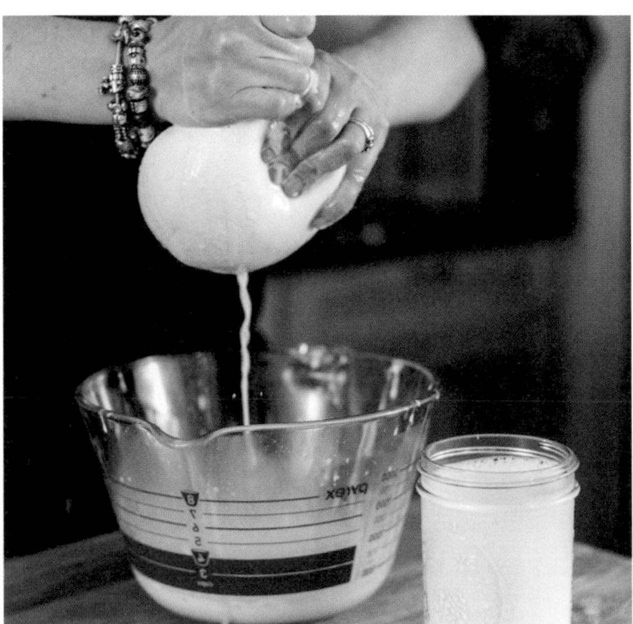

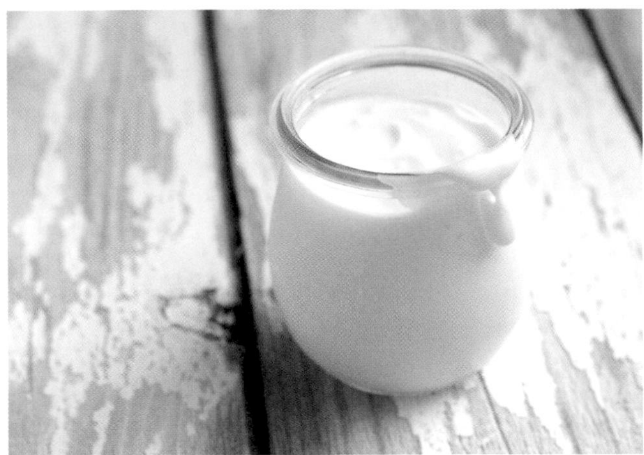

COCONUT MILK YOGURT

 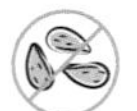 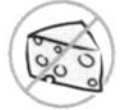 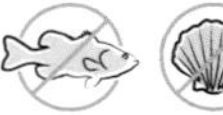  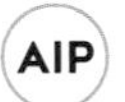 AIP

PREP TIME: 5 minutes, plus time to incubate and chill

COOK TIME: 5 minutes   YIELD: 1 3/4 cups

- 1 batch Coconut Milk (opposite), or 1 (13½-ounce) can full-fat coconut milk
- 1¼ teaspoons gelatin
- 2 teaspoons honey
- *Lactobacillus*-based probiotic capsule(s), 15 to 20 billion PFU (aka CFU)

1. Thoroughly clean or sterilize the jars you'll be using to make the yogurt.

2. Pour the coconut milk into a heatproof glass container to heat the milk in the microwave, or into a saucepan to heat the milk on the stovetop. Sprinkle the gelatin over the surface of the milk and wait 2 to 3 minutes for the gelatin to bloom (or absorb liquid). Stir the gelatin into the milk.

3. Heat the coconut milk to 120°F in the microwave or on the stovetop. (If you make this yogurt frequently, you'll quickly find out just how many seconds it takes to heat the milk perfectly—in my microwave, it takes 75 seconds.)

4. Stir thoroughly to make sure the gelatin is completely dissolved. Let the milk cool to 105°F. (Anywhere between 100°F and 110°F will work, but don't add your probiotic until the coconut milk is below 110°F.)

5. Stir in the honey. Open the probiotic capsule(s) and sprinkle the contents into the milk. Stir well.

6. Pour into the sterilized jar(s) and incubate in the yogurt maker for about 12 hours. (If the yogurt is too sour, incubate for a shorter period next time; if it's not sour enough, incubate it longer.)

7. Refrigerate the yogurt until the gelatin has set, 2 to 3 hours. Stir and enjoy! Store in the refrigerator for up to 10 days.

NUT & SEED MILKS

  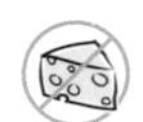 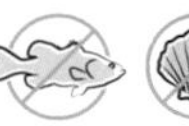 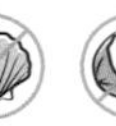  

PREP TIME: 15 minutes, plus time to soak

YIELD: about 4 cups

- 1 cup raw nuts or seeds, such as almonds, cashews, walnuts, or shelled sunflower seeds
- ½ teaspoon sea salt
- 4 cups water

1. Place the nuts or seeds in a bowl and pour enough water over them to cover by at least 1 inch. Add the salt. Cover the bowl and let soak at room temperature overnight or for up to 2 days.

2. Drain the nuts or seeds and rinse well.

3. Combine the soaked nuts or seeds with the water in a blender. Blend on high for 3 to 5 minutes.

4. Pour the pulp into a nut milk bag, yogurt cheese bag, paint-straining bag, or fine-mesh strainer set over a glass bowl, mason jar, or measuring cup. Either let the milk strain out by gravity or squeeze the pulp through the bag.

5. If not using immediately, store the milk in a jar in the refrigerator for up to a week or in the freezer for up to 3 months. Shake or blend before using, if desired.

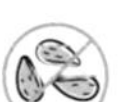 *use shelled sunflower seeds or pepitas*

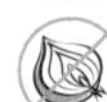 *avoid cashews or pistachios*

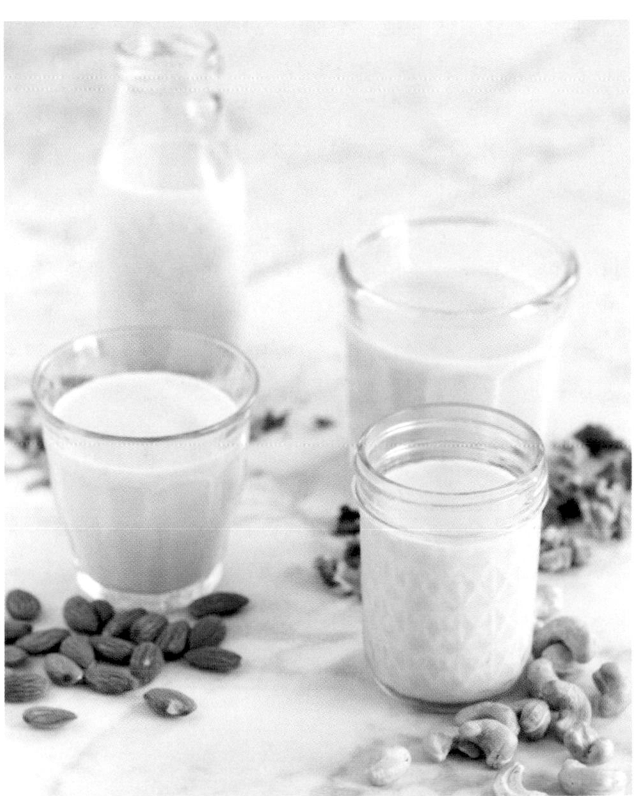

SPICE BLENDS

SIMPLE GREEK SEASONING

 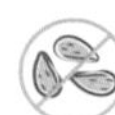 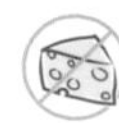 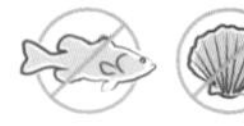 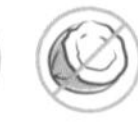  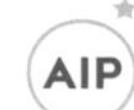 AIP

YIELD: 7 tablespoons

2 tablespoons dried lemon zest

2 tablespoons dried oregano leaves

2 tablespoons granulated garlic

1 tablespoon sea salt

1 teaspoon cracked black pepper

AIP *omit pepper*

ITALIAN SEASONING

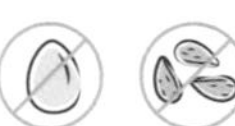  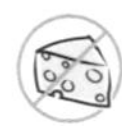 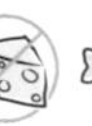 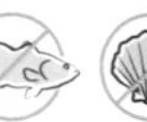 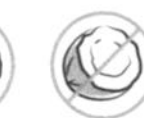  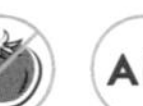 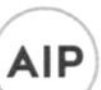

YIELD: 7 tablespoons

1 tablespoon dried marjoram leaves

1 tablespoon dried oregano leaves

1 tablespoon dried rosemary leaves

1 tablespoon dried savory

1 tablespoon dried thyme leaves

1 tablespoon granulated garlic

1 tablespoon sea salt

 *omit garlic*

ADOBO SEASONING

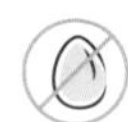 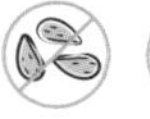 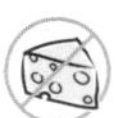 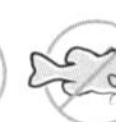  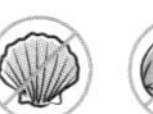 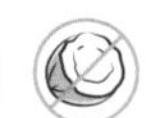  

YIELD: 10 tablespoons

3 tablespoons dried oregano leaves

2 tablespoons granulated garlic

2 tablespoons granulated onion

2 tablespoons sea salt

1 tablespoon cracked black pepper

AIP *omit pepper*

MONTREAL STEAK SEASONING

 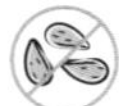 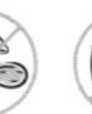 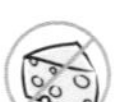 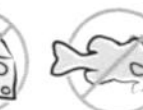  

YIELD: 10 tablespoons

2 tablespoons paprika

2 tablespoons sea salt

1½ tablespoons cracked black pepper

1 tablespoon dried dill

1 tablespoon granulated garlic

1 tablespoon granulated onion

1 tablespoon ground coriander

½ to 1 tablespoon red pepper flakes, to taste

AIP POULTRY SEASONING

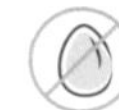 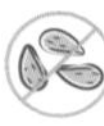 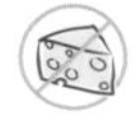  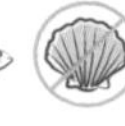 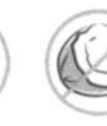  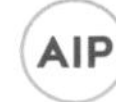

YIELD: 13 tablespoons

3 tablespoons dried savory

3 tablespoons granulated garlic

3 tablespoons sea salt

2 tablespoons dried thyme leaves

1 tablespoon dried marjoram leaves

1 tablespoon granulated onion

AIP HERBES DE PROVENCE

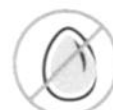 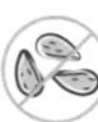 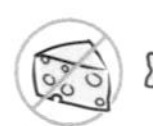 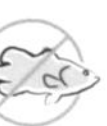  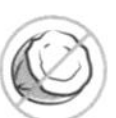 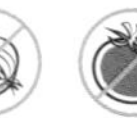 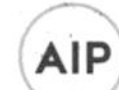

YIELD: 10 tablespoons

3 tablespoons dried marjoram leaves

3 tablespoons dried savory

3 tablespoons dried thyme leaves

1 teaspoon dried oregano leaves

1 teaspoon dried rosemary leaves

1 teaspoon dried tarragon

½ teaspoon dried rubbed sage

AIP STEAK SEASONING

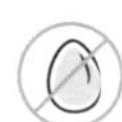  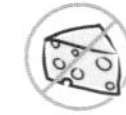 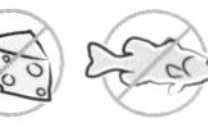  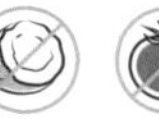 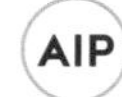

YIELD: 5 tablespoons

3 tablespoons truffle salt

1 tablespoon turmeric powder

1 teaspoon granulated garlic

1 teaspoon granulated onion

1 teaspoon dried oregano leaves

KOWLOON CURRY

 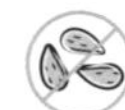 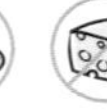 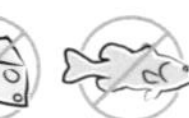 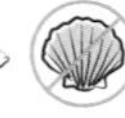 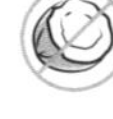 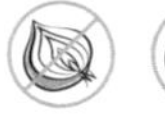 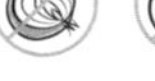

YIELD: about 3/4 cup

5 tablespoons ground coriander

2 tablespoons turmeric powder

1 tablespoon anise seeds, ground

1 tablespoon fenugreek seeds, ground

1 tablespoon ginger powder

1 tablespoon ground cumin

2 teaspoons ground cinnamon

2 teaspoons red mustard seeds, ground

1 teaspoon ground black pepper

NIGHTSHADE-FREE CURRY POWDER

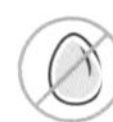 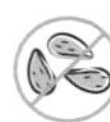 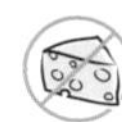 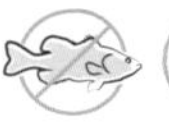 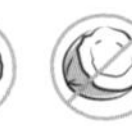 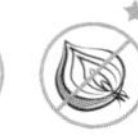 

YIELD: about 1/2 cup

- 2 tablespoons turmeric powder
- 1 tablespoon ground coriander
- 1 tablespoon ground cumin
- 1 tablespoon ginger powder
- 1½ teaspoons ground cardamom
- 1½ teaspoons mustard powder
- 1½ teaspoons sea salt
- ¾ teaspoon anise seeds, ground
- ¾ teaspoon caraway seeds, ground
- ¾ teaspoon granulated garlic
- ¾ teaspoon ground black pepper
- ¾ teaspoon ground cinnamon

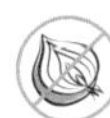 *omit garlic*

PORK SEASONING

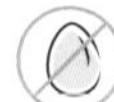  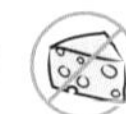 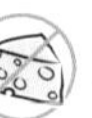 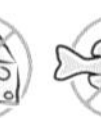 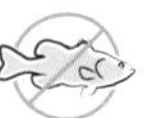  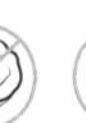 

YIELD: 1/2 cup

- 3 tablespoons sea salt
- 1 tablespoon anise seeds, ground
- 2 tablespoons fennel seeds, ground
- 2 tablespoons dried tarragon

JERK SPICE

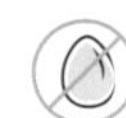 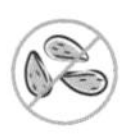 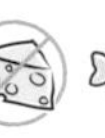 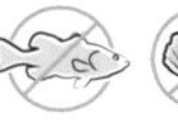  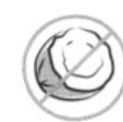 

YIELD: about 1/2 cup

- 2 tablespoons dried ground thyme
- 1½ tablespoons sea salt
- 1 tablespoon ground allspice
- 1 tablespoon ground coriander
- 1 tablespoon ginger powder
- 2 teaspoons ground dried Scotch bonnet or habanero peppers (optional)
- 1½ teaspoons ground cinnamon
- 1½ teaspoons granulated onion
- 1 teaspoon granulated garlic
- ¼ teaspoon ground cloves

1. Combine the spices in a spice shaker or spice jar. (If you don't have a spice shaker, you can sprinkle the blends into food by hand or dust with a sieve.)

2. Store in the pantry for up to 6 months or freeze for up to 2 years.

TIP: For spices that need to be ground before being added to your spice blend, use a spice grinder, mini food processor, or mortar and pestle to grind them.

 *omit hot peppers*

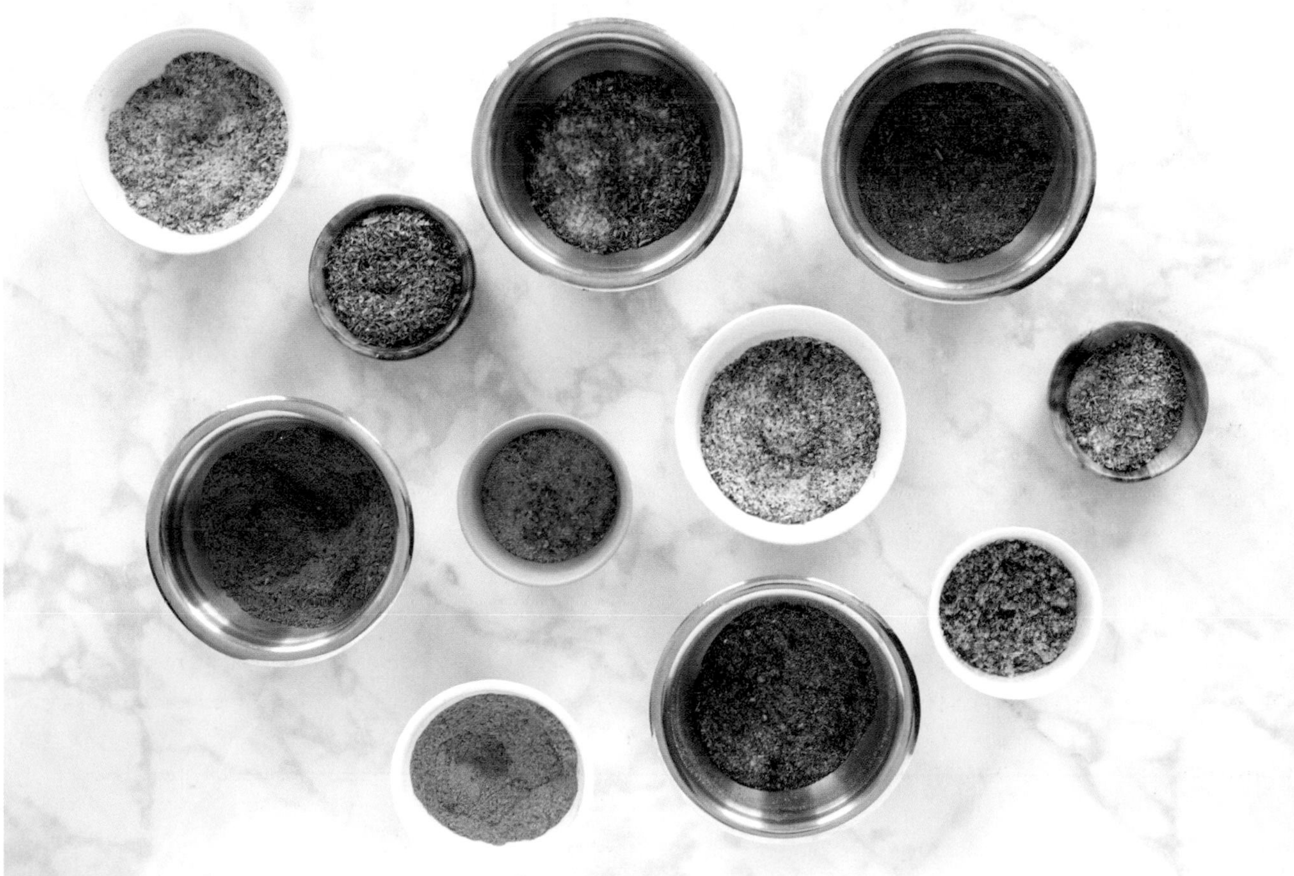

SALAD DRESSINGS

BASIC VINAIGRETTE

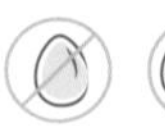 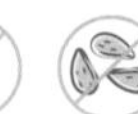 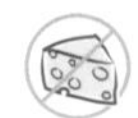 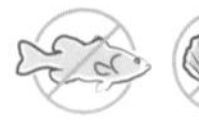 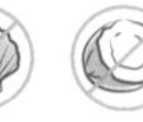 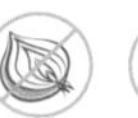  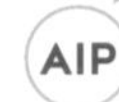 AIP*

YIELD: 1/3 cup

3 tablespoons oil, such as olive, avocado, walnut, or macadamia nut

2 tablespoons acidic liquid, such as lemon juice, lime juice, apple cider vinegar, balsamic vinegar, coconut water vinegar, or white or red wine vinegar

⅛ teaspoon ground black pepper (optional)

Pinch of sea salt

AIP *omit pepper; use olive oil or avocado oil*

HONEY-MUSTARD VINAIGRETTE

 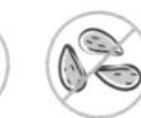 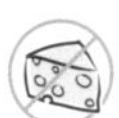 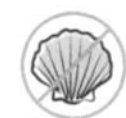 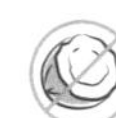 

YIELD: 1/2 cup

3 tablespoons olive oil

2 teaspoons honey

2 teaspoons Dijon mustard

2 tablespoons lemon juice

2 tablespoons white wine, kombucha, or white wine vinegar

1 anchovy

GREEN GODDESS DRESSING

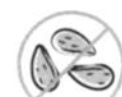 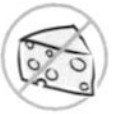  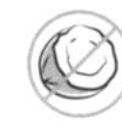 

YIELD: 1 cup

½ cup Mayonnaise (page 487)

½ cup chopped fresh parsley

¼ cup full-fat coconut milk, homemade (page 480) or canned

1½ tablespoons red wine vinegar

1 teaspoon anchovy paste

¼ teaspoon cracked black pepper (optional)

THAI SALAD DRESSING

 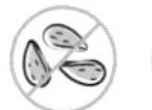 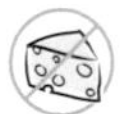 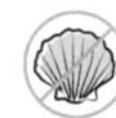 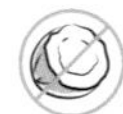  AIP

YIELD: scant 1/2 cup

¼ cup lime juice (about 2 limes)

2 tablespoons fish sauce

2 tablespoons chopped fresh cilantro

1 tablespoon chopped fresh mint

1 clove garlic, crushed to a coarse paste

½ teaspoon honey

CREAMY BALSAMIC DRESSING

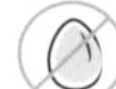 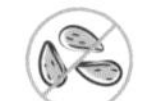 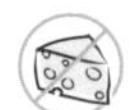  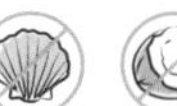 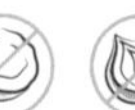 

YIELD: 3/4 cup

½ cup balsamic vinegar

¼ cup olive oil

1 tablespoon Dijon mustard

Pinch of sea salt or truffle salt

GREEK SALAD DRESSING

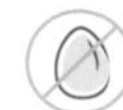 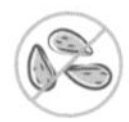 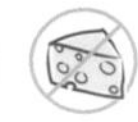  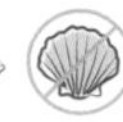 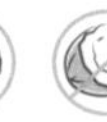 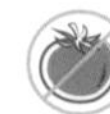 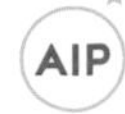

YIELD: 1 cup

½ cup olive oil

⅓ cup apple cider vinegar or red wine vinegar

1 teaspoon finely grated lemon zest

2 tablespoons lemon juice

2 cloves garlic, crushed to a coarse paste

1 teaspoon dried oregano leaves

⅛ teaspoon sea salt

Pinch of cracked black pepper

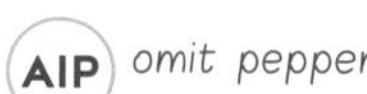 *omit pepper*

ITALIAN VINAIGRETTE

 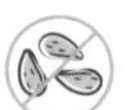 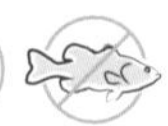 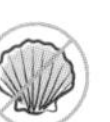 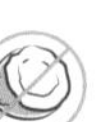 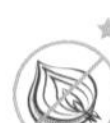 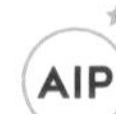

YIELD: 2/3 cup

6 tablespoons olive oil

¼ cup apple cider vinegar

¼ teaspoon dried marjoram leaves

¼ teaspoon dried oregano leaves

¼ teaspoon dried rosemary leaves

¼ teaspoon dried savory

¼ teaspoon dried thyme leaves

1 clove garlic, crushed to a coarse paste

Pinch of sea salt

Pinch of cracked black pepper

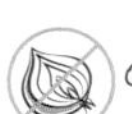 *omit garlic*

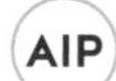 *omit pepper*

CAESAR SALAD DRESSING

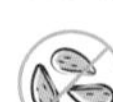 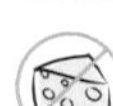  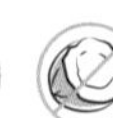 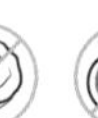

YIELD: 1/2 cup

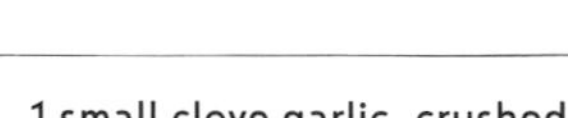

⅓ cup Mayonnaise (page 487)

2 tablespoons lemon juice

1 teaspoon anchovy paste

1 small clove garlic, crushed to a coarse paste

⅛ teaspoon cracked black pepper

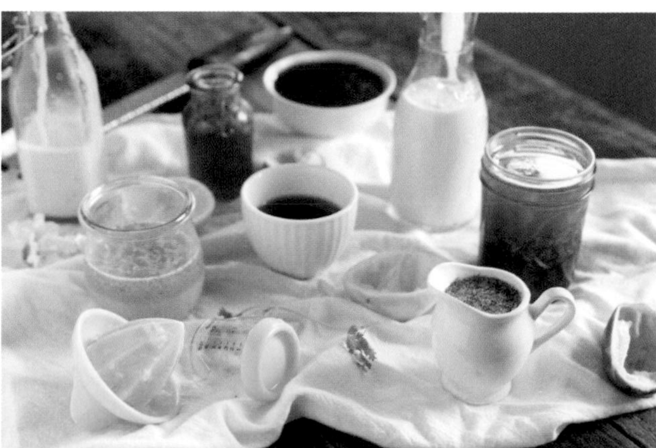

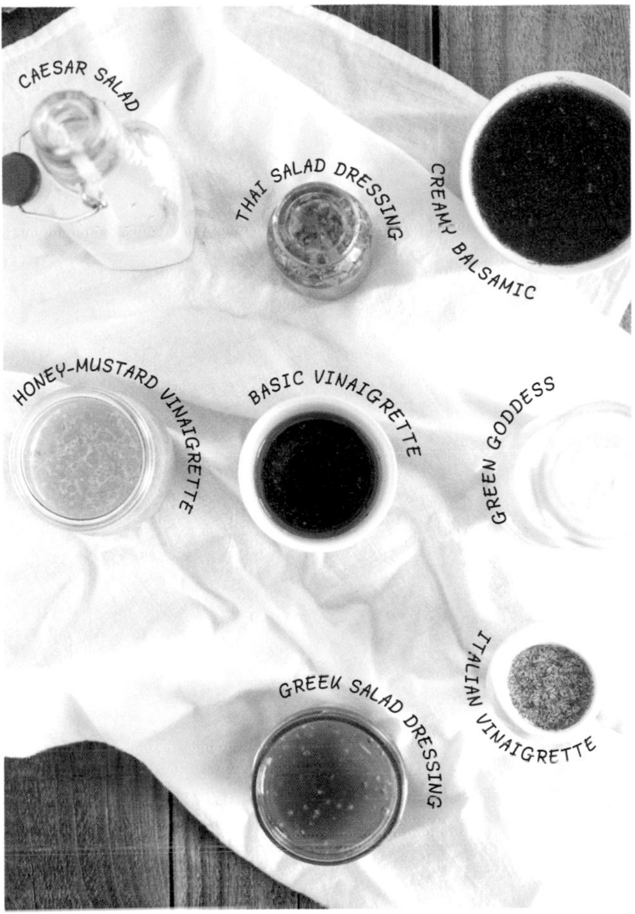

1. Combine all the ingredients in a blender and blend until thoroughly combined. (If making the Basic Vinaigrette, simply combine the ingredients in a jar and shake before serving.)

2. Pour the dressing into a bottle or jar. Serve immediately or place in the refrigerator until ready to use. Allow the dressing to warm to room temperature before serving (take the bottle out of the fridge about 30 minutes before mealtime). Shake before serving.

3. The Thai Salad Dressing will keep in the refrigerator for up to 4 days. The other dressings will keep for about a month.

TIP: It's usually best to dress a salad right before serving it. For recipes like Paleo Caesar Salad (page 520), you may choose to assemble half the batch and store the leftover components separately until you plan to eat the remaining servings.

LARD OR TALLOW

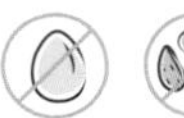  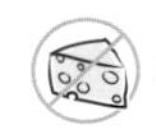 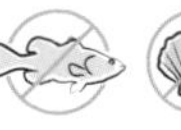 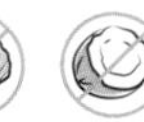   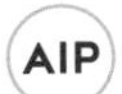 AIP

PREP TIME: 5 minutes
COOK TIME: 1 hour per pound of fat
YIELD: 1 pint tallow or lard per pound of fat

1 to 5 pounds animal fat, ground or cut into 1-inch or smaller cubes

1. Place the fat in a large, heavy pot and cover with a lid. Set on the stovetop over low heat.

2. Cook for about 1 hour per pound of fat, stirring every 30 to 45 minutes to dislodge any sticky bits from the bottom of the pot. The lard or tallow is ready when all the fat has melted. (There will be some bits that look like ground beef as well.) The exact cooking time will vary depending on the type of fat and the size of the pieces.

3. Place a metal sieve over a jar, measuring cup, or glass bowl. Line the sieve with a single sheet of paper towel. Pour the tallow or lard through the lined sieve into the jar. The strained bits can be added to scrambled eggs, soup, or stew for extra flavor or discarded. Let the lard or tallow cool before putting the lid on the jar.

4. Store at room temperature out of direct sunlight for up to 3 months or in the refrigerator or freezer for up to 2 years.

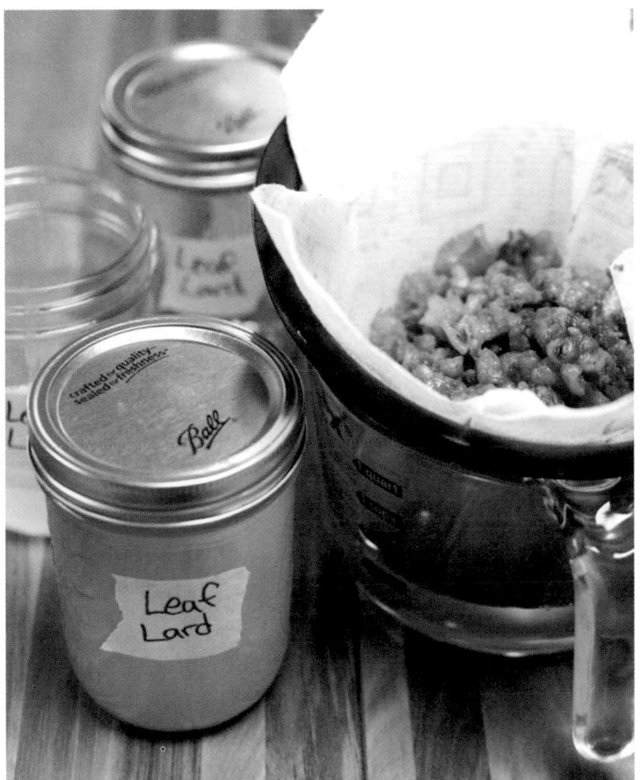

BONE STOCK

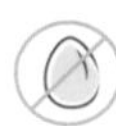  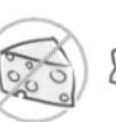  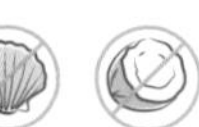   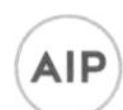 AIP

 *omit garlic and onion (all varieties)*

PREP TIME: 10 minutes COOK TIME: 4 hours to 5 days

YIELD: 8 to 10 cups

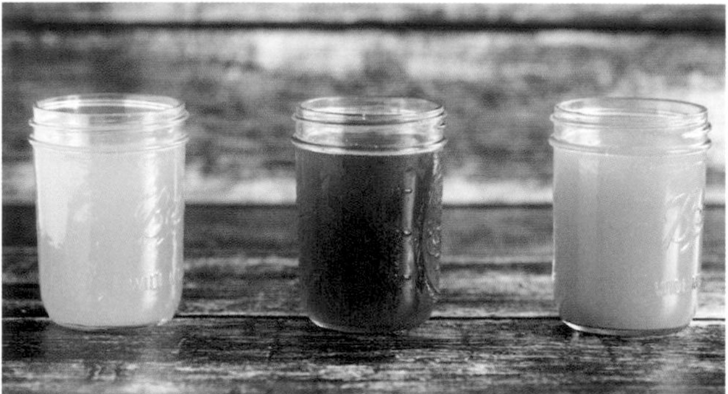

FISH STOCK

2 to 4 pounds fish heads, tails, and bones

1 gallon water, or enough to cover the bones by 1 to 2 inches

1 tablespoon apple cider vinegar

1 medium-sized yellow onion or 2 medium leeks, roots cut off, quartered

3 to 4 stalks celery, cut into thirds

1 to 2 carrots, cut in half

1. Combine all the ingredients in a stockpot. Bring to a boil over high heat, then reduce the heat to maintain a simmer. Alternatively, cook under high pressure in a pressure cooker, or bring to a boil and then reduce the heat to low in a slow cooker.

2. During the first hour of cooking, skim off any foam that rises to the surface. (This improves the flavor of the final stock.) You don't need to do so if you're using a pressure cooker.

3. Simmer, covered, for 3 to 4 hours (or 1 to 2 hours in a pressure cooker or 6 to 8 hours in a slow cooker). Periodically stir and check the water level, topping off with additional water if needed to keep the ingredients covered by an inch or two of water.

4. Strain the stock and discard the bones and vegetables. Store the stock in the refrigerator for up to 5 days or in the freezer for up to 6 months.

TIPS: You can substitute 1 cup of white wine for 1 cup of the water in the fish stock if you like.

When a recipe calls for bone stock but doesn't specify which kind, you can use any of the above varieties that you have on hand.

CHICKEN OR TURKEY STOCK

2 to 3 pounds chicken or turkey bones (from 2 to 3 roasting chickens or 1 turkey; include giblets and feet if desired)

1 gallon water, or enough to cover the bones by 1 to 2 inches

1 tablespoon apple cider vinegar

2 medium-sized yellow onions, roots cut off, quartered

6 to 8 stalks celery, cut into thirds

4 to 5 carrots, cut in half

6 to 8 cloves garlic

3 bay leaves

1 teaspoon sea salt

BEEF, BISON, LAMB, OR PORK STOCK

2 to 3 pounds beef, bison, lamb, or pork bones

1 gallon water, or enough to cover the bones by 1 to 2 inches

1 tablespoon apple cider vinegar

2 medium-sized yellow onions, roots cut off, quartered

1 teaspoon whole cloves (omit for pork stock)

3 bay leaves

1 teaspoon sea salt

1. Combine the bones, water, and vinegar in a stockpot. Bring to a boil over high heat, then reduce the heat to maintain a simmer. Alternatively, cook under high pressure in a pressure cooker, or bring to a boil and then reduce the heat to low in a slow cooker.

2. During the first hour of cooking, skim off any foam that rises to the surface. (This improves the flavor of the final stock.) You don't need to do so if you're using a pressure cooker.

3. Simmer, covered, for 24 to 48 hours (or 6 to 12 hours in a pressure cooker or 2 to 5 days in a slow cooker). Periodically stir and check the water level, topping off with additional water if needed to keep the ingredients covered by an inch or two of water.

4. Add the remaining ingredients. Simmer for an additional 4 to 6 hours (or 1 to 2 hours in a pressure cooker or 6 to 8 hours in a slow cooker).

5. Strain the stock and discard the bones and vegetables. Store the stock in the refrigerator for up to 5 days or in the freezer for up to 6 months.

DIPS AND SPREADS

MAYONNAISE

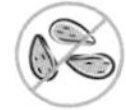 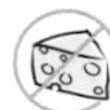 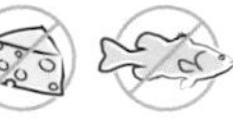 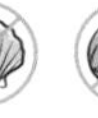 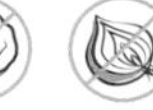 

PREP TIME: 5 minutes *YIELD: a little over 1 cup*

- ½ cup avocado oil
- ½ cup olive oil
- 1 tablespoon lemon juice
- 1½ teaspoons apple cider vinegar
- 1 tablespoon Dijon mustard
- 2 large egg yolks

IN A BLENDER OR FOOD PROCESSOR:

1. Combine the avocado oil and olive oil in a measuring cup with a pour spout.

2. Place the lemon juice, vinegar, mustard, and egg yolks in a food processor or blender. Process until creamy, about 15 seconds.

3. With the blender or food processor running, very slowly drizzle in the oil. It should take at least 3 minutes to add all the oil. The mixture should thicken and gradually lighten in color as you add the oil.

4. If you see any oil that isn't well incorporated, pour the mayonnaise into a bowl and whip it by hand with a whisk. (If you have a really good food processor, you probably won't need to do so.)

5. Store in the refrigerator for up to 5 days.

WITH AN IMMERSION BLENDER:

1. Combine the lemon juice, vinegar, mustard, and egg yolks in the immersion blender jar.

2. Place the immersion blender in the jar, covering the ingredients added in Step 1, then pour the avocado oil and olive oil into the jar.

3. Turn on the immersion blender and slowly pull it upward. Take 15 to 20 seconds to lift it to the surface. The ingredients will turn to mayonnaise nearly instantly.

4. Store in the refrigerator for up to 5 days.

TIP: The CDC estimates that only 1 in 20,000 eggs is contaminated with salmonella. To reduce your risk of salmonella poisoning, use pasteurized eggs in this recipe.

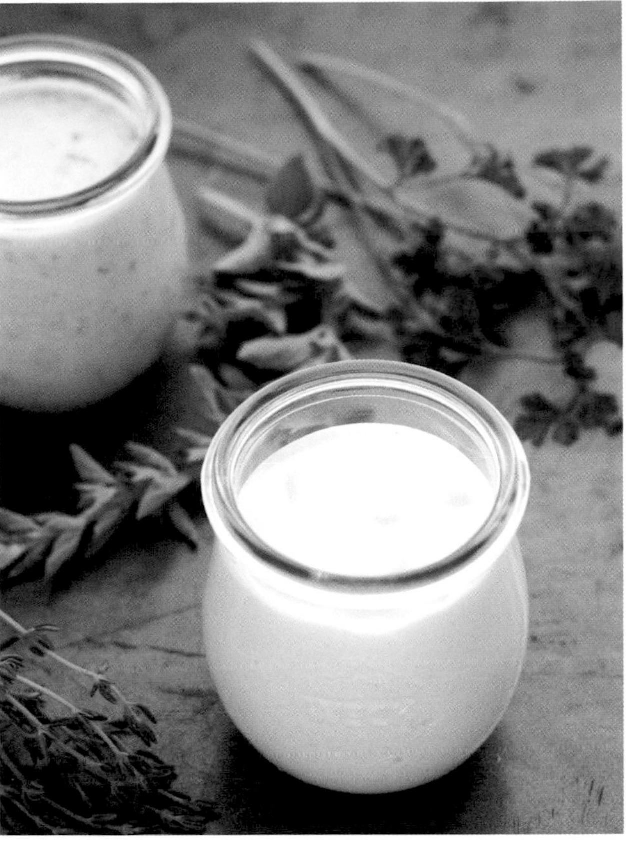

RANCH DIP

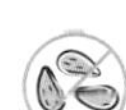 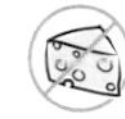 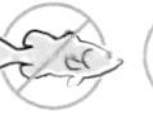  

PREP TIME: 5 minutes *YIELD: about 1 cup*

- ¼ cup coconut cream, homemade (page 480) or store-bought
- 1 tablespoon fresh oregano, chopped
- 1 tablespoon fresh parsley, chopped
- ½ teaspoon fresh thyme
- ½ teaspoon granulated garlic
- ¼ teaspoon sea salt
- ⅛ teaspoon ground black pepper
- ½ cup Mayonnaise (at left)

1. Combine the coconut cream, herbs, granulated garlic, salt, and pepper in a blender and blend until smooth.

2. Transfer the dip to a bowl. Place in the refrigerator to chill for 20 minutes if there is any residual heat from blending.

3. Stir in the mayonnaise and serve. Store in the refrigerator for up to 5 days.

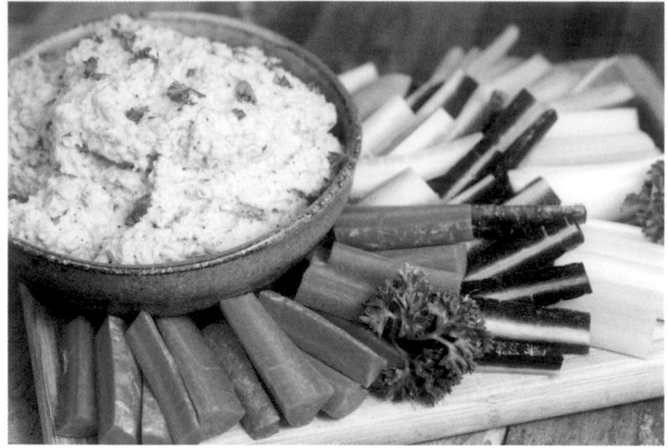

CAULIFLOWER HUMMUS

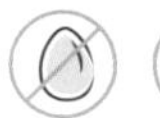 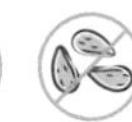 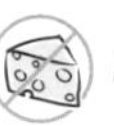 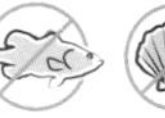 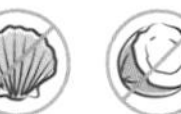 

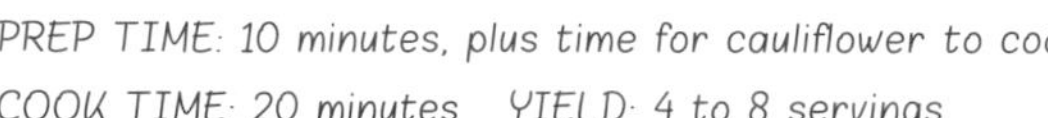

PREP TIME: 10 minutes, plus time for cauliflower to cool
COOK TIME: 20 minutes YIELD: 4 to 8 servings

- 6 cups cauliflower florets
- ¼ cup plus 2 tablespoons olive oil, divided
- ⅓ cup tahini
- Juice of 2 lemons
- 1 clove garlic, crushed to a coarse paste
- ½ teaspoon sea salt
- ¼ teaspoon ground cumin

1. Preheat the oven to 425°F.

2. In a bowl, toss the cauliflower florets with 2 tablespoons of the olive oil. Place on a rimmed baking sheet and roast until tender and starting to brown, about 20 minutes. Let cool completely.

3. Combine the roasted cauliflower with the remaining ingredients in a blender or food processor. Process until the mixture reaches hummus consistency. Taste and add more salt, if desired. If the hummus is too thick, add more olive oil or water to thin it.

4. Pour the hummus into a bowl and serve. Store in the refrigerator for up to a week.

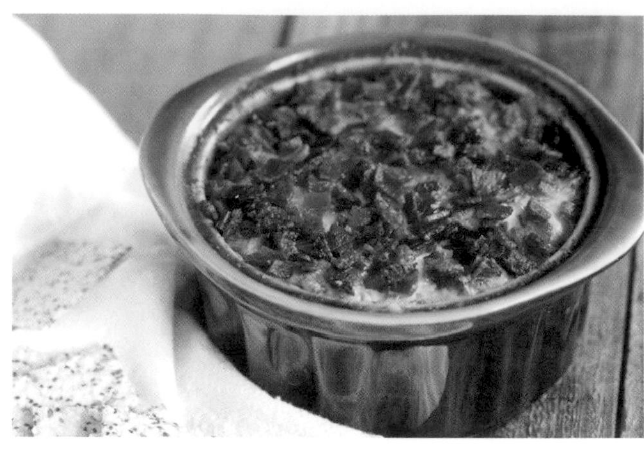

HOT ARTICHOKE DIP

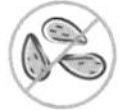 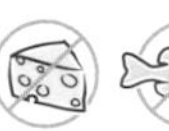 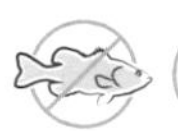  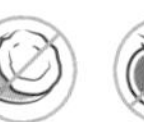

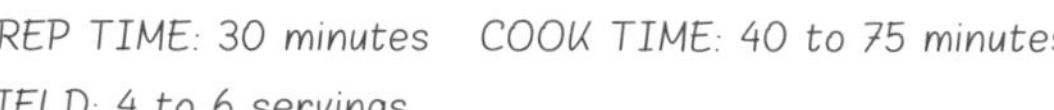

PREP TIME: 30 minutes COOK TIME: 40 to 75 minutes
YIELD: 4 to 6 servings

- 4 large fresh artichokes or 8 ounces jarred or canned artichoke hearts
- 2 tablespoons bacon fat or olive oil
- 1 small yellow onion, finely chopped
- 3 cloves garlic, minced
- 2 cups fresh spinach
- 4 ounces bacon, cooked until crispy (see page 502)
- ⅔ cup Mayonnaise (page 487)
- 1 tablespoon lemon juice

1. If using fresh artichokes, boil or steam them in a stockpot until tender, 25 to 30 minutes. If using jarred or canned artichoke hearts, drain and dice them, then skip to Step 3.

2. Drain the artichokes and let cool to room temperature. Remove the inner leaves and scrape off the meat for the filling. Remove and discard the choke. Finely chop the hearts.

3. Meanwhile, heat a skillet over medium-high heat. Add the bacon fat and onion and cook, stirring occasionally, until the onion is soft and a little browned, about 10 minutes. Add the garlic and spinach and cook until the spinach is wilted, 2 to 3 minutes. Stir in the artichoke meat. Set aside and let cool.

4. Preheat the oven to 375°F.

5. Pulse the cooled bacon in a food processor until you have awesome homemade bacon bits. (You can also chop the bacon by hand.) Set aside.

6. Stir the mayonnaise and lemon juice into the artichoke mixture. Spoon the mixture into an oven-safe dish. Sprinkle the bacon bits over the top.

7. Bake for 25 to 30 minutes, until bubbly around the edges, then serve.

CHOCOLATE HAZELNUT SPREAD

 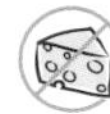 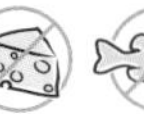 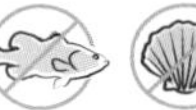  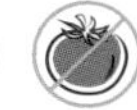

PREP TIME: 10 minutes *COOK TIME: 5 minutes*
YIELD: 1 cup

- 1 cup unsalted hazelnuts (aka filberts)
- 3 ounces bittersweet chocolate
- 2 tablespoons coconut oil

1. Place the hazelnuts in a food processor or blender and process for 2 to 3 minutes, until a paste begins to form.

2. Melt the chocolate and coconut oil in a small saucepan over low heat, or microwave on low power, checking and stirring every 20 seconds, until melted.

3. Add the melted chocolate mixture to the hazelnuts and process for an additional 2 to 3 minutes, until completely smooth. Place in a jar, cover, and let cool. Store at room temperature for up to 3 days or in the refrigerator for up to 3 months.

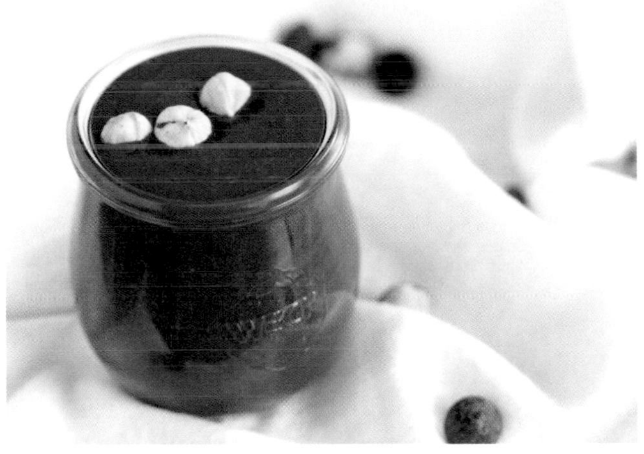

BABA GHANOUSH

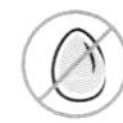  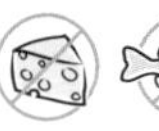 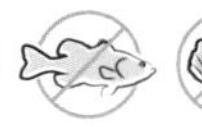 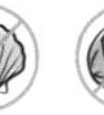

PREP TIME: 10 minutes, plus time to chill
COOK TIME: 20 minutes *YIELD: 6 to 10 servings*

- 2 large eggplants, peeled and sliced into 1-inch-thick rounds
- 3 tablespoons olive oil, divided
- ½ teaspoon sea salt
- 2 cloves garlic, crushed to a coarse paste
- 2 tablespoons lemon juice
- 2 tablespoons tahini
- ½ teaspoon ground cumin

1. Preheat the oven to 400°F.

2. In a bowl, toss the eggplant rounds with 2 tablespoons of the olive oil and the salt. Place on a rimmed baking sheet and roast for 20 minutes.

3. Place the roasted eggplant in a blender or food processor with the remaining ingredients and blend until smooth. Taste and add more salt, if desired.

4. Pour the baba ghanoush into a bowl and place in the refrigerator to chill before serving. Drizzle with additional olive oil and and sprinkle with cumin, if desired. Store in the refrigerator for up to a week.

GUACAMOLE

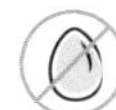  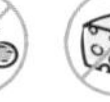 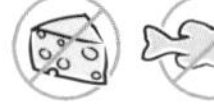 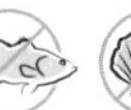  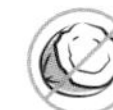  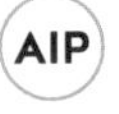

PREP TIME: 10 minutes *YIELD: 8 to 10 servings*

- 1½ large or 2 smaller ripe avocados
- ½ cup finely chopped fresh cilantro
- 1 tablespoon lime juice
- ½ teaspoon sea salt or truffle salt
- ¼ teaspoon cracked black pepper

1. Cut the avocados in half and scoop the flesh into a bowl.

2. Add the remaining ingredients, mash with a fork to mix thoroughly, and serve. Store in the refrigerator for up to a week.

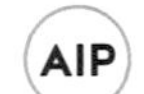 *omit pepper*

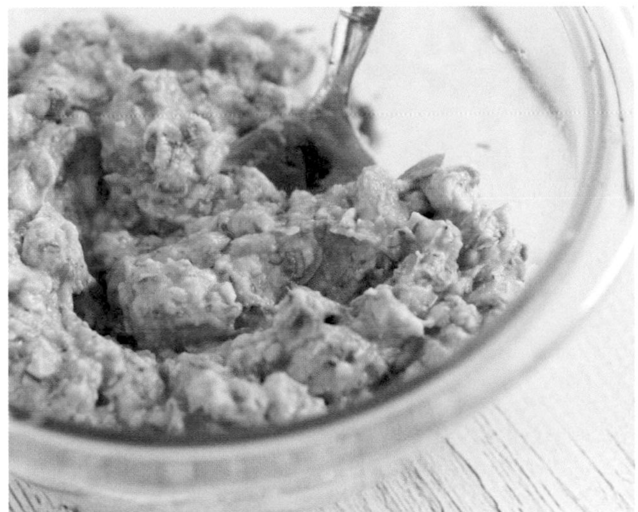

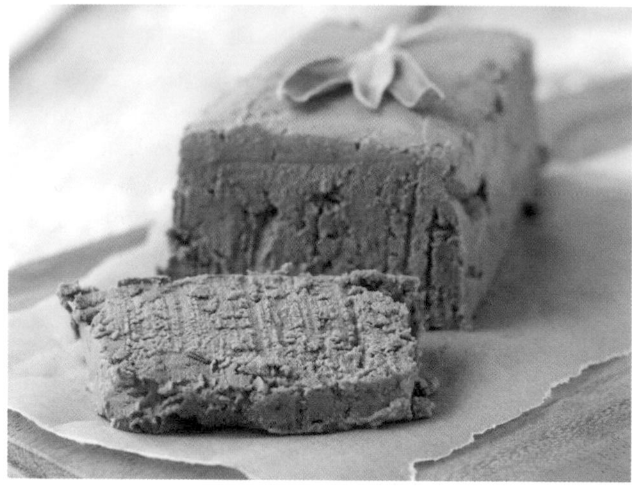

LIVER PÂTÉ

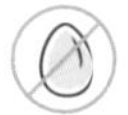 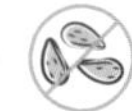 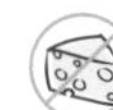 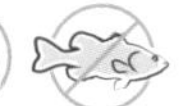 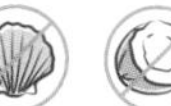  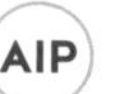 AIP

PREP TIME: 10 minutes, plus time to chill
COOK TIME: 30 minutes YIELD: 8 to 12 servings

- 1 pound liver
- ½ cup tallow, coconut oil, lard, ghee, or unsalted butter, divided
- 1 small yellow onion, finely chopped
- 2 cloves garlic
- 6 or 7 fresh sage leaves, or 1 tablespoon dried rubbed sage
- 3 to 4 sprigs thyme, or ¾ teaspoon dried thyme leaves
- 1 small sprig rosemary, or 2 teaspoons dried rosemary leaves
- 1 bay leaf
- ⅛ teaspoon ground mace
- ⅓ cup dry sherry or cognac
- ¼ teaspoon sea salt

1. Slice the liver into 2-inch chunks. (You don't need to do so if you are using chicken livers.) Remove any vessels that the butcher missed. Set aside.

2. Line a 7½ by 3½-inch loaf pan with parchment paper. (This optional step makes removing the pâté easier; you could use a glass or ceramic serving dish instead.)

3. Heat ¼ cup of the tallow in a large skillet over medium-high heat. Add the onion, garlic, sage, thyme, rosemary, bay leaf, and mace. Cook, stirring frequently, until the onion is well cooked, about 10 minutes.

4. Add the liver to the skillet and cook, stirring frequently, until browned on the outside and still pink in the middle, 3 to 4 minutes.

5. Add the sherry to the skillet and bring to a boil, increasing the heat to high if you prefer. Boil for 2 to 3 minutes, until you can't smell alcohol in the steam.

6. Remove from the heat. Remove the rosemary and thyme stems and bay leaf. Add the salt and remaining ¼ cup of tallow.

7. Pour the hot liver mixture into a blender or food processor and pulse until smooth. Taste and add more salt, if needed. Pour the mixture into the prepared loaf pan.

8. Once the pâté is cool enough to touch, cover with plastic wrap and press it tightly across the entire surface (the plastic wrap should be touching the pâté with no air bubbles) to prevent oxidation. You'll still get some, which is okay, but this step helps the pâté retain more of its nice pinkish color.

9. Refrigerate overnight or up to a few days before serving. Consume within 5 days.

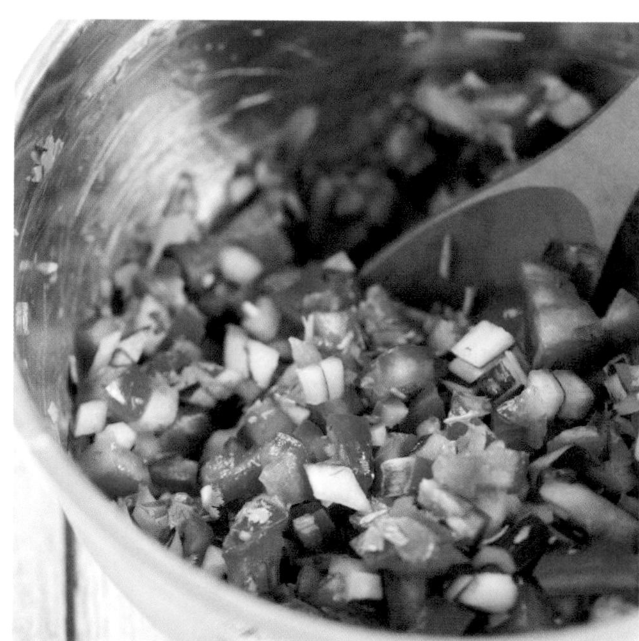

PICO DE GALLO

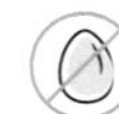 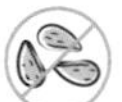 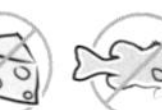 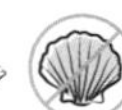 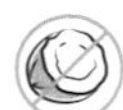

PREP TIME: 15 minutes YIELD: 4 to 8 servings

- 1½ pounds ripe tomatoes
- ½ large red onion, finely diced
- ½ cup finely chopped fresh cilantro leaves
- 1 tablespoon lime juice
- 1 jalapeño pepper, finely diced (optional)
- ¼ teaspoon sea salt

1. Cut the tomatoes in half and remove the pulp and embedded seeds. Dice the tomato flesh and place in a bowl.

2. Stir in the remaining ingredients. Taste and add more salt, if desired, then serve. Store in the refrigerator for up to a week.

SAUERKRAUT

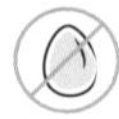  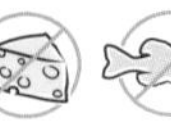  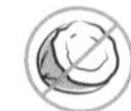 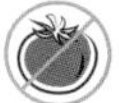 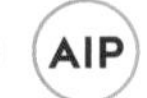 AIP

PREP TIME: 20 minutes
FERMENT TIME: 5 days to 5 months
YIELD: 30-plus servings

3 pounds cabbage (1 large head or 2 smaller heads)

4½ tablespoons unrefined sea salt, pink, pickling, or other non-iodized salt

1. Peel a few of the outer leaves from each head of cabbage and set aside.

2. Slice the rest of the cabbage as thinly as possible using a food processor, mandoline, or knife.

3. Place the sliced cabbage in a large bowl; if you don't have a bowl big enough for all 3 pounds, you can work in batches. Sprinkle the cabbage with the salt. Massage the cabbage with your hands to thoroughly distribute the salt and start the process of breaking down the cabbage. Keep massaging until the cabbage is well wilted.

4. Make sure your fermentation crock or vessel is very clean (see Tip for vessel recommendations). Pack the cabbage tightly into the vessel, handful by handful, pressing down firmly after each handful.

5. Place the large outer leaves from Step 1 over the top of the sliced cabbage. (You may have to tear or fold the leaves to cover the entire surface.) This ensures that the sliced cabbage stays submerged.

6. Weight down the cabbage. If you are using a fermentation crock, use the weight that comes with it. Otherwise, a clean glass jar, slightly smaller in diameter than the mouth of your fermentation vessel, filled with water works well.

7. If using a fermentation crock, put on the lid. Otherwise, cover the vessel with a breathable barrier (a paint-straining bag, nut milk bag, coffee filter, linen towel, several layers of cheesecloth, or even paper towels) and secure with a rubber band (unless you are using something like a paint-straining bag that has elastic around the opening).

8. Check the level of the liquid in the fermentation vessel over the next 24 hours. If it is not at least 1 inch above the top of the cabbage, dissolve 1 teaspoon of salt into 1 cup of water. Then pour the salty water into the fermentation vessel until the liquid is at least 1 inch above the top of the cabbage.

9. The sauerkraut will be ready in as little as 5 days but can ferment for up to 5 months (check the liquid level periodically and top up with salted water as needed). A little bubbling or foaming is normal. Once the sauerkraut is fermented to your liking, transfer to smaller jars (if desired) and store in the refrigerator for up to 6 months.

TIP: You don't need special equipment to make sauerkraut. A large glass cracker or cookie jar with a wide mouth, a slightly smaller jar that fits inside the mouth of the larger jar, a tea towel, and a knife are really the only "equipment" you need. Of course, if you want a foolproof way to ferment vegetables and think you will be doing a lot of fermenting, a fermentation crock is a worthwhile investment.

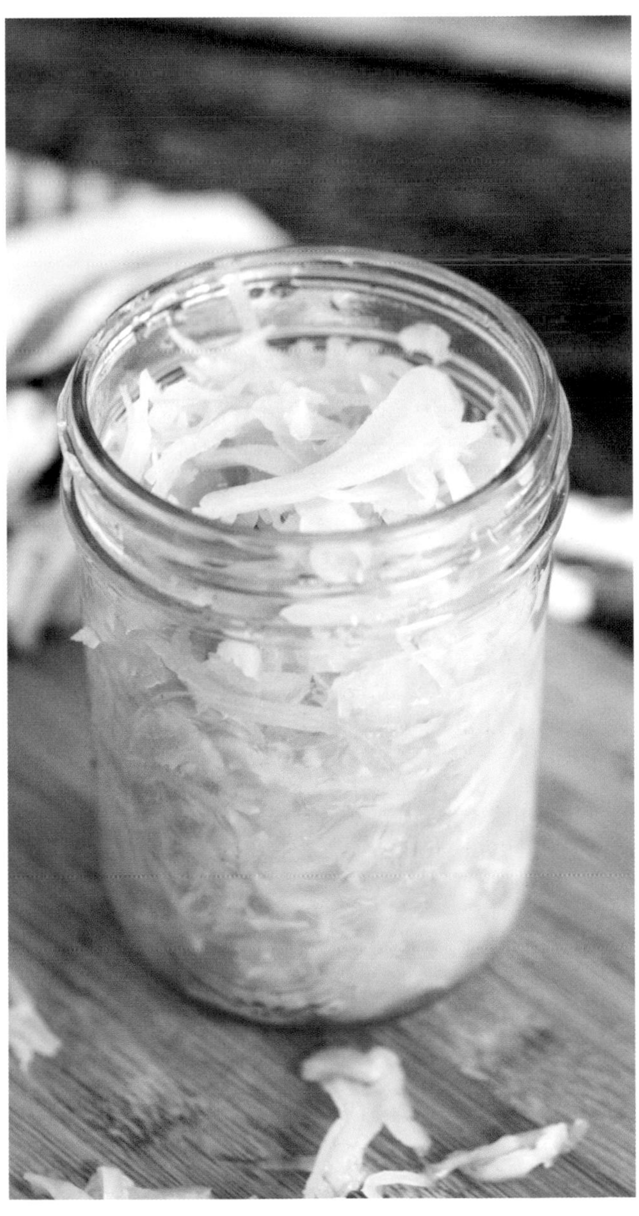

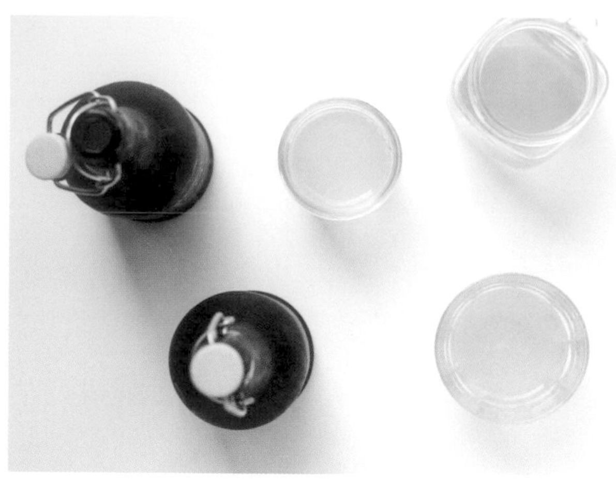

KOMBUCHA

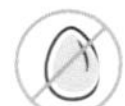 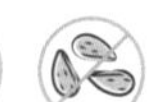 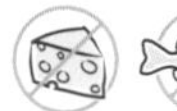  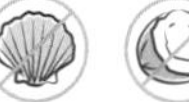   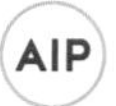 AIP

PREP TIME: 20 minutes FERMENT TIME: 14 to 17 days
YIELD: 4 to 6 servings

5 black or green tea bags, or about 5 teaspoons loose-leaf tea

8 cups filtered water, 6 cups boiling and the rest at room temperature

¾ cup white sugar

1 kombucha scoby

½ cup kombucha from a previous batch

1. Place the tea bags or loose-leaf tea in a large teapot and pour the 6 cups of boiling water over the tea bags or leaves.

2. Steep the tea for about 20 minutes, then stir in the sugar until dissolved.

3. Allow the tea to cool to room temperature. Remove the tea bags or pour the tea through a sieve to remove the leaves.

4. Pour the tea into a half-gallon jar, then place the scoby in the tea. (It's okay if the scoby sinks; it will typically float up in a couple of days.) Add the ½ cup of kombucha from a previous batch to the jar (this helps the culture get going quicker). Top with room-temperature filtered water until just before the jar narrows at the top.

5. Cover with cheesecloth, a tea towel, or a paper towel and secure with a rubber band. Allow to ferment at room temperature and out of direct sunlight for 14 to 17 days.

6. With clean hands, remove the scoby from the jar and start a new culture by following the directions above (remembering to add ½ cup of this batch to the new batch of kombucha). Stir the remaining kombucha, pour into bottles or jars, and place in the refrigerator (or follow the directions below for an optional second fermentation). Store in the fridge for up to 6 months.

TIP: When you purchase a scoby, it comes with 1/2 to 1 cup of kombucha to help get your first batch started. You can also grow your own scoby by adding a bottle of unflavored kombucha from the store to room-temperature sweet tea as directed above; it typically takes 3 to 4 weeks to grow a scoby, and you'll want to toss your first batch of kombucha (it won't taste very good).

OPTIONAL SECOND FERMENTATION

You may do a second, optional fermentation to flavor your kombucha or to increase the fizziness of unflavored kombucha:

1. If making flavored kombucha, place up to 3 tablespoons of a flavoring liquid such as lemon or other fruit juice or ginger juice in each 12- to 16-ounce bottle. Sliced fresh ginger and fruits and whole spices like cinnamon bark or cloves can be added to the bottles as well. Otherwise, have empty bottles on hand for unflavored kombucha.

2. Pour the stirred kombucha into the bottles. Tighten the caps on the bottles and allow to ferment at room temperature and out of direct sunlight for 3 to 5 days.

3. Store the flavored kombucha in the refrigerator until you are ready to enjoy it!

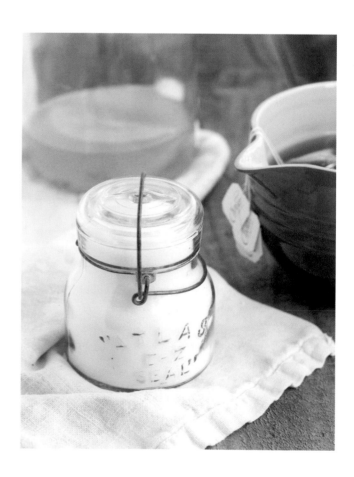

SAUCES, MARINADES, AND OTHER INDISPENSABLE FLAVOR ENHANCERS

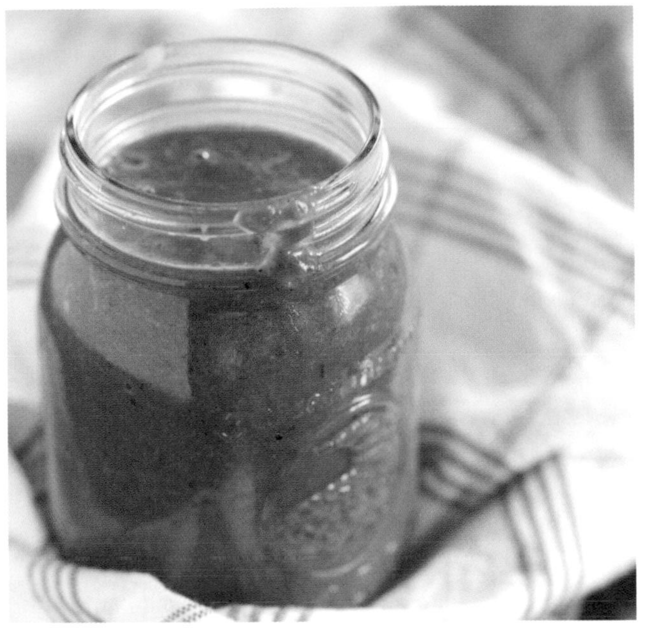

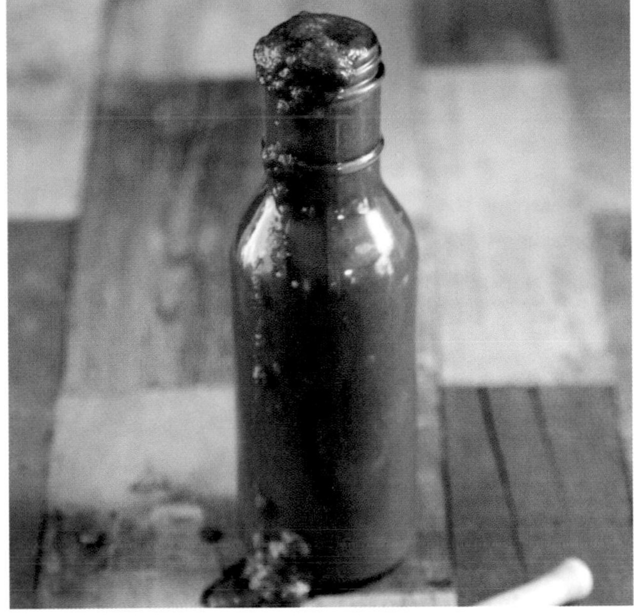

BASIC BARBECUE SAUCE

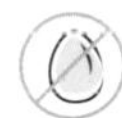 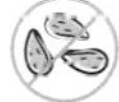 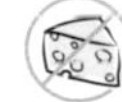 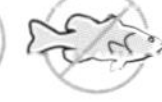  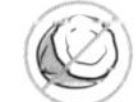

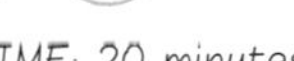

PREP TIME: 10 minutes *COOK TIME: 20 minutes*

YIELD: 4 cups

½ cup unsalted butter, ghee, or olive oil

1 medium-sized sweet onion, chopped

1 (15-ounce) can crushed tomatoes

1 cup water

½ cup red wine vinegar

Juice of 1 lemon

3 tablespoons honey

1 tablespoon blackstrap molasses

1½ teaspoons mustard powder

1 teaspoon red pepper flakes (optional)

1 teaspoon smoked paprika

1 teaspoon sea salt

¼ teaspoon ground black pepper

1. Heat the butter in a skillet over medium-high heat. Add the onion and sauté until caramelized, about 8 minutes.

2. Add the remaining ingredients and reduce the heat to medium-low. Simmer, stirring occasionally, for 10 minutes.

3. Blend the sauce with an immersion blender or countertop blender until smooth. Store in the refrigerator for up to 2 weeks.

TIP: Use either version of barbecue sauce as a marinade for red meat or chicken before grilling or as a serving sauce.

AIP BARBECUE SAUCE

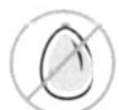 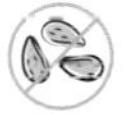 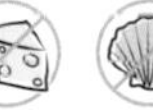 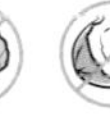  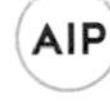 AIP

PREP TIME: 15 minutes *COOK TIME: 30 minutes*

YIELD: about 3 cups

2 tablespoons red palm oil

1 large sweet onion, diced

1 apple, peeled, cored, and grated

⅓ cup apple cider vinegar

¼ cup molasses

1½ tablespoons fish sauce

1 clove garlic, crushed to a coarse paste

1 tablespoon peeled and finely grated fresh ginger

1 teaspoon turmeric powder

¼ teaspoon ground mace

Pinch of ground cinnamon

1. Heat the oil in a saucepan over medium-high heat. Add the onion and sauté until caramelized, 10 to 15 minutes.

2. Add the remaining ingredients and stir to combine. Bring to a boil, then reduce the heat to maintain a simmer. Simmer, uncovered, for 15 minutes.

3. Remove from the heat and puree the sauce with an immersion blender or countertop blender. Store in the refrigerator for up to 2 weeks.

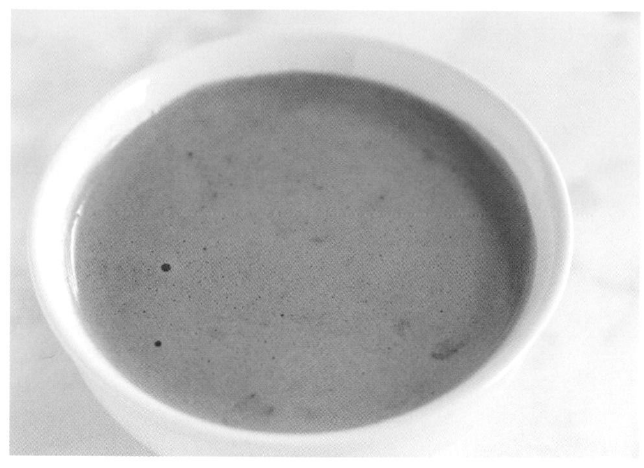

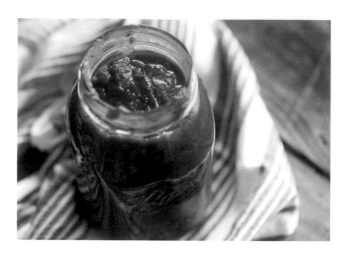

HOISIN SAUCE

 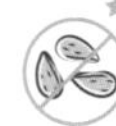 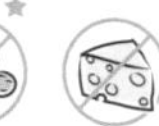 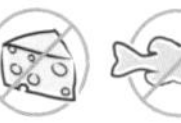  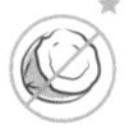 

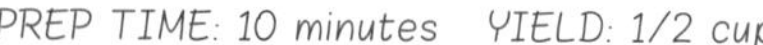

PREP TIME: 10 minutes YIELD: 1/2 cup

¼ cup coconut aminos

2 tablespoons smooth sunflower seed butter or cashew butter

2 tablespoons coconut water vinegar

1 tablespoon blackstrap molasses

2 teaspoons toasted (dark) sesame oil

1 clove garlic, crushed to a coarse paste

⅛ teaspoon ground black pepper

1 to 2 teaspoons minced hot pepper (optional)

Whisk all the ingredients together to create a smooth paste. Store in the refrigerator for up to 2 weeks.

TIP: Use as a stir-fry sauce or marinade for beef before grilling.

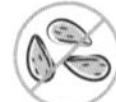 *use sunflower seed butter*

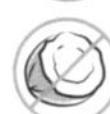 *use apple cider vinegar*

 *omit hot pepper*

CLASSIC PIZZA SAUCE

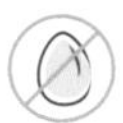  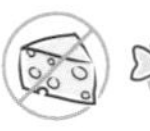 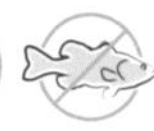  

PREP TIME: 5 minutes COOK TIME: 5 minutes
YIELD: about 3 cups

1 tablespoon olive oil

2 to 3 cloves garlic, crushed to a coarse paste

1 (28-ounce) can crushed tomatoes

1 (6-ounce) can tomato paste

1 tablespoon honey

1 tablespoon red wine vinegar

1 teaspoon dried basil

1 teaspoon dried oregano

1 teaspoon dried thyme leaves

Sea salt and ground black pepper

1. Heat a medium saucepan over medium-high heat. Add the olive oil and garlic and cook for 30 seconds, until fragrant and starting to brown.

2. Add the remaining ingredients and bring just to a simmer. Remove from the heat and season to taste with salt and pepper.

3. Store in the refrigerator for up to a week or in the freezer for up to 3 months.

TERIYAKI MARINADE

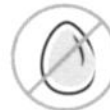 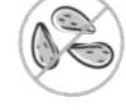 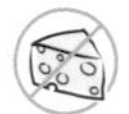 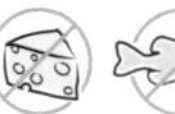   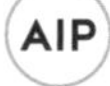

PREP TIME: 5 minutes YIELD: 3/4 cup

1 teaspoon finely grated orange zest (optional)

½ cup fresh orange juice

¼ cup coconut aminos

4 cloves garlic, crushed to a coarse paste

2 teaspoons peeled and finely grated fresh ginger

In a small bowl, combine all the ingredients. Store in the refrigerator for up to 2 weeks.

TIP: Use this marinade to poach fish, to marinate chicken or red meat before grilling, or as a stir-fry sauce.

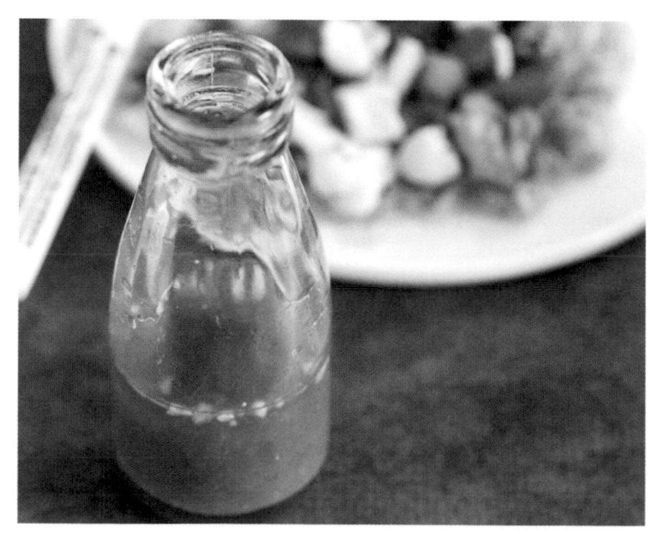

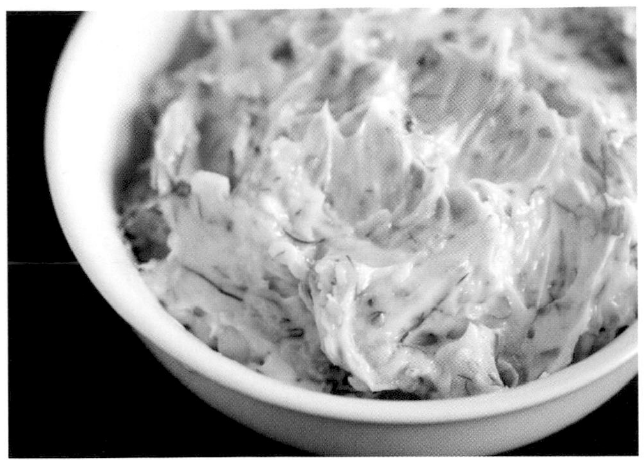

MAÎTRE D' BUTTER

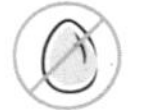 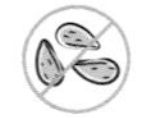 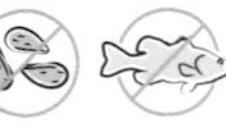  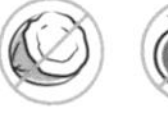 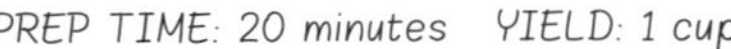

PREP TIME: 20 minutes YIELD: 1 cup

- 1 cup unsalted butter or ghee, softened
- ½ cup chopped fresh dill
- ⅓ cup chopped fresh parsley
- 4 cloves garlic, crushed to a coarse paste
- Finely grated zest of 1 lemon
- ½ teaspoon sea salt
- ¼ teaspoon ground black pepper

Place all the ingredients in a bowl and mix with a fork until thoroughly combined. Store in the refrigerator for up to a month or in the freezer for up to 6 months.

TIP: Maître d' Butter pairs well with fish, shellfish, and red meat.

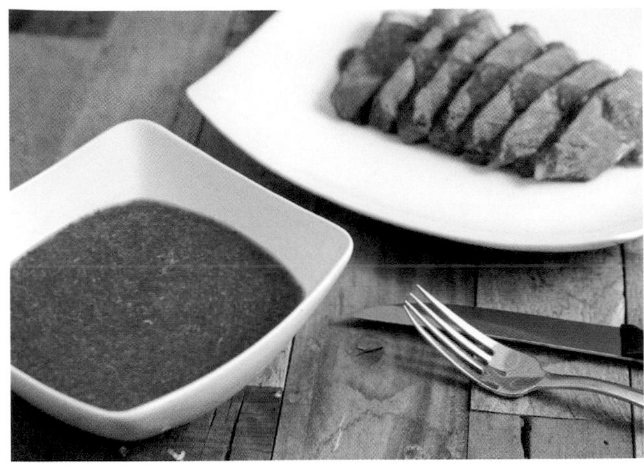

CHIMICHURRI

  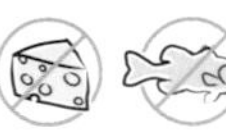     AIP

PREP TIME: 10 minutes YIELD: 1 cup

- ⅔ cup chopped fresh cilantro
- ⅔ cup chopped fresh parsley
- ½ cup olive oil
- ⅓ cup red wine vinegar
- 2 cloves garlic, crushed to a coarse paste
- ¼ teaspoon ground cumin
- ¼ teaspoon sea salt
- ½ teaspoon red pepper flakes (optional)

Place all the ingredients in a blender and blend until smooth. Store in the refrigerator for up to 2 weeks.

TIP: Chimichurri pairs well with red meat and poultry, especially grilled, as well as fried eggs.

 *omit red pepper flakes*

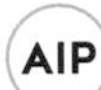 AIP *omit cumin and red pepper flakes*

AIP PESTO

 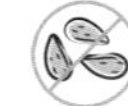 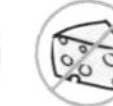 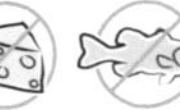   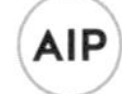 AIP

PREP TIME: 10 minutes YIELD: 3/4 cup

- 2 cups fresh basil leaves
- ¾ cup fresh cilantro leaves
- 4 cloves garlic, crushed to a coarse paste
- ½ cup olive oil
- 1 teaspoon apple cider vinegar
- ½ teaspoon sea salt

Place all the ingredients in a blender and blend until smooth. Store in the refrigerator for up to 2 weeks.

TIP: Serve with "pasta" (pages 549, 551, and 553), on pizza (page 529), or as a serving sauce for red meat or chicken.

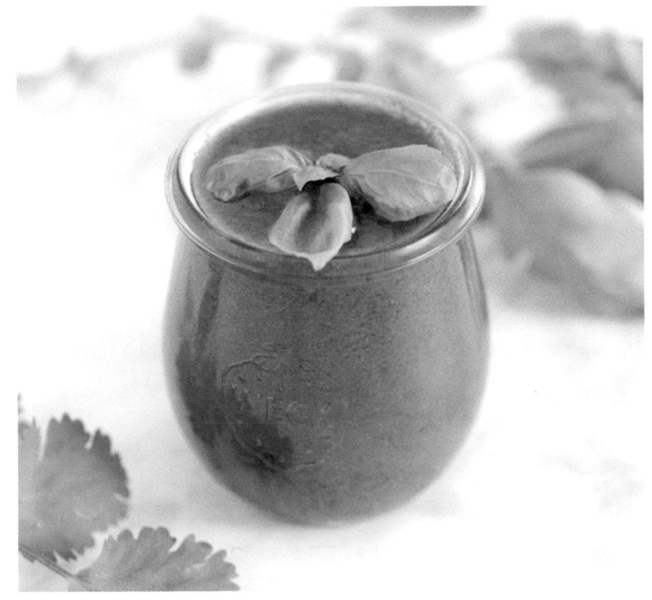

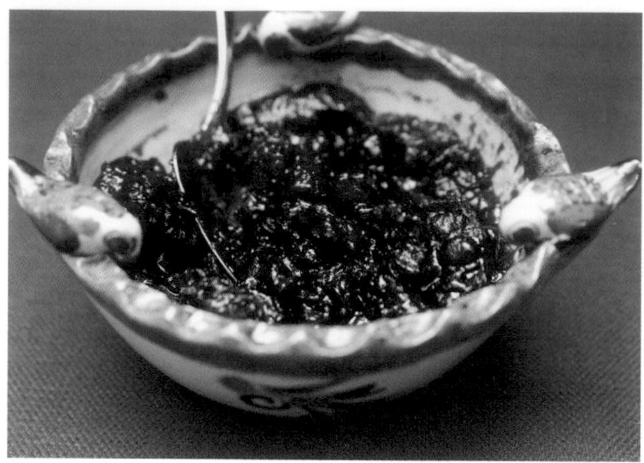

MAPLE CRANBERRY SAUCE

 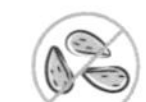 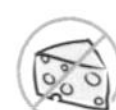  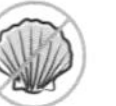  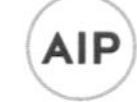 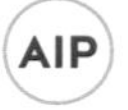

PREP TIME: 5 minutes, plus at least 1 hour to chill
COOK TIME: 10 minutes YIELD: 2 cups

2 cups fresh or frozen cranberries
½ cup maple syrup
¼ cup water

1. Combine all the ingredients in a small saucepan. Bring to a boil over high heat, then reduce the heat to maintain a simmer. Simmer, uncovered, for 8 to 10 minutes, stirring occasionally, until most of the berries have popped and the sauce has thickened.

2. Transfer to a serving bowl and refrigerate for at least 1 hour before serving. Store in the refrigerator for up to 3 months.

TIP: This sauce pairs well with poultry and pork.

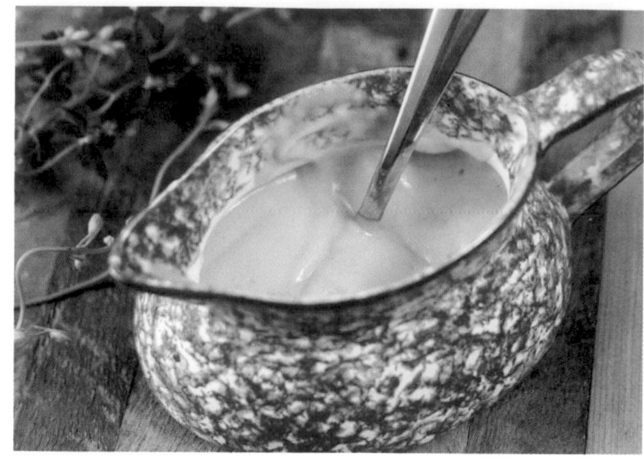

CAULIFLOWER GRAVY

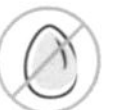 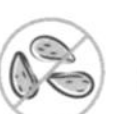 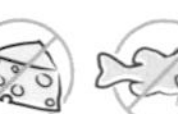 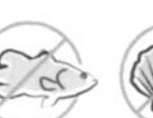 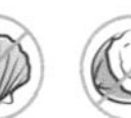  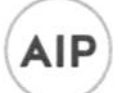

PREP TIME: 10 minutes COOK TIME: 30 minutes
YIELD: 6 to 8 servings

½ medium head cauliflower, cut into florets
1½ cups Bone Stock (page 486)
1 clove garlic
Sea salt

1. Place the cauliflower, stock, and garlic in a saucepan. Bring to a boil, then reduce the heat to maintain a simmer. Simmer for 15 to 20 minutes, until the cauliflower is overcooked.

2. Pour the mixture into a blender. Cover the lid with a tea towel to make sure you don't burn yourself. Blend on high for 1 minute, until completely smooth. Season to taste with salt. If the gravy is too thick, thin it with additional stock or water. Store in the refrigerator for up to 5 days.

PAN GRAVY

 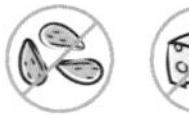 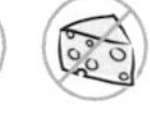 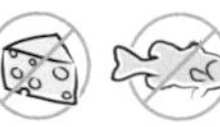  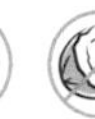 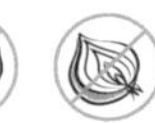  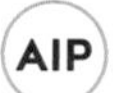

PREP TIME: 5 minutes COOK TIME: 8 minutes
YIELD: about 2 cups

Pan juices from roasting meat
2 cups Bone Stock (page 486)
¼ cup kuzu starch or arrowroot powder
¼ cup cold water
Sea salt

1. Place your roasting pan with the pan juices on a burner on the stovetop. Add the stock and bring to a simmer over medium-high heat.

2. In a small bowl, combine the kuzu starch with the water. Stir until smooth, then pour into the hot stock while stirring constantly. Keep stirring gently until the gravy thickens; it will be opaque when you first add the starch but will become more translucent as the starch cooks. Season to taste with salt. Store in the refrigerator for up to 5 days.

HOLLANDAISE

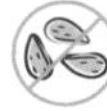 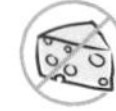 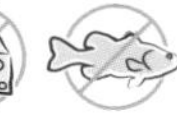 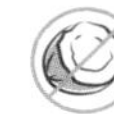 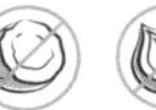 

PREP TIME: 5 minutes COOK TIME: 5 minutes
YIELD: 1/2 cup

2 large egg yolks

1 tablespoon lemon juice

¼ cup lard, ghee, or unsalted butter, 1 tablespoon cold and 3 tablespoons melted

1. Combine the egg yolks, lemon juice, and 1 tablespoon of cold lard in a small saucepan. Mix vigorously.

2. If you have an electric range, preheat a burner to low heat. Place the saucepan over low heat and stir constantly for 1 to 2 minutes, just until the lard is melting and the mixture is thinning out.

3. Very slowly dribble in the 3 tablespoons of melted lard, mixing constantly. It should take 1 to 2 minutes to add all the lard.

4. Remove from the heat and continue to stir for another minute. Hollandaise is best served immediately, but you can keep it warm in a Thermos or travel mug for up to 1 hour after making it.

TIPS: If your hollandaise separates, remove the saucepan from the heat, add an ice cube to the sauce, and whisk vigorously.

To reheat leftover hollandaise, place in a microwave-safe bowl, microwave for 10 seconds, and then stir thoroughly; repeat (heating, then stirring) until warmed through.

Hollandaise pairs well with eggs, fish, and vegetables.

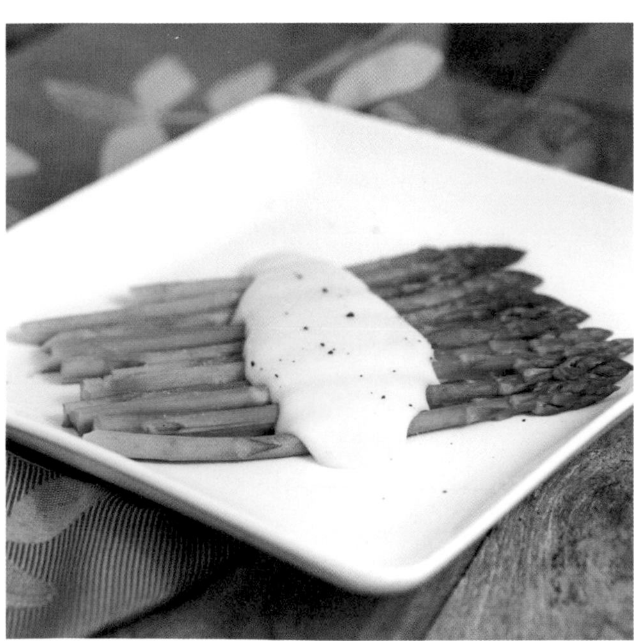

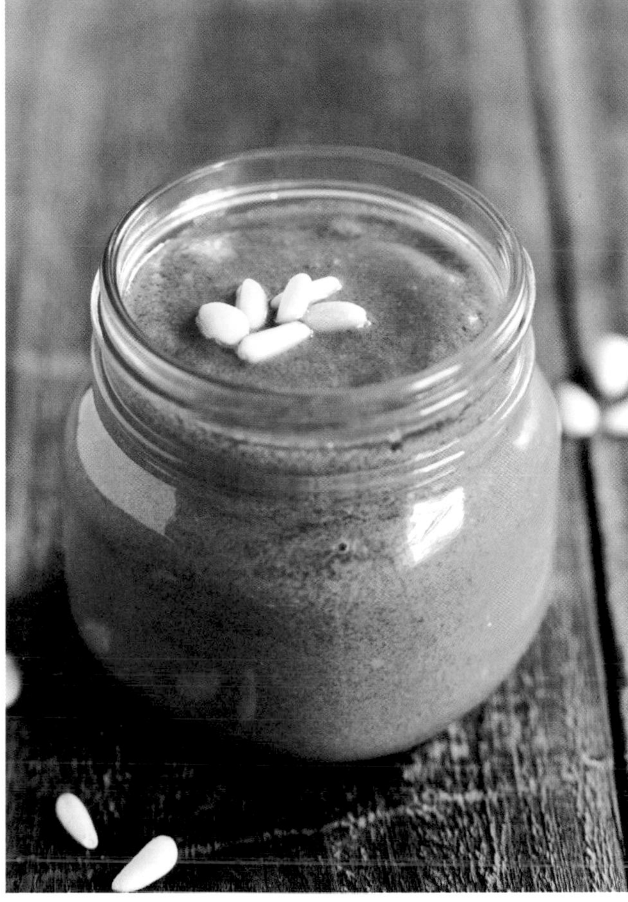

LEMON BASIL PESTO

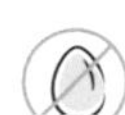 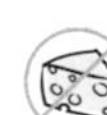 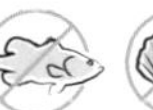  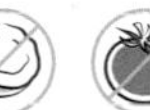 

PREP TIME: 10 minutes COOK TIME: 15 minutes
YIELD: 1 cup

4 large cloves garlic (do not peel)

¼ cup pine nuts

2 cups lemon or lime basil

7 tablespoons olive oil

¼ teaspoon sea salt

1. Heat a well-seasoned cast-iron skillet over medium heat. Add the garlic still in the peel to the pan. Stir or shake the skillet frequently so the garlic rotates and cooks on all sides. Cook until the garlic is starting to brown and feels fairly soft to the touch, 7 to 8 minutes.

2. Remove the garlic from the skillet and add the pine nuts. Again, stir or shake the skillet frequently so the pine nuts get toasted on all sides. Cook until starting to brown and become fragrant, 5 to 6 minutes.

3. Remove the pine nuts from the skillet and let cool. Peel the now-cool garlic. Place all the ingredients in a blender or food processor and pulse until the pesto is a paste. Store in the refrigerator for up to 2 weeks.

TIP: Replace the lemon basil with sweet basil for a more traditional pesto!

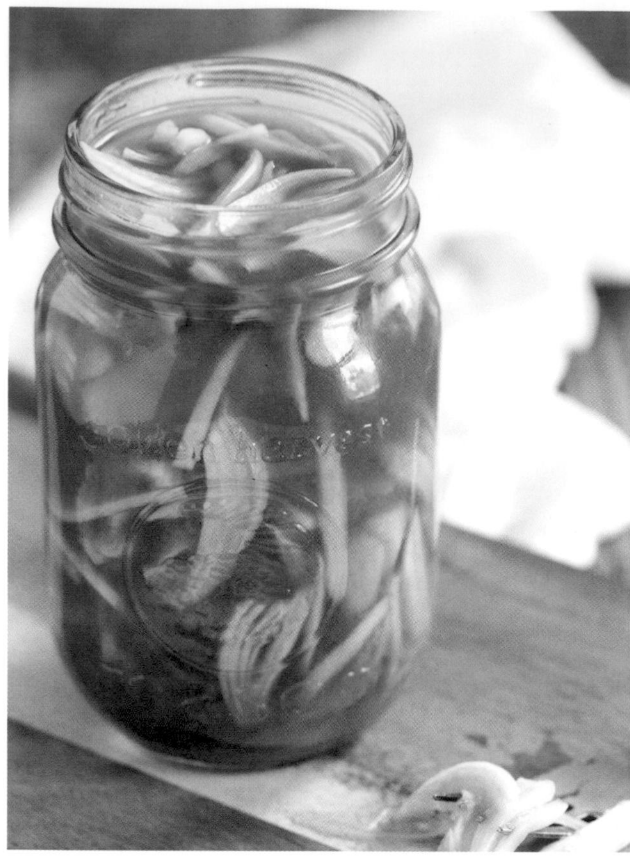

EASY PICKLED SHALLOTS

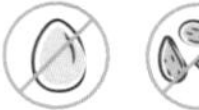 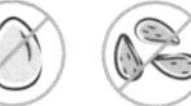 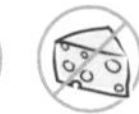 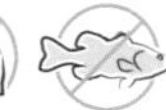 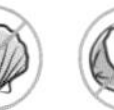  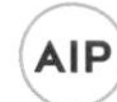 AIP

PREP TIME: 5 minutes, plus time to marinate *YIELD: 2 cups*

- 4 to 5 shallots, or 1 medium-sized red onion (2 cups sliced)
- ¾ cup apple cider vinegar or coconut water vinegar
- 2 tablespoons lemon juice
- 2 teaspoons sea salt

1. Slice the shallots into half-moons, making them as thin as possible. Place in a pint-sized mason jar.

2. In a bowl, combine the vinegar and lemon juice. Add the salt and stir to dissolve. Pour the liquid over the shallots and top off the jar with water, filling the jar to the brim. Secure the lid and shake well.

3. Leave on the counter for at least 8 hours; 24 hours is better. Store in the refrigerator for up to 6 months.

"SNEAKY LIVER" GROUND BEEF

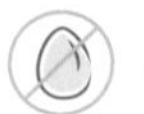 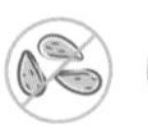 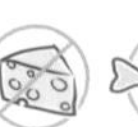 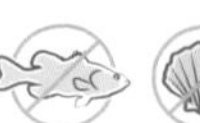 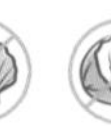 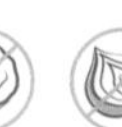 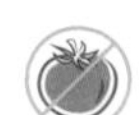 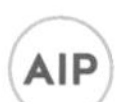 AIP

PREP TIME: 10 minutes, plus 1 hour to soften liver
YIELD: 5 pounds ground meat

- 1 pound liver, frozen
- 4 pounds ground beef, thawed

1. Place the frozen liver in the refrigerator for 1 hour to soften slightly but not thaw. Grate the mostly frozen liver using a box grater.

2. Mix the grated liver thoroughly with the ground beef. Divide the meat mixture into five 1-pound portions.

3. Use immediately or place in one or more freezer-safe containers or bags and refreeze for up to 3 months.

TIP: Use in any recipe in place of ground beef.

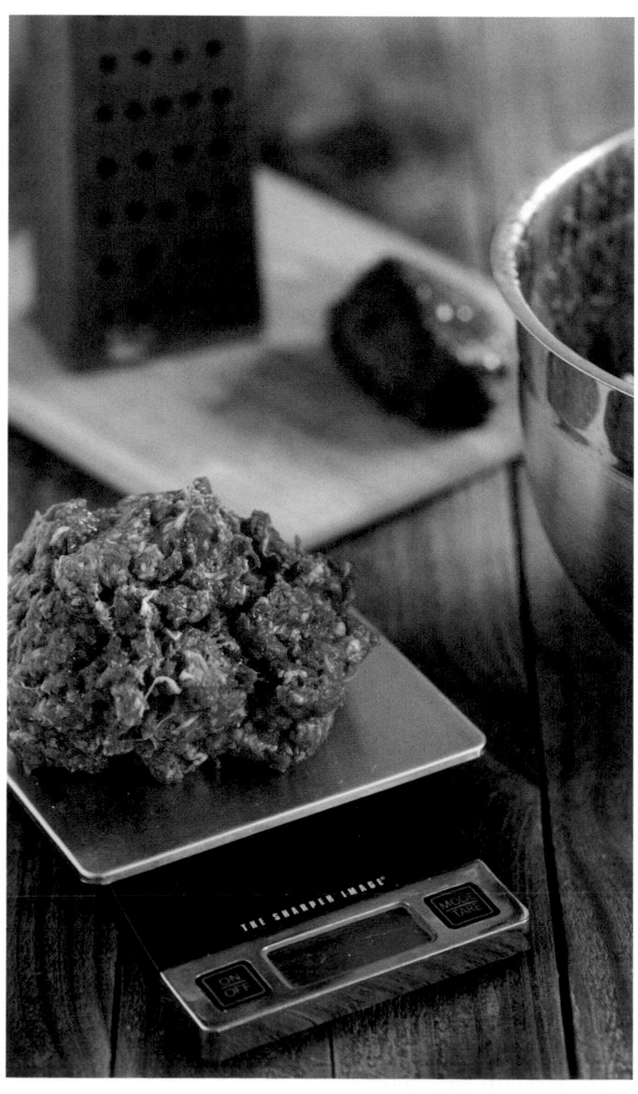

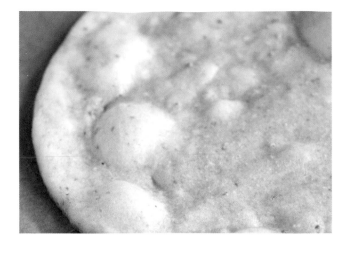

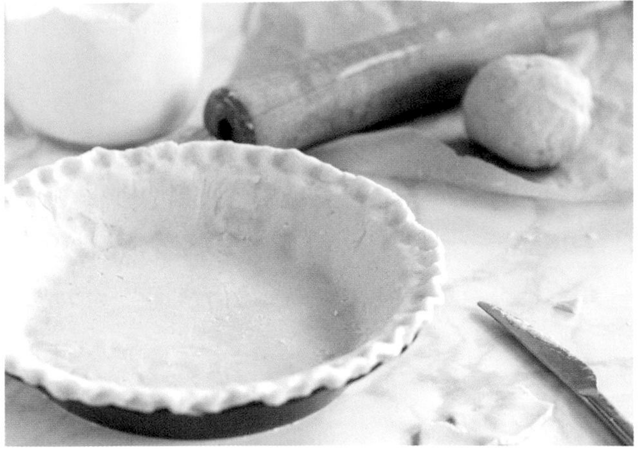

CASSAVA FLOUR PIE CRUST

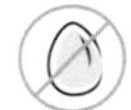  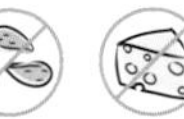 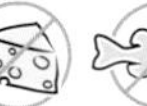  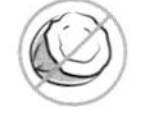 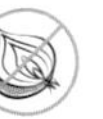 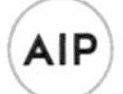

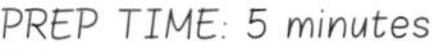

PREP TIME: 5 minutes
YIELD: one double crust for an 8- or 9-inch pie

- 2 cups cassava flour
- ⅛ teaspoon sea salt
- 1 cup cold lard or unsalted butter
- 1 tablespoon apple cider vinegar
- 5 to 6 tablespoons ice water

1. In a mixing bowl, combine the cassava flour and salt. Add the lard, then use a pastry blender or 2 knives to cut the lard into the flour until the mixture resembles dry oatmeal; the largest pieces of lard should be no bigger than peas.

2. Add the vinegar and then the ice water 1 tablespoon at a time and work it into the dough. Stop adding water as soon as the dough holds together easily.

3. Place the dough in the refrigerator to keep it cold while you prepare the pie filling.

PIZZA CRUST

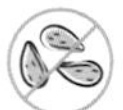 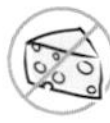  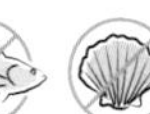 

PREP TIME: 10 minutes *YIELD: one 10-inch-round crust*

- 1 cup tapioca starch
- ¼ cup sifted coconut flour (measure after sifting)
- 1 teaspoon dried oregano leaves (omit if making flatbread)
- ½ teaspoon granulated garlic (omit if making flatbread)
- ½ teaspoon sea salt
- ½ cup full-fat coconut milk, homemade (page 480) or canned, warmed
- ½ cup olive oil or avocado oil
- 1 large egg, beaten

1. In a large mixing bowl, whisk the tapioca starch, coconut flour, oregano (if using), granulated garlic (if using), and salt until well combined.

2. In a separate bowl, whisk together the coconut milk, oil, and egg. Pour over the tapioca starch mixture and stir to combine. Let sit for 3 to 5 minutes to thicken before using to make DIY Pizza (page 529) or Flatbread (page 572).

ALMOND FLOUR PIE CRUST

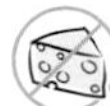 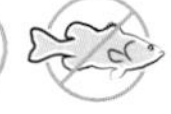 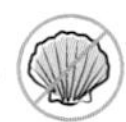  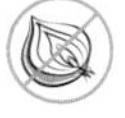 

PREP TIME: 5 minutes
YIELD: one double crust for an 8- or 9-inch pie

- 4 cups blanched almond flour
- ½ cup arrowroot powder
- 2 large egg whites
- ¼ teaspoon sea salt

Combine all the ingredients in a mixing bowl and work together with your hands to form a dough.

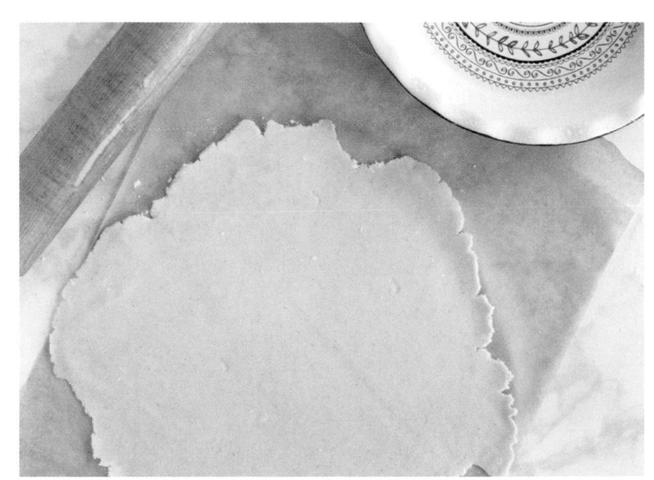

Chapter 40: BREAKFAST

DIY PANCAKES

 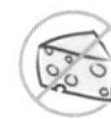 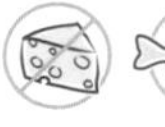 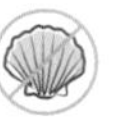 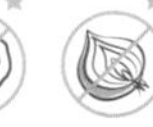 

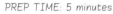

PREP TIME: 5 minutes

COOK TIME: 10 to 20 minutes, depending on the size of your skillet

YIELD: six 5- to 6-inch pancakes

2 large green plantains (about 2 cups pureed)

4 large eggs

2 teaspoons vanilla extract

3 tablespoons coconut oil, plus more for the pan

½ teaspoon baking soda

⅛ teaspoon sea salt

1. Peel and chop the plantains. Place in a blender with the eggs and blend until smooth; if your blender has a smoothie setting, that works well here.

2. Add the rest of the ingredients to the blender and blend on high for an additional minute. Fold in any add-ins (see suggestions, above right).

3. Heat 1 tablespoon of coconut oil in a skillet or on a griddle over medium-high heat. Pour the batter into the skillet until your pancake is the desired size.

4. Cook for 4 to 5 minutes on the first side, until the top looks fairly dry with little bubbles in it (just like a regular pancake). Flip and cook on the second side for 1½ to 2 minutes.

5. Repeat Steps 3 and 4 with the remaining batter, adding more coconut oil to the pan as needed. Serve the pancakes warm or cooled.

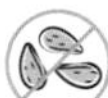 *don't make the banana nut version*

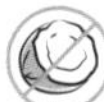 *use avocado oil or olive oil instead of coconut oil*

 *stick with plain or strawberry*

ADD-INS

Chocolate Chip Pancakes: Add ½ cup bittersweet chocolate chips.

Blueberry Pancakes: Add 1 cup fresh, frozen, or freeze-dried blueberries.

Banana Nut Pancakes: Add 1 large banana, chopped (not mashed), and ½ cup chopped walnuts or pecans.

Strawberry Pancakes: Add 1 cup chopped fresh or sliced freeze-dried strawberries.

Apple Cinnamon Pancakes: Add 1 large apple, peeled, cored, and finely diced, and 2 teaspoons ground cinnamon.

TIP: Sometimes this batter thickens while it sits; if it does, simply blend it for an additional 10 seconds.

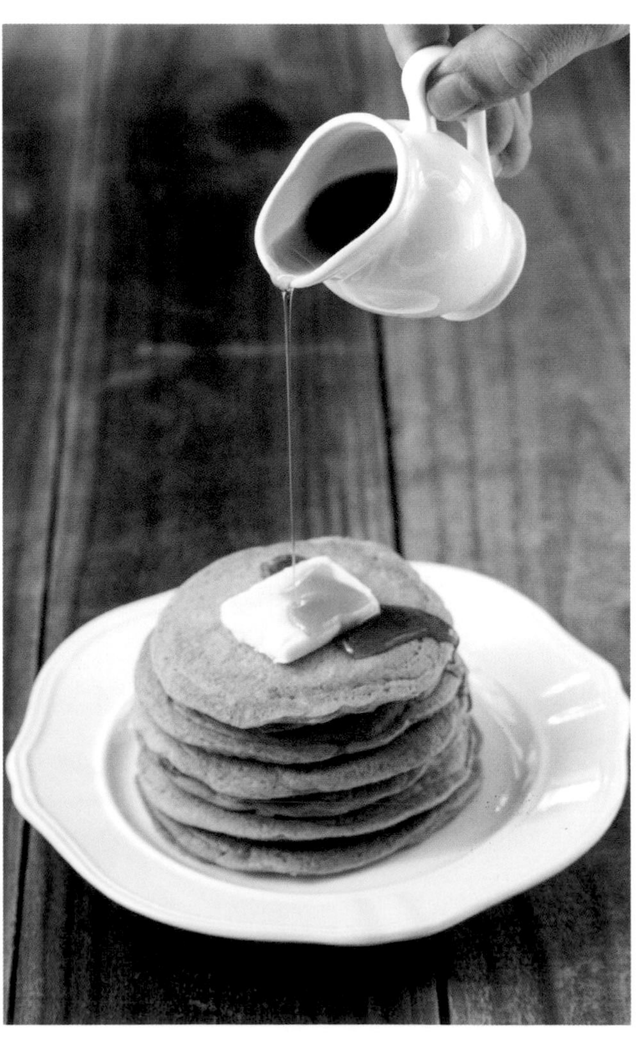

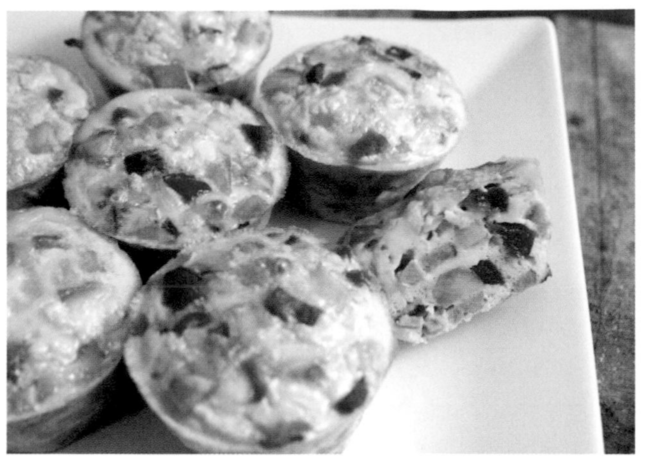

HAM & SWEET POTATO EGG MUFFINS

 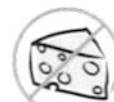 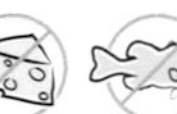  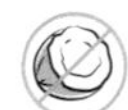

PREP TIME: 10 minutes   COOK TIME: 22 minutes
YIELD: 12 egg muffins (2 per serving)

2 tablespoons olive oil

2 cups diced peeled sweet potatoes (about 1 medium)

1½ cups diced red and green bell pepper (about ½ large each)

½ cup diced white onions (about ½ small)

10 ounces smoked uncured ham, diced

12 large eggs

¾ teaspoon sea salt

⅛ teaspoon ground black pepper

1. Preheat the oven to 350°F. Grease a standard-size 12-cup muffin pan or use a silicone muffin pan.

2. Heat a skillet over medium-high heat. Add the olive oil, sweet potatoes, bell peppers, and onions. Sauté, stirring frequently, until the veggies start to soften and caramelize, about 8 minutes. Remove from the heat and stir in the diced ham. Set aside.

3. Thoroughly whisk or blend the eggs with the salt and pepper.

4. Spoon the ham and veggie mixture into the muffin cups. Pour the eggs over the veggies, which will nearly fill the cups.

5. Bake for 20 to 22 minutes, until set. Immediately remove the egg muffins from the pan and enjoy!

OVEN SCRAMBLED EGGS

 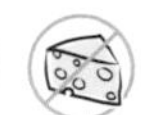 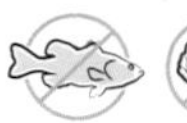 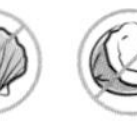 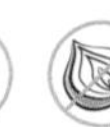 

PREP TIME: 5 minutes   COOK TIME: 40 minutes
YIELD: 8 to 12 servings

24 large eggs

½ cup cooking fat of choice (I like to use ¼ cup ghee and ¼ cup coconut oil)

2 cups cool water

2 teaspoons sea salt

1. Preheat the oven to 350°F.

2. Place all the ingredients in a blender and blend on high for 20 to 30 seconds. (Depending on the size of your blender, you may need to do this in 2 batches; you can blend 12 eggs with the fat, then 12 eggs with the water and salt, then mix in your baking dish.)

3. Pour the egg mixture into a 13 by 9-inch glass or ceramic baking dish. Bake, stirring at the 10-minute, 20-minute, 25-minute, and 30-minute marks. Remove from the oven when the eggs are just slightly underdone (a bit gooey underneath when you stir them), typically after about 30 minutes. If the eggs are not cooked enough at 30 minutes, check them every 3 to 4 minutes, until done. It shouldn't take more than 40 minutes total.

4. Stir the eggs to break up the bigger pieces, then let them sit in the baking dish for 3 to 4 minutes to finish cooking before serving.

TIP: To store leftovers, let the eggs cool, then transfer them to a covered dish. If the eggs release water while they cool, discard the water (it'll make the eggs turn green during storage).

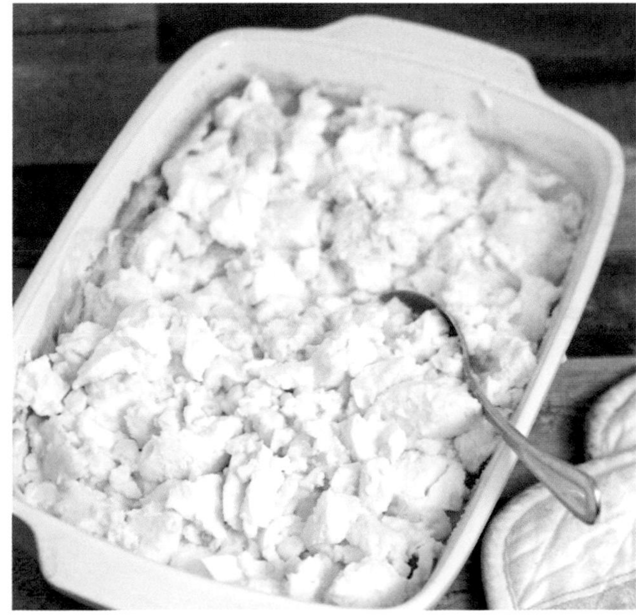

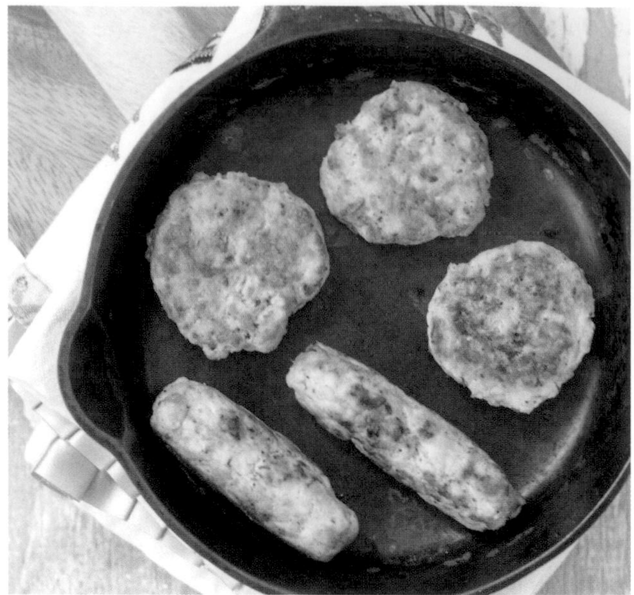

SAUSAGE PATTIES

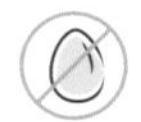  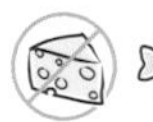  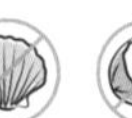 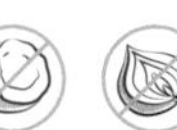  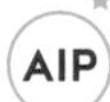 AIP

PREP TIME: 10 minutes COOK TIME: 25 minutes
YIELD: 10 to 20 servings

BREAKFAST SAUSAGE

2 teaspoons sea salt

2 teaspoons dried rubbed sage

1 teaspoon ground mace

1 teaspoon dried thyme leaves

1 teaspoon ground black pepper (optional)

¼ teaspoon ginger powder

½ teaspoon baking soda

¼ cup water

3 pounds ground pork

BRATWURST

2 teaspoons sea salt

2 teaspoons ginger powder

1 teaspoon ground caraway seed

1 teaspoon granulated garlic

1 teaspoon granulated onion

1 teaspoon ground white pepper (optional)

½ teaspoon ground mace

½ teaspoon dried savory

1 tablespoon maple syrup

½ teaspoon baking soda

¼ cup water

3 pounds ground pork

SWEET ITALIAN SAUSAGE

1 teaspoon sea salt

2 teaspoons dried tarragon

¼ teaspoon dried oregano

¼ teaspoon dried rosemary

¼ teaspoon ground black pepper

4 to 5 cloves garlic, crushed to a coarse paste

¾ teaspoon minced fresh basil

3 tablespoons minced fresh parsley

3 pounds ground pork

1. Combine the salt, spices, and baking soda, if called for, in a spice grinder and grind to a fine powder. You can also grind them with a mortar and pestle, clean coffee grinder, mini blender, or mini food processor.

2. Add the powdered spices to the water or garlic and minced fresh herbs, then add the mixture to the ground pork. Mix to completely incorporate the spices into the meat. Cover with plastic wrap and refrigerate overnight or up to 24 hours, if desired.

3. Preheat the oven to 400°F.

4. Use your hands to form 4- to 8-ounce patties (how big you make the patties will depend on how large a serving size you are aiming for). Place the patties on a rimmed baking sheet, spacing them about 1 inch apart. You may need 2 baking sheets, depending on how thick you make your patties.

5. Bake the sausage patties for 15 to 25 minutes (depending on how thick they are), until the internal temperature reaches a minimum of 160°F. Alternatively, you can fry the patties in a skillet or on a griddle over medium-high heat.

6. To freeze the sausage, place the patties on a baking sheet in the freezer overnight, then transfer to a resealable plastic freezer bag or container for storage. Reheat from frozen in the microwave or fry in a skillet.

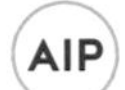 *omit pepper; make breakfast or Italian sausage*

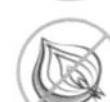 *make breakfast sausage*

CRISPY BACON

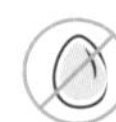 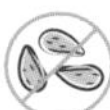 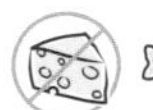 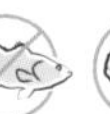  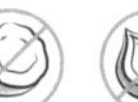  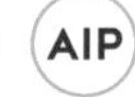 AIP

PREP TIME: 5 minutes COOK TIME: about 20 minutes
YIELD: varies

Bacon slices

1. Lay the slices of bacon in a baking dish with at least a 1½-inch rim (an extra-large roasting pan or lasagna pan works well, too). Place in a cold oven, then turn the oven on to 365°F.

2. Most of the bacon will be perfectly cooked, lightly browned, and crispy around the time your oven reaches temperature. If your bacon is thinly sliced, watch it, because it may be done before your oven beeps. Very thickly cut bacon may need 3 to 5 minutes more after the oven comes to temperature. If you like your bacon on the soft side, remove it from the oven a few minutes earlier.

TIP: To make bacon bits, simply chop the crispy bacon with a knife or break it apart with your fingers. Store in an airtight container in the refrigerator until ready to use.

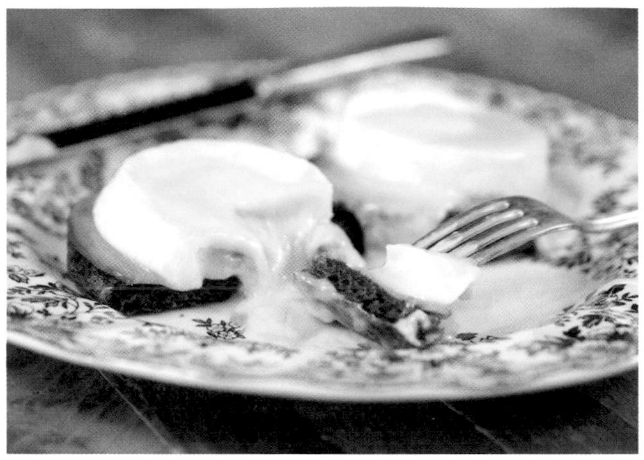

EGGS BENEDICT

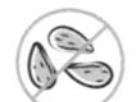 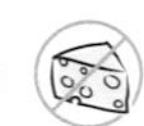 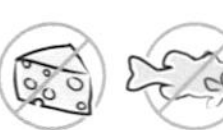 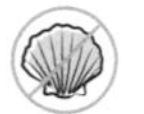 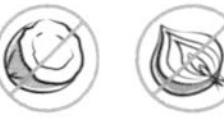 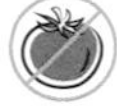

PREP TIME: 1 hour COOK TIME: 20 minutes
YIELD: 4 servings

4 large eggs
4 slices Canadian bacon
2 English Muffins (page 567)
1 batch Hollandaise (page 497)
Special equipment: egg poacher

1. Poach the eggs using an egg poacher. Gently grease the wells of the poacher with lard or coconut oil, then crack the eggs into the wells. Bring some water to a boil in a lidded skillet. Place the poacher in the water, cover the skillet, and cook the eggs for 6 minutes.

2. Meanwhile, warm the Canadian bacon in a skillet over medium heat for 1 to 2 minutes per side.

3. Gently cut down the middle of each of the English muffins and toast the halves in a toaster or toaster oven or under the broiler.

4. To assemble, place a toasted English muffin half cut side up on a plate. Lay a slice of Canadian bacon on top. Gently transfer a poached egg on top of the Canadian bacon. Then pour a few spoonfuls of hollandaise over the whole thing. Repeat with the remaining ingredients and serve!

WAFFLES

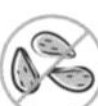 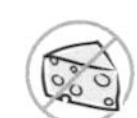 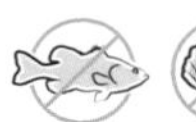 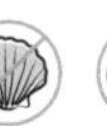  

PREP TIME: 5 minutes COOK TIME: 15 minutes
YIELD: eight to ten 4-inch square Belgian-style (thick) waffles

2 large green plantains (2½ to 3 cups chopped)
4 large eggs (or 5 eggs if the plantains are extra-large)
3 tablespoons coconut oil
2 teaspoons vanilla extract
½ teaspoon baking soda
⅛ teaspoon sea salt

1. Peel and chop the plantains. Place in a blender with the eggs and blend until smooth. Add the rest of the ingredients and blend on high for an additional minute.

2. Heat a waffle maker to high. Pour the batter into the waffle maker and cook for about 4½ minutes for Belgian-style (thick) waffles (follow the manufacturer's directions). Remove the waffle from the waffle maker.

3. Repeat with the remaining batter and serve.

TIPS: Sometimes this batter thickens while it sits; if it does, simply blend it for an additional 10 seconds.

To freeze the waffles, let them cool on a cooling rack, then place in a single layer on a baking sheet. Freeze for 4 to 6 hours or overnight. Remove from the baking sheet and transfer to an airtight container or freezer bag for long-term storage. Reheat from frozen in the microwave for 30 to 45 seconds or in a toaster or toaster oven if you enjoy them crispy.

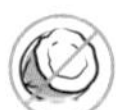 *use avocado oil or olive oil instead of coconut oil*

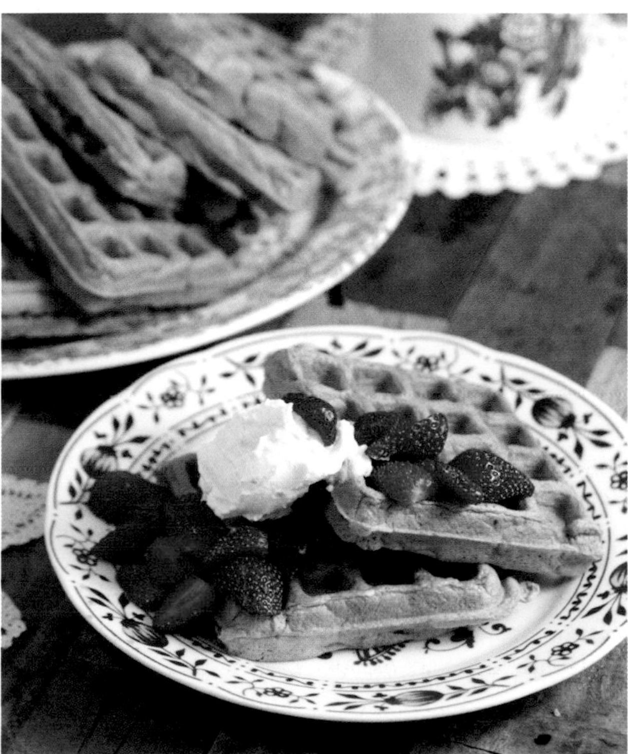

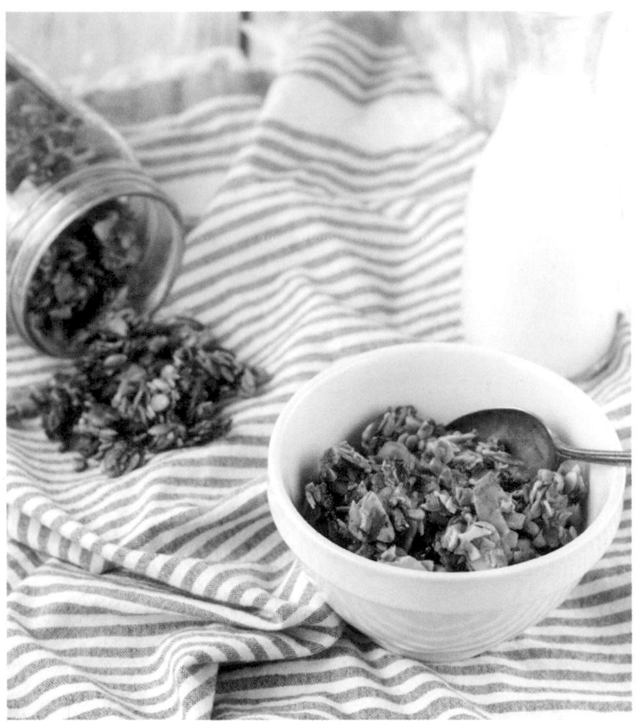

GRANOLA

 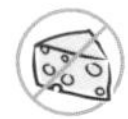 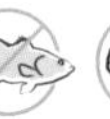 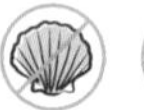 

PREP TIME: 5 minutes COOK TIME: 30 minutes
YIELD: 12 servings

2 cups sliced almonds

2 cups unsweetened coconut flakes

1 cup raw shelled sunflower seeds

1 cup raw pepitas

1 teaspoon ground cinnamon

1 teaspoon ground nutmeg

⅓ cup coconut oil

¼ cup honey

2 teaspoons vanilla extract

1 to 2 cups dried fruit, such as dried pineapple, raisins, or dried cranberries (optional)

1. Preheat the oven to 300°F. Line a large rimmed baking sheet with parchment paper.

2. Combine the almonds, coconut flakes, sunflower seeds, and pepitas in a large bowl. Add the cinnamon and nutmeg and stir to coat the nuts and seeds.

3. Melt the coconut oil and honey in a small saucepan over low heat or in the microwave. Stir in the vanilla.

4. Pour the coconut oil mixture over the nuts and seeds, then stir to coat. Pour the granola onto the prepared baking sheet and spread it out evenly. Bake for 30 minutes, until golden brown.

5. Remove from the oven and sprinkle the dried fruit over the top, if using. Let the granola cool completely in the pan (for larger chunks), then pour into a container for storage. Store at room temperature for up to a month.

CLAFOUTIS

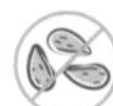  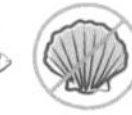 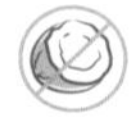 

PREP TIME: 20 minutes COOK TIME: 35 minutes
YIELD: 8 servings

3 cups whole cherries

1 very large green plantain or 1½ medium green plantains (1 cup puree)

3 large eggs

½ cup unsalted butter, plus more for greasing the baking dish

3 tablespoons honey

2 tablespoons lemon juice

1 tablespoon vanilla extract

⅛ teaspoon sea salt

1. Preheat the oven to 375°F. Grease a 10-inch baking dish or skillet with butter.

2. Pit the cherries and place in the greased baking dish (this amount should be perfect to cover the dish in a single layer).

3. Peel the plantain and combine with the remaining ingredients in a blender or food processor. Blend until completely smooth, 3 to 5 minutes, depending on your blender or food processor. Pour the batter over the cherries.

4. Bake for 35 minutes or until the middle doesn't jiggle and a toothpick inserted in the center comes out clean. Let cool for 15 to 20 minutes before serving.

TIP: Clafoutis is best served warm, but leftovers are great, too. Store covered on the counter.

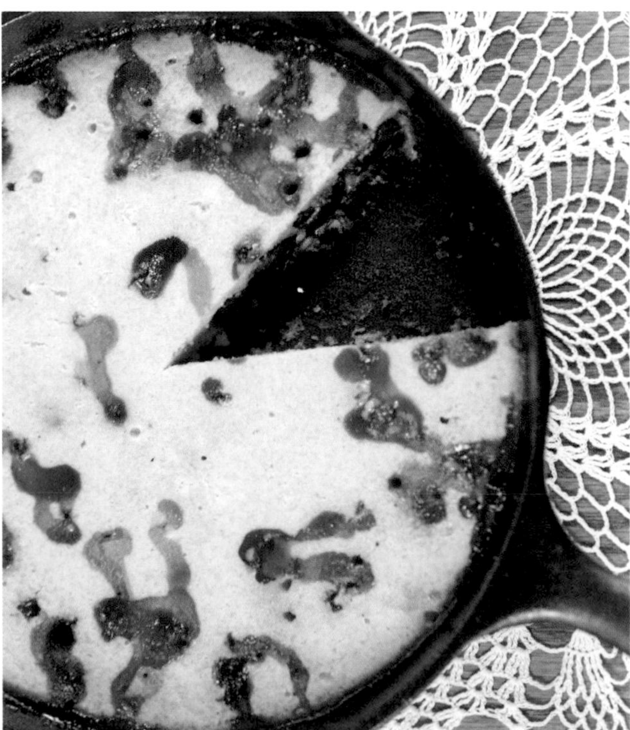

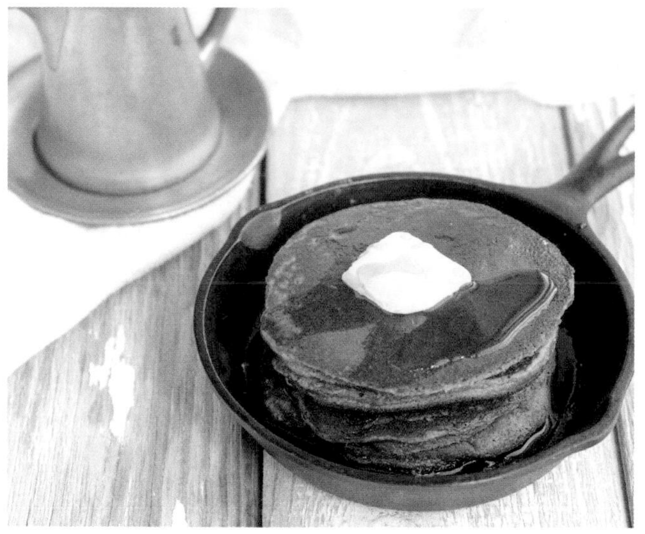

PUMPKIN PANCAKES

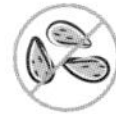 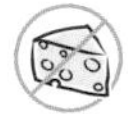 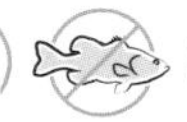   

PREP TIME: 10 minutes COOK TIME: 30 minutes
YIELD: twelve 3- to 4-inch pancakes

½ cup pumpkin powder

2 tablespoons honey (optional)

5 large eggs

½ teaspoon ground allspice

½ teaspoon ginger powder

½ teaspoon ground nutmeg

⅛ teaspoon ground cinnamon

⅛ teaspoon ground cloves

½ teaspoon baking soda

1 teaspoon cream of tartar

Coconut oil or other cooking fat, for the pan

1. Place all the pancake ingredients in a blender and blend for about 30 seconds, until smooth.

2. Heat about 2 tablespoons of coconut oil in a skillet or griddle over medium heat. Pour about 3 tablespoons of the batter into the pan, spacing the pancakes far enough apart that they won't touch as they spread.

3. Cook for 6 to 8 minutes on the first side, until the batter starts to look a little dry around the edges and is more solid on top. If you use a spatula to get a sneak peek at the underside of a pancake, it should be nicely browned but not too dark. Carefully flip the pancakes.

4. Cook for 2 to 4 minutes on the other side, until the pancakes are browned and feel solid when you press gently with your spatula or finger.

5. Repeat Steps 3 and 4 with the remaining batter, adding a little more coconut oil to the pan as needed. Enjoy the pancakes warm or cooled.

TIP: Pumpkin powder is simply dehydrated ground pumpkin. (It is not the same thing as pumpkin protein powder or pumpkin seed powder.) Jansal Valley and Barry Farms brands are available online.

CREPES

 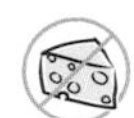 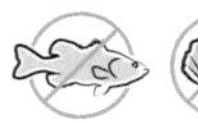 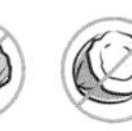 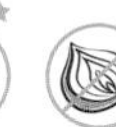 

PREP TIME: 10 minutes COOK TIME: 15 minutes
YIELD: 7 or 8 crepes

1 large green plantain

3 large eggs

3 tablespoons water

2 tablespoons coconut oil, plus more for frying

⅛ teaspoon sea salt

1. Peel the plantain and place in a blender or food processor with the rest of the ingredients. Puree for 2 minutes or until the batter is completely smooth.

2. Heat a crepe maker, crepe pan, or omelet pan over medium to medium-high heat.

3. Add 1 teaspoon of coconut oil to the pan (just enough that the crepe doesn't stick, but not so much that the batter can't spread when you swirl the pan). Add 3 to 4 tablespoons of the batter (you could use a ¼-cup scoop or just eyeball it) and immediately hold the pan up over the element while you swirl/angle the pan so that the batter spreads out into a uniform circle. (If you have a crepe pan, use the spreader to spread the batter; if you have a crepe maker, follow the manufacturer's directions.)

4. Cook the crepe for 45 to 75 seconds on the first side, until the top looks dry. Flip and cook on the second side for 15 to 30 seconds.

5. Repeat Steps 3 and 4 with the remaining batter, adding more coconut oil to the pan as needed. If the batter does not spread easily, add another tablespoon of water to it before cooking the rest of the crepes.

TIP: For sweet crepes, serve with fruit and Coconut Whipped Topping (page 480) or spread 2 to 3 tablespoons Chocolate Hazelnut Spread (page 489) over one side of the crepe and roll or fold, as shown. For savory crepes, serve with sautéed veggies, sausage, bacon, and/or scrambled eggs.

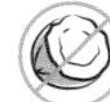 *use avocado oil or olive oil instead of coconut oil*

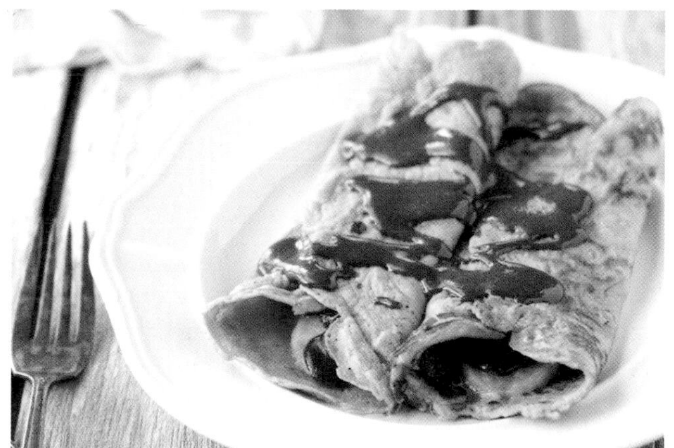

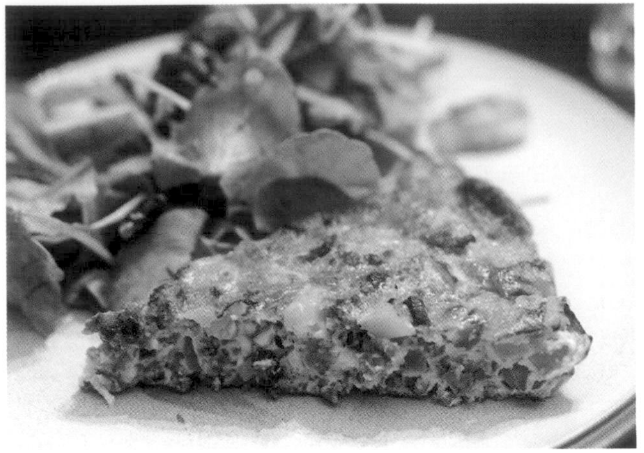

PORK & WINTER SQUASH FRITTATA

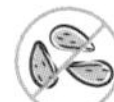 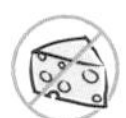 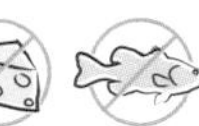 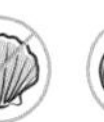 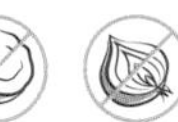 

PREP TIME: 15 minutes *COOK TIME: 40 minutes*
YIELD: 6 servings

3 to 4 slices thick-cut bacon, chopped

1 pound ground pork

1 tablespoon fresh sage, chopped

2 sprigs thyme

½ teaspoon sea salt or truffle salt

¼ teaspoon ground mace

3 cups winter squash, peeled, seeded, and cut into ¼- to ½-inch dice

10 large eggs, beaten

1. Place the chopped bacon in a cold large ovenproof skillet, then turn on the heat to medium-high. Cook until crisp, 8 to 10 minutes.
2. Preheat the oven broiler to high.
3. Add the ground pork, sage, thyme, salt, and mace to the skillet. Cook, stirring frequently with a wooden spoon or spatula to break up the pork, until the pork is fully browned, 8 to 10 minutes.
4. Carefully remove the sprigs of thyme, then add the squash. Cook until the squash is tender, 5 to 6 minutes. The cooking time will depend on the variety of squash you are using and how finely diced it is.
5. Add the beaten eggs. Cook for 1 to 2 minutes, stirring a couple of times.
6. Transfer the skillet to the oven and broil until the eggs are completely cooked, puffed up, and starting to brown on top, 7 to 10 minutes (the broiling time varies from oven to oven, so watch it carefully). Serve immediately. Store in the refrigerator for up to 5 days.

BACON, SPINACH & OLIVE FRITTATA

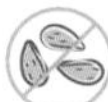 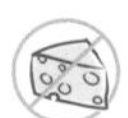 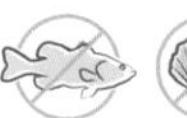   

PREP TIME: 10 minutes *COOK TIME: 30 minutes*
YIELD: 3 to 4 servings

6 ounces bacon (6 to 7 thick-cut slices), cut into small pieces

½ medium-sized yellow onion, finely diced

1½ cups diced red bell peppers (about 1 large)

1 cup sliced black olives, or 1 (3.8-ounce) can sliced black olives

4 cups chopped fresh spinach

8 large eggs, beaten

1. Heat a large ovenproof skillet over medium-high heat and preheat the oven broiler to high.
2. Place the bacon and onion in the skillet and cook, stirring occasionally, until the bacon is crisp and the onion is fully cooked and caramelized, 8 to 10 minutes.
3. Add the peppers and olives to the skillet and sauté, stirring occasionally, until the peppers are cooked, 4 to 5 minutes. Add the spinach and stir until wilted, about 1 minute.
4. Add the beaten eggs. Cook for 1 to 2 minutes, stirring a couple of times.
5. Transfer the skillet to the oven and broil until the eggs are completely cooked, puffed up, and starting to brown on top, 7 to 10 minutes (the broiling time varies from oven to oven, so watch it carefully). Serve immediately. Store in the refrigerator for up to 5 days.

 *omit onion*

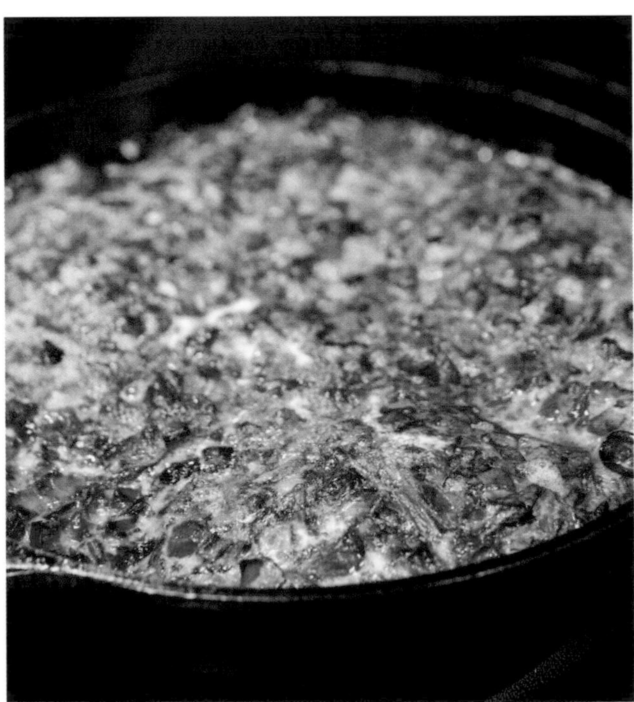

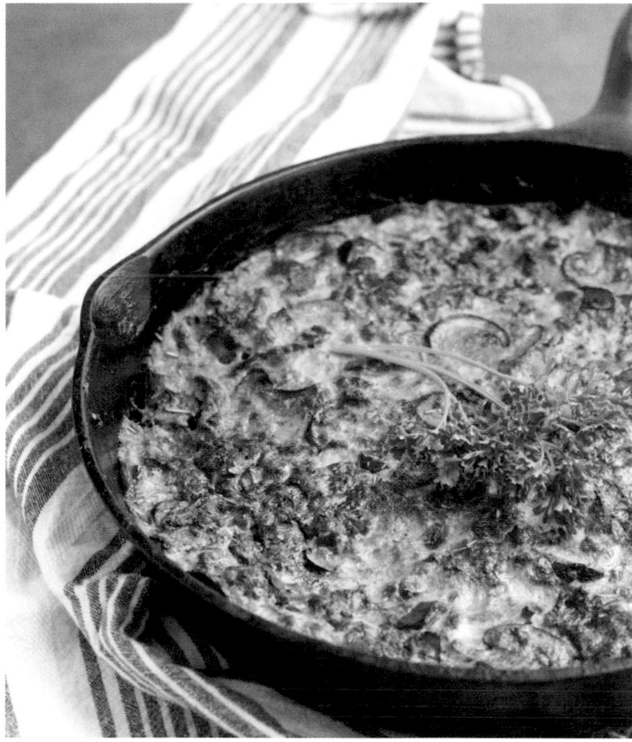

SAUSAGE & MUSHROOM FRITTATA

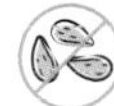 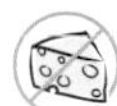 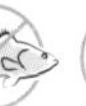  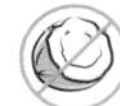

PREP TIME: 10 minutes *COOK TIME: 25 to 30 minutes*
YIELD: 4 servings

- 6 to 8 ounces bulk pork sausage
- ½ medium-sized yellow onion, diced
- ½ red bell pepper, diced
- 3 cups mushrooms, thinly sliced (about 1 pound)
- 8 large eggs, beaten

1. Heat a large ovenproof skillet over medium-high heat and preheat the oven broiler to high.
2. Place the sausage in the pan and use a wooden spoon or spatula to break up the clumps as it cooks. (No oil is necessary if you have a nice fatty sausage; if you are using a very lean sausage, add a tablespoon of coconut oil to the pan to prevent sticking.)
3. Add the onion, bell pepper, and mushrooms and sauté, stirring occasionally, until the vegetables are cooked, 8 to 10 minutes.
4. Add the beaten eggs. Cook for 1 to 2 minutes, stirring a couple of times.
5. Transfer the skillet to the oven and broil until the eggs are completely cooked, puffed up, and starting to brown on top, 7 to 10 minutes (the broiling time varies from oven to oven, so watch it carefully). Serve immediately. Store in the refrigerator for up to 5 days.

VEGGIE FRITTATA

 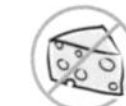 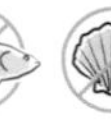  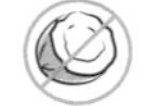

PREP TIME: 5 minutes *COOK TIME: 15 minutes*
YIELD: 3 to 4 servings

- 1 tablespoon coconut oil, olive oil, or other cooking fat
- ½ medium-sized yellow onion, finely chopped
- ½ red bell pepper, finely chopped
- 1½ cups mushrooms, thinly sliced
- 2 cups chopped kale (tough stems removed)
- 2 cups fresh spinach, chopped
- 8 large eggs, beaten

1. Heat a large ovenproof skillet over medium-high heat and preheat the oven broiler to high.
2. Place the oil in the pan. Add the onion, bell pepper, and mushrooms and sauté, stirring occasionally, until the vegetables are starting to soften, 3 to 4 minutes.
3. Add the kale and continue to sauté until all the vegetables are cooked, 8 to 10 minutes.
4. Add the spinach and stir until the spinach is wilted.
5. Add the beaten eggs. Cook for 1 to 2 minutes, stirring a couple of times.
6. Transfer the skillet to the oven and broil until the eggs are completely cooked, puffed up, and starting to brown on top, 7 to 10 minutes (the broiling time varies from oven to oven, so watch it carefully). Serve immediately. Store in the refrigerator for up to 5 days.

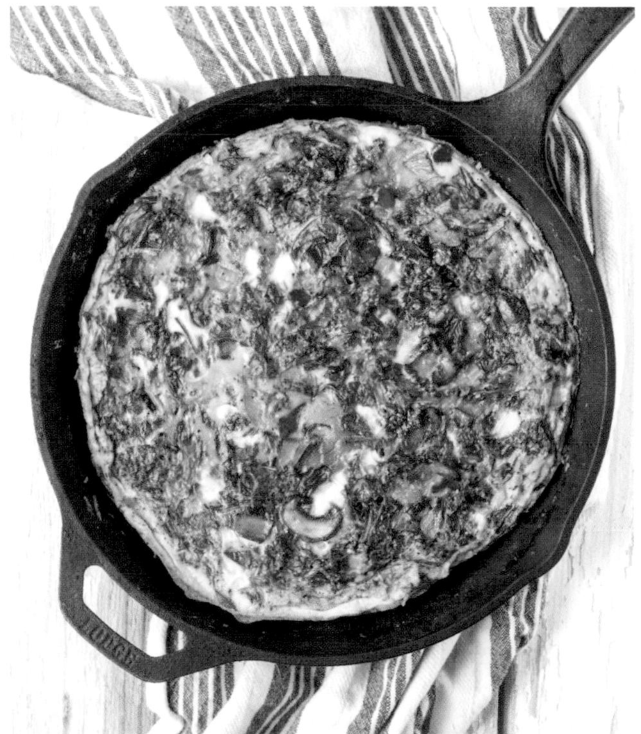

DIY OMELET

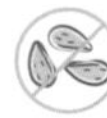 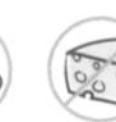   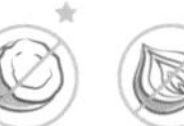 

PREP TIME: 2 minutes *COOK TIME: 5 minutes*
YIELD: 1 serving

Filling of choice (see below)
1 tablespoon coconut oil
2 large eggs
2 tablespoons water
Dash of sea salt

1. Prepare the filling (see some fun combinations at right!). This may involve sautéing a few veggies or simply chopping up and reheating some leftovers.

2. Heat the coconut oil in an omelet pan or 8-inch skillet over medium heat.

3. Blend the eggs, water, and salt with a hand mixer (or whisk thoroughly by hand), then pour into the hot pan. Cook for 4 to 5 minutes, until the egg mixture looks fairly solid.

4. Lay the filling over half of the omelet. Wiggle a spatula underneath the half that does not have the filling on it and flip that half over the filling. Slide onto a plate and enjoy!

FILLING OPTIONS

- Sautéed mushrooms and fresh spinach
- Pico de Gallo (page 490) and chopped avocado (do not heat)
- Fried leftover Mashed Plantains (page 554) and bacon
- Fried bulk sausage and chopped plantain or winter squash
- DIY Baked Chicken Breast (page 541), Pesto (page 495 or 497), chopped canned artichoke hearts, and sliced black olives
- DIY Baked Chicken Breast (page 541), Hollandaise (page 497), and capers
- Leftover Simple Steak (page 547) and Chimichurri (page 495)
- Steamed asparagus and Hollandaise (page 497)
- Sautéed onion and sweet peppers with fresh, seeded Roma tomato
- Sweet peppers, butternut squash, and chopped fresh parsley

 *avoid*

 *avoid*

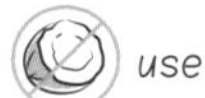 *use olive oil or avocado oil*

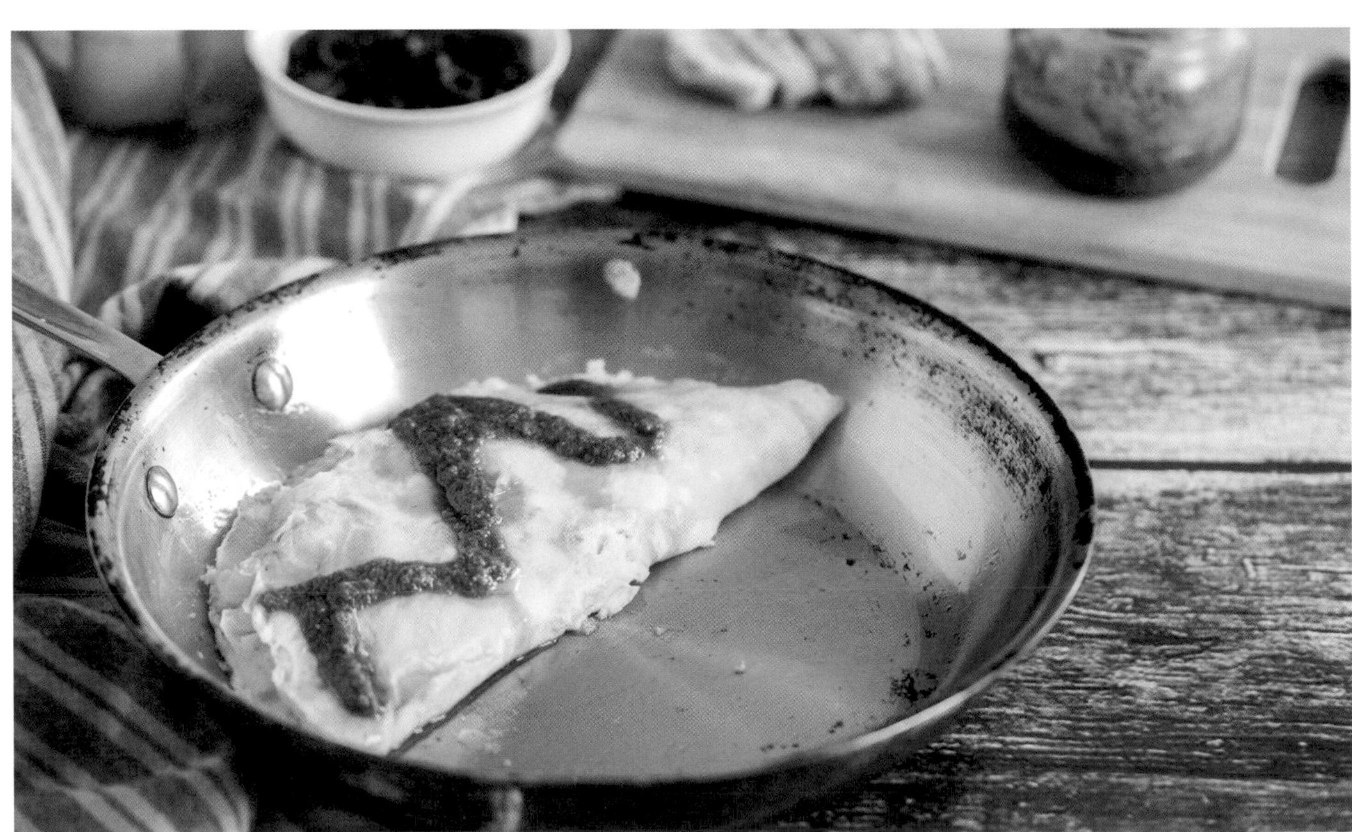

DIY PALEO PORRIDGE

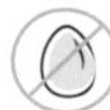 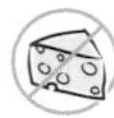 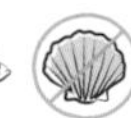 

PREP TIME: 10 minutes *COOK TIME: 10 minutes*
YIELD: 1 large serving

- ¼ cup unsweetened shredded coconut
- ¼ cup raw almonds
- ¼ cup raw walnuts
- 3 tablespoons raw pepitas
- ½ cup boiling water
- 1½ teaspoons honey (optional)

1. Combine the coconut, almonds, walnuts, and pepitas in a blender or food processor and blend until the ingredients are finely ground and the blade starts to seize.

2. Boil some water in a kettle or in the microwave. Pour ½ cup into a microwave-safe container and mix in the honey, if using.

3. Stir the ground nuts into the hot honey water. Microwave on high for 30 seconds; stir once more. Alternatively, heat the porridge in a small saucepan over medium-low heat, stirring constantly, for 4 to 5 minutes, until it almost simmers.

4. Let sit for 3 to 5 minutes to thicken. Stir in add-ins (at right), if using. Serve immediately.

ADD-IN SUGGESTIONS

Spiced Porridge: Stir in ½ teaspoon ground nutmeg and ½ teaspoon ground cinnamon.

Apple-Cinnamon Porridge: Stir in 2 tablespoons freeze-dried apple pieces (or applesauce) and ½ teaspoon ground cinnamon.

Maple-Nut Porridge: Use 1 tablespoon maple syrup instead of the honey and sprinkle 2 tablespoons chopped pecans over the top.

Banana-Nut Porridge: Omit the honey and mash in half of a ripe banana instead. Sprinkle 2 tablespoons chopped pecans over the top.

Blueberry Porridge: Stir in ⅓ cup fresh or frozen blueberries (or any other berries you like).

Peaches & Cream Porridge: Stir in ⅓ cup chopped fresh or preserved peaches and 1 to 2 tablespoons coconut milk or unsalted butter.

Pumpkin Pie Porridge: Stir in ¼ cup fresh or canned pumpkin puree and ⅛ teaspoon each of ground allspice, ground cinnamon, ground cloves, ginger powder, and ground nutmeg.

Butter & Salt Porridge: Stir in ½ teaspoon salt (or to taste) and melt 2 tablespoons unsalted butter or ghee over the top.

Chocolate Porridge: Stir in 1 tablespoon cocoa powder.

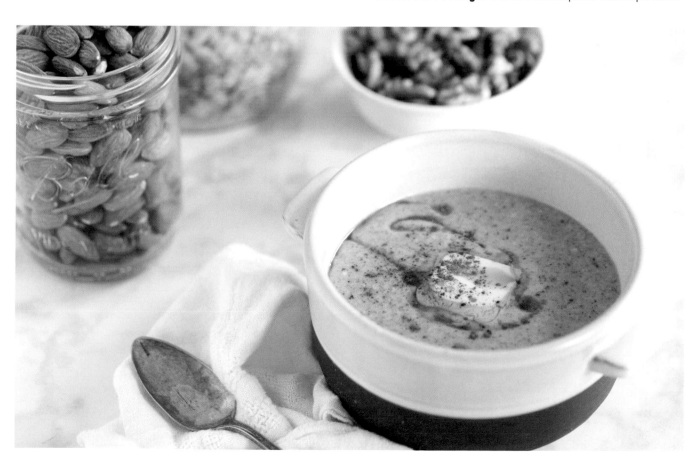

Chapter 41: SOUPS, STEWS, AND SALADS

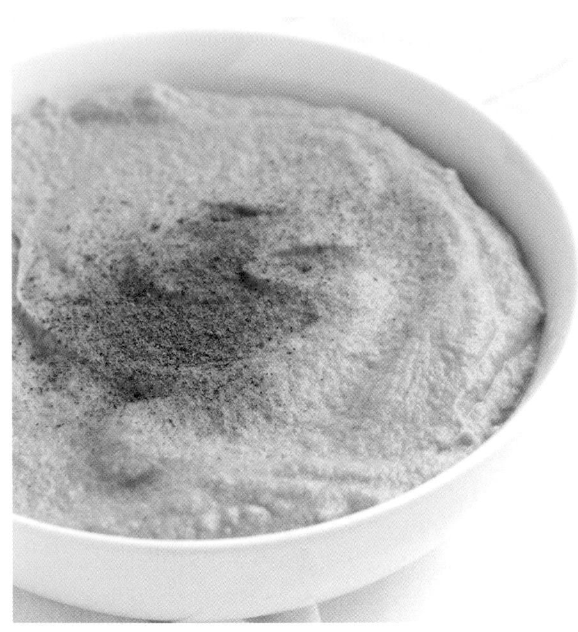

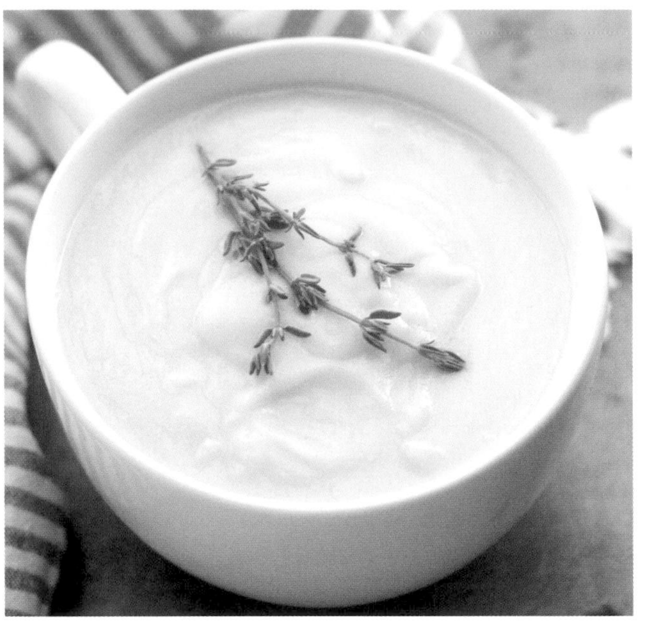

"CREAM" OF BROCCOLI SOUP

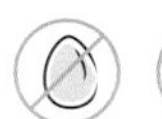 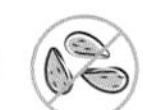 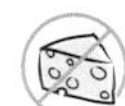 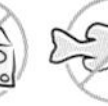 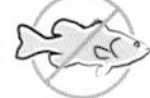 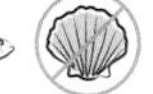 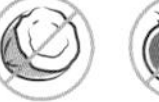 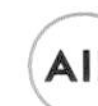 

PREP TIME: 10 minutes COOK TIME: 30 minutes
YIELD: 2 to 3 servings

1 to 2 large heads broccoli

1 small avocado

2 cups Bone Stock (page 486)

½ teaspoon ground nutmeg

Sea salt and ground black pepper (optional)

1. Cut the broccoli into florets. Peel the stems if they're tough, then slice them. (You should get about 4 cups of florets and stems.) Peel and pit the avocado and cut it into medium-sized chunks.

2. Bring the stock to a simmer in a stockpot over medium-high heat. Add the broccoli and steam until dark green and tender, 7 to 8 minutes.

3. Reduce the heat to low. Add the nutmeg and avocado chunks and continue to cook for 3 to 4 more minutes, until the avocado is warm.

4. Puree the soup with an immersion blender, or use a blender or food processor, being careful not to burn yourself. Taste and season with salt and pepper, if desired.

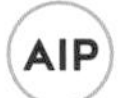 *omit pepper and replace nutmeg with 1/4 teaspoon mace*

"CREAM" OF CELERY ROOT SOUP

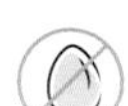 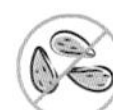 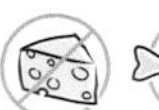  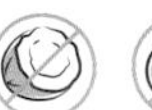 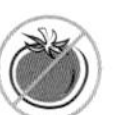

PREP TIME: 15 minutes COOK TIME: 30 minutes
YIELD: 3 to 4 servings

4 cups Chicken Stock (page 486)

2 large celery roots, peeled and cut into ½-inch dice

½ yellow onion, chopped

2 cloves garlic, chopped

2 sprigs thyme, or ½ teaspoon dried thyme leaves

2 tablespoons unsalted butter, ghee, or olive oil

½ cup dry white wine

Sea salt and ground black pepper (optional)

1. Combine the stock, celery roots, onion, garlic, and thyme in a large saucepan or small stockpot. Bring to a boil, then reduce the heat to a simmer. Simmer, uncovered, for 20 to 25 minutes, until the celery roots are soft when pierced with a knife.

2. Remove the thyme sprigs and puree the soup using an immersion blender. You could also do this in a conventional blender, but be careful not to burn yourself!

3. Stir in the butter and wine and simmer for another 3 to 5 minutes. Taste and season with salt and pepper, if desired.

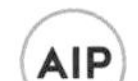 *omit pepper*

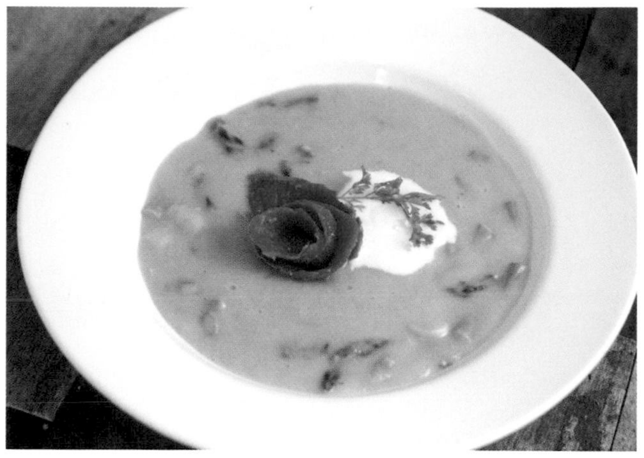

ASPARAGUS SOUP

 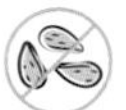 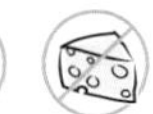 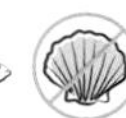 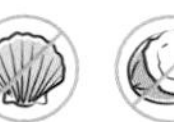  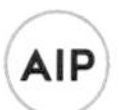 AIP

PREP TIME: 10 minutes *COOK TIME: 25 minutes*
YIELD: 6 servings

- 2 bunches asparagus (about 2½ pounds)
- 6 cups Chicken Stock (page 486), divided
- 1½ cups cubed green plantains (about 1 large or 1½ medium)
- 2 cups cauliflower florets (about ½ small head)
- Juice of 1 lemon
- 1 teaspoon sea salt
- 8 to 12 ounces lox, for garnish (optional)
- 1 cup Coconut Milk Yogurt (page 481) or kefir, for garnish (optional)

1. Snap the tough stems off the asparagus. Add the tough stems to a large soup pot with 5 cups of the stock, the plantains, and cauliflower. Bring to a boil, then reduce the heat to maintain a simmer. Simmer for 15 to 20 minutes, until the asparagus stems are soft when pierced with a knife and the cauliflower is overcooked. (For very tough stems, you may need to simmer longer.)

2. Meanwhile, slice the tender asparagus tips into ½-inch pieces.

3. In a blender in 2 batches or with an immersion blender, puree the contents of the pot until completely smooth (this takes 1 to 2 minutes in a blender, but may take longer with an immersion blender).

4. Bring the remaining 1 cup of stock and the asparagus tips to a simmer on the stovetop (do this in a separate small pot if you opted to puree with an immersion blender, or in the same pot if you used a countertop blender). Simmer for 3 to 5 minutes, until the asparagus is tender but not too soft.

5. Add the tender asparagus tips and stock to the puree in the soup pot. Stir in the lemon juice and salt. Stir and taste for seasoning. Add more salt, if needed.

6. Ladle into bowls and garnish with lox and a dollop of coconut milk yogurt, if desired.

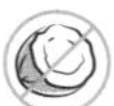 *omit coconut yogurt*

CHUNKY NOTATO LEEK SOUP

 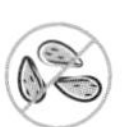 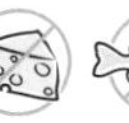 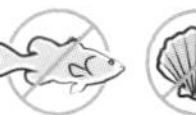 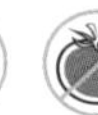 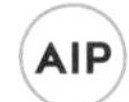 AIP

PREP TIME: 20 minutes *COOK TIME: 40 minutes*
YIELD: 5 to 6 servings

- 3 slices thick-cut bacon, chopped
- 2 pounds turnips, cut into 1-inch cubes (5 to 6 cups)
- 1 green plantain, peeled and grated
- 1 bunch leeks, sliced (5 to 6 cups)
- 4 cups Chicken Stock (page 486)
- 1 cup coconut cream or full-fat coconut milk, homemade (page 480) or canned
- ¼ cup chopped fresh parsley leaves (optional)
- ½ teaspoon sea salt or truffle salt (optional)

1. Place the bacon in a large saucepan or small stockpot over medium-high heat. Cook, stirring occasionally, until browned, about 10 minutes.

2. Add the turnips, plantain, leeks, and stock. Bring to a boil, then reduce the heat to maintain a rapid simmer for 20 to 25 minutes.

3. Stir in the coconut cream and parsley, if using. Cook for 2 to 3 minutes. Taste and add the salt, if needed, and serve.

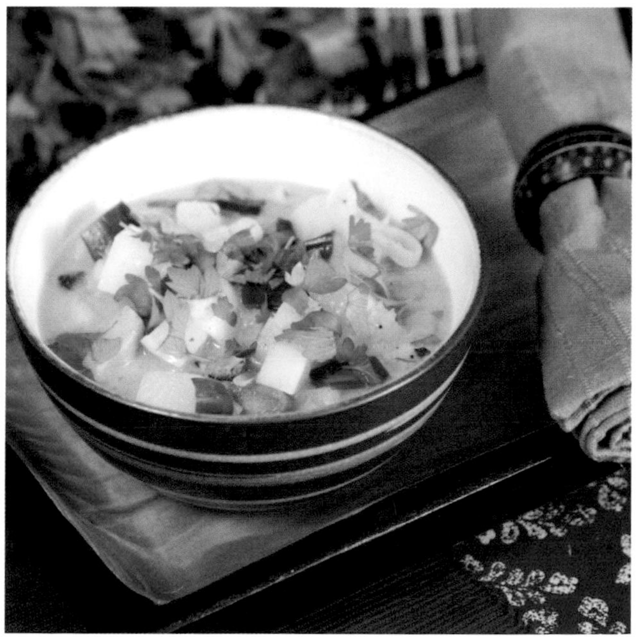

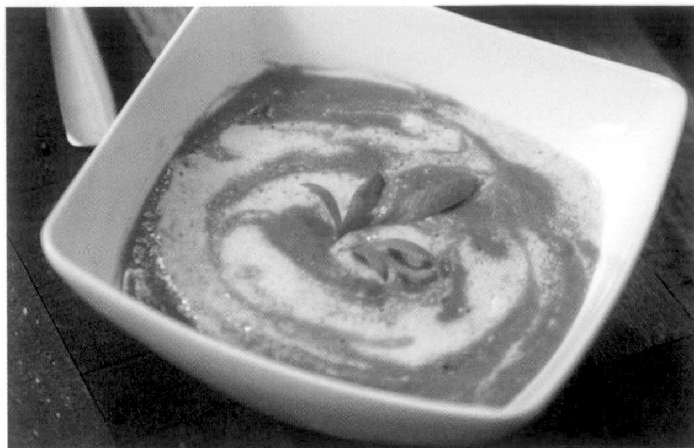

LETTUCE SOUP

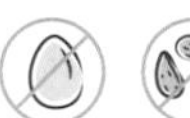 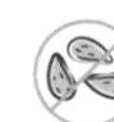 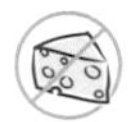 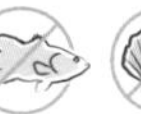 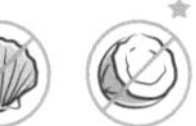   AIP

PREP TIME: 10 minutes *COOK TIME: 30 minutes*
YIELD: 2 to 4 servings

- 3 tablespoons olive oil
- 1 cup chopped shallots (about 3 large shallots)
- 1 clove garlic, chopped
- ¾ teaspoon ground coriander
- ⅛ teaspoon ground cardamom
- ¼ teaspoon ground black pepper
- ¾ teaspoon sea salt
- 1 pound lettuce (about 2 large heads), roughly chopped
- 4 cups Chicken Stock (page 486)
- 1 green plantain, peeled and cut into 1-inch chunks
- Coconut Milk Yogurt (page 481), for serving (optional)

1. Heat the olive oil in a large soup pot over medium-high heat. Add the shallots and cook, stirring frequently, until beginning to soften, about 5 minutes.

2. Add the garlic, spices, and salt. Cook, stirring frequently, for another minute or until fragrant.

3. Add the lettuce. Stir constantly for 2 to 3 minutes to wilt the lettuce.

4. Add the stock and plantain. Bring to a boil, then reduce the heat to maintain a simmer for 20 minutes.

5. Puree the soup by transferring the entire contents of the pot into a blender and blending on high for 1 minute (do this in batches if you have a small blender). An immersion blender can also be used, but it will be harder to get that perfect creamy consistency. Taste for seasoning and add more salt, if desired.

6. Ladle into bowls and garnish with a dollop of coconut milk yogurt, if desired.

TIPS: If you can't find green plantains, you can use a russet potato, a white sweet potato, or 2 medium parsnips instead.

Boston and Bibb lettuce are traditionally used for lettuce soup, but any variety you have on hand will work.

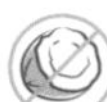 *omit coconut milk yogurt*  *omit shallots*

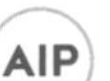 *omit coriander, cardamom, pepper, and yogurt; can replace spices with 1/8 teaspoon mace or a pinch of ground cloves*

NEW ENGLAND CLAM CHOWDER

  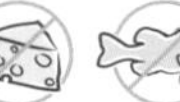 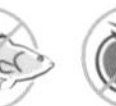 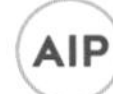 AIP

PREP TIME: 20 minutes *COOK TIME: 35 minutes*
YIELD: 6 to 8 servings

- 4 slices thick-cut bacon, chopped
- 1 onion, diced
- 2 to 3 stalks celery, thinly sliced
- 1 large carrot, diced
- 1 large turnip, cut into ¾-inch cubes
- 3 cups Bone Stock (page 486)
- 3 (5- to 6-ounce) cans clams, drained
- 1 green plantain, peeled and grated
- 2 bay leaves
- 4 to 5 sprigs thyme, leaves only
- 2 cups coconut cream, homemade (page 480) or store-bought
- 3 tablespoons chopped fresh parsley
- Sea salt or truffle salt (optional)

1. Place the bacon in a medium stockpot, then turn on the heat to medium-high. Cook, stirring occasionally, until the bacon is crisp.

2. Add the onion, celery, carrot, and turnip and cook until fragrant, stirring occasionally, about 5 minutes.

3. Add the stock, clams, plantain, bay leaves, and thyme. Bring to a boil, then reduce the heat to maintain a simmer for 20 minutes, stirring occasionally.

4. Add the coconut cream and parsley. Taste and season with salt, if desired. Cook for 1 to 2 minutes and serve.

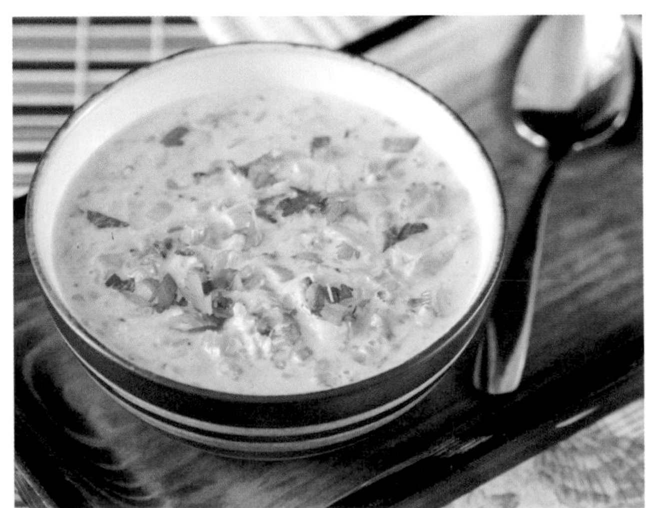

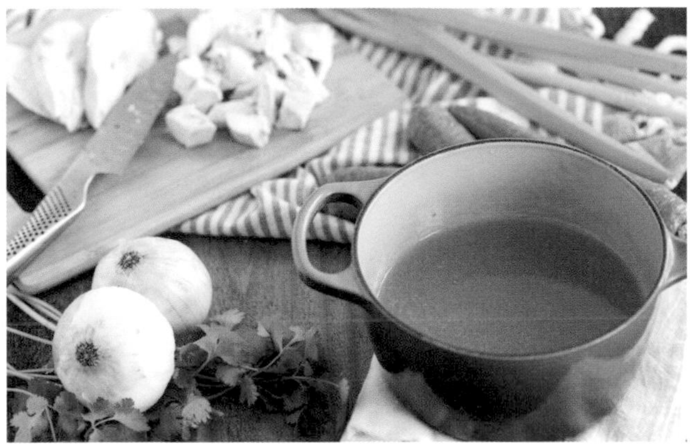

DIY SOUP

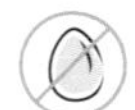 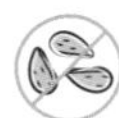 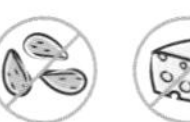 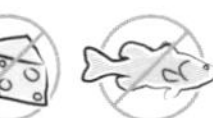 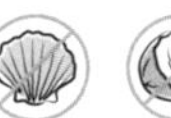 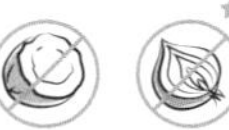   AIP

PREP TIME: 10 minutes COOK TIME: 20 minutes
YIELD: varies

2 parts Bone Stock (page 486)

2 to 3 parts mixed vegetables and vegetable-like fruits (onion, celery, carrots, turnips, rutabaga, radishes, kohlrabi, leeks, broccoli, sea vegetables, parsnip, green plantain, cauliflower, winter squash, mushrooms, zucchini, sweet potato, spinach, kale, collard greens), cut into bite-sized pieces

Fresh herbs (thyme, rosemary, sage, garlic, ginger, oregano, basil, parsley, chives; optional)

1 part leftover or precooked meat (chicken, pork, beef, lamb, or sausage), cut into bite-sized pieces

Sea salt

1. Pour the stock into a large soup pot and bring to a simmer over medium heat.
2. Add the vegetables. If you have leafy greens or sea vegetables, add them at the same time as the meat. If using a tough fresh herb like rosemary or thyme, add it now; otherwise, add herbs with the leafy greens and meat.
3. Once the veggies are cooked, 10 to 15 minutes, add the meat, leafy greens, tender herbs, and/or seaweed. Cook for 2 to 3 more minutes.
4. Taste and add salt, if needed, before serving.

GREAT COMBINATIONS

Chicken Vegetable Soup: Chicken Stock, leftover chicken, carrots, celery, onion, sweet potato, fresh parsley

Steak & Potato Soup: Beef Stock, leftover roast beef or steak, carrots, celery, onion, mushrooms, potato or green plantain or parsnip, rosemary, thyme

Asian Chicken Soup: Chicken Stock, leftover chicken, carrots, snap peas, bamboo shoots or water chestnuts, shiitake mushrooms, finely grated fresh ginger, and seaweed

Pork Vegetable Soup: Pork Stock, leftover pork roast or chop, carrots, celery, onion, winter squash, kale, canned tomatoes, crushed garlic, Italian seasoning (page 482)

Sausage & Broccoli Soup: Chicken or Pork Stock, leftover sausage, broccoli, onion, carrots, green plantain, a splash of white wine, thyme

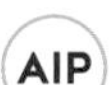 *avoid non-AIP options*

 *avoid*

 *avoid*

CURRY CARROT SOUP

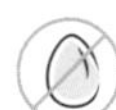 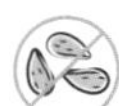 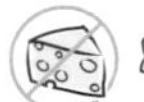  

PREP TIME: 10 minutes COOK TIME: 50 minutes
YIELD: 3 to 4 servings

6 cups Chicken Stock (page 486)

¼ medium-sized onion, finely chopped

1 pound carrots, roughly chopped

1 teaspoon finely grated fresh ginger

1 teaspoon curry powder, homemade (page 483) or store-bought

2 tablespoons coconut butter (aka coconut cream concentrate)

1. In a stockpot, bring the stock to a simmer over medium-high heat. Add the onion and carrots and simmer until the carrots are very soft, 35 to 40 minutes.
2. Add the ginger and curry powder and cook for another 5 minutes.
3. Puree the soup with an immersion blender until smooth. You can also use a blender, being careful not to burn yourself!
4. Stir in the coconut butter and serve.

 *use Nightshade-Free Curry Powder (page 483)*

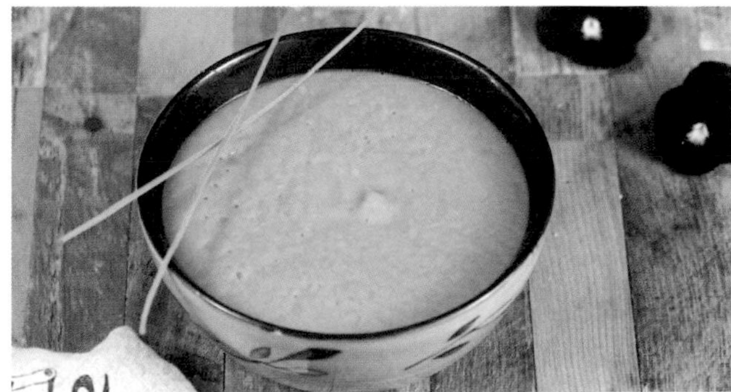

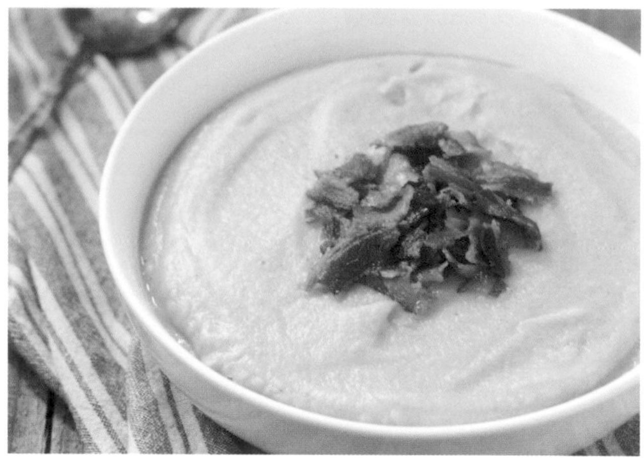

RUSTIC BACON & PUMPKIN SOUP

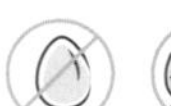 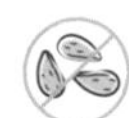 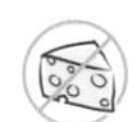  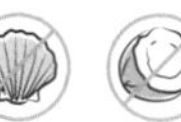 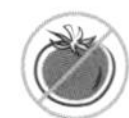  AIP

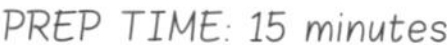

PREP TIME: 15 minutes
COOK TIME: 1 hour (including time to roast pumpkins)
YIELD: 4 to 6 servings

1 pound bacon

3 pounds pie pumpkin or other winter squash

2 medium-sized yellow onions, diced

2 to 3 cloves garlic

2 cups Chicken Stock (page 486)

¼ teaspoon ground nutmeg

1. Cook the bacon in the oven or on the stovetop until crispy. My preferred method is to lay the bacon strips on 2 rimmed baking sheets. Place in a cold oven and turn the oven on to 400°F. Around the time the oven reaches temperature, the bacon will be ready. Remove the bacon from the baking sheets and reserve the fat. Once the bacon has cooled, cut or crumble into large bits.

2. Preheat the oven to 375°F; if you do this immediately after cooking the bacon, it's fine if your oven starts out a little hot.

3. Carefully cut the pumpkins in half and scoop out the seeds. Place the pumpkin halves on a rimmed baking sheet; it doesn't matter whether they're cut side up or down. Bake for 35 to 45 minutes, until soft. Remove from the oven and let cool.

4. Spoon the pumpkin "meat" out of the peel. Mash with a fork or potato masher (this gives a more uneven texture, which is part of the rustic nature of this soup; use a potato ricer or immersion blender for a finer-textured soup). Set aside.

5. Heat 2 to 3 tablespoons of the reserved bacon fat in a medium stockpot over medium-high heat. Add the onions and garlic and sauté until the onions are fully cooked and caramelized.

6. Add the stock to deglaze the pot. Add the mashed pumpkin, nutmeg, and 2 to 3 more tablespoons of bacon fat (you want 4 to 5 tablespoons total; it's a good idea to add a little less and then taste your soup and decide whether you want it to be more bacon-y).

7. Reduce the heat to medium-low and bring to a simmer. Remove from the heat.

8. Serve the soup by ladling into bowls and generously topping with bacon bits.

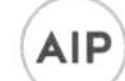 *replace nutmeg with 1/8 teaspoon mace*

WATERMELON GAZPACHO

 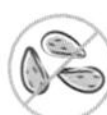 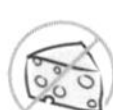 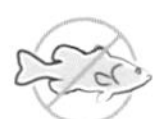 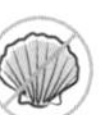 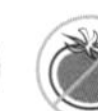 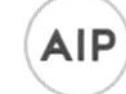 AIP

PREP TIME: 20 minutes, plus time to chill
YIELD: 4 to 6 servings

5 cups cubed seedless watermelon (or remove seeds if using a seeded watermelon)

2 teaspoons red or white wine vinegar

1 tablespoon olive oil

¼ teaspoon sea salt

¼ red onion, finely diced (about ½ cup)

½ cucumber, finely diced (about ¾ cup)

½ jicama, finely diced (about 1½ cups)

2 tablespoons chopped fresh cilantro

1 tablespoon chopped fresh mint

1. Combine the watermelon, vinegar, olive oil, and salt in a blender and pulse until smooth. (It's okay if it remains a little pulpy.)

2. Stir the onion, cucumber, jicama, cilantro, and mint into the watermelon mixture.

3. Pour into a container, cover, and place in the fridge to chill for 2 hours (or up to overnight) before serving.

TIP: If you can't find jicama, a finely diced Granny Smith apple is a great substitute.

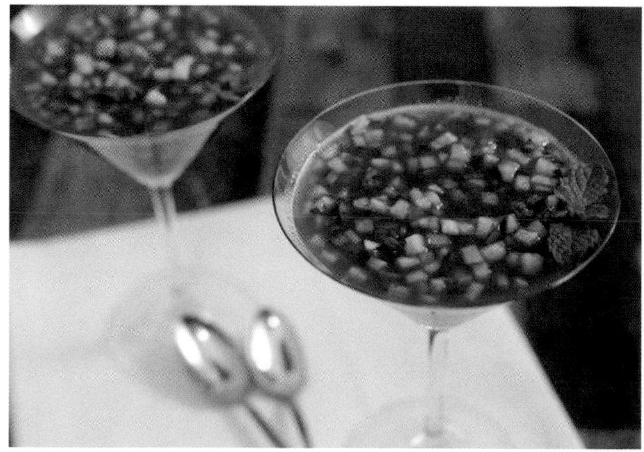

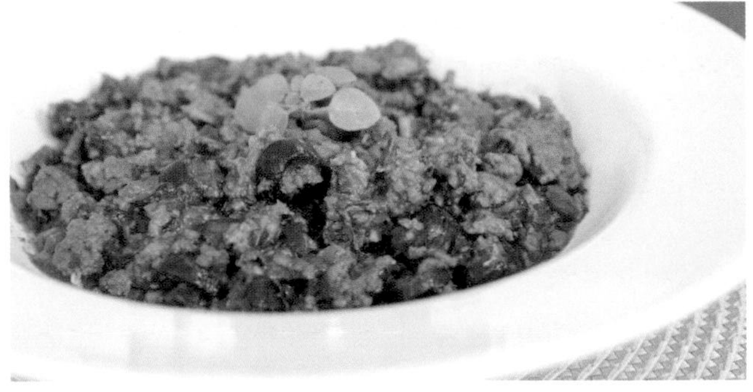

SPANISH PICADILLO

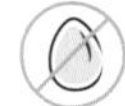  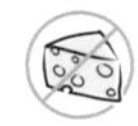 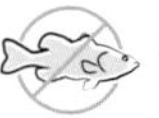 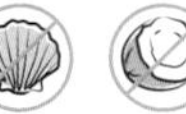  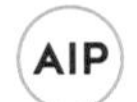 AIP

PREP TIME: 30 minutes COOK TIME: 2 1/2 hours
YIELD: 8 to 10 servings

- 4 ounces bacon or pancetta, diced
- ½ large white onion, finely diced
- 1 large (2 medium) carrot, finely diced
- 3 stalks celery, finely diced
- 7 to 8 cloves garlic
- 3 pounds ground beef or other red meat (lamb is particularly good)
- 1½ teaspoons sea salt
- 2 cups Bone Stock (page 486)
- 1 (16-ounce) can or box pumpkin puree
- 10 ounces mushrooms, chopped into ¼-inch pieces
- 1 can sliced olives (drained weight 12 ounces)
- 5 to 6 ounces fresh spinach, chopped
- 1 large bunch fresh basil (2 to 2½ ounces), chopped

1. Place the bacon in a large saucepan and turn on the heat to medium-high. Once the bacon starts to release some fat, add the onion, carrot, and celery. Sauté together for 10 minutes, until the onion is starting to caramelize. Add the garlic and stir to combine.

2. Add the ground beef to the pan, 1 pound at a time with ½ teaspoon of salt added with each pound of ground beef. Break up the beef with a spoon or spatula, and once it's browned, add the next pound.

3. Once all the beef is browned, add the stock and pumpkin puree and reduce the heat to low. Simmer, uncovered, for 1 to 2 hours, stirring occasionally. If the mixture begins to get dry and stick to the bottom, reduce the heat even further and add a little more stock or water. The longer the mixture simmers, the better; if you want to simmer it all day, go ahead.

4. Add the mushrooms and olives to the pot and stir to incorporate. Simmer for 10 more minutes, until the mushrooms are cooked.

5. Stir in the spinach and basil and cook for 5 more minutes. Taste and add more salt, if needed, before serving.

VARIATION: ***Spanish Rice.*** *Mix 1 part picadillo with 1 part steamed white rice (if you include rice in your diet) or cooked cauli-rice (page 555) just prior to serving. This is a great way to stretch this dish even further!*

CREAMY COLESLAW

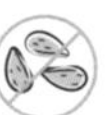 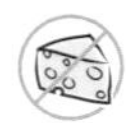  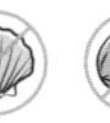 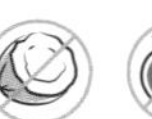 *

PREP TIME: 15 minutes YIELD: 6 to 8 servings

- ½ head green cabbage (about 1 pound)
- 2 tablespoons sea salt
- 2 medium carrots (see Tip)
- ½ cup Mayonnaise (page 487)
- 1 tablespoon Dijon mustard
- 1½ tablespoons apple cider vinegar
- ¼ cup finely chopped fresh dill
- ¼ teaspoon turmeric powder
- ¼ teaspoon paprika

1. Slice the cabbage as thinly as you can (I use my mandoline set to 1/16 inch thick). Put the cabbage in a colander and toss with the salt. Place the colander in the sink and let sit for at least 1 hour and up to 3 hours; let it sit longer if your cabbage is not very thinly sliced.

2. Rinse the cabbage very thoroughly (taste it to make sure you rinsed off all the salt) and let drain, or dry in a salad spinner. Transfer to a large bowl.

3. Coarsely grate the carrots and combine with the cabbage.

4. In a small bowl, mix together the mayonnaise, mustard, vinegar, dill, turmeric, and paprika. Pour the mixture over the cabbage and carrots and toss until thoroughly coated. It's best to cover with plastic wrap and refrigerate for at least 1 hour before serving. Stir before serving, as the dressing tends to settle.

TIP: If you purchase a coleslaw mix with preshredded cabbage and carrots already included, you can salt the carrots along with the cabbage.

 *omit paprika*

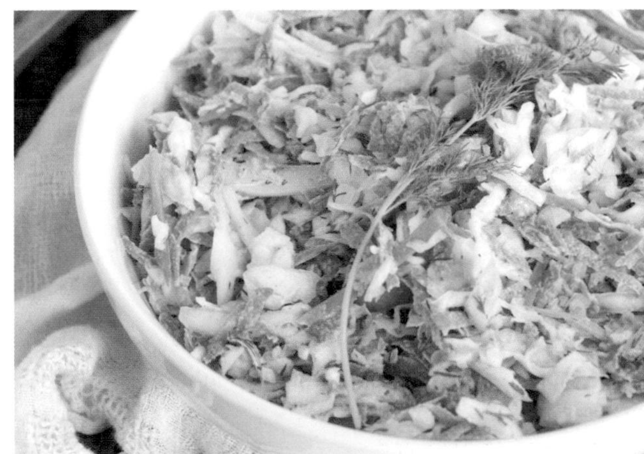

HAMBURGER STEW

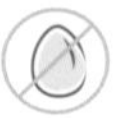 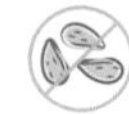 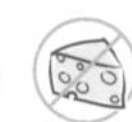  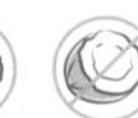  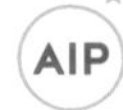 AIP*

PREP TIME: 15 minutes COOK TIME: 50 minutes
YIELD: 5 to 6 servings

- 3 tablespoons olive oil, divided
- 2 medium zucchini, peeled and roughly chopped
- 3 cups Beef Stock (page 486)
- 1 medium white onion, roughly chopped
- 3 medium carrots, sliced into ½-inch rounds
- 3 stalks celery, sliced into ½-inch slices
- 2 pounds ground beef
- 1 bay leaf
- 1 sprig rosemary
- 5 sprigs thyme
- 2 teaspoons sea salt
- ¼ teaspoon ground black pepper
- 8 ounces mushrooms, sliced
- 2 green plantains, peeled and cut into ½-inch chunks
- Chopped fresh parsley, for garnish (optional)

1. Heat 2 tablespoons of the olive oil in a stockpot or Dutch oven over medium-high heat. Add the zucchini and sauté, stirring frequently, until browned and soft, 8 to 10 minutes.

2. Transfer the zucchini to a blender and pour in the stock. Blend on high until completely smooth, 1 to 2 minutes. Set aside.

3. Add the remaining tablespoon of olive oil to the pot. Add the onion, carrots, and celery and sauté, stirring frequently, until the onion is starting to caramelize, 7 to 8 minutes.

4. Add the ground beef, bay leaf, rosemary, and thyme to the vegetables, breaking up the meat with a spoon or spatula. Season with the salt and pepper. Brown the meat, stirring infrequently to avoid breaking it up too much, 8 to 10 minutes.

5. Add the mushrooms, plantains, and zucchini puree to the pot and bring to a simmer. Reduce the heat to medium-low and cook, uncovered, for 20 minutes, stirring occasionally. Taste for seasoning and add more salt, if desired.

6. Remove the thyme and rosemary stems and the bay leaf before serving. Garnish with parsley, if desired.

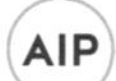 *omit pepper*

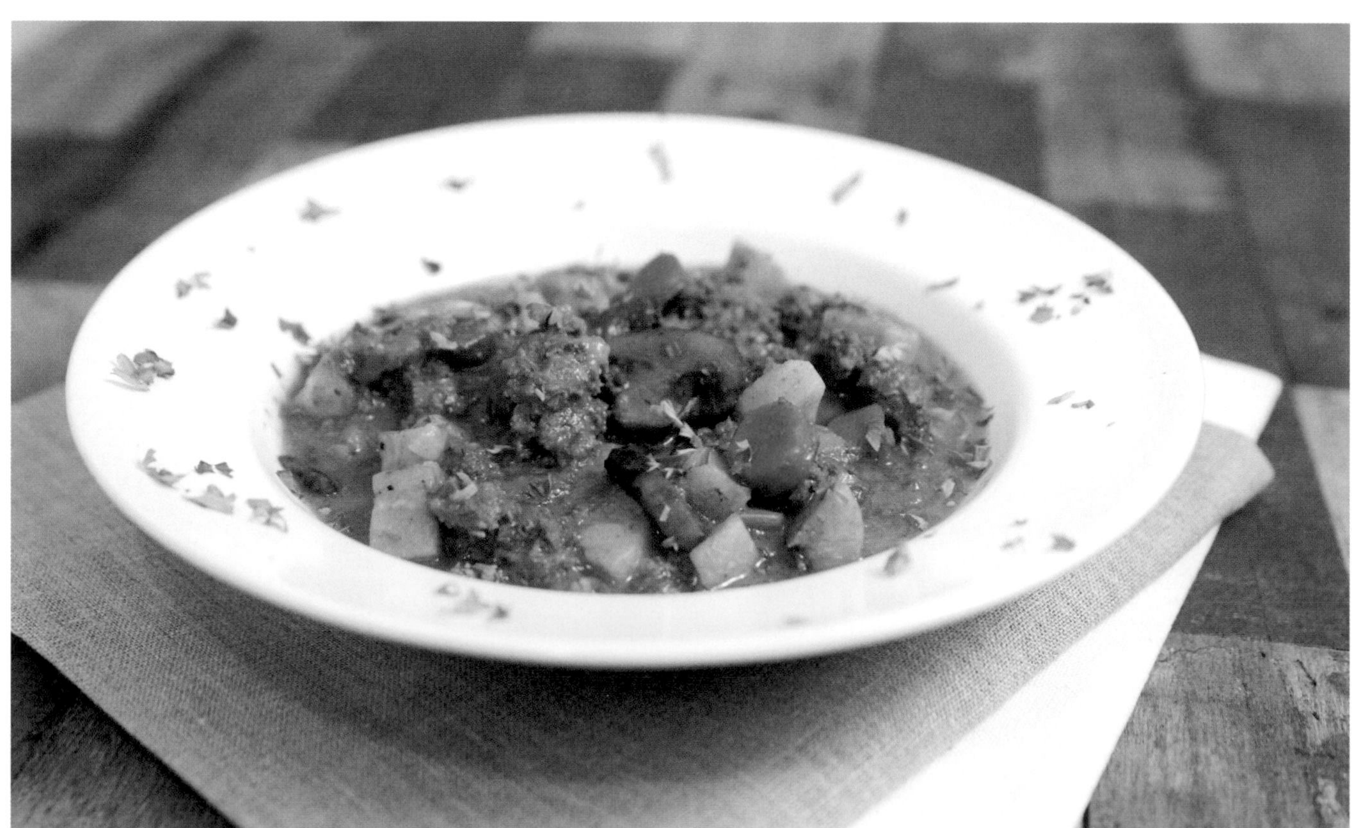

PUMPKIN CHILI

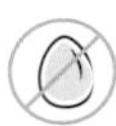 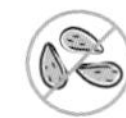 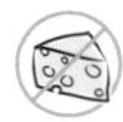  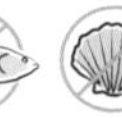 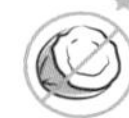

PREP TIME: 15 minutes *COOK TIME: 1 hour 20 minutes*
YIELD: 6 to 8 servings

- 1 medium pie pumpkin, peeled and cut into ½-inch dice
- 1 large sweet potato, peeled and cut into ½-inch dice
- 2 tablespoons coconut oil, melted
- 2 pounds ground turkey
- 1 pound ground beef
- 2 onions, finely chopped
- 6 to 8 stalks celery, chopped
- 8 to 10 cloves garlic, chopped
- 3 bay leaves
- 2½ to 3 tablespoons chili powder
- 1½ tablespoons ground cumin
- 1 teaspoon ground cinnamon
- 1 teaspoon ground nutmeg
- 2 teaspoons cocoa powder
- ¼ teaspoon cayenne pepper (optional, or substitute fresh hot peppers for more heat)
- 3 (15-ounce) cans diced tomatoes
- 1 (6-ounce) can tomato paste
- 2 cups pumpkin puree (fresh puree can be made by blending some extra roasted pumpkin, or use canned)
- ½ teaspoon sea salt
- ⅛ teaspoon ground black pepper
- 1½ tablespoons chopped fresh basil
- 1½ tablespoons chopped fresh oregano
- 3 tablespoons chopped fresh cilantro
- 10 ounces fresh spinach, chopped

1. Preheat the oven to 350°F.
2. In a bowl, toss the pumpkin and sweet potato with the coconut oil. Spread on a rimmed baking sheet lined with aluminum foil and bake for 30 minutes or until soft and starting to brown. Turn on the broiler to get the vegetables a bit browner with some crispy bits, 6 to 7 minutes. Set aside.
3. Meanwhile, brown the turkey and beef with the onions, celery, garlic, and bay leaves in a large pot over medium-high heat. Stir only occasionally so that you don't break up the meat into too-small pieces.
4. When the meat is browned, add the chili powder, cumin, cinnamon, nutmeg, cocoa powder, and cayenne, if using. Stir and cook until fragrant, 3 to 4 minutes.
5. Add the diced tomatoes, tomato paste, pumpkin puree, salt, and pepper. Bring to a simmer, then reduce the heat to medium-low. Simmer for 15 minutes, stirring occasionally, until the celery is soft.
6. Stir in the fresh herbs and spinach. Add the roasted pumpkin and sweet potato and stir to incorporate. Taste and season with more salt and pepper if needed before serving.

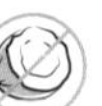 *use olive oil or avocado oil instead of coconut oil*

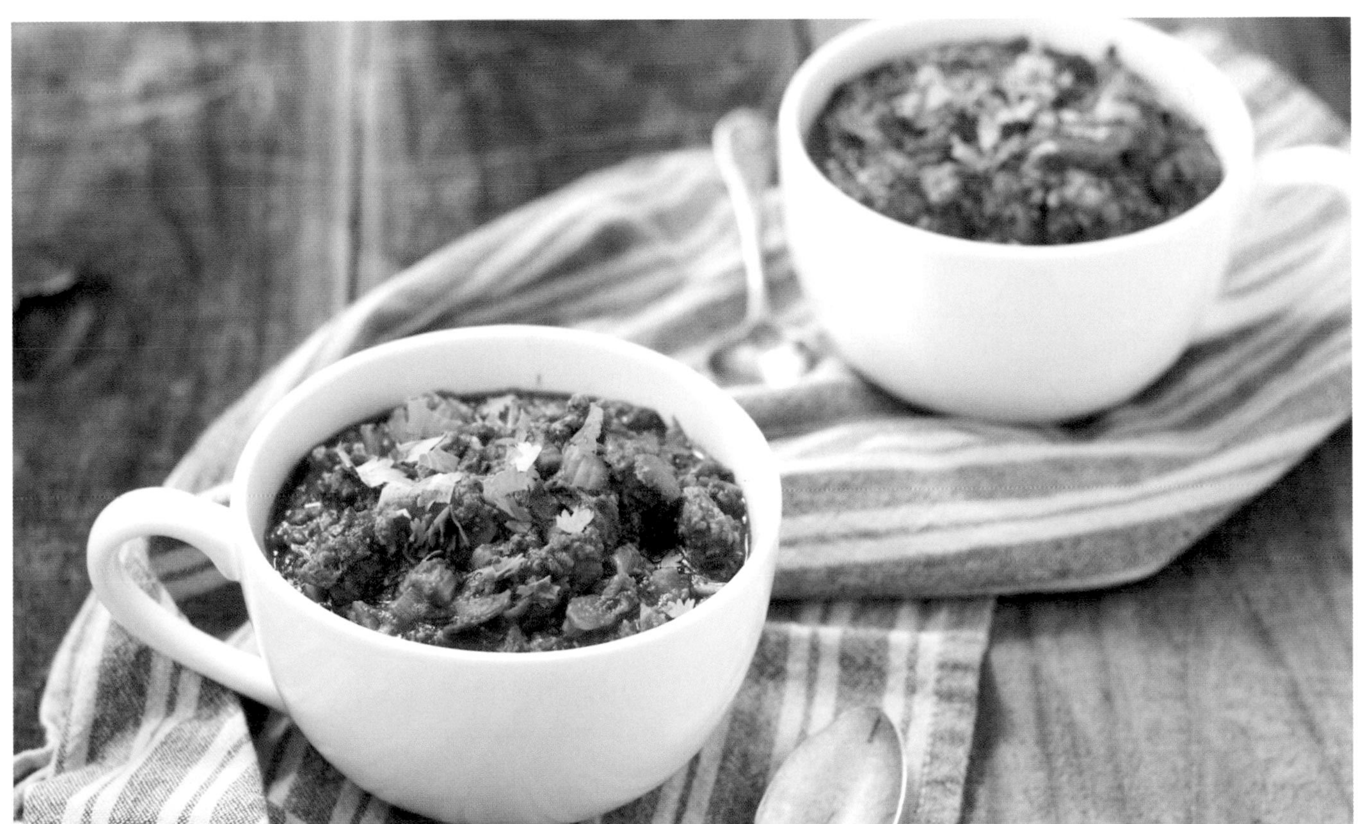

MOROCCAN LAMB STEW

 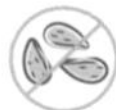 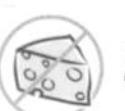  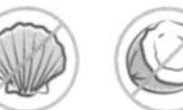 

PREP TIME: 20 minutes, plus time to marinate
COOK TIME: 2 1/2 hours   YIELD: 5 to 6 servings

3 pounds lamb hearts or lamb stew meat
1 teaspoon fennel seeds
1 teaspoon ground coriander
1 teaspoon ground cumin
1 teaspoon finely grated fresh ginger
1 teaspoon turmeric powder
4 cloves garlic, minced
½ cup red palm oil
2 tablespoons lemon juice
2 medium-sized yellow onions, sliced
⅓ cup Kalamata olives, pitted and sliced
½ cup dried apricots, finely chopped
4 small sweet potatoes, peeled and cut into 1-inch cubes
2 cups Bone Stock (beef, lamb, or chicken) (page 486)
1 cinnamon stick
2 bay leaves
½ teaspoon sea salt
½ teaspoon ground black pepper
Chopped fresh cilantro, for garnish

1. Cut the lamb hearts into 1- to 2-inch cubes. The only trimming you need to do is to remove any large vessels, and even those will be tender enough to eat at the end. Place the lamb in a bowl or resealable plastic bag.

2. Grind the fennel seeds (and any other whole spices you are using) in a spice grinder, mini food processor, or mortar and pestle. Combine with the coriander, cumin, ginger, turmeric, garlic, palm oil, and lemon juice. Whisk to combine.

3. Pour the palm oil mixture over the lamb and stir to coat. Cover the bowl with plastic or reseal the plastic bag and place in the refrigerator to marinate for 4 to 6 hours or overnight (up to 24 hours).

4. Preheat the oven to 300°F.

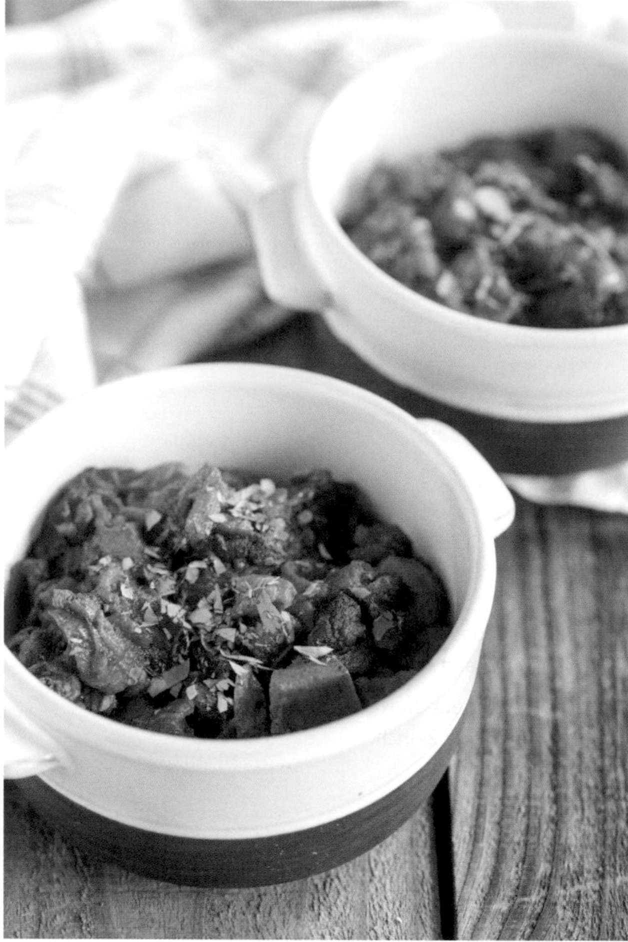

5. Heat a stockpot over medium-high heat. Brown the lamb pieces in batches. There should be enough oil on the lamb to brown without sticking, but if the pieces start to stick, add an extra 1 to 2 tablespoons of palm oil (or marinade). It should take only 3 to 4 minutes to brown each batch. Remove the browned lamb to a bowl.

6. Add the onion to the pot and cook until soft and caramelized, about 10 minutes. If you do not have enough fat in the pot left from browning the lamb, you may choose to add 1 to 2 tablespoons of palm oil.

7. Place all the lamb and any leftover marinade back in the pot. Add the olives, apricots, sweet potato, stock, cinnamon stick, bay leaves, salt, and pepper.

8. Cook uncovered in the oven for 2 hours. Taste and season with more salt and pepper, if needed. Serve in a bowl on its own or over cauli-rice, garnished with chopped cilantro.

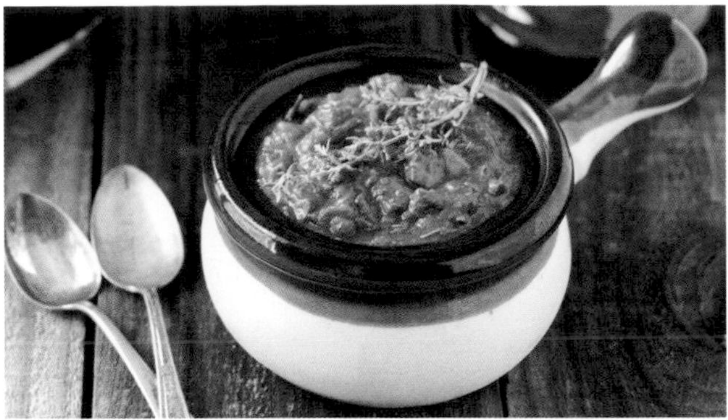

HEARTY BEEF STEW

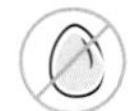  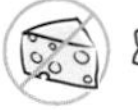  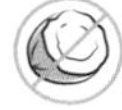

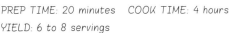

PREP TIME: 20 minutes *COOK TIME: 4 hours*
YIELD: 6 to 8 servings

2 to 3 tablespoons olive oil, avocado oil, or tallow

3 pounds beef chuck stew meat, cut into 1- to 2-inch chunks

2 medium-sized yellow onions, peeled, halved, and sliced into ¼-inch semicircles

¾ pound carrots (about 2 large), roughly chopped into ½- to ¾-inch rounds

8 stalks celery, roughly chopped into ½- to ¾-inch pieces

¾ pound parsnips (about 2 large), roughly chopped into ½- to ¾-inch pieces

8 cloves garlic, chopped

1 generous sprig rosemary (about 2 tablespoons chopped)

1½ tablespoons chopped fresh thyme

1 bay leaf

2 cups Bone Stock (page 486)

2 cups dry red wine

½ (6-ounce) can tomato paste

½ teaspoon sea salt

⅛ teaspoon ground black pepper

1. Preheat the oven to 300°F.

2. Heat 2 tablespoons of olive oil in a large oven-safe pot over medium-high heat. Add half of the beef and stir frequently until browned. Remove the meat from the pot. Brown the other half of the beef and remove it from the pot, too. Set aside.

3. Add the vegetables and garlic to the pot. Add 1 tablespoon oil, if needed (this will depend on the fat content of the beef).

4. Cook, stirring relatively frequently, until the vegetables are starting to soften, about 10 minutes.

5. Return the meat to the pot. Add the rosemary, thyme, and bay leaf, then add the stock, wine, tomato paste, salt, and pepper. Bring to a simmer over medium heat, then cover and place in the oven.

6. Cook for 3 hours. Taste and add more salt and pepper if needed before serving.

DIY SALAD

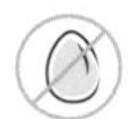 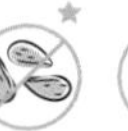 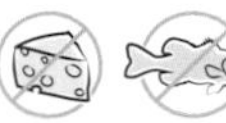 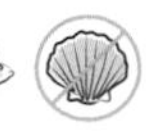 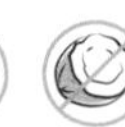    AIP

PREP TIME: 15 minutes *YIELD: varies*

Leafy greens (arugula, baby collards, beet greens, broccoli leaves, cabbage, carrot tops, celery leaves, chard, endive, kale, kohlrabi greens, lettuce, mizuna, mustard greens, pea leaves, radicchio, radish tops, sorrel, spinach, sweet potato leaves, turnip greens, watercress)

Veggies (asparagus [raw, broiled, grilled], avocado, beets [raw, roasted, steamed], broccoli florets [raw or steamed], broccoli slaw, carrots [sliced, shredded], celery root, cucumber, fennel, jicama, kelp noodles, kohlrabi, mushrooms, olives, onion, radish sprouts, radishes, sea vegetables, sunflower sprouts, sweet peppers, tomato, turnips, wakame noodles, zucchini and other summer squash; optional)

Fresh herbs (basil, chervil, chives, cilantro, dill, fennel, mint, oregano, parsley, tarragon; optional)

Fresh or dried fruit (apples, apricots, Asian pears, berries, citrus segments, fresh figs, halved grapes, mangoes, melon, pears, pomegranate seeds, peaches, raisins, dried cranberries, dried apricots; optional)

Nuts and seeds (sliced almonds, chopped Brazil nuts, pecans, pine nuts, pistachios, walnuts, pepitas, shelled sunflower seeds; optional)

Protein (bacon bits, shrimp, salmon, tuna, scallops, sliced steak, leftover chicken, sliced leftover sausage; optional)

Salad dressing of choice (pages 484 to 485)

Toss your selected leafy greens with veggies, herbs, fruit, nuts, and/or seeds in a large bowl. Add protein, if using. Drizzle with dressing immediately before serving.

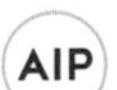 *avoid non-AIP options*

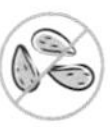 *don't use*

 *avoid*

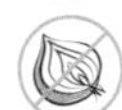 *avoid*

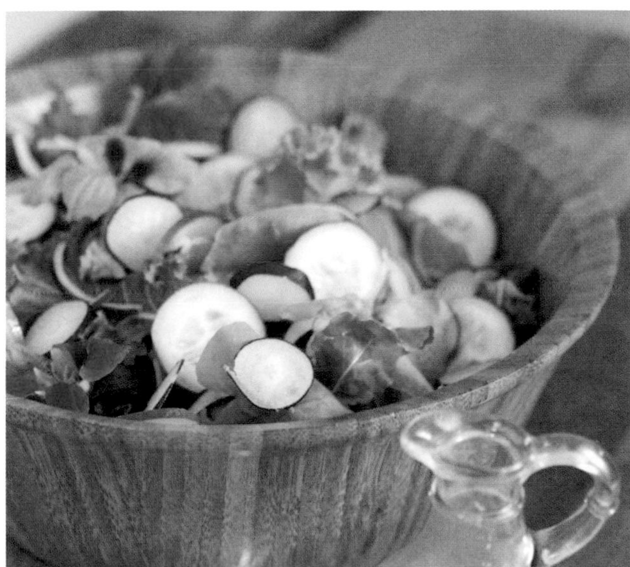

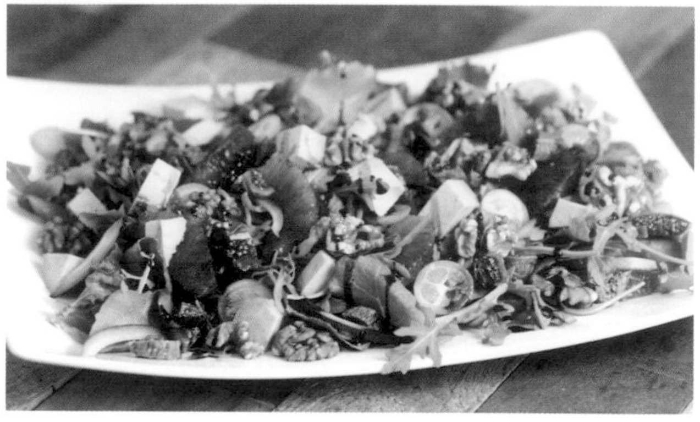

CITRUS, FIG & WALNUT SALAD

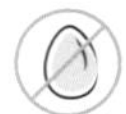 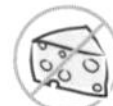 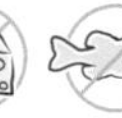 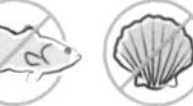 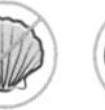 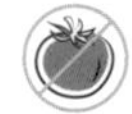

PREP TIME: 10 minutes *YIELD: 1 to 2 servings*

- 2 cups fresh arugula
- 2 cups baby kale (see Tip)
- 3 tablespoons thinly sliced red onions
- 1 large orange, segmented
- 4 kumquats, thinly sliced (discard the seeds but leave the peels on)
- 3 dried figs, cut into ½-inch pieces
- ½ avocado, peeled and cut into ½- to ¾-inch dice
- ½ cup walnut halves or large pieces
- 2 tablespoons Basic Vinaigrette made with balsamic vinegar (page 484)

Gently toss the salad ingredients together. Drizzle the dressing over the salad immediately before serving.

TIP: You can also use regular kale to make this salad; remove and discard the stems and tear the leaves into bite-sized pieces. If you can't find kumquats, use 2 oranges instead.

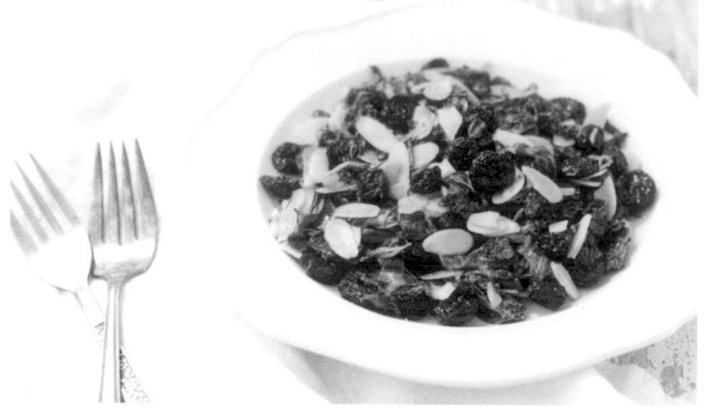

WILTED SPINACH SALAD WITH ALMONDS & CRANBERRIES

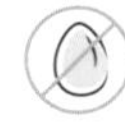  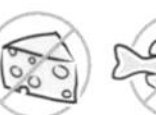  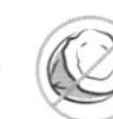  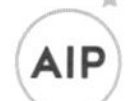 AIP

PREP TIME: 5 minutes *COOK TIME: 7 minutes*
YIELD: 2 to 4 servings

- 1½ tablespoons coconut oil
- 2 cups chopped kale (tough stems removed)
- 1 to 2 tablespoons water
- ¼ cup dried cranberries
- 3 cups fresh spinach
- 2 tablespoons sliced almonds

1. Heat the coconut oil in a cast-iron or other heavy skillet over medium-high heat.

2. Add the kale and 1 tablespoon of water. Cook, stirring frequently, until the kale has softened, 3 to 4 minutes.

3. Add the cranberries and cook for 2 to 3 more minutes.

4. Add the spinach. If the kale is starting to stick, also add another tablespoon of water. Cook, stirring, until the spinach has wilted. Stir in the almonds and serve.

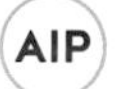 *omit almonds*

 *omit almonds*

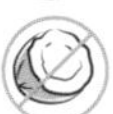 *use olive or avocado oil*

PALEO CAESAR SALAD

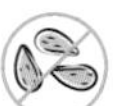 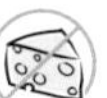  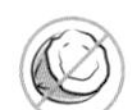 

PREP TIME: 10 minutes *YIELD: 4 to 5 servings*

- 4 to 5 slices bacon
- 1 small head romaine lettuce, or 1 large romaine heart
- 1 batch Caesar Salad Dressing (page 484)
- Cracked black pepper

1. Fry the bacon in a skillet (or bake in the oven; see page 502) until crispy. Drain on paper towels. When cool, break the bacon into small pieces.

2. Tear or chop the lettuce into large bite-sized pieces. Wash and dry using a salad spinner or paper towels.

3. Place the lettuce in a bowl and toss with the dressing until evenly coated. Top with the bacon and sprinkle with pepper to taste. Serve as a side salad or add grilled chicken or shrimp to make it a dinner salad.

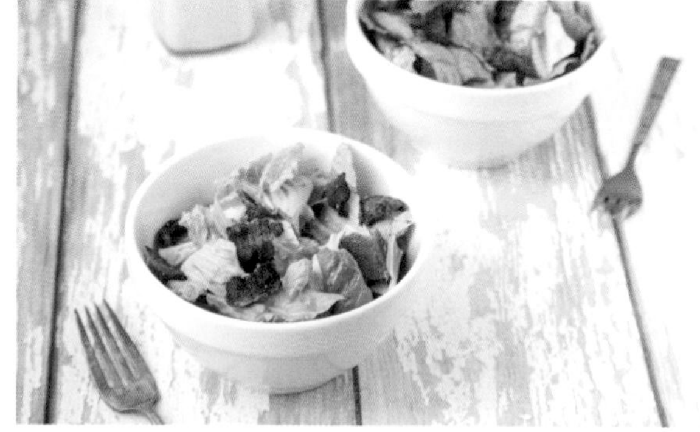

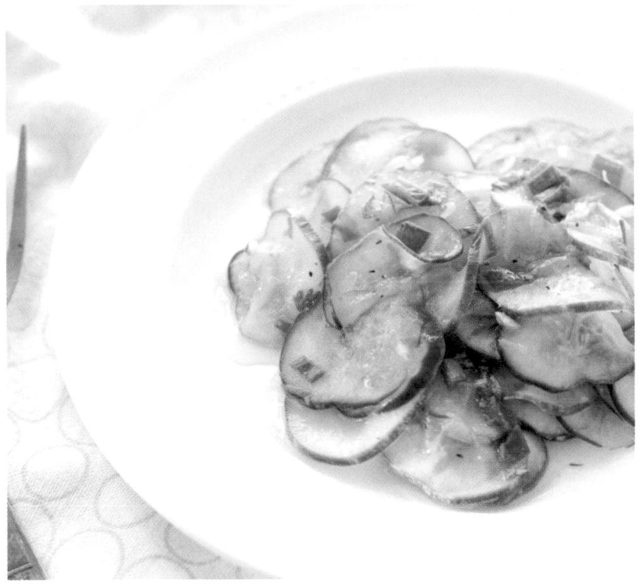

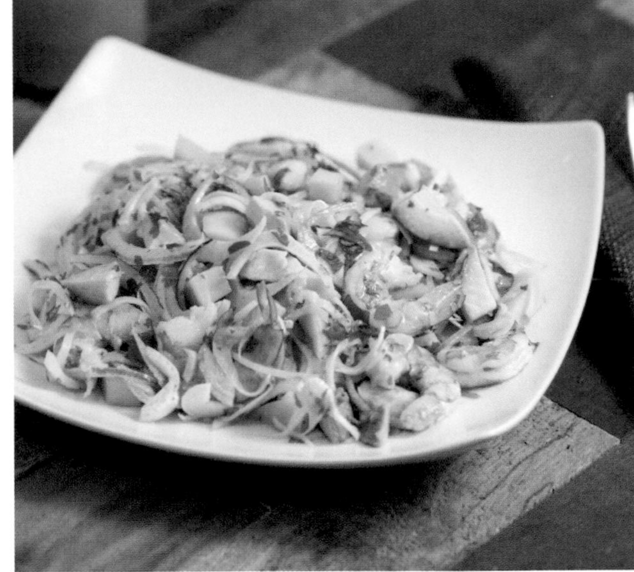

SIMPLE CUCUMBER SALAD

 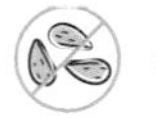 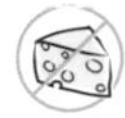 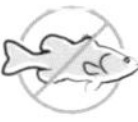 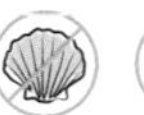 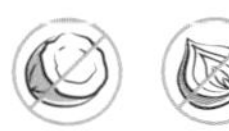  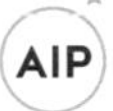 AIP

PREP TIME: 10 minutes, plus 1 hour to salt cucumbers
YIELD: 4 servings

1½ large English cucumbers, finely sliced

1 to 2 teaspoons sea salt

4 large green onions, sliced

2 tablespoons finely chopped fresh cilantro

1 teaspoon finely grated lemon zest

¼ cup lemon juice (about 2 lemons)

¼ cup olive oil

⅛ teaspoon cracked black pepper

1. Place the cucumber slices in a colander and sprinkle liberally with the salt. Place the colander in the sink and let sit for 1 hour.

2. Rinse the cucumber slices very thoroughly (taste a piece to make sure you've rinsed off all the salt). Let the cucumbers drain on paper towels or a clean tea towel to dry completely.

3. To make the dressing, combine the onions, cilantro, lemon zest, lemon juice, olive oil, and pepper and stir to combine.

4. Transfer the cucumbers to a bowl, pour the dressing on top, stir to incorporate, and serve!

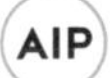 *omit pepper*

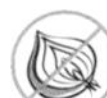 *use green parts of green onions only*

SHRIMP SALAD

  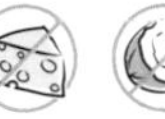  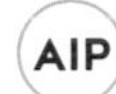 AIP

PREP TIME: 20 minutes
YIELD: 2 to 3 servings

½ cup chopped fresh cilantro

3 tablespoons lime juice (about 2 limes)

3 tablespoons olive oil

2 tablespoons fish sauce

1 pound precooked shrimp

½ large fennel bulb, sliced extremely thin, about 3 cups

1 medium mango, peeled and diced

½ cup very finely sliced red onion

1 large avocado, peeled and diced

1. To make the dressing, stir together the cilantro, lime juice, olive oil, and fish sauce in a bowl or measuring cup. Set aside.

2. Toss the shrimp, fennel, mango, and onion in a bowl. Drizzle the dressing over the shrimp salad and toss to coat completely.

3. Add the diced avocado and gently toss to incorporate. If you're making this salad ahead of time, keep the avocado separate until just before serving.

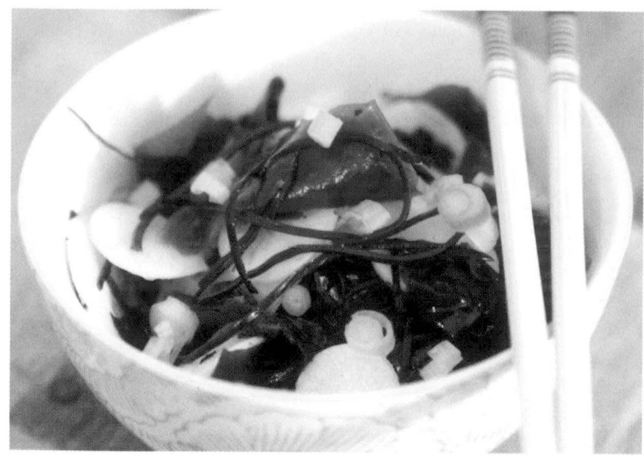

SEAWEED SALAD

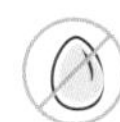 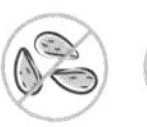 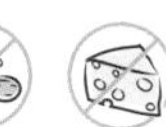  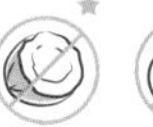 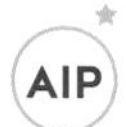 AIP

PREP TIME: 10 minutes YIELD: 8 servings

3 tablespoons lemon juice

2 tablespoons coconut water vinegar

1 tablespoon toasted (dark) sesame oil

2 teaspoons fish sauce

2 teaspoons honey

1 teaspoon fresh ginger juice (see Tip)

2 ounces dried seaweed, such as wakame, arame, dulse, agar, or a mix

2 cups finely sliced cucumbers (remove the peel if it's tough) (about 1 medium cucumber)

2 cups finely sliced Japanese turnips or daikon (about 8 ounces)

1 avocado, peeled and diced (optional)

2 green onions, finely chopped, for garnish

1. To make the dressing, combine the lemon juice, vinegar, sesame oil, fish sauce, honey, and ginger juice.

2. Soak the seaweed in cold water for 5 minutes (taste it, and if it's still quite tough, soak for an additional 2 to 5 minutes, tasting again every minute or two).

3. Rinse and drain the seaweed. If there are any very large pieces, give them a rough chop. Combine the rehydrated seaweed, cucumbers, turnips, and dressing. Gently toss in the avocado, if using. Garnish with green onions.

TIP: To make fresh ginger juice, finely grate fresh ginger with a Microplane or box grater and then squeeze the grated ginger with your fingers over a measuring spoon or cup to catch the juice. A thumb's length of fresh ginger should be more than enough for the required 1 teaspoon of ginger juice.

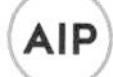 *substitute more fish sauce for the sesame oil*

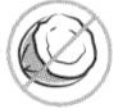 *use white wine vinegar instead of coconut water vinegar*

STRAWBERRY & ARUGULA SALAD WITH CANDIED PECANS

 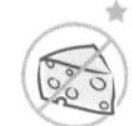 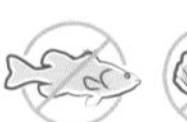 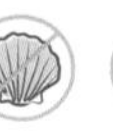 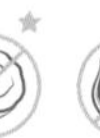 

PREP TIME: 10 minutes COOK TIME: 6 minutes
YIELD: 2 servings

1 tablespoon coconut oil

2 teaspoons honey

1 cup raw pecan halves

1 teaspoon ground nutmeg

½ teaspoon ground allspice

¼ teaspoon ground cardamom

¼ teaspoon ground cinnamon

2½ ounces fresh arugula

½ pound fresh strawberries, sliced

¼ cup crumbled goat cheese (optional)

1 batch Basic Vinaigrette made with lime juice and olive oil (page 484)

1. Heat a skillet over medium-high heat. Add the coconut oil and honey, then add the pecans and stir to coat.

2. Sprinkle the spices over the pecans and stir to coat evenly. Continue to cook, stirring constantly, until the pecans have browned and are fragrant, 5 to 6 minutes. Watch carefully to make sure they don't burn! Pour the candied pecans onto a plate and let cool.

3. Toss the arugula, strawberries, and pecans together in a bowl. Top the salad with the crumbled goat cheese, if using.

4. Drizzle the vinaigrette over the salad just before serving.

 *use olive oil or avocado oil*

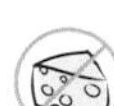 *omit goat cheese*

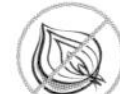 *omit goat cheese and use maple syrup instead of honey*

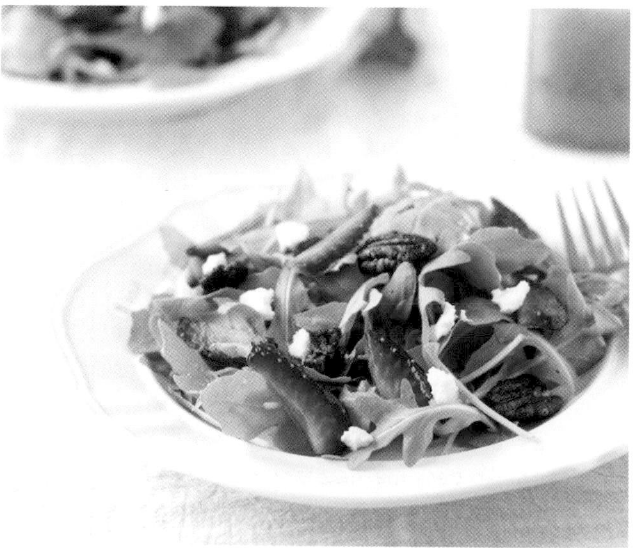

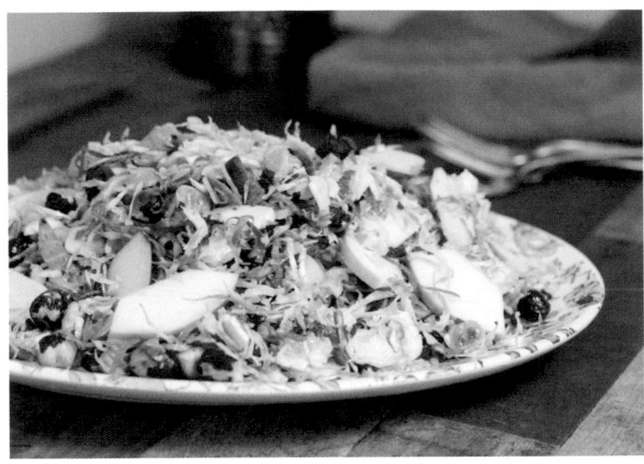

SHAVED BRUSSELS SLAW WITH HAZELNUTS, APPLE & MINT

 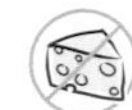 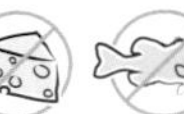  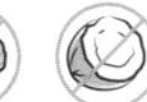 

PREP TIME: 10 minutes *COOK TIME: 15 minutes*
YIELD: 5 to 8 servings

- 1 cup raw hazelnuts
- 4 ounces pancetta, diced
- 2 pounds Brussels sprouts
- 1 clove garlic, minced
- Finely grated zest and juice of 1 lemon
- 2 tablespoons olive oil
- ½ teaspoon sea salt
- 1 Granny Smith apple, cored and thinly sliced
- ⅓ cup mint chiffonade (see Tips)

1. To toast the hazelnuts, preheat the oven to 375°F. Place the hazelnuts on a rimmed baking sheet and bake for 10 minutes.

2. While the hazelnuts are in the oven, place the pancetta in a cold skillet and turn the heat to medium. Sauté, stirring occasionally, until browned, about 8 minutes. Remove the pancetta from the skillet and set aside to cool.

3. Remove the hazelnuts from the oven and immediately pour into a clean tea towel. Fold the towel over the hazelnuts and let them sit for 1 to 2 minutes. With the tea towel still covering the hazelnuts, rub the hazelnuts with the towel to start removing the skins. You can open up the towel and see how it's going (at this point, the towel is really just to protect your hands from those hot nuts!). Pick out the hazelnuts from which the skins have been removed (it's fine if there's a little skin left on them) and continue until you've removed all the skins. (Don't worry if some stubborn skins remain.) Let the hazelnuts cool completely.

4. Slice the Brussels sprouts very thinly, discarding the stems. An easy method is to trim off the stems and shave them with a mandoline or a food processor with a slicer attachment. Two pounds of whole Brussels sprouts will give you about 12 ounces shaved.

5. Combine all the ingredients in a bowl and mix thoroughly. Serve immediately. If you are not going to serve all of the slaw, use the hazelnuts as a garnish instead of mixing them in, because they'll go a bit soft when stored in the refrigerator. Leftover slaw can be stored in the fridge for up to 5 days.

TIPS: I recommend that you buy raw hazelnuts and toast them yourself—the flavor of freshly toasted hazelnuts is so much better! But to save time, you can purchase toasted hazelnuts and use them in this recipe; if you do so, skip Steps 1 through 4 and begin at Step 5.

You can use bacon instead of pancetta if you prefer.

To save time, purchase a 10- to 12-ounce bag of shaved Brussels sprouts instead of whole Brussels sprouts. If you buy them preshaved, skip Step 5.

To chiffonade mint, stack several mint leaves on top of each other and slice very thin strips across the leaves all the way down. Measure 1/3 cup after you chiffonade the mint; it will be close to 1 cup of loosely packed leaves before you chiffonade.

SIMPLE FENNEL SALAD

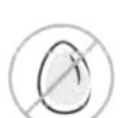 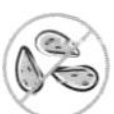 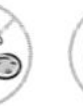 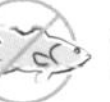  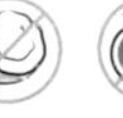 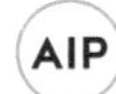 AIP

PREP TIME: 5 minutes *YIELD: 3 to 4 servings*

- Juice of 1 lemon (about 3 tablespoons)
- 1 tablespoon olive oil
- ¼ teaspoon sea salt
- 1 pound fennel (bulb, stems, and leaves)

1. To make the dressing, mix together the lemon juice, olive oil, and salt in a small bowl. Set aside.

2. Thinly slice the fennel bulb and chop the stems and leaves. A mandoline makes this job go very quickly!

3. Gently toss the fennel with dressing and serve.

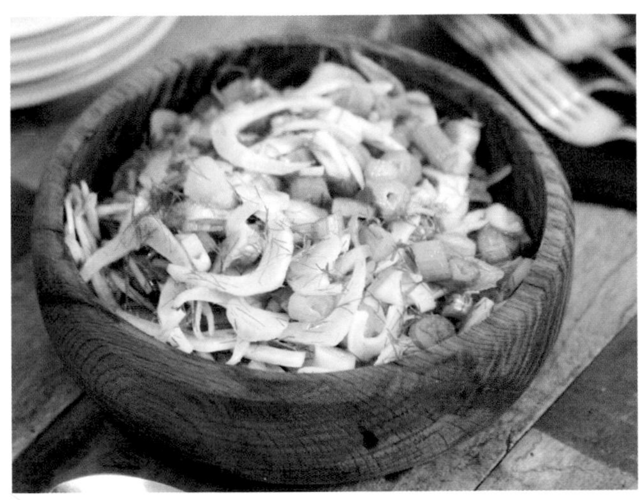

Chapter 42:
MAIN DISHES

DIY STIR-FRY

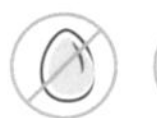 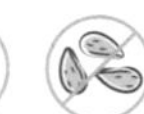 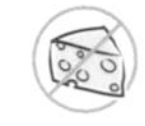 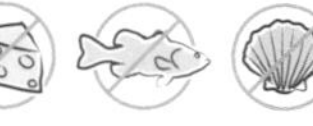  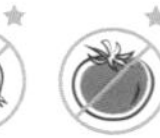 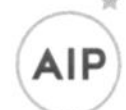

PREP TIME: 20 minutes *COOK TIME: 20 minutes*
YIELD: 2 to 3 servings

3 to 5 tablespoons coconut oil, avocado oil, or olive oil, divided

½ to 1 tablespoon minced garlic (optional)

½ to 1 tablespoon minced fresh ginger or galangal (optional)

1 pound chicken, pork, beef, lamb, shrimp, raw or cooked, cut into bite-sized pieces

3 to 5 cups mixed vegetables (carrots, onions, broccoli, broccoli rabe, cauliflower, bok choy, tatsoi, sliced bamboo shoots, sliced water chestnuts, sui choi cabbage, snap peas, broccoli slaw, asparagus, fennel bulb, kohlrabi, bell peppers, tomato [seeded], mushrooms, celery, seaweed), cut into bite-sized pieces

2 to 3 cups kelp, sweet potato (boil first), or wakame noodles (optional)

Flavoring liquid (see below)

Sea salt

Chopped green onions, for garnish (optional)

FLAVORING LIQUID OPTIONS:

½ cup Teriyaki Marinade (page 494) plus 1 tablespoon arrowroot powder or kuzu starch

½ cup Bone Stock (page 486) plus 1 tablespoon coconut water vinegar and 1 tablespoon arrowroot powder or kuzu starch

1 tablespoon coconut aminos, ½ cup Bone Stock (page 486), and 1 tablespoon arrowroot powder or kuzu starch

3 tablespoons Hoisin Sauce (page 494), 2 tablespoons ketchup or tomato paste, 1 tablespoon chili paste or chopped chilies, or 2 teaspoons coconut aminos

1. Heat a wok or large skillet over medium-high heat. Add 2 to 3 tablespoons of coconut oil to the hot wok. If you're using ginger and garlic, add it now and cook for 1 minute.

2. If using raw meat, add the meat to the hot coconut oil. Cook, stirring frequently, until fully cooked. Remove the cooked meat from the wok and set aside.

3. Add the mixed vegetables to the hot coconut oil. (If you cooked meat and there's not much oil left in the wok, add a little more before adding your veggies.) Cook, stirring frequently, until the vegetables are cooked to your liking. Add the veggies that take longer to cook first (such as broccoli, carrots, cauliflower, mushrooms, onions, or peppers), then add the veggies that cook faster or are cut into very small pieces (such as seaweed, leafy greens, broccoli slaw, bok choy, or snap peas) after the larger veggies are most of the way cooked. If the veggies are releasing a lot of liquid into the wok, turn the heat up.

4. Add your flavoring liquid to the mostly cooked veggies.

5. Add the cooked meat (whether you just cooked it or are using precooked meat) to the wok as well as the noodles, if using. Keep stirring. Taste and season with salt, if needed. Once the flavoring liquid has thickened, serve. Garnish with chopped green onions, if desired.

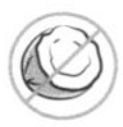 *avoid*

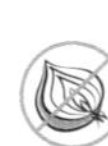 *avoid*

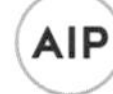 *avoid non-AIP options*

 *avoid*

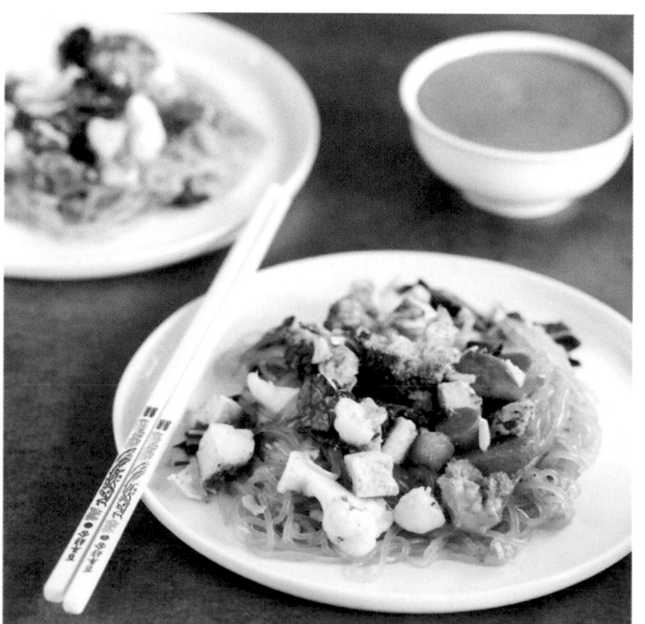

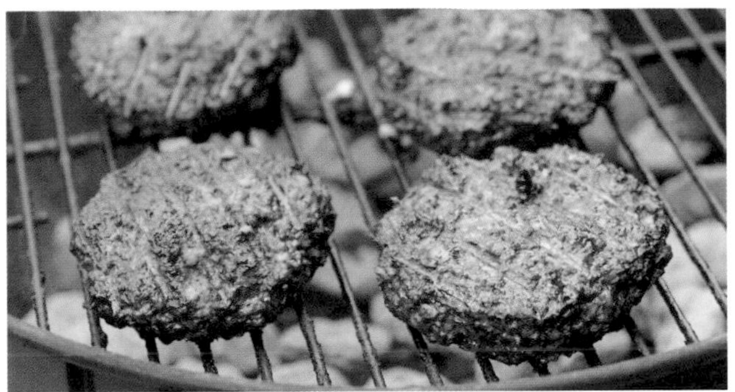

50/50/50 BURGERS

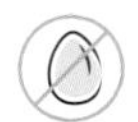 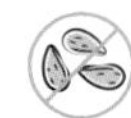 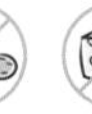 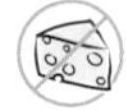  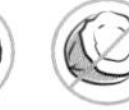 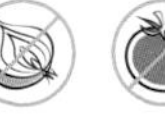 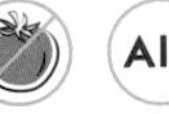 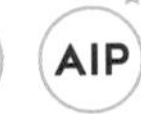

PREP TIME: 15 minutes
COOK TIME: 12 to 24 minutes, depending on method
YIELD: 8 patties

1 pound ground beef (see Tip)

1 pound liver (bison, chicken, duck, or other liver of choice)

1 pound bacon

4 Sesame Seed Buns (page 565), 8 Choux Pastry Buns (page 564), or 8 Grilled Portobello Mushroom Caps (page 552), or lettuce for wrapping

Burger toppings of choice

1. Grind the liver and bacon separately or together. There are a bunch of different ways to do this. Some butchers will do it for you. You can grate frozen liver following the directions for "Sneaky Liver" Ground Beef on page 498. You can use a meat grinder attachment for a stand mixer. You can buy an inexpensive tabletop hand-crank meat grinder or a deluxe electric countertop meat grinder. And most food processors will do a pretty acceptable job of grinding meat. Bacon grinds more easily when it's cold; I like to grind both the bacon and the liver when I'm using a food processor (which seems to keep both from being ground too finely). No matter which kitchen tool you use, the goal is the texture of ground beef. Liver has a lot of moisture in it and tends to liquefy a little in food processors. The bacon will make the mixture a little thicker.

2. Mix your ground bacon and liver with the ground beef, using your hands. Form 6-ounce patties. The liver can make the patties sticky; try wetting your hands with cold water before forming the patties.

3. To grill: Preheat a grill pan or gas or charcoal grill to medium-high heat. Place the patties on the heated grill. Grill for 6 to 8 minutes per side for medium, or until cooked to your liking.

4. To pan-fry: Heat a couple tablespoons of a good cooking fat (tallow, lard, coconut oil) over medium-high heat. Place the patties in a hot pan. Cook for 8 to 12 minutes per side, until cooked to your liking.

5. To bake: Preheat the oven to 400°F. Place the patties on a rimmed baking sheet or in a roasting pan. Bake for 18 to 22 minutes, until cooked to your liking.

6. Serve with your favorite burger toppings on a bun, between Grilled Portobello Mushroom Caps, or in a lettuce wrap.

TIP: If you are using a stronger-flavored liver like beef or pork or you strongly dislike the taste of liver, you can use 2 pounds of ground beef to dilute the flavor further.

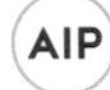 *avoid non-AIP options*

GREMOLATA-TOPPED FISH FILLETS

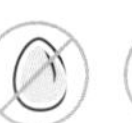 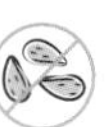 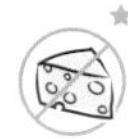  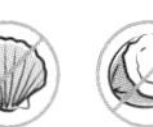  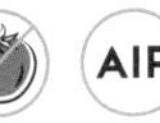

PREP TIME: 15 minutes *COOK TIME: 20 minutes*
YIELD: 4 servings

2 tablespoons olive oil (optional)

¼ cup crumbled plantain chips

¼ cup chopped fresh parsley

1 clove garlic, crushed to a coarse paste

Finely grated zest and juice of 1 lemon

1 tablespoon unsalted butter or ghee, melted

1 to 1½ pounds medium-firm fish fillets (such as sea bass, mahi mahi, halibut, or swordfish), cut into 4 pieces

¼ teaspoon sea salt

⅛ teaspoon ground black pepper

1. Preheat the oven to 425°F. Line a rimmed baking sheet with aluminum foil and spread the olive oil over the top. Alternatively, use a silicone baking mat and skip the olive oil.

2. Mix the plantain chip crumbs with the parsley, garlic, lemon zest, and melted butter.

3. Place the fish fillets on the prepared baking sheet. Drizzle with the lemon juice and sprinkle with the salt and pepper.

4. Evenly coat the tops of the fish fillets with the crumb mixture from Step 2.

5. Bake for 15 to 20 minutes, until the fish is fully cooked.

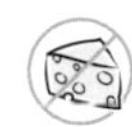 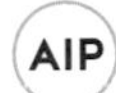 *use olive oil instead of butter; omit pepper* 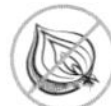 *omit garlic*

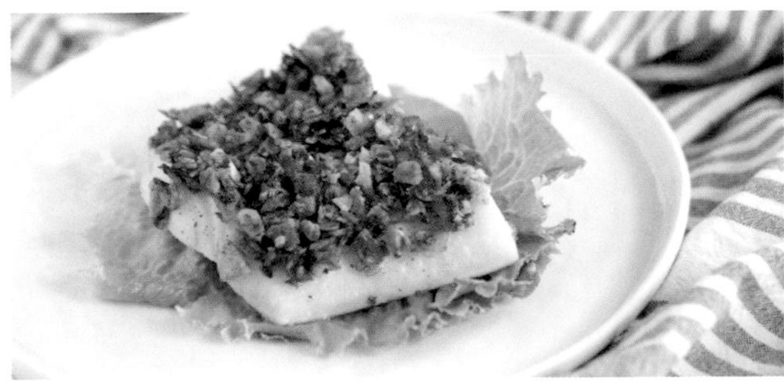

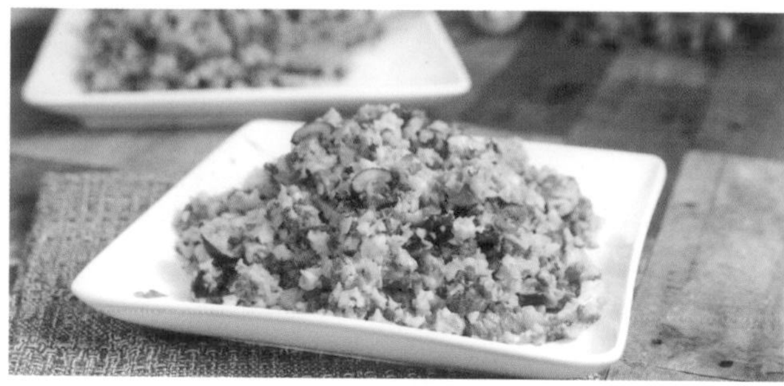

BEEF & MUSHROOM RISOTTO

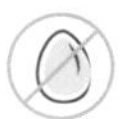 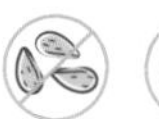 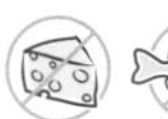 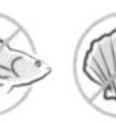  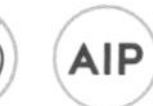 AIP

PREP TIME: 15 minutes COOK TIME: 30 minutes YIELD: 3 servings

2 pounds parsnips (5 to 6 medium parsnips)

1 tablespoon olive oil

½ medium white onion, diced

1 carrot, diced

1 pound ground beef

8 ounces cremini mushrooms, sliced

2 cups Beef Stock (page 486), divided

1 tablespoon apple cider vinegar, or ¼ cup red or white wine

1½ teaspoons sea salt

1 tablespoon finely chopped fresh tarragon, or 1 teaspoon dried tarragon

½ cup full-fat coconut milk, homemade (page 480) or canned

Chopped fresh parsley, for garnish

1. To rice the parsnips, peel the parsnips and chop into big chunks. Place in a food processor and pulse until the pieces are fairly uniform in size and about the size of a large grain of rice. (You should have 6 to 7 cups of riced parsnips.)
2. Heat a large skillet over medium-high heat. Add the olive oil, onion, and carrot. Sauté until the vegetables are tender, about 5 minutes.
3. Add the ground beef to skillet and cook, stirring to break up the beef, until browned, about 3 to 5 minutes.
4. Add the mushrooms, 1 cup of stock, vinegar, and salt. Increase the heat to high and cook until the liquid is mostly evaporated, about 5 to 8 minutes.
5. Add the riced parsnips and remaining 1 cup of stock to pan and stir just to mix. Reduce the heat to medium-low and cover. Cook for 8 to 10 minutes, until the parsnips are tender and mushy, stirring once or twice. If the vegetables start to stick because the pan is becoming dry, add another few tablespoons of stock or water. If your largest skillet isn't big enough for all these ingredients, you can remove the beef mixture before adding the parsnips, then mix the beef mixture back in right before serving.
6. Add the coconut milk and tarragon and stir to incorporate. Turn off the heat and let sit on the stovetop covered for 2 to 3 minutes more. Taste and add more salt, if needed.
7. Garnish with chopped parsley, if desired. Serve!

THAI BEEF LETTUCE WRAPS

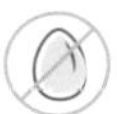 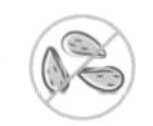 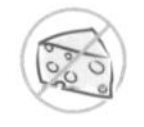  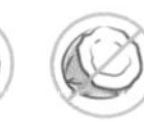  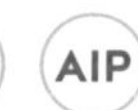

PREP TIME: 10 minutes COOK TIME: 20 minutes
YIELD: 4 to 6 servings

2 pounds lean ground beef (or ground pork, chicken, or turkey)

2 cups Beef Stock (page 486) (or Chicken Stock if using ground pork, chicken, or turkey)

½ teaspoon sea salt (optional)

3 cloves garlic, minced

⅓ cup lime juice (2 to 3 limes)

3 tablespoons fish sauce

⅔ cup minced cilantro (about 1 bunch)

⅔ cup minced chopped mint (about 1 bunch)

1 head romaine lettuce, for serving

1. Brown the ground beef in a large skillet over medium-high heat, breaking up frequently with a spoon or spatula to achieve a fine cooked ground beef texture (small pieces), 8 to 10 minutes.
2. Add the stock to beef. If the stock is unseasoned, add the salt. Let simmer, stirring occasionally, until stock has completely boiled away, about 6 to 8 minutes.
3. Combine the garlic, lime juice, and fish sauce in a bowl. Then combine the cilantro and mint in a separate bowl. Separate the lettuce leaves and cut in half if they are very large.
4. Once the stock has boiled off completely, stir in the lime juice mixture. Simmer, stirring constantly, until the lime juice mixture has also boiled away, about 2 to 3 minutes.
5. Stir in the herbs, immediately remove the beef from the heat, and serve.
6. Serve with a generous spoonful of beef mixture into a lettuce leaf, wrap the lettuce leaf up around the edges (taco style!) and enjoy! You can also serve as a salad on a bed of shredded lettuce.

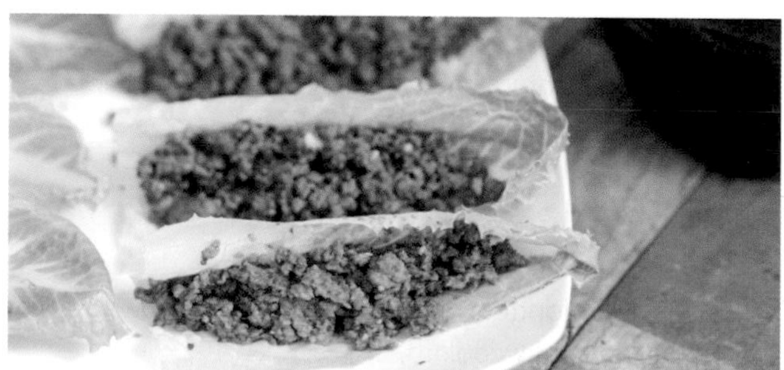

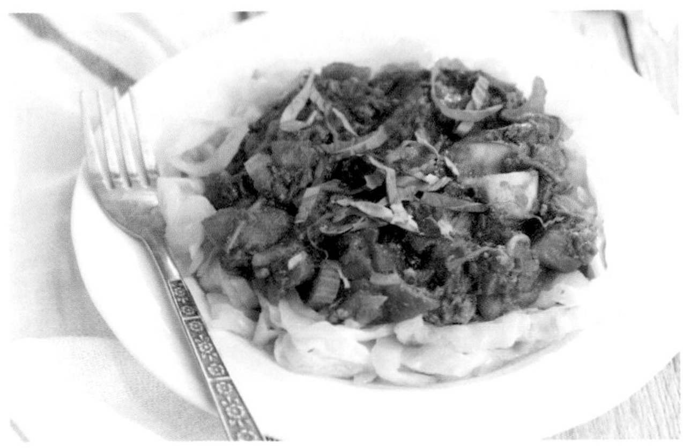

MEATY RATATOUILLE PASTA SAUCE

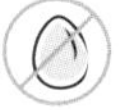 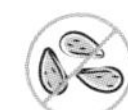 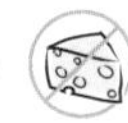 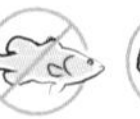 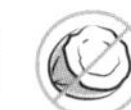

PREP TIME: 15 minutes, plus time to salt eggplant
COOK TIME: 1 hour YIELD: 6 to 8 servings

- 2 eggplants, peeled and cut into ½-inch dice
- 2 tablespoons sea salt (for salting eggplant)
- 2 pounds ground turkey or ground beef
- 2 medium-sized yellow onions, diced
- 6 to 8 stalks celery, cut into ¼-inch slices
- 8 to 10 cloves garlic, finely chopped
- 5 (15-ounce) cans diced tomatoes
- 1 (6-ounce) can tomato paste (you can use 2 cans for a thicker sauce)
- 4 medium zucchini, quartered and cut into ¼-inch slices
- 1 pound mushrooms, sliced
- 2 tablespoons fresh basil and/or oregano, finely chopped
- 1 (10-ounce) bag fresh spinach, roughly chopped

1. Put the eggplant in a colander and toss with the salt. Place the colander in the sink for 1 to 3 hours.

2. Rinse the eggplant thoroughly, then place on layers of paper towel on a rimmed baking sheet or the counter. Cover with more paper towel and press the excess water out. Set aside.

3. Heat a very large pot over medium-high heat. Add the turkey, onions, celery, and garlic. Cook, stirring frequently, until the turkey is browned and the onions and celery are starting to soften, about 15 minutes.

4. Add the canned tomatoes and tomato paste. Stir well and bring to a simmer.

5. Add the zucchini, mushrooms, and eggplant. Stir to incorporate and cover. Bring to a simmer, then reduce the heat to medium-low. Simmer, covered, for about 10 minutes, until the vegetables are starting to soften.

6. Remove the lid and simmer, uncovered, for 20 to 30 minutes (or longer), stirring occasionally, until the vegetables are fully cooked.

7. Add the basil and/or oregano and spinach. Stir to incorporate and cook for 2 to 3 more minutes, until fragrant.

8. Serve as a stew over Zoodles (page 553), Sweet Potato or Butternut Squash "Linguine" (page 551), Spaghetti Squash Noodles (page 549), sweet potato noodles, wakame noodles, or kelp noodles.

PULLED PORK LETTUCE WRAPS WITH LIME-BASIL PESTO & PICKLED SHALLOTS

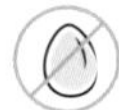  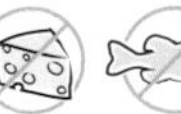  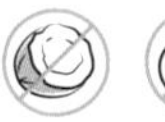 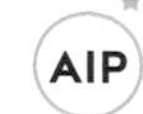 AIP*

PREP TIME: 30 minutes COOK TIME: 10 hours
YIELD: 10 to 16 servings

- 3 to 4 tablespoons Adobo Seasoning (page 482)
- 1 (6- to 8-pound) pork shoulder (bone-in or boneless; this just affects the number of servings)
- 10 to 16 large lettuce leaves or double batch Tortillas (page 567)
- 1 batch Lemon Basil Pesto (page 497)
- 1 batch Easy Pickled Shallots (page 498)

1. Preheat the oven to 250°F.

2. Rub the Adobo Seasoning over the entire surface of the pork shoulder. Place on a roasting pan and roast, uncovered, for 8 to 10 hours.

3. Remove from the oven and let rest for 10 minutes. Slice or pull the pork apart. To pull, place the pork shoulder in a large casserole dish. Use 2 sturdy forks, moving in opposite directions, to pull the meat apart into strands.

4. Place a healthy serving of pork in a lettuce leaf or tortilla, dribble pesto sparingly on top, and add a spoonful of pickled shallots. Wrap it all together and enjoy!

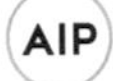 *use AIP Pesto; omit pepper in Adobo Seasoning*

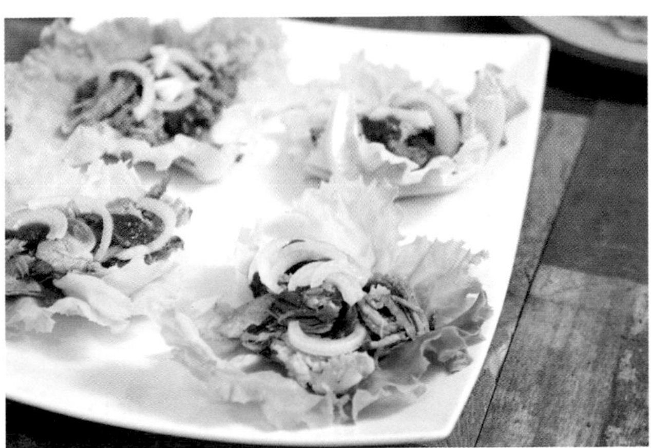

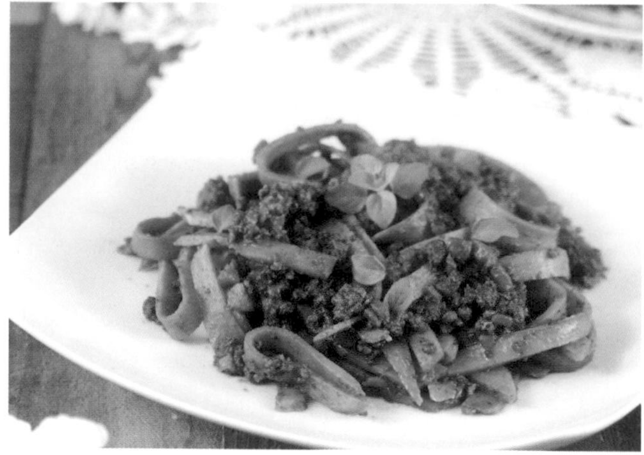

"SPAGHETTI" BOLOGNESE

 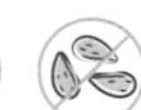 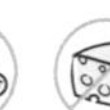 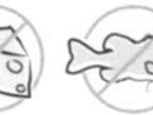    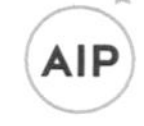

PREP TIME: 20 minutes COOK TIME: 4 1/2 hours
YIELD: 6 to 8 servings

2 tablespoons tallow or other cooking fat

1 large onion, finely diced

4 carrots, finely diced

4 stalks celery, finely diced

4 cloves garlic, minced

1½ teaspoons sea salt, divided

4 ounces pancetta, ham, or Canadian bacon, finely diced

2 pounds lean ground beef or a combination of veal, pork, and beef

1 cup dry white wine

2 cups Beef Stock (page 486)

1 batch Coconut Milk (page 480), or 1 (13½-ounce) can full-fat coconut milk

⅓ cup each umeboshi paste and tamarind paste, or 1 (15-ounce) can crushed tomatoes

1. Heat the tallow in a large saucepan over medium heat. Once hot, add the onion, carrots, celery, garlic, and ½ teaspoon of the salt. Sauté for 5 minutes, stirring often.

2. Add the pancetta and cook for another 10 minutes, until the vegetables are softened and the pancetta is golden.

3. Increase the heat to high and add one-third of the ground beef at a time, stirring and breaking up clumps with a spoon after each addition.

4. Once the meat is fully browned, continue to cook for 15 minutes, stirring frequently, to caramelize.

5. Reduce the heat to medium and add the white wine. With a wooden spoon, scrape up all the brown bits stuck to the bottom of the pan.

6. Add the stock, coconut milk, umeboshi and tamarind pastes, and remaining 1 teaspoon of salt. Bring to a boil, then reduce the heat to low and simmer very gently, half-covered, for 4 hours. Stir every once in a while. If the sauce starts to stick before the end of the cooking time, add a bit of stock or water.

7. Taste and add a little more salt, if desired.

8. Serve over noodles: Zoodles (page 553), Sweet Potato or Butternut Squash "Linguine" (page 551), Spaghetti Squash Noodles (page 549), sweet potato noodles, wakame noodles, or kelp noodles.

 *use umeboshi paste and tamarind paste*

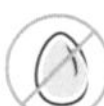 *use umeboshi paste and tamarind paste*

TARRAGON-SEARED FISH FILLETS

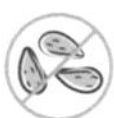 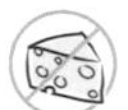  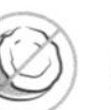 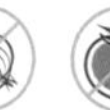 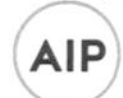

PREP TIME: 10 minutes COOK TIME: 15 minutes
YIELD: 4 servings

2 to 3 tablespoons olive oil, avocado oil, or coconut oil

2 (6- to 8-ounce) medium or firm fish steaks or fillets (such as mahi mahi, amberjack, grouper, or halibut)

3 tablespoons finely chopped fresh tarragon

Finely grated zest and juice of 1 lemon

⅛ teaspoon sea salt or truffle salt

¼ teaspoon cracked or ground black pepper

1. Heat the oil in a large nonstick or well-seasoned cast-iron skillet over medium to medium-high heat.

2. Pat the fish dry with a paper towel. Coat both sides of the fillets with the chopped tarragon, lemon zest, salt, and pepper

3. Place the fish in the pan and cook for 5 to 6 minutes on the first side, until the edges are turning opaque.

4. Flip and cook the other side for 4 to 5 minutes, until the fish is opaque throughout and the segments flake apart (adjust the cook time for thicker or thinner fillets).

5. Squeeze the lemon juice over the fish and serve.

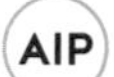 *omit pepper*

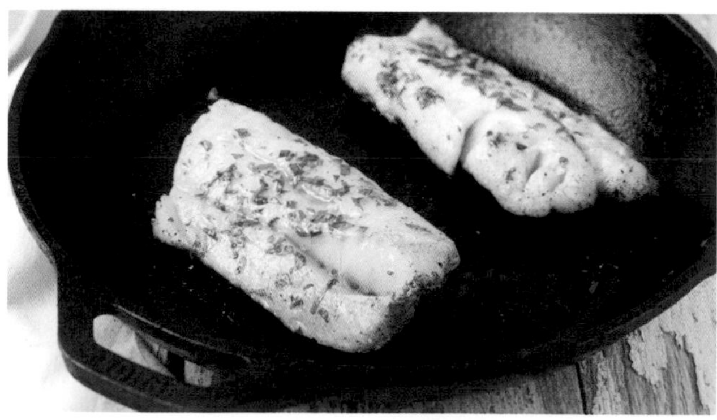

DIY PIZZA

 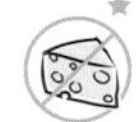 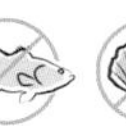  

PREP TIME: 5 minutes *COOK TIME: 10 minutes*
YIELD: 2 servings

1 tablespoon olive oil

1 batch Pizza Crust (page 499)

Sauce of choice (see below)

Shredded mozzarella cheese (optional)

TOPPING OPTIONS: pepperoni, salami, ham, chicken, bacon, sausage, smoked salmon, Canadian bacon, anchovies, bell peppers, artichoke hearts, mushrooms, sliced black or green olives, pineapple, steamed broccoli, spinach, sautéed onion, thinly sliced or diced steamed asparagus

SAUCE OPTIONS:

Classic Pizza Sauce (page 494)

Pesto (page 495 or 497)

Cauliflower Gravy (page 496). Suggestion: Make it with 4 to 6 cloves of garlic instead of just one.

Ranch Dip (page 487)

Hollandaise (page 497)

Chimichurri (page 495)

Crushed garlic and olive oil or melted unsalted butter or ghee

Barbecue Sauce (page 493)

1. Rub a pizza stone or large well-seasoned cast-iron skillet with the olive oil and place in the oven to heat. Preheat the oven to 450°F.

2. Remove the hot pizza stone or skillet from the oven. Pour the pizza crust dough into the heated pan and spread it with a spatula to a 9- to 10-inch circle of even thickness (it should be about ¼ inch thick).

3. Bake for about 9 minutes, depending on how crispy you like the crust, then remove from the oven and lower the oven temperature to 400°F.

4. If making more than one pizza, you may transfer the baked pizza crusts to a baking sheet.

5. Spread 3 to 4 tablespoons of sauce over the crust, or to your liking. Sprinkle shredded cheese over the sauce, if using. Spread your toppings of choice evenly over the top.

6. Return the pizza to the oven and bake for another 8 to 10 minutes and serve!

GREAT FLAVOR COMBINATIONS WITHOUT CHEESE!

- Leftover chicken, diced canned artichoke hearts, sliced black olives, and Pesto
- Bacon, sausage, mushrooms, sliced black olives, and either Classic Pizza Sauce or Ranch Dip
- Leftover chicken, broccoli, spinach, and Hollandaise, Ranch Dip, or crushed garlic and olive oil
- Leftover Simple Steak (page 547), spinach, sautéed mushrooms, fresh basil, and Chimichurri
- Smoked salmon, steamed asparagus, and Hollandaise
- Ham, bacon, pineapple, and either Classic Pizza Sauce or Cauliflower Gravy
- Leftover pork, pineapple, bell peppers, and Barbecue Sauce

TIP: You can par-bake the crust and then store it in the freezer for an extra-quick weeknight meal later. Bake the crust for 7 minutes, let it cool completely, wrap it in plastic wrap, and place it in a freezer-safe container. Par-baked crusts will keep in the freezer for up to 6 months. When you're ready to make a pizza, you can use the crust directly from the freezer; simply increase the baking time to 12 to 14 minutes after adding toppings.

 *avoid* 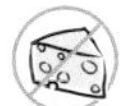 *avoid*

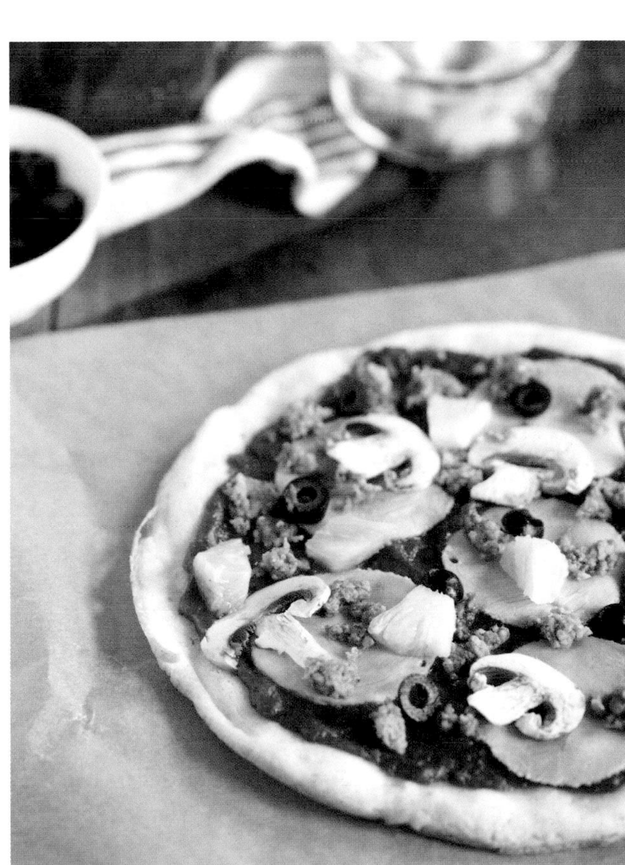

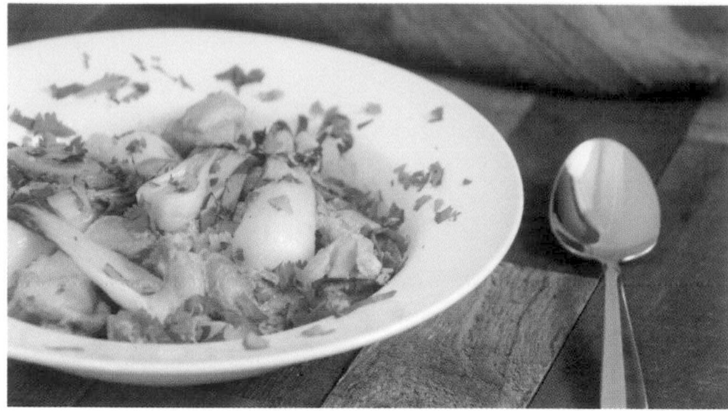

THAI GREEN CURRY

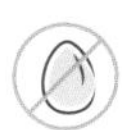 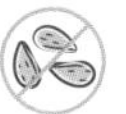 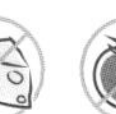 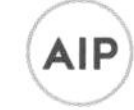 AIP

PREP TIME: 25 minutes COOK TIME: 25 minutes
YIELD: 4 to 6 servings

GREEN CURRY PASTE

(Makes 1½ to 2 cups)

3 shallots, chopped (about ⅔ cup)

9 cloves garlic, crushed

1 inch fresh galangal, or 2 medium slices dried galangal rehydrated in ¼ cup hot water

1 stalk lemongrass (white part only), chopped

1 teaspoon finely grated kaffir lime or lime zest

2 tablespoons kaffir lime juice or regular lime juice

1 teaspoon sea salt

1 teaspoon shrimp paste

1 tablespoon fish sauce

⅓ cup chopped fresh cilantro stems

¼ teaspoon wasabi powder (optional)

CURRY

2 tablespoons coconut oil

1 scant cup Green Curry Paste (from left)

1 batch Coconut Milk (page 480), or 1 (13½-ounce) can full-fat coconut milk

2 pounds boneless, skinless chicken thigh meat, chopped into 1-inch pieces

2 large carrots, sliced

½ bunch radishes, sliced

1 pound bok choy, leaves separated and roughly chopped if very large

½ cup Thai basil leaves (optional)

1 batch Cauli-rice (page 555), for serving

½ cup chopped fresh cilantro leaves, for garnish

1. To make the curry paste, put all the ingredients in a blender and blend until a completely smooth paste forms, 1 to 2 minutes. If it's not blending well, add a little bit of water to help the ingredients to incorporate.

2. Heat the coconut oil over medium-high heat in a 10- to 12-inch sauté pan.

3. Add the curry paste and cook for 2 to 3 minutes, stirring constantly, until curry paste has deepened in color slightly and become very fragrant.

4. Add one-third of the can of coconut milk. Continue to cook the curry paste for another 3 to 4 minutes, stirring constantly.

5. Add the chicken and another one-third of the can coconut milk. Cook uncovered, stirring occasionally, until chicken is fully cooked, 10 to 12 minutes.

6. Add the carrots and radishes. Cook uncovered, stirring occasionally, for 5 minutes. Add the bok choy and cook 4 to 5 more minutes, until all the vegetables are cooked al dente.

7. Add the remaining coconut milk and stir in just to heat. Add the Thai basil leaves, if using.

8. To serve, pour over cauli-rice and sprinkle chopped cilantro generously over the top.

TIPS: This recipe makes more curry paste than you'll need for this dish. You could always make a half batch, but it is so delicious and stores so well that I suggest you make a full batch so you can whip up another dish of green curry on a whim. Store the leftover curry paste in the refrigerator for up to a week or in the freezer for up to 6 months.

For a creamier curry, use 1 2/3 cups coconut cream in place of the coconut milk.

CEVICHE

  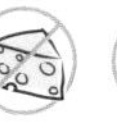 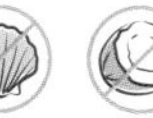  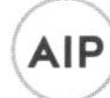 AIP

PREP TIME: 30 minutes, plus time to marinate
YIELD: 2 to 3 servings

¾ pound sushi-grade ahi tuna, sliced into very thin strips

½ red onion, thinly sliced

⅔ cup lime juice (about 6 limes)

1 teaspoon finely grated lime zest

¼ teaspoon sea salt

½ cup chopped fresh cilantro

1 large avocado, peeled and diced

1. Combine the tuna, onion, lime juice and zest, and salt in a bowl. Cover and refrigerate to marinate for 1 hour, stirring every 15 to 20 minutes.

2. Stir in the cilantro and avocado immediately before serving. Serve with plantain chips, if desired.

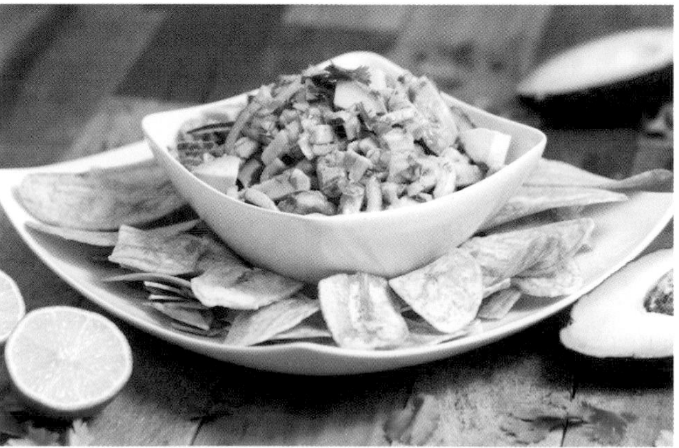

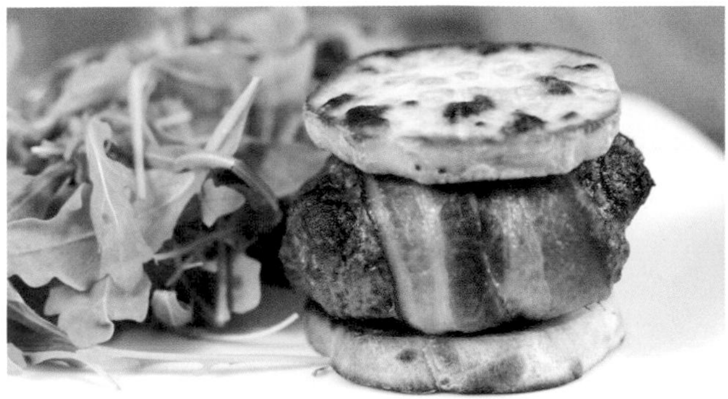

BACON-WRAPPED CURRY BURGERS WITH SWEET POTATO "BUNS"

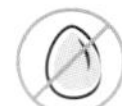 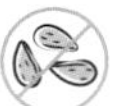 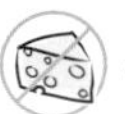 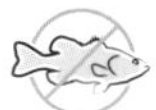 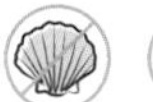 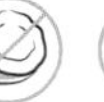 

PREP TIME: 15 minutes *COOK TIME: 30 minutes*
YIELD: 8 servings

3 pounds ground beef or pork

2 tablespoons curry powder, homemade (page 483) or store-bought

16 to 24 slices bacon

2 to 3 very large sweet potatoes (ideally 3 to 4 inches in circumference)

3 to 4 tablespoons coconut oil, lard, unsalted butter, or ghee

1. Place the oven racks in the middle of the oven, spaced at least a few inches apart. Preheat the oven to 375°F. Set a metal rack inside a rimmed baking sheet.

2. Combine the ground meat with the curry powder. Mix with your hands until evenly distributed. Cover and refrigerate the meat until ready to cook (optional).

3. Form 8 patties with the meat, about 6 ounces each. Wrap 2 or 3 slices of bacon around each patty and place on the rack inside the baking sheet. Fold the ends of the bacon under the patties so they stay in place.

4. Peel the sweet potatoes and slice into ½-inch-thick rounds. Place the sweet potato rounds on a second baking sheet and toss liberally with the oil. (If using a solid fat like butter, melt it before tossing.)

5. Place both baking sheets in the oven and bake for 25 to 30 minutes. At the 15-minute mark, pull the sweet potato rounds out of the oven and flip them (no need to flip the burgers). Bake until the sweet potatoes are lightly browned (probably closer to 25 minutes, depending on their exact size), the burgers are cooked to an internal temperature of 160°F, and the bacon is an appetizing brown color (probably closer to 30 minutes).

6. To serve, place each bacon-wrapped burger between 2 sweet potato rounds as a "bun."

 *use Nightshade-Free Curry Powder (page 483)*

SPATCHCOCKED CHICKEN

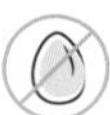  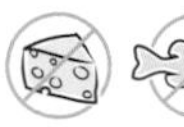 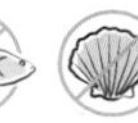 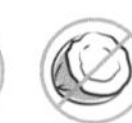 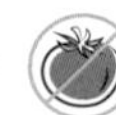 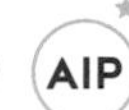 AIP

PREP TIME: 10 minutes
COOK TIME: 45 minutes
YIELD: 5 to 8 servings

4 cloves garlic, minced

Finely grated zest and juice from 1 lemon

2 tablespoons chopped fresh oregano

½ teaspoon chopped fresh rosemary

½ teaspoon chopped fresh thyme

1 teaspoon sea salt

¼ teaspoon ground black pepper

2 tablespoons avocado oil, divided

1 (4- to 5-pound) whole chicken

1. Prepare the seasoning slurry by mixing together the garlic, lemon zest and juice, oregano, rosemary, thyme, salt, pepper, and 1 tablespoon of the avocado oil.

2. Rub the remaining tablespoon of avocado oil over the bottom of a cast-iron or stainless-steel skillet (a 10-inch or larger skillet will fit most chickens).

3. Preheat the oven to 425°F.

4. Using poultry shears, cut along the right side of the chicken's backbone (so you're cutting through the ribs and not the vertebrae) all the way down the spine. Repeat down the left side to remove the backbone entirely. Turn the chicken over (back to breast side up) and open it up to begin to lie flat. You can more thoroughly flatten the chicken by pulling up on one side while pushing down on the other; this breaks the ribs.

5. Place the chicken skin side up in the prepared skillet. Pat dry with paper towel. Rub the seasoning slurry all over the skin of the chicken.

6. Roast the chicken for 45 minutes. Let rest in the pan for 5 to 10 minutes before serving.

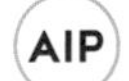 *omit pepper*

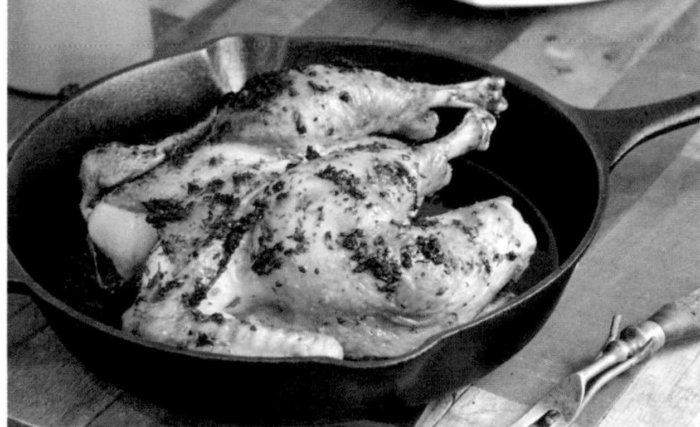

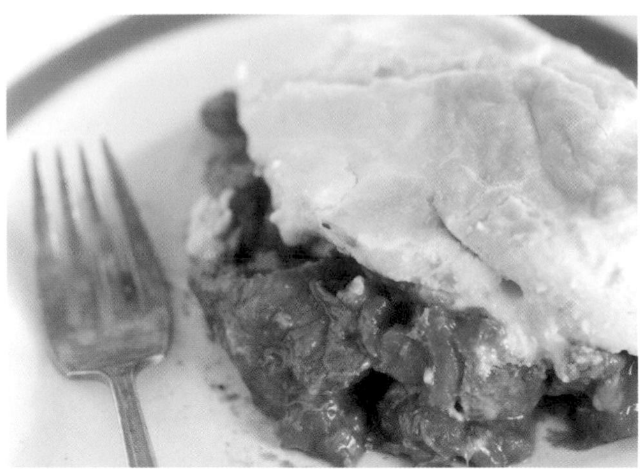

STEAK & KIDNEY POT PIE

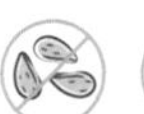 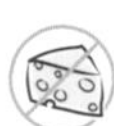 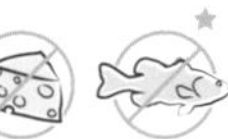  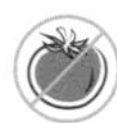

PREP TIME: 30 minutes, plus time to cool
COOK TIME: 3 hours YIELD: 10 to 12 servings

- 3 pounds steak
- 1½ pounds lamb kidneys
- 3 medium carrots
- 6 ounces portobello mushrooms
- 1 large sweet onion
- 4 to 5 tablespoons olive oil, avocado oil, or tallow, divided
- ½ teaspoon sea salt
- ½ teaspoon ground black pepper
- 2 tablespoons arrowroot powder
- 2 cups Beef Stock (page 486)
- 1½ teaspoons fish sauce
- 1 bay leaf
- 1 batch Choux Pastry dough (page 564)

1. Slice the steak and kidneys into ¼-inch-thick slices. Slice the carrots into ½-inch-thick rounds. Slice the mushrooms into ½-inch dice. Cut the onion in half, then slice into ¼-inch-thick half-moons.

2. Heat 3 tablespoons of the oil in a large pot over medium-high heat. Season the steak and kidneys with the salt and pepper, then brown separately in batches. Set aside.

3. Add 1 to 2 tablespoons more oil to the pan, if needed. Brown the onion for 7 to 8 minutes. Add the carrots and mushrooms and sauté for 3 to 4 more minutes.

4. Return the meat to the pot. Whisk the arrowroot powder into the beef stock and add to the pot. Add the fish sauce and bay leaf. Simmer, uncovered, for 1½ hours. Taste and season with salt and pepper as needed.

5. Pour the steak and kidney filling into a large casserole or lasagna dish. Let cool to room temperature (if it's a little warmer than room temperature when the choux pastry is ready, that's okay).

6. While the filling is cooling, prepare the choux pastry dough by completing Steps 1 through 4 on page 564. Preheat the oven to 425°F.

7. Immediately pour the dough over the cooled steak and kidney filling. Spread with a spoon or spatula to evenly cover the entire surface.

8. Bake for 25 to 30 minutes, until lightly browned on top. You might want to put a rimmed baking sheet under the casserole dish just in case it bubbles over a little. Enjoy!

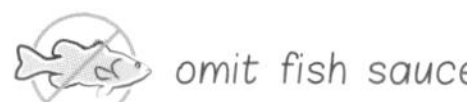 *omit fish sauce*

BROILED PORK CHOPS

 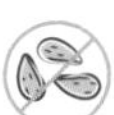 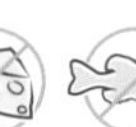 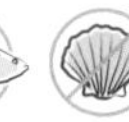 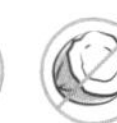 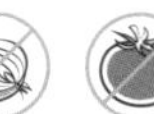 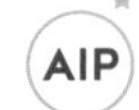 AIP

PREP TIME: 10 minutes COOK TIME: 15 minutes
YIELD: 4 servings

- 1 to 2 tablespoons Pork Seasoning (page 483)
- 4 (1- to 1½-inch-thick) bone-in or boneless pork chops, about 8 ounces each

1. Turn the broiler to high and let the oven preheat for about 10 minutes.

2. Sprinkle the pork seasoning liberally over both sides of the pork chops.

3. Place the pork chops on a roasting pan, using the rack insert that came with the pan.

4. Broil the pork chops on the first side for 6 to 8 minutes, depending on the thickness. Flip and broil on the second side for another 6 to 8 minutes.

5. Let the chops rest for 5 minutes before serving.

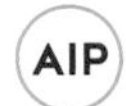 *substitute AIP Herbes de Provence (page 482) for Pork Seasoning*

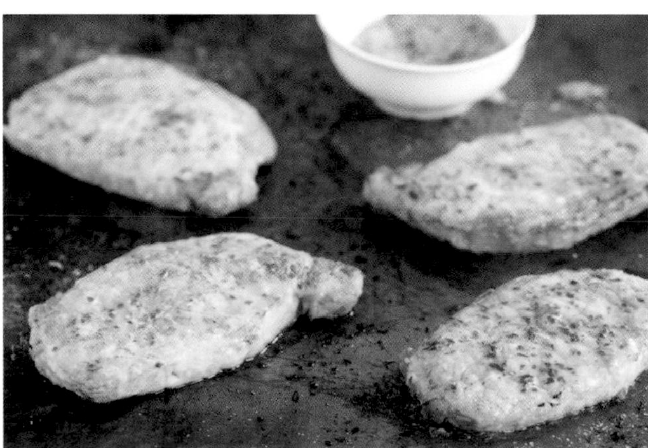

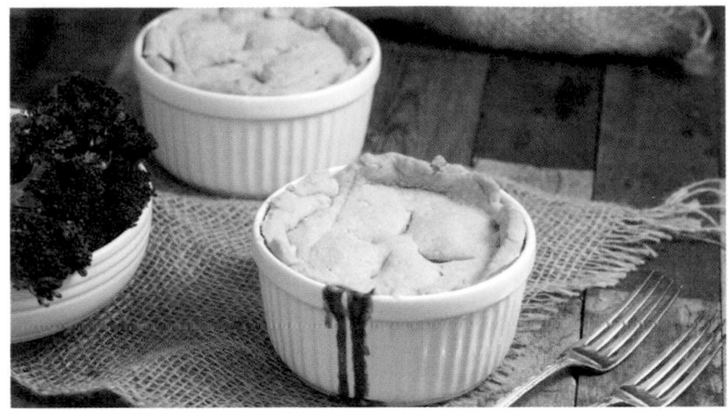

CHICKEN OR BEEF POT PIE

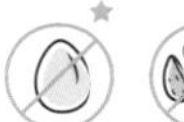 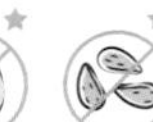 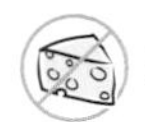 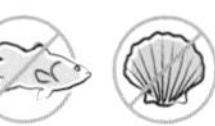 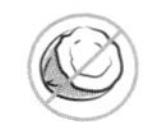  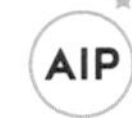 AIP

PREP TIME: 20 minutes *COOK TIME: 1 hour 40 minutes*
YIELD: 6 to 8 servings

- 2 tablespoons olive oil
- 2 pounds flank steak or other inexpensive tougher steak or chicken breasts or thighs, cut into ½-inch pieces
- ½ large white onion, diced
- 4 stalks celery, diced
- 3 carrots, diced
- 4 cups Bone Stock (beef for beef pot pie or chicken for chicken pot pie; page 486)
- 2 tablespoons apple cider vinegar, or 3 tablespoons tomato paste
- 2 teaspoons sea salt
- 2 bay leaves
- 1 green plantain, peeled and grated
- 1 cup fresh or frozen peas (optional)
- 1 batch Pie Crust (page 499)

1. Heat a large skillet over medium-high heat. Add the olive oil and meat. Brown the meat, 6 to 8 minutes for steak or 8 to 10 minutes for chicken, stirring occasionally.

2. Add the onion, celery, and carrots to the skillet and cook until starting to brown, another 7 to 8 minutes, stirring occasionally.

3. Add the stock, vinegar, salt, bay leaves, and grated plantain. Reduce the heat to maintain a simmer. Cook until the plantain dissolves into the stock, about 20 minutes. As the stock thickens, stir more frequently to make sure it's not burning on the bottom (add more water if needed to prevent scorching).

4. Taste and add salt, if needed. Spoon the filling into ramekins for individual pot pies or into a large casserole dish. Allow to cool before adding the crust.

5. Preheat the oven to 375°F.

6. Prepare the pie crust and roll between 2 sheets of parchment paper to a thickness of ¼ to ⅜ inch, trying to roughly mimic the size and shape of your chosen dish(es). Carefully transfer the crust onto the filling. Use any leftover crust to fill any gaps or make decorations for the top. Using a sharp knife, pierce a few slits through the crust.

7. Bake for 50 to 60 minutes, until the crust is starting to brown. Serve!

AIP *use vinegar; omit peas; use Cassava Flour Pie Crust*

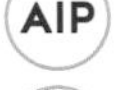 *use vinegar*

 *use Cassava Flour Pie Crust*

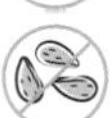 *use Cassava Flour Pie Crust*

 *use Cassava Flour Pie Crust*

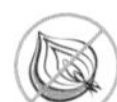 *omit onion*

SHRIMP PAD THAI

 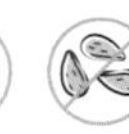 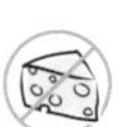   AIP

PREP TIME: 10 minutes *COOK TIME: 10 minutes*
YIELD: 2 to 4 servings

- 2 tablespoons coconut oil or avocado oil
- 4 cloves garlic, minced
- ¼ cup lime juice (about 2 limes)
- 3 tablespoons fish sauce
- 1 tablespoon coconut aminos (or use 1 additional tablespoon fish sauce)
- 1½ teaspoons coconut water vinegar
- 1 (12-ounce) bag broccoli slaw
- 2 medium carrots, cut into thin julienne strips
- 1 to 1¼ pounds salad shrimp, precooked, tails removed
- 4 to 5 green onions, finely chopped
- 5 tablespoons chopped fresh cilantro
- ⅓ cup chopped roasted unsalted cashews, for garnish (optional)

1. Heat a large skillet or wok over medium-high heat. Add the oil and garlic. Cook for 1 minute, until the garlic is starting to brown and become fragrant.

2. Add the lime juice, fish sauce, coconut aminos, vinegar, broccoli slaw, and carrots. Cook, stirring frequently, until the slaw and carrots are cooked al dente, 5 to 7 minutes.

3. Add the shrimp and cook for 1 to 2 more minutes, stirring frequently, just until the shrimp are warmed.

4. Add the green onions and cilantro and cook for 30 seconds. Garnish with the cashews, if using, and serve.

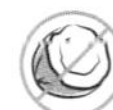 *use avocado oil and apple cider vinegar; omit coconut aminos*

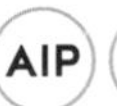 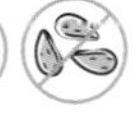 *omit cashews*

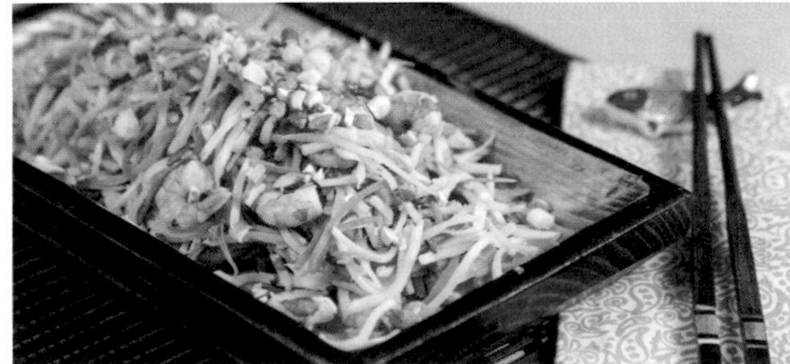

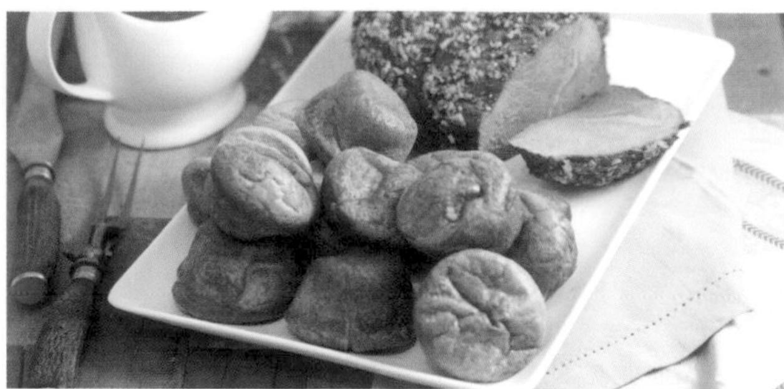

HERB-CRUSTED ROAST BEEF WITH PALEO YORKSHIRE PUDDINGS & PAN GRAVY

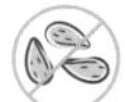 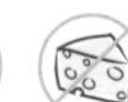 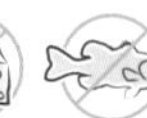  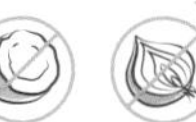  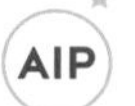 AIP

PREP TIME: 15 minutes COOK TIME: 2 hours
YIELD: 6 to 8 servings

- 1 tablespoon fennel seeds
- 4 to 5 cloves garlic, minced
- 1 teaspoon truffle salt, or 1 teaspoon each sea salt and ground black pepper
- 1 tablespoon chopped fresh rosemary
- 1 (2- to 3-pound) boneless beef roast
- ⅓ cup high-smoke-point cooking fat (ghee, palm shortening, or avocado oil)
- 2 large green plantains (1½ to 1¾ cups pureed)
- 6 large eggs, room temperature
- 1 teaspoon sea salt
- 1 batch Pan Gravy (page 496)

1. Preheat the oven to 300°F.

2. Grind the fennel seeds in a spice grinder, mini food processor, clean coffee grinder, or mortar and pestle. Combine with the garlic, truffle salt, and rosemary. Rub the herbs all over the roast.

3. Place the roast on a roasting pan and insert a meat thermometer. Bake for 1½ to 1¾ hours, or until the internal temperature reaches 145°F (for medium-rare).

4. Let the roast rest for at least 10 minutes before carving. If waiting for the Yorkshire puddings to cook, cover the roast with aluminum foil to keep warm.

5. To prepare the Yorkshire puddings, put about 1½ teaspoons of fat in each cup of a standard-size 12-cup metal muffin pan (a silicone pan can't handle heat this high). Put the muffin pan in the oven and turn up the temperature to 450°F.

6. Peel the plantains. Place in a blender with the eggs and salt and blend on high for 3 to 5 minutes, until smooth and airy.

7. Remove the hot pan from the oven and pour the plantain batter into the muffin cups. Put in the oven immediately and bake for 20 minutes.

8. While the Yorkshire puddings are baking, prepare the pan gravy.

9. Remove the Yorkshire puddings from the oven and invert muffin pan to remove them. Serve immediately with roast beef and pan gravy.

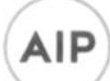 *don't make Yorkshire puddings and substitute 3 tablespoons fresh tarragon for fennel seeds*

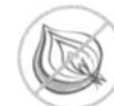 *use AIP Herbes de Provence (page 482) to season roast beef*

LAMB CURRY

 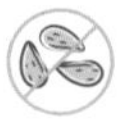 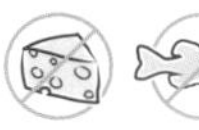  

PREP TIME: 15 minutes COOK TIME: 1 hour
YIELD: 5 or 6 servings

- 3 tablespoons red palm oil, tallow, lard, or coconut oil, divided
- 3 pounds lamb stew meat, cubed
- 2 medium-sized yellow onions, diced
- 2 medium carrots, chopped
- 2½ tablespoons curry powder, homemade (page 483) or store-bought
- 1 tablespoon lemon juice
- 1 cup Chicken Stock (page 486)
- ⅓ cup coconut butter (aka coconut cream concentrate)
- 4 cups fresh spinach

1. In a stockpot, heat 2 tablespoons of the oil over medium-high heat. Brown the meat in 2 or 3 batches, setting the browned meat aside in a large bowl.

2. Add another tablespoon of oil to the pot. Add the onion and carrots and cook until the onions are starting to turn translucent, 7 to 8 minutes.

3. Return the meat to the pot. Add the curry powder, lemon juice, and stock. Cover, reduce the heat to medium, and simmer for 1 hour.

4. Remove the lid and continue to simmer uncovered for 30 to 40 minutes.

5. Stir in the coconut butter and spinach. When the spinach has wilted (about 1 minute), serve.

 *use Nightshade-Free Curry Powder (page 483)*

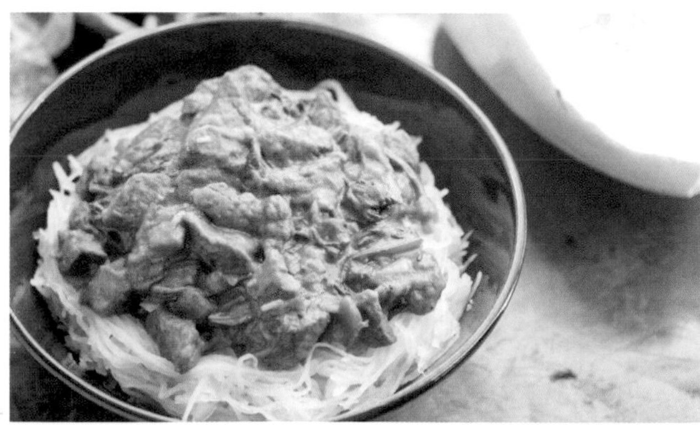

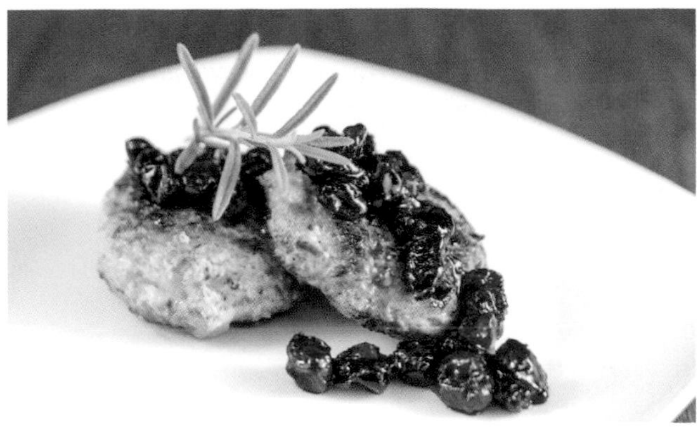

BACON-APPLE CHICKEN BURGERS WITH MAPLE CRANBERRY SAUCE

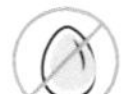 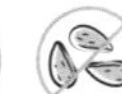 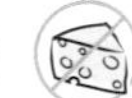 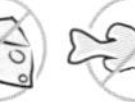  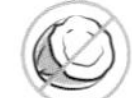  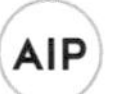

PREP TIME: 15 minutes *COOK TIME: 1 hour 15 minutes*
YIELD: 5 to 7 servings

8 to 10 ounces bacon (if using 2½ pounds ground chicken, use 10 ounces bacon)

1 medium onion, minced

1 large Granny Smith or Fuji apple, peeled, cored, and minced

2 teaspoons minced fresh rosemary

2 to 2½ pounds ground chicken

½ teaspoon sea salt or truffle salt

¼ teaspoon ground black pepper (optional)

1 tablespoon bacon fat or other cooking fat, if needed

Maple Cranberry Sauce (page 496), for serving

1. Place the bacon in a cold skillet, then turn on the heat to medium-high. Cook, flipping once or twice, until the bacon is crispy.

2. When the bacon is crispy, remove it from the pan and add the onion to the bacon fat in the pan. Sauté for 5 minutes over medium-high heat, stirring occasionally, until the onion is starting to soften. Add the apple and rosemary and continue sautéing until the onion is browned and both the onion and apple are soft, 5 to 8 more minutes. Remove from the pan with a slotted spoon and allow to cool slightly. Do not clean the pan; you will use it to cook the burgers.

3. When the bacon is cool enough to handle, chop into small pieces (think bacon bit size).

4. Combine the ground chicken, bacon, apple and onion mix, and salt in a bowl. Mix well with your hands and form into 6- to 8-ounce patties.

5. Preheat the pan over medium heat. If there is no bacon fat left in the pan, add a tablespoon of bacon fat. Fry the patties in the pan, in batches if needed to prevent overcrowding, until fully cooked, 15 to 25 minutes total, flipping once. To ensure that the burgers are fully cooked, check the internal temperature with a meat thermometer: it should read 160°F.

6. Serve with chilled maple-cranberry sauce.

BROILED SALMON WITH DILL-CAPER SAUCE

 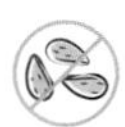 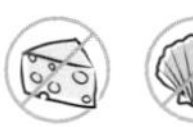  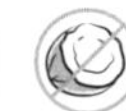 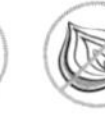  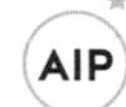

PREP TIME: 15 minutes *COOK TIME: 10 minutes*
YIELD: 4 servings

½ cup Mayonnaise (page 487)

3 tablespoons chopped fresh dill

2 to 3 tablespoons capers (if they are large, give them a bit of a chop)

1 to 2 tablespoons olive oil or avocado oil

4 (6- to 8-ounce) salmon fillets

½ teaspoon truffle salt, or ½ teaspoon sea salt and ¼ teaspoon ground black pepper

1½ teaspoons fresh thyme leaves (from 5 to 6 sprigs)

1. To make the dill-caper sauce, combine the mayonnaise, dill, and 2 tablespoons of capers. Taste and add an additional tablespoon of capers, if desired. Store the sauce in the refrigerator until you are ready to serve the salmon.

2. Place a rack high up in the oven so that the surface of the salmon will be 6 to 8 inches from the top element. Turn the broiler to high and let it preheat for about 10 minutes before putting the salmon in the oven. Coat a rimmed baking sheet with the olive oil.

3. Place the salmon fillets skin side down on the oiled baking sheet. Sprinkle with the truffle salt and thyme.

4. Broil for 8 to 9 minutes, until the segments flake apart easily and the salmon is opaque throughout. Serve with the dill-caper sauce.

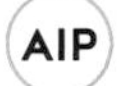 *don't make dill-caper sauce; omit pepper*

 *don't make dill-caper sauce*

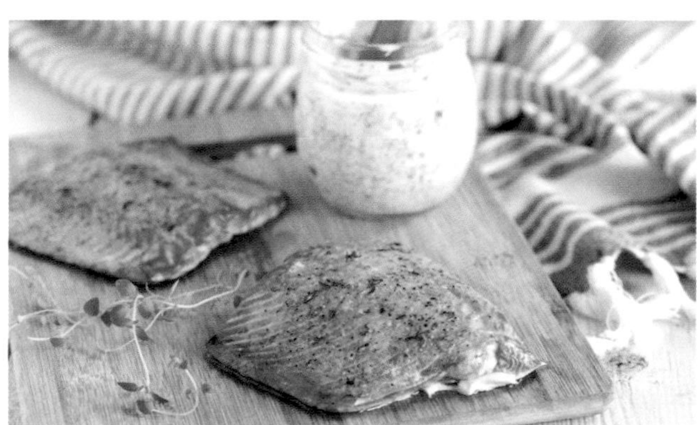

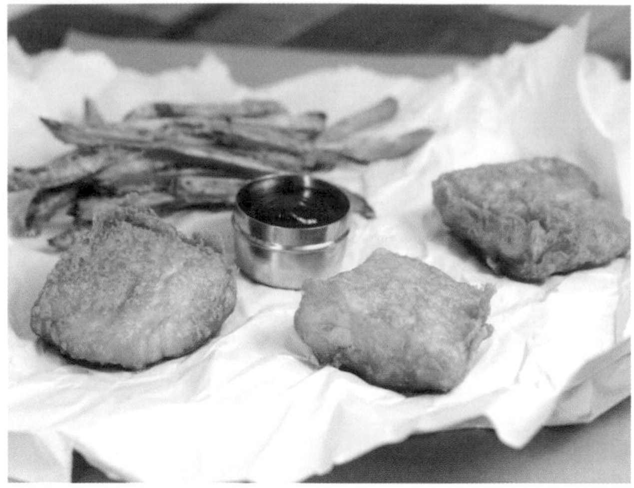

FISH N' CHIPS

 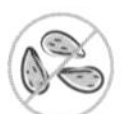 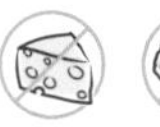  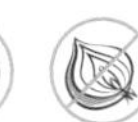  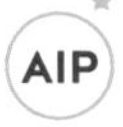 AIP

PREP TIME: 10 minutes COOK TIME: 20 minutes
YIELD: 3 to 5 servings

1½ pounds white fish fillets (such as cod or halibut), cut to the desired shape

Lard, tallow, or other high-smoke-point fat, for deep-frying

TEMPURA-STYLE BATTER

3 large egg whites, room temperature

½ cup tapioca starch, plus an extra ½ cup or so for dredging

½ teaspoon sea salt

"BEER" BATTER

½ cup cassava flour

½ teaspoon sea salt

¼ teaspoon baking soda

⅔ cup sparkling water or unflavored kombucha, store-bought or homemade (page 492)

1 batch Cassava Oven Fries (page 554) or Oven-Baked Sweet Potato Fries (page 557), for serving

1. Pat the fish dry with a paper towel and set aside.

2. Heat the fat in a countertop deep-fryer or in a large heavy-bottomed pan to between 350°F and 375°F, staying at least 5°F below the fat's smoke point.

FOR TEMPURA-STYLE BATTER:

3. Use a hand mixer to beat the egg whites until stiff. Fold in the tapioca and salt to completely combine. (You will lose a little of the air you beat into the egg whites, but that's okay.)

4. When the fat is at temperature, dredge the fish fillets in the tapioca, then dip in the batter. Use your fingers to spread the batter over the fish; don't worry if it's not completely evenly coated. The coating should end up about ¼ inch thick or slightly less before you fry it.

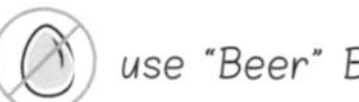 *use "Beer" Batter*

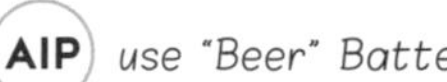 *use "Beer" Batter*

FOR "BEER" BATTER:

3. Combine the cassava flour, salt, and baking soda in a bowl. Pour the sparkling water into the bowl and mix for a smooth batter.

4. When the fat reaches temperature, dip the fish into the batter to coat completely.

TO FRY THE FISH:

5. Carefully place the battered fish in the deep fryer; 4- to 5-ounce fillets will take 5 to 6 minutes total. Gently flip the fillets after 3 to 4 minutes. Tempura-style batter should be a very light golden brown; "beer" batter will be a deeper golden brown. The fish should be opaque throughout.

6. Carefully lift the pieces out of the deep-fryer with a fry basket and place them on paper towels or a cooling rack. Serve with the fries.

TIP: Both of these batter recipes work well for other deep-frying applications, like shrimp, calamari, and zucchini, mushrooms, or other veggies.

COCONUT OIL-POACHED TILAPIA WITH ASIAN PEAR SLAW

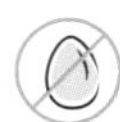  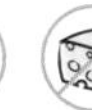   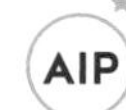

PREP TIME: 20 minutes COOK TIME: 22 minutes
YIELD: 3 to 4 servings

½ cup coconut oil, or more as needed to be ¼ inch deep in the pan

Pinch of sea salt

3 or 4 (6- to 7-ounce) tilapia or other white fish fillets

1 batch Asian Pear Slaw (page 559)

1. Heat the coconut oil and salt in a skillet over medium-low heat until hot and just starting to bubble, but not at a rolling simmer. Add the tilapia to the pan.

2. Cover and cook until the top edges of the fish are opaque, 10 to 12 minutes. Flip each piece of fish and cook for another 8 to 10 minutes, until the fish is fully cooked and opaque throughout.

3. Serve with the slaw and enjoy!

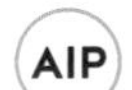  *do not make slaw*

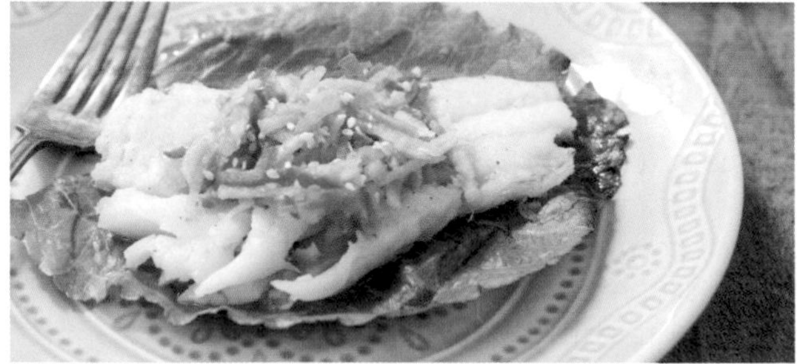

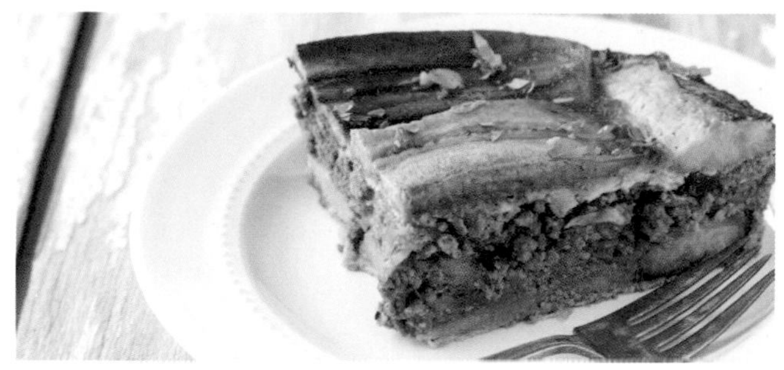

PUERTO RICAN LASAGNA

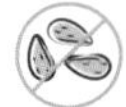 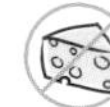 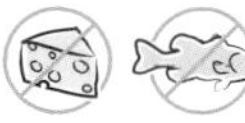  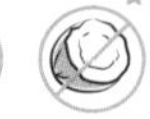

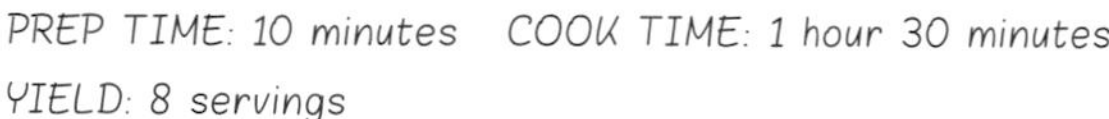
PREP TIME: 10 minutes COOK TIME: 1 hour 30 minutes
YIELD: 8 servings

- 3 to 4 tablespoons coconut oil, divided
- 2 pounds ground beef
- 1 medium-sized yellow onion
- ½ cup red bell pepper, diced
- ½ cup green bell pepper, diced
- 4 to 5 cloves garlic, finely chopped
- 2 bay leaves
- ½ cup Chicken Stock (page 486)
- ½ cup dry white or red wine
- 1 (6-ounce) can tomato paste
- ½ teaspoon sea salt
- 6 very ripe plantains (should be almost completely black)
- 8 large eggs
- Ground black pepper

1. Heat a large saucepan or small stockpot over medium-high heat. Add 1 tablespoon of the coconut oil and the ground beef, onion, bell peppers, garlic, and bay leaves. Brown the beef, breaking it up with a large spoon, 8 to 10 minutes.

2. Add the stock, wine, tomato paste, and salt. Reduce the heat to a simmer and cook, uncovered, for 10 to 20 minutes, stirring occasionally. Taste and add more salt, if desired.

3. Preheat the oven to 350°F.

4. Cut the plantains in half crosswise and peel. Then cut each half lengthwise into ¼-inch-thick strips (about 8 slices per plantain—it's okay if they aren't all evenly thick).

5. Heat 1 to 2 tablespoons of coconut oil in a skillet or griddle. Place the plantain slices in the hot oil and fry for 3 to 4 minutes on both sides to lightly brown. Set aside. (You will probably have to work in batches, adding more oil to the pan after each batch.)

6. Beat or whisk 4 of the eggs with a dash of salt and pepper. Pour into a large rectangular casserole dish or lasagna pan. Bake for 6 to 7 minutes, until set but not completely cooked. Remove from the oven and prick the surface of the eggs several times with a fork. (Alternatively, you can microwave the eggs for about 1 minute.)

7. Lay half of the fried plantain slices over the eggs in a solid layer, like lasagna noodles. Pour all the meat sauce over the plantain layer. Spread out to a uniform layer. Then place the rest of the plantain slices over the top of the meat sauce (like your second layer of noodles).

8. Beat or whisk the remaining 4 eggs with a dash of salt and pepper and pour over the top of the lasagna.

9. Bake for 45 to 50 minutes. Let the lasagna rest for 5 minutes before serving. Store leftovers in the refrigerator for up to 5 days.

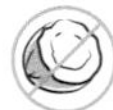 *use olive oil or avocado oil instead of coconut oil*

CHICKEN FINGERS

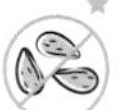 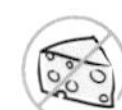 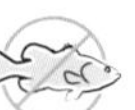  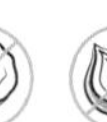 

PREP TIME: 10 minutes COOK TIME: 18 minutes
YIELD: 4 servings

- ½ cup almond meal or ground sunflower seeds
- ½ teaspoon sea salt
- ¾ teaspoon paprika
- ¼ teaspoon ground coriander
- ¼ teaspoon ground cumin
- 1 large egg
- 1 pound chicken tenders or boneless, skinless chicken breast, cut into strips

1. Preheat the oven to 425°F. Line a large rimmed baking sheet with parchment paper.

2. Combine the almond meal with the salt and spices on a plate or shallow dish. Beat the egg in a separate shallow dish.

3. Dry the chicken with a paper towel. Dip a chicken tender in the egg, then in the almond meal mixture, coating all sides. Place on the lined baking sheet. Repeat until all the chicken is coated.

4. Bake for 16 to 18 minutes, turning once in the middle of baking, until completely cooked; the internal temperature should reach 180°F. Serve with Ranch Dip (page 487), Barbecue Sauce (page 493), or a mixture of half honey and half Dijon mustard for dipping.

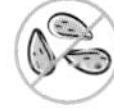 *use ground sunflower seeds*  *omit paprika*

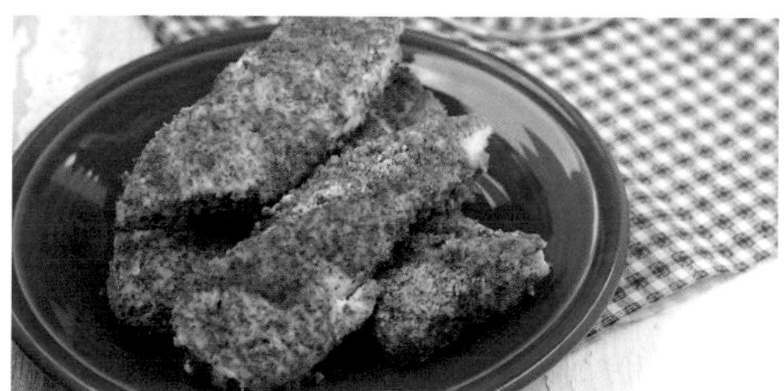

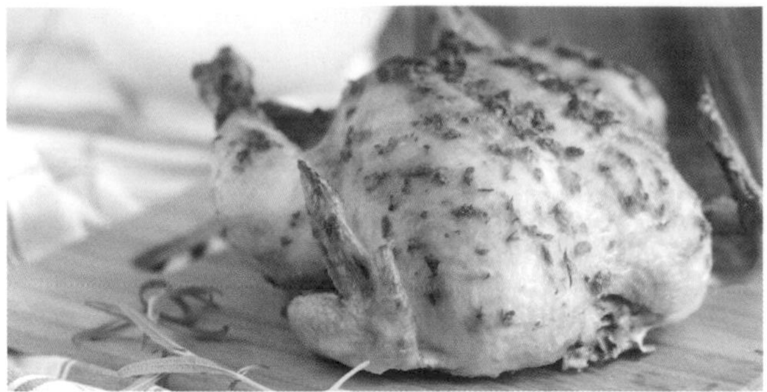

MUSTARD & ROSEMARY ROASTED CHICKEN WITH PAN SAUCE

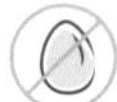  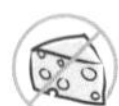 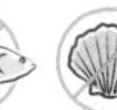 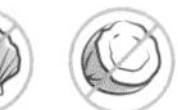  

PREP TIME: 15 minutes *COOK TIME: 2 hours*
YIELD: 10 to 14 servings

2 (4- to 5-pound) whole chickens

2 tablespoons lard, coconut oil, or unsalted butter

2 tablespoons Dijon mustard

1½ tablespoons chopped fresh rosemary, or 1 tablespoon dried rosemary

¼ cup arrowroot powder or kuzu starch

¼ cup cold water

1. Preheat the oven to 350°F.

2. Remove the chickens from the packaging, pat dry with paper towels, and remove any giblets (save these for making bone stock!). Place the chickens on a roasting pan, using the rack insert that comes with the pan.

3. Melt the lard and mix with the mustard and rosemary. Baste the entire surface of both chickens with the mustard sauce.

4. Roast the chickens for 20 minutes per pound (or until a meat thermometer reads at least 165°F—it's standard to cook chicken until the breast meat reads 180°F). Set the chickens aside to rest.

5. To make the pan gravy, place the roasting pan onto a large element on the stovetop. Turn to medium-high heat and bring the juices to a simmer.

6. Mix the arrowroot powder with the cold water.

7. Pour the starchy water into the pan while whisking with a wire whisk. Keep whisking until the gravy has thickened, about 3 to 4 minutes. If it's too thin, repeat with additional arrowroot powder. If the gravy is too thick, thin it out with a little hot water. If there are any lumps, simply pour the gravy through a strainer before serving.

8. Carve the chickens and serve with gravy. Store leftovers in the refrigerator for up to 5 days.

MIDDLE EASTERN DUKKAH-CRUSTED LAMB CHOPS

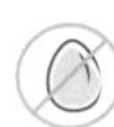 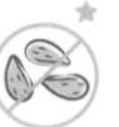 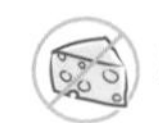  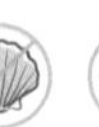 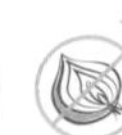 

PREP TIME: 10 minutes *COOK TIME: 30 minutes*
YIELD: 4 to 5 servings

1 tablespoon honey

1 tablespoon pomegranate molasses

½ cup raw unsalted pepitas or pistachios

2½ tablespoons sesame seeds

1 tablespoon ground coriander

2 teaspoons ground cumin

¼ teaspoon sea salt

1 to 3 tablespoons red palm oil

4 pounds lamb chops (rib or loin)

1. Combine the honey and pomegranate molasses. Set aside.

2. Heat a skillet over medium heat. Add the pepitas and sesame seeds to the pan and toast the seeds, shaking or stirring occasionally, until fragrant and starting to brown. Remove from the heat and let cool. Place the seeds in a food processor and grind until the consistency of coarse sand.

3. Combine the ground, toasted pepitas and sesame seeds with the coriander, cumin, and salt. Place on a plate and set aside.

4. Heat a large skillet over medium-high heat. Add 1 to 2 tablespoons of palm oil to the pan. Fry the lamb chops in the oil in batches, 2 minutes per side for medium-rare (or 3 minutes per side for medium). You can adjust the cooking time for the thickness of the chops and your desired doneness.

5. As the chops are cooked, set aside and cover with aluminum foil or place in a warm oven (set to its lowest temperature) to keep warm.

6. Take each cooked lamb chop and dip into the ground pepitas mixture on each side to give it a nice coating. Drizzle with the pomegranate molasses mixture and serve.

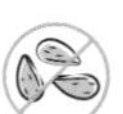 *use pepitas*

 *omit honey and use pepitas*

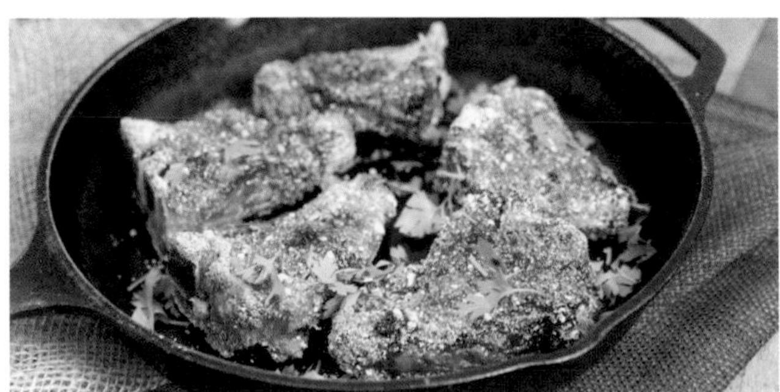

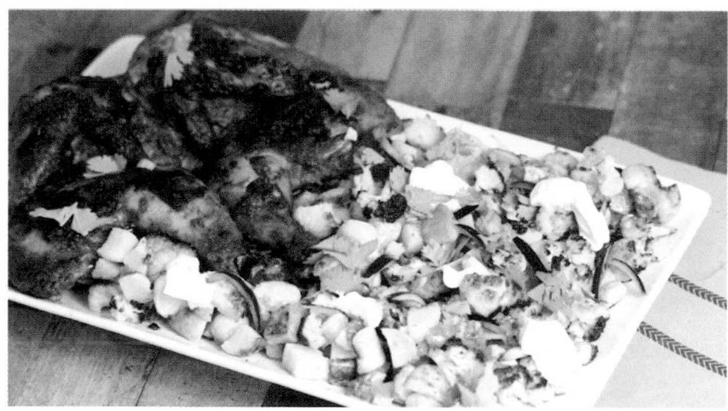

BENGALI TANDOORI CHICKEN WITH ALOO GOBI

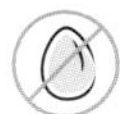  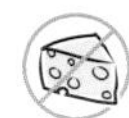 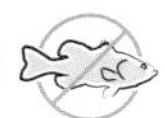 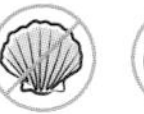 

PREP TIME: 15 minutes, plus time to marinate
COOK TIME: 45 minutes *YIELD: 4 to 6 servings*

1 tablespoon granulated garlic
2 teaspoons granulated onion
2 teaspoons ginger powder
1 teaspoon ground coriander
1 teaspoon ground cumin
1 teaspoon fennel seeds
1 teaspoon garam masala
½ teaspoon turmeric powder
¼ teaspoon fenugreek seeds
2 teaspoons sea salt
1 tablespoon Dijon mustard
2 tablespoons ghee or other fat
2 tablespoons lemon juice
¼ cup Coconut Milk Yogurt (page 481)
1 (3-pound) whole chicken, spatchcocked (see page 531) or cut into pieces
1 batch Potatoless Aloo Gobi (page 558), uncooked
Chopped fresh cilantro, for garnish (optional)

SERVING SUGGESTIONS (OPTIONAL)

¼ cup Easy Pickled Shallots (page 498)
Additional Coconut Milk Yogurt (page 481)

1. Using a blender or spice grinder, blend the spices and salt together to grind the whole-seed spices and fully combine.

2. Add the mustard, ghee, lemon juice, and yogurt to the blender with the spices and blend to form a smooth, thick puree.

3. Thoroughly coat the chicken in the marinade. Refrigerate for 3 to 4 hours or up to 24 hours.

4. Preheat the oven to 425°F.

5. Place the Aloo Gobi in a rimmed baking sheet or large roasting pan, pushing it to the sides to make room for the chicken in the center. Place the chicken in the middle of the pan, surrounded by the Aloo Gobi. Use any remaining marinade from the chicken to coat the top of the chicken thoroughly.

6. Roast for 45 minutes, until the chicken reaches an internal temperature of 160°F and the vegetables are browned.

7. Garnish with fresh cilantro and serve with pickled shallots and additional coconut milk yogurt, if desired.

HONEY-GARLIC CHICKEN WINGS

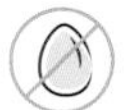  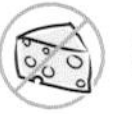  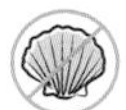 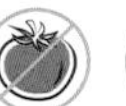 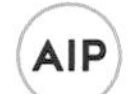

PREP TIME: 5 minutes, plus time to marinate
COOK TIME: 30 minutes to 1 hour, depending on method
YIELD: 6 to 8 servings

⅓ cup honey
¼ cup lemon juice (about 2 lemons)
¼ cup water
2 tablespoons coconut aminos
2 tablespoons apple cider vinegar
2 teaspoons granulated garlic
¾ teaspoon ginger powder
3 pounds chicken wings, separated

1. Bring the honey, lemon juice, water, coconut aminos, vinegar, garlic, and ginger to a simmer in a small saucepan over medium-high heat. Reduce the heat to low and simmer for 5 minutes. Remove from the heat and let cool.

2. Place the chicken wings in a large resealable plastic bag or bowl and pour the marinade over them. Let the wings marinate in the refrigerator for at least 2 hours.

3. If grilling, preheat a gas or charcoal grill to medium-high heat. Drain the excess marinade off the wings, then place on the hot grill. Grill the wings until fully cooked, turning once (about 20 minutes total, depending on the temperature of your grill). The internal temperature should reach 165°F.

Alternatively, preheat the oven to 400°F, place the wings in a greased baking dish, and bake for 45 to 60 minutes, turning once, until fully cooked; the internal temperature should reach 165°F.

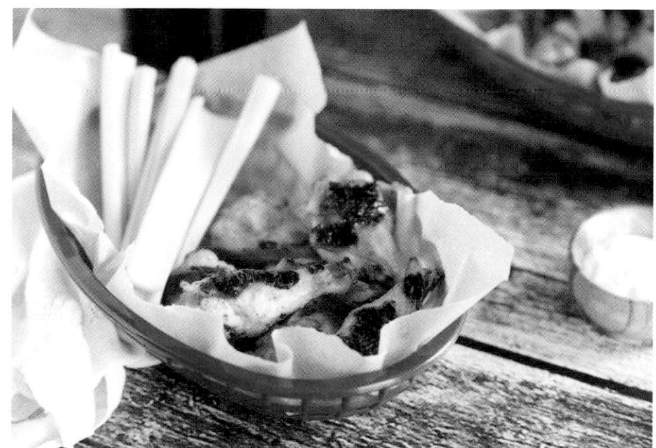

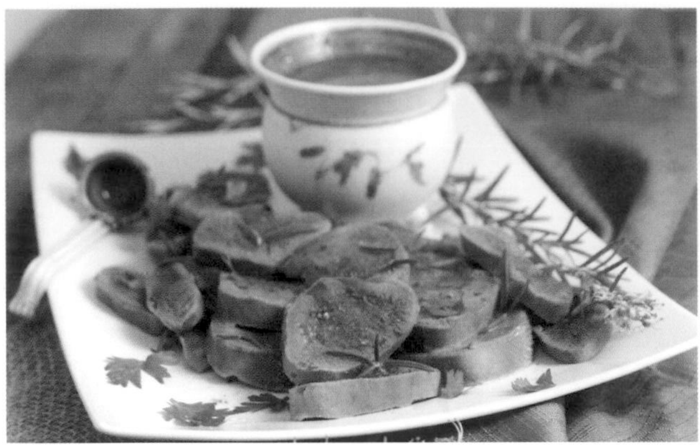

BEEF TONGUE WITH ROSEMARY-MUSTARD REDUCTION

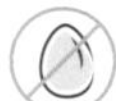 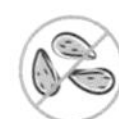 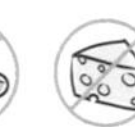   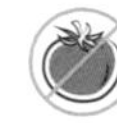 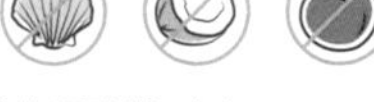

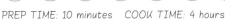

PREP TIME: 10 minutes COOK TIME: 4 hours
YIELD: 6 to 8 servings

- 2½ to 3 pounds beef tongue
- 1 teaspoon sea salt
- 3 stalks celery, roughly chopped
- 2 carrots, roughly chopped
- 1 medium onion, quartered
- 5 to 6 sprigs fresh thyme, or 2 teaspoons dried thyme
- 1 large sprig fresh rosemary
- 8 cloves garlic
- 6 cups water
- 1 teaspoon finely chopped fresh rosemary
- 2 tablespoons prepared brown or Dijon mustard
- 2 teaspoons lemon juice
- ¼ cup unsalted butter, ghee, or lard

1. Season the beef tongue with the salt and place in a stockpot. Place the vegetables, thyme, rosemary sprig, and garlic around the tongue. Ideally, the pot should be a tightly packed. Pour the water over the top, just enough to cover the tongue.

2. Bring to a boil over high heat. Reduce the heat to a simmer and simmer, uncovered, for 3 to 3½ hours. Check the water level every half hour or so and top off with more water as needed.

3. Remove the tongue from the pot and let cool. Pour the stock through a fine-mesh sieve (or a few layers of cheesecloth) into a smaller pot and discard the vegetables and other bits.

4. Bring the stock to a boil. Maintain a rolling boil until it has reduced to 1½ cups or less (10 to 15 minutes, depending on how much liquid you started with).

5. As soon as the tongue is cool enough to touch, peel off the white leathery skin (you might need a knife to get it started, but then it should come off easily) and discard. Slice the tongue as desired. If your liquid still needs a few more minutes to reduce, cover the tongue with aluminum foil to keep warm.

6. Add the chopped rosemary to the stock and boil for another 2 to 3 minutes. Remove from the heat. Add the mustard, lemon juice, and butter and whisk to combine.

7. Pour the rosemary-mustard reduction over the sliced tongue and serve!

HERB-CRUSTED PORK LOIN

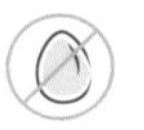 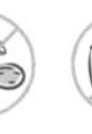 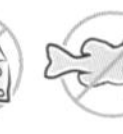 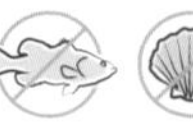 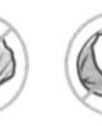  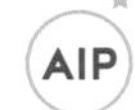 AIP

PREP TIME: 10 minutes, plus time to marinate
COOK TIME: 1 hour 30 minutes YIELD: 6 to 8 servings

- 8 to 9 cloves garlic
- 2 tablespoons chopped fresh rosemary
- 2 tablespoons chopped fresh thyme
- 2 teaspoons finely grated lemon zest
- ½ teaspoon cracked black pepper
- ½ teaspoon paprika
- ½ teaspoon sea salt
- 3 to 4 pounds pork center loin or sirloin

1. Preheat the oven to 350°F.

2. Blend the garlic, herbs, lemon zest, spices, and salt in a small food processor. Alternatively, you could chop the herbs extremely finely and then grind the rub ingredients in a mortar and pestle.

3. Rub the garlic-herb mixture evenly over the entire pork loin. If desired, you can wrap the pork in plastic wrap, place in the refrigerator, and let the meat "marinate" in the herbs for a few hours or overnight.

4. Place the pork loin fat side up in a roasting pan. Cook for 20 minutes per pound, until the internal temperature reaches 160°F.

5. Remove the roast from the oven and let rest for 5 to 10 minutes before serving.

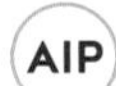 *omit paprika and pepper*  *omit paprika*

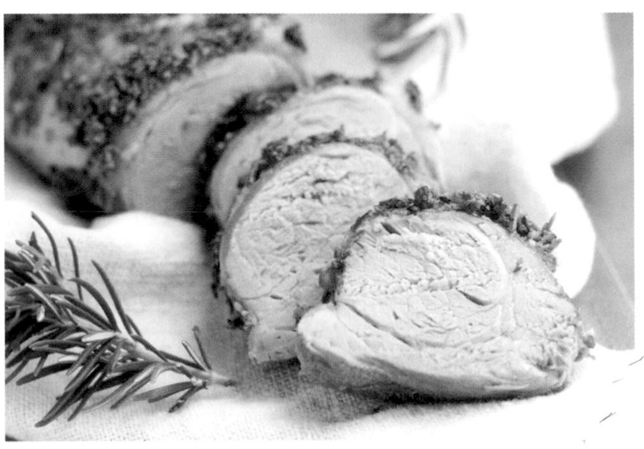

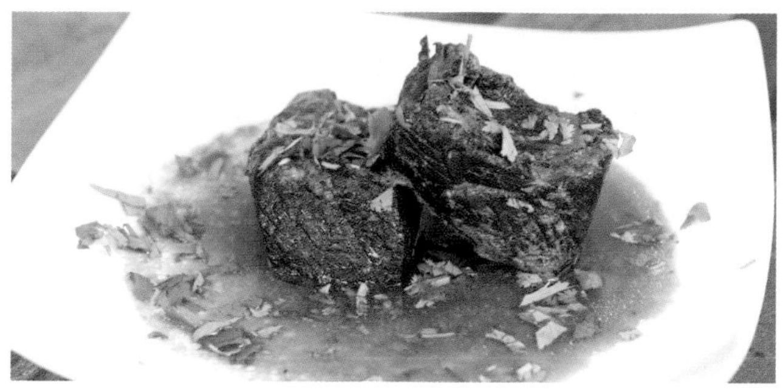

KOREAN SHORT RIBS

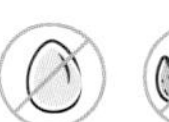 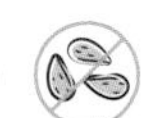 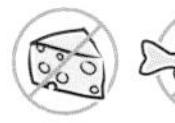  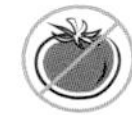  AIP

PREP TIME: 20 minutes COOK TIME: 2 hours 30 minutes
YIELD: 5 to 8 servings

6 pounds English style beef short ribs

2 teaspoons sea salt or truffle salt

1 pear, cubed or chopped

6 cloves garlic, smashed with the side of a knife

3 green onions, chopped

1 (1-inch) piece fresh ginger, peeled and chopped

Juice of 1 lime

1 cup Beef Stock or Chicken Stock (page 486)

2 tablespoons honey

1 tablespoon coconut aminos

1 tablespoon fish sauce

1 tablespoon toasted (dark) sesame oil

1 tablespoon apple cider vinegar

¼ cup chopped fresh cilantro, for garnish

1. Preheat the oven broiler to high.
2. Pat the short ribs dry with paper towels. Sprinkle the salt all over the ribs.
3. Place the short ribs on a rimmed baking sheet. Broil until the ribs are starting to brown, 4 to 5 minutes. Flip and brown on the other side for 4 to 5 minutes.
4. Combine the pear, garlic, green onions, ginger, lime juice, stock, honey, coconut aminos, fish sauce, sesame oil, and vinegar in a blender. Blend to form a smooth puree.
5. Place the browned short ribs in a pressure cooker, packing them tightly.
6. Pour the puree over the short ribs and cook on high pressure for 2 hours according to the manufacturer's directions and safety protocols.
7. Remove the short ribs from the pressure cooker and let cool for 5 to 10 minutes.
8. To make the sauce, either simmer the remaining liquid using the sauté function on your pressure cooker, or transfer the liquid to a saucepan and simmer on the stovetop over high heat until the liquid is reduced by three-quarters.
9. Pour the sauce over the short ribs and garnish with the chopped cilantro.

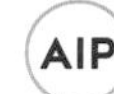 *omit sesame oil* 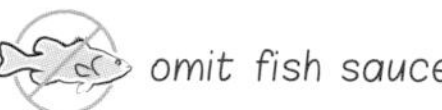 *omit fish sauce*

DIY BAKED CHICKEN BREAST

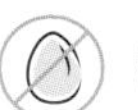 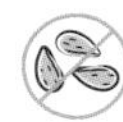 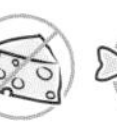 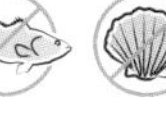 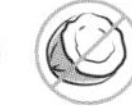 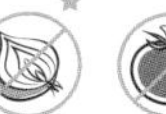  AIP

PREP TIME: 5 minutes COOK TIME: 40 minutes
YIELD: varies

Boneless, skinless chicken breast (see Tip)

Olive oil (about 1 tablespoon per chicken breast)

Seasoning mix of choice (pages 482 and 483) (1 to 2 teaspoons per chicken breast)

Sea salt (if using a seasoning mix without salt)

1. Preheat the oven to 350°F.
2. Coat the chicken with the olive oil. Place on a rimmed baking sheet and sprinkle liberally on both sides with the seasoning mix. If using a mix that does not contain salt, sprinkle a little salt on the chicken as well, ⅛ to ¼ teaspoon per chicken breast.
3. Bake for 30 to 40 minutes, until the internal temperature reaches 165°F (the exact cooking time will depend on the thickness of the chicken).
4. Enjoy as is, serve with your favorite sauce (see Chapter 39), or use for making soup (page 513), salad (page 519), or stir-fry (page 524).

TIP: You can use any chicken pieces for this recipe, with or without the bone and skin, including wings, legs, thighs, or a mix. Adjust the cooking time accordingly using the guide on page 641.

VARIATION: ***Jerk Chicken.*** *Mix equal parts olive oil, honey, and lime juice in a dish. Add chicken pieces (bone-in, skin-on chicken is traditional) and turn to coat, then season the chicken generously with Jerk Spice (1 to 2 tablespoons per breast), coating it completely. It's best to let the chicken marinate in the refrigerator overnight before baking. Once cooked through, broil on high for 4 to 5 minutes or finish on the grill.*

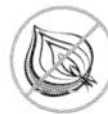 *use low-FODMAP spice mix* 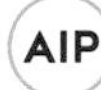 *use AIP spice mix*

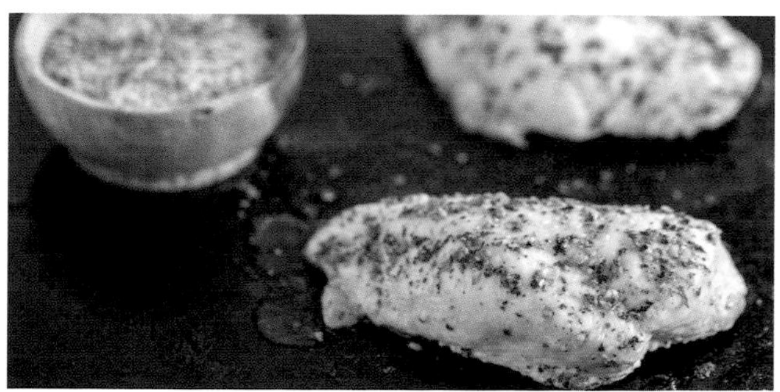

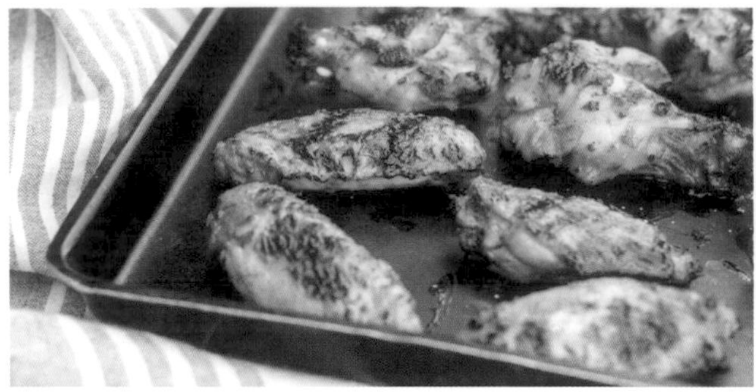

ASIAN-INSPIRED CHICKEN WINGS

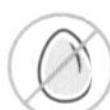 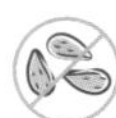 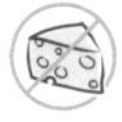  

PREP TIME: 5 minutes, plus time to marinate
COOK TIME: 30 minutes to 1 hour, depending on method
YIELD: 6 to 8 servings

3 pounds chicken wings, separated

2 tablespoons coconut oil

4 cloves garlic, chopped

1 tablespoon chopped fresh ginger

1 teaspoon anise seeds

1 teaspoon fennel seeds

½ cup coconut aminos

2 tablespoons honey

1 tablespoon coconut water vinegar or apple cider vinegar

1 tablespoon fish sauce

2 tablespoons toasted (dark) sesame oil

1. Place the chicken wings in a large bowl (if overly wet, pat dry with paper towel) and set aside.

2. Heat the coconut oil in a small saucepan over medium heat. Add the garlic, ginger, anise seeds, and fennel seeds and cook, stirring so that the spices don't burn, until fragrant, 2 to 3 minutes.

3. Add the coconut aminos, honey, vinegar, and fish sauce. Bring to a boil and simmer for 1 minute.

4. Remove from the heat and stir in the sesame oil.

5. Pour the mixture over the chicken wings and stir to coat. Once the wings have cooled enough to handle, cover and place in the refrigerator to marinate overnight (or up to 24 hours). Stir the wings once or twice while marinating to ensure that they are evenly coated.

6. If grilling, preheat a grill pan or a gas or charcoal grill to medium-high heat. Drain the excess marinade off the wings, then place on the hot grill. Grill the wings until cooked, turning once (about 20 minutes total, depending on the temperature of your grill). The internal temperature should reach 165°F.

Alternatively, preheat the oven to 400°F. Place the wings on a rimmed baking sheet lined with greased aluminum foil. Bake for 45 to 60 minutes, turning once, until the internal temperature reaches 165°F. Serve immediately.

CASHEW CHICKEN

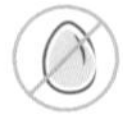 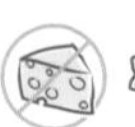 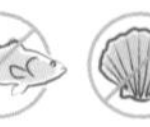 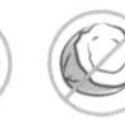 

PREP TIME: 10 minutes COOK TIME: 20 minutes
YIELD: 4 to 6 servings

3 tablespoons avocado oil or coconut oil

3 cloves garlic, finely chopped

2 teaspoons finely chopped fresh galangal or ginger, or 1 teaspoon galangal powder

2 pounds boneless, skinless chicken thighs or breasts, chopped into ½-inch pieces

8 ounces mushrooms, sliced

1 (5-ounce) can sliced bamboo shoots, drained and rinsed

1 (5-ounce) can sliced water chestnuts, drained and rinsed

4 to 6 bunches bok choy, tatsoi, or similar vegetable (about 1½ pounds or 14 to 16 cups chopped)

8 ounces whole raw cashews (about 1½ cups)

1 cup Bone Stock (page 486), divided

2 tablespoons arrowroot powder or kuzu starch

1 tablespoon coconut water vinegar or apple cider vinegar

2 teaspoons sea salt

1 batch Cauli-rice (page 555), for serving

1. Heat a wok or very large sauté pan over medium-high heat. Add the oil, garlic, and galangal and cook for about 1 minute, until fragrant.

2. Add the chicken and cook, stirring frequently, until thoroughly done, 5 to 8 minutes.

3. Add the mushrooms, bamboo shoots, and water chestnuts and cook for 3 to 4 more minutes, stirring frequently, until the mushrooms are mostly cooked.

4. Add the bok choy, cashews, and ½ cup of the stock. Cook, stirring frequently, until the greens start to wilt, 3 to 4 minutes.

5. In a small bowl, mix the arrowroot powder, vinegar, and salt with the remaining ½ cup of stock to make a slurry. Add the slurry to the wok and stir until the sauce has thickened, about 2 minutes. Taste and add more salt, if needed, before serving.

6. Serve over cauli-rice.

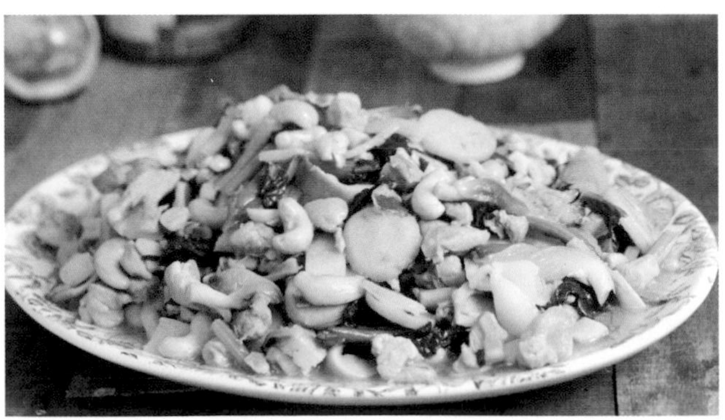

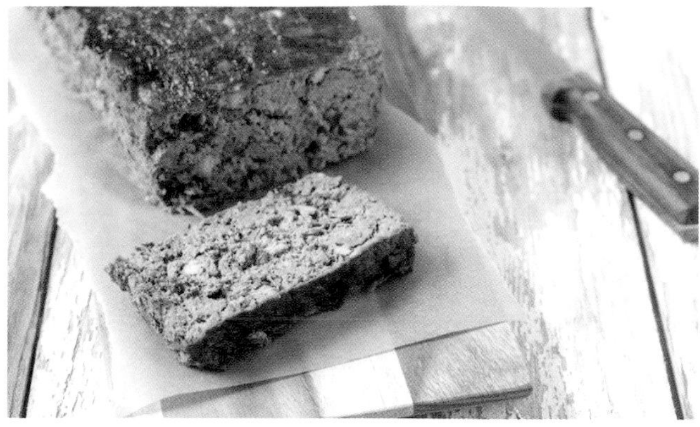

MEATLOAF

 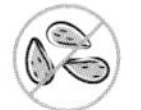 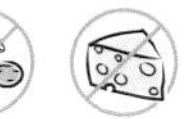 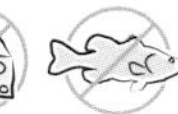     AIP

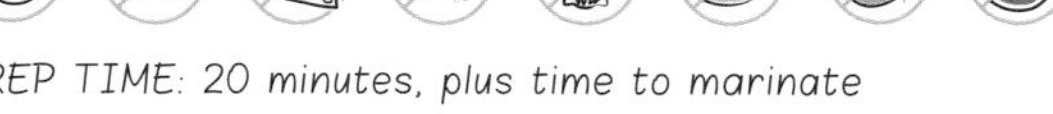

PREP TIME: 20 minutes, plus time to marinate
COOK TIME: 1 hour 40 minutes   YIELD: 6 to 8 servings

- 2 to 3 tablespoons tallow, olive oil, or avocado oil
- 1 medium-sized yellow onion, minced
- 2 stalks celery, minced
- 1 medium carrot, minced
- 1 teaspoon fennel seeds
- 1 pound frozen liver or ground beef
- 1 pound ground beef
- 1 pound ground pork
- 2 large eggs (optional, for a denser loaf)
- 4 cloves garlic, minced
- ¼ cup chopped fresh parsley
- 3 tablespoons chopped fresh basil
- 3 tablespoons chopped fresh oregano
- 1 tablespoon chopped fresh chives
- 1 tablespoon chopped fresh thyme
- 3 tablespoons apple cider vinegar
- 2 tablespoons coconut aminos
- 1 tablespoon blackstrap molasses
- 1 tablespoon fish sauce
- 2 teaspoons paprika
- ½ teaspoon ground black pepper
- ¼ teaspoon cayenne pepper

1. Heat the tallow in a skillet over medium-high heat. Add the onion, celery, and carrot and sauté until soft and starting to brown, 8 to 10 minutes. Set aside to cool before adding to the meat mixture in Step 4.

2. Grind the fennel seeds in a spice grinder, clean coffee grinder, or mortar and pestle.

3. If adding frozen liver, grate the liver with a box grater.

4. Combine all the ingredients in a large bowl and mix very thoroughly. Cover and refrigerate for 4 to 6 hours or up to overnight to let the flavors combine.

5. Preheat the oven to 350°F.

6. Press the meat mixture into a 9 by 5-inch loaf pan. Place the loaf pan on a cookie sheet or in a larger baking pan before placing in the oven.

7. Bake for 1 hour 40 minutes, or until the internal temperature reaches 160°F. Let the meatloaf sit for 5 to 10 minutes before serving.

 *omit*

 *omit onion and garlic*

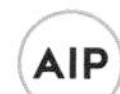 *omit cayenne, paprika, fennel seeds, pepper, and eggs*

 *omit cayenne and paprika*

SALMON EN PAPILLOTE WITH MAÎTRE D' BUTTER

 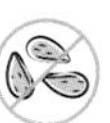  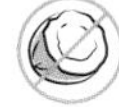 

PREP TIME: 10 minutes   COOK TIME: 20 minutes
YIELD: 4 servings

- 6 tablespoons Maître d' Butter (page 495)
- 4 (6- to 8-ounce) salmon or trout fillets

1. Preheat the oven to 350°F.

2. Prepare the parchment envelope for the fish by placing a large sheet of aluminum foil or parchment paper on a rimmed baking sheet. The foil or parchment should measure a little over twice the length of your fish fillets when placed side by side.

3. Place the fish on one half of the foil or parchment, leaving 3 to 4 inches of space (in addition to one long side) around it for folding the foil or parchment over. Spoon 1½ tablespoons of Maître d' Butter onto each fillet. Also add about 1 tablespoon of water around the fillets. Fold over the long side of the foil or parchment to cover the fish. Then triple-fold all 3 open sides to form a seal.

4. Place on a baking sheet and bake for 20 minutes, or until the fish is opaque throughout and the segments flake apart easily. Serve.

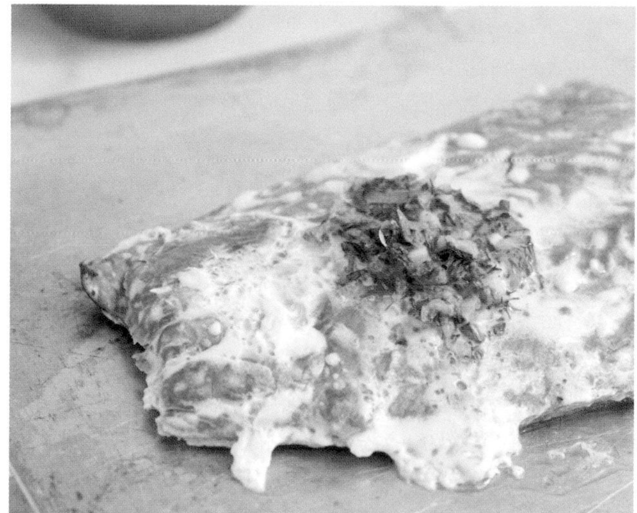

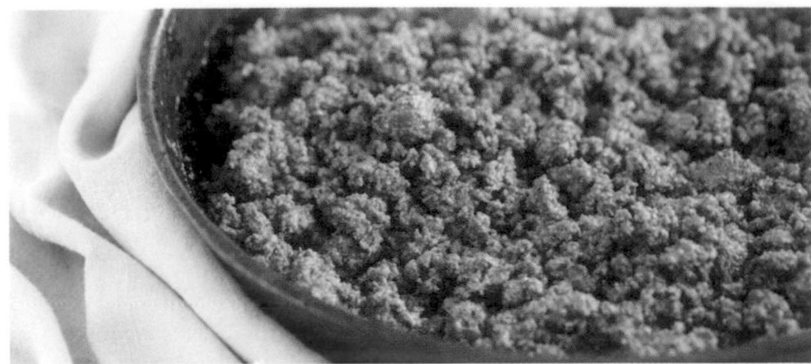

TACOS

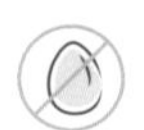 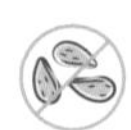 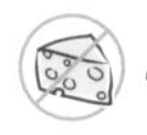 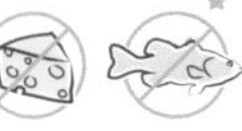 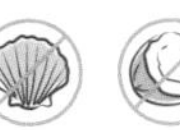  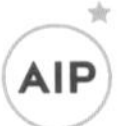 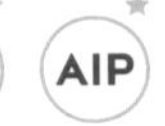

PREP TIME: 10 minutes *COOK TIME: 20 minutes*
YIELD: 5 or 6 servings

TACO MEAT

- 2 pounds ground beef
- 1 cup Bone Stock (page 486)
- 1 tablespoon gelatin (optional)
- 2 tablespoons chili powder
- 1 tablespoon granulated onion
- 1 tablespoon ground cumin
- 2 teaspoons granulated garlic
- 2 teaspoons paprika
- ¼ teaspoon cayenne pepper (optional)
- ½ teaspoon dried oregano
- 1 teaspoon sea salt
- 1 teaspoon ground black pepper
- Taco toppings of choice

AIP TACO MEAT

- 2 pounds ground beef
- 1 cup Bone Stock (page 486)
- 1 tablespoon gelatin (optional)
- 1 tablespoon dried oregano
- 1½ teaspoons granulated garlic
- 1¼ teaspoons granulated onion
- 1 teaspoon dried marjoram
- 1 teaspoon ginger powder
- 1 teaspoon turmeric powder
- ¼ teaspoon ground cinnamon
- 1 teaspoon sea salt
- 1 tablespoon fish sauce
- Taco toppings of choice

1. Heat a skillet over medium-high heat. Add the ground beef and cook, stirring frequently to break up the meat, until fully cooked, 7 to 8 minutes. If the beef is very fatty, use a spoon to remove the excess fat from the pan.
2. Blend the stock and gelatin together. Add to the beef, along with all the spices (and fish sauce if making AIP taco meat). Stir to fully incorporate.
3. Reduce the heat to medium and cook for another 10 to 12 minutes, stirring occasionally, until the stock has entirely evaporated.
4. Serve with Guacamole (page 489), Pico de Gallo (page 490), Cauli-rice (page 555), Tortillas (page 567), lettuce (as lettuce wraps or shredded), and/or chopped fresh cilantro and your favorite taco toppings.

 *make AIP recipe* 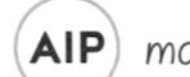 *make AIP recipe*

 *omit fish sauce from AIP recipe*

BARBECUE CHICKEN WITH ARUGULA PESTO

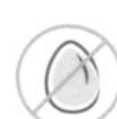 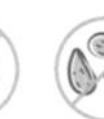 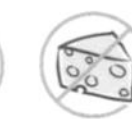 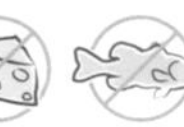  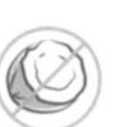 

PREP TIME: 15 minutes *COOK TIME: 30 minutes*
YIELD: 8 to 10 servings

- 6 cloves garlic (do not peel)
- 4 cups fresh arugula
- ¼ cup olive oil
- 1 teaspoon lemon juice
- 1¼ teaspoons sea salt, divided
- 2 teaspoons granulated garlic
- 2 teaspoons paprika
- 1 teaspoon ground coriander
- 1 teaspoon ground cumin
- ½ teaspoon cracked black pepper
- 10 boneless, skinless chicken thighs (about 4 pounds)

1. Heat a nonstick or well-seasoned cast-iron skillet over medium heat. Place the garlic still in the peel in the pan and cook, stirring or shaking the pan frequently so the garlic cooks on all sides, until the garlic is starting to brown and feels fairly soft to the touch, 7 to 8 minutes.
2. Let the garlic cool, then peel. Place the garlic in a blender or food processor with the arugula, olive oil, lemon juice, and ¼ teaspoon of the salt. Pulse until the mixture is a paste.
3. Preheat a grill pan or gas or charcoal grill to medium-high heat.
4. Mix the remaining 1 teaspoon of salt with the granulated garlic, paprika, coriander, cumin, and pepper in a bowl. Toss with the chicken and rub around with your hands to thoroughly coat each piece.
5. Place the chicken on the grill. Cook for about 10 minutes on the first side and 8 minutes on the second side, or until completely cooked (internal temperature should read 180°F). You may have to adjust your cooking time depending on the temperature of your grill. Top each thigh with arugula paste and serve!

 *omit paprika*

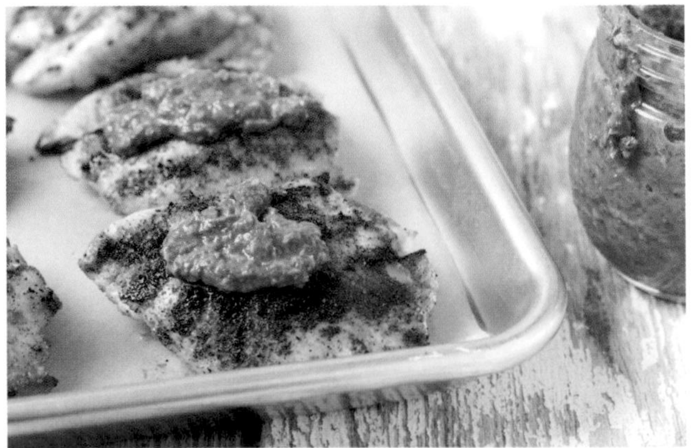

MILD BARBACOA

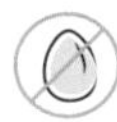 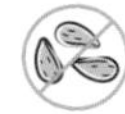  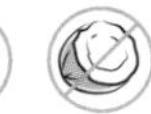  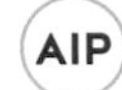 AIP

PREP TIME: 30 minutes, plus optional dry rub overnight

COOK TIME: 2 1/2 hours in a pressure cooker or 10 1/2 hours in a slow cooker   YIELD: 10 to 16 servings

5 to 7 pounds beef shoulder or brisket

2 tablespoons dried oregano

1 tablespoon granulated garlic

1 tablespoon granulated onion

1 tablespoon dried thyme

1 tablespoon turmeric powder

2 teaspoons ginger powder

1 tablespoon sea salt, divided

1 medium bunch cilantro, roughly chopped

1 medium-sized red onion, roughly chopped

Cloves from 1 head garlic, peeled and smashed

5 bay leaves

2 cinnamon sticks (preferably Mexican cinnamon)

3 tablespoons fish sauce

1 tablespoon blackstrap molasses

Juice of 4 limes

½ cup apple cider vinegar

4 cups Beef Stock (page 486)

1. Pat the beef shoulder dry with paper towels.

2. Combine the oregano, granulated garlic, granulated onion, thyme, turmeric, ginger, and 1 teaspoon of the salt in a bowl. Then rub the spices all over shoulder. If you'd like, you can wrap the seasoned shoulder in plastic wrap and refrigerate overnight or up to 24 hours.

3. Place the cilantro, onion, and garlic in a pressure cooker or slow cooker. Wrap the bay leaves and cinnamon sticks in butcher's twine to make a little bouquet garni and place in the pressure cooker or slow cooker.

4. Place the seasoned beef shoulder on top of the herbs.

5. Add the fish sauce, molasses, lime juice, vinegar, and remaining salt. Pour the stock into the pressure cooker or slow cooker until the beef is just covered. If you run out of stock, top off with water.

6. Cook the beef for 2 hours on high pressure in a pressure cooker, according to the manufacturer's directions and following all safety protocols, or cook for 8 to 10 hours on low in a slow cooker.

7. Remove the beef from the pressure cooker or slow cooker and let cool for 5 to 10 minutes.

8. Remove the bouquet garni, then simmer the cooking liquid, uncovered, until it is reduced by half. If you're using a slow cooker, transfer the liquid to a saucepan to simmer on the stovetop until reduced.

9. After the beef has rested and while the liquid is simmering, shred the beef by using 2 forks and pulling in opposite directions, repeatedly.

10. Once the liquid is reduced, place in a blender and blend on high for 30 seconds to form a smooth puree. You should end up with about 5 cups of puree.

11. Pour the puree over the pulled beef and mix to evenly coat. Alternatively, you can pour only a few cups first and then taste to see how you like it. Continue to add a little more puree until the beef is to your liking.

12. Serve in lettuce wraps or Tortillas (page 567), with Guacamole (page 489), Pico de Gallo (page 490), and fresh limes!

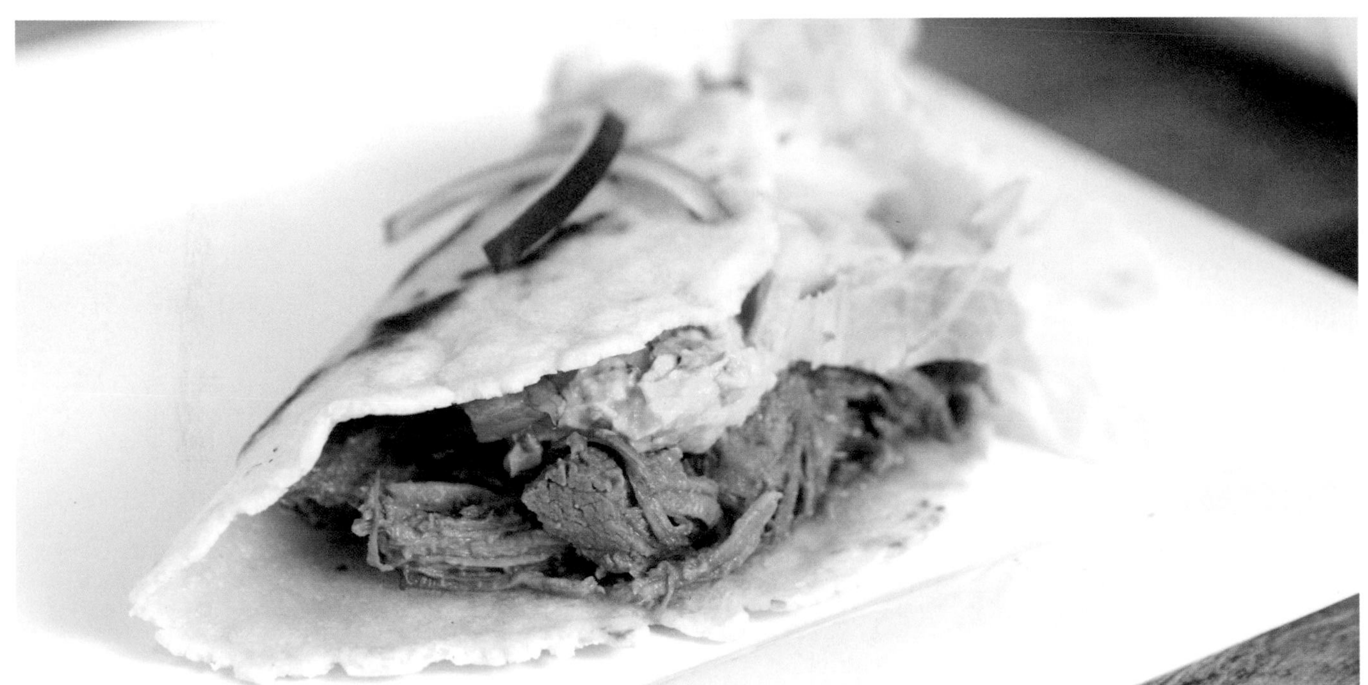

MEATBALLS WITH ASIAN DIPPING SAUCE

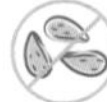 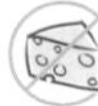  

PREP TIME: 20 minutes COOK TIME: 25 minutes
YIELD: 40 meatballs (4 to 6 servings)

DIPPING SAUCE

¼ cup coconut aminos

1½ teaspoons fish sauce

1 teaspoon granulated garlic

⅛ teaspoon ground cloves

⅛ teaspoon ground cinnamon

⅛ teaspoon fennel seeds, ground to a powder

1 tablespoon honey

¼ cup toasted (dark) sesame oil

1 cup Mayonnaise (page 487)

MEATBALLS

2 tablespoons coconut oil

1 medium-sized yellow onion, finely chopped

1 cup shelled sunflower seeds

2 pounds ground beef

1 teaspoon granulated garlic

1 teaspoon fresh thyme, chopped

1 teaspoon dry rubbed sage, or 2 teaspoons chopped fresh sage

¼ teaspoon cracked black pepper

¼ teaspoon sea salt

2 large eggs

1. To make the dipping sauce, put the coconut aminos and fish sauce in a small saucepan. Whisk in the granulated garlic, cloves, cinnamon, and ground fennel seeds. Bring to a simmer over high heat, then reduce the heat to low and simmer for 5 minutes. Add the honey and whisk to dissolve. Remove from the heat and let cool completely.

2. Stir the cooled sauce mixture and sesame oil into the mayonnaise. Transfer the sauce to a bowl or serving dish and refrigerate until the meatballs are ready to serve.

3. To make the meatballs, preheat the oven to 400°F. Line a rimmed baking sheet with parchment paper.

4. Heat the coconut oil in a skillet over medium-high heat (cast iron is great here). Sauté the onion until soft and nicely browned, then let cool.

5. Grind the sunflower seeds in a food processor or blender until the texture of coarse sand.

6. Mix the sunflower seeds and onion with the ground beef, spices, salt, and egg.

7. Form the meat mixture into 1-inch balls and place on prepared baking sheet. You should get about 40 meatballs.

8. Bake for 14 to 16 minutes, until fully cooked. Serve with the dipping sauce.

TIP: The dipping sauce can be made ahead and stored in the refrigerator for up to 5 days.

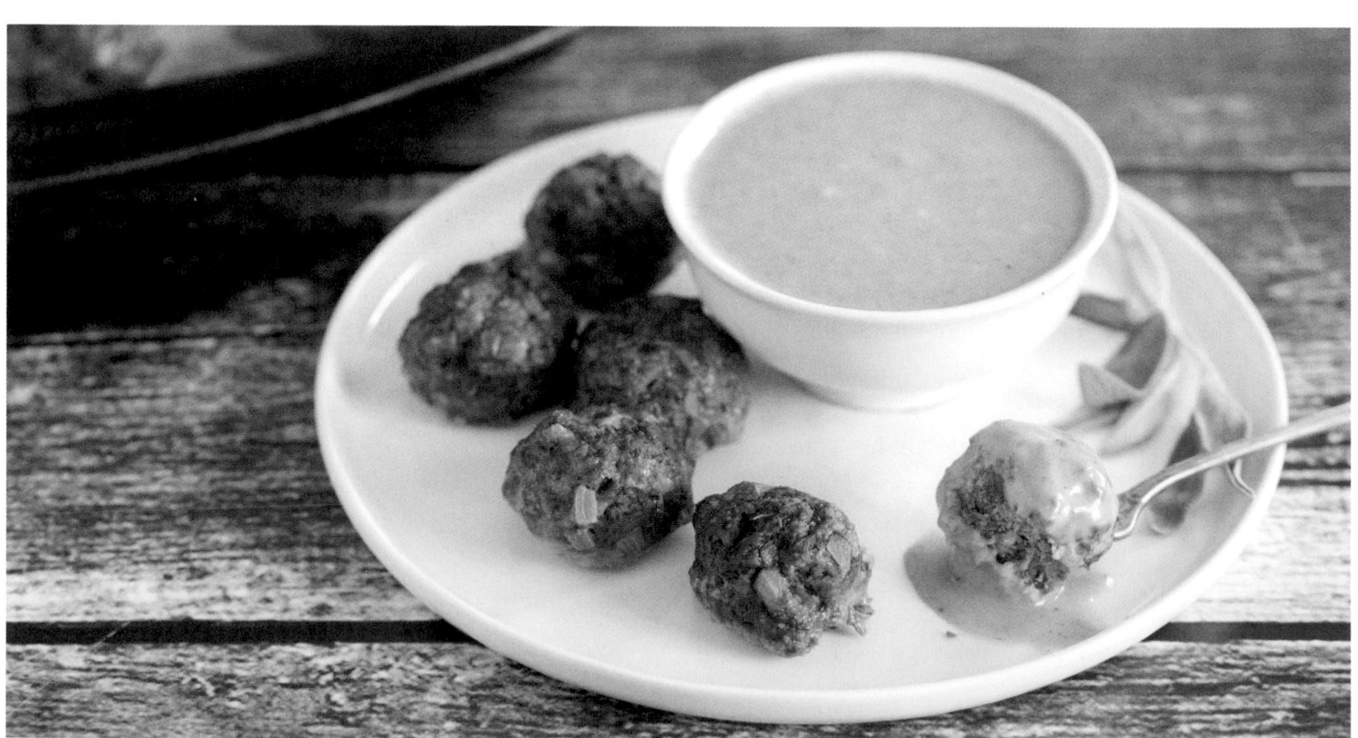

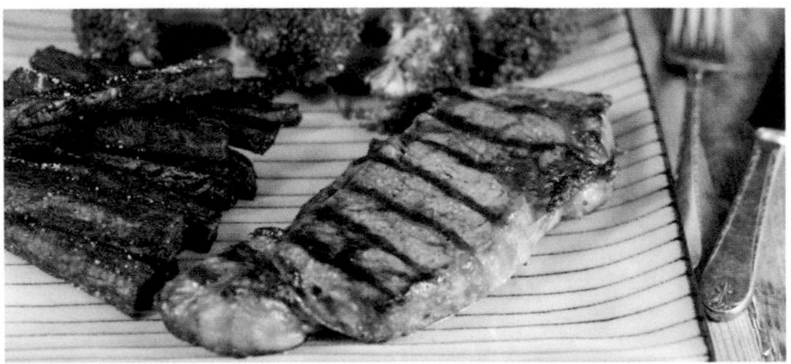

SIMPLE STEAK

 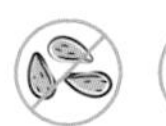 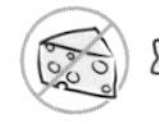 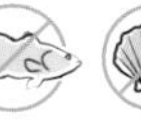 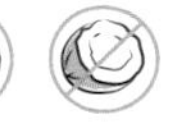 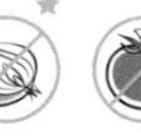  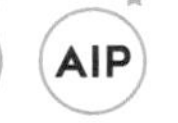 AIP

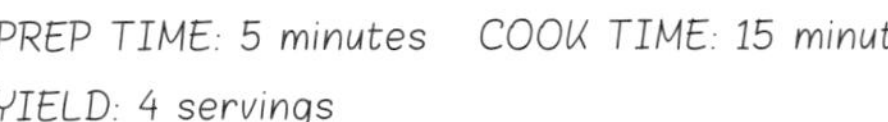

PREP TIME: 5 minutes *COOK TIME: 15 minutes*
YIELD: 4 servings

4 (6- to 8-ounce) steaks, about 1 inch thick (bone-in or boneless)

1 to 2 tablespoons Steak Seasoning (page 482), or 1 to 2 teaspoons sea salt and ½ teaspoon ground black pepper, or 1 to 2 teaspoons truffle salt

2 tablespoons olive oil, avocado oil, or tallow (if pan-searing)

TO GRILL:

1. Pat the steaks dry with paper towels and season with the steak seasoning.
2. Preheat a grill pan or gas or charcoal grill to medium-high heat. Place the steaks on the heated grill. Grill 3 to 5 minutes per side, depending on the exact thickness of the steaks and how you want the steaks cooked. (Three minutes per side will result in rare steaks.)
3. Remove the steaks from the grill and let rest for at least 5 minutes before serving.

TO PAN-SEAR:

1. Preheat the oven to 350°F.
2. Pat the steaks dry with paper towels and season with the steak seasoning.
3. Heat the olive oil in a large ovenproof skillet over medium-high heat. Place the steaks, separated at least 1 inch apart, in skillet. Sear on the first side for 3 minutes. Flip and sear the second side for 3 minutes.
4. Place skillet in oven. Cook for 4 to 8 minutes, depending on the thickness of the steaks and how you want the steaks cooked. When in doubt, insert a meat thermometer into the middle of one steak and monitor the temperature (see page 640).
5. Remove the steaks from the skillet and let rest at least 5 minutes before serving.

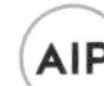 *use AIP Steak Seasoning*  *use salt and pepper*

 *use AIP Steak Seasoning*

BALSAMIC PRESSURE COOKER ROAST BEEF

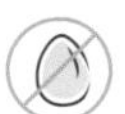 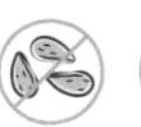 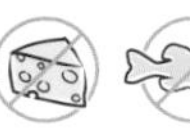 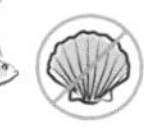 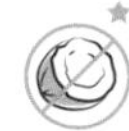  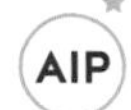 AIP

PREP TIME: 5 minutes *COOK TIME: 1 hour 15 minutes*
YIELD: 6 to 10 servings

3 to 4 pounds beef chuck roast, shoulder roast, cheek, brisket, or any other tough roast (bone-in or boneless; this just affects the number of servings)

1½ teaspoons sea salt or truffle salt

½ teaspoon ground black pepper

1 tablespoon olive oil

1 cup Beef Stock (page 486)

½ cup balsamic vinegar

1 tablespoon coconut aminos

1 tablespoon fish sauce

1 tablespoon honey

4 cloves garlic, minced

½ teaspoon dried lavender or rosemary or a mix (optional)

Coarse finishing salt and chopped parsley, for garnish

1. Pat the chuck roast dry with paper towels and rub the salt and pepper on all sides of roast.
2. If your pressure cooker has a sear or sauté function, add the olive oil to the pressure cooker. Sear the roast on all sides, 2 to 3 minutes per side. Otherwise, sear the roast in the olive oil in a large skillet over medium-high heat and transfer to the pressure cooker afterward.
3. Add the remaining ingredients to the pressure cooker.
4. Place the lid on the pressure cooker and cook on high pressure for 45 minutes according to the manufacturer's directions and following all safety protocols.
5. Remove the roast from the pressure cooker, and let rest for 5 to 10 minutes. (You can tent with aluminum foil to keep it warm.)
6. Reduce the liquid by about two-thirds either in the pressure cooker using the sauté function or in a saucepan on the stovetop over high heat.
7. Slice the roast and pour the juices on top. Garnish with coarse finishing salt and chopped parsley, if desired, before serving.

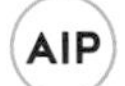 *omit pepper*  *omit fish sauce*

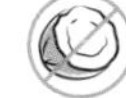 *omit coconut aminos*

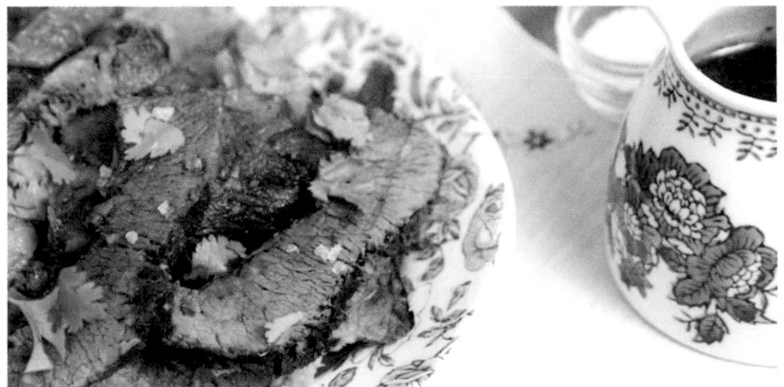

Chapter 43:
SIDE DISHES

DIY STEAMED VEGGIES

  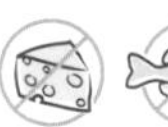    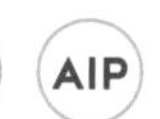 AIP

PREP TIME: 5 to 10 minutes COOK TIME: 3 to 40 minutes, depending on vegetable YIELD: varies

Vegetable of choice

1. Fill a saucepan with enough water so that the water just barely reaches the bottom of the steamer insert or steamer basket.

2. Bring the water to a boil over high heat. Once boiling, add the vegetables to the steamer insert or basket. Cover the saucepan with a loose-fitting lid. If using a steamer insert, position the lid so that one side hangs over the insert just enough to let steam escape.

3. Cook until the desired tenderness is reached, using the cooking times below as a guide.

STEAMING TIMES

Artichoke: 35 to 40 minutes for a whole artichoke, 20 minutes for baby artichokes, 10 minutes for artichoke hearts

Asparagus: 4 minutes for thin spears; add another minute or two for thicker spears

Beets: 30 to 40 minutes for whole medium-sized beets or wedges of larger beets

Broccoli: 5 minutes for florets; add another minute or two if florets are large

Brussels sprouts: 10 to 12 minutes for whole, 7 to 8 minutes if cut in half

Cabbage: 20 to 23 minutes for quartered, 8 to 10 minutes for shredded

Carrots: 8 minutes for ¼-inch-thick rounds

Cauliflower: 6 to 8 minutes for medium florets

Kohlrabi: 30 to 35 minutes for wedges

Leafy greens: 3 to 5 minutes, just until wilted

Turnips: 15 minutes for ¼-inch-thick slices

Winter squash: 5 to 10 minutes for 1-inch pieces

Zucchini and other summer squash: 8 to 10 minutes for ¼-inch-thick slices, 15 to 20 minutes for whole pattypan squash

VARIATIONS: Want to add a little pizzazz? Add your favorite spice blends (pages 482 to 483) to your vegetables before steaming. Alternatively, drizzle your favorite salad dressing (pages 484 to 485) over the top after steaming.

TIPS: Adding a tablespoon of lemon juice, white wine vinegar, or coconut water vinegar to the water under the steamer basket will help retain nutrients in your vegetables.

Don't have a steamer insert or steamer basket? You can also "steam" vegetables by adding about 1/2 inch of salted water to a saucepan, placing the vegetables in the water once it comes to a boil (you can add lemon juice or vinegar, too), and covering the pan with a lid.

If you plan on using the microwave, the steaming times are typically a few minutes longer, depending on the wattage of your microwave. Simply rinse your vegetables and place in a microwave-safe container with a vented lid or a loose-fitting lid that you can leave open at one corner (and no additional water other than what clings to your veggies after rinsing).

The steaming times for frozen vegetables are usually a bit shorter, but check the packaging for directions.

 *avoid*

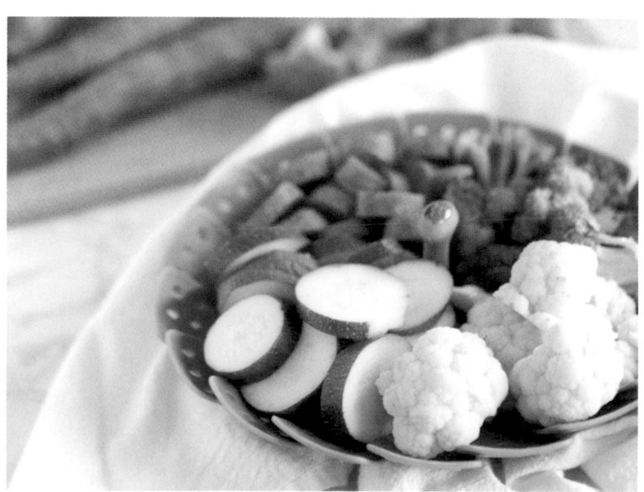

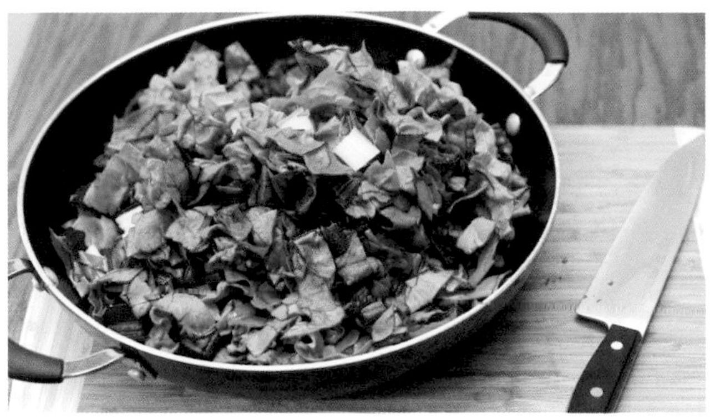

DIY BRAISED GREENS

 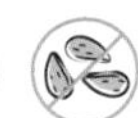 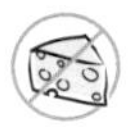 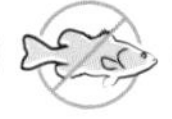 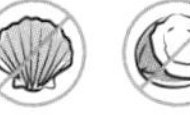  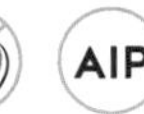 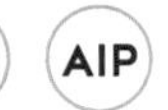 AIP

PREP TIME: 5 minutes COOK TIME: 3 to 15 minutes, depending on vegetable YIELD: 2 to 4 servings

2 tablespoons olive oil, ghee, unsalted butter, avocado oil, coconut oil, tallow, or lard

4 to 12 cups chopped greens (less for substantial greens and more for tender greens)

1 tablespoon to 2 cups Bone Stock (page 486)

Sea salt

1. Heat the oil in a large skillet or wok over medium-high heat. Add the greens and 1 to 3 tablespoons of the stock, adding less for tender greens or more for tougher greens. Stir relatively frequently. If the stock evaporates before the greens are fully cooked, add a little more. For tender greens, you probably won't have to add more liquid. For tougher greens, you may need to add liquid several times during cooking.

2. When the greens are done to your liking, taste and season with salt, if desired. Ideally, serve just as the liquid is fully evaporated. Otherwise, you can serve with tongs or a slotted spoon, leaving the liquid in the pan.

VARIATIONS: You can keep braised greens super-simple, or you can play with adding herbs and other seasonings. Crushed garlic, grated ginger, and citrus zest should be added with the greens (if cooking very tender greens, you may want to add the garlic and ginger to the oil 1 to 2 minutes before adding the greens). Woody herbs like rosemary, savory, and thyme can be added with the greens. Tender herbs like cilantro, parsley, tarragon, marjoram, basil, oregano, chives, and green onion can be added right at the end of the cooking time.

TIPS: The more tender the greens, the less time they take to braise. Very tender greens that might also be used as salad greens, like spinach, lamb's quarter, sorrel, mizuna, sweet potato greens, and celery leaves, cook very quickly—as little as 3 to 4 minutes.

Mustard greens, turnip greens, radish tops, carrot tops, baby collards, beet greens, kohlrabi greens, chard, and some more tender varieties of kale are more substantial greens and take longer to braise—5 to 10 minutes.

The greens that take the longest to cook are those with the thickest and most substantial leaves, such as cabbage, kale, bok choy, broccoli leaves, cauliflower leaves, Brussels sprouts, and collards, which more typically take 10 to 15 minutes to braise. The longer the cooking time, the more stock is typically used.

As a general rule, the more tender the greens, the more the greens will shrink during cooking. So, for tender greens like spinach, you'll want to start out with more leaves. If cooking a large amount of a tougher green, use 3 to 4 tablespoons of cooking fat and be prepared to use as much as 2 cups of liquid.

If using a tougher green, remove the stems before cooking.

 *avoid*

SPAGHETTI SQUASH NOODLES

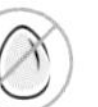 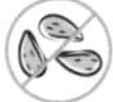  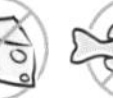  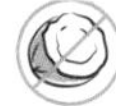 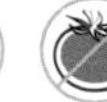 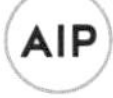 AIP

PREP TIME: 10 minutes
COOK TIME: 10 minutes to 1 hour, depending on method
YIELD: 4 to 8 servings

3 to 4 pounds spaghetti squash (2 small or 1 large)

1. If using the oven, preheat the oven to 375°F.

2. Pierce the spaghetti squash all over with a fork. Bake the squash whole for 45 to 60 minutes, or cook the squash whole in the microwave for 10 to 15 minutes.

3. Let the squash cool enough to handle. Cut in half lengthwise. Spoon out the seeds and discard. Scrape out the noodlelike strings with a fork.

4. Serve with Meaty Ratatouille Pasta Sauce (page 527), "Spaghetti" Bolognese (page 528), or DIY Baked Chicken Breast (page 541) and pesto (page 495 or 497).

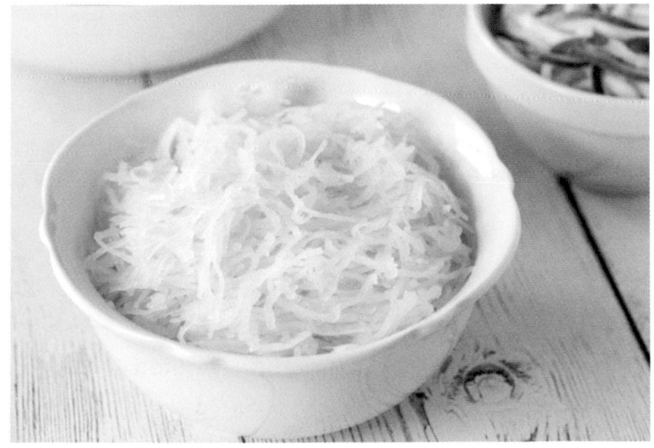

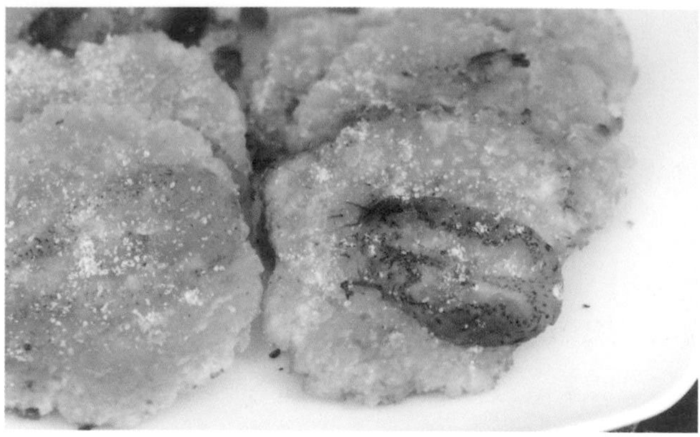

TOSTONES

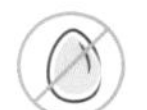 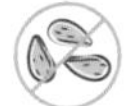 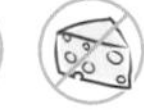 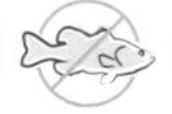    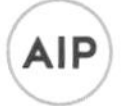 AIP

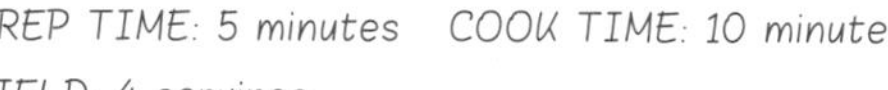

PREP TIME: 5 minutes COOK TIME: 10 minutes
YIELD: 4 servings

2 green plantains (see Tip)
½ cup duck fat, lard, or coconut oil
Sea salt

1. Peel the plantains and slice at an angle into 1-inch-thick slices.

2. Preheat a large stainless-steel skillet over medium heat (skip this step if using a gas stove).

3. Add a big dollop of duck fat to the hot skillet, then arrange the plantain slices in the skillet in a single layer (if your skillet is too small to fit them all at once, cook them in batches).

4. Fry the plantain slices for 2 to 3 minutes on each side, until they are golden in color. (I prefer to flip 3 times as opposed to once to make sure they don't get too brown.) If the plantains are browning too quickly, reduce the heat. Maintain at least ⅛ inch of fat in the bottom of the skillet to prevent the plantains from sticking; add more fat as needed.

5. Remove the fried plantain slices from the skillet with tongs or a slotted spoon. Traditionally, they are pounded flat with a hinged utensil made for the task, called a tostonera, but any kitchen utensil that has a large enough flat surface (such as a bowl, cup, or plate) will do the trick. I flatten mine on a cutting board with a 4-cup measuring cup and then peel the mashed plantain off the bottom of the measuring cup with a spatula directly into the hot skillet. Be inventive: there are probably a dozen different items in your kitchen that will flatten the fried plantain slices!

6. Fry the plantain slices a second time, this time about 1 minute per side, until crisp and golden brown, adding more duck fat as needed to maintain about ⅛ inch of fat in the pan. You'll almost certainly have to fry the plantains in 2 or even 3 batches, unless you own the world's biggest skillet.

7. Remove the tostones from the skillet and place on a serving plate or cutting board lined with paper towels to drain the excess fat. Sprinkle liberally with salt while the tostones are still warm. Serve immediately; tostones are best enjoyed right when you make them.

TIP: Peel green plantains by slicing just through the peel (not the fruit), lengthwise from tip to tip, then prying off the peel with your thumbs. Sometimes the plantain is easier to peel if you make more than one slice down the length of the plantain.

DIY ROASTED ROOTS

 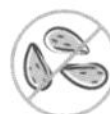 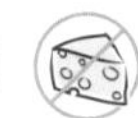 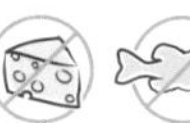  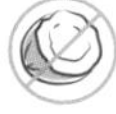 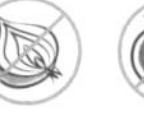 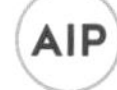 AIP

PREP TIME: 10 minutes COOK TIME: 35 minutes
YIELD: 4 to 6 servings

2 pounds root vegetables (sweet potatoes, green plantains, winter squash, parsnips, carrots, beets, turnips, rutabaga, boniato, celery root, or a mix), peeled and cut into 1-inch chunks

2 tablespoons melted coconut oil, unsalted butter, or ghee, or avocado oil or olive oil

¼ to ½ teaspoon sea salt

1. Preheat the oven to 350°F. Line a rimmed baking sheet with aluminum foil, parchment paper, or a silicone baking mat.

2. Place the root vegetables in a big bowl. Toss with the coconut oil and salt until evenly coated. Arrange in a single layer on the prepared baking sheet.

3. Bake for 20 minutes, then remove from the oven and toss.

4. Bake for another 10 to 15 minutes, until completely cooked and slightly browned. Enjoy!

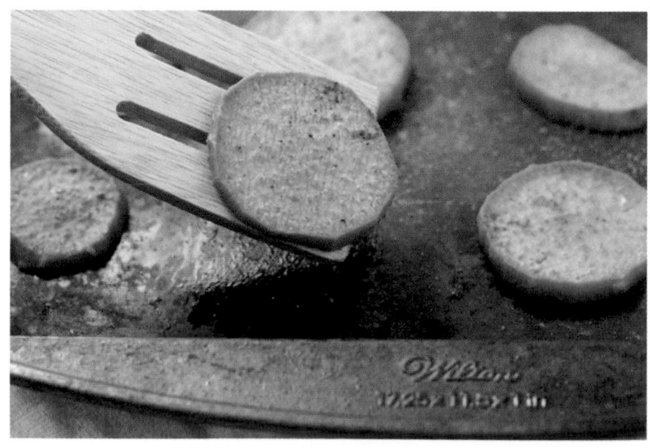

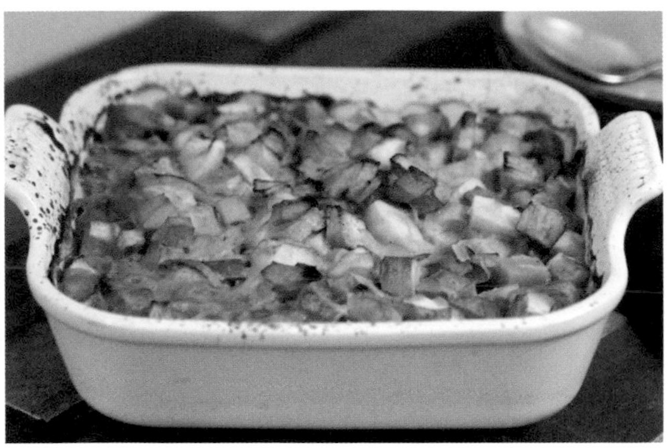

ROOT VEGETABLE CASSEROLE

 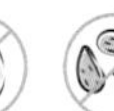 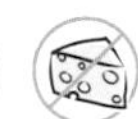 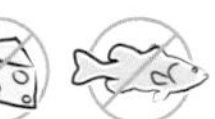 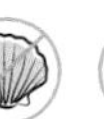   AIP*

PREP TIME: 15 minutes   COOK TIME: 1 hour 30 minutes
YIELD: 8 to 10 servings

- 3 to 4 tablespoons olive oil or avocado oil, divided
- 1 medium-sized yellow onion, sliced into half-moons
- 1 pound yellow summer squash or peeled zucchini, diced
- 2 cloves garlic, minced
- 2 cups Chicken Stock (page 486)
- 1 cup white wine
- 1 teaspoon sea salt
- 1/8 teaspoon ground black pepper
- 4 pounds (about 10 cups diced) root vegetables (use at least 4 different varieties, such as sweet potatoes, winter squash, green plantains, parsnips, carrots, or boniato), diced into 3/4-inch pieces

1. Heat 1 to 2 tablespoons of the oil in a skillet over medium-high heat, then add the onion. Cook, stirring occasionally, until browned, about 10 minutes.

2. Remove the onion from the skillet and place in a 9-inch square casserole dish; set aside. Add another 1 to 2 tablespoons of oil and the summer squash to the pan. Cook, stirring occasionally, until browned, about 10 minutes. Add the garlic and cook for 2 more minutes.

3. Add the stock and wine to the squash. Simmer until the liquid is reduced by two-thirds, about 15 minutes. Add the salt and pepper.

4. Preheat the oven to 400°F.

5. Carefully pour the contents of the skillet into a blender. Blend on high for 30 seconds to 1 minute, until completely smooth. Taste and add more salt, if needed. This sauce should be a little salty.

6. Toss the root vegetables with the caramelized onion in the casserole dish. Pour the sauce from the blender all over the vegetables.

7. Bake, uncovered, for 50 to 60 minutes, until the vegetables are fully cooked. Let sit for 5 to 10 minutes before serving.

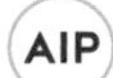 *omit pepper*

SWEET POTATO OR BUTTERNUT SQUASH "LINGUINE"

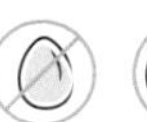 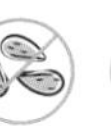 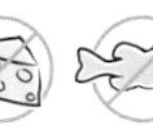 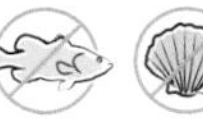  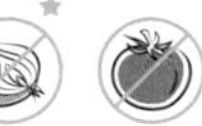 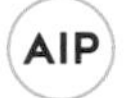 AIP

PREP TIME: 15 minutes   COOK TIME: 5 minutes
YIELD: 6 to 8 servings

- 6 to 8 (long) sweet potatoes, or 2 medium butternut squash
- 1/2 cup coconut oil

1. If using sweet potatoes, peel the sweet potatoes and slice lengthwise as thinly as possible (a mandoline works well for this task, but you can do it with a sharp chef's knife or vegetable peeler, too). Then cut each slice into long, thin strips 1/4 to 1/2 inch wide. The longer your sweet potatoes, the longer your "linguine" will be.

If using butternut squash, peel the squash, cut off the stems, and slice in half crosswise just above the bulge. Use the lower section (the section with seeds) for another dish, like DIY Roasted Roots (opposite) or Maple & Sage Roasted Winter Squash (page 559). Slice the upper section lengthwise as thinly as possible, then cut each slice into long, thin strips 1/4 to 1/2 inch wide.

2. Heat the coconut oil in a large skillet over medium heat. Add the sweet potato or squash strips to the oil and cook, stirring gently, until tender, 3 to 5 minutes.

3. Serve with Meaty Ratatouille Pasta Sauce (page 527), "Spaghetti" Bolognese (page 528), or DIY Baked Chicken Breast (page 541) and pesto (page 495 or 497).

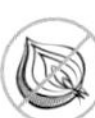 *use butternut squash*

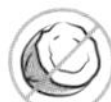 *use olive oil or avocado oil instead of coconut oil*

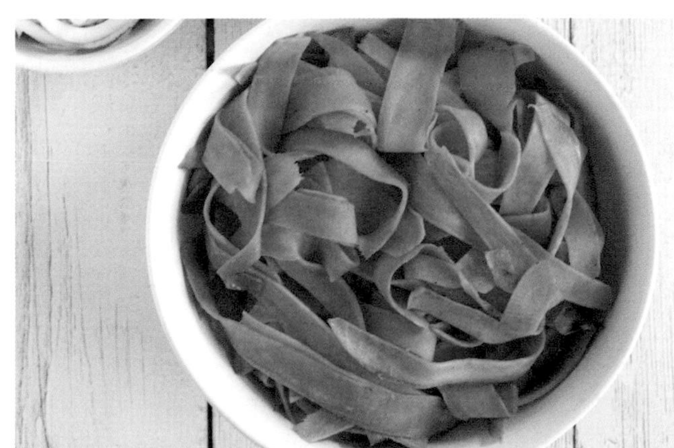

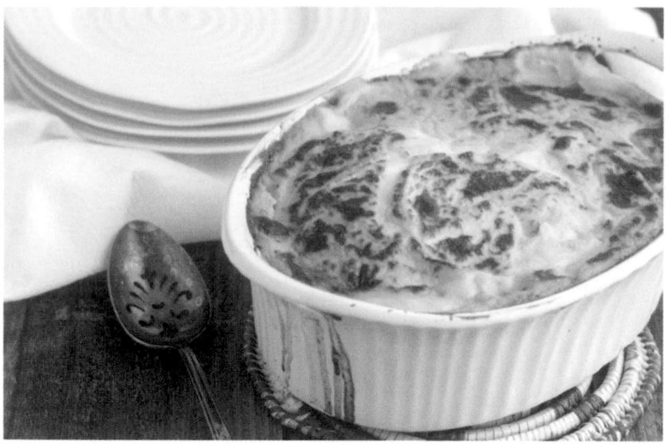

SCALLOPED NOTATOES

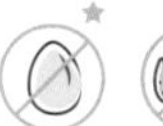 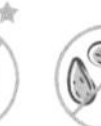 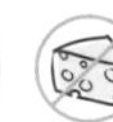 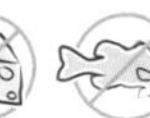 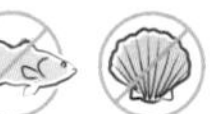  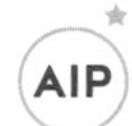 AIP

PREP TIME: 15 minutes *COOK TIME: 50 minutes*
YIELD: 6 to 8 servings

1½ pounds turnips (large radishes such as daikon or rutabaga work well, too)

1 small head cauliflower (5 to 6 cups florets)

4 ounces thick-sliced ham or pancetta

2 cups Bone Stock (page 486)

¼ cup plus 1 tablespoon ghee, unsalted butter, or lard, divided

1 large egg

Sea salt and ground black pepper

1. Slice the turnips into very thin rounds, about ⅛ inch thick (a mandoline makes this job quick and easy). Cut the cauliflower into florets. You can also use the cauliflower stems by cutting them into small pieces. Cut the ham into ¼-inch dice.

2. Bring the stock to a simmer in a large pot over medium-high heat. Add the cauliflower and simmer until slightly overcooked, about 15 minutes.

3. In a skillet over medium-high heat, sauté the ham with 1 tablespoon of the ghee until browned, about 5 minutes. Set aside.

4. Preheat the oven to 375°F.

5. Pour the stock and cauliflower into a blender. Add the remaining ¼ cup of ghee and blend on high until you have a completely smooth puree (20 seconds to a minute, depending on your blender).

6. Beat the egg slightly in a bowl, then temper the egg. To temper the egg, add a spoonful of the hot cauliflower puree to the egg while stirring vigorously. Add another spoonful the same way. Then a third spoonful.

7. Add the tempered egg to the cauliflower puree and blend to combine. Taste the puree. If needed, add salt and pepper (it should be just a bit too salty, because the turnips will dilute the seasoning once baked).

8. Toss the turnips with the ham, then lay the turnips and ham in a 9-inch square baking dish or similar-sized casserole dish (it doesn't need to be neat). Pour the cauliflower puree over the top. Stir to coat the turnip slices well with the sauce, then smooth it out to make sure the turnip slices are all lying flat.

9. Bake for 30 minutes, until bubbling and the turnips are soft with just a little bit of give when pierced with a knife. To brown the top layer, broil for 3 to 5 minutes at the end of baking, then serve.

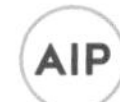 *use lard and omit egg and pepper*

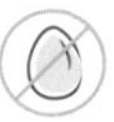 *omit*

GRILLED PORTOBELLO MUSHROOM CAPS

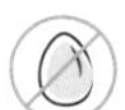  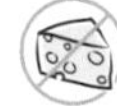  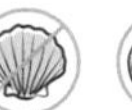 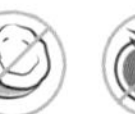  AIP

PREP TIME: 5 minutes *COOK TIME: 5 minutes*
YIELD: 2 or 3 servings

3 tablespoons avocado oil

3 tablespoons balsamic vinegar

4 to 6 portobello mushroom caps, stems removed

1. Preheat a grill pan or a gas or charcoal grill to medium-high heat.

2. Mix the oil and vinegar in a small bowl and use a pastry brush to brush both sides of each mushroom cap, being more generous on the lamella (or gill) side.

3. Grill the mushroom caps for 3 to 5 minutes per side, until grill marks form and the mushrooms are fully cooked.

4. Serve with a main dish or use in place of hamburger buns for 50/50/50 Burgers (page 525).

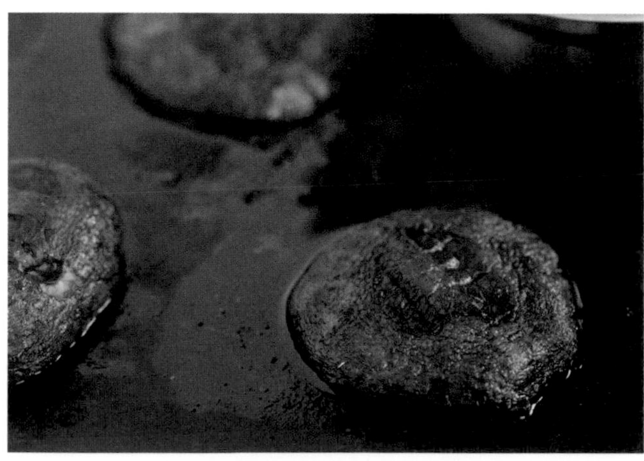

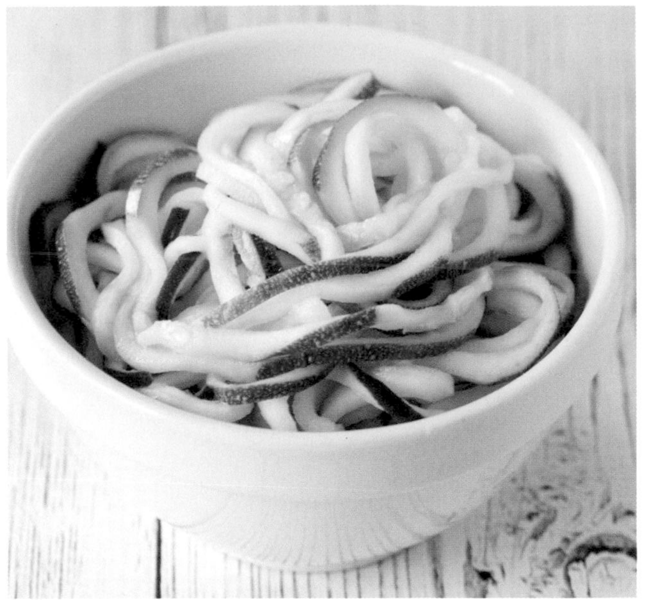

ZOODLES

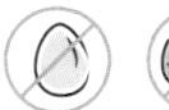 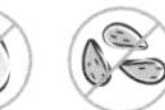 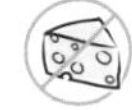  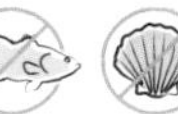 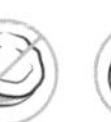 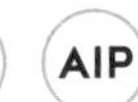 AIP

PREP TIME: 15 minutes, plus time to salt zucchini
COOK TIME: 5 minutes
YIELD: 3 to 4 servings

4 large zucchini (about 2 pounds)

2 teaspoons sea salt

2 to 3 tablespoons olive oil or avocado oil

1. Finely julienne the zucchini lengthwise to create long "matchstick" strips, or use a spiral slicer.

2. Place the zucchini in a colander and toss with the salt. Set the colander in the sink and let sit for 1 hour.

3. Rinse the zucchini very, very thoroughly (have a taste to make sure there's no salt left at all). Drain on a tea towel or paper towels to get rid of as much moisture as possible.

4. Heat the oil in a large skillet over medium-high heat. Add the zucchini and cook, stirring gently but frequently, until the zoodles are cooked al dente, 4 to 5 minutes. If there's a lot of liquid in the pan, turn up the heat.

5. Serve with Meaty Ratatouille Pasta Sauce (page 527), "Spaghetti" Bolognese (page 528), or pesto (page 495 or 497) and DIY Baked Chicken Breast (page 541).

PARSNIP & FENNEL PUREE

 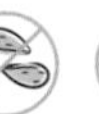 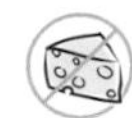   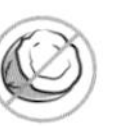  AIP*

PREP TIME: 10 minutes   COOK TIME: 35 minutes
YIELD: 4 to 6 servings

3 tablespoons olive oil

1 medium onion, peeled and chopped

1 pound fennel bulb, chopped (about 1 large bulb)

1½ pounds parsnips, cut into 1-inch pieces

4 cups Chicken Stock (page 486)

2 tablespoons duck fat, unsalted butter, ghee, or additional olive oil

Sea salt and ground black pepper (optional)

1. Heat the olive oil in a large skillet or saucepan over medium heat. Add the onion and fennel bulb and cook, covered, stirring occasionally, for 15 minutes.

2. Add the parsnips and stock. Increase the heat to maintain a rapid simmer and simmer, uncovered, for 20 minutes. Ideally, there should be almost no liquid left in the pan by the time the vegetables are done cooking. If the stock evaporates too soon, add a little extra stock or water.

3. Drain the vegetables and place in a blender or food processor, reserving the liquid to thin the puree. Add the duck fat and process on high until a smooth puree forms, adding some of the reserved liquid, if needed.

4. Taste and add salt and pepper, if desired.

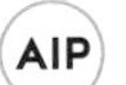 *omit pepper*

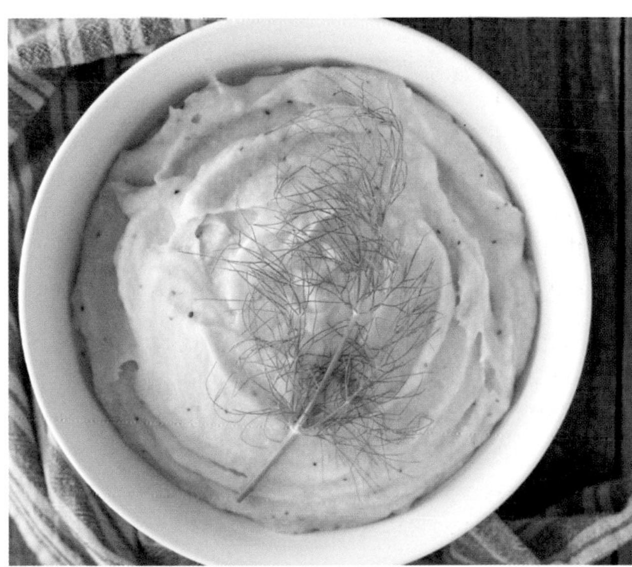

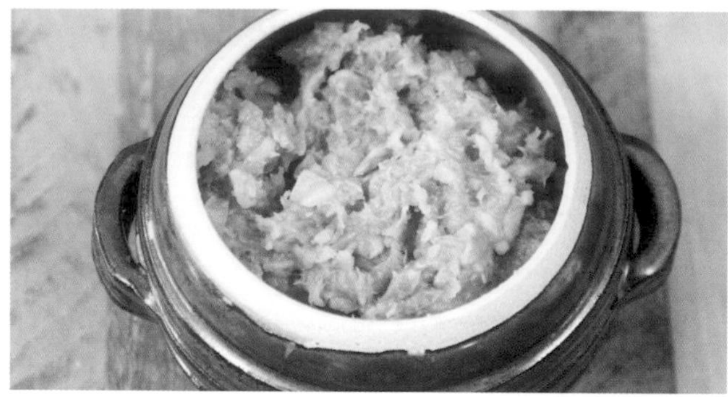

MASHED PLANTAINS

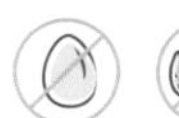 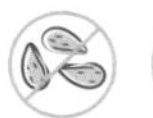 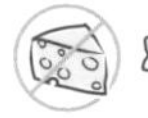 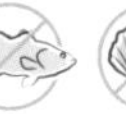 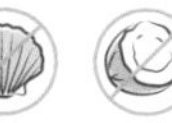  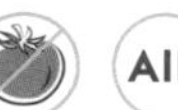 

PREP TIME: 15 minutes COOK TIME: 25 minutes
YIELD: 4 to 6 servings

3 green or fully ripe plantains, peeled and cut into 1-inch-thick semicircles

6 ounces bacon, cut into small pieces

1 medium-sized yellow onion, diced

4 cloves garlic, minced

Extra bacon fat, lard, or unsalted butter

Sea salt and ground black pepper (optional)

1. Place the plantains in a pot with 2 inches of water. Bring to a boil over high heat, then reduce the heat to maintain a simmer. Simmer, covered, until the plantains are tender when pierced with a knife. If using green plantains, this will take about 20 minutes. If using fully ripe plantains, it will take about 10 minutes.
2. Place the bacon in a cold skillet, then turn on the heat to medium-high. Cook for 5 minutes, then add the onion and garlic. Continue cooking, stirring occasionally, until the bacon is crisp and the onion is soft and caramelized, about 15 minutes.
3. Drain the plantains, reserving the cooking liquid. Place the plantains in a bowl along with ½ cup of the cooking liquid. Mash with a wire potato masher to the desired consistency. Add the bacon, onion, garlic, and all the fat from the pan. Stir to incorporate. Taste and season with salt and pepper, if desired.
4. If you prefer a thinner mash, you can add more of the cooking liquid or additional bacon fat before serving.

TIP: This dish tastes similar to mashed potatoes when you use green plantains. If you use ripe plantains, the mash will be sweeter with a slight apple flavor. Green plantains tend to thicken as they sit, so if you have leftovers, you will likely need to add some more liquid to them before reheating. For extra flavor, simmer the plantains in Bone Stock (page 486) instead of water.

 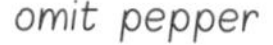 *omit pepper*  *omit onion and garlic*

CASSAVA OVEN FRIES

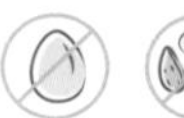 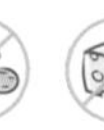 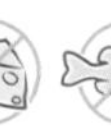 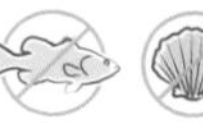 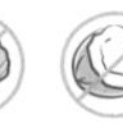 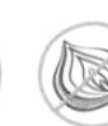  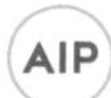 AIP

PREP TIME: 15 minutes COOK TIME: 1 hour
YIELD: 4 to 6 servings

2½ pounds cassava (aka yuca, manioc, or tapioca root)

½ cup melted lard or duck fat (see Tip)

1½ teaspoons sea salt

1. Bring 3 inches of water to a boil in a large pot.
2. Peel the cassava. Cut big cylinders, about 3 to 4 inches long, down the length of the cassava. Cut each cylinder in half lengthwise, then cut each half lengthwise again 2 or 3 times to make large wedges. Cassava can have a long, stringy thread running down the middle—if you see that, trim it off.
3. Add the cassava wedges to the pot and boil, uncovered, for 10 minutes.
4. Preheat the oven to 375°F.
5. Drain the cassava wedges completely. Toss with the lard on a rimmed baking sheet. Bake for 40 minutes, stirring and flipping at the 15-minute mark, 25-minute mark, and 35-minute mark. The cooking time will vary based on the thickness of the wedges. The fries may be done in 35 minutes. They should be turning golden brown and be crisp on the outside. If you aren't sure, put them back in the oven for a few more minutes (these fries are fairly forgiving, especially if the wedges are thick).
6. Sprinkle and toss with the salt.

TIP: Utilize the heat of your oven to melt the lard: Place the lard in a rimmed baking sheet and place in the oven while it's preheating. A preheated pan also shortens the cooking time a bit. Just be careful when you add the cassava wedges to the pan and toss them in the melted lard. It will be hot!

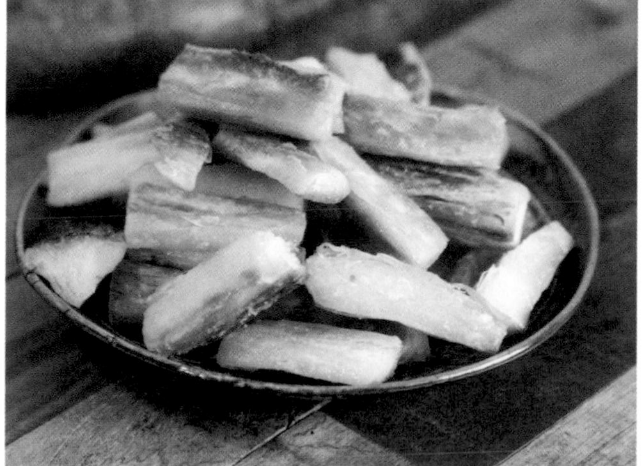

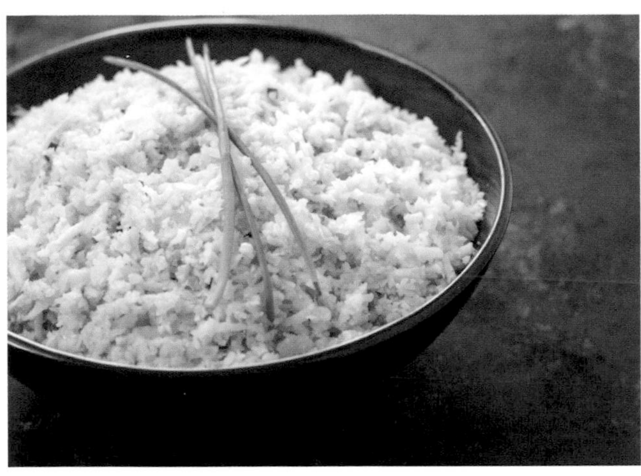

CAULI-RICE

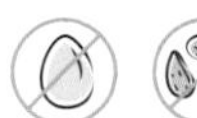 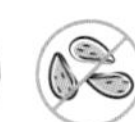 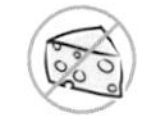 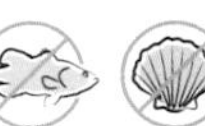   AIP*

PREP TIME: 10 minutes COOK TIME: 10 minutes
YIELD: 4 to 6 servings

1 small head cauliflower (about 2 pounds)

3 to 4 tablespoons avocado oil, olive oil, or coconut oil

⅛ teaspoon sea salt

ASIAN CAULI-RICE

1 (1-inch) piece fresh ginger, sliced

3 to 4 cloves garlic, crushed to a coarse paste

⅛ teaspoon sea salt

1 tablespoon coconut water vinegar or apple cider vinegar

1 tablespoon chopped fresh chives

LEMON PARSLEY CAULI-RICE

1 clove garlic, crushed to a coarse paste

⅛ teaspoon sea salt

⅛ teaspoon ground black pepper

1 tablespoon finely grated lemon zest

1 tablespoon lemon juice

¼ cup chopped fresh parsley

CUMIN CAULI-RICE

¾ teaspoon ground cumin

¼ teaspoon sea salt

1. Core the cauliflower and place the florets in a food processor (you may have to do this in batches). Pulse until chopped to rice-grain size. Set aside. Alternatively, you can grate the cauliflower with a box grater. Also, many stores sell fresh or frozen cauli-rice!

2. Heat 3 tablespoons of the oil in a large skillet or wok over medium-high heat.

3. If making the Asian-inspired cauli-rice, add the ginger slices to the oil and cook until fragrant and browned, 3 to 4 minutes. Remove the ginger slices and discard.

4. Add the cauliflower to the pan as well as the salt, pepper, garlic, or cumin, depending on the variation you're making. Cook, stirring frequently, until the cauliflower is cooked al dente (about 6 to 8 minutes, or less if using frozen store-bought cauli-rice). If the rice starts sticking to the pan or the pan looks very dry, add another tablespoon of oil.

5. Stir in the remaining ingredients and cook for 1 minute. Enjoy!

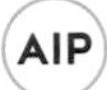 *don't make cumin variation; omit pepper*

MOROCCAN "COUSCOUS"

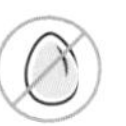 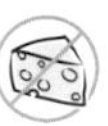 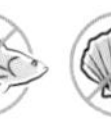 

PREP TIME: 15 minutes
COOK TIME: 7 minutes, plus 1 hour to refrigerate
YIELD: 3 to 4 servings

1 small head cauliflower

2 tablespoons coconut oil

¼ teaspoon sea salt

½ teaspoon ground cinnamon

½ teaspoon ground cumin

½ teaspoon turmeric powder

¾ cup whole cashews

½ cup raisins

⅓ cup Medjool dates (about 4 dates), pitted and chopped

2 tablespoons chopped crystallized ginger

1 bunch parsley (about 1 cup chopped)

1 large orange (about 2 tablespoons finely grated zest and ½ cup juice)

2 tablespoons apple cider vinegar

1. Pulse the cauliflower florets and stems in a food processor until it resembles small rice grains or large couscous grains (depending on your food processor, you might want to do this in batches). Note that this does not work very well with frozen cauliflower.

2. Heat the coconut oil in a large skillet over medium-high heat. Add the cauliflower, salt, cinnamon, cumin, and turmeric. Cook, stirring frequently, until the cauliflower is cooked al dente, 6 to 7 minutes.

3. Pour the cauliflower into a large bowl. Stir in the cashews, raisins, dates, ginger, parsley, and orange zest until combined. Pour the orange juice and vinegar over the top and stir to coat.

4. Refrigerate for at least 1 hour before serving.

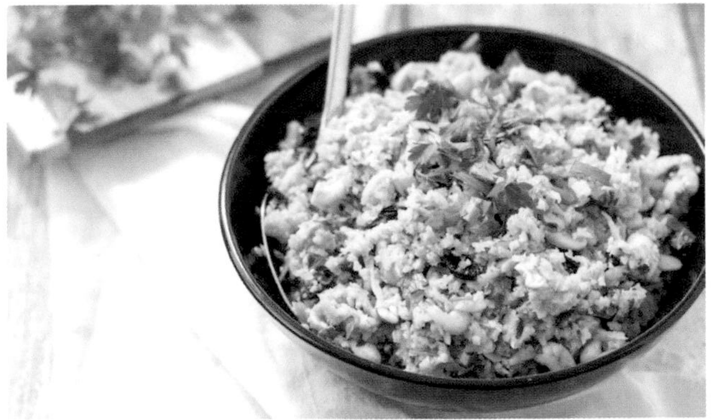

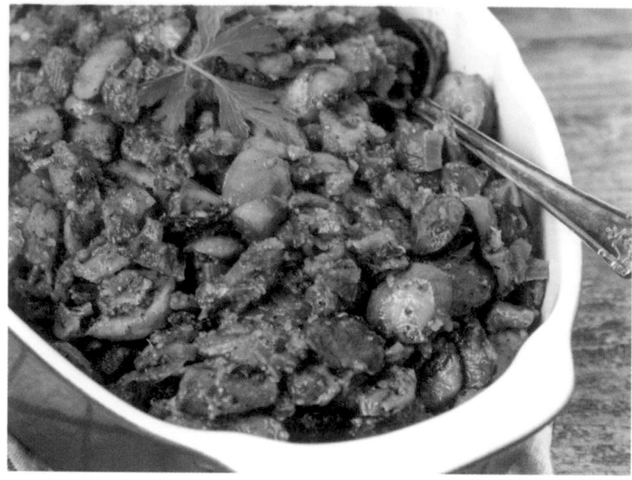

EGGPLANT & WILD MUSHROOM DRESSING

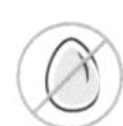 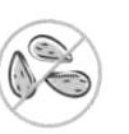 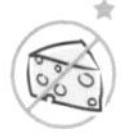 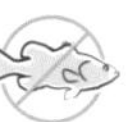 

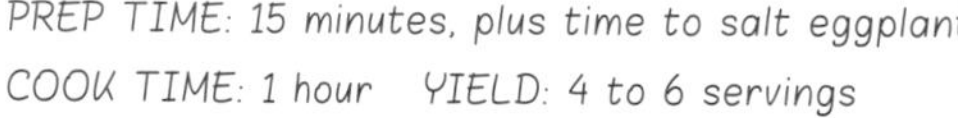

PREP TIME: 15 minutes, plus time to salt eggplant
COOK TIME: 1 hour   YIELD: 4 to 6 servings

- 2 large eggplants, peeled and cut into ½-inch dice
- 2 tablespoons sea salt
- 6 ounces bacon, chopped
- 2 to 3 tablespoons unsalted butter, ghee, olive oil, or lard
- 1 medium-sized yellow onion, finely chopped
- 2 to 3 stalks celery, cut into ¼-inch slices
- 2 pounds assorted mushrooms
- 1 tablespoon fresh parsley, finely chopped
- 1 tablespoon dried savory
- Sea salt and ground black pepper (optional)
- 1 cup Bone Stock (page 486)

1. Put the eggplant in a colander and sprinkle liberally with the salt. Place the colander in the sink and let sit for at least 1 hour. This step is critical for getting the eggplant to hold its shape and not turn to mush.

2. Rinse the salt off the eggplant, then place the eggplant on several paper towels on the counter or a rimmed baking sheet. Cover with more paper towels and gently squeeze the excess water out of the eggplant. Set aside.

3. Add the bacon to a cold skillet, then heat the skillet over medium-high heat, stirring fairly frequently. When the bacon is mostly cooked, add the eggplant and cook, stirring frequently, until the eggplant is starting to brown. If the eggplant starts to stick to the pan, add 1 tablespoon of butter.

4. Set the bacon and eggplant aside in a large bowl and return the skillet to the stovetop. Add 1 tablespoon of butter to the skillet with the onion and celery and cook until softened.

5. Add the mushrooms to the skillet (you may need to do this in 2 batches, depending on the size of your skillet). If the vegetables start to stick, add another tablespoon of butter. Cook until the mushrooms are nicely sautéed but still firm. Add the mushrooms to the eggplant and bacon in the bowl.

6. Toss the vegetables with the savory and parsley until well combined. Taste and add salt and pepper, if desired.

7. Preheat the oven to 325°F.

8. Place the dressing in a casserole dish and pour the stock over the top. Bake for 30 minutes. Serve.

TIP: If using this dressing to stuff a turkey, omit the stock and cook the turkey as per the guide on page 640.

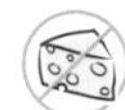 *avoid*

CELERY ROOT PUREE

 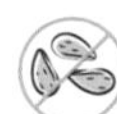 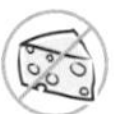 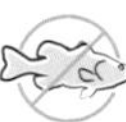 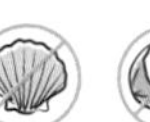 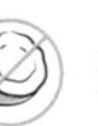 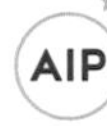

PREP TIME: 10 minutes   COOK TIME: 15 minutes
YIELD: 4 to 6 servings

- ¼ cup duck fat, unsalted butter, or ghee
- 2 large celery roots, peeled and cut into ½-inch dice
- 2 cups Chicken Stock (page 486)
- Sea salt and ground black pepper (optional)

1. Heat the duck fat in a large skillet or saucepan over medium-high heat. Add the celery roots and sauté, stirring frequently, until browned, 8 to 9 minutes.

2. Add the stock, ¼ cup at a time, stirring frequently, adding the next ¼ cup only when the stock has almost completely evaporated. After adding the last of the stock, immediately remove the pan from the heat.

3. Puree using an immersion blender, countertop blender, or food processor. Taste and add salt and pepper, if desired.

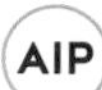 *omit pepper*

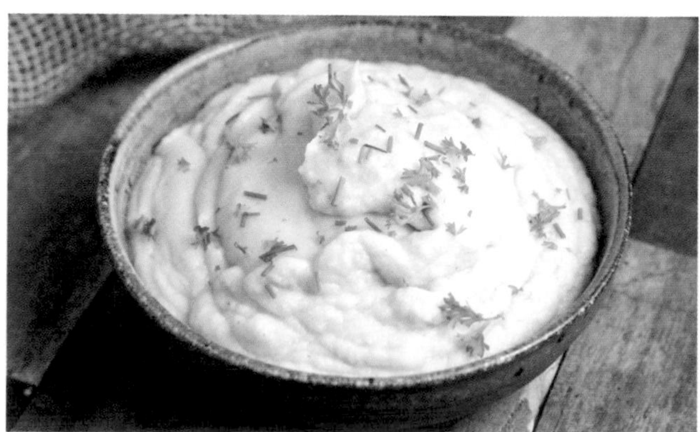

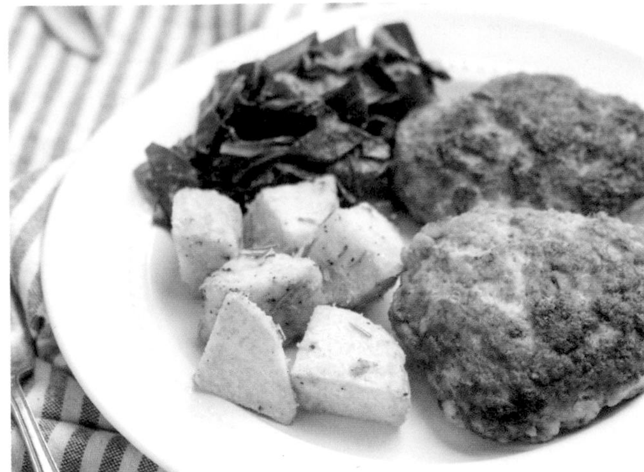

SAVORY-ROASTED TARO

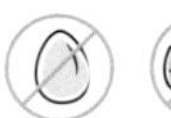 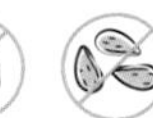 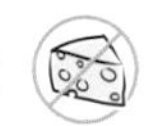 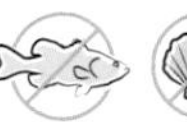 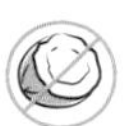 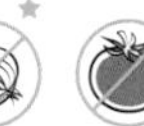 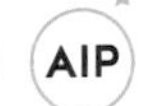 AIP

PREP TIME: 15 minutes COOK TIME: 25 minutes
YIELD: 2 to 4 servings

2 pounds fresh taro (8 to 10 small tubers)

3 tablespoons tallow, lard, or duck fat, melted

2 teaspoons dried savory

2 cloves garlic, crushed to a coarse paste

½ teaspoon sea salt

¼ teaspoon ground black pepper

1. Fill a saucepan with enough water so that the water just barely reaches the bottom of the steamer insert or steamer basket. Bring to a boil over high heat.

2. Once the water comes to a boil, place the whole unpeeled taro tubers in the steamer basket or steamer insert and cover with a loose-fitting lid. Steam for 10 to 15 minutes (depending on the size of the tubers), until you can pierce them easily with a knife but before they get too soft (think of not-quite-cooked potatoes). Remove from the heat and let cool until you can handle them.

3. Preheat the broiler for 10 minutes (set to high, and with a rack placed 6 to 8 inches from the broiler element). Line a rimmed baking sheet with aluminum foil or parchment paper.

4. Peel off the barklike skin of the taro with a paring knife (it should come off fairly easily). Cut the peeled taro into quarters or ½-inch-thick rounds and place in a large bowl. Pour the tallow, savory, garlic, salt, and pepper over the taro and toss to coat. Spread the taro on the prepared baking sheet.

5. Broil for 10 minutes, flipping or stirring every 3 to 5 minutes, until browned and slightly crisp on the outside.

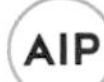 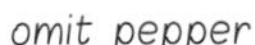 *omit pepper*

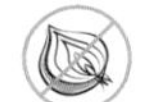 *omit garlic*

OVEN-BAKED SWEET POTATO FRIES

  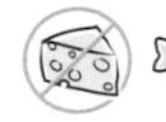 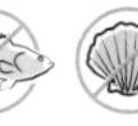 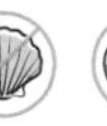 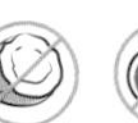 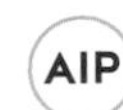 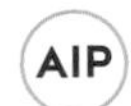 AIP

PREP TIME: 10 minutes COOK TIME: 30 minutes
YIELD: 4 servings

1½ pounds sweet potatoes

3 tablespoons arrowroot powder

3 tablespoons ghee or lard, melted

½ teaspoon sea salt

SERVING SUGGESTION

1 teaspoon maple sugar

½ teaspoon ground cinnamon

1. Preheat the oven to 400°F. Line a rimmed baking sheet with parchment paper.

2. Peel the sweet potatoes and cut into french fry-like strips (4 to 6 inches long and ¼ to ⅜ inch thick).

3. In a bag or bowl, toss the sweet potatoes with the arrowroot powder to completely coat. Discard any arrowroot powder that didn't stick to the sweet potatoes. Toss the coated sweet potatoes with the melted ghee and salt.

4. Arrange the sweet potato strips on the prepared baking sheet in a single layer, taking the time to separate the strips so they aren't touching each other.

5. Bake for 15 minutes, then flip each strip over and bake for an additional 10 to 15 minutes, until browned with crispy edges.

6. Sprinkle the warm fries with the maple sugar and cinnamon, if desired, and serve. (Or serve with ketchup, as pictured.)

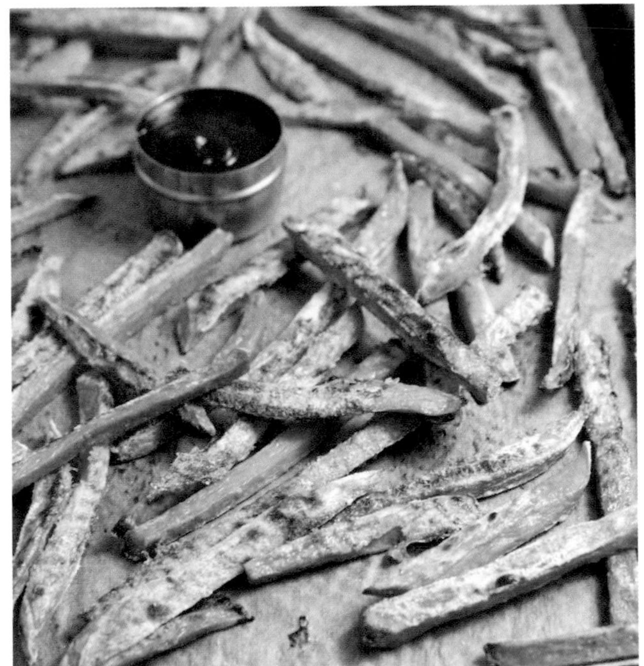

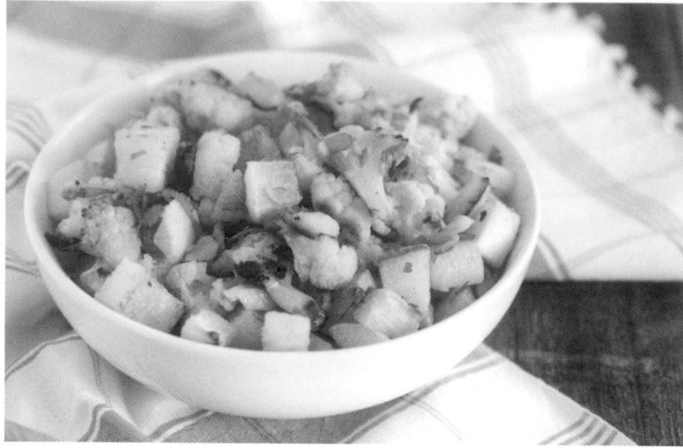

POTATOLESS ALOO GOBI

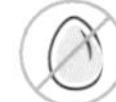 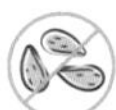 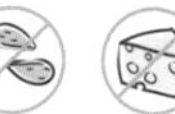 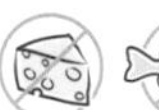  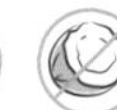 

PREP TIME: 10 minutes COOK TIME: 45 minutes
YIELD: 4 to 6 servings

½ medium head cauliflower, cut into ¾-inch-thick florets

1 pound turnips or daikon, cut into ¾-inch cubes

½ teaspoon sea salt

½ teaspoon ground cumin

3 tablespoons olive oil

1. Preheat the oven to 425°F.
2. Toss all the ingredients together to completely coat the vegetables.
3. Bake for 35 to 45 minutes, until browned, and serve.

TIP: If you include potatoes in your diet, you can replace the turnips with potatoes.

ROASTED GREEN BEANS

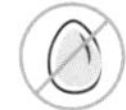 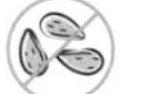 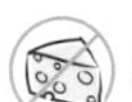  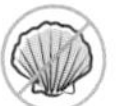 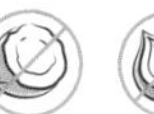 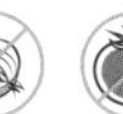

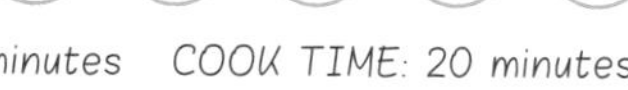

PREP TIME: 5 minutes COOK TIME: 20 minutes
YIELD: 4 servings

3 tablespoons olive oil, ghee, or avocado oil

1½ pounds green beans, trimmed

1 teaspoon sea salt or truffle salt

⅛ teaspoon ground black pepper

1 to 2 tablespoons lemon juice

1. Preheat the oven to 450°F. Line a rimmed baking sheet with aluminum foil or parchment paper.
2. Toss the green beans with the oil (if using ghee, melt it first) and sprinkle liberally with the salt and pepper.
3. Roast for 18 to 20 minutes (or longer if you have thicker beans), stirring the beans at the 10-minute mark. They're done when they start browning and getting a little crisp on the outside and are soft but not mushy on the inside.
4. Place the green beans in a serving bowl and toss with the lemon juice before serving.

TIP: Okra can be cooked the same way; simply cut whole fresh okra into 2-inch pieces.

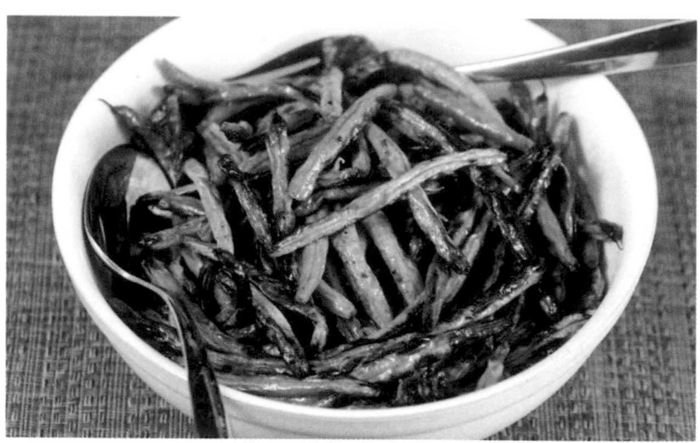

BROILED ASPARAGUS

 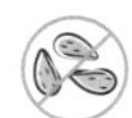 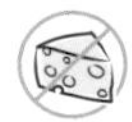     AIP

PREP TIME: 5 minutes COOK TIME: 8 minutes
YIELD: 2 to 4 servings

1 pound asparagus, tough ends snapped off and discarded

2 tablespoons avocado oil

¼ teaspoon sea salt or truffle salt

⅛ teaspoon ground black pepper

1. Position an oven rack 6 inches below the broiler and preheat the broiler to high for 10 to 15 minutes.
2. Place the asparagus on a rimmed baking sheet. Drizzle with the oil and sprinkle with the salt and pepper; toss to combine.
3. Broil for 6 to 8 minutes, until starting to brown.

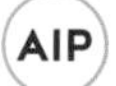 *omit pepper*

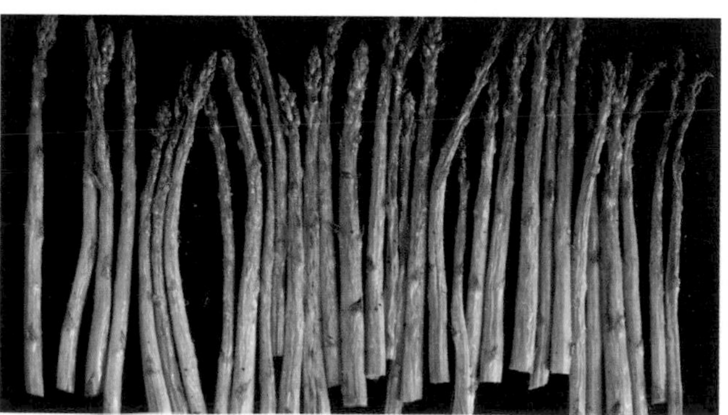

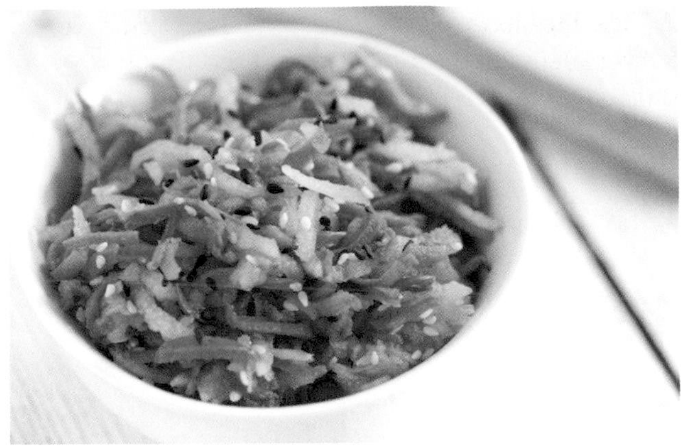

ASIAN PEAR SLAW

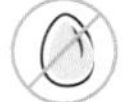 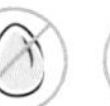 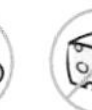 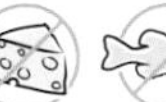 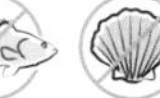 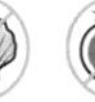 

PREP TIME: 10 minutes, plus time to marinate
YIELD: 2 to 4 servings

1 medium Asian pear
1 large carrot
1 tablespoon coconut water vinegar
1 teaspoon toasted (dark) sesame oil
1 tablespoon sesame seeds

1. Finely julienne the Asian pear and carrot using a mandoline or sharp knife (a julienne cut is like a long matchstick). You should end up with a 50/50 mix of Asian pear and carrot, 3 to 4 loosely packed cups.

2. Toss the Asian pear and carrot with the vinegar, sesame oil, and sesame seeds. Let marinate at room temperature for 20 minutes (or longer in the refrigerator) before serving.

MAPLE & SAGE ROASTED WINTER SQUASH

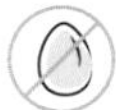 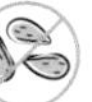 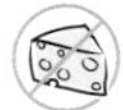 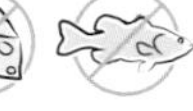 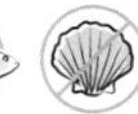 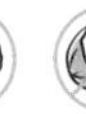 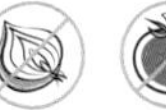 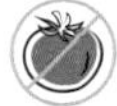 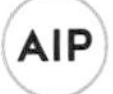 AIP

PREP TIME: 10 minutes COOK TIME: 35 minutes
YIELD: 4 to 6 servings

2 pounds winter squash, peeled, seeded, and cut into 1½-inch pieces
3 tablespoons coconut oil, melted
2 tablespoons maple sugar
1 tablespoon chiffonade fresh sage
½ teaspoon sea salt

1. Preheat the oven to 425°F. Line a rimmed baking sheet with aluminum foil or parchment paper.

2. In a large bowl, toss the squash with the coconut oil, maple sugar, sage, and salt. Spread out onto the prepared baking sheet.

3. Roast for 30 to 35 minutes, until slightly browned and tender. Shake the pan (and maybe toss the squash chunks) every 10 minutes during baking.

 *use lard instead of coconut oil*

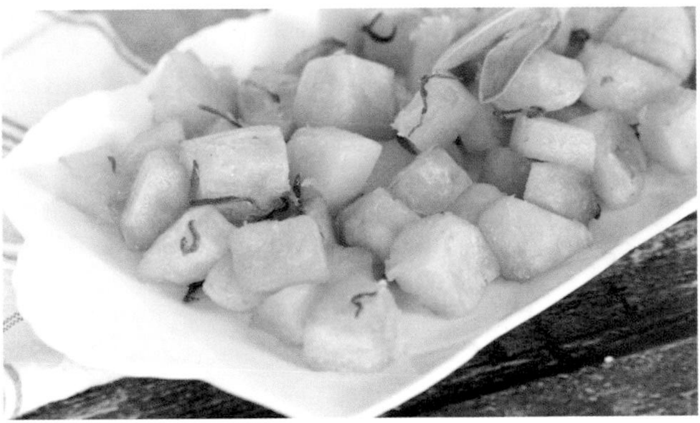

ROSEMARY & SAGE ROASTED PARSNIPS

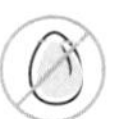 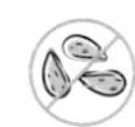 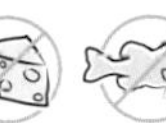 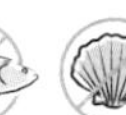  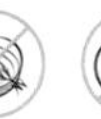 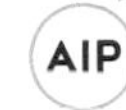 AIP

PREP TIME: 10 minutes COOK TIME: 40 minutes
YIELD: 3 to 6 servings

2 pounds parsnips, cut into ½-inch-wide rounds or ½-inch-thick wedges
3 tablespoons lard or duck fat, melted
1 tablespoon chopped fresh rosemary
1 tablespoon chopped fresh sage
¼ teaspoon sea salt or truffle salt
⅛ teaspoon ground black pepper

1. Preheat the oven to 350°F.

2. In a large bowl, toss the parsnips with the lard, herbs, salt, and pepper. Place in a single layer on the baking sheet.

3. Roast for 40 minutes, until golden brown, stirring at the 20-minute and 30-minute marks.

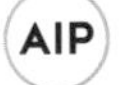 *omit pepper*

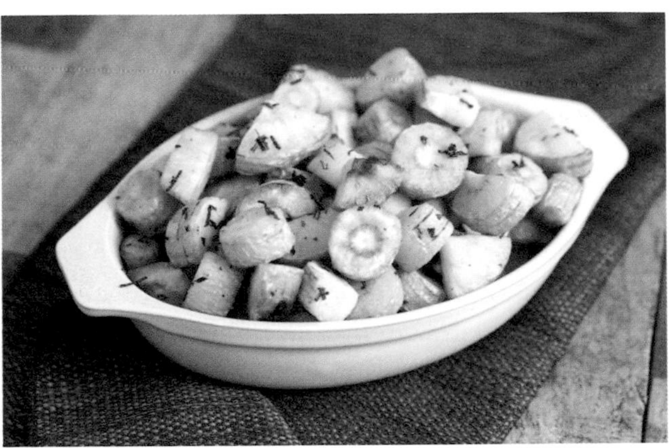

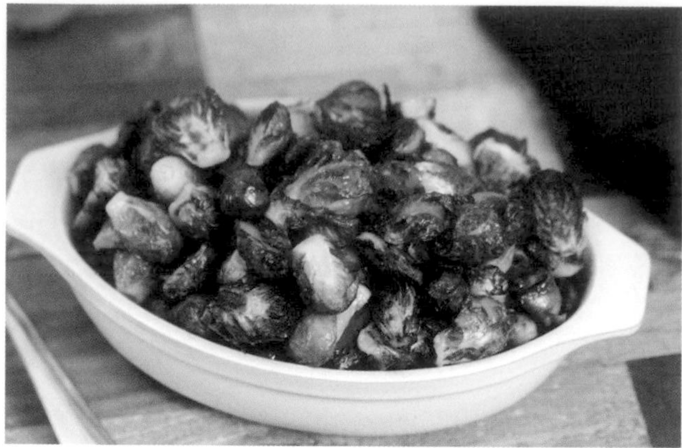

ROASTED BRUSSELS SPROUTS

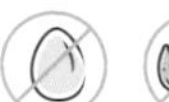 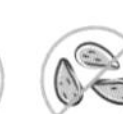 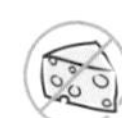 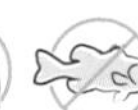  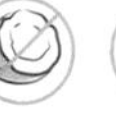 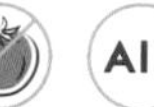 AIP

PREP TIME: 10 minutes COOK TIME: 35 minutes
YIELD: 4 to 6 servings

4 pounds Brussels sprouts

¼ cup olive oil or melted lard or ghee

1 teaspoon sea salt

1. Preheat the oven to 375°F
2. Trim any brown parts off the Brussels sprouts. Slice medium-sized sprouts in half, slice large sprouts into quarters, or leave small sprouts whole. Any leaves that fall off can be added to the Brussels sprouts.
3. Toss the Brussels sprouts with the oil and salt. Place on a rimmed baking sheet, spreading out in a uniform layer.
4. Roast for 30 to 35 minutes, stirring once halfway through cooking, until browned.

BACON-BRAISED KALE

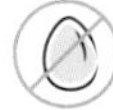 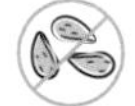 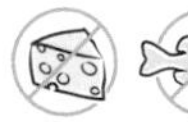 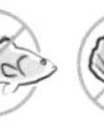 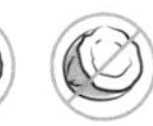  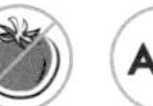 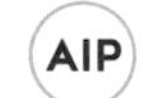 AIP

PREP TIME: 5 minutes COOK TIME: 8 minutes
YIELD: 4 servings

3 ounces bacon, chopped into small pieces

1 large bunch kale, chopped and tough stems removed

¼ to ½ cup Bone Stock (page 486), divided

1 tablespoon lemon juice

1 clove garlic, crushed to a coarse paste

1. Place the bacon in a cold skillet. Cook over medium-high heat, stirring occasionally, until the bacon is crispy. If the bacon releases a lot of fat, drain enough to leave 2 to 3 tablespoons in the pan.
2. Add the kale and 2 tablespoons of the stock. Cook, stirring, until the stock has evaporated. Add another 2 tablespoons of stock and cook, stirring occasionally, until the stock has evaporated. Continue until the kale is completely cooked, 3 to 5 minutes.
3. Stir in the garlic and lemon juice and cook for 1 more minute. Serve.

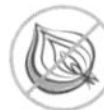 *omit garlic*

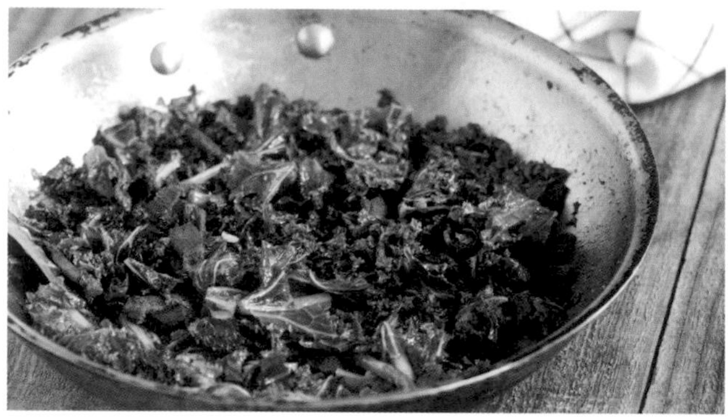

MINTED ZUCCHINI

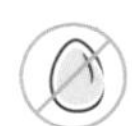 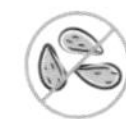 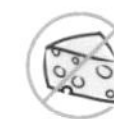 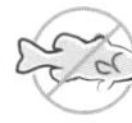  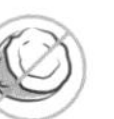 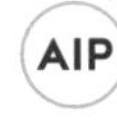 AIP

PREP TIME: 5 minutes COOK TIME: 6 minutes
YIELD: 2 to 4 servings

1 tablespoon olive oil

2 medium zucchini, cut into ¼-inch semicircles

2 tablespoons chopped fresh mint

¼ teaspoon sea salt

Pinch of ground black pepper

1. Heat a skillet over medium heat. Add the oil and zucchini and sauté, stirring frequently, until the zucchini is soft and just starting to brown, 5 to 6 minutes. If the zucchini releases a lot of liquid, increase the heat.
2. Add the mint, salt, and pepper and continue to cook for 1 minute. Serve.

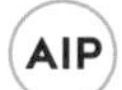 *omit pepper*

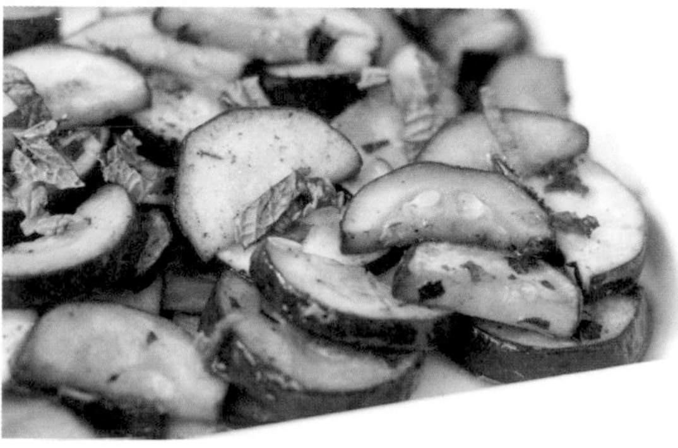

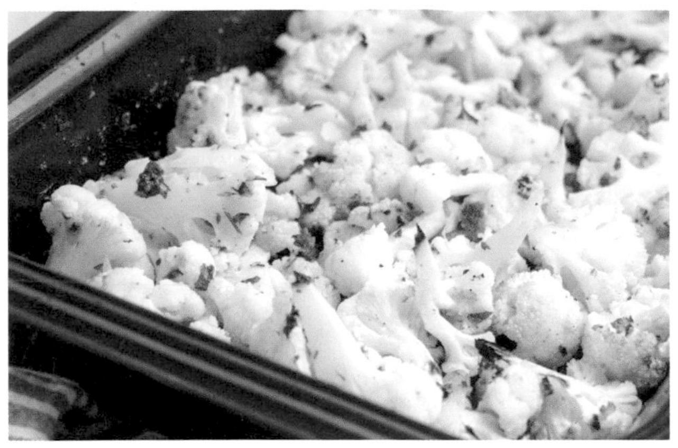

ROASTED BROCCOLI OR CAULIFLOWER

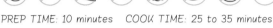

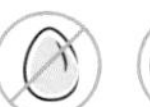 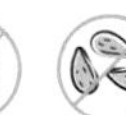 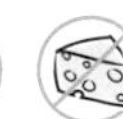 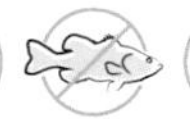 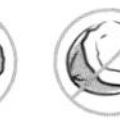   AIP

PREP TIME: 10 minutes COOK TIME: 25 to 35 minutes
YIELD: 4 to 8 servings

- 8 cups broccoli and/or cauliflower florets and cubed stems (about 2 pounds)
- ¼ cup avocado oil or olive oil
- 6 to 8 cloves garlic, minced
- 1 tablespoon finely grated lemon zest
- ¼ teaspoon sea salt or truffle salt
- ⅛ teaspoon ground black pepper
- ¼ cup chopped fresh parsley

1. Preheat the oven to 450°F.
2. In a casserole dish, toss the broccoli and/or cauliflower florets and stems with the oil, garlic, lemon zest, salt, and pepper.
3. Roast for 25 to 35 minutes, until the broccoli and cauliflower are fully cooked (it depends on how big the florets are and how soft you like them), stirring once halfway through cooking.
4. Toss with the fresh parsley and serve.

TIP: For a little extra zing, reserve the juice from the lemon and squeeze it over the broccoli right before serving.

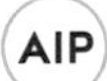 *omit pepper*

BALSAMIC-ROASTED BEETS

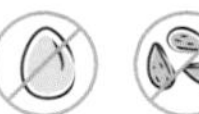 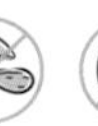 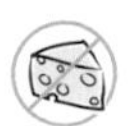 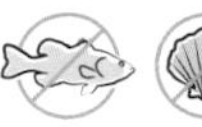 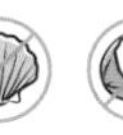  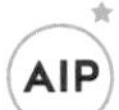 AIP

PREP TIME: 10 minutes COOK TIME: 1 hour
YIELD: 4 to 6 servings

- 6 to 8 medium beets, quartered
- 2 tablespoons balsamic vinegar
- 1 tablespoon extra-virgin coconut oil, melted, or olive oil
- ¼ teaspoon sea salt or truffle salt
- ⅛ teaspoon ground black pepper

1. Preheat the oven to 350°F. If using a baking dish with a lid, grease the inside of the dish. Alternatively, lay a large piece of aluminum foil in a baking dish or on a rimmed baking sheet, lifting the sides to create an edge all the way around.
2. Combine the beets, vinegar, coconut oil, and salt in a bowl, then pour into the prepared baking dish or into the foil. Cover the baking dish with its lid or fold the edges of the foil up and over the beets to make a "packet" for the beets to cook in, sealing the edges closed.
3. Bake for 45 to 60 minutes, until the beets are tender. The exact cooking time will depend on the size of the beets.

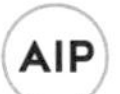 *omit pepper*

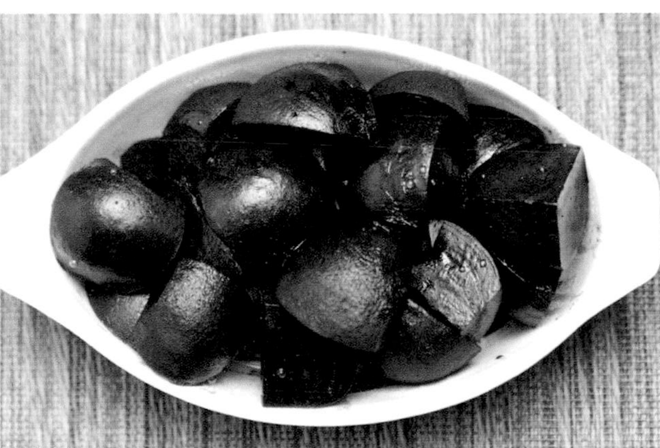

Chapter 44: BREADS, MUFFINS, AND SNACK FOODS

YEAST BREAD

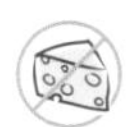   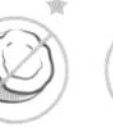 

PREP TIME: 15 minutes, plus 1 hour to rise
COOK TIME: 1 hour YIELD: 14 to 16 slices

7/8 cup sparkling water

3 large eggs

1 teaspoon sea salt

2 tablespoons apple cider vinegar

2 tablespoons honey

¼ cup coconut oil, melted

3 cups finely milled blanched almond flour

3 cups almond meal

⅔ cup tapioca starch

⅔ cup arrowroot powder

2 teaspoons active dry yeast

BREAD MACHINE DIRECTIONS:

1. Mix the water, eggs, salt, vinegar, and honey in your bread machine pan.
2. Place the coconut oil, almond flour, almond meal, tapioca, and arrowroot powder on top of the wet ingredients. Sprinkle the yeast on top of the dry ingredients (or follow the manufacturer's directions).
3. Use the whole-wheat cycle on your bread machine if it has one; if not, use a regular cycle.
4. Very Important: Check during the initial knead that the ingredients are mixing well and are not sticking to the edge of the pan. If they are, use a spatula to gently push them down into the rest of the dough and maybe help mix the dough, depending on your machine.
5. As soon as the bread is done, remove promptly from the bread machine.

OVEN DIRECTIONS:

1. Proof the yeast by warming the water (105°F to 110°F) and then adding the yeast and honey to the water. It should start to foam in 5 to 10 minutes.
2. Add the remaining wet ingredients to the proofed yeast and stir.
3. Add the dry ingredients and stir to fully incorporate by hand or in a stand mixer with the paddle attachment.
4. Pour the dough into a greased 9 by 5-inch loaf pan. Smooth out the top.
5. Let the dough rise in a warm spot in your kitchen, 45 to 60 minutes. Unlike wheat-based bread, the dough won't double in size, but it should still rise noticeably, at least 25 percent.
6. When the dough has about 15 minutes of rising time left, preheat the oven to 350°F.
7. Bake for 55 to 65 minutes, until golden brown on top and a toothpick comes out clean. Let cool until cool enough to handle, then remove from the pan.

TIP: To store, wrap a sheet of paper towel around the loaf and place in a plastic bag. Store in the refrigerator for up to a week. For longer storage, slice the loaf before freezing to make it easy to thaw a few slices at a time. It will keep in the freezer for up to 6 months.

 *use avocado oil instead of coconut oil*

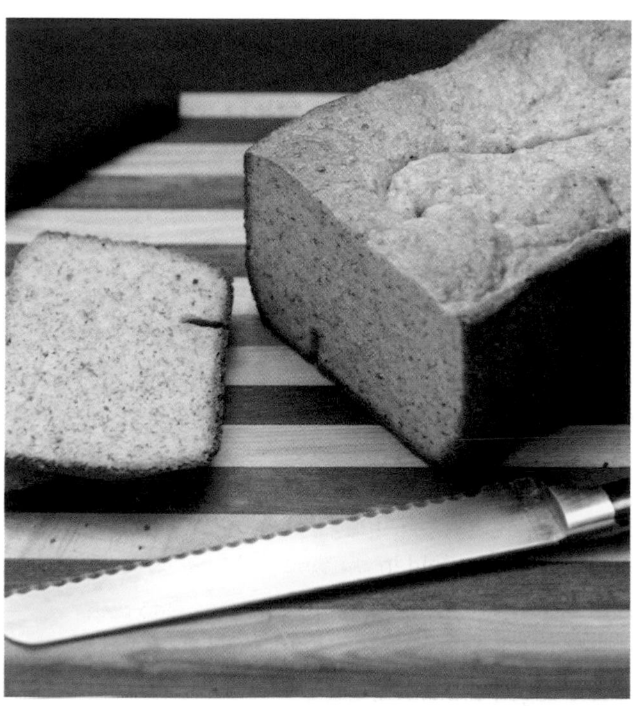

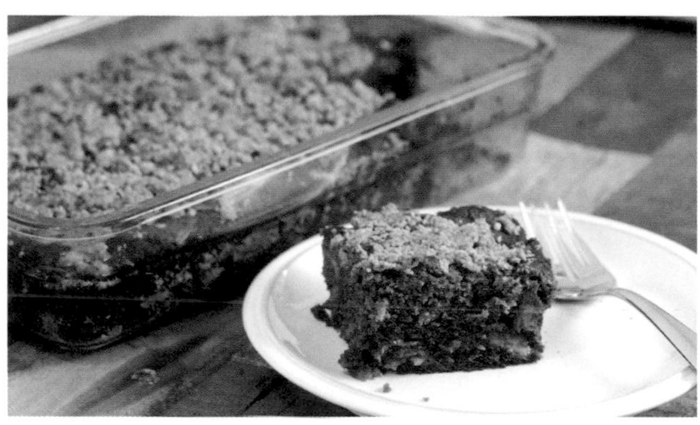

RHUBARB COFFEE CAKE

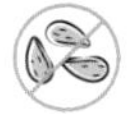 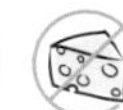 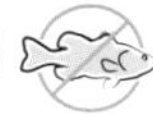  

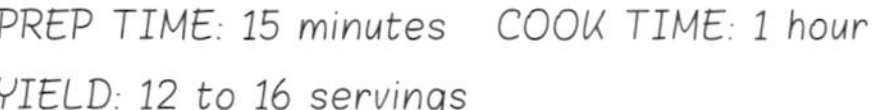
PREP TIME: 15 minutes COOK TIME: 1 hour
YIELD: 12 to 16 servings

½ cup lard

¾ cup honey

1 large egg

1 tablespoon apple cider vinegar

¾ cup less 1 tablespoon coconut cream, homemade (page 480) or store-bought

2 teaspoons baking soda, divided

1⅔ cups plus ¼ cup cassava flour, divided

½ teaspoon ground allspice

½ teaspoon ground cardamom

½ teaspoon sea salt

3 cups finely diced rhubarb

2 tablespoons ghee, unsalted butter, or lard, melted

2 tablespoons maple sugar

½ teaspoon ground cinnamon

½ cup chopped pecans (optional)

1. Preheat the oven to 325°F. Grease a 10 by 7-inch or an 8-inch square baking dish with lard, coconut oil, or ghee.
2. Add the lard, honey, and egg to the bowl of a stand mixer. With whisk attachment at a medium speed, cream together until light and fluffy, 3 to 4 minutes.
3. Combine the apple cider vinegar and coconut cream (tip: add vinegar to the bottom of a measuring cup, then pour in coconut cream to the ¾ cup line). Add 1 teaspoon baking soda and let sit for 2 minutes. (Caution: it will froth and expand, so use at least a 2-cup measuring cup or do this step in a mixing bowl.)
4. Combine the 1⅔ cups cassava flour, allspice, cardamom, remaining baking soda, and salt.
5. With the mixer on low, add thirds of the flour mixture and then the coconut cream mixture, alternately. Once fully incorporated, remove whisk attachment and fold in rhubarb by hand.
6. Pour the batter into the prepared baking dish.
7. To make the crumb topping: Combine the ghee, maple sugar, cinnamon, and the remaining ¼ cup of cassava flour in a small bowl. With your fingers, gently drop the crumb topping onto the surface of the cake batter, breaking up any bigger pieces as you go.
8. Sprinkle the pecans over the top of the cake, if using.
9. Bake for 10 minutes. After 10 minutes, increase the oven temperature to 350°F. Bake for an additional 50 minutes, until a toothpick inserted in the center comes out clean.
10. Remove from the oven and let cool before serving. Store in an airtight container on the counter for up to 3 days, in the refrigerator for up to a week, or in the freezer for up to 6 months.

KALE CHIPS

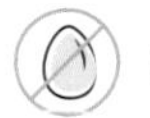 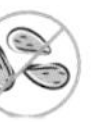 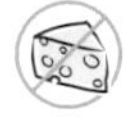 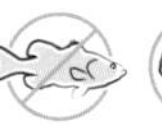 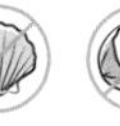 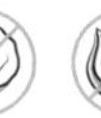  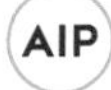 AIP

PREP TIME: 5 minutes COOK TIME: 40 minutes
YIELD: 2 to 4 servings

8 loosely packed cups kale, torn into 1- to 1½-inch pieces, tough stems removed

2 tablespoons olive oil, avocado oil, or melted coconut oil

¼ teaspoon sea salt

1. Preheat the oven to 275°F.
2. Wash and dry kale. Place the kale in a large bowl with a lid.
3. Pour the oil over the kale, then cover with the lid. Shake the bowl to coat the kale with oil. Alternatively, stir to coat or place the kale directly on the baking sheet and give it a good massage with your hands.
4. Spread out onto a rimmed baking sheet. Sprinkle with the salt.
5. Bake for 30 to 40 minutes, until crisp.

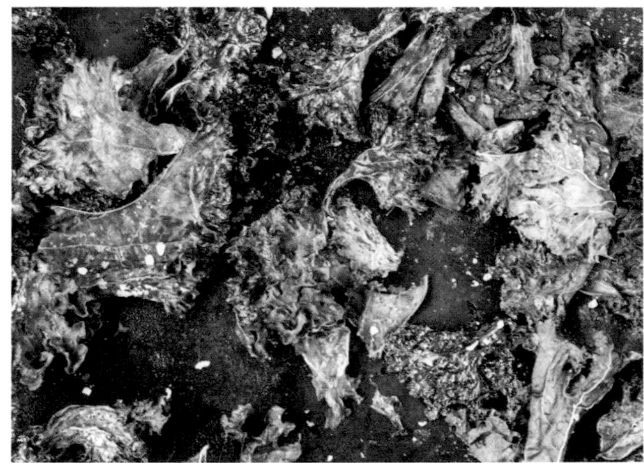

CHOUX PASTRY BUNS

 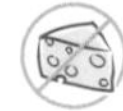  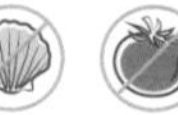

PREP TIME: 15 minutes, plus time to cool

COOK TIME: 30 minutes

YIELD: eight to ten 3-inch "buns"

- ⅓ cup sifted coconut flour
- ⅓ cup tapioca starch
- ⅓ cup arrowroot powder
- Pinch of sea salt
- 4 large eggs
- 1 large egg yolk
- 1 cup full-fat coconut milk, homemade (page 480) or canned
- ½ cup palm shortening or unsalted butter

1. Measure all the ingredients before you begin. It's very important that they be exact and ready to use. Combine the flour, tapioca starch, arrowroot powder, and salt in a bowl. Crack the eggs into 4 separate bowls, then add the egg yolk to one of the bowls (so that one bowl has one whole egg plus one egg yolk).

2. Preheat the oven to 425°F. Line 2 rimmed baking sheets with silicone baking mats or parchment paper.

3. Heat the coconut milk and shortening in a large saucepan over medium heat until the mixture just starts to simmer. Remove the pan from the heat and pour all the dry ingredients into the pot. Stir constantly and vigorously until the mixture is thick and fully combined.

4. With the pot still off the heat, add the eggs one at a time and rapidly stir with each addition. Each time you add an egg, the dough will seem to separate, and then, as you stir, it will come together again. Wait until it comes together before adding the next egg. When all the eggs are added, you will have a very thick and sticky cream-colored dough.

5. To form the pastry dough into buns, scoop the dough into a pastry bag or a resealable plastic bag with a 1-inch diameter hole cut off of one corner. Pipe into bun shapes onto the prepared cookie sheet. For example, if using as sandwich bread or hamburger buns, pipe 3-inch-diameter circles, spacing them at least 1 inch apart. If using as hotdog buns, pipe into 6-inch-long oblong shapes.

6. Immediately place the buns in the oven and bake for 18 to 20 minutes. They will puff up to be about 1 inch high and will be light golden in color.

7. Remove from the oven and gently turn each one upside down. Let them cool upside down on the cookie sheet for 20 minutes. Then move them to a cooling rack to cool completely.

8. Use one each as a top and bottom of a hamburger or hotdog bun. Store in an airtight container or bag in the refrigerator for up to a week.

TIP: The baked choux pastry buns can double as cream puffs or éclairs (see page 576)! Simply cut the pastries in half using a sharp knife; each pastry is quite thin, so you can just trace around the circumference without cutting all the way through the pastry. Then pipe chilled pastry cream or spoon Coconut Whipped Topping (see page 480) into the middle of the cooled buns and enjoy!

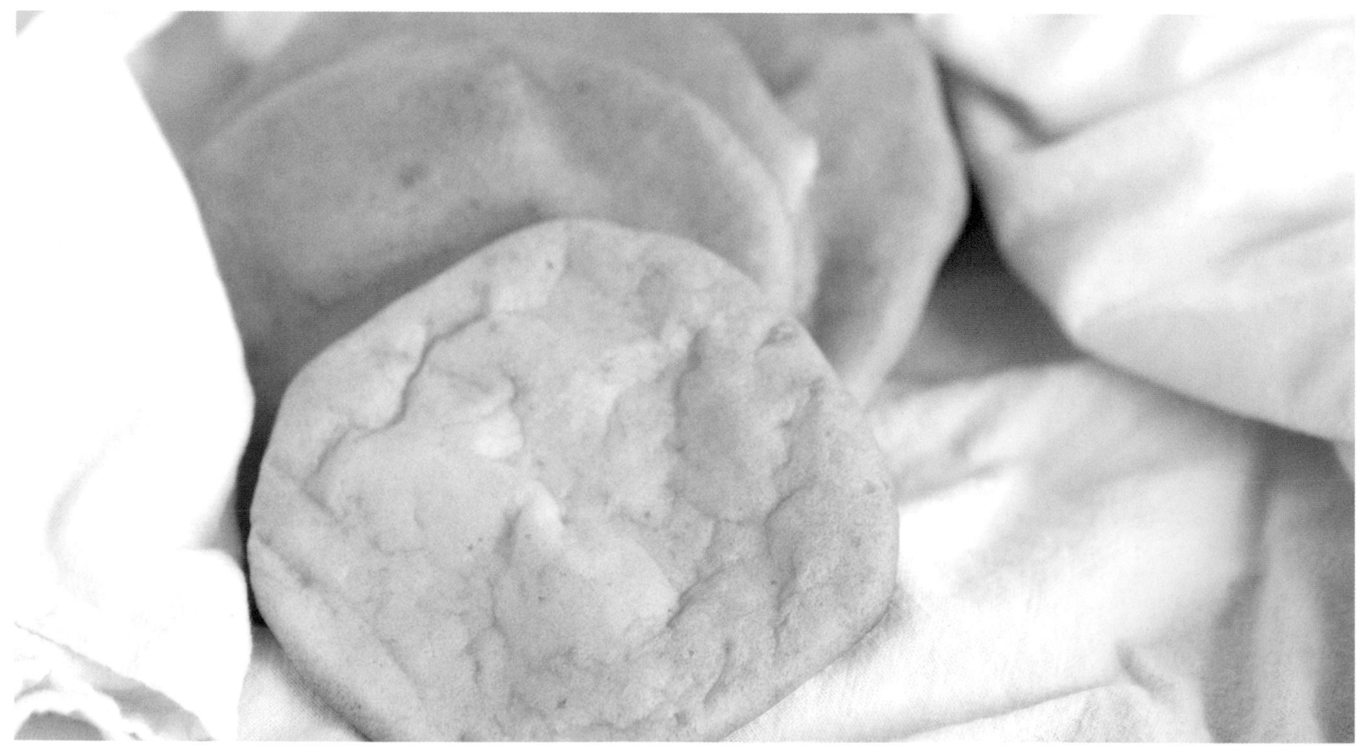

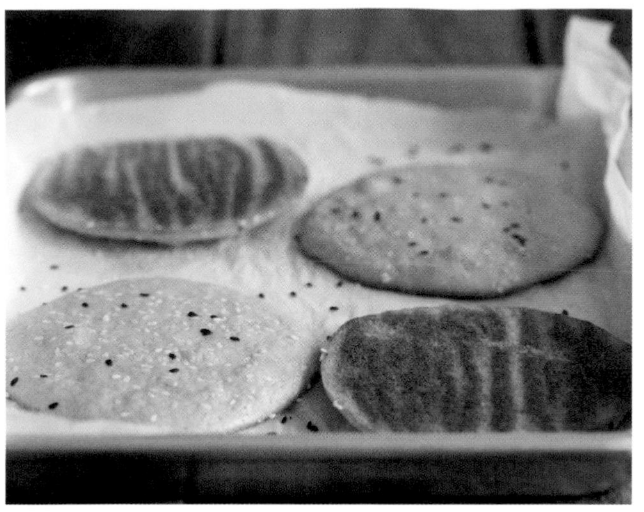

SESAME SEED BUNS

 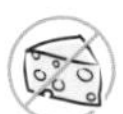 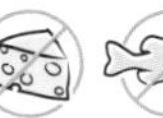  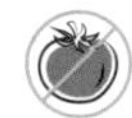

PREP TIME: 10 minutes *COOK TIME: 12 minutes*
YIELD: 2 buns

2 tablespoons sesame seeds, plus extra for sprinkling on top

2 tablespoons palm shortening, unsalted butter, ghee, or lard

2 large eggs

2 tablespoons arrowroot powder

2 tablespoons sifted coconut flour

¼ teaspoon baking soda

¼ teaspoon cream of tartar

½ teaspoon apple cider vinegar

½ teaspoon honey

Pinch of sea salt

1. Grind the sesame seeds in a spice grinder or mini food processor until finely ground.

2. Line a rimmed baking sheet with parchment paper and grease the paper lightly with palm shortening. Preheat the oven to 350°F.

3. Place all the ingredients in a blender or food processor and blend until smooth, about 30 seconds. Let the batter sit to thicken slightly, about 2 minutes.

4. Spoon into 4 globs of batter, spacing them at least 4 inches apart on the prepared baking sheet. Using the back of your spoon or a rubber spatula, spread out the dough, forming a uniform circle about 3 inches in diameter and ½ inch thick. (You are making 2 buns, or 2 tops and 2 bottoms.)

5. Sprinkle the extra sesame seeds over two of your batter circles, which will be the top halves of the buns.

6. Bake for 12 minutes. Enjoy warm or make ahead and cool on a wire rack. Store in a plastic bag in the refrigerator for up to a week.

DINNER ROLLS

 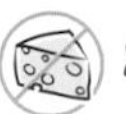 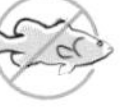  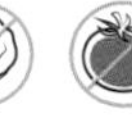

PREP TIME: 15 minutes, plus 1 hour to rise
COOK TIME: 22 minutes *YIELD: 12 rolls*

1 tablespoon active dry yeast

½ cup warm water (105°F to 110°F)

1 tablespoon honey

4 large eggs

¼ cup ghee, unsalted butter, or lard, plus another 2 tablespoons, melted for brushing

2¼ cups cassava flour

1 teaspoon sea salt

1. Proof the yeast by stirring into warm water with the honey. Let sit for 5 minutes, until foamy.

2. Place the eggs and ghee in a blender and blend on high for 1 minute, until light and foamy.

3. Combine the cassava flour and salt in a mixing bowl. Pour the egg mixture and yeast mixture into the cassava flour. Work into a stiff dough (if your dough doesn't hold together, add another tablespoon of water; or if your dough is too sticky, add another tablespoon or two of cassava flour).

4. Divide the dough into twelve parts, and roll each part into a ball (about 2 inches in diameter). Line a 9-inch square baking pan with parchment paper. Arrange the rolls in the baking pan, with about ½ inch of space between them.

5. Place the rolls in a warm spot in your kitchen (or if you have a warming/proofing feature on your oven, that's even better!) and let rise for 1 hour.

6. Preheat the oven to 375°F.

7. Brush the top of the rolls with melted ghee.

8. Place the rolls in the oven and bake for 20 to 22 minutes.

9. Serve these rolls warm or room temperature. Store the rolls in an airtight container on the countertop for up to a couple of days (they will dry out a bit over that time), or freeze for up to 6 months.

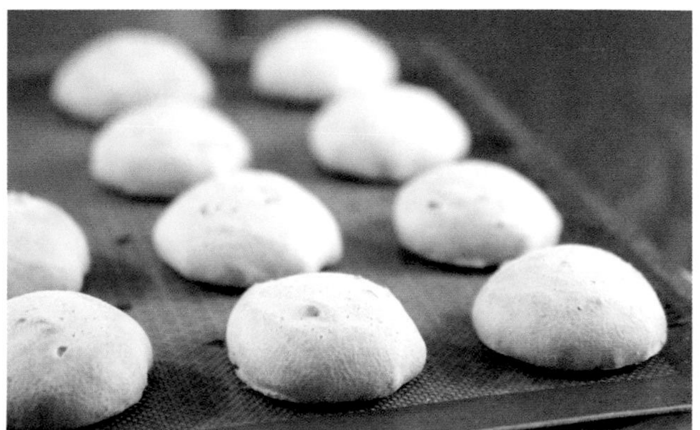

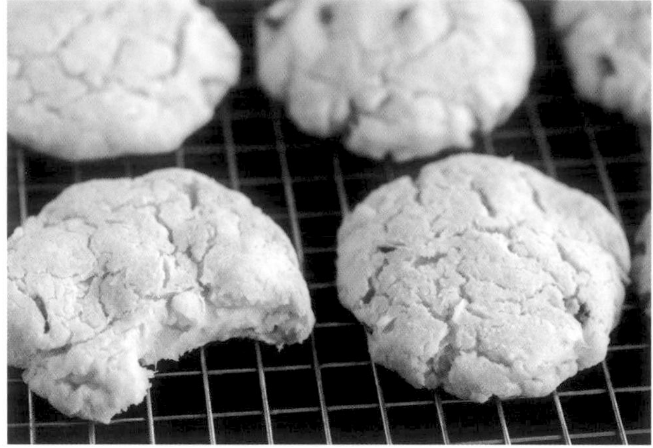

YUCA BISCUITS

 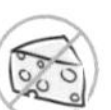 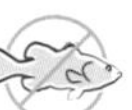  

PREP TIME: 15 minutes *COOK TIME: 25 minutes*
YIELD: 9 or 10 biscuits

- 1¾ cups mashed yuca (aka cassava, manioc, or tapioca root; about 1 pound)
- 4 tablespoons lard, unsalted butter, or ghee, divided
- ½ cup arrowroot powder
- 2 tablespoons sifted coconut flour
- ½ teaspoon sea salt
- 1 large egg
- ¼ teaspoon baking soda
- ½ teaspoon cream of tartar
- 2 tablespoons minced fresh chives (or scant 2 tablespoons dried chives)

1. To make the mashed yuca, cut away the wax-covered peel and cut the yuca into 1- to 2-inch cubes, discarding the tough stringy vein that runs down the middle. Boil the yuca cubes in salted water for about 30 minutes, until the pieces are tender enough to easily slide off a paring knife when speared. Drain and mash the cubes in a bowl using a wire potato masher (do not use a blender, immersion blender, or food processor). Let the mashed yuca cool.

2. Preheat the oven to 400°F. Line a cookie sheet with parchment paper.

3. Melt 3 tablespoons of the lard in the microwave or in a small pot on the stove.

4. Mix all the ingredients together in a bowl. The dough will be very stiff, so it might be easier to knead it together with your hands.

5. Pour the dough onto a sheet of parchment paper. Using your hands or a rolling pin, mold it into a rough circle about ½ inch thick. Use a 2-inch biscuit cutter to cut out circles of the dough and place the rounds on the prepared cookie sheet. Keep re-forming the dough to cut out more biscuits until all the dough is used.

6. Melt the remaining tablespoon of lard and use a pastry brush to brush it on the tops of the biscuits.

7. Bake for 23 to 25 minutes, until just starting to turn golden brown on the top.

8. Enjoy warm or let cool on a wire cooling rack. Store in an airtight container on the counter for up to 2 days, or freeze for up to 6 months.

PUMPKIN COFFEE CAKE

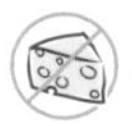 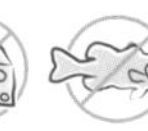 

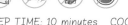

PREP TIME: 10 minutes *COOK TIME: 40 minutes*
YIELD: 10 to 12 servings

- 1½ cups pumpkin puree
- 3 large eggs
- ¼ cup honey
- ¼ cup maple syrup
- 2 tablespoons ghee or unsalted butter
- 1 teaspoon vanilla extract
- 1½ cups chestnut flour
- 2 tablespoons sifted coconut flour
- 2 tablespoons tapioca starch
- ½ teaspoon sea salt
- ¾ teaspoon baking soda
- 1 teaspoon ginger powder
- ¾ teaspoon ground allspice
- ¾ teaspoon ground cardamom
- ¾ teaspoon ground cloves
- ¾ teaspoon ground nutmeg
- ¾ cup chopped raw walnuts

1. Preheat the oven to 350°F. Grease a 12-cup tube pan or Bundt pan.

2. Combine all the ingredients except the walnuts in a blender and blend until smooth. Fold in the walnuts.

3. Pour the batter into the prepared pan and bake for 40 minutes or until a toothpick comes out clean. Store in an airtight container on the counter for up to 2 days, in the refrigerator for up to a week, or in the freezer for up to 6 months.

TIP: You can bake this coffee cake in a standard-size loaf pan; it will take 55 minutes to cook through. You can also make muffins, which will take 20 minutes to bake.

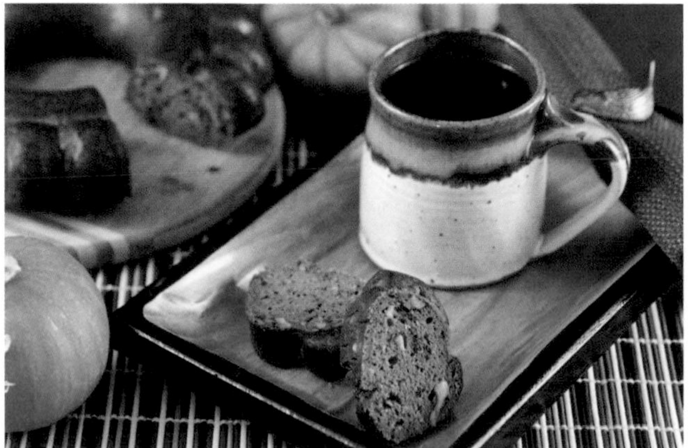

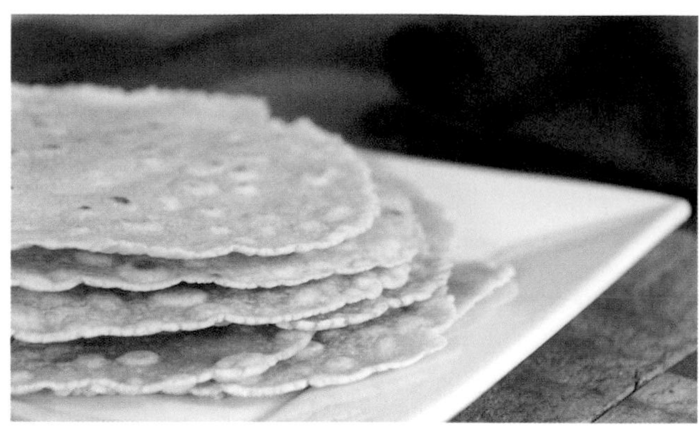

TORTILLAS

 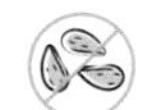 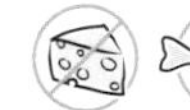  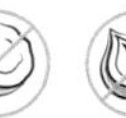 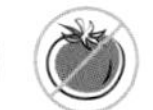 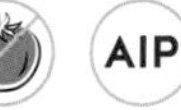 AIP

PREP TIME: 15 minutes COOK TIME: 25 minutes
YIELD: 8 tortillas

1½ cups cassava flour	⅛ teaspoon baking soda
¾ teaspoon sea salt	¾ cup warm water
¼ teaspoon cream of tartar	6 tablespoons olive oil or avocado oil

1. Combine the flour, salt, cream of tartar, and baking soda in a mixing bowl. Add the water and oil and mix with a wooden spoon or your hands until a stiff dough forms. If the dough is sticky, use a bit more flour. If the dough is crumbly, add a bit more oil.

2. Divide the dough in half, then in half again, then in half again to create 8 fairly equal portions. Form each piece into a ball.

3. Place a dough ball on a silicone baking mat or sheet of parchment paper or wax paper and flatten as much as possible with the palm of your hand. Cover the flattened dough with a sheet of parchment paper or wax paper. Roll the dough into a very flat rough circle, 8 to 10 inches in diameter. Carefully remove the bottom mat or paper so the rolled-out tortilla is stuck to one sheet of parchment paper or wax paper. Set aside and roll out the remaining dough balls. (When they're stuck to the parchment or wax paper, you can easily stack them in preparation for cooking.)

4. Preheat a 10-inch or larger skillet (well-seasoned cast iron or enameled cast iron works well here) over medium heat (or medium-high heat if using a stainless-steel skillet).

5. When the skillet is hot, peel a rolled-out raw tortilla off its parchment or wax paper and place in the skillet. Cook for about 1 minute, until the bottom has a few pale brown spots. The top will begin to show a few little bubbles. Flip and cook for 30 to 45 seconds. (Ideally, the tortilla will be soft, with a few small pale golden brown spots on the surface. If the tortilla is browning too fast, reduce the heat a bit. If it's taking longer than a minute to see a few pale golden brown spots on the underside, increase the heat a bit.) Remove from the skillet with tongs and stack in a covered container. Repeat until all the tortillas are cooked.

6. Serve warm or let cool for later use. Store in an airtight container or resealable plastic bag at room temperature for up to 24 hours. To freeze, separate the tortillas with sheets of parchment paper or wax paper and place in a resealable plastic bag; they can be frozen indefinitely.

ENGLISH MUFFINS

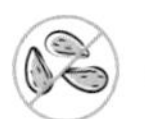 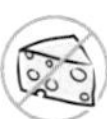 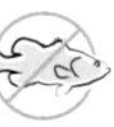    

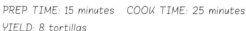

PREP TIME: 10 minutes, plus 45 minutes to rise
COOK TIME: 12 minutes YIELD: 4 English muffins

1 large green plantain	1 tablespoon avocado oil
1 large egg	¼ teaspoon sea salt
1 teaspoon active dry yeast	½ teaspoon baking soda

1. Peel the plantain and give it a rough chop. Place in a blender with the egg, yeast, avocado oil, and salt. (If your blender has a smaller jar, you'll want to use that.) Blend on high until a completely smooth puree forms.

2. Pour the batter into a bowl and let sit in a warm spot to rise for 45 minutes.

3. Preheat the oven to 425°F. Line a cookie sheet with parchment paper or a silicone baking mat. Place 4 English muffin rings on the parchment. Lightly grease the insides of the rings with lard. (Alternatively, you can grease 4 wells of a muffin top pan.)

4. Add the baking soda to the batter and whisk by hand just to combine. Spoon the batter into the prepared English muffin rings, dividing it equally among the rings.

5. Bake for 12 minutes, until browned on top. Let cool slightly before popping out of the rings.

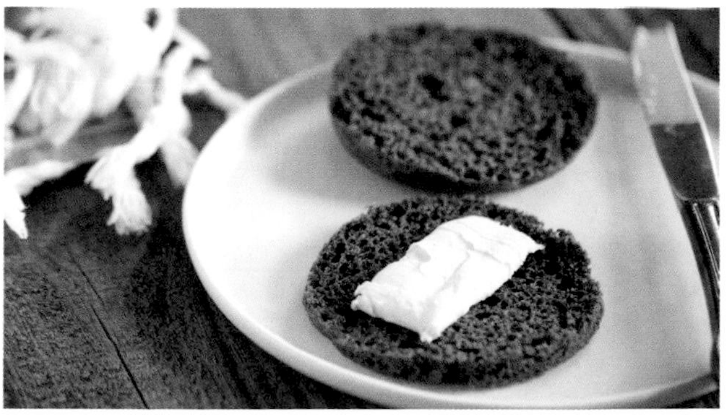

GRAHAM CRACKERS

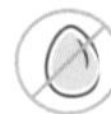 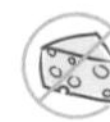 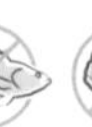  

PREP TIME: 25 minutes COOK TIME: 14 minutes
YIELD: about 3 dozen crackers

- 3 tablespoons sifted coconut flour
- ¼ cup tapioca starch
- 2 cups blanched almond flour
- 1½ teaspoons ground cinnamon
- ½ teaspoon sea salt
- ½ teaspoon cream of tartar
- ¾ teaspoon baking soda
- ½ cup palm shortening
- ⅓ cup honey

1. Place all the dry ingredients in a small bowl or measuring cup. Stir to combine.

2. In a bowl, mix together the shortening and honey with a rubber spatula or wooden spoon.

3. Add the dry ingredients to the shortening and honey mixture. Work in until fully incorporated and a stiff ball of dough holds together.

4. Split the dough in half. Roll out half of the dough between 2 sheets of parchment paper, aiming for a thickness of slightly less than ⅛ inch. Peel off the top sheet of parchment paper.

5. Use a straight-blade pastry wheel or pastry scraper to cut the dough into 2-inch squares. Remove the edge pieces that don't form squares and add them to the second half of the dough.

6. Do not try to peel the dough off the parchment paper. Instead, grab the entire sheet of parchment paper and slide it onto a cookie sheet. Put it in the freezer for 1 hour (or until you have some free time to bake it). You can stack 3 or 4 sheets of parchment paper with scored dough squares on top of them in the freezer.

7. When you're ready to bake the graham crackers, preheat the oven to 300°F. Line a cookie sheet with parchment paper.

8. Take the dough squares out of the freezer one sheet at a time. Peel the frozen squares off the parchment and place them on the prepared cookie sheet, spaced about ½ inch apart.

9. Let the squares sit at room temperature for about 5 minutes. Then prick all over the surface of each cracker with the tines of a fork. Aim to prick about halfway through the dough.

10. Bake for 13 to 14 minutes, until golden brown. Let cool on the cookie sheet for a few minutes, then remove to a wire cooling rack. Store in an airtight container at room temperature for up to a week.

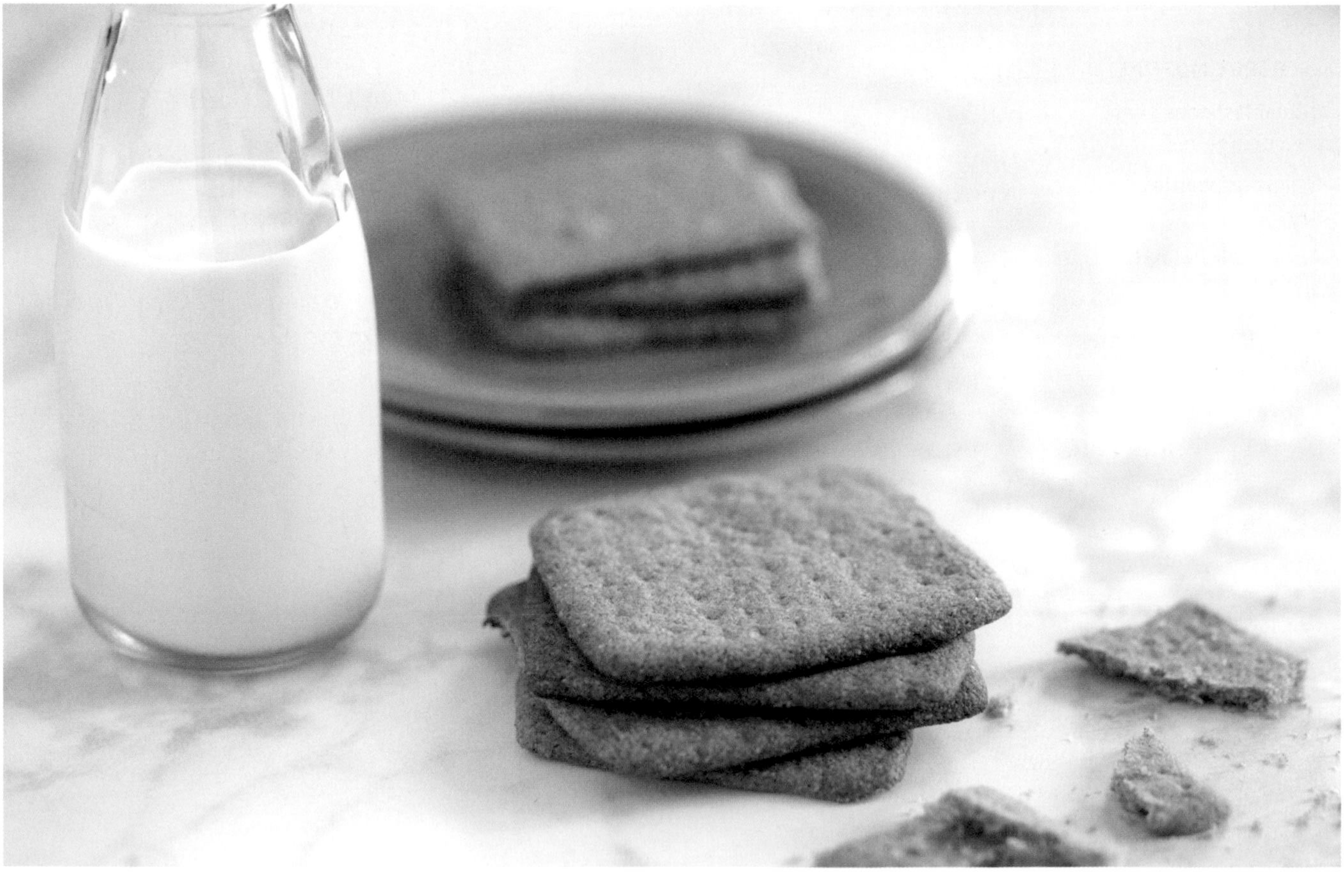

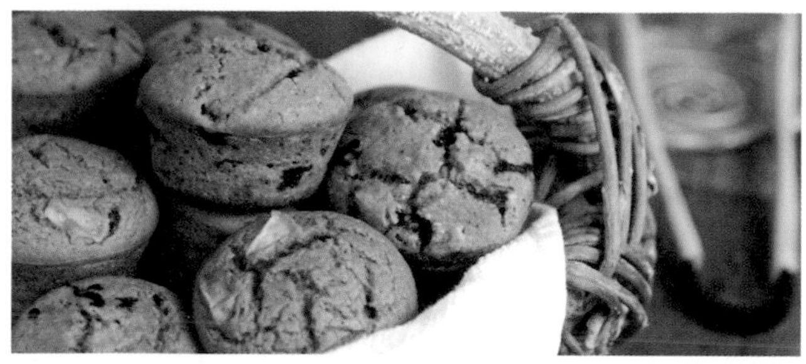

DIY MUFFINS

 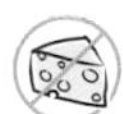 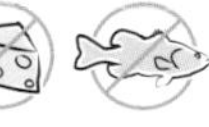 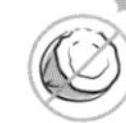  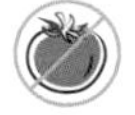

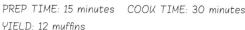

PREP TIME: 15 minutes *COOK TIME: 30 minutes*
YIELD: 12 muffins

2 large green plantains (1½ to 2 cups pureed)

5 large eggs

⅓ cup coconut oil, melted

1 tablespoon vanilla extract

¼ cup maple sugar or evaporated cane juice

½ teaspoon sea salt

⅓ cup cassava flour

½ teaspoon baking soda

BLUEBERRY MUFFINS

¼ teaspoon ground cinnamon

1½ cups blueberries, fresh or frozen

RASPBERRY MUFFINS

1 to 2 tablespoons finely grated orange zest

1½ cups raspberries, fresh or frozen

WALNUT OR PECAN MUFFINS

1 cup chopped toasted walnuts or pecans

¼ teaspoon ground cinnamon or nutmeg

1 to 2 tablespoons additional maple sugar (optional)

APPLE SPICE MUFFINS

1 large Granny Smith apple, peeled, cored, and diced

½ teaspoon ground cinnamon

¼ teaspoon ground cardamom

¼ teaspoon ground nutmeg

Pinch of ground cloves

LEMON POPPY SEED MUFFINS

3 tablespoons finely grated lemon zest

3 tablespoons poppy seeds

1 to 2 tablespoons additional maple sugar (optional)

CHOCOLATE CHIP MUFFINS

1 cup bittersweet chocolate chips

Reduce the maple sugar to 2 tablespoons (optional)

1. Preheat the oven to 350°F. Grease a standard-size 12-cup muffin pan or line with silicone or paper liners.

2. Peel the plantains and place in a blender with the eggs, coconut oil, vanilla, sugar, and salt. If the variation you are making requires additional sugar, add it during this step.

3. Blend for 1 to 2 minutes, until completely smooth, scraping the sides once or twice. Pour the mixture into a mixing bowl.

4. Add the cassava flour and baking soda and mix until thoroughly combined. Fold in the ingredients for your chosen variation.

5. Spoon the batter into the prepared muffin pan, filling the cups about three-quarters full. Bake for 27 to 30 minutes, until a toothpick inserted in the middle of one of the center muffins comes out clean. Store in an airtight container on the counter for up to 3 days, in the refrigerator for up to a week, or in the freezer for up to 6 months.

TIP: You can make these muffins with 2 yellow plantains or 5 green-tipped bananas instead of green plantains; if you do, increase the cassava flour to 2/3 cup.

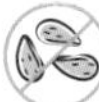 *don't make walnut or pecan muffins*

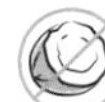 *use avocado oil or olive oil instead of coconut oil*

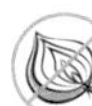 *don't make blueberry or apple spice muffins*

NUT-FREE QUICK BREAD

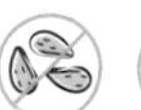 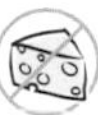 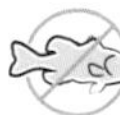 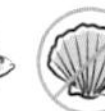 

PREP TIME: 10 minutes *COOK TIME: 35 minutes*
YIELD: 10 to 12 slices

4 large eggs

¼ cup unsalted butter, coconut oil, ghee, or palm shortening, melted

¼ cup tapioca starch

¼ cup sifted coconut flour

1 teaspoon apple cider vinegar

½ teaspoon cream of tartar

¼ teaspoon baking soda

1. Preheat the oven to 350°F. Line a 7½ by 3½-inch loaf pan with wax paper and generously grease the paper with coconut oil or lard. Alternatively, use a silicone loaf pan.

2. Beat the eggs in a blender or food processor until frothy, about 30 seconds. Add the remaining ingredients and process until smooth. Let the batter sit for a minute to thicken.

3. Pour the batter into the prepared loaf pan and smooth out the top. Bake for 35 minutes.

4. Store in a resealable plastic bag in the refrigerator for up to a week. For longer storage, slice the loaf before freezing to make it easy to thaw a few slices at a time. It will keep in the freezer for up to 6 months.

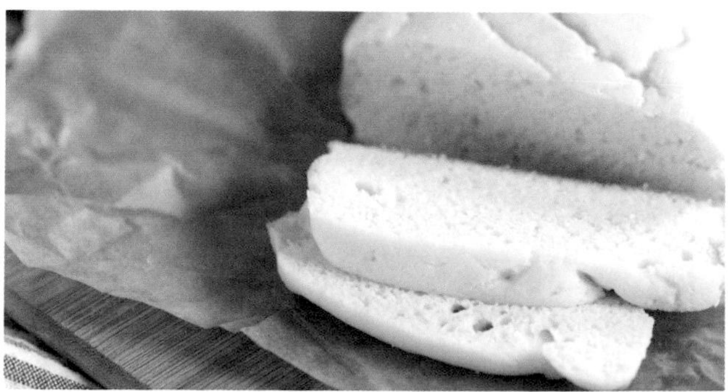

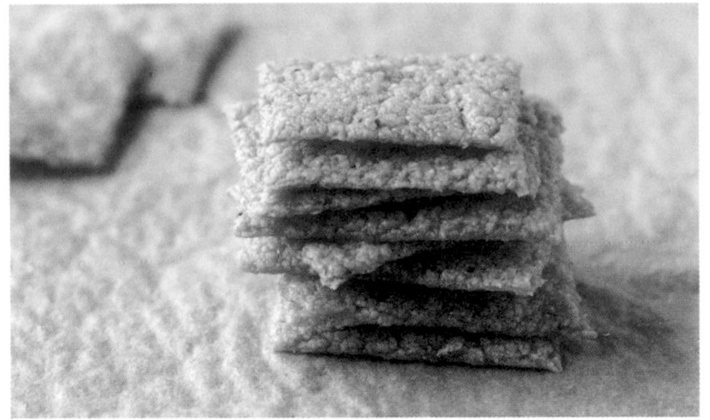

PLANTAIN CRACKERS

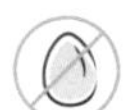 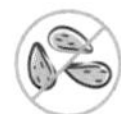 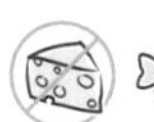 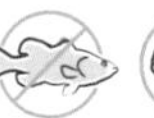 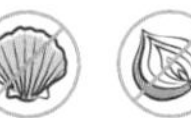  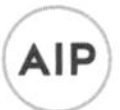 AIP

PREP TIME: 10 minutes *COOK TIME: 1 hour 30 minutes*
YIELD: 6 to 8 servings

2 large green plantains
½ cup coconut oil, melted
½ teaspoon sea salt

1. Preheat the oven to 300°F. Line a rimmed baking sheet with parchment paper, making sure the parchment goes right up to each edge of the pan.

2. Place all the ingredients in a food processor and process until a completely smooth puree forms, 2 to 4 minutes. The mixture is easier to blend if the plantains are at room temperature.

3. Pour the puree onto the lined baking sheet. Use a rubber spatula to smooth it out and cover the entire sheet uniformly. The puree should be about ⅛ inch thick.

4. Bake for 10 minutes. Remove from the oven and use a pastry wheel, pizza cutter, or pastry scraper to cut into crackers (whatever size you like). The crackers will pull away from each other slightly and shrink up a bit while baking.

5. Bake for another 50 to 80 minutes, until golden brown. Keep an eye on them and don't pull them out of the oven until they are a nice medium shade of brown. Let cool slightly on the pan, then move to a cooling rack. Once completely cool, break apart any crackers that are stuck together.

6. Store in an airtight container at room temperature for up to a week.

TIP: The baking time can vary quite a bit depending on how green the plantains are and how much volume of plantain you have in the recipe. Crackers made from greener plantains take longer to bake (and typically taste better, too), as do crackers made with slightly larger plantains.

CARROT-PARSNIP MUFFINS

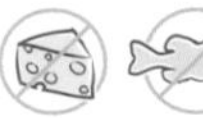 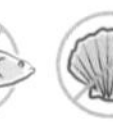  

PREP TIME: 15 minutes *COOK TIME: 35 minutes*
YIELD: 12 muffins

4 large eggs
⅓ cup evaporated cane juice
1½ cups grated carrots
1½ cups grated parsnips
2 tablespoons coconut oil, melted
½ teaspoon vanilla extract
1½ cups blanched almond flour
1 tablespoon coconut flour
¾ teaspoon baking soda
½ teaspoon cream of tartar
1 teaspoon ground nutmeg
½ teaspoon ground allspice
¼ teaspoon ginger powder
¼ teaspoon ground cardamom
½ cup chopped raw walnuts (optional)

1. Preheat the oven to 350°F. Grease a standard-size muffin pan or line the cups with silicone or paper liners.

2. Combine the eggs, evaporated cane juice, carrots, parsnips, coconut oil, and vanilla in a large bowl. Stir to form a batter.

3. Combine the almond flour, coconut flour, baking soda, cream of tartar, and spices in a small bowl. Add the dry ingredients to the wet ingredients and stir until combined into a very thick batter. Fold in the walnuts, if using.

4. Spoon the batter into the prepared muffin cups and bake for 35 minutes, until a toothpick inserted in the middle of one of the center muffins comes out clean.

5. Let cool in the pan for a few minutes before removing. Store in an airtight container on the counter for up to 2 days, in the refrigerator for up to a week, or in the freezer for up to 6 months.

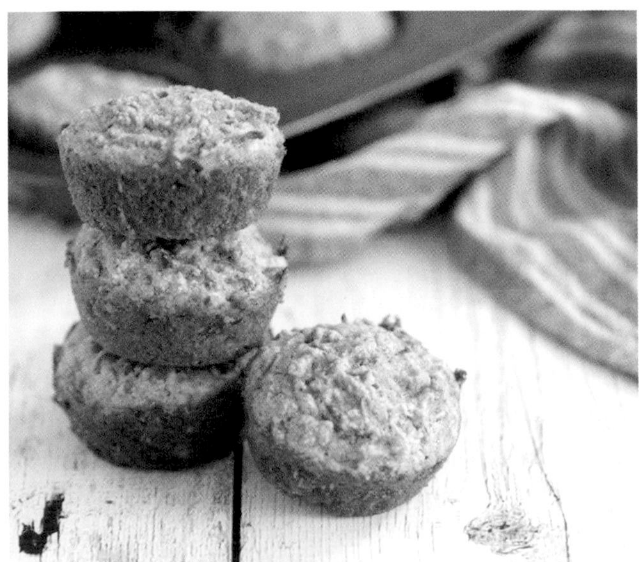

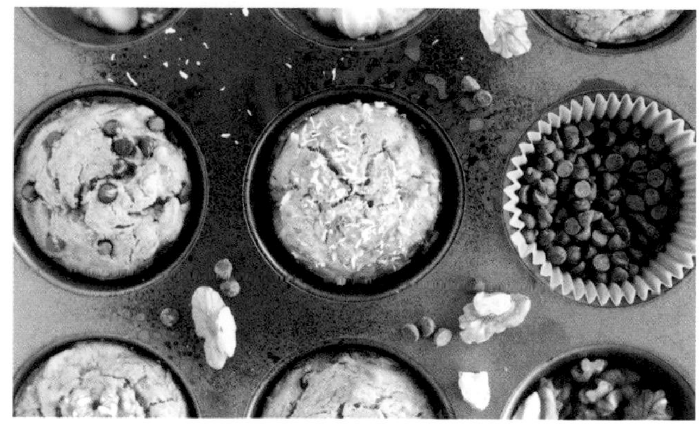

BANANA MUFFINS

 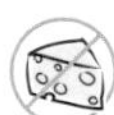 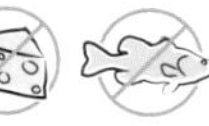 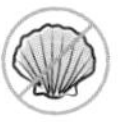 

PREP TIME: 15 minutes COOK TIME: 30 minutes
YIELD: 12 muffins

4 medium overripe bananas

⅓ cup ghee, unsalted butter, or coconut oil, melted

½ cup coconut cream or full-fat coconut milk, homemade (page 480) or canned

2 large eggs

1 cup cassava flour

¾ teaspoon baking soda

½ teaspoon sea salt

BANANA-NUT MUFFINS

¾ cup chopped raw walnuts or pecans

CHOCOLATE CHIP BANANA MUFFINS

1 cup bittersweet chocolate chips

COCONUT-MACADAMIA BANANA MUFFINS

⅔ cup macadamia nuts, chopped

⅔ cup unsweetened coconut flakes, chopped

1. Preheat the oven to 350°F. Grease a standard-size muffin pan or line the cups with silicone or paper liners.

2. If making Coconut-Macadamia Banana Muffins, toast the macadamia nuts and coconut flakes on a rimmed baking sheet in the oven until starting to brown, 6 to 8 minutes, stirring every 2 to 3 minutes.

3. In a large mixing bowl, mash the bananas with a fork to form a lumpy puree (do not use a food processor or blender).

4. Add the melted ghee, coconut cream, and eggs. Stir to completely combine.

5. In a separate bowl, combine the cassava flour, baking soda, and salt. Add the dry ingredients to the banana mixture and stir to fully combine.

6. Fold in the ingredients for the variation you are making, if desired. (These muffins are tasty plain, too!)

7. Spoon the batter into the prepared muffin cups, filling them about three-quarters full. Bake for 27 to 30 minutes, until a toothpick inserted in the middle of one of the center muffins comes out clean. Store in an airtight container on the counter for up to 3 days, in the fridge for up to a week, or in the freezer for up to 6 months.

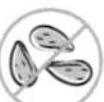 *don't make banana-nut muffins*

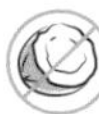 *don't make coconut-macadamia banana muffins; use butter, ghee, or olive oil*

CHEWY GRANOLA BARS

 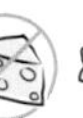 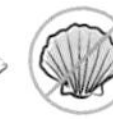 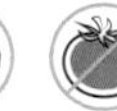

PREP TIME: 10 minutes COOK TIME: 25 minutes
YIELD: 10 to 16 servings

½ cup coconut flakes, chopped

2 large eggs

1 tablespoon honey

1 teaspoon vanilla extract

Pinch of sea salt

Pinch of ground cinnamon

½ cup finely unsweetened shredded coconut

½ cup raw pepitas, chopped

⅓ cup shelled sunflower seeds

3 tablespoons sesame seeds

⅓ cup dried apricots, chopped

⅓ cup dried cranberries, chopped

¼ cup mini bittersweet chocolate chips

1. Preheat the oven to 350°F. Grease a 9-inch square baking pan with coconut oil or palm shortening.

2. If desired, toast the coconut flakes in a skillet over medium-high heat for 6 to 7 minutes, until lightly browned.

3. Place the eggs, honey, vanilla, salt, and cinnamon in a blender and blend for about 20 seconds.

4. Combine the remaining dry ingredients in a bowl. Pour the egg mixture over the dry ingredients and mix thoroughly. Pour the granola into the prepared baking pan and press down evenly.

5. Bake for 18 minutes. Let cool completely, then cut into bars or squares. Store in an airtight container in the refrigerator for up to a week.

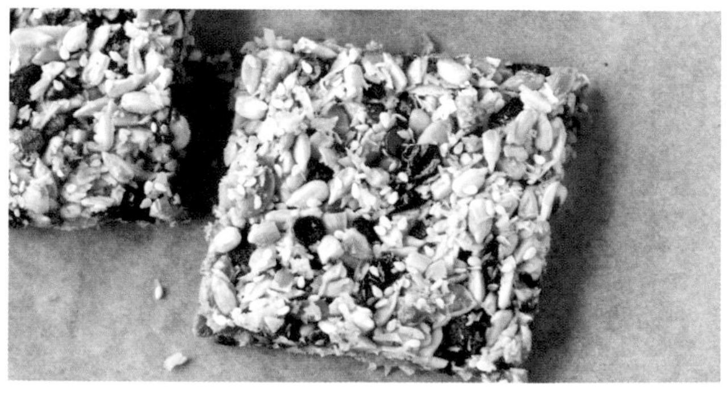

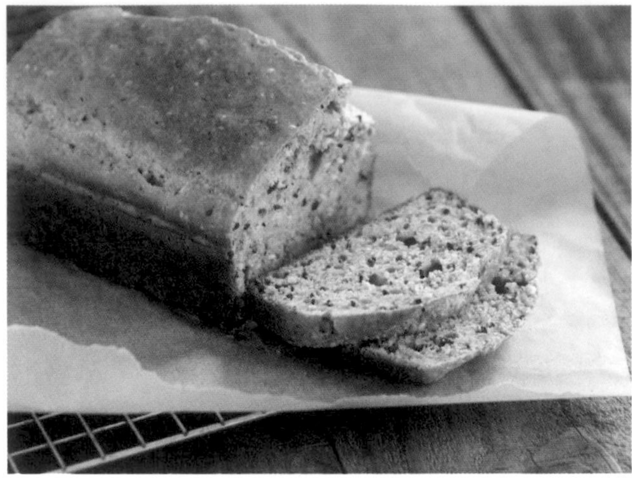

"MULTIGRAIN" QUICK BREAD

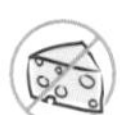 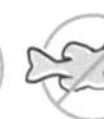  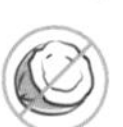 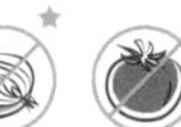

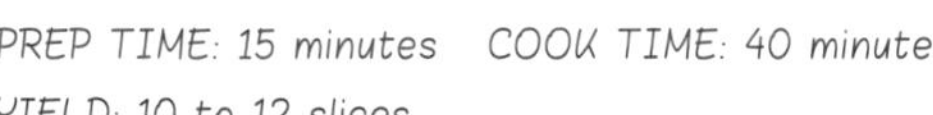

PREP TIME: 15 minutes COOK TIME: 40 minutes
YIELD: 10 to 12 slices

- 1½ cups blanched almond flour
- ½ cup arrowroot powder
- ¼ cup tapioca starch
- ½ teaspoon baking soda
- ½ teaspoon sea salt
- 4 large eggs
- 1 teaspoon honey
- 1 teaspoon apple cider vinegar
- ¼ cup raw pepitas, roughly chopped
- ¼ cup raw shelled sunflower seeds
- 2 tablespoons white sesame seeds
- 2 tablespoons black sesame seeds

1. Preheat the oven to 350°F. Grease a 7½ by 3½-inch loaf pan very generously with coconut oil, or use a silicone loaf pan.

2. In a small bowl or measuring cup, combine the almond flour, arrowroot powder, tapioca starch, baking soda, and salt.

3. In a large bowl, beat the eggs with a hand mixer until thick and frothy, 4 to 5 minutes. Stir in the honey and vinegar.

4. Fold the dry ingredients into the egg mixture until well combined. Fold in the pepitas and other seeds.

5. Pour the batter into the prepared loaf pan. Bake for 40 minutes. Let cool for 10 to 15 minutes before removing from the pan to slice.

6. Store in a plastic bag in the refrigerator for up to a week. For longer storage, slice the loaf before freezing to make it easy to thaw a few slices at a time. It will keep in the freezer for up to 6 months.

 *use maple syrup instead of honey*

FLATBREAD

 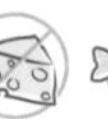 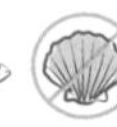 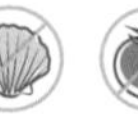

PREP TIME: 10 minutes COOK TIME: 11 minutes
YIELD: one 10-inch round flatbread (about 2 servings)

- 1 tablespoon olive oil, for the pizza stone/skillet
- 1 batch Pizza Crust (page 499), made without oregano and granulated garlic
- 1 teaspoon chopped fresh rosemary
- 2 cloves garlic, crushed to a coarse paste
- ½ teaspoon Maldon sea salt or other coarse salt

FOR SERVING (OPTIONAL)

- 3 tablespoons olive oil
- 1 tablespoon balsamic vinegar
- ⅛ teaspoon cracked black pepper
- Pinch of sea salt

1. Rub a pizza stone or large well-seasoned cast-iron skillet with 1 tablespoon of olive oil and place in the oven to heat. Preheat the oven to 450°F.

2. Remove the hot pizza stone or skillet from the oven. Pour the pizza crust dough onto the hot stone or into the hot pan, using a spatula to spread it into a 9- to 10-inch circle of even thickness (about ¼ inch thick). Sprinkle the rosemary, garlic, and salt over the top.

3. Bake for 9 to 11 minutes, depending on how crispy you like it.

4. Remove the flatbread from the pizza stone or skillet to a cutting board. Cut in half, then slice into 1-inch strips.

5. If desired, mix the olive oil with the balsamic vinegar, pepper, and salt as a dip for the flatbread.

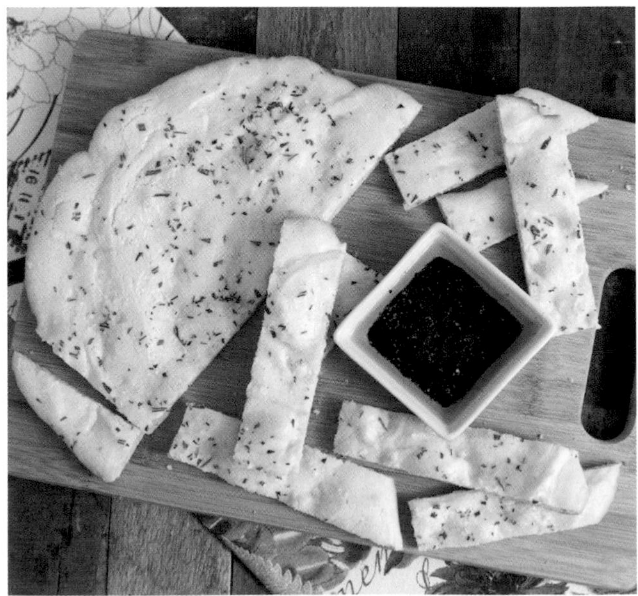

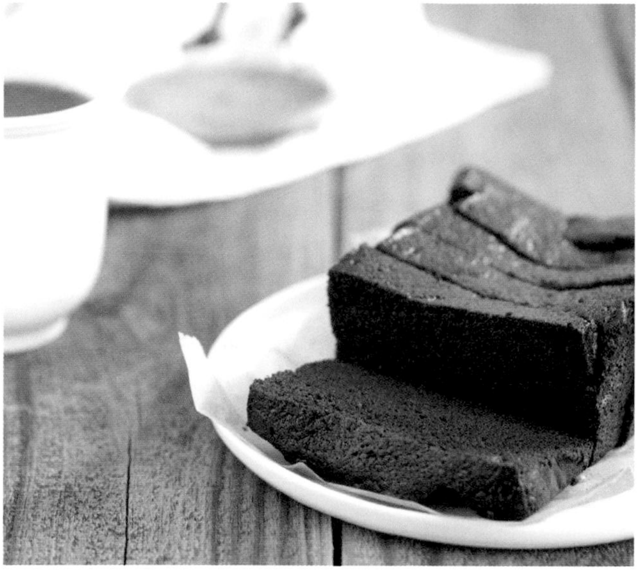

MEXICAN CHOCOLATE COFFEE CAKE

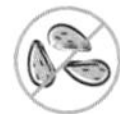 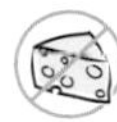 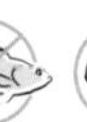  

PREP TIME: 10 minutes *COOK TIME: 1 hour*
YIELD: 10 to 12 servings

⅓ cup plus 1 tablespoon coconut flour

⅓ cup cacao powder

1 teaspoon ground cinnamon

½ teaspoon cayenne pepper

½ teaspoon baking soda

½ teaspoon sea salt

6 large eggs

½ cup honey

½ cup blackstrap molasses

2 teaspoons vanilla extract

½ cup coconut oil, melted

3 ounces unsweetened chocolate, melted

1. Preheat the oven to 325°F. Line a 9 by 5-inch loaf pan with wax paper. Grease the wax paper with coconut oil.

2. Sift the coconut flour, cacao powder, cinnamon, cayenne, baking soda, and salt into a small bowl.

3. In a food processor or blender, combine the eggs, honey, molasses, and vanilla. Pulse a few times to combine. Add the melted coconut oil and chocolate and process for 1 minute.

4. Add the dry ingredients to the food processor or blender and pulse to combine.

5. Pour the batter into the prepared loaf pan and bake for 55 to 60 minutes (test at the 55-minute mark).

6. Let the coffee cake cool completely in the pan. Remove from the pan and carefully remove the wax paper. Store in an airtight container on the counter for up to 3 days, in the refrigerator for up to a week, or in the freezer for up to 6 months.

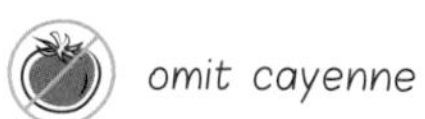 *omit cayenne*

MONKEY BARS

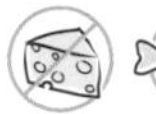 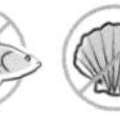 

PREP TIME: 15 minutes *COOK TIME: 18 minutes*
YIELD: 20 large squares

2 large overripe bananas

½ cup crunchy almond butter

3 large eggs

¼ cup coconut oil, melted

1 cup almond meal or almond flour

3 tablespoons sifted coconut flour

½ teaspoon baking soda

¼ teaspoon sea salt

⅓ cup mini bittersweet chocolate chips

DRIZZLE TOPPING (OPTIONAL)

1 ounce bittersweet chocolate

1½ teaspoons unsalted butter, lard, palm shortening, or ghee

1. Preheat the oven to 350°F. Grease a 13 by 9-inch baking pan with coconut oil.

2. Peel the bananas and place in a mixing bowl. Mash the bananas with a fork until mushy and smooth. Add the almond butter, eggs, melted coconut oil, almond meal, coconut flour, baking soda, and salt. Mix thoroughly to form a batter. Fold in the chocolate chips.

3. Pour the batter into the prepared baking pan and spread it evenly with a spatula or spoon.

4. Bake for 17 to 18 minutes, until a toothpick inserted in the center comes out clean. Let cool, then cut into squares.

5. To make the optional drizzle topping, melt the chocolate and butter together. Use a spoon to drizzle the chocolate mixture over the tops of the bars. You can let the topping harden at room temperature or pop the bars in the refrigerator if you're feeling impatient. Store in an airtight container in the fridge for up to a week or in the freezer for up to 6 months.

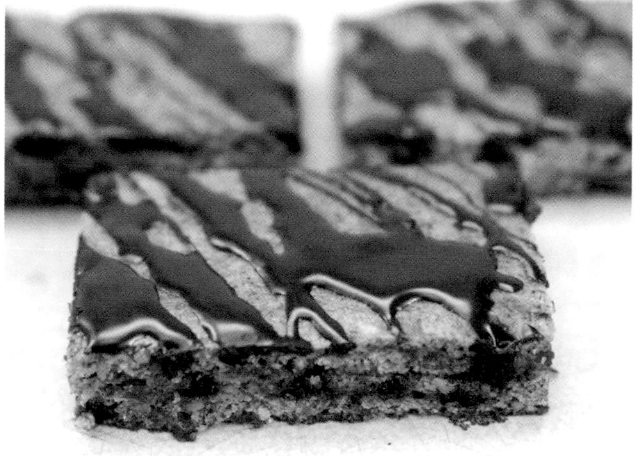

Chapter 45:
DESSERTS

SPICE CAKE WITH MAPLE CASHEW FROSTING

 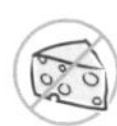 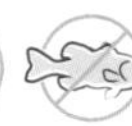  

PREP TIME: 30 minutes COOK TIME: 30 minutes
YIELD: one 8- or 9-inch cake

CAKE

12 large eggs, room temperature

1 cup honey

½ cup coconut oil, melted

½ cup palm shortening or unsalted butter

¾ cup sifted coconut flour

½ cup arrowroot powder

2 teaspoons ginger powder

1 teaspoon ground cinnamon

1 teaspoon sea salt (see Tip)

½ teaspoon baking soda

½ teaspoon ground allspice

½ teaspoon ground cloves

½ teaspoon ground cardamom

½ teaspoon ground nutmeg

FROSTING

1 cup smooth cashew butter

1 cup palm shortening or unsalted butter

⅓ cup maple syrup

Ground cinnamon or nutmeg, for dusting (optional)

1. Grease three 8- or 9-inch round cake pans with palm shortening. Cut out circles of wax paper and line the bottom of each pan, then grease the wax paper. Dust the pans with 1 or 2 tablespoons of arrowroot powder and tap and swish it around to coat. Discard any leftover powder in the pans and set aside.

2. Preheat the oven to 350°F.

3. Combine all the cake ingredients in the bowl of a stand mixer and whip for 3 to 4 minutes, until thoroughly mixed and smooth.

4. Divide the batter among the 3 pans. Spread the batter to the edges of each pan.

5. Place the cakes in the oven on 2 racks, spacing them out so that they bake evenly. Bake for 27 to 28 minutes, rotating the pans halfway through, until a toothpick inserted in the middle of a cake comes out clean.

6. Let cool on wire racks until the cakes are room temperature. Invert each cake over a plate or cutting board.

7. Prepare the frosting: Whip the cashew butter, shortening, and maple syrup in the bowl of a stand mixer for 1 to 2 minutes, until fluffy. Store in the refrigerator but allow to come to room temperature before frosting the cake.

8. Place the first cake layer on a cake plate or serving dish, cover the top of the cake with frosting, add the second layer, cover it with frosting, and then add the third layer. Cover the whole cake with frosting. Dust the top with cinnamon or nutmeg, if desired.

TIP: If using salted cashew butter to make the frosting, use just 1/2 teaspoon salt in the cake batter.

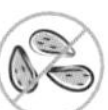 *use sunflower seed butter for frosting*

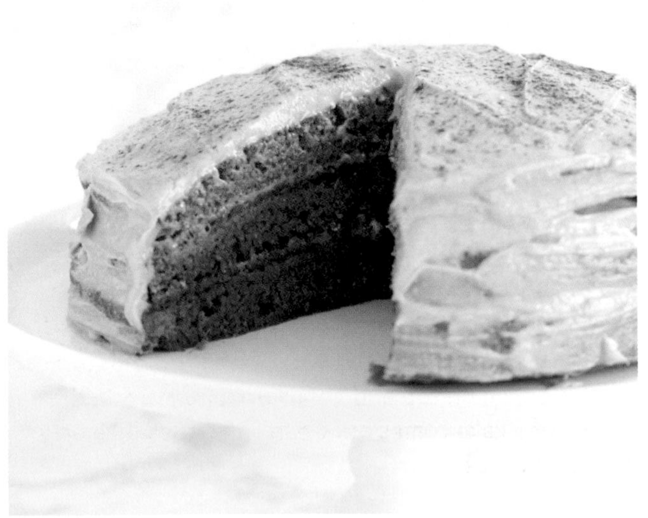

VANILLA CAKE WITH WHIPPED CHOCOLATE FROSTING

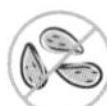 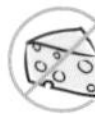 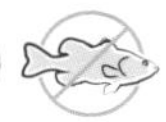 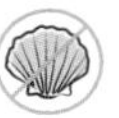 

PREP TIME: 20 minutes, plus time to chill frosting
COOK TIME: 28 minutes YIELD: 1 cake or 2 dozen cupcakes

12 large eggs, room temperature

1 cup honey

¾ cup palm shortening or unsalted butter

¼ cup coconut oil, melted

1 tablespoon vanilla extract

Seeds scraped from 1 (8-inch) Madagascar vanilla bean (see Tips)

¾ cup sifted coconut flour

½ cup arrowroot powder

½ teaspoon baking soda

1 teaspoon sea salt

FROSTING

8 ounces semisweet to bittersweet chocolate

1 cup palm shortening or unsalted butter

1. Preheat the oven to 350°F. Prepare the cake pans or muffin pans, if needed:

If using three 8- or 9-inch round cake pans to make a layer cake, trace the bottom of a pan on a piece of wax paper and cut out the circle. Repeat twice more so you have 3 wax paper circles. Grease the pans with palm shortening, lay a wax paper circle on the bottom of each pan, and then grease the wax paper. Add 1 to 2 tablespoons of arrowroot powder to each pan and tap and swish it around to coat. Discard any leftover powder in the pans and set aside.

If using muffin pans to make cupcakes, line each muffin cup with a paper or silicone liner.

If using silicone cake pans or muffin pans, no additional prep work is necessary.

2. Beat the eggs in the bowl of a stand mixer for 1 minute. Add the honey, shortening, coconut oil, and vanilla extract and seeds and beat to combine.

3. In a separate bowl, combine the coconut flour, arrowroot powder, baking soda, and salt. Add the dry ingredients to the wet ingredients and beat on high for 1 to 2 minutes, until the batter is smooth. Allow the batter to sit for 1 to 2 minutes to thicken.

4. Divide the batter evenly between the prepared pans. Use a rubber spatula to spread the batter to the edges. If making cupcakes, fill each liner about two-thirds full.

5. Stagger the pans in the oven. Bake round layers for 27 to 28 minutes, until the cakes are starting to turn golden brown on top and a toothpick inserted in the middle of a cake comes out clean. Cupcakes take only about 22 minutes.

6. Let cool completely on a wire rack before removing from the pans. The cupcakes can be removed earlier.

7. To remove cake layers from round cake pans, run a knife around the edge of each cake. Put one hand over the top of the cake and invert the pan. The cake should fall into your hand (if it doesn't, try putting the pan upside down on a cutting board and tap the bottom gently). Put a plate or cutting board where the pan used to be and flip it right side up again.

8. To make the frosting, melt the chocolate and shortening in a saucepan on the stovetop or in a microwave-safe bowl in the microwave, being careful not to burn it. Mix to completely combine. Let the frosting cool to room temperature; this takes several hours, but you can speed up the process by placing it in the refrigerator.

9. Once cool, the frosting is ready to use as a ganache-style frosting. If you prefer a lighter frosting, whip the frosting in the bowl of a stand mixer fitted with the whisk attachment for 3 to 4 minutes, until light and fluffy.

10. Using an offset spatula, frost the cake or cupcakes. For the layer cake, place the first layer on a cake plate or serving dish, cover the top with frosting, add the second layer, cover it with frosting, add the third layer, and then cover the whole cake with frosting.

TIPS: To scrape the seeds from a vanilla bean, slice the vanilla bean pod open lengthwise with a sharp knife, then scrape the seeds out of each half of the pod with a knife.

Instead of using frosting between the cake layers, try fruit preserves or jam instead!

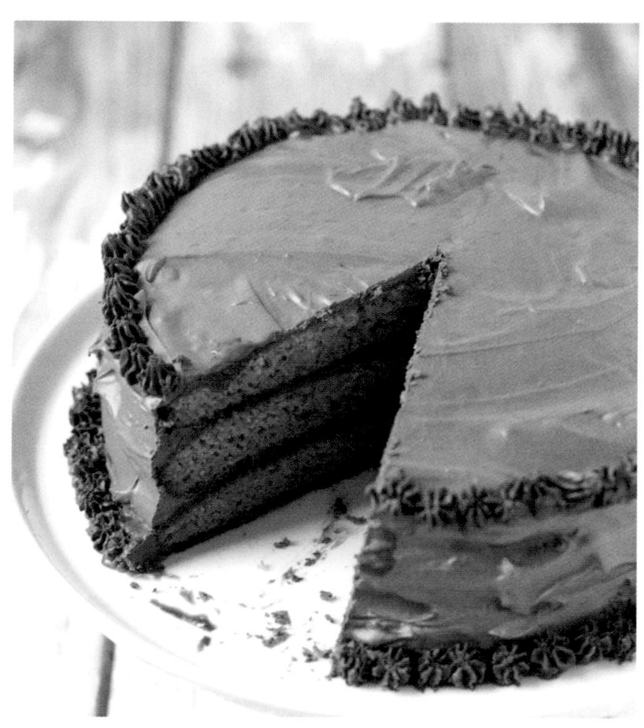

CHOCOLATE ÉCLAIRS

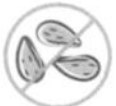 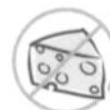 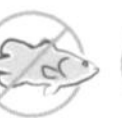  

PREP TIME: 30 minutes, plus time to cool
COOK TIME: 30 minutes
YIELD: sixteen to twenty 4-inch-long éclairs

3 cups coconut cream, homemade (page 480) or store-bought (see Tip)

8 large egg yolks

1 cup arrowroot powder

¾ cup honey

1½ tablespoons vanilla extract

Seeds scraped from 2 (8-inch) Madagascar vanilla beans

1 batch Choux Pastry dough (page 564)

CHOCOLATE GLAZE

1¾ ounces bittersweet chocolate

1 tablespoon palm shortening or unsalted butter

1. To make the pastry cream, combine the coconut cream, egg yolks, arrowroot powder, honey, and vanilla extract and seeds in a large saucepan and whisk together.

2. Put the saucepan over medium-low heat; bring the mixture to just below the boiling point, whisking constantly. The pastry cream will start to steam slightly and then start to thicken. Once it becomes thick and gooey, remove it from the heat. It takes 7 to 8 minutes if you put it on a preheated element.

3. Pour the pastry cream into a bowl or measuring cup and cover the surface with wax paper to prevent a skin from forming on top. Let cool to room temperature before piping the cream into the éclairs.

4. While the pastry cream is cooling, make the choux pastry dough by completing Steps 1 through 5 on page 564. Pipe the dough onto the prepared cookie sheets into 4 by 1-inch rectangles, spacing them at least 1 inch apart.

5. Bake and cool the pastries following Steps 6 and 7 on page 564.

6. Once cool, cut the pastries in half using a sharp knife (the pastry is quite thin, so you can just trace around the circumference without cutting all the way through the whole pastry). Pipe the cooled pastry cream into the middle. Make sure to cut and fill the pastries relatively promptly after they have cooled. They have a habit of getting soft if they sit too long and are then much harder to cut open cleanly.

7. Melt the chocolate and shortening together on the stovetop or in your microwave. Spread over the tops of the éclairs with a spatula or the back of a spoon. Serve. Store in the refrigerator for up to a week.

TIP: For this much coconut cream, it's easiest to buy coconut cream. But please do not confuse coconut cream with creamed coconut or coconut cream concentrate, both of which are the same thing as coconut butter. You can also make your own cream from homemade coconut milk, following the instructions on page 480, but you'll need to make 4 1/2 batches of coconut milk. Alternatively, you can chill cans of full-fat coconut milk overnight and scoop the cream off the top. You'll need four or five 13 1/2-ounce cans to get this much cream.

PASTRY CREAM VARIATIONS:

Lighter pastry cream. *Fold in 1 cup softly whipped heavy cream or coconut cream to the cooled pastry cream.*

Chocolate pastry cream. *Add 4 ounces finely grated bittersweet or unsweetened chocolate to the hot pastry cream. Stir until melted.*

Coffee pastry cream. *Add 1 to 2 tablespoons very finely ground coffee powder to the saucepan with the rest of the ingredients.*

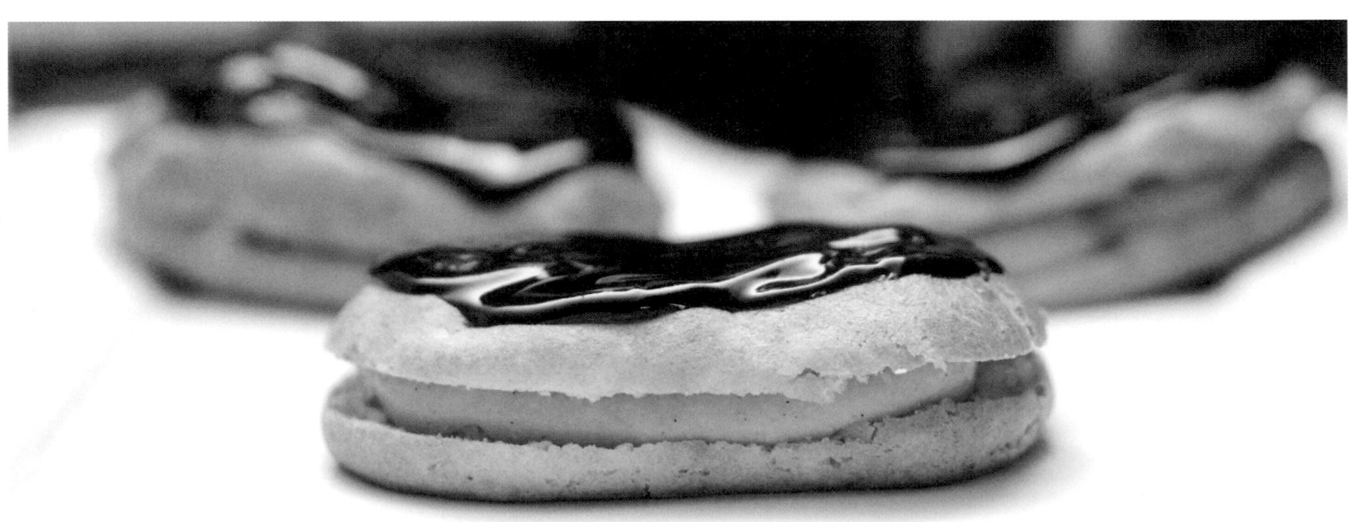

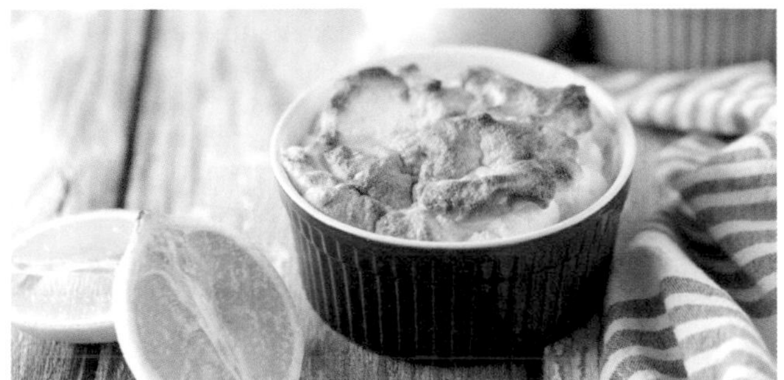

MEYER LEMON CUSTARD SOUFFLÉ

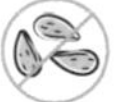 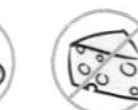   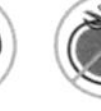 

PREP TIME: 30 minutes COOK TIME: 25 minutes
YIELD: 4 servings

1 large whole egg, plus 3 room-temperature eggs, separated

6 tablespoons evaporated cane juice or maple sugar, blended to a superfine powder (measure after blending; see Tips), divided

Juice and finely grated zest of 2 large Meyer lemons (3 to 4 tablespoons juice and 1 to 1½ tablespoons zest), divided

1 teaspoon arrowroot powder

2 tablespoons unsalted butter, lard, palm shortening, or ghee

1. Combine the whole egg, 2 tablespoons of the evaporated cane juice, the juice and zest from one of the lemons, and the arrowroot powder in a small saucepan. Whisk well.

2. Place the saucepan over medium heat and whisk fairly constantly until the mixture thickens (3 to 4 minutes, depending on how long it takes your element to heat up). Remove the pan from the heat.

3. Whisk in the butter. If the butter isn't incorporating well, pour the custard into a blender and blend for 30 seconds. Divide the custard evenly between four 6-ounce or 8-ounce ramekins. Place the ramekins on a cookie sheet and let the custard cool while you prepare the soufflé.

4. Preheat the oven to 350°F.

5. In a small bowl, combine the 3 egg yolks and the juice and zest of the remaining lemon. Set aside.

6. In a medium bowl, whip the 3 egg whites using a hand mixer (or small stand mixer) until soft peaks form (basically until it's foamy and starting to hold its shape). Gradually add the remaining 4 tablespoons of evaporated cane juice, 1 tablespoon at a time, while continuing to whip the egg whites. Whip until all the sugar is incorporated and stiff peaks form (basically until it holds its shape completely).

7. Spoon a large amount of the egg whites into the egg yolk mixture. Fold until completely combined (this thickens the yolks before you fold into the rest of the whites so that you retain more of the air you whipped into the whites).

8. Fold the thickened egg yolk mixture into the rest of the whites. Gently fold until just barely incorporated. Spoon over the custard in the ramekins.

9. Immediately place in the oven. Bake for 15 to 17 minutes, until golden brown. Serve immediately.

TIPS: To get the right consistency before measuring, place the evaporated cane juice in a blender and blend for about 1 minute, until it is a superfine powder.

If you want to use regular lemons instead of Meyer lemons, add an extra tablespoon of evaporated cane juice to both the custard and the soufflé.

Soufflés do fall after they are removed from the oven, so ideally you would time this dessert to be served fairly soon after they come out of the oven (within 5 minutes). But really, don't worry if your soufflé falls while cooking. It will still taste good!

CHOCOLATE SHELL TOPPING

 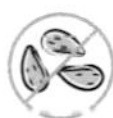 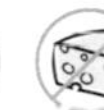 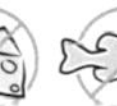 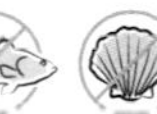  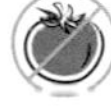

PREP TIME: 5 minutes COOK TIME: 5 minutes YIELD: 1 cup

6 ounces bittersweet chocolate

½ cup coconut oil

1. Melt the chocolate and coconut oil in a small saucepan over low heat or on medium power in the microwave. Stir well, then let cool.

2. Store in a glass jar at room temperature.

3. Pour over Vanilla Ice Cream (page 585), or use for Monkey's Lunch Ice Cream Bars (page 582) or Chocolate-Dipped Ice Cream Sandwiches (page 579).

TIP: Before using the shell topping, make sure it hasn't solidified during storage. To re-liquefy it, gently heat it in the microwave for about 30 seconds.

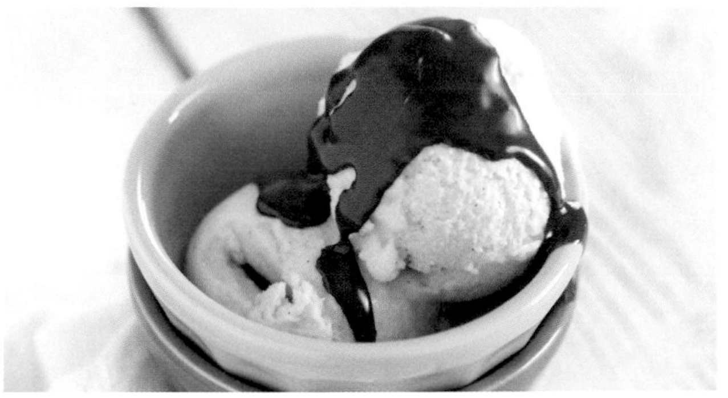

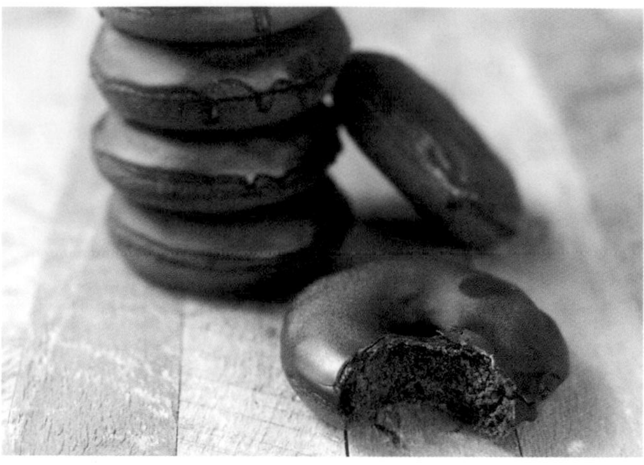

CHOCOLATE-GLAZED CHOCOLATE DOUGHNUTS

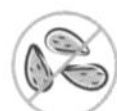 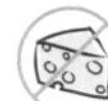 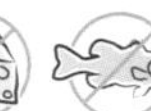  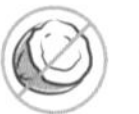 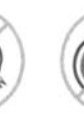 

PREP TIME: 15 minutes
COOK TIME: 6 minutes
YIELD: 12 mini doughnuts

1 large green plantain

2 large eggs

4 ounces bittersweet chocolate

2 tablespoons lard, unsalted butter, ghee, or palm shortening

½ teaspoon ground vanilla bean (optional)

¼ teaspoon baking soda

Generous pinch of sea salt

CHOCOLATE GLAZE

2 ounces semisweet chocolate

1 tablespoon unsalted butter, ghee, or palm shortening

Special equipment: mini doughnut maker

1. Peel and quarter the plantain and put in a blender with the eggs. Puree until completely smooth.

2. Melt the chocolate and lard together (you can do this in a double boiler on the stovetop or in a microwave-safe bowl on medium power in the microwave). Preheat the mini-doughnut maker.

3. Add the vanilla bean, baking soda, and salt to the plantain-egg mixture in the blender. Blend for a few seconds to combine.

4. Turn the blender on low and remove the lid insert. Slowly pour the melted chocolate-lard mixture into the blender and keep blending until it's fully incorporated.

5. Once the mini-doughnut maker is preheated, pour the batter into each well, filling to exactly level with the top of the well. Close the lid and cook for 6 minutes or according to the manufacturer's directions.

6. Carefully remove the doughnuts and let cool on a wire cooling rack before glazing. Repeat with the remaining batter.

7. To glaze the doughnuts, melt the chocolate and ghee in a saucepan, stirring well. Place in a shallow bowl.

8. Carefully dip one side of each doughnut into the melted chocolate (if it starts to cool, it will coat the doughnuts more thickly and end up more like a frosting than a glaze). Place the doughnuts, glaze side up, on a baking sheet lined with parchment paper, wax paper, or a silicone baking mat.

9. Let cool to room temperature and enjoy! Store in the refrigerator for up to 2 days or in the freezer for up to 6 months.

CINNAMON-APPLE 2-MINUTE MUG CAKE

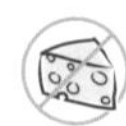 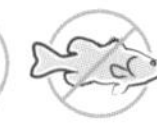  

PREP TIME: 5 minutes *COOK TIME: 2 minutes*
YIELD: 1 small cake

1 large egg

½ apple, peeled, cored, and finely chopped

3 tablespoons almond flour

2 tablespoons chopped raw walnuts

1 tablespoon unsweetened shredded coconut

2 tablespoons honey

¼ teaspoon ground cinnamon

Pinch of sea salt

Vanilla Ice Cream (page 585), for serving (optional)

1. Combine all the ingredients in a microwave-safe mug and stir to combine.

2. Microwave on high power for 1 minute 45 seconds to 2 minutes (less if you have a high-powered microwave, more if you have a lower-powered microwave).

3. Enjoy warm. Serve with ice cream, if desired.

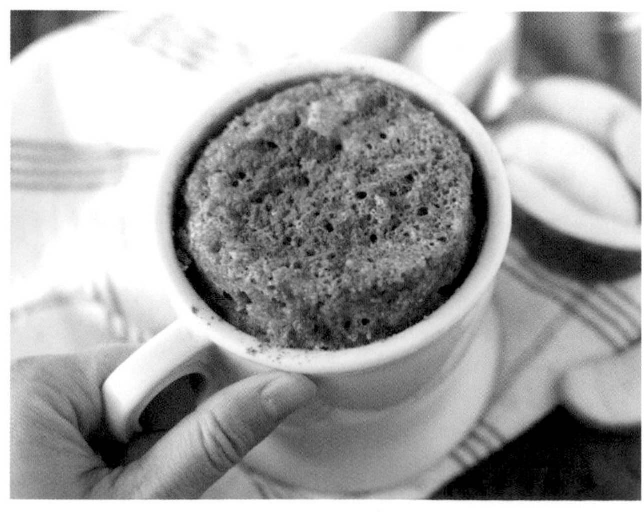

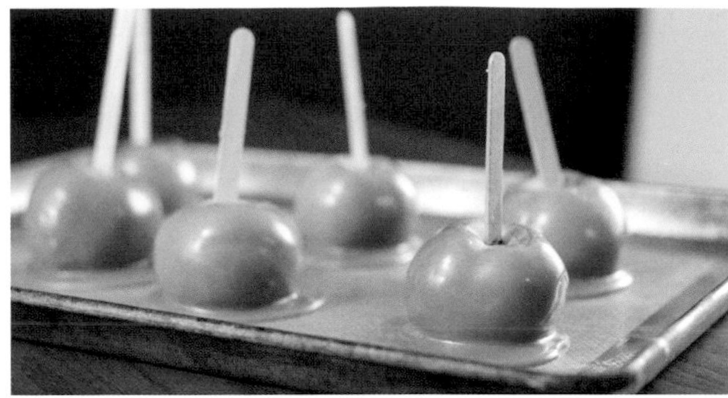

CARAMEL APPLES

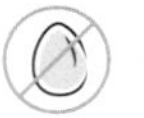 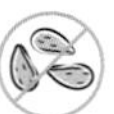 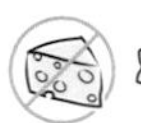 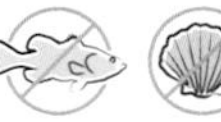  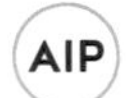 AIP

PREP TIME: 10 minutes, plus an hour to cool
COOK TIME: 30 minutes
YIELD: 8 to 10 apples

1 cup honey

1 cup coconut cream, homemade (page 480) or store-bought

Dash of sea salt

8 to 10 apples, chilled

Special equipment: 8 to 10 ice pop sticks or cake pop sticks

1. Combine the honey, coconut cream, and salt in a medium heavy-bottomed saucepan. Whisk to thoroughly combine. Attach a candy thermometer to the side of the pan.

2. Turn the heat on to medium-low. Heat the mixture until it reaches 245°F (don't let it go over 248°F); there is no need to stir. At around 220°F, it will start to bubble. If it looks like it's going to bubble over, stir a little to pop some of the bubbles. This step should take 20 to 30 minutes and is pretty hands-off, so be patient.

3. Once the temperature of the caramel reaches 245°F, remove from the heat. Let the caramel cool to under 200°F before dipping the apples. Around 180°F works best for a thick coating.

4. While waiting for the caramel to cool, skewer the apples with the sticks. Line a rimmed baking sheet with wax paper, parchment paper, or a silicone baking mat and grease the paper or liner.

5. Once the caramel is cool, dip the apples in the caramel to evenly coat. Place the apples on the prepared baking sheet, then place the baking sheet in the refrigerator for at least 1 hour to allow the caramel to harden. (I know, it's difficult to wait!) Peel off the paper or mat and enjoy.

TIP: This caramel is nice and sticky, so if you want to roll your caramel apples in some chopped nuts, go right ahead! Walnuts and pecans are my favorite.

CHOCOLATE-DIPPED ICE CREAM SANDWICHES

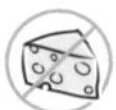 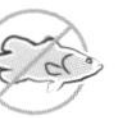 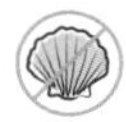 

PREP TIME: 40 minutes COOK TIME: 10 minutes
YIELD: 18 sandwiches

1 batch Graham Crackers (page 568)

½ batch Vanilla Ice Cream (page 585)

1 batch Chocolate Shell Topping (page 577)

1. Find pairs of graham crackers that are similar in size and shape. Line a cookie sheet with wax paper.

2. If the ice cream isn't freshly churned, set it on the counter to soften for 30 minutes. Gently spread a ½- to ¾-inch layer of the ice cream on a graham cracker. Place a second cracker on top and gently squeeze together. Place the ice cream sandwich on the lined cookie sheet.

3. Working quickly, repeat Step 2 with the remaining graham crackers and ice cream, then put the cookie sheet in the freezer until the ice cream sandwiches harden, at least 20 minutes.

4. Remove the ice cream sandwiches from the freezer one at a time. Holding one end, dip it into the chocolate mixture, then allow to drip while the chocolate hardens. Turn it around and dip the other side, overlapping the chocolate with the first dip. Dip as many times as you want for the thickness of chocolate coating you like.

5. Place back in the freezer (again on wax paper) and repeat with the rest of the ice cream sandwiches.

6. Keep in the soft zone of your freezer or allow to sit for about 5 minutes after taking out of the freezer. To store, individually wrap in wax paper or toss into a freezer-safe storage container.

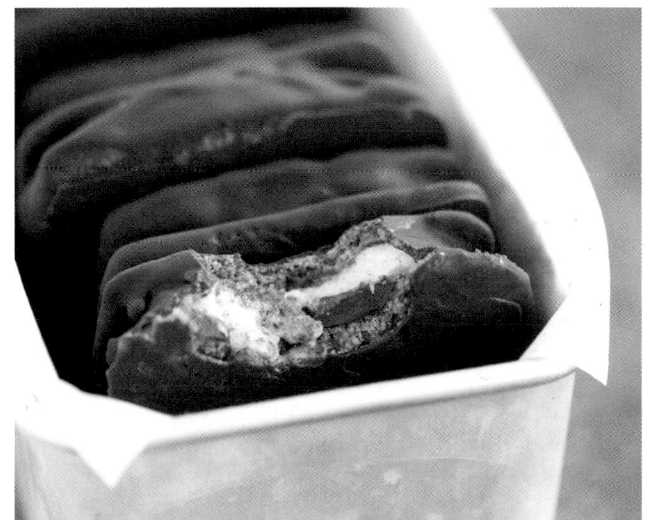

DARK CHOCOLATE GELATO

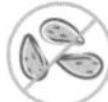 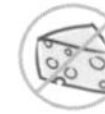 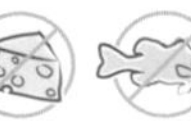  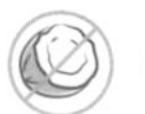 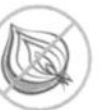 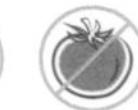

PREP TIME: 20 minutes, plus time to freeze
COOK TIME: 5 minutes YIELD: 1 quart

10 ounces bittersweet chocolate

1 cup hot or room-temperature water

6 large egg yolks

2 teaspoons vanilla extract

Pinch of sea salt

1 cup ice water

1. Melt the chocolate and hot or room-temperature water (you can do this in a double boiler on the stovetop or in a microwave-safe bowl on medium power in the microwave). Stir to completely combine.

2. Place the egg yolks in a bowl. Temper the yolks: while stirring, add a small ladleful of the chocolate-water mixture to the yolks. Keep stirring and add a second ladleful. Then add the yolk mixture to the rest of the chocolate-water mixture and mix thoroughly.

3. Place the chocolate-egg mixture in a blender. Add the vanilla and salt and blend on low. Either add the 1 cup ice water a little bit at a time, blending for a few seconds after each addition, or drizzle the ice water through the lid by removing the lid insert.

IF USING AN ICE CREAM MAKER:

1. Pour the custard mixture into your ice cream maker and churn, following the manufacturer's directions.

2. Scoop the churned ice cream into a freezer-safe container and freeze for 1 to 4 hours to harden a little more before serving.

IF USING A HIGH-POWERED BLENDER (SUCH AS A BLENDTEC OR VITAMIX):

1. Place the custard mixture in a freezer-safe bowl and freeze until mostly solid, 4 to 6 hours.

2. Scoop the frozen custard into your blender and press the ice cream button. It works best if you blend the custard before it is 100 percent solid. Put it back in the freezer for another hour or two before serving.

3. Store in the soft zone of your freezer or remove from the freezer and place in the refrigerator for about an hour or on the kitchen counter for 20 minutes before serving.

VARIATIONS:

Mocha gelato. *Use 1 cup hot strong coffee (or even espresso!) to melt the chocolate instead of water.*

Double chocolate gelato. *Add Chocolate Shell Topping (page 577).*

Grown-up gelato. *Replace an ounce or two of the water with rum.*

Chocolate-mint gelato. *Replace the vanilla with peppermint oil.*

Chocolate-cherry or chocolate-nut gelato. *Add chopped cherries and/or walnuts right at the end of churning.*

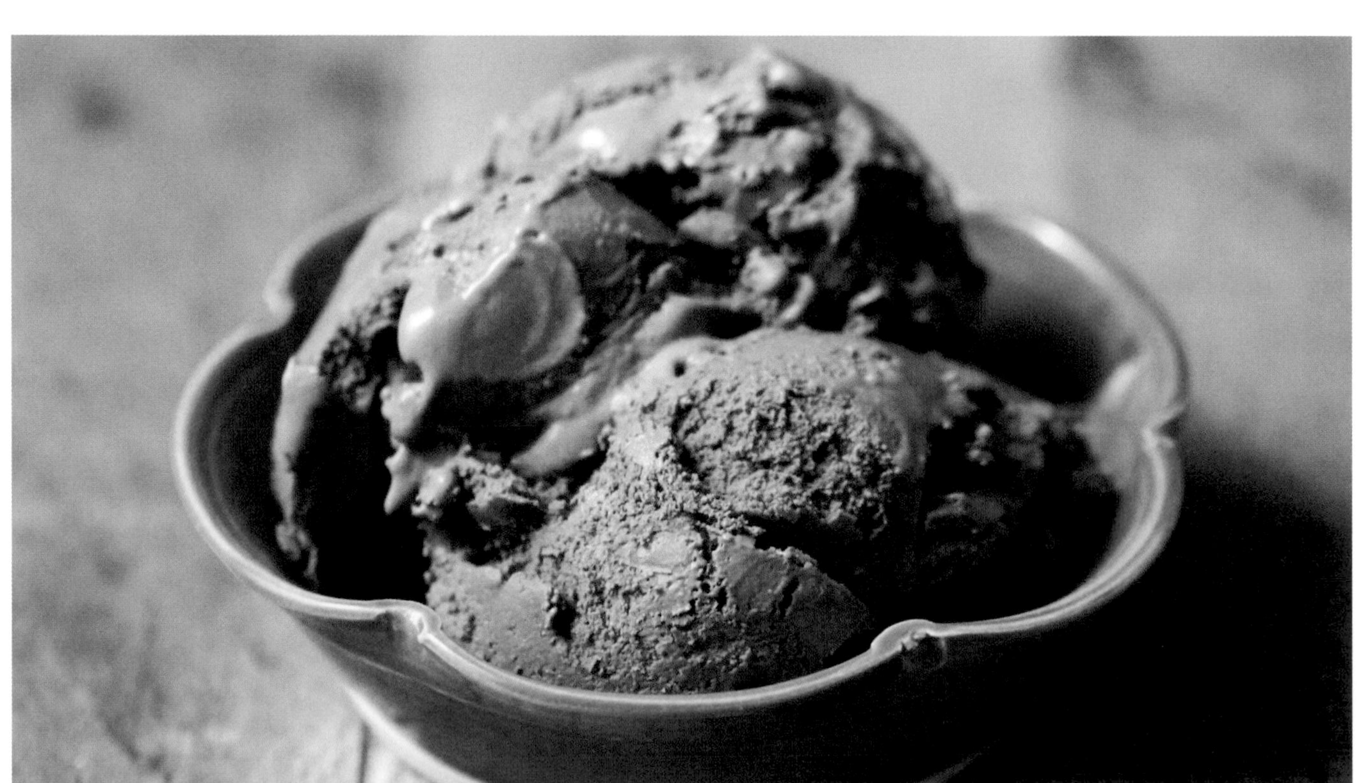

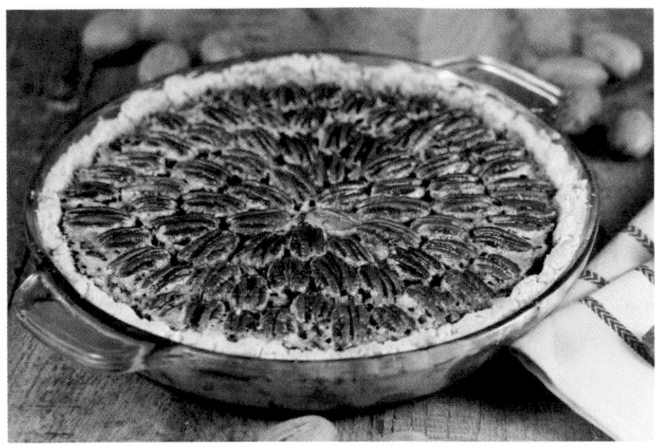

PECAN PIE

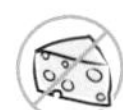 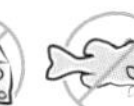   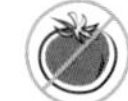

PREP TIME: 20 minutes *COOK TIME: 1 hour*
YIELD: one 9-inch pie (8 to 10 servings)

½ batch Pie Crust (page 499)

2 cups chopped raw pecans

1¼ cups raw pecan halves, for the top

¾ cup honey

¾ cup maple syrup

4 large whole eggs

1 large egg yolk (left over from making your crust)

6 tablespoons ghee, unsalted butter, or lard

1½ teaspoons vanilla extract

⅛ teaspoon sea salt

1. Preheat the oven to 375°F.
2. Place the pie crust dough on a sheet of parchment paper and roll out to ¼ inch thick or slightly thinner. Carefully transfer the dough to a 9-inch pie plate. Make sure the dough lines the plate well; take the time to fill in any cracks that form during the transfer. Make a nice edge.
3. Par-bake the crust for 15 minutes, until starting to turn golden brown. Remove from the oven.
4. Toast the pecans on a rimmed baking sheet for 5 to 8 minutes (you can do this while your pie crust is baking), until fragrant (pecan pieces take about 5 minutes; halves take a little longer).
5. Once the pecans and crust are out of the oven, reduce the oven temperature to 350°F.
6. Bring the honey and maple syrup to a rapid simmer in a small saucepan over medium-high heat.
7. Beat the whole eggs and egg yolk together. Temper the eggs: add a little bit of the very hot honey-maple syrup mixture to the eggs while you stir quickly, then add the eggs to honey-maple syrup mixture and remove from the heat.
8. Stir in the ghee, vanilla, salt, and chopped pecans. Pour into the pie crust.
9. Arrange the pecan halves to cover the top of the pie. Bake for 20 to 25 minutes, until set. (You'll know it's set when you move the pie a little and the middle doesn't jiggle.) Let cool completely before serving.

PINEAPPLE AND LYCHEE GRANITA

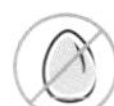 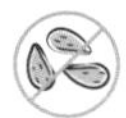 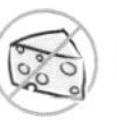 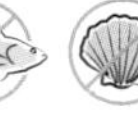 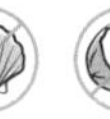  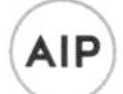 AIP

PREP TIME: 3 hours *YIELD: 8 servings*

2 pounds fresh lychee, rambutan, or longan

2 limes

4 cups (about 1½ pounds) fresh pineapple chunks

¼ teaspoon sea salt

1. Peel and pit the lychee.
2. Zest the limes and reserve the zest for garnish, then cut the remaining peel off the limes.
3. Place the peeled limes, lychee, pineapple, and salt in a blender and blend until completely smooth.
4. Pour the puree onto a rimmed baking sheet or into a sheet pan or lasagna pan and place in the freezer.
5. After 1 hour, remove the baking sheet from the freezer and scrape and mash the fruit with a fork to make little ice crystals. Return the baking sheet to the freezer.
6. After another hour, remove the baking sheet from freezer and mash the fruit a second time. Return the baking sheet to the freezer.
7. After a third hour, remove the baking sheet from the freezer and mash the fruit a final time. Transfer the granita to a freezer-safe container and store in the freezer until ready to serve.

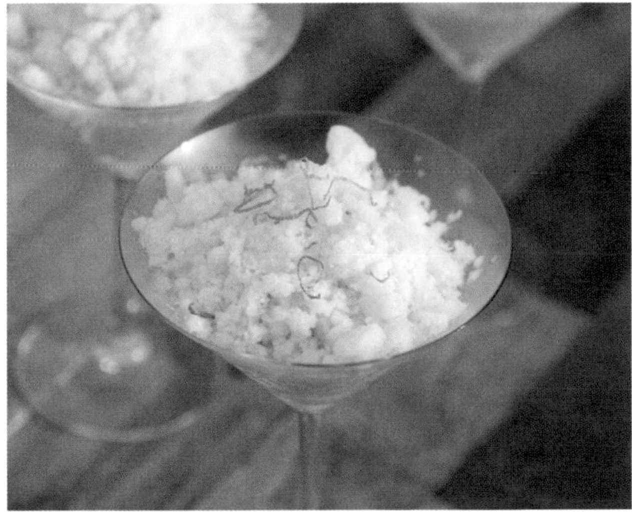

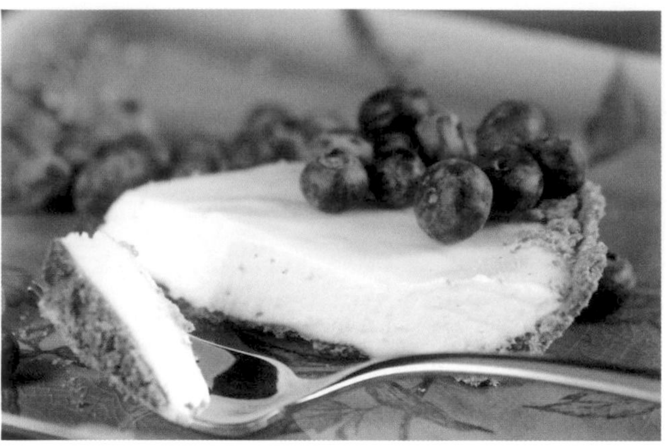

LEMON "CHEESE" CAKE

 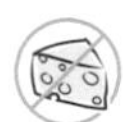 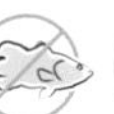 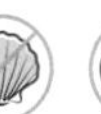 

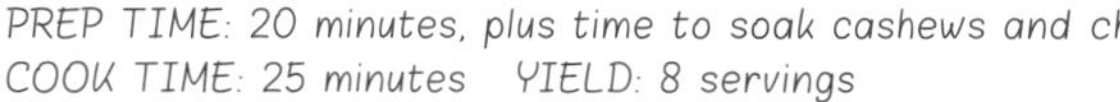

PREP TIME: 20 minutes, plus time to soak cashews and chill
COOK TIME: 25 minutes YIELD: 8 servings

2 cups raw cashews

2 tablespoons palm shortening, lard, unsalted butter, or ghee, melted

1½ tablespoons honey

¾ cup chestnut flour

¼ teaspoon ground cinnamon

Sea salt

1 tablespoon gelatin

1 cup full-fat coconut milk, homemade (page 480) or canned, or Coconut Milk Yogurt (page 481), or coconut milk kefir

⅛ teaspoon baking soda

⅛ teaspoon cream of tartar

¼ cup honey

1 tablespoon finely grated lemon zest

3 tablespoons lemon juice

Fresh berries or sliced stone fruit (such as blueberries, raspberries, peaches, or apricots), for serving

1. Soak the cashews in enough cool water to cover for at least 2 hours. Drain before adding in Step 6.

2. Preheat the oven to 300°F.

3. Combine the shortening, honey, chestnut flour, cinnamon, and a pinch of salt in a shallow 8- or 9-inch pie plate. Use your fingers to work it into a crust (it will be quite dry and crumbly, and that's okay). Pat it down to line the pie plate; it will be quite thin. Take a fork and poke little holes all over the crust.

4. Bake the crust for 13 to 14 minutes, until starting to brown on the bottom. Let cool completely.

5. Place the coconut milk in a small saucepan and sprinkle the gelatin over the top. Wait for the gelatin to become translucent as it absorbs the milk. Heat the milk and gelatin over medium heat until just starting to simmer, then remove from the heat. (If you're using yogurt or kefir and want to protect the probiotics, place a thermometer in your pot. Gelatin dissolves at 82°F. As long as you keep the temperature below 100°F, your probiotics will survive.)

6. Pour the coconut milk mixture, drained cashews, and remaining ingredients into a blender. Blend on high until completely creamy (this will take about a minute in a high-powered blender).

7. Pour the filling into the crust and spread it out evenly. Chill until set, 3 to 4 hours in the refrigerator or about an hour in the freezer.

8. Serve with fresh berries or stone fruit.

MONKEY'S LUNCH ICE CREAM BARS

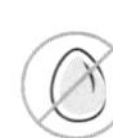 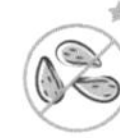 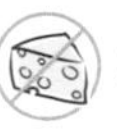 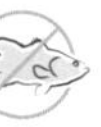  

PREP TIME: 5 minutes, plus 3 hours to freeze
COOK TIME: 10 minutes YIELD: ten 1/4-cup ice pops

3 overripe bananas

¾ cup smooth almond butter or other nut or seed butter of choice

½ batch Chocolate Shell Topping (page 577)

Special equipment:
10 (2-ounce) ice pop molds

1. Blend the bananas and almond butter together with an immersion blender. Spoon the mixture into the ice pop molds. Insert the sticks into the molds and put in the freezer until frozen, 3 to 4 hours.

2. To serve, remove an ice cream bar from its mold (running hot water over the outside is helpful). Dip the bar in the chocolate shell topping. Remove and hold over the jar of shell topping to catch the drips. For a thicker chocolate shell, dip again after the first coat solidifies. Enjoy immediately.

TIP: A fun variation is to roll the ice cream bars in chopped nuts (walnuts and pecans are especially tasty) immediately after dipping them in the shell topping.

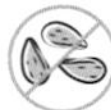 *use a seed butter*

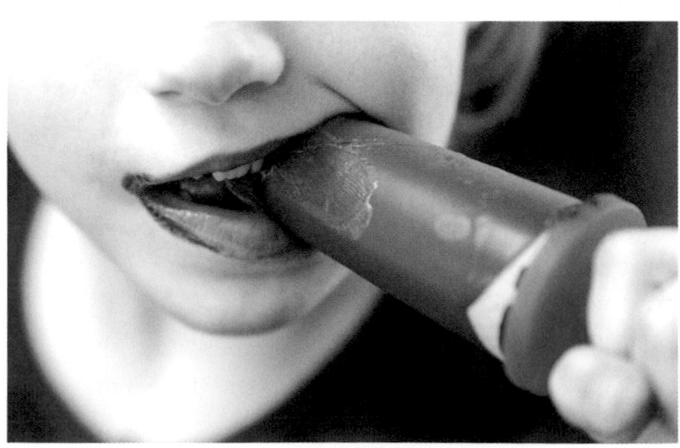

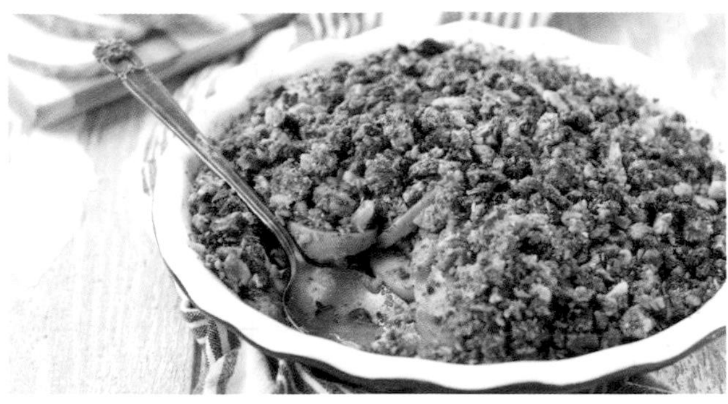

APPLE CRISP

 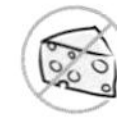 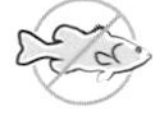  

PREP TIME: 1 hour 30 minutes (including 1 hour to chill topping)
COOK TIME: 45 minutes   YIELD: 6 generous servings

¾ cup chopped raw pecans (see Tip)

¾ cup chopped raw walnuts (see Tip)

¼ cup almond meal

¼ cup finely shredded unsweetened coconut

3 tablespoons muscovado sugar or evaporated cane juice

½ teaspoon ground allspice

½ teaspoon ground nutmeg

Pinch of sea salt

⅓ cup coconut oil, melted

6 medium to large apples (about 2½ pounds)

1 teaspoon finely grated lemon zest

2 tablespoons lemon juice

½ teaspoon ground cinnamon

¼ teaspoon ground cardamom

1 batch Vanilla Ice Cream (page 585), for serving (optional)

1. Pour the pecans and walnuts into a bowl. Add the almond meal, shredded coconut, sugar, allspice, nutmeg, and salt and mix to combine.
2. Pour the melted coconut oil over the nut mixture and stir to fully combine. Pat down the crisp topping slightly and place in the refrigerator to harden for at least 20 minutes (1 hour is better).
3. Preheat the oven to 375°F.
4. Peel and core the apples, then cut into large bite-sized pieces.
5. Toss the apple pieces with the lemon zest, lemon juice, cinnamon, and cardamom.
6. Place the apple mixture in a casserole dish, 8- or 9-inch square baking dish, or 9-inch deep-dish pie plate.
7. Remove the crisp topping from refrigerator. Use a knife or your fingers to crumble it, making sure there are some big pieces and some small ones. Cover the surface of the apples with the crisp topping crumbs.
8. Bake for 40 minutes, then increase the oven temperature up to 425°F for 5 minutes to brown the crisp a little more (watch carefully to make sure it doesn't burn).
9. Remove from the oven and let cool slightly. Serve warm with ice cream, if desired.

TIP: Chop the nuts by hand for the best texture.

MAPLE-WALNUT DARK CHOCOLATE CHUNK COOKIES

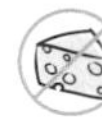 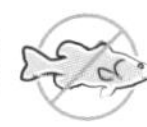  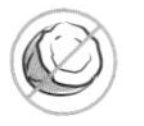 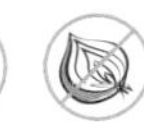 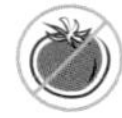

PREP TIME: 15 minutes   COOK TIME: 20 minutes
YIELD: 18 to 20 cookies

¼ cup palm shortening, unsalted butter, ghee, or lard

¼ cup walnut oil, avocado oil, or coconut oil

⅔ cup maple sugar

1 large egg

1 teaspoon maple extract

2 cups blanched almond flour

¾ teaspoon baking soda

¼ teaspoon sea salt

Pinch of ground cinnamon

¾ cup chopped raw walnuts or pecans

1 (3½-ounce) bar dark chocolate (80% to 90% cacao), chopped, or ⅔ cup dark chocolate chunks

1. Preheat the oven to 350°F.
2. In a bowl, vigorously stir together the shortening, oil, and maple sugar until well combined (or beat in the bowl of a stand mixer). Add the egg and stir vigorously to fully combine. Add the maple extract and stir again.
3. Add the almond flour, baking soda, salt, and cinnamon and stir to incorporate. Fold in the nuts and chocolate.
4. Scoop rounded tablespoons of the dough with a spoon or form 1½-inch balls of dough (for more uniformly shaped cookies) and place on an ungreased cookie sheet.
5. Bake for 10 minutes. Let cool on the cookie sheet. Repeat with the remaining dough. Store in an airtight container at room temperature for up to a week or in the freezer for up to 6 months.

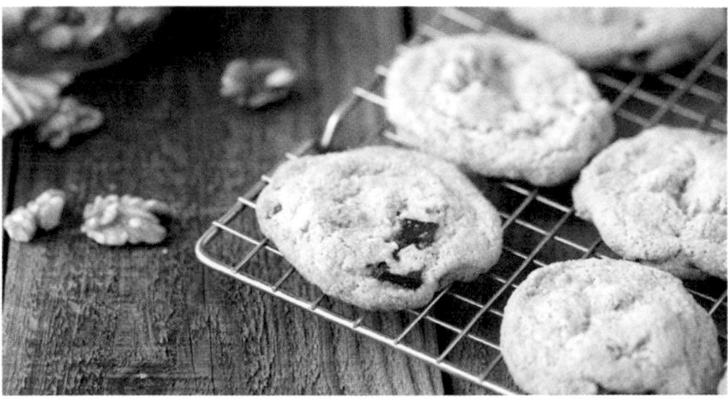

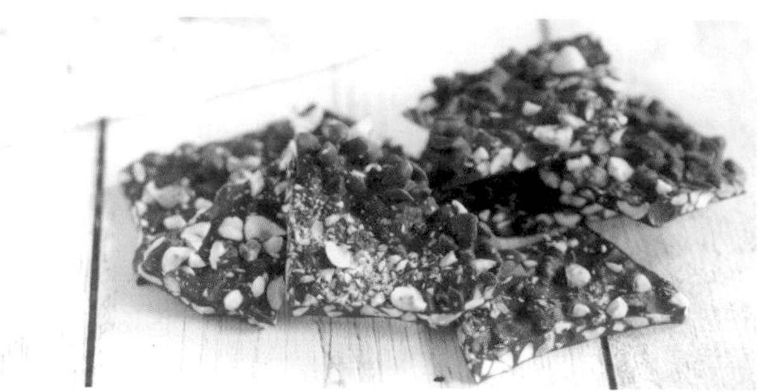

SALTED HAZELNUT DARK CHOCOLATE BARK

 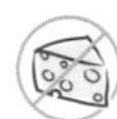 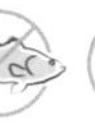  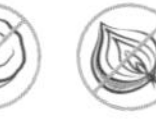 

PREP TIME: 15 minutes, plus time to chill
COOK TIME: 20 minutes YIELD: 18 to 20 pieces

3 cups raw hazelnuts

12 ounces bittersweet chocolate

2 tablespoons coconut oil, unsalted butter, ghee, lard, or palm shortening

½ teaspoon coarse unrefined sea salt (optional)

1. Preheat the oven to 350°F.

2. Place the hazelnuts on a rimmed baking sheet. Bake for 15 minutes. Remove from the oven and immediately pour into a clean tea towel. Fold the towel over the nuts and let them sit for 1 to 2 minutes.

3. With the tea towel still covering the hazelnuts, rub the top of the towel to start removing the skins. Pick out the nuts that have the skins removed (it's fine if there's a little skin left on them) and continue until you've removed all the skins from the nuts.

4. Discard the skins and place the nuts back on the tea towel (you could also do this on a cutting board or in a large resealable plastic bag). Crush the nuts with a rolling pin, until the pieces are pea-sized or a little smaller.

5. Melt the chocolate and coconut oil in a double boiler or in a microwave-safe bowl in the microwave on medium power.

6. Line a rimmed baking sheet with parchment paper, wax paper, or a silicone baking mat.

7. Mix the crushed hazelnuts into the melted chocolate mixture and pour onto the prepared baking sheet. Spread to ¼ to ⅜ inch thick. Sprinkle the salt over the top.

8. Refrigerate until the chocolate bark is cold and hard. Remove from the refrigerator and break into pieces (however big or small you like). Store in an airtight container at room temperature for up to a month or in the fridge for up to 6 months.

FREEZER FUDGE

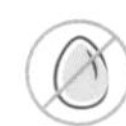  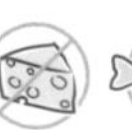 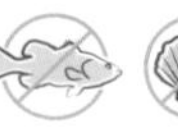 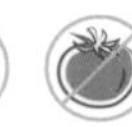 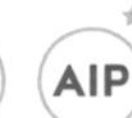 AIP

PREP TIME: 10 minutes COOK TIME: 2 minutes
YIELD: 2 dozen pieces

1½ cups smooth nut or seed butter of choice

6 tablespoons coconut oil, melted

¼ cup honey

¼ teaspoon sea salt (use half this amount if your nut or seed butter is salted)

CHOCOLATE TOPPING

2 ounces bittersweet chocolate

3 tablespoons coconut oil

Maldon sea salt, for garnish (optional)

1. Grease a 9 by 5-inch glass baking dish with coconut oil, or use candy molds.

2. In a bowl, whisk together the nut or seed butter, coconut oil, honey, and salt until fully combined. (If it isn't coming together well, gently warm the mixture on low power in the microwave or in a double boiler.) Pour the fudge into the prepared dish or molds. Freeze for at least 1 hour, until set.

3. To make the topping, melt the chocolate and coconut oil on low power in the microwave or in a double boiler.

4. Once frozen, remove the fudge from the dish to a cutting board and cut into squares. If using candy molds, simply pop out of the molds. Place on a rimmed baking sheet lined with parchment paper or wax paper.

5. Drizzle the chocolate topping over the fudge. Let the topping start to solidify before sprinkling with the salt, if using. Put back in the freezer for 5 minutes to fully set.

6. Transfer to a freezer-safe container and store for up to 6 months. Consume straight from the freezer.

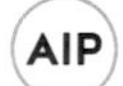 *use coconut butter; omit chocolate topping*

 *use a seed butter*

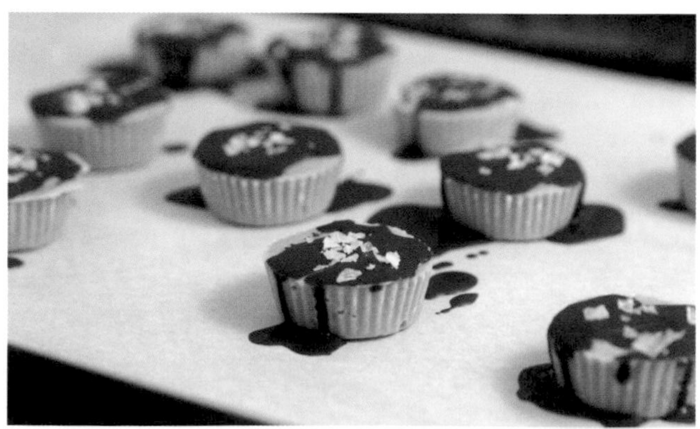

VANILLA ICE CREAM

 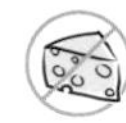 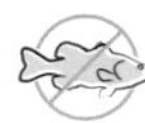   

PREP TIME: 20 minutes, plus time to chill
COOK TIME: 20 minutes YIELD: 1 quart

2 cups almond, cashew, or sunflower seed milk (page 481)

1 batch Coconut Milk (page 480), or 1 (13½-ounce) can full-fat coconut milk

1 (8-inch) Madagascar vanilla bean

1 teaspoon gelatin

6 large egg yolks

¼ cup honey

1. Place the milks in a medium saucepan. Slice the vanilla bean in half with a sharp knife and add the halves to the pan. Sprinkle the gelatin over the top. Place over medium-low heat, stirring constantly, until hot and steaming but just short of a simmer (do not let it simmer!).

2. Place the egg yolks in a heat-safe container. Temper the yolks by adding a ladleful of hot milk to the yolks while stirring. Then add the tempered yolks to the saucepan, again stirring constantly.

3. Heat the mixture, stirring constantly and never letting it simmer, until it thickens (it should coat the back of a wooden spoon and be about as thick as heavy cream), 6 to 8 minutes. (If the mixture boils, the eggs will curdle. If this happens, it's still salvageable: remove from the heat immediately and pulse in a blender until smooth.)

4. Remove from the heat and pour into a bowl or measuring cup. Let cool to room temperature.

5. Remove the vanilla bean halves and scrape the seeds off the pod with a spoon or the back of a sharp knife. Add the vanilla seeds back to the ice cream and discard the pod. Stir in the honey.

IF USING AN ICE CREAM MAKER:

1. Chill the ice cream mixture in the fridge until cold.

2. Place the chilled mixture in your ice cream maker and churn, following the manufacturer's directions.

3. Pour the churned ice cream into a freezer-safe container and freeze for 1 to 4 hours to harden a little more before serving.

IF USING A HIGH-POWERED BLENDER (SUCH AS A BLENDTEC OR VITAMIX):

1. Place the ice cream mixture in a freezer-safe bowl and freeze until mostly solid, 4 to 6 hours.

2. Scoop the ice cream into your blender and press the ice cream button. It works best if you blend it before the ice cream is 100 percent solid. Put it back in the freezer for another hour or two before serving.

3. Store in the soft zone of your freezer, or remove from the freezer and place in the fridge for about an hour or on the kitchen counter for 20 minutes before serving.

TIP: Want a sweeter ice cream? Add up to an extra 1/2 cup of honey.

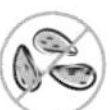 *use a seed milk*

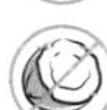 *use a nut or seed milk instead of coconut milk*

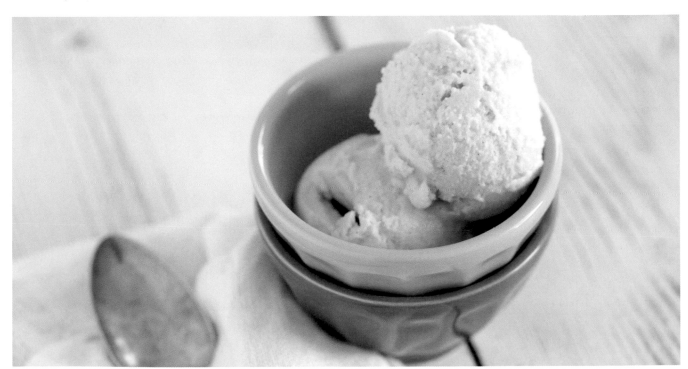

OLIVE OIL ICE CREAM

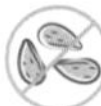 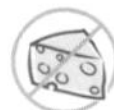  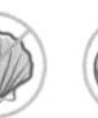 

PREP TIME: 10 minutes, plus time to chill
COOK TIME: 20 minutes YIELD: 3 cups

- 1 batch Coconut Milk (page 480), or 1 (13½-ounce) can full-fat coconut milk
- 3 large egg yolks
- ⅔ cup high-quality olive oil (see Tip)
- ⅓ cup honey
- ½ teaspoon vanilla extract
- ¼ teaspoon sea salt
- High-quality balsamic vinegar, for serving (optional)

1. Heat the coconut milk in a saucepan over medium-low heat, stirring constantly, until hot and steaming but just short of a simmer (do not let the milk simmer!).

2. Place the egg yolks in a glass measuring cup or other heat-safe container.

3. Temper the egg yolks by adding a ladleful of hot coconut milk to the yolks while stirring. Add the tempered yolks to the saucepan, again stirring constantly.

4. Heat the mixture, stirring constantly without letting it simmer, until it thickens (it should coat the back of a wooden spoon and be about as thick as heavy cream), 6 to 8 minutes. (If the mixture boils, the eggs will curdle. If this happens, it's still salvageable: remove from the heat immediately and pulse in a blender until smooth.)

5. Remove from the heat and pour into a bowl or measuring cup. Let cool to room temperature.

6. Add the remaining ingredients; I think it's best to blend them for a minute to fully incorporate, but you can whisk them together, too.

IF USING AN ICE CREAM MAKER:

1. Chill the ice cream mixture in the refrigerator until cold.

2. Place the chilled mixture in your ice cream maker and churn, following the manufacturer's directions.

3. Pour the churned ice cream into a freezer-safe container and freeze for 1 to 4 hours to harden a little more before serving.

IF USING A HIGH-POWERED BLENDER (SUCH AS A BLENDTEC OR VITAMIX):

1. Place the ice cream mixture in a freezer-safe bowl and freeze until mostly solid, 4 to 6 hours.

2. Scoop the mixture into your blender and press the ice cream button. It works best if you blend the ice cream before it is 100 percent solid. Put it back in the freezer for another hour or two before serving.

3. To serve, drizzle with a high-quality balsamic vinegar, if desired.

4. Store in the soft zone of your freezer, or remove from the freezer and place in the fridge for about an hour or on the kitchen counter for 20 minutes before serving.

TIP: The incredible flavor of this ice cream hinges on using the best-quality olive oil you can find, ideally one that's very peppery (indicating a high polyphenol content) with a rich, full-bodied flavor. For an even richer ice cream, use coconut cream instead of full-fat coconut milk.

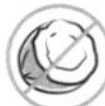 *use a nut or seed milk instead of coconut milk*

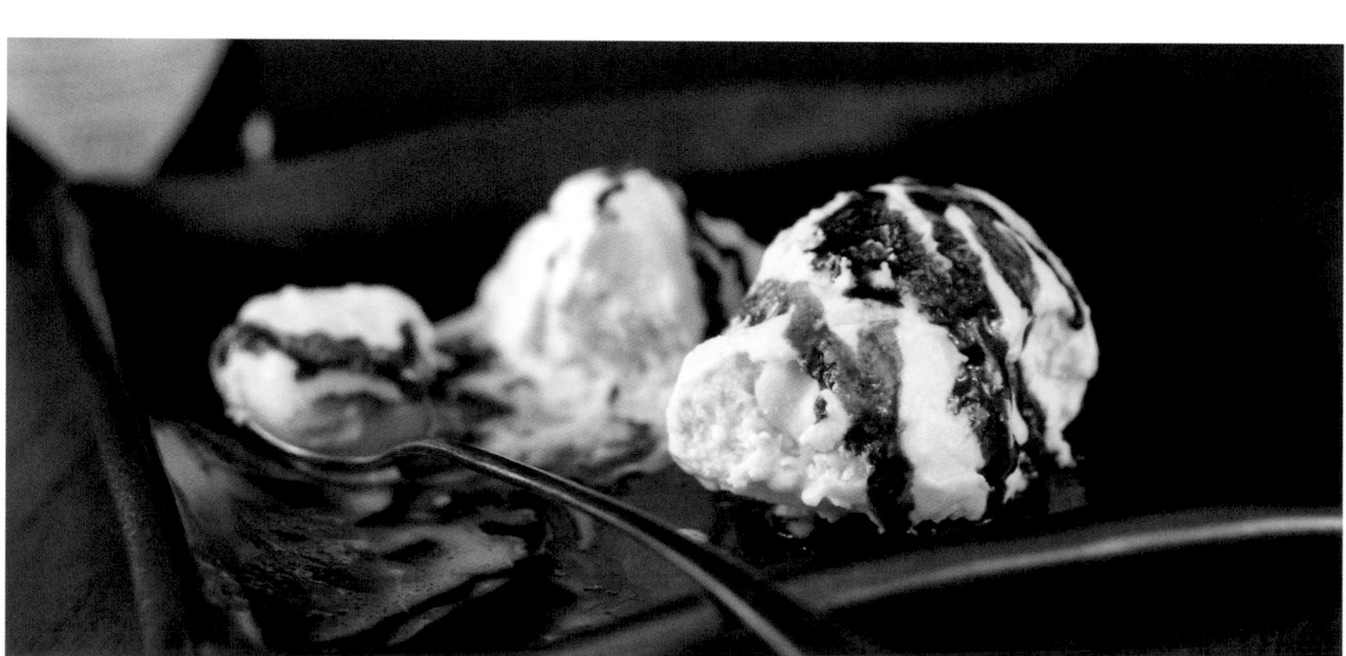

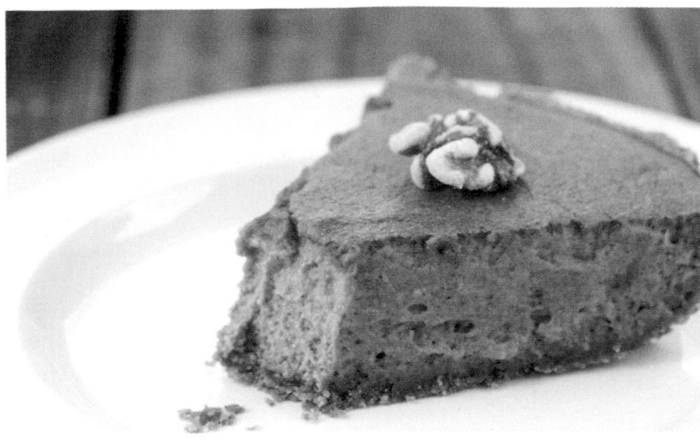

PUMPKIN PIE

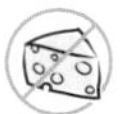 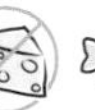  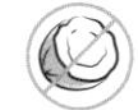 

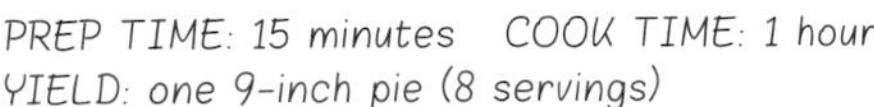

PREP TIME: 15 minutes COOK TIME: 1 hour
YIELD: one 9-inch pie (8 servings)

- ½ batch Pie Crust (page 499)
- ⅔ cup raw walnut halves
- ⅓ cup raw or roasted unsalted cashews
- 3 large eggs, plus 1 large egg yolk
- ¼ cup honey
- ¼ cup maple syrup
- ½ cup water
- 1¾ cups homemade pumpkin puree, or 1 (15-ounce) can pumpkin puree
- 1 teaspoon ginger powder
- 1 teaspoon ground allspice
- 1 teaspoon ground nutmeg
- ½ teaspoon ground cardamom
- ½ teaspoon ground cloves
- ¼ teaspoon sea salt

1. Preheat the oven to 375°F.

2. Place the pie crust dough on a sheet of parchment paper and roll out with a rolling pin to ¼ inch thick or slightly thinner. Carefully transfer the dough to a 9-inch pie plate. Make sure the dough lines the plate well; take the time to fill in any cracks that form during the transfer. Make a nice edge.

3. Par-bake the crust for 15 minutes, until starting to turn golden brown. Let cool for at least 10 minutes before pouring the custard in.

4. Reduce the oven temperature to 350°F.

5. Place the walnuts and cashews in a food processor or blender and pulse until finely ground. Add the eggs, honey, and maple syrup and blend for 2 to 3 minutes, until completely smooth (you can add some of the water if it's too thick for your food processor or blender to puree well). It is important to blend until *completely* smooth; otherwise, the custard will be watery.

6. Add the water, pumpkin puree, spices, and salt and blend until combined.

7. Pour the custard into the cooled par-baked crust (it doesn't need to be room temperature, just cool enough to touch). Spread the top evenly with a spatula.

8. Bake for 40 to 45 minutes, until the custard is completely set. Allow to cool completely before serving.

MOLTEN LAVA CHOCOLATE CAKE

 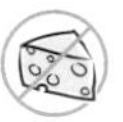 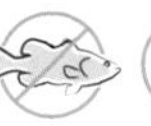 

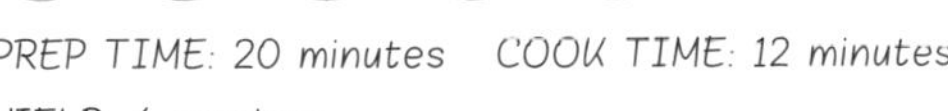

PREP TIME: 20 minutes COOK TIME: 12 minutes
YIELD: 4 servings

- ¼ cup coconut oil
- 4 ounces semisweet or bittersweet chocolate
- 2 large eggs
- ½ teaspoon vanilla extract
- 2 tablespoons muscovado sugar or evaporated cane juice
- ⅛ teaspoon sea salt
- 1 teaspoon coconut flour
- 2 teaspoons cacao powder
- Vanilla Ice Cream (page 585), for serving (optional)

1. Preheat the oven to 375°F. Grease four 6-ounce ramekins with coconut oil.

2. In a 4-cup measuring cup or medium microwave-safe bowl, melt the coconut oil and chocolate in the microwave on low power. Stir until smooth and let cool.

3. In a small bowl, beat the eggs, vanilla, sugar, and salt with a hand mixer until light and frothy, about 5 minutes. (Doing this with a hand mixer seems to take an eternity, but hang in there; it's worth it!)

4. Pour the egg mixture over melted chocolate. Sift the coconut flour and cacao powder over the top. Then gently fold all the ingredients together.

5. Pour the batter into the prepared ramekins, filling them to within ½ inch of the top. Place the ramekins on a rimmed baking sheet and bake for 10 to 11 minutes.

6. Remove from the oven and serve immediately.

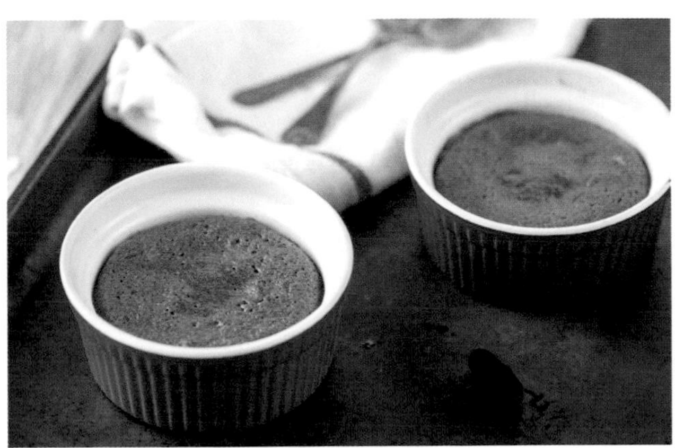

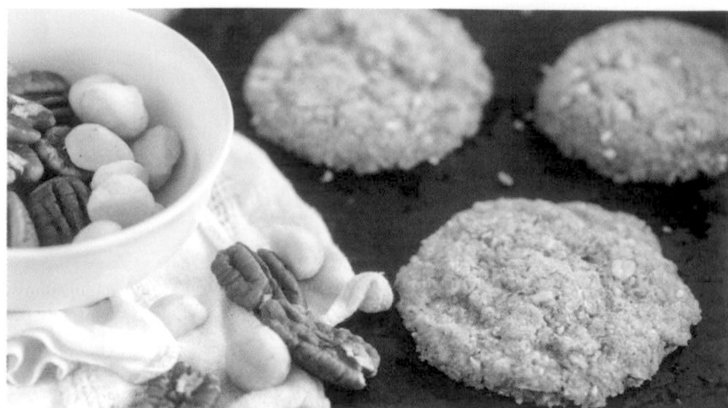

N'OATMEAL COOKIES

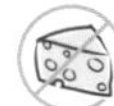  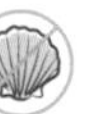 

PREP TIME: 15 minutes *COOK TIME: 20 minutes*
YIELD: 30 cookies

- ¾ cup coconut oil, melted and cooled
- ⅔ cup muscovado sugar
- 1 large egg
- 1 teaspoon vanilla extract
- 1½ cups blanched almond flour
- ¾ teaspoon baking soda
- ½ teaspoon cream of tartar
- ½ teaspoon sea salt
- ¼ cup macadamia nuts
- ¼ cup raw pecans
- 2 tablespoons raw shelled sunflower seeds
- ¼ cup sliced almonds
- ½ cup finely shredded unsweetened coconut
- 1 tablespoon sesame seeds
- Pinch of ground cinnamon
- ½ cup bittersweet mini chocolate chips or raisins (optional)

1. Preheat the oven to 350°F.
2. In a medium bowl, mix together the coconut oil, sugar, egg, and vanilla. Add the almond flour, baking soda, cream of tartar, and salt and mix well to form a dough.
3. Pulse the macadamia nuts in a food processor until they resemble coarse sand, then pour into a mixing bowl. Pulse the pecans to a similar texture, then pour into the bowl with the macadamia nuts. Pulse the sunflower seeds to a similar texture, then pour into the same bowl. Pulse the almonds to a slightly coarser texture, resembling quick oats, and pour into the same bowl.
4. Add the shredded coconut, sesame seeds, and processed nuts to the dough and stir to combine. Fold in the chocolate chips or raisins, if using.
5. Drop 1-inch balls of the dough onto an ungreased cookie sheet. Bake for 9 to 10 minutes, until slightly underdone. Let cool completely on the cookie sheet. Repeat with the remaining dough. Store in an airtight container at room temperature for up to 3 days or in the freezer for up to 6 months.

HIDDEN SPINACH BROWNIES

 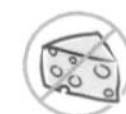 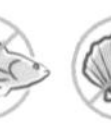  

PREP TIME: 15 minutes *COOK TIME: 40 minutes*
YIELD: about 2 dozen brownies

- ½ cup coconut oil
- 6 ounces semisweet chocolate
- 1 tablespoon vanilla extract
- ½ cup cocoa powder
- ¼ teaspoon baking soda
- ½ teaspoon cream of tartar
- ½ teaspoon sea salt
- Pinch of ground cinnamon
- 1¼ cups frozen chopped spinach (measured frozen)
- 1 cup pureed green plantains (about 1 large or 1½ medium)
- 6 large eggs
- 1 tablespoon honey
- 1 tablespoon molasses
- ½ cup lard, palm shortening, unsalted butter, or ghee

1. Preheat the oven to 325°F. Line a 13 by 9-inch baking pan with wax paper or use a silicone baking pan.
2. Melt the coconut oil and chocolate in a saucepan over low heat or in a microwave-safe bowl at medium power in the microwave. Add the vanilla and stir to incorporate. Let cool.
3. Mix the cocoa powder, baking soda, cream of tartar, salt, and cinnamon in a bowl.
4. Blend the spinach, plantains, eggs, honey, and molasses in a food processor or blender until completely smooth, 2 to 4 minutes. Add the lard and process until full incorporated.
5. Slowly add the melted chocolate mixture to the spinach mixture while processing or blending constantly. Mix in the dry ingredients and process or stir to fully incorporate.
6. Pour the batter into the prepared baking pan and spread out with a spatula. Bake for 40 minutes.
7. Let cool completely in the pan, then cut into squares. Store in an airtight container in the refrigerator for up to a week.

TIP: These brownies are extra-tasty with 3/4 cup chopped walnuts folded into the batter before baking.

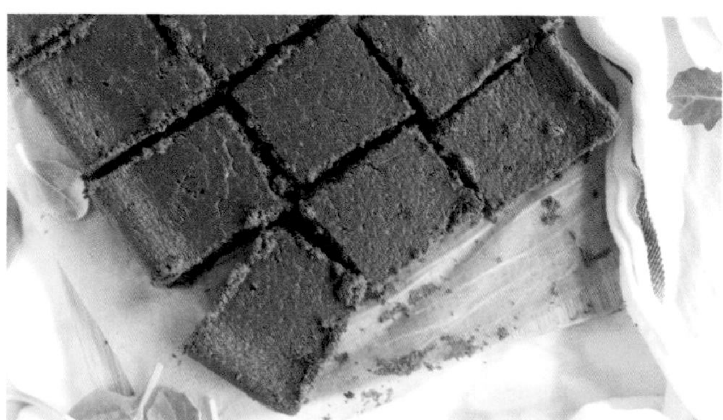

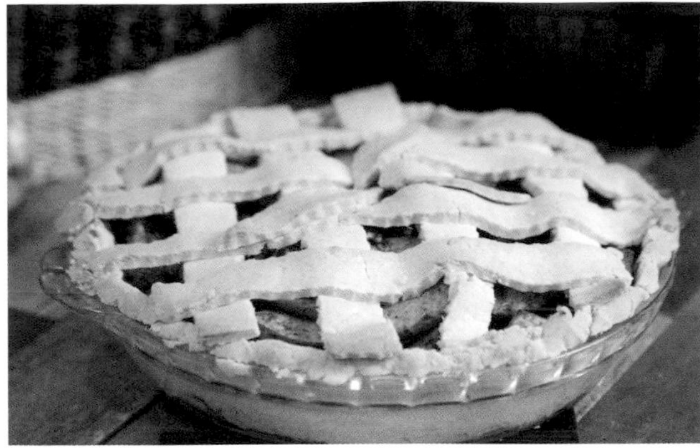

APPLE PIE

  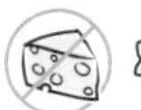 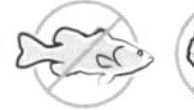 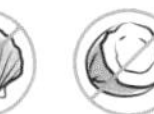  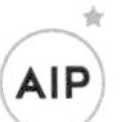 AIP

PREP TIME: 30 minutes COOK TIME: 1 hour
YIELD: one 9-inch pie (8 servings)

6 cups peeled and sliced Granny Smith apples (5 to 6 apples)

¼ cup evaporated cane juice or maple sugar

2 tablespoons lemon juice

1 teaspoon finely grated lemon zest

½ teaspoon ground allspice

½ teaspoon ground cinnamon

⅛ teaspoon ground cardamom

Pinch of ground cloves

½ cup chopped raw walnuts

Pinch of sea salt

1 batch Pie Crust (page 499)

Vanilla Ice Cream (page 585), for serving (optional)

1. Combine the apples, evaporated cane juice, lemon juice, lemon zest, spices, walnuts, and salt in a bowl. Toss to thoroughly coat the apples.
2. Preheat the oven to 350°F.
3. Divide the pie crust dough in half. Place one half on a sheet of parchment paper and roll out with a rolling pin to ¼ inch thick or slightly thinner. Carefully transfer the dough to a 9-inch pie plate. Make sure the dough lines the plate well; take the time to fill in any cracks that form during the transfer. Make a nice edge.
4. Pour the filling into the pie crust.
5. Roll out the other half of the pie crust dough. You can cut strips of dough for a crosshatch pattern on the top, as shown, or simply cover for a double-crust pie (remember to cut a couple slits in the top crust for venting).
6. Bake for 1 hour. Serve warm with ice cream, if desired.

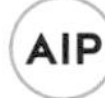 *replace allspice and cardamom with 1/4 teaspoon mace and additional 1/4 teaspoon cinnamon; omit walnuts*

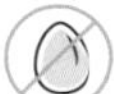 *use Cassava Flour Pie Crust*

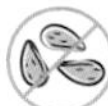 *omit walnuts; use Cassava Flour Pie Crust*

GRILLED STUFFED BANANAS

 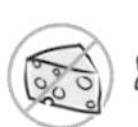 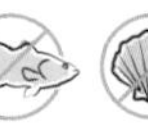 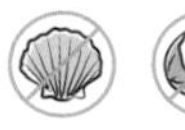  

PREP TIME: 5 minutes COOK TIME: 18 minutes
YIELD: 2 to 4 servings

¼ cup chopped raw pecans

¼ cup chopped raw walnuts

½ teaspoon ground cinnamon

¼ teaspoon ground allspice

¼ teaspoon ginger powder

¼ teaspoon ground nutmeg

⅛ teaspoon ground cardamom

⅛ teaspoon ground cloves

Dash of sea salt

2 large or 3 medium-sized very ripe bananas, unpeeled

1. Combine the nuts with spices and salt and mix to evenly coat.
2. Slice the bananas lengthwise about three-quarters of the way through the banana (careful not to cut the peel underneath). Spread the banana open and fill the groove with the nut mixture.
3. Preheat a grill pan or gas or charcoal grill to medium to moderately hot. Grill the stuffed bananas for 14 to 18 minutes (the time will vary depending on the size of the bananas and the temperature of your grill). The peels will darken (and maybe turn completely black), which is normal. You know they're done when the peels are dark, the bananas are bubbling away, and they smell fantastic! Alternatively, you can place the stuffed bananas on a rimmed baking sheet lined with parchment paper or aluminum foil and bake in the middle of a 425°F oven for 12 to 14 minutes.
4. Remove from the grill (or oven) and enjoy warm. Eat with a spoon scooping right out of the peel!

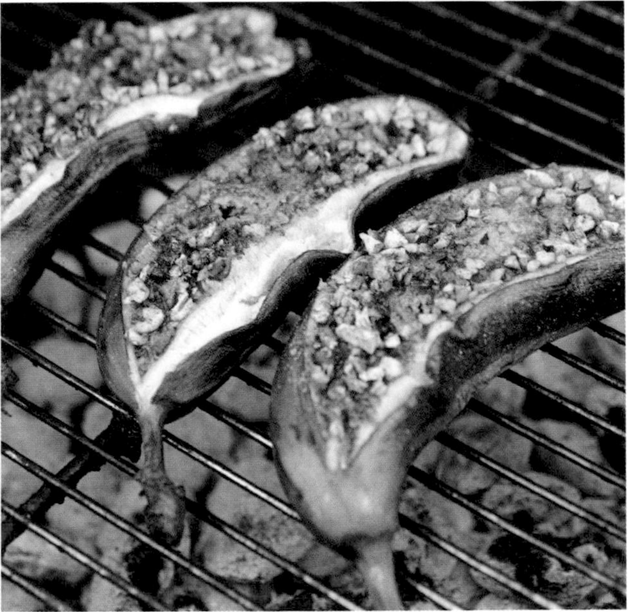

STRAWBERRY-RHUBARB COBBLER

 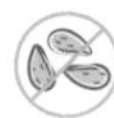 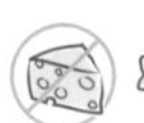 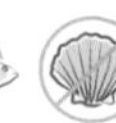 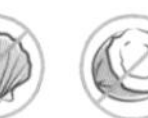 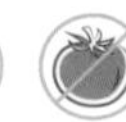 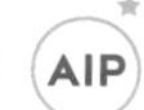 AIP

PREP TIME: 20 minutes COOK TIME: 30 minutes
YIELD: 9 to 12 servings

- 1½ cups cassava flour
- 1 teaspoon baking soda
- 1 teaspoon cream of tartar
- ¼ teaspoon sea salt
- ¼ teaspoon ground cardamom
- ¼ teaspoon ground cinnamon
- ¼ cup lard, cold
- ¾ cup coconut cream, homemade (page 480) or store-bought
- 1½ pounds rhubarb, chopped
- ½ cup maple syrup
- 3 tablespoons arrowroot powder
- 3 tablespoons water
- 1½ pounds strawberries, sliced
- 2 teaspoons grated orange zest
- ½ teaspoon vanilla extract
- 1 tablespoon maple sugar
- 1 teaspoon ground cinnamon

1. Mix together the cassava flour, baking soda, cream of tartar, salt, cardamom, and cinnamon in a large bowl.

2. Add the lard, then use a whisk or 2 knives to cut the lard into the flour mixture until it resembles dry oatmeal; the largest pieces of lard should be no bigger than peas.

3. Add the coconut cream and mix until the dough is soft and pulls away from the side of the bowl. If the dough is still dry or crumbly, add water a tablespoon at a time until the dough comes together.

4. Roll out the dough to a thickness of ¾ inch. Use a 2-inch biscuit cutter to cut out 9 to 12 biscuits.

5. Preheat the oven to 400°F.

6. Put the rhubarb and maple syrup in a saucepan and bring to a simmer over medium-high heat. Simmer until the rhubarb is soft but not mushy, about 8 minutes.

7. Mix the arrowroot powder with the water and pour into the rhubarb mixture. Stir constantly until it thickens, about 1 minute.

8. Remove from the heat and fold the strawberries, orange zest, and vanilla into the warm rhubarb mixture.

9. Pour the rhubarb mixture into a 9-inch square baking dish. Arrange the biscuits on top of the rhubarb mixture. Mix together the maple sugar and cinnamon and sprinkle over the top of each biscuit.

10. Bake for 20 minutes. Let cool for at least 15 minutes before serving. Store in the refrigerator for up to a week.

TIP: The biscuits are delicious on their own, too! Arrange them on a rimmed baking sheet lined with parchment paper and bake in a 400°F oven for 15 minutes. Make savory biscuits by replacing the cinnamon and cardamom with 2 to 3 tablespoons of chopped fresh herbs.

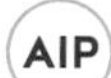 *replace cardamom with cinnamon or mace*

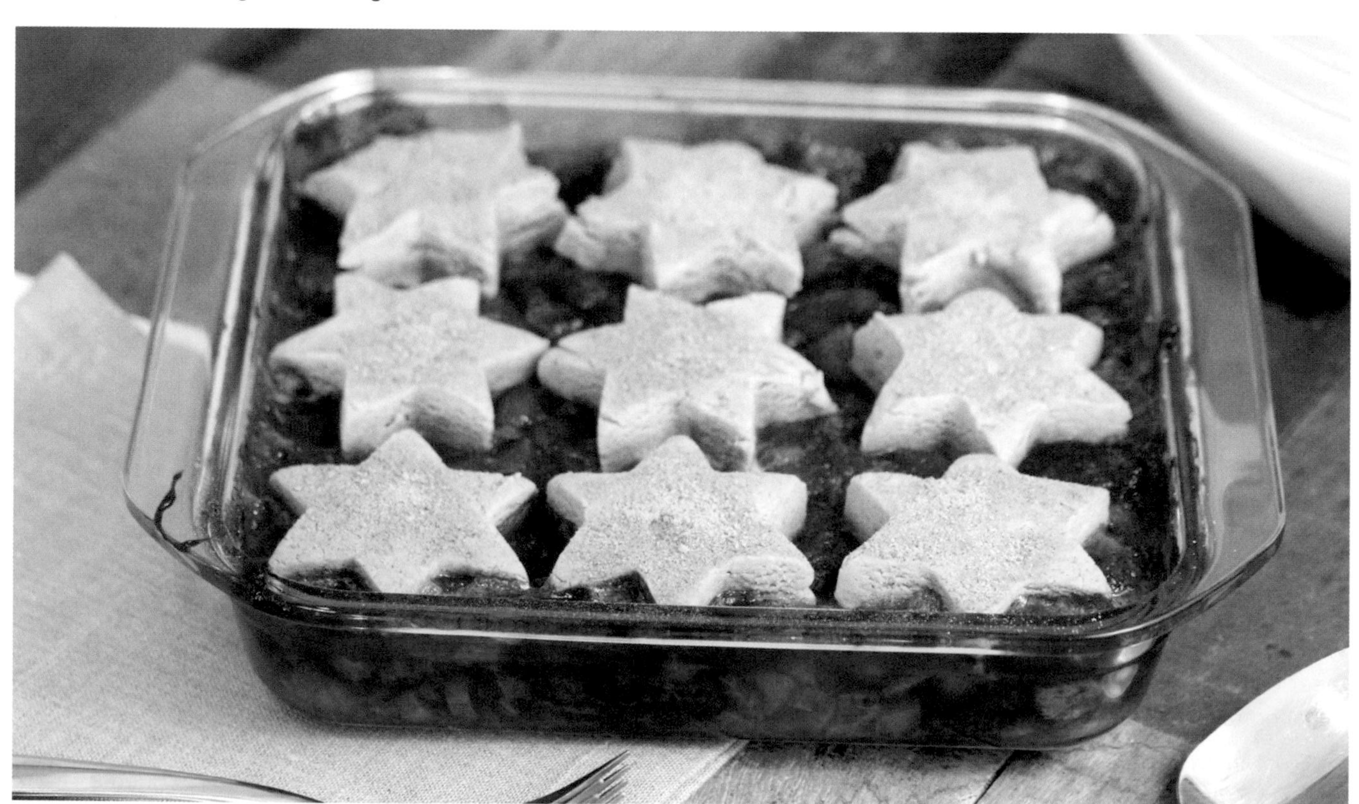

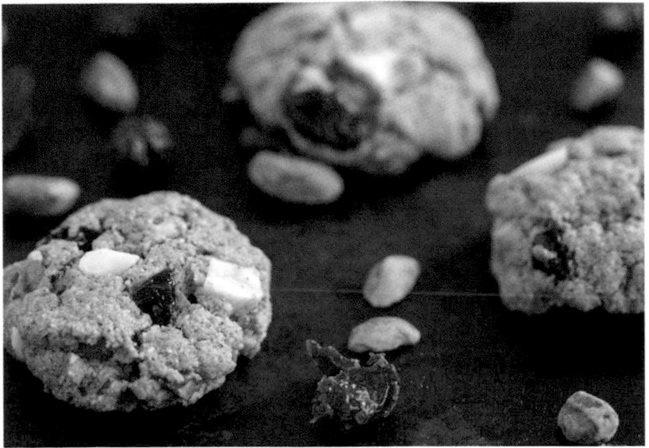

HOLIDAY HERMIT COOKIES

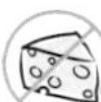   

PREP TIME: 20 minutes *COOK TIME: 10 minutes*
YIELD: 2 dozen cookies

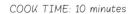

- ¼ cup coconut oil, melted
- ¼ cup smooth almond butter
- ¼ cup muscovado sugar
- 1 large egg
- 1 teaspoon vanilla extract
- 1½ cups blanched almond flour
- ½ teaspoon sea salt
- ½ teaspoon ground allspice
- ½ teaspoon ground cinnamon
- ½ teaspoon ground nutmeg
- ¼ teaspoon ground cloves
- 1 teaspoon baking soda
- ⅓ cup chopped macadamia nuts
- ⅓ cup unsalted pistachios (if they are on the large side, give them a rough chop)
- ⅓ cup chopped raw walnuts
- ¼ cup chopped dried cherries
- ¼ cup chopped dried cranberries
- ¼ cup chopped golden raisins
- ¼ cup chopped Medjool dates

1. Preheat the oven to 350°F.
2. Put the coconut oil, almond butter, sugar, egg, and vanilla in a mixing bowl and stir to combine. Add the almond flour, salt, spices, and baking soda. Mix to fully incorporate and form a thick dough.
3. Add the nuts and dried fruits to the dough and stir to combine.
4. Drop rounded tablespoons of the dough onto an ungreased cookie sheet. Flatten to a thickness of about ½ inch or slightly less. (These cookies don't spread, so whatever shape you make them is the shape they will be after being baked.)
5. Bake for 9 to 10 minutes. Let cool on the cookie sheet for at least a couple of minutes before moving to a cooling rack. Repeat with the remaining dough.
6. Store in an airtight container at room temperature for up to 3 days or freeze for up to 6 months.

CHOCOLATE CHIP COOKIES

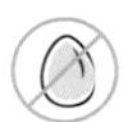 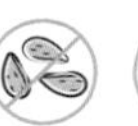 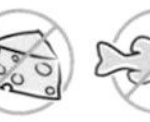 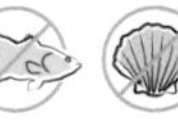 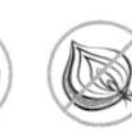 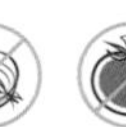 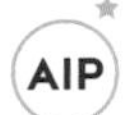 AIP*

PREP TIME: 15 minutes *COOK TIME: 33 minutes*
YIELD: about 3 dozen cookies

- ½ cup palm shortening or unsalted butter
- ½ cup coconut oil
- ⅓ cup maple syrup
- ½ cup muscovado sugar, evaporated cane juice, or maple sugar
- 1 tablespoon vanilla extract
- 1½ cups cassava flour
- 3 tablespoons gelatin
- 1 teaspoon baking soda
- 1 teaspoon sea salt
- ¼ teaspoon ground cinnamon
- 1 (10-ounce) bag bittersweet chocolate chips

1. Preheat the oven to 350°F.
2. Combine the shortening, coconut oil, maple syrup, sugar, and vanilla in a large mixing bowl. Stir vigorously until completely combined and creamy.
3. In a separate bowl, combine the cassava flour, gelatin, baking soda, salt, and cinnamon and mix to incorporate. Add the flour mixture to sugar mixture and stir to form a dough. Fold in the chocolate chips.
4. Use your hands to form 1-inch or slightly larger balls and place the one-third of the balls on an ungreased cookie sheet, spaced at least 1½ inches apart. Flatten the cookies slightly, to about ⅜ inch thick.
5. Bake for 10 to 11 minutes. Allow to cool completely on the cookie sheet before transferring to a cooling rack so the gelatin can set. Repeat with the remaining dough.
6. Store in an airtight container at room temperature for up to 3 days or freeze for up to 6 months.

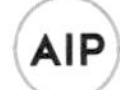 *use palm shortening; replace chocolate chips with dried fruit*

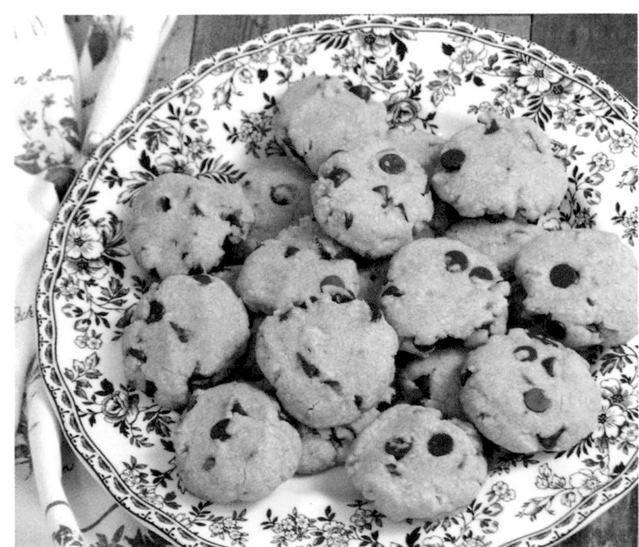

GINGERBREAD CUTOUTS WITH ROYAL ICING

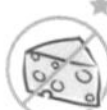 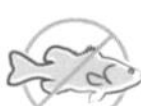  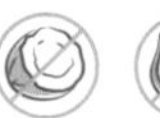  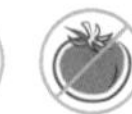

PREP TIME: 20 minutes, plus time for dough to rest and time to decorate

COOK TIME: 18 minutes

YIELD: about 3 dozen cookies

1 cup smooth almond butter

⅓ cup blackstrap molasses

⅓ cup maple sugar or evaporated cane juice

2 tablespoons ghee

½ cup tapioca starch

2 teaspoons ginger powder

1½ teaspoons ground cinnamon

¼ teaspoon ground cloves

¼ teaspoon baking soda

¼ teaspoon sea salt

ROYAL ICING

2 cups evaporated cane juice, maple sugar, or white sugar

1 tablespoon arrowroot powder

1 large egg white

1 teaspoon lemon juice

1. Combine the almond butter, molasses, sugar, and ghee in a bowl and stir until completely smooth.

2. Mix the tapioca starch, ginger, cinnamon, cloves, baking soda, and salt in a small bowl or measuring cup, then add to the almond butter mixture. Knead to form a stiff dough. It's easiest to stick your hands right into the bowl and work the dough together that way.

3. Form the dough into a ball and let it sit at room temperature for 1 hour.

4. Preheat the oven to 300°F. Line a cookie sheet with parchment paper or a silicone baking mat.

5. Place the dough on a sheet of wax paper or parchment paper and roll it out to ⅛ inch thick. Use cookie cutters to cut out shapes and transfer to the prepared cookie sheet. If the shapes aren't transferring easily, put the rolled-out dough in the refrigerator for 10 or more minutes or in the freezer for 5 minutes.

6. Bake for 16 to 18 minutes, depending on the size of your cookies. Repeat with the remaining dough. Let the cookies cool before decorating.

7. Prepare the royal icing: First, make a grain-free confectioners' sugar. Blend the 2 cups of evaporated cane juice (or maple or white sugar) in a blender or food processor until it's a fine powder; this typically takes 30 seconds to a minute. Measure out 1½ cups of this finely ground sugar (save the remainder for other uses). Pour this sugar back into your blender or food processor and add the arrowroot powder. Pulse to combine to finish the confectioners' sugar.

8. Whip the egg white and lemon juice in a bowl (you can do this by hand or with a hand mixer). Slowly add the confectioners' sugar, whip to combine, add a little more, whip to combine, until all the sugar has been added and the royal icing is smooth and glossy.

9. Place the royal icing in a piping bag or a resealable plastic bag with a corner cut off. Pipe the icing decorations onto your gingerbread cutouts. Store in an airtight container on the counter for up to 3 days, in the refrigerator for up to a week, or in the freezer for up to 6 months.

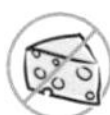 *replace ghee with palm shortening*

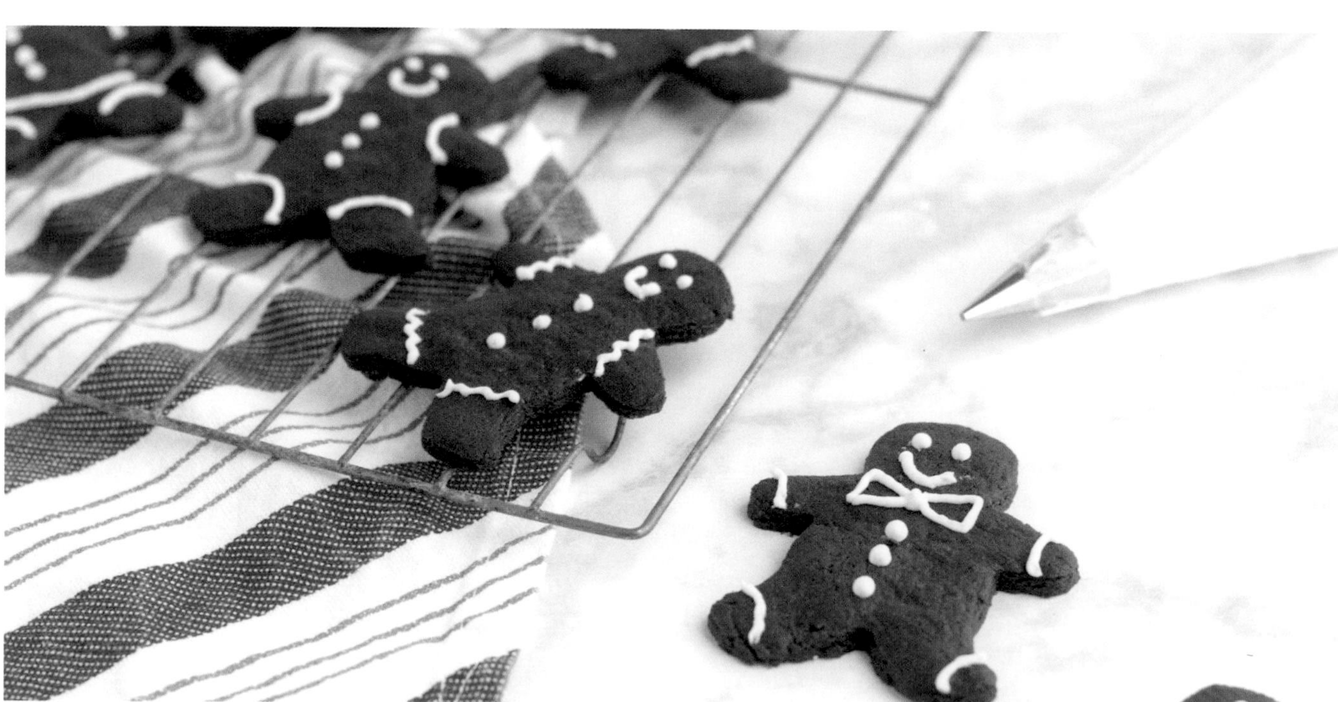

ALMOND-COCONUT BARS

 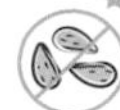 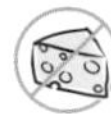 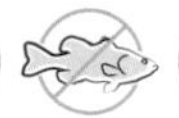 

PREP TIME: 10 minutes, plus 1 hour to set

COOK TIME: 5 minutes YIELD: 12 to 16 bars

- ⅔ cup coconut oil
- 2 cups whole raw almonds
- 1 cup unsweetened shredded coconut
- ½ cup smooth almond butter
- 1½ tablespoons blackstrap molasses
- 1 tablespoon coconut flour
- 1 tablespoon vanilla extract
- ½ teaspoon sea salt
- 3 ounces bittersweet chocolate

1. Melt the coconut oil in a microwave-safe bowl in the microwave on low power or in a small saucepan on the stovetop over low heat.

2. Line a 9-inch square baking pan with wax paper.

3. Pulse the almonds in a food processor until they resemble coarse sand (the goal is something a little coarser than almond meal). Add the remaining ingredients except the chocolate and pulse until a textured paste forms. Finish with a good stir by hand to make sure all the ingredients are evenly incorporated.

4. Pour the mixture into the prepared baking pan and smooth it out to the corners. Refrigerate until set, at least 1 hour.

5. Melt the chocolate either in the microwave on low power or in a heatproof bowl set over a pan of simmering water (aka double boiler). Drizzle the melted chocolate over the almond-coconut base and spread with a spoon or rubber spatula until the base is evenly coated. Place the bars back in the refrigerator for about 5 minutes, until the chocolate is solid but still a little soft (for ease of cutting). Cut into bars and store in a plastic container in the fridge for up to a month or in the freezer for up to 6 months.

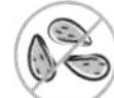 *replace almonds with sunflower seeds and almond butter with sunflower butter*

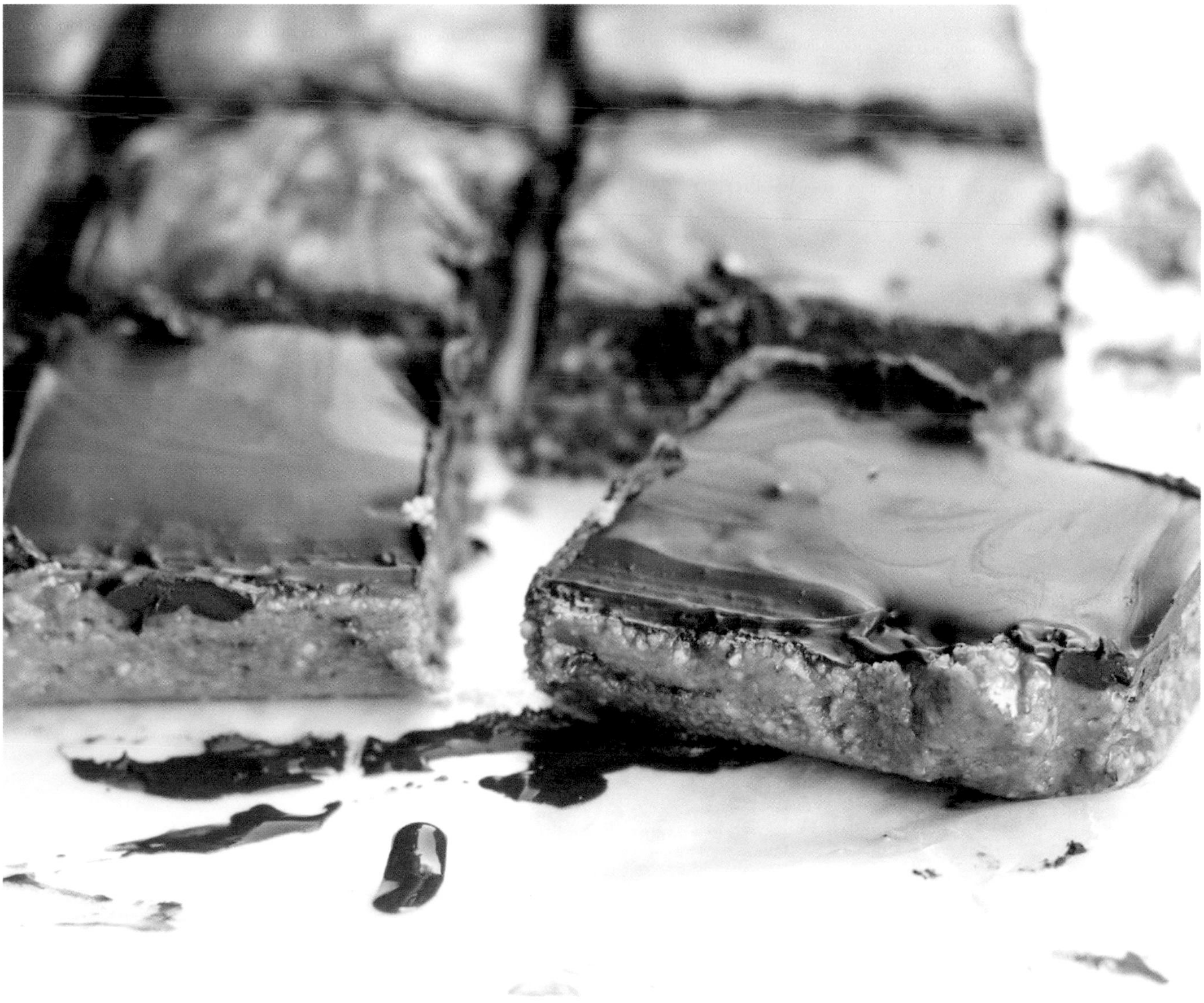

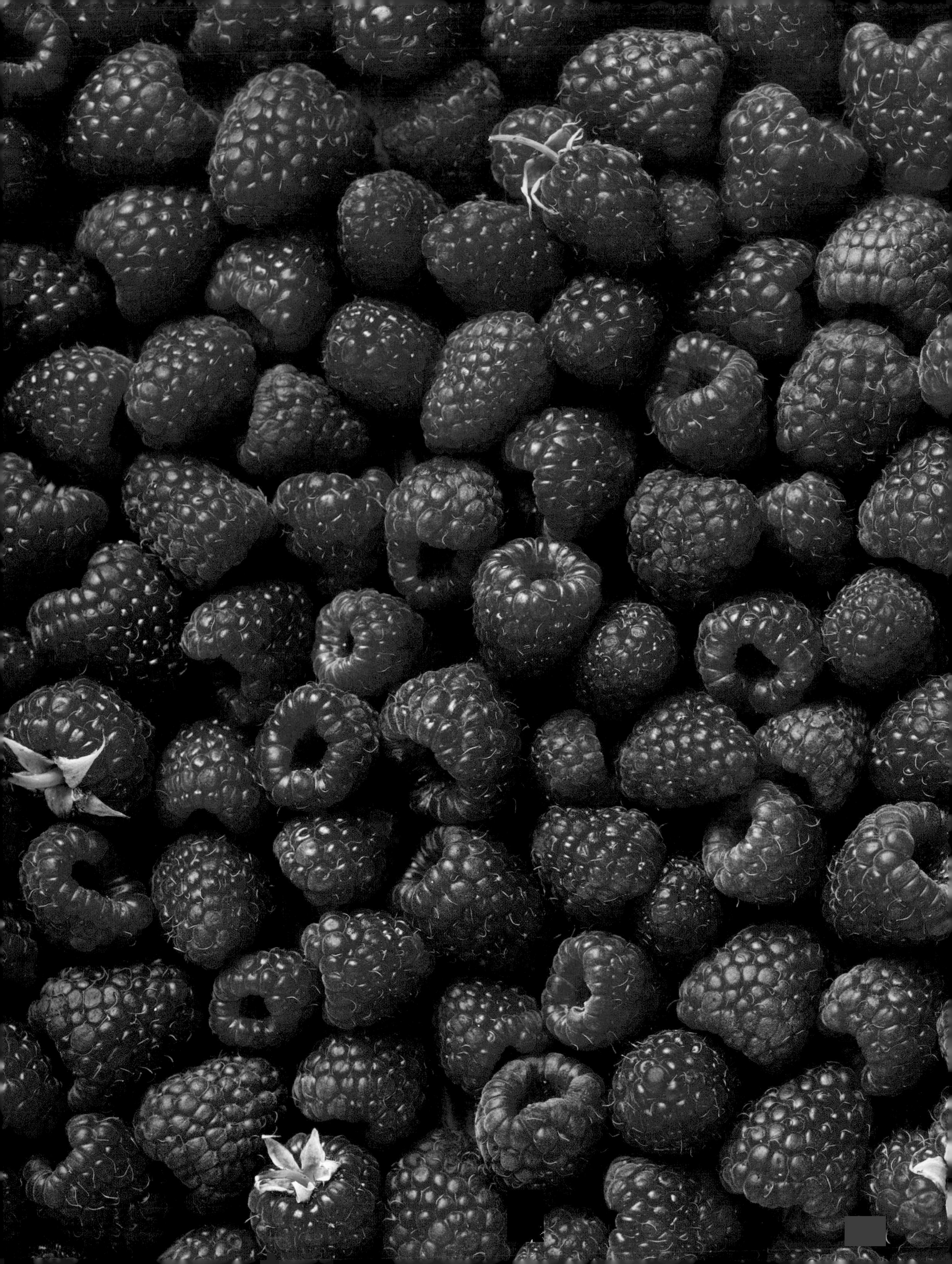

9.

MEAL PLANS

Following a meal plan can be an amazing tool for successfully sticking to dietary priorities. In fact, planning ahead can make all the difference in the world, taking the overwhelm out of learning to eat using Paleo principles. To help you get started, I've included a whopping twenty 1-week meal plans for you to choose from!

Meal plans start on Sundays. This day generally includes more involved recipes as well as efforts to prepare items you may need throughout the week, like a big batch of sausage patties, bone stock, or salad dressing. Weeknight meals are generally more straightforward, with less prep time and shorter cook times to accommodate a typical busy weeknight schedule. If a weeknight meal requires a bit more of a time commitment, it will come with the awesome trade-off of lots of leftovers.

The meal plans assume that you will shop on Saturday and have everything in house by the time you're cooking breakfast on Sunday morning. Though the shopping lists are designed for one big weekly shopping trip (which may or may not include more than one stop), you can break it up into two or more trips to the grocery store if that makes more sense for you. You may want to do a bigger shop on Saturday morning and another smaller shop on Wednesday afternoon, for example. This is actually a better way to organize your week from a nutrient density standpoint, because your produce will be fresher. Have a look at which fresh vegetables and fruits are used in the recipes later in the week and save those items for your midweek supplemental shopping trip.

If your weekend falls on different days, go ahead and do your shopping on the first day of your weekend and start cooking on the second day of your weekend.

The meal plans were constructed assuming that you are feeding two adults. If you'll simply be feeding yourself, you may either halve the recipes, skip a few recipes and eat more leftovers, or freeze the extra portions. If you're cooking for a family of more than two, you'll want to double or triple each recipe in order to have enough for the leftover meals that are built into each plan.

You'll also notice several meals composed of leftovers each week. Sometimes leftovers are reinvented (used to make soup or salad wraps, for example) and sometimes they're just straight up enjoying the same meal again. You'll often have a day in between when you enjoy a meal for the first time and when you eat the leftovers, so your meals shouldn't feel too repetitive. If they do, feel free to spruce them up with a new sauce (see Chapter 40) or a new side dish (see Chapter 44). Generally, you will have a couple meals' worth of leftovers for your freezer by the end of the week. (These extra portions are built in to help you stock your freezer with emergency meals and to accommodate those who need larger portion sizes.)

Don't like eating leftovers and don't mind spending more time in the kitchen? Or are you cooking for a horde so that even a triple batch is unlikely to provide leftovers? Go ahead and substitute new meals instead of leftovers in the plans. Remember to adjust the quantities in your shopping list accordingly.

Among the twenty meal plans are six weeks of general meal plans (Everyday Meal Plan Weeks 1 through 6) and fourteen themed meal plans. Most of the themed meal plans are appropriate for everyone (although you may not wish to follow the Weight-Loss Meal Plan if you are extremely active or underweight, and you may not wish to follow the Performance Meal Plan if you're quite sedentary), so even if you have no particular risk factors for cancer, cardiovascular disease, diabetes, mental health challenges, or autoimmune disease, you can still follow those meal plans and enjoy the recipes featured in them.

Once you've selected which meal plan you intend to follow, read through the calendar for that plan and have a look at each of the recipes and the corresponding shopping list. If any food jumps out at you as being a strong dislike or sensitivity, plan a substitute for either that ingredient or the entire dish. You may need to make substitutions to accommodate seasonal availability, too. If you know that it's going to be difficult to get blood oranges, for example, you can choose regular oranges instead. Or maybe you know that your local farmer will have Brussels sprouts this week, so you can swap Roasted Brussels Sprouts for the planned Broiled Asparagus. You may also choose to substitute simpler meals for breakfasts and lunches. If you know that you'd rather just have a can of salmon with some salad for lunch than a meal that requires preparation, that's fine. There are also opportunities to customize your meals. For example, the DIY recipes have a lot of flexibility built right in, so go ahead and choose your favorite options. Also make sure to adjust the plan if you are feeding more or fewer than two adults.

Determine if and how you want to modify the plan, and update the shopping list to reflect those modifications. Next, compare the items on your shopping list with what's in your pantry, fridge, and freezer. Strike off the list any foods that you already have on hand. Also figure out if you will need to order any ingredients online. For those items, you'll want to order well in advance to make sure that they arrive in time. Finally, make a plan of which items you are going to buy from which stores, farm stands, or farmers markets.

Before you go shopping, have a look at the "Make Ahead" list for your meal plan. This list includes recipes that can be made ahead of time on the weekend to save you time during the week. You may wish to tackle these recipes on Saturday afternoon before you start your meal plan week. It's not essential to do all or any of these tasks during a big cooking session, but if you typically find yourself pressed for time on weekdays, you will appreciate the effort you put in over the weekend. You can also save yourself some time by looking for quality versions of common make-ahead recipes at the store:

- **Mayonnaise:** Look for options that use only avocado and/or olive oil.
- **Sauerkraut:** Look for raw, unpasteurized options.
- **Bone broth:** Check out page 638 for favorite brands and where to buy them.
- **Salad dressing:** Look for olive oil or avocado oil-based dressings with no added preservatives.
- **Coconut milk yogurt:** Look for yogurt or kefir with short ingredient lists and few or no emulsifiers.
- **Coconut and nut milk:** Look for milks with only coconut or nuts and water as the ingredients.
- **Coconut cream:** Look for options with only coconut and water as the ingredients.
- **Kombucha:** Look for raw, unpasteurized options and pay attention to the flavoring ingredients used.

You can also substitute store-bought versions of some whole recipes, but make sure to read ingredients thoroughly. For example, you can save time by purchasing:

- Siete tortillas or coconut wraps instead of making homemade tortillas
- Simple Mills crackers instead of making homemade crackers
- Legit Bread Company or Simple Mills bread mix instead of making bread from scratch

Most importantly, have fun. These meal plans are designed to make things easier for you. If they aren't achieving that goal, nothing is forcing you to stick with them. Go ahead and devise your own plans! Or skip the meal plans altogether and buy whatever inspires you at the farmers market on Saturday morning; you can decide what to make from those ingredients when you get home. The point is to figure out how to make this approach work for you, and meal plans are only one tool in your toolbox.

THE BEST SNACKS

The meal plans in this book don't include snacks because it's generally better to avoid snacking. However, if you have kids or your schedule or health history mean that snacking is part of your day, think of a snack as an opportunity to up your nutrient intake. There are plenty of snack options that include organ meat, seafood, and veggies. It's also best to think of a snack as a mini meal, meaning that you want a balance of protein, carbohydrates, and healthy fats.

Here are some of my favorite nutrient-packed snacks:

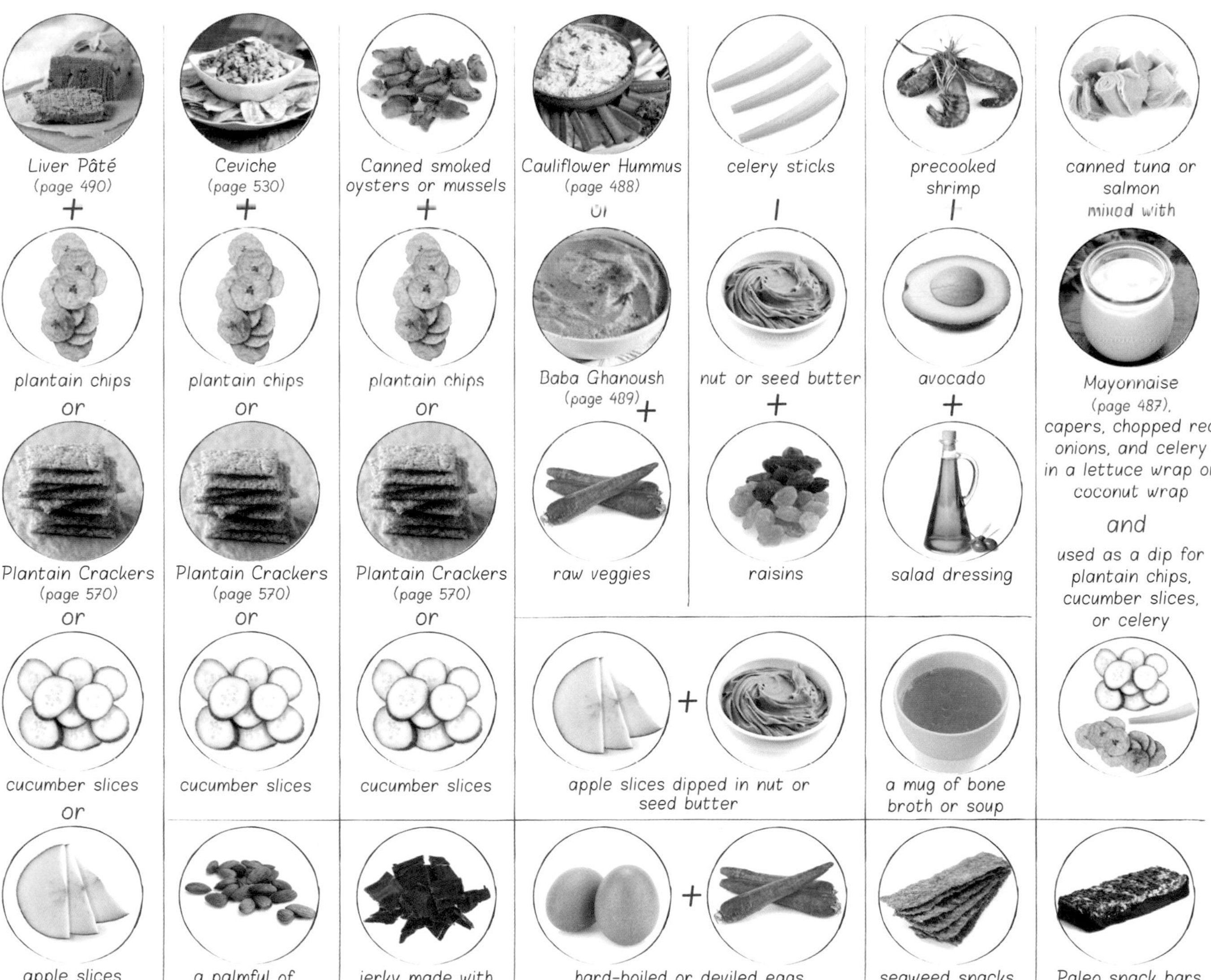

Chapter 46:
MEAL PLANS

EVERYDAY MEAL PLAN Week 1

SHOPPING LIST

PRODUCE
arugula – 2 cups
avocados – 2½
baby kale – 2 cups
basil – 2 tablespoons
berries of choice – 2 pounds
bok choy – 4 to 6 bunches
cassava – 2½ pounds
cauliflower – 1 head
celery – 8 stalks
chives – 1 tablespoon
cilantro – 1¾ cups
cucumber – ½ cup
dill – 3 tablespoons
eggplants – 2
fennel bulb – ½
garlic – 4 heads
ginger root – 1 inch plus 1 tablespoon
jalapeño pepper – 1
jicama – ½ cup
kale – 2 cups
kumquats – 4
lemons – 1½
lime juice – 5 tablespoons
mangoes – 2
mint – 1 tablespoon
mushrooms – 28 ounces
orange – 1
oregano – 1 tablespoon
parsley – 1 tablespoon
plantains, green – 3
portobello mushroom caps – 6
red bell pepper – ½
red onions – ½ plus 1 cup
romaine lettuce – 2 heads
spaghetti squash – 4 pounds
spinach – 12 ounces
thyme – 2 teaspoons
tomatoes – 1½ pounds
watermelon – 5 cups
yellow onions – 2½
zucchini – 4
salad veggies of choice for DIY Salad (page 519) – 2 meals

MEAT & SEAFOOD
bacon – 2 pounds
Canadian bacon – 4 slices
chicken tenders – 1 pound
chicken thighs – 2 pounds
chicken wings – 3 pounds
ground beef – 3 pounds
ground turkey – 2 pounds
liver – 1 pound
salmon fillets – 4 (6 to 8 ounces each)
shrimp, precooked – 1 pound

EGGS & DAIRY
eggs – 44

DELI & PREPARED FOODS
bone stock – 2 cups (or ingredients to make homemade, page 486)

DRIED HERBS & SPICES
anise seed
black pepper
cayenne pepper
chili powder
fennel seeds
galangal
garlic powder
granulated onion
ground coriander
ground cumin
oregano
paprika
sea salt
truffle salt
ingredients for salad dressing of choice (pages 484 to 485)

VINEGARS & OILS
apple cider vinegar
avocado oil
balsamic vinegar
coconut oil
coconut water vinegar
duck fat
lard
olive oil
sesame oil
white wine vinegar
ingredients for salad dressing of choice (pages 484 to 485)

BULK
dried figs – 3
raw cashews – 8 ounces
raw walnut halves – ½ cup

SWEETENERS & BAKING SUPPLIES
active dry yeast – 1 teaspoon
almond flour – ½ cup
arrowroot powder – 2 tablespoons
baking soda – 1¼ teaspoons
cassava flour – 1½ cups
cream of tartar – ¼ teaspoon
gelatin – 1 tablespoon
honey – 2 tablespoons
vanilla extract – 2 teaspoons

CANNED & JARRED GOODS
anchovy paste – 1 teaspoon
capers – 3 tablespoons
coconut aminos – ½ cup
coconut cream – ¼ cup (or ingredients to make homemade, page 480)
diced tomatoes – 5 (15-ounce) cans
mayonnaise – 1½ cups (or ingredients to make homemade, page 487)
tomato paste – 1 can

ASIAN FOODS
bamboo shoots – 1 (5-ounce) can
fish sauce – 3 tablespoons
water chestnuts – 1 (5-ounce) can

MAKE AHEAD OR PURCHASE QUALITY OPTIONS
salad dressing, bone stock, mayonnaise

	BREAKFAST	LUNCH	DINNER
SUNDAY	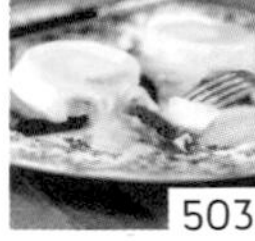 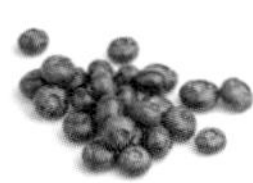 503 Eggs Benedict and berries	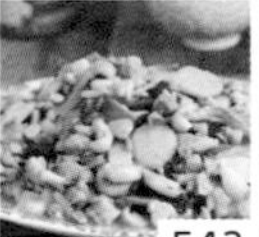 542 555 Cashew Chicken and Asian Cauli-rice	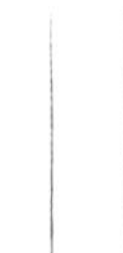 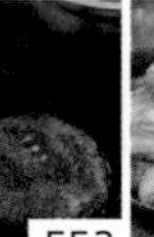 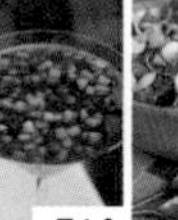 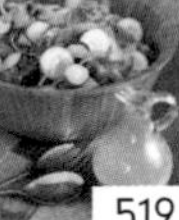 525 552 554 514 519 50/50/50 Burgers, Grilled Portobello Mushroom Caps, Cassava Oven Fries, Watermelon Gazpacho, and DIY Salad
MONDAY	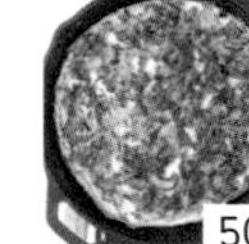 507 502 Veggie Frittata and Crispy Bacon	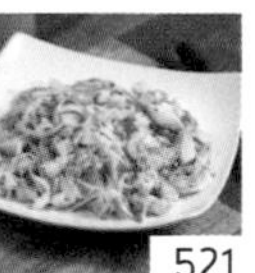 521 Shrimp Salad	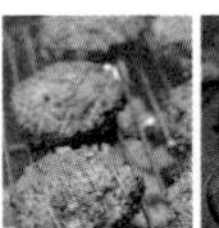 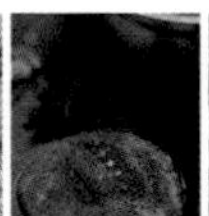 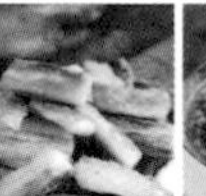 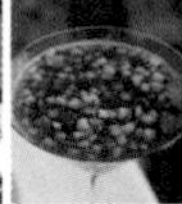 LEFTOVER LEFTOVER LEFTOVER LEFTOVER Leftover 50/50/50 Burgers, Grilled Portobello Mushroom Caps, Cassava Oven Fries, and Watermelon Gazpacho
TUESDAY	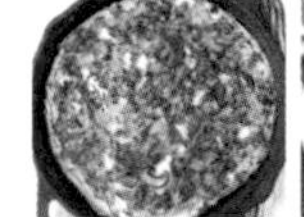 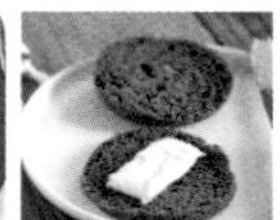 LEFTOVER LEFTOVER Leftover Veggie Frittata and English Muffins and berries	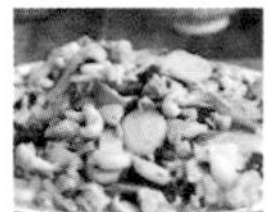 LEFTOVER LEFTOVER Leftover Cashew Chicken and Asian Cauli-rice	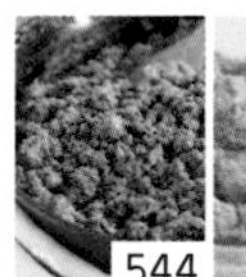 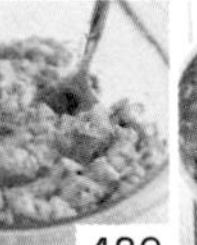 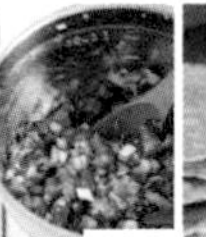 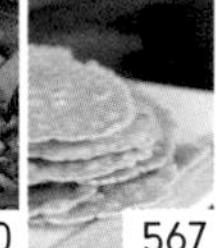 544 489 490 567 Taco Meat, Guacamole, Pico de Gallo, and Tortillas Serve with shredded romaine lettuce.
WEDNESDAY	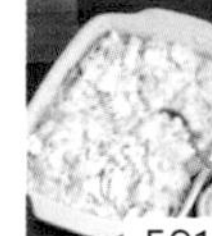 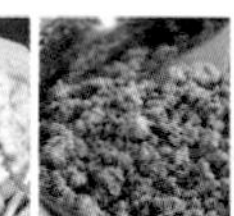 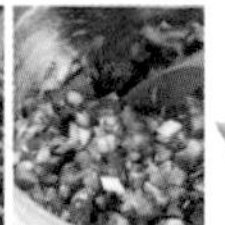 501 LEFTOVER LEFTOVER Oven Scrambled Eggs with leftover Taco Meat and Pico de Gallo and mango	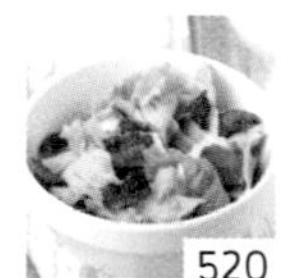 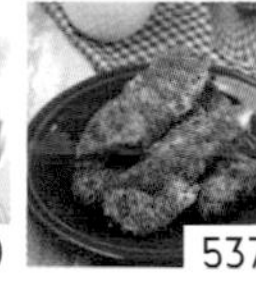 520 537 Paleo Caesar Salad and Chicken Fingers Use leftover Crispy Bacon in Caesar Salad. Wrap in leftover Tortilla.	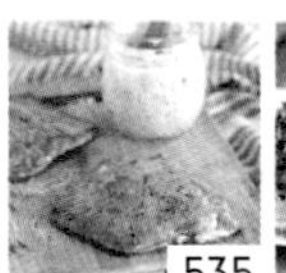 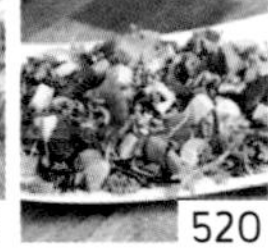 535 520 Broiled Salmon with Dill-Caper Sauce and Citrus, Fig & Walnut Salad
THURSDAY	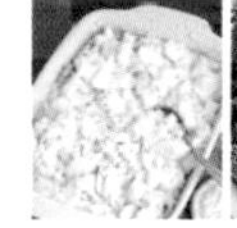 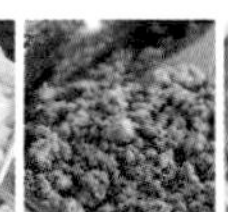 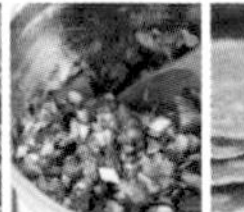 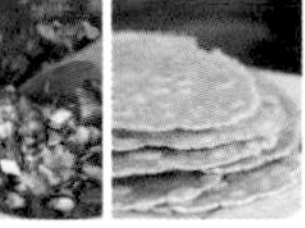 LEFTOVER LEFTOVER LEFTOVER LEFTOVER Breakfast tacos made with leftover Oven Scrambled Eggs, Taco Meat, Pico de Gallo, and Tortillas	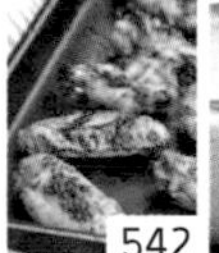 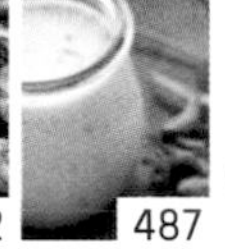 542 487 Asian-Inspired Chicken Wings, Ranch Dip, and raw veggies for dipping	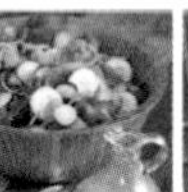 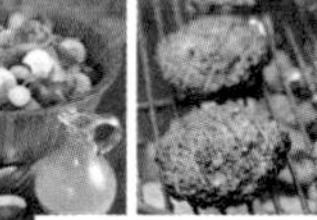 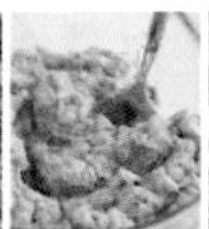 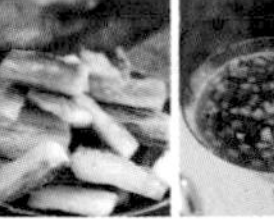 519 LEFTOVER LEFTOVER LEFTOVER LEFTOVER DIY Salad and leftover 50/50/50 Burgers, Guacamole, Cassava Oven Fries, and Watermelon Gazpacho
FRIDAY 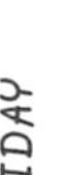 	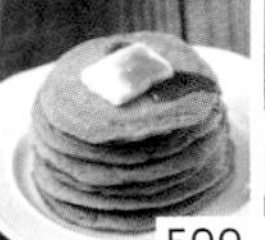 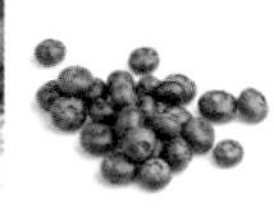 500 LEFTOVER DIY Pancakes, leftover Oven Scrambled Eggs, and berries	LEFTOVER LEFTOVER Leftover Broiled Salmon with Dill-Caper Sauce and Paleo Caesar Salad	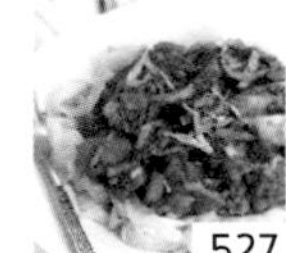 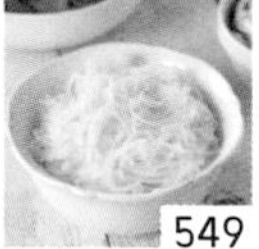 527 549 Meaty Ratatouille Pasta Sauce over Spaghetti Squash Noodles
SATURDAY	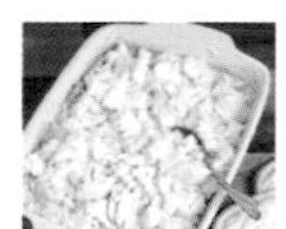 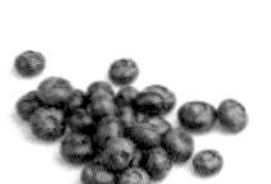 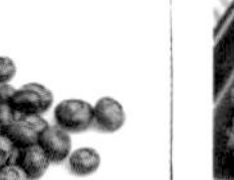 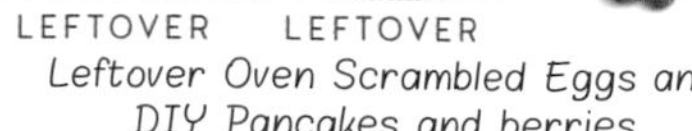 LEFTOVER LEFTOVER Leftover Oven Scrambled Eggs and DIY Pancakes and berries	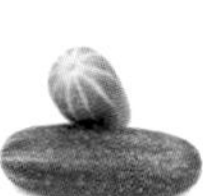 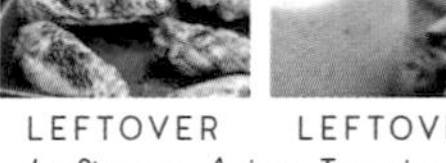 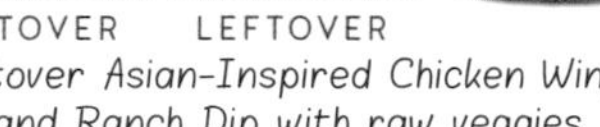 LEFTOVER LEFTOVER Leftover Asian-Inspired Chicken Wings and Ranch Dip with raw veggies	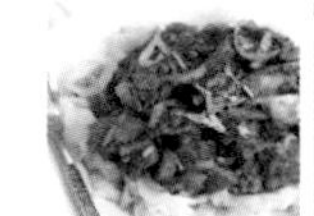 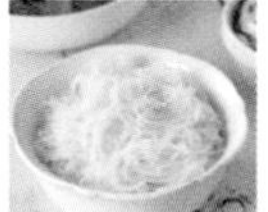 LEFTOVER LEFTOVER Leftover Meaty Ratatouille Pasta Sauce over Spaghetti Squash Noodles

EVERYDAY MEAL PLAN Week 2

SHOPPING LIST

PRODUCE

asparagus - 2 bunches
bananas - 2
berries of choice - 12 pounds
broccoli slaw - 1 package
carrots - 5
cauliflower - 2 heads
celery - 4 stalks
cilantro - 1 cup
dill - ½ cup
fennel bulb - 1 pound
garlic - 2 heads
grapefruit - 1
green onions - 5
lemons - 6
limes - 3
mint - 2 tablespoons
mushrooms - 3 cups
oranges - 2
parsley - 1¼ cups
plantains, green - 6
red bell pepper - ½
romaine lettuce - 1 head
sage - 2 teaspoons
shallots - 5
turnips - 1 pound
white onion - ½
yellow onion - ½
zucchini - 2
salad veggies of choice for DIY Salad (page 519) - 4 meals
veggies of choice for DIY Steamed Veggies (page 548) - 1 meal
veggies of choice for DIY Omelet (page 508) - 2 meals

MEAT & SEAFOOD

bacon - 5 slices
chicken - 1 whole (3 pounds)
flank steak or chicken thighs (for Pot Pie) - 2 pounds
ground pork - 3 pounds
lox - 1½ pounds
salad shrimp, precooked - 1 pound
salmon fillets - 4 (6 to 8 ounces each)
steaks - 4 (6 to 8 ounces each)
meat of choice for DIY Omelet (page 508) - 2 meals

EGGS & DAIRY

butter - 1 cup
eggs - 21
ghee - 2 tablespoons

DRIED HERBS & SPICES

bay leaf
black pepper
coarse sea salt
fennel seeds
fenugreek
garam masala
garlic powder
ground coriander
ground cumin
ginger powder
ground mace
onion powder
red pepper flakes
sea salt
thyme
truffle salt
turmeric powder
ingredients for salad dressing of choice (pages 484 to 485)

VINEGARS & OILS

apple cider vinegar
avocado oil
coconut oil
coconut water vinegar
duck fat
olive oil
red wine vinegar
ingredients for salad dressing of choice (pages 484 to 485)

DELI & PREPARED FOODS

bone stock - 2½ quarts (or ingredients to make homemade, page 486)

BULK

roasted unsalted cashews - ⅓ cup

SWEETENERS & BAKING SUPPLIES

baking soda - 1 teaspoon
cassava flour - ⅓ cup
evaporated cane juice - ¼ cup
gelatin - 1¼ teaspoons
honey - 2 teaspoons
vanilla extract - 1 tablespoon
ingredients for pie crust of choice (page 499)

CANNED & JARRED GOODS

anchovy paste - 1 teaspoon
coconut aminos - 1 tablespoon
coconut milk - 1¾ cups (or ingredients to make homemade, page 480)
mayonnaise - ½ cup (or ingredients to make homemade, page 487)
mustard - 1 tablespoon

ASIAN FOODS

fish sauce - 3 tablespoons

FROZEN FOODS

frozen peas - 1 cup

SUPPLEMENTS

Lactobacillus-based probiotic supplement capsules or non-dairy yogurt starter

OTHER

add-ins of choice for DIY Muffins (page 569)

MAKE AHEAD OR PURCHASE QUALITY OPTIONS

salad dressing, coconut milk yogurt, mayonnaise, bone stock

	BREAKFAST	LUNCH	DINNER
SUNDAY	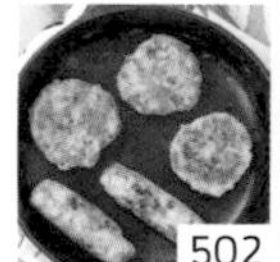 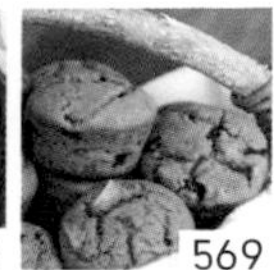 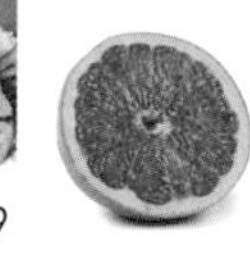 502 569 Breakfast Sausage, DIY Muffins, and half a grapefruit *Reserve 8 ounces of Breakfast Sausage mix for frittata later in the week.*	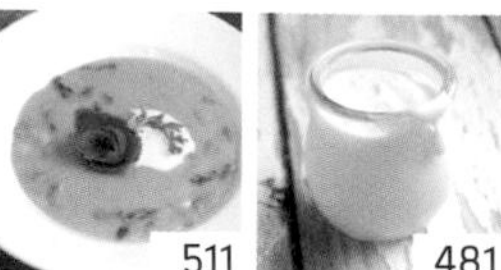 511 481 Asparagus Soup, Coconut Milk Yogurt, and lox	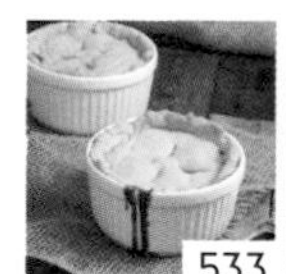 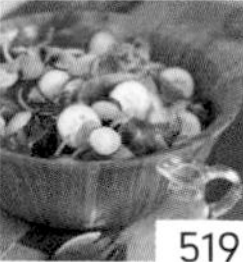 533 519 Chicken or Beef Pot Pie and DIY Salad
MONDAY	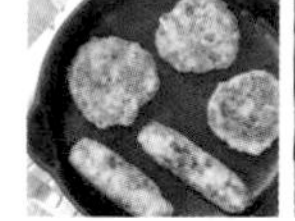 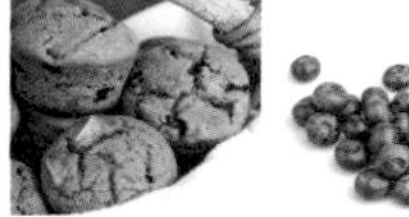 LEFTOVER LEFTOVER Leftover Breakfast Sausage and DIY Muffins and berries	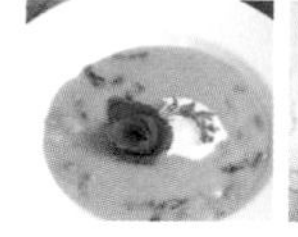 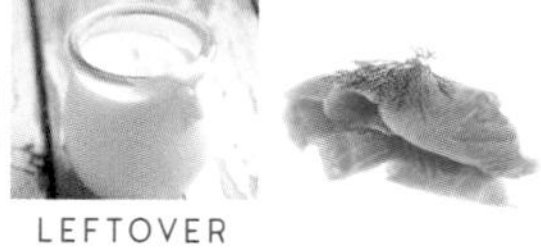 LEFTOVER LEFTOVER Leftover Asparagus Soup, Coconut Milk Yogurt, and lox	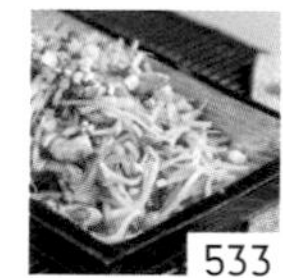 533 Shrimp Pad Thai
TUESDAY	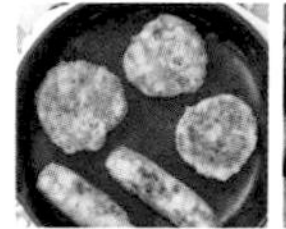 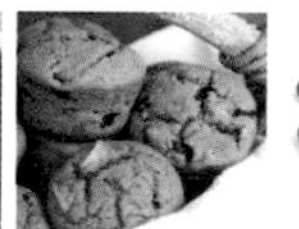 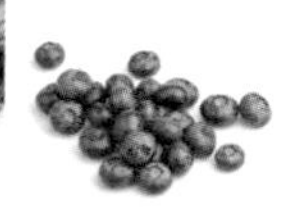 LEFTOVER LEFTOVER Leftover Breakfast Sausage and DIY Muffins and berries	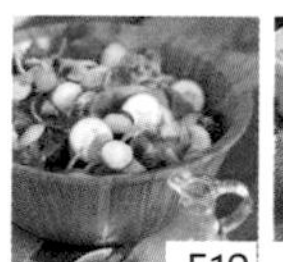 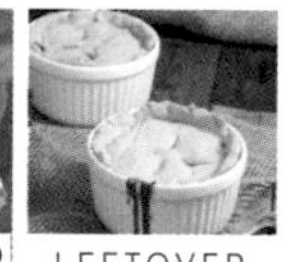 519 LEFTOVER DIY Salad and leftover Chicken or Beef Pot Pie	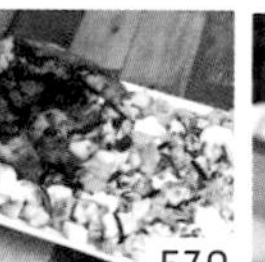 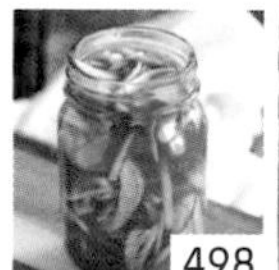 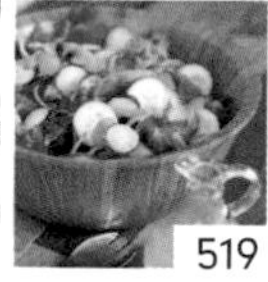 539 498 519 Bengali Tandoori Chicken with Aloo Gobi, Easy Pickled Shallots, and DIY Salad
WEDNESDAY	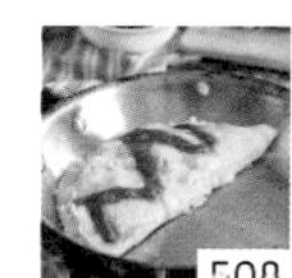 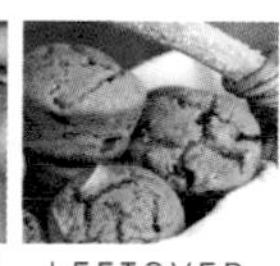 508 LEFTOVER DIY Omelet and leftover DIY Muffins	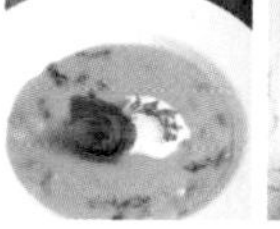 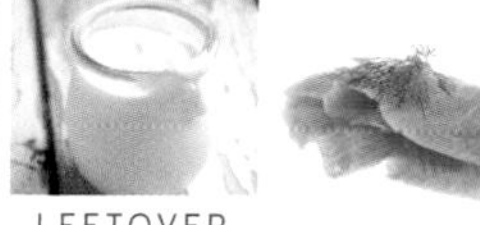 LEFTOVER LEFTOVER Leftover Asparagus Soup, Coconut Milk Yogurt, and lox	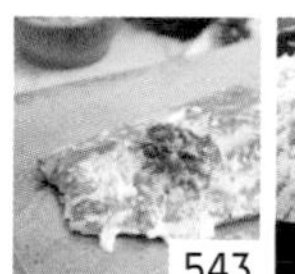 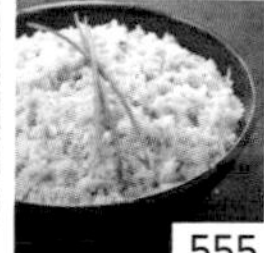 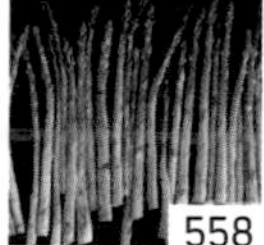 543 555 558 Salmon en Papillote with Maître d' Butter, Lemon Parsley Cauli-rice, and Broiled Asparagus
THURSDAY	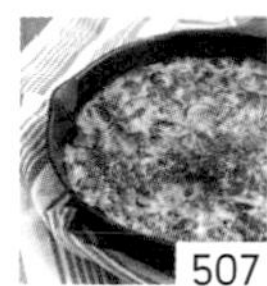 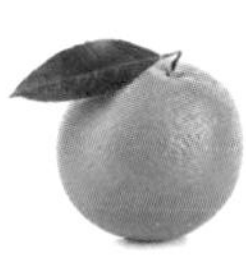 507 Sausage & Mushroom Frittata and an orange *Use reserved Breakfast Sausage mix.*	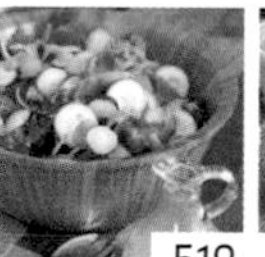 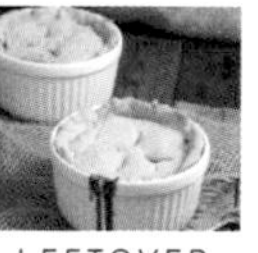 519 LEFTOVER DIY Salad and leftover Chicken or Beef Pot Pie	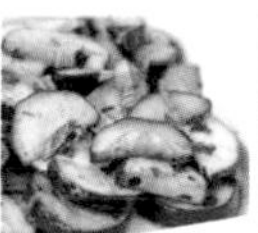 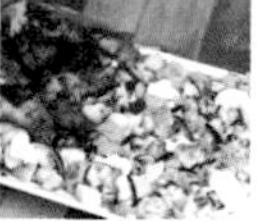 560 LEFTOVER Minted Zucchini and leftover Bengali Tandoori Chicken with Aloo Gobi
FRIDAY	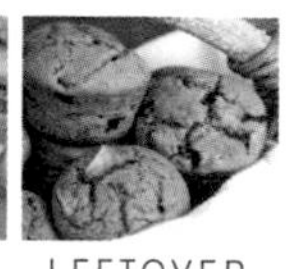 508 LEFTOVER DIY Omelet and leftover DIY Muffins	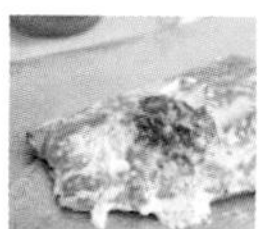 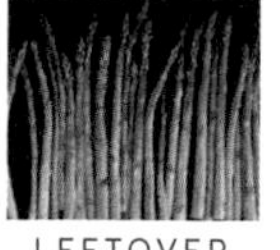 LEFTOVER LEFTOVER LEFTOVER Leftover Salmon en Papillote with Maître d' Butter, Lemon Parsley Cauli-rice, and Broiled Asparagus	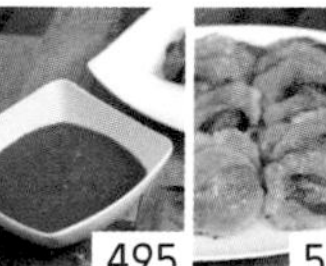 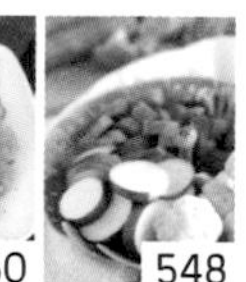 547 495 550 548 Simple Steak, Chimichurri, Tostones, and DIY Steamed Veggies
SATURDAY	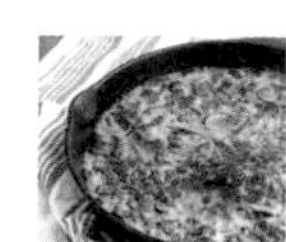 LEFTOVER Leftover Sausage & Mushroom Frittata and a banana	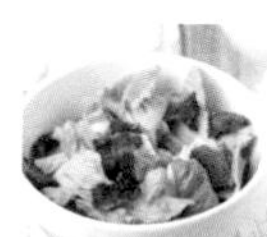 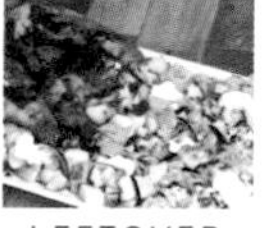 520 LEFTOVER Paleo Caesar Salad and leftover Bengali Tandoori Chicken with Aloo Gobi	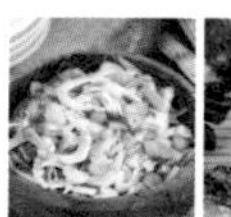 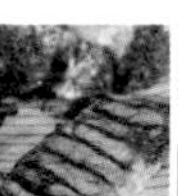 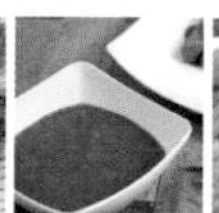 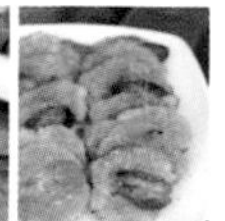 523 LEFTOVER LEFTOVER LEFTOVER Simple Fennel Salad and leftover Simple Steak, Chimichurri, and Tostones

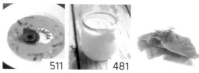

EVERYDAY MEAL PLAN Week 3

SHOPPING LIST

PRODUCE
arugula - 2 cups
asparagus - 1 pound
avocado - ½
bananas - 2
berries of choice - 2 pounds
Brussels sprouts - 2 pounds
broccoli florets - 8 cups
carrots - ¾ pound
cauliflower - 1 head
celery - 8 stalks
chives - 2 tablespoons
fennel bulb - 1 pound
garlic - 3 heads
Granny Smith apples - 2
green bell pepper - 1
kale - 4 cups
kumquats - 4
lemons - 2
mint - ⅓ cup
mushrooms - 1½ cups
orange - 1
parsley - ½ cup
parsnips - 2¼ pounds
peaches - 2
plantain, green - 1
red bell pepper - 2
red onion - ⅓
rosemary - 1 sprig plus 3 tablespoons
sage - 1 tablespoon
spinach - 2 cups
sweet potatoes - 2 cups
thyme - 3½ tablespoons
turnips - 1½ pounds
white onions - 3
winter squash - 2 pounds
yellow onions - 2½
yuca - 1 pound
fruit of choice for Crepes (page 505) - 1 meal
salad veggies of choice for DIY Salad (page 519) - 5 meals
veggies of choice for DIY Omelet (page 508) - 1 meal
veggies of choice for DIY Steamed Veggies (page 548) - 2 meals

MEAT & SEAFOOD
bacon - 8 ounces
duck fat - 2 tablespoons
fish fillets (such as sea bass, mahi mahi, halibut, or swordfish) - 1 to 1½ pounds
ground chicken - 2 pounds
ham - 14 ounces
pancetta - 4 ounces
pork center loin - 4 pounds
steaks - 4 (6 to 8 ounces each)
stew meat - 3 pounds
meat of choice for DIY Omelet (page 508) and/or Crepes (page 505) - 1 meal

EGGS & DAIRY
butter - 1 tablespoon
eggs - 29
ghee - 5 tablespoons

DRIED HERBS & SPICES
bay leaf
black pepper
paprika
sea salt
truffle salt
ingredients for steak seasoning of choice (page 482)
ingredients for salad dressing of choice (pages 484 to 485)

VINEGARS & OILS
avocado oil
balsamic vinegar
coconut oil
duck fat
lard
olive oil
ingredients for salad dressing of choice (pages 484 to 485)

DELI & PREPARED FOODS
bone stock - 1 quart (or ingredients to make homemade, page 486)

BULK
dried figs - 3
raw hazelnuts - 1 cup
raw walnuts - ½ cup

SWEETENERS & BAKING SUPPLIES
arrowroot powder - ½ cup
baking soda - ¼ teaspoon
coconut flour - 2 tablespoons
cream of tartar - ½ teaspoon
maple syrup - ½ cup
maple sugar - 2 tablespoons

CANNED & JARRED GOODS
tomato paste - ½ can

FROZEN FOODS
frozen cranberries - 2 cups

DRINKS
dry red wine - 2 cups

OTHER
plantain chips - ¼ cup

MAKE AHEAD OR PURCHASE QUALITY OPTIONS
salad dressing, bone stock, lard

	BREAKFAST	LUNCH	DINNER
SUNDAY	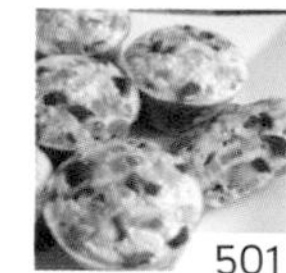 501 Ham & Sweet Potato Egg Muffins and berries	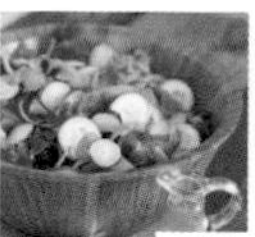 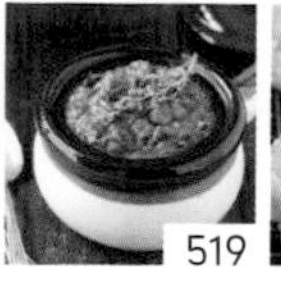 519 519 566 DIY Salad, Hearty Beef Stew, and Yuca Biscuits *Freeze half of the stew and biscuits for later in the week.*	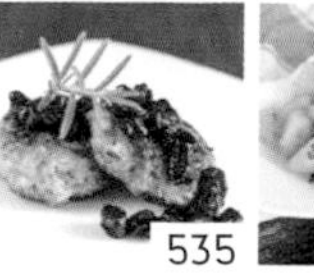 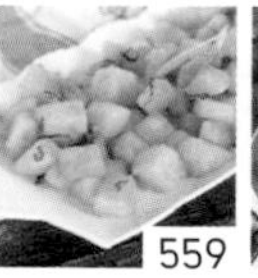 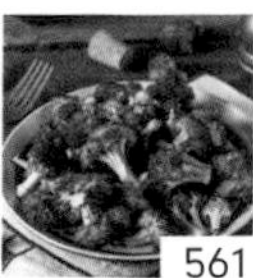 535 559 561 Bacon-Apple Chicken Burgers with Maple Cranberry Sauce, Maple & Sage Roasted Winter Squash, and Roasted Broccoli
MONDAY 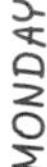	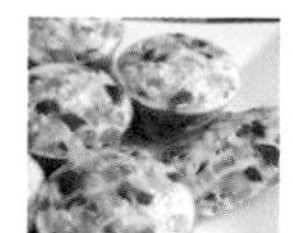 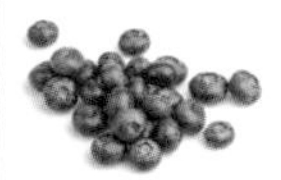 LEFTOVER Leftover Ham & Sweet Potato Egg Muffins and berries	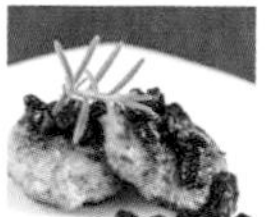 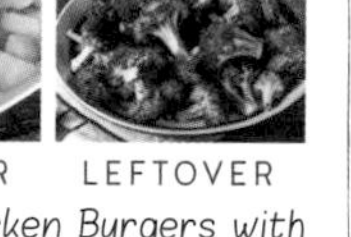 LEFTOVER LEFTOVER LEFTOVER Leftover Bacon-Apple Chicken Burgers with Maple Cranberry Sauce, Maple & Sage Roasted Winter Squash, and Roasted Broccoli	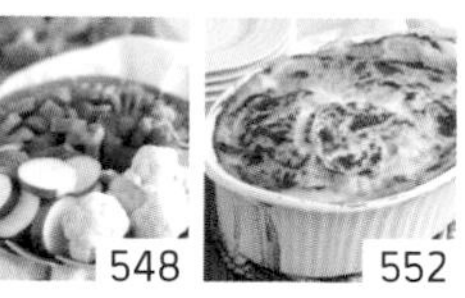 525 548 552 Gremolata-Topped Fish Fillets, DIY Steamed Veggies, and Scalloped Notatoes
TUESDAY	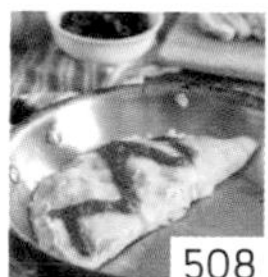 508 DIY Omelet	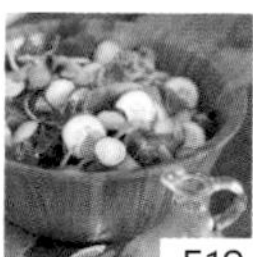 519 LEFTOVER LEFTOVER DIY Salad and leftover Hearty Beef Stew and Yuca Biscuits	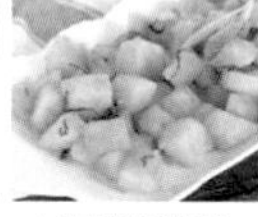 558 LEFTOVER LEFTOVER Broiled Asparagus and leftover Bacon-Apple Chicken Burgers with Maple Cranberry Sauce and Maple & Sage Roasted Winter Squash
WEDNESDAY	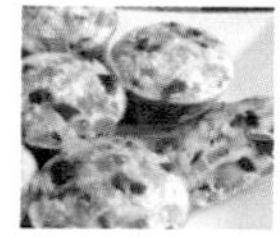 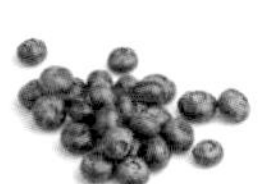 LEFTOVER Leftover Ham & Sweet Potato Egg Muffins and berries	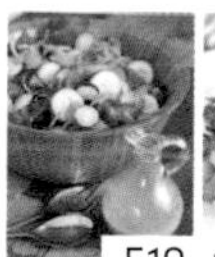 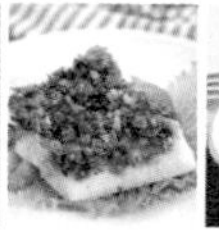 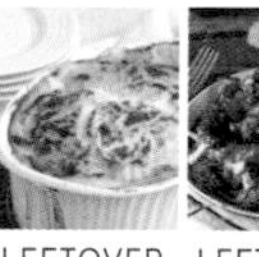 519 LEFTOVER LEFTOVER LEFTOVER DIY Salad and leftover Gremolata-Topped Fish Fillets, Scalloped Notatoes, and Roasted Broccoli	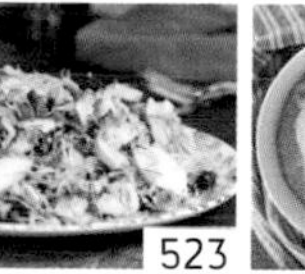 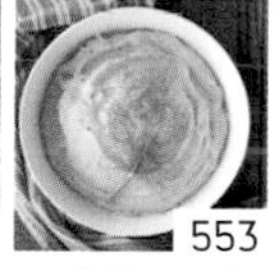 540 523 553 Herb-Crusted Pork Loin, Shaved Brussels Slaw with Hazelnuts, Apple & Mint, and Parsnip & Fennel Puree
THURSDAY	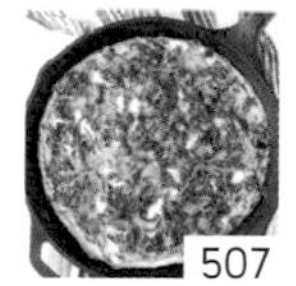 507 Veggie Frittata and a banana	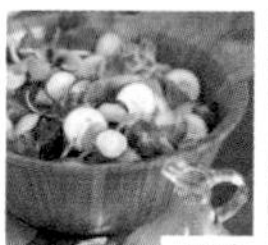 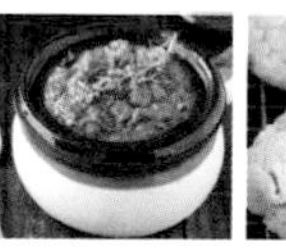 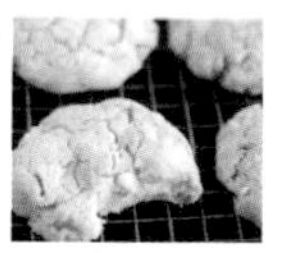 519 LEFTOVER LEFTOVER DIY Salad and leftover Hearty Beef Stew and Yuca Biscuits	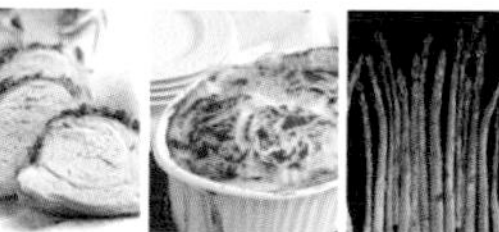 LEFTOVER LEFTOVER LEFTOVER LEFTOVER Leftover Herb-Crusted Pork Loin, Scalloped Notatoes, Broiled Asparagus, and Shaved Brussels Slaw with Hazelnuts, Apple & Mint
FRIDAY	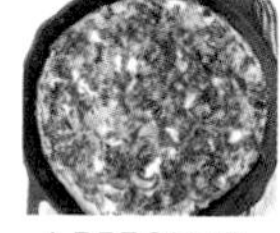 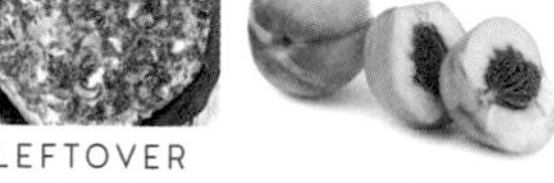 LEFTOVER Leftover Veggie Frittata and a peach	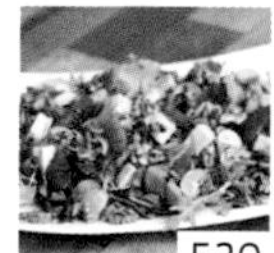 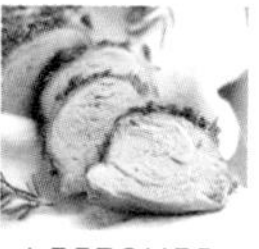 520 LEFTOVER Citrus, Fig & Walnut Salad and leftover Herb-Crusted Pork Loin	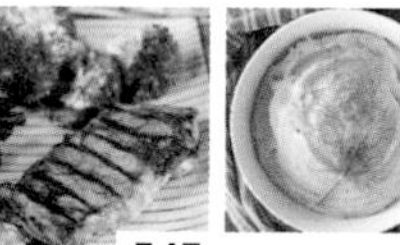 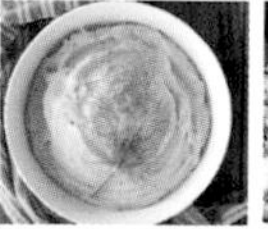 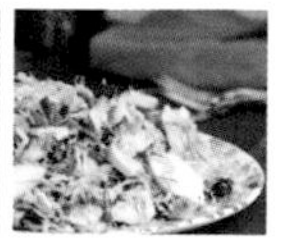 547 LEFTOVER LEFTOVER Simple Steak and leftover Parsnip & Fennel Puree and Shaved Brussels Slaw with Hazelnuts, Apple & Mint
SATURDAY	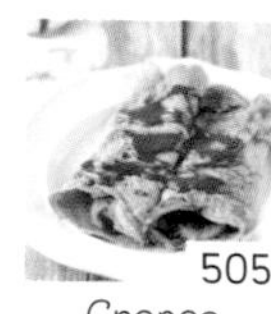 505 Crepes	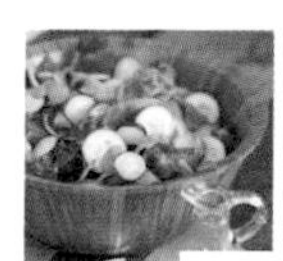 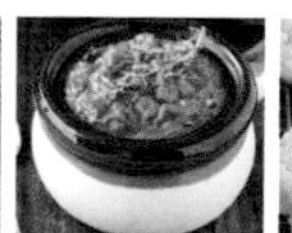 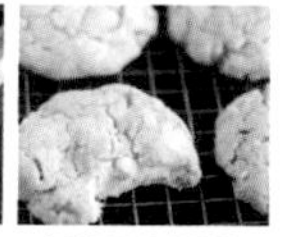 519 LEFTOVER LEFTOVER DIY Salad and leftover Hearty Beef Stew and Yuca Biscuits	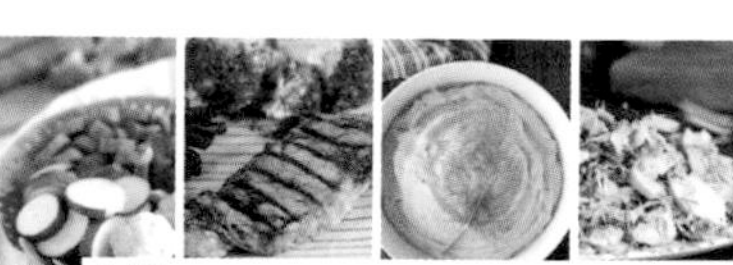 548 LEFTOVER LEFTOVER LEFTOVER DIY Steamed Veggies and leftover Simple Steak, Parsnip & Fennel Puree, and Shaved Brussels Slaw with Hazelnuts, Apple & Mint

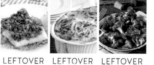

EVERYDAY MEAL PLAN Week 4

SHOPPING LIST

PRODUCE

Asian pear - 1
avocado - 1
berries of choice - 2 pounds
Brussels sprouts - 4 pounds
carrot - 1
cauliflower - 2 heads
celery - 3 stalks
celery root - 2
chives - 1 tablespoon
cilantro - 1¼ cups
eggplants - 2
fennel bulb - ½
garlic - 1 head
ginger root - 1 inch
grapefruit - 1
kiwi - 2
leek - 1 bunch
lemons - 2
limes - 4
mango - 1
mint - ⅔ cup
mushrooms (mix of varieties) - 3 pounds
oranges - 2
parsley - 1 bunch
plantains, green - 4
red bell pepper - ½
red onions - ½ cup
romaine lettuce - 2 heads
rosemary - 1½ tablespoons
turnips - 2 pounds
yellow onions - 1½
greens of choice for DIY Braised Greens - 1 meal
root vegetables of choice for DIY Roasted Roots (page 550) - 2 pounds
salad veggies of choice for DIY Salad (page 519) - 2 meals
veggies of choice for DIY Steamed Veggies (page 548) - 1 meal

MEAT & SEAFOOD

bacon - 14 ounces
Canadian bacon - 4 slices
chickens - 2 whole (4 to 5 pounds each)
crabmeat - 8 ounces
ground beef - 2 pounds
ground pork - 3 pounds
lamb chops - 4 pounds
shrimp, precooked - 1 pound
smoked salmon - 8 ounces
tilapia or other white fish fillets - 4 (6 to 7 ounces each)

EGGS & DAIRY

eggs - 23

DRIED HERBS & SPICES

black pepper
caraway seeds
garlic powder
ginger powder
ground cinnamon
ground coriander
ground cumin
ground mace
ground white pepper
onion powder
savory
sea salt
truffle salt
turmeric powder
ingredients for salad dressing of choice (pages 484 to 485)

VINEGARS & OILS

apple cider vinegar
avocado oil
coconut oil
coconut water vinegar
duck fat
lard
olive oil
red palm oil
sesame oil
ingredients for salad dressing of choice (pages 484 to 485)

DELI & PREPARED FOODS

beef stock - 2 cups (or ingredients to make homemade, page 486)
bone stock - 3¼ cups (or ingredients to make homemade, page 486)
chicken stock - 1 quart (or ingredients to make homemade, page 486)
Medjool dates - ⅓ cup

BULK

cashews - ¾ cup
crystallized ginger - 2 tablespoons
pepitas - ½ cup
raisins - ½ cup
sesame seeds - 3½ tablespoons

SWEETENERS & BAKING SUPPLIES

active dry yeast - 1 teaspoon
arrowroot powder - ¼ cup
baking soda - 1½ teaspoons
honey - 1 tablespoon
maple syrup - 1 tablespoon
vanilla extract - 2 teaspoons

CANNED & JARRED GOODS

anchovy paste - 1 teaspoon
coconut cream - 1 cup (or ingredients to make homemade, page 480)
Dijon mustard - 2 tablespoons
mayonnaise - ½ cup (or ingredients to make homemade, page 487)
pomegranate molasses - 1 tablespoon

ASIAN FOODS

fish sauce - 5 tablespoons

MAKE AHEAD OR PURCHASE QUALITY OPTIONS

salad dressing, bone stock, mayonnaise

	BREAKFAST	LUNCH	DINNER
SUNDAY	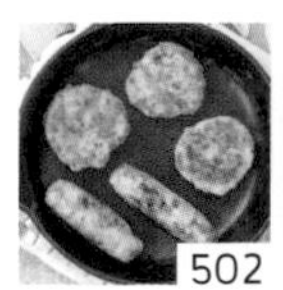 502 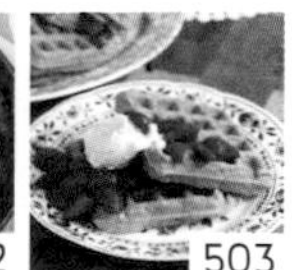 503 Bratwurst and Waffles with berries *Reserve 8 ounces of Bratwurst mix for frittata later in the week.*	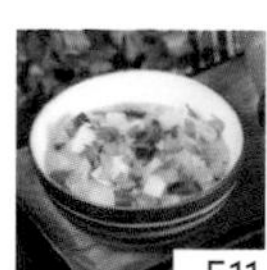 511 Chunky Notato Leek Soup with crabmeat	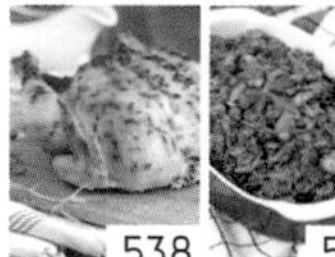 538 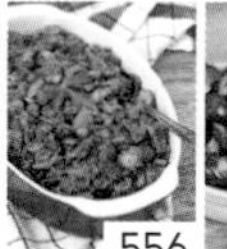 556 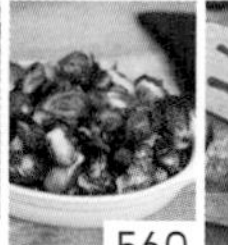 560 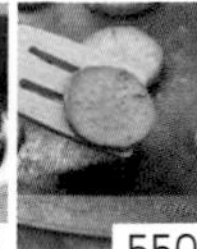 550 Mustard & Rosemary Roasted Chicken with Pan Sauce, Eggplant & Wild Mushroom Dressing, Roasted Brussels Sprouts, and DIY Roasted Roots
MONDAY	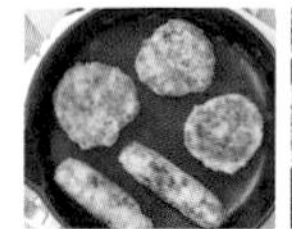 LEFTOVER 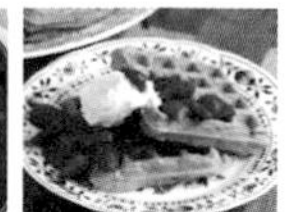 LEFTOVER Leftover Bratwurst and Waffles with berries	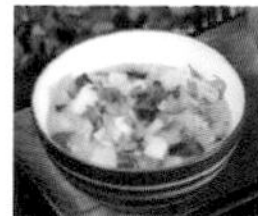 LEFTOVER LEFTOVER Leftover Chunky Notato Leek Soup and Mustard & Rosemary Roasted Chicken with Pan Sauce	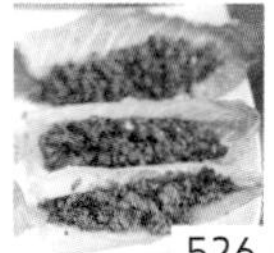 526 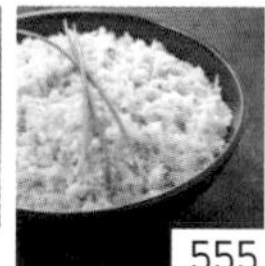 555 Thai Beef Lettuce Wraps and Asian Cauli-rice
TUESDAY	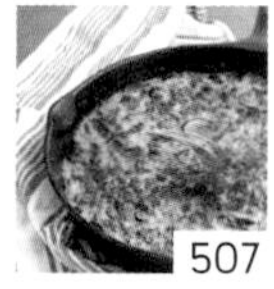 507 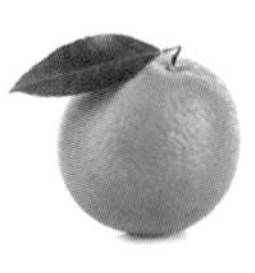 Sausage & Mushroom Frittata and an orange *Use reserved Bratwurst mix.*	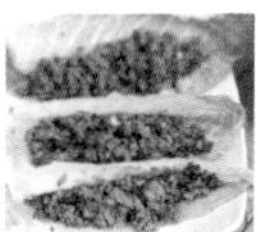 LEFTOVER LEFTOVER Leftover Thai Beef Lettuce Wraps and Asian Cauli-rice	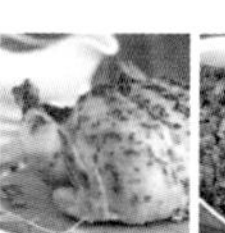 LEFTOVER 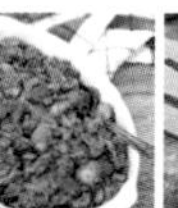 LEFTOVER 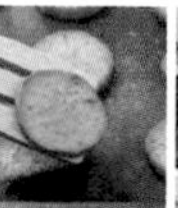 LEFTOVER 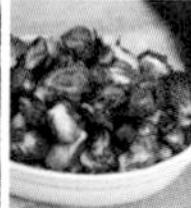 LEFTOVER Leftover Mustard & Rosemary Roasted Chicken with Pan Sauce, Eggplant & Wild Mushroom Dressing, DIY Roasted Roots, and Roasted Brussels Sprouts
WEDNESDAY	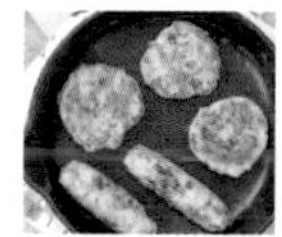 LEFTOVER 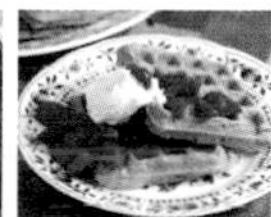 LEFTOVER Leftover Bratwurst and Waffles with berries	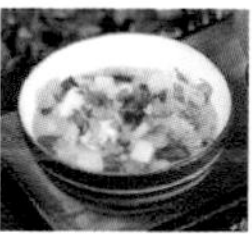 LEFTOVER Leftover Chunky Notato Leek Soup with smoked salmon	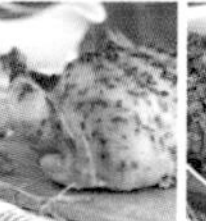 LEFTOVER 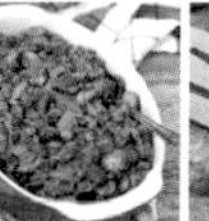 LEFTOVER 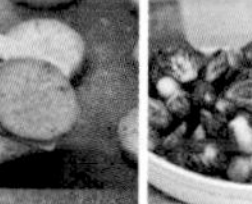 LEFTOVER LEFTOVER Leftover Mustard & Rosemary Roasted Chicken with Pan Sauce, Eggplant & Wild Mushroom Dressing, DIY Roasted Roots, and Roasted Brussels Sprouts
THURSDAY	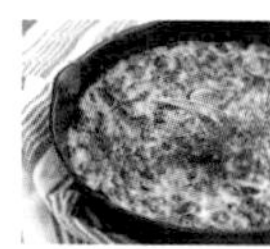 LEFTOVER 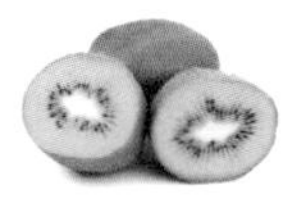 Leftover Sausage & Mushroom Frittata and a kiwi	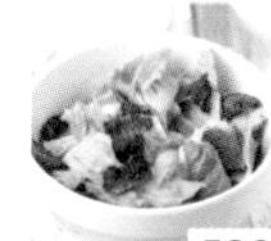 520 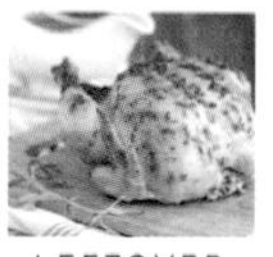 LEFTOVER Paleo Caesar Salad and leftover Mustard & Rosemary Roasted Chicken with Pan Sauce *Wrap in coconut wraps or Tortillas, if desired.*	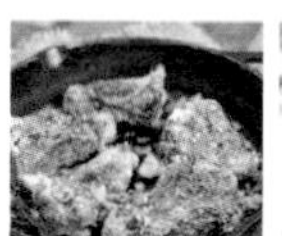 538 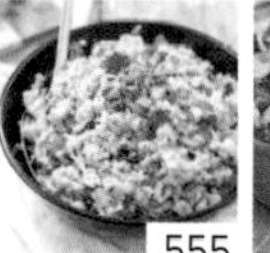 555 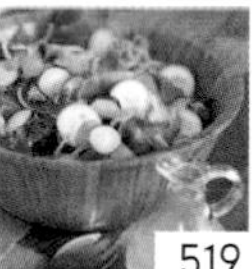 519 Middle Eastern Dukkah-Crusted Lamb Chops, Moroccan "Couscous," and DIY Salad
FRIDAY	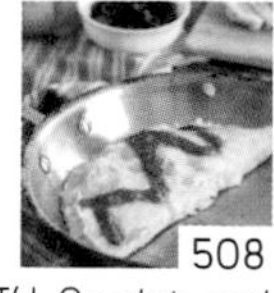 508 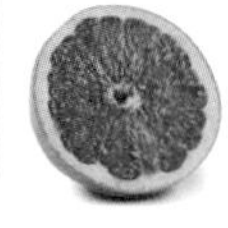 DIY Omelet and half a grapefruit	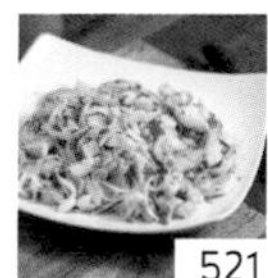 521 Shrimp Salad	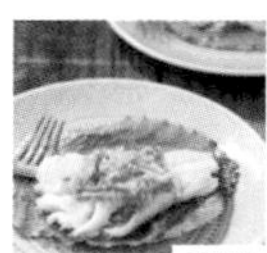 536 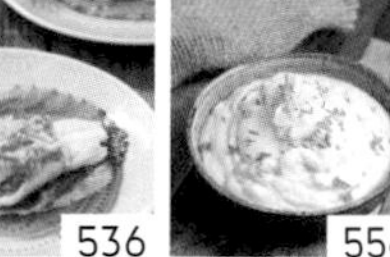 556 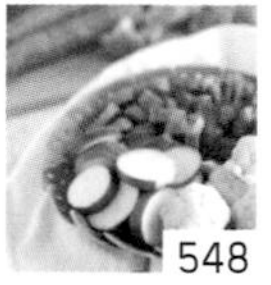 548 Coconut Oil-Poached Tilapia with Asian Pear Slaw, Celery Root Puree, and DIY Steamed Veggies
SATURDAY 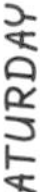	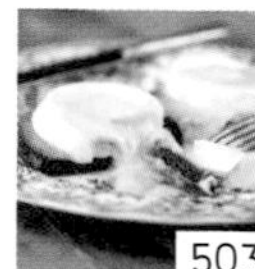 503 Eggs Benedict	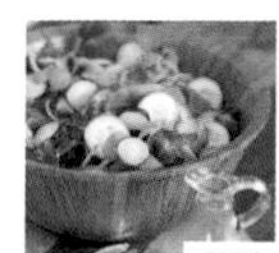 519 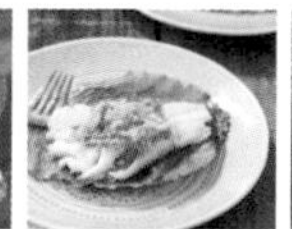 LEFTOVER 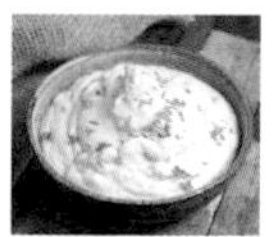 LEFTOVER DIY Salad and leftover Coconut Oil-Poached Tilapia with Asian Pear Slaw and Celery Root Puree	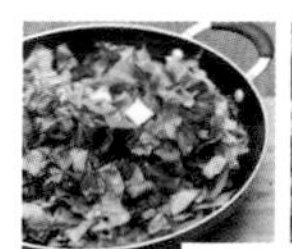 549 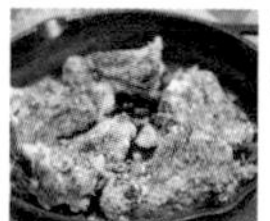 LEFTOVER 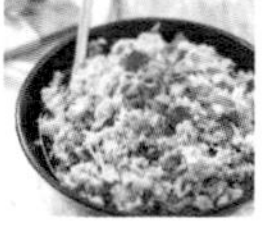 LEFTOVER DIY Braised Greens and leftover Middle Eastern Dukkah-Crusted Lamb Chops and Moroccan "Couscous"

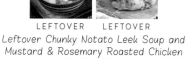

EVERYDAY MEAL PLAN Week 5

SHOPPING LIST

PRODUCE

asparagus - 1 pound
avocado - 1
berries of choice - 1 pound
Brussels sprouts - 2 pounds (save time by purchasing already shaved)
carrots - 5
cauliflower - 1 head
celery - 3 stalks
cilantro - ½ cup
fennel bulb - ½
garlic - 1 head
Granny Smith apple - 1
kale - 2 cups
lettuce (romaine, butter, or Bibb) - 2 heads
lemon or lime basil - 2 cups (or use sweet basil)
lemons - 2
limes - 3
mango - 1
mint - ⅓ cup
mushrooms - 1½ pounds
parsley - ½ cup
plantains, green - 4
red bell pepper - 1
red onions - ½ cup
rosemary - 1 sprig
sage - 1 tablespoon
shallots - 5
spinach - 6 cups
taro root - 2 pounds
thyme - 5 sprigs
white onion - 1
winter squash - 2 pounds
yellow onions - 3
zucchini - 2
salad veggies of choice for DIY Salad (page 519) - 1 meal
veggies of choice for DIY Omelet (page 508) - 2 meals
veggies of choice for DIY Soup (page 513) - 1 meal

MEAT & SEAFOOD

bacon - 1 pound
chicken breasts - 4 pounds
fish fillets (such as sea bass, mahi mahi, halibut, or swordfish) - 1 to 1½ pounds
ground beef - 2 pounds
lamb stew meat - 3 pounds
pancetta - 4 ounces
pork sausage (loose) - 8 ounces
pork shoulder - 6 to 8 pounds
shrimp, precooked - 1 pound
tallow - 3 tablespoons

EGGS & DAIRY

butter - 1 tablespoon
eggs - 38

DRIED HERBS & SPICES

bay leaf
black pepper
curry powder (or ingredients to make homemade, page 483)
ginger powder
granulated garlic
granulated onion
ground allspice
ground cinnamon
ground cloves
ground cumin
ground nutmeg
oregano
savory (or use rosemary or thyme)
sea salt
truffle salt
ingredients for salad dressing of choice (pages 484 to 485)
ingredients for seasoning of choice for DIY Baked Chicken Breast (pages 482 to 483)

VINEGARS & OILS

apple cider vinegar
avocado oil
coconut oil
olive oil
red palm oil
ingredients for salad dressing of choice (pages 484 to 485)

DELI & PREPARED FOODS

beef bone stock - 3 cups (or ingredients to make homemade, page 486)
bone stock - 3 to 4 cups (or ingredients to make homemade, page 486)

BULK

pine nuts - ¼ cup
raw hazelnuts - 1 cup

SWEETENERS & BAKING SUPPLIES

baking soda - 1 teaspoon
cassava flour - ⅓ cup
cream of tartar - 1 teaspoon
evaporated cane juice - ¼ cup
honey - 2 tablespoons
maple sugar - 2 tablespoons
pumpkin powder - ½ cup (may need to order online)
vanilla extract - 1 tablespoon

CANNED & JARRED GOODS

coconut cream concentrate - ⅓ cup

ASIAN FOODS

fish sauce - 2 tablespoons

OTHER

plantain chips - ¼ cup
add-ons of choice for DIY Muffins (page 569)

MAKE AHEAD OR PURCHASE QUALITY OPTIONS

salad dressing, bone stock, pickled shallots

	BREAKFAST	LUNCH	DINNER
SUNDAY	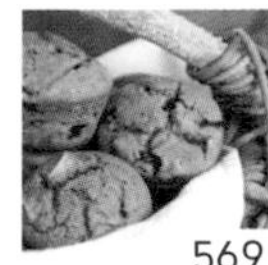 569 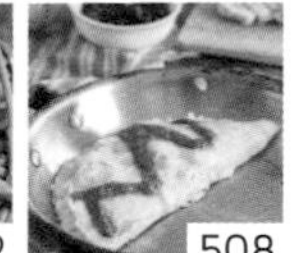 508 DIY Muffins and DIY Omelet	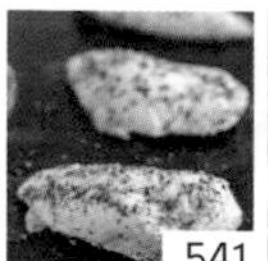 541 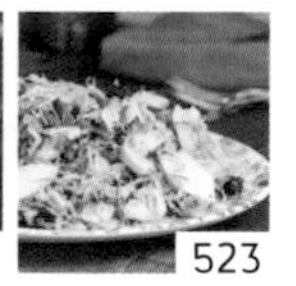 523 DIY Baked Chicken Breast and Shaved Brussels Slaw with Hazelnuts, Apple & Mint Make enough chicken for 4 meals.	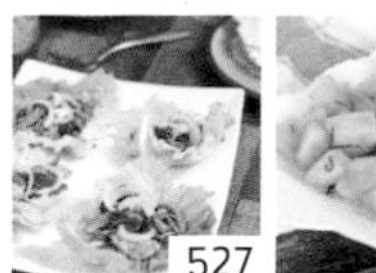 527 559 Pulled Pork Lettuce Wraps with Lemon Basil Pesto & Easy Pickled Shallots and Maple & Sage Roasted Winter Squash
MONDAY 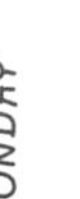	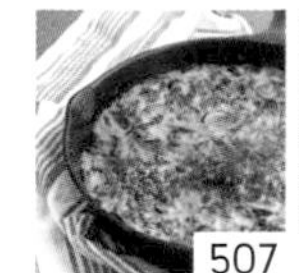 507 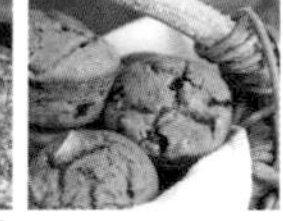 LEFTOVER 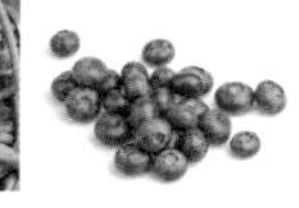 Sausage & Mushroom Frittata, leftover DIY Muffins, and berries	LEFTOVER LEFTOVER Leftover DIY Baked Chicken Breast and Shaved Brussels Slaw with Hazelnuts, Apple & Mint	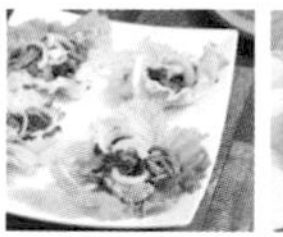 LEFTOVER 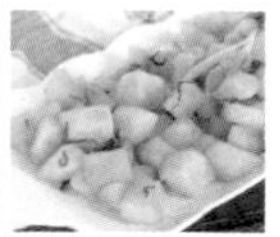 LEFTOVER Leftover Pulled Pork Lettuce Wraps with Lemon Basil Pesto & Pickled Shallots and Maple & Sage Roasted Winter Squash
TUESDAY	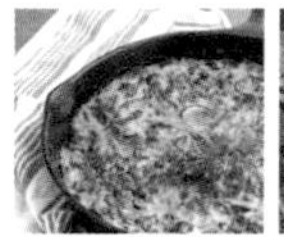 LEFTOVER 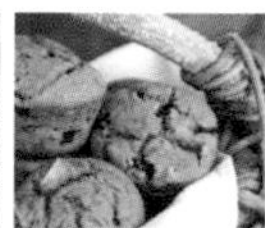 LEFTOVER 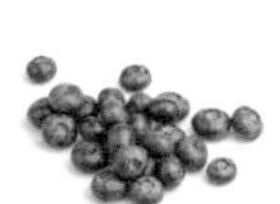 Leftover Sausage & Mushroom Frittata and DIY Muffins and berries	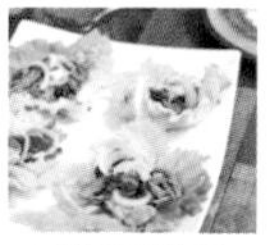 LEFTOVER Leftover Pulled Pork Lettuce Wraps with Lemon Basil Pesto & Easy Pickled Shallots	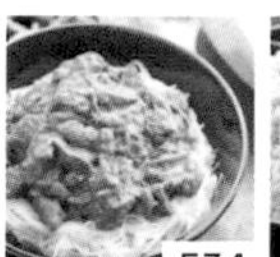 534 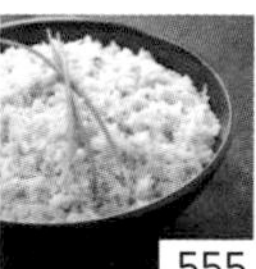 555 Lamb Curry and Cumin Cauli-rice
WEDNESDAY	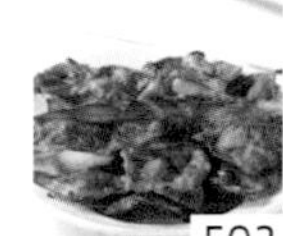 502 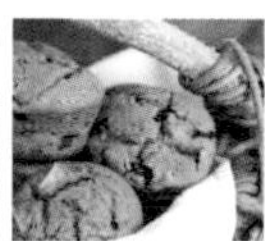 LEFTOVER 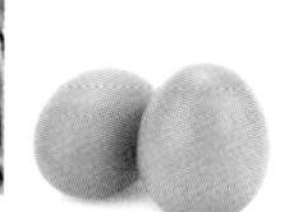 Crispy Bacon, leftover DIY Muffins, and 2 eggs, any style	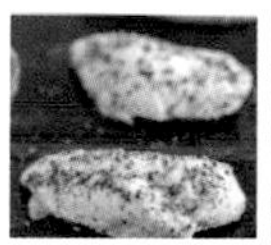 LEFTOVER LEFTOVER Leftover DIY Baked Chicken Breast and Shaved Brussels Slaw with Hazelnuts, Apple & Mint	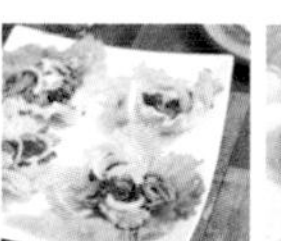 LEFTOVER 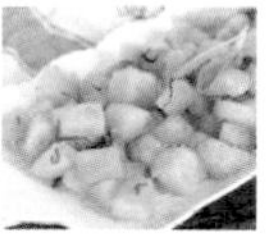 LEFTOVER Leftover Pulled Pork Lettuce Wraps with Lemon Basil Pesto & Easy Pickled Shallots and Maple & Sage Roasted Winter Squash
THURSDAY	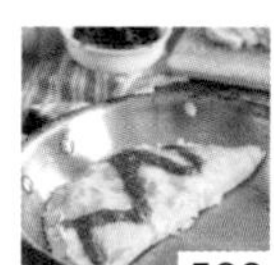 508 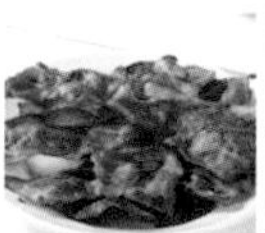 LEFTOVER 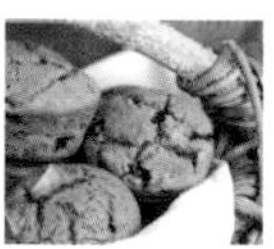 LEFTOVER DIY Omelet and leftover Crispy Bacon and DIY Muffins	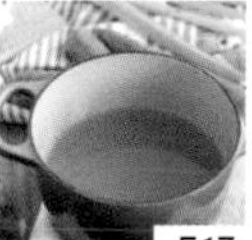 513 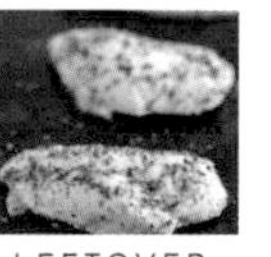 LEFTOVER DIY Soup made with leftover DIY Baked Chicken Breast	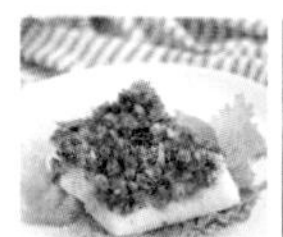 525 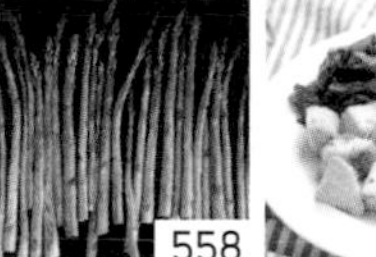 558 557 Gremolata-Topped Fish Fillets, Broiled Asparagus, and Savory-Roasted Taro
FRIDAY	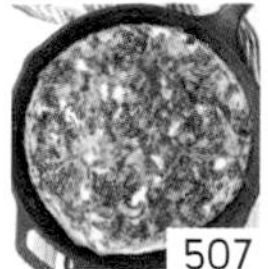 507 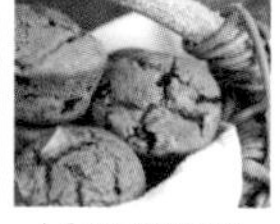 LEFTOVER Veggie Frittata and leftover DIY Muffins	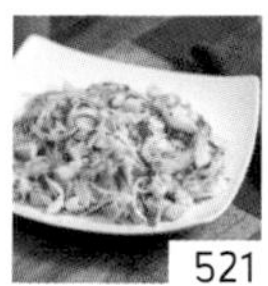 521 Shrimp Salad	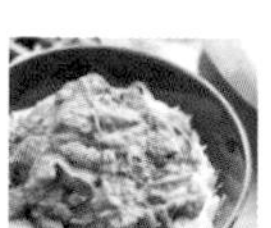 LEFTOVER 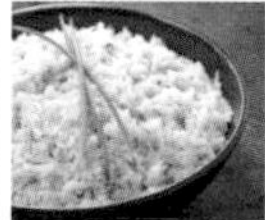 LEFTOVER Leftover Lamb Curry and Cumin Cauli-rice
SATURDAY 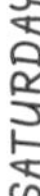	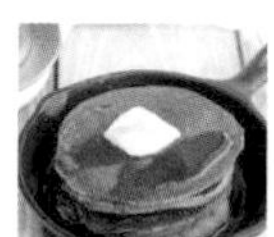 505 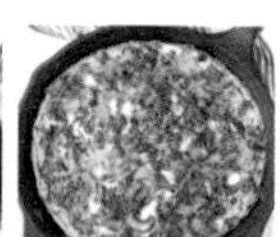 LEFTOVER Pumpkin Pancakes and leftover Veggie Frittata	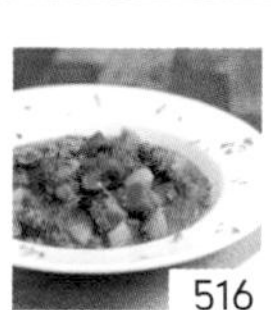 516 Hamburger Stew	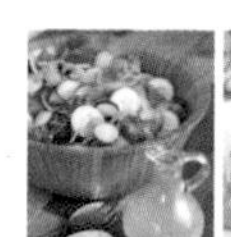 519 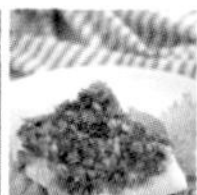 LEFTOVER 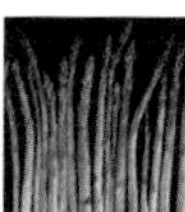 LEFTOVER 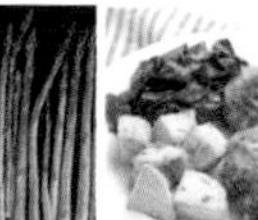 LEFTOVER DIY Salad and leftover Gremolata-Topped Fish Fillets, Broiled Asparagus, and Savory-Roasted Taro

EVERYDAY MEAL PLAN Week 6

SHOPPING LIST

PRODUCE
arugula - 2 cups
avocado - 1
baby kale - 2 cups
basil - 1½ tablespoons
berries of choice - 1 pound
bok choy - 4 to 6 bunches
cantaloupe - 1
carrot - 1
cauliflower - 1 head
celeriac - 2
celery - 8 stalks
chives - 1 tablespoon
cilantro - 3 tablespoons
cremini mushrooms - 8 ounces
garlic - 3 heads
ginger root - 1 inch
kabocha squash (or other winter squash) - 3 cups
kumquats - 4
lemons - 2
lime basil - 2 cups (or use regular basil)
mushrooms - 8 ounces
orange - 1
oregano - 1½ tablespoons
parsnips - 2 pounds
pie pumpkin - 1
plantains, green - 4
portobello mushroom caps - 6
red onion - ¼
romaine lettuce - 1 head
sage - 1 tablespoon
spinach - 10 ounces
sweet potatoes - 2½ pounds
tarragon - ¼ cup
thyme - 4 sprigs
white onions - 3
yellow onion - ½
zucchini - 4
salad veggies of choice for DIY Salad (page 519) - 6 meals

MEAT & SEAFOOD
bacon - 1½ pounds
chicken breasts - 4 pounds
chicken thighs - 2 pounds
fish steaks or fillets (such as mahi mahi, amberjack, grouper, or halibut) - 2 (6 to 8 ounces each)
ground beef - 3 pounds
ground pork - 1 pound
ground turkey - 2 pounds
liver - 1 pound

EGGS & DAIRY
eggs - 39
ghee or butter - 2 tablespoons (or use olive oil)

DRIED HERBS & SPICES
bay leaf
black pepper
cayenne pepper
chili powder
galangal (or use grated ginger root)
granulated garlic
ground cinnamon
ground cumin
ground mace
ground nutmeg
oregano
sea salt
truffle salt
ingredients for salad dressing of choice (pages 484 to 485)
ingredients for seasoning of choice for DIY Baked Chicken Breast (pages 482 to 483)

VINEGARS & OILS
apple cider vinegar
avocado oil
balsamic vinegar
coconut oil
coconut water vinegar
lard
olive oil
ingredients for salad dressing of choice (pages 484 to 485)

DELI & PREPARED FOODS
beef bone stock - 2 cups (or ingredients to make homemade, page 486)
bone stock - 5 cups (or ingredients to make homemade, page 486)

BULK
dried figs - 3
pine nuts - ¼ cup
raw cashews - 8 ounces
raw walnut halves - ½ cup

SWEETENERS & BAKING SUPPLIES
arrowroot powder - 5 tablespoons
baking soda - ½ teaspoon
cocoa powder - 2 teaspoons
coconut flour - ¼ cup
tapioca starch - 1 cup
vanilla extract - 2 teaspoons

CANNED & JARRED GOODS
anchovy paste - 1 teaspoon
black olives, sliced - 1 can
coconut milk - 1 cup (or ingredients to make homemade, page 480)
diced tomatoes - 3 (15-ounce) cans
marinated artichoke hearts - 1 can or jar
mayonnaise - ½ cup (or ingredients to make homemade, page 487)
pumpkin puree - 2 cups
tomato paste - 1 can

ASIAN FOODS
bamboo shoots - 1 (5-ounce) can
water chestnuts - 1 (5-ounce) can

DRINKS
dry white wine - ½ cup

OTHER
coconut wraps or ingredients to make Tortillas (page 567) (optional)

MAKE AHEAD OR PURCHASE QUALITY OPTIONS
salad dressing, bone stock, plantain crackers

	BREAKFAST	LUNCH	DINNER
SUNDAY	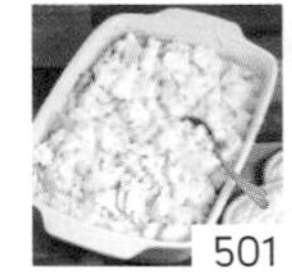 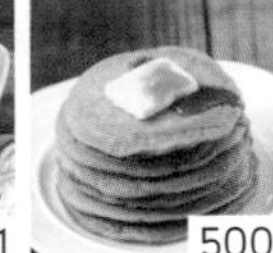 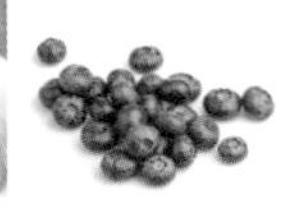 501 500 Oven Scrambled Eggs, DIY Pancakes, and berries	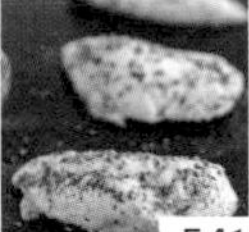 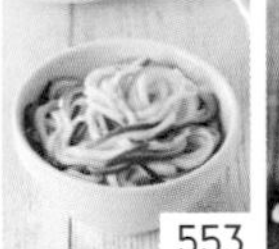 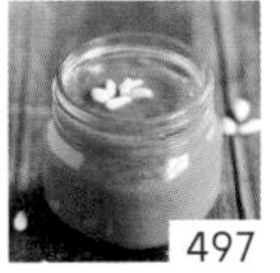 541 553 497 DIY Baked Chicken Breast, Zoodles, and Lemon Basil Pesto Make enough chicken for 4 meals.	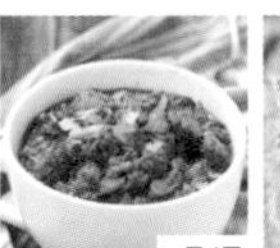 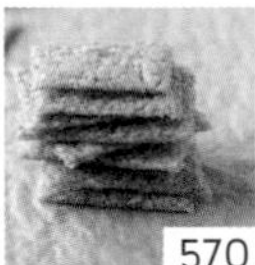 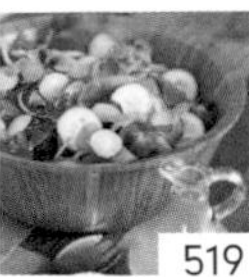 517 570 519 Pumpkin Chili, Plantain Crackers, and DIY Salad
MONDAY	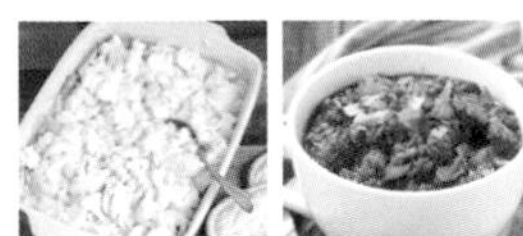 LEFTOVER LEFTOVER Leftover Oven Scrambled Eggs and Pumpkin Chili	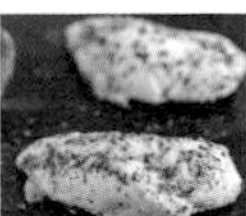 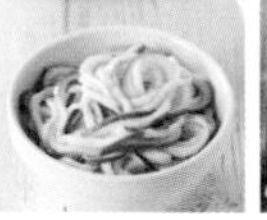 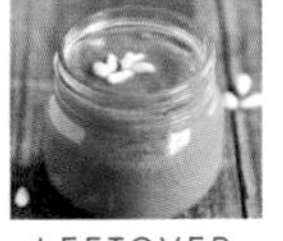 LEFTOVER LEFTOVER LEFTOVER Leftover DIY Baked Chicken Breast, Zoodles, and Lemon Basil Pesto	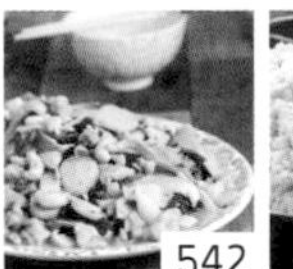 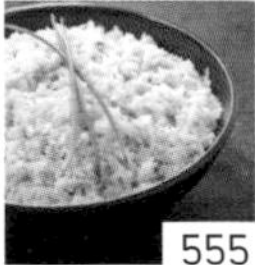 542 555 Cashew Chicken and Asian Cauli-rice
TUESDAY	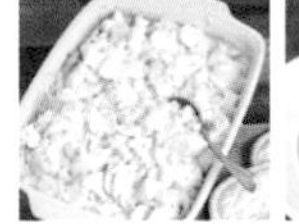 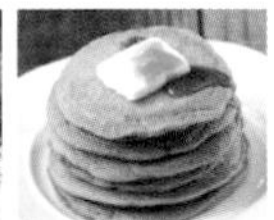 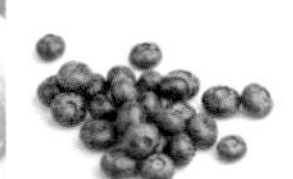 LEFTOVER LEFTOVER Leftover Oven Scrambled Eggs and DIY Pancakes and berries	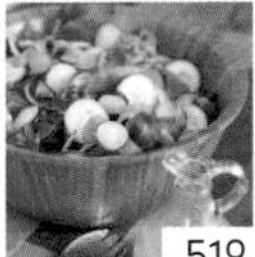 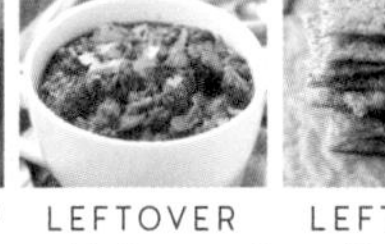 519 LEFTOVER LEFTOVER DIY Salad and leftover Pumpkin Chili and Plantain Crackers	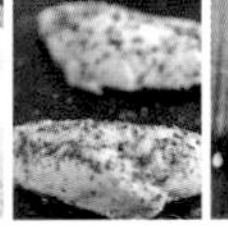 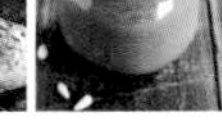 499 520 LEFTOVER LEFTOVER Pizza Crust and Paleo Caesar Salad Make pizza with leftover DIY Baked Chicken, Lemon Basil Pesto, chopped artichoke hearts, and sliced black olives.
WEDNESDAY	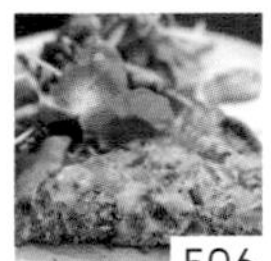 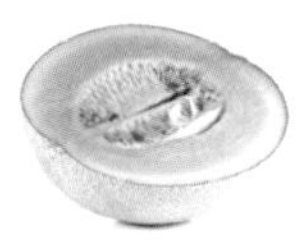 506 Pork & Winter Squash Frittata and cantaloupe	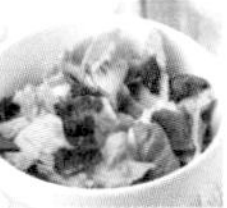 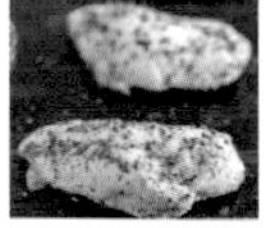 LEFTOVER LEFTOVER Leftover Paleo Caesar Salad with DIY Baked Chicken Breast Wrap in coconut wraps or Tortillas, if desired.	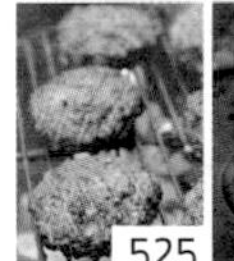 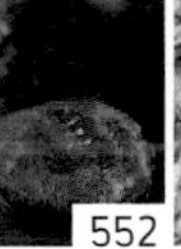 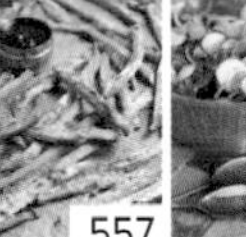 525 552 557 519 50/50/50 Burgers, Grilled Portobello Mushroom Caps, Oven-Baked Sweet Potato Fries, and DIY Salad
THURSDAY	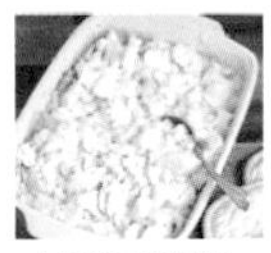 LEFTOVER LEFTOVER Leftover Oven Scrambled Eggs and Pumpkin Chili	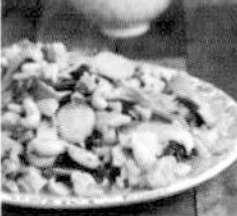 LEFTOVER LEFTOVER Leftover Cashew Chicken and Asian Cauli-rice	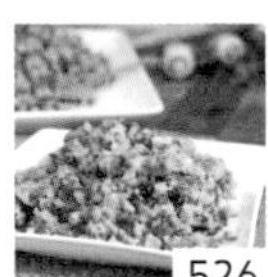 526 Beef & Mushroom Risotto
FRIDAY	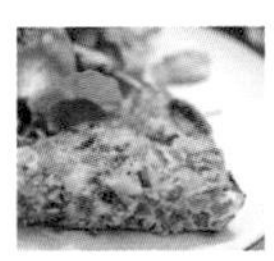 LEFTOVER Leftover Pork & Winter Squash Frittata and cantaloupe	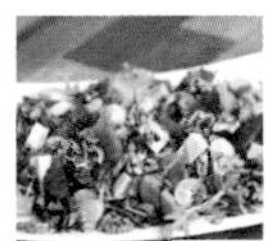 520 LEFTOVER Citrus, Fig & Walnut Salad and leftover 50/50/50 Burgers	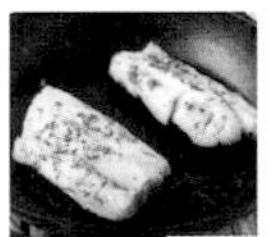 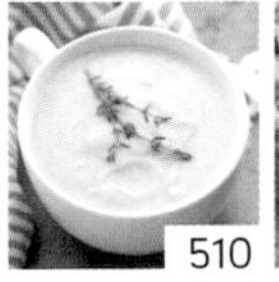 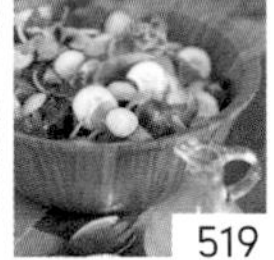 528 510 519 Tarragon-Seared Fish Fillets, "Cream" of Celery Root Soup, and DIY Salad
SATURDAY	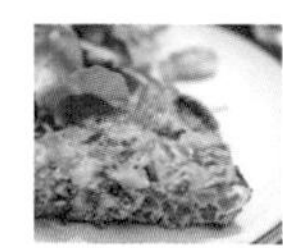 LEFTOVER Leftover Pork & Winter Squash Frittata and cantaloupe	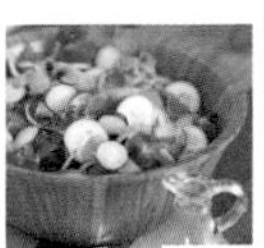 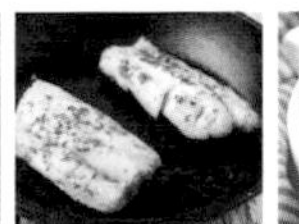 519 LEFTOVER LEFTOVER DIY Salad and leftover Tarragon-Seared Fish Fillets and "Cream" of Celery Root Soup	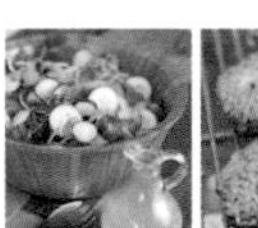 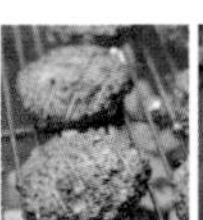 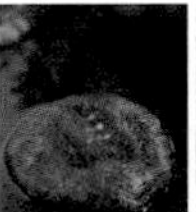 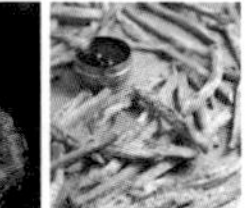 519 LEFTOVER LEFTOVER LEFTOVER DIY Salad and leftover 50/50/50 Burgers, Grilled Portobello Mushroom Caps, and Oven-Baked Sweet Potato Fries

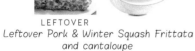

JUST GETTING STARTED MEAL PLAN

This meal plan takes advantage of easy recipes, familiar flavors, and a few Paleo adaptations of American staples to ease you into this new way of eating! Pair this plan with a close look at your sleep, movement throughout the day, and stress levels and take steps toward better lifestyle habits.

SHOPPING LIST

PRODUCE

asparagus - 1 pound
avocado - 1
berries of choice - 2 pounds
cantaloupe - 1
cauliflower - 2 heads
cilantro - ½ cup
fennel bulb - 1¼ pounds
garlic - 2 heads
grapefruit - 1
green and red bell peppers - 1½ cups
green beans - 1½ pounds
lemons - 4
limes - 2
mango - 1
onion - 1
oranges - 2
parsley - ½ cup
parsnips - 1½ pounds
plantains, green - 5
red onions - ½ cup
rosemary - 1½ tablespoons
sweet potatoes - 2 cups
white onions - ½ cup
yellow onion - 1
root vegetables of choice for DIY Roasted Roots (page 550) - 2 pounds
salad veggies of choice for DIY Salad (page 519) - 5 meals
veggies of choice for DIY Steamed Veggies (page 548) - 2 meals

MEAT & SEAFOOD

bacon - 1¼ pounds
beef shoulder or chuck roast - 4 pounds
chicken tenders - 1 pound
chickens - 2 whole (4 to 5 pounds each)
duck fat - 2 tablespoons
fish fillets (such as sea bass, mahi mahi, halibut, or swordfish) - 1 to 1½ pounds
ham - 10 ounces
pork chops - 2 pounds
shrimp, precooked - 1 pound

EGGS & DAIRY

butter - 1 tablespoon
eggs - 46

DRIED HERBS & SPICES

black pepper
granulated garlic
ground coriander
ground cumin
lavender (or use rosemary)
oregano
paprika
sea salt
truffle salt
ingredients for salad dressing of choice (pages 484 to 485)

VINEGARS & OILS

apple cider vinegar
avocado oil
balsamic vinegar
coconut oil
olive oil
ingredients for salad dressing of choice (pages 484 to 485)

DELI & PREPARED FOODS

beef bone stock - 1 cup (or ingredients to make homemade, page 486)
bone stock - 1 quart (or ingredients to make homemade, page 486)

BULK

black sesame seeds - 2 tablespoons
raw pepitas - ¼ cup
sesame seeds - 2 tablespoons
sunflower seeds - ¼ cup

SWEETENERS & BAKING SUPPLIES

almond flour - 2 cups
arrowroot powder - ¾ cup
baking soda - 1 teaspoon
honey - 2 tablespoons
coconut flour - ¼ cup
tapioca starch - 1¼ cups
vanilla extract - 2 teaspoons

CANNED & JARRED GOODS

coconut aminos - 1 tablespoon
coconut milk - ½ cup (or ingredients to make homemade, page 480)
Dijon mustard - 2 tablespoons
tahini - ⅓ cup

ASIAN FOODS

fish sauce - 3 tablespoons

OTHER

plantain chips - ¼ cup

MAKE AHEAD OR PURCHASE QUALITY OPTIONS

salad dressing, bone stock, "multigrain" quick bread

	BREAKFAST	LUNCH	DINNER
SUNDAY	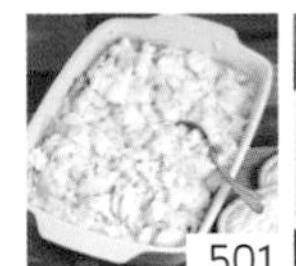 501 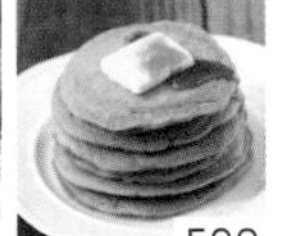 500 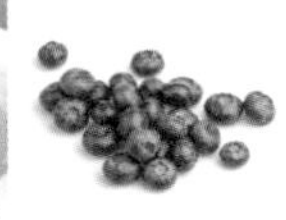 Oven Scrambled Eggs, DIY Pancakes, and berries	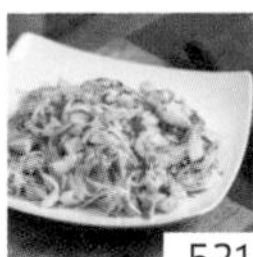 521 Shrimp Salad	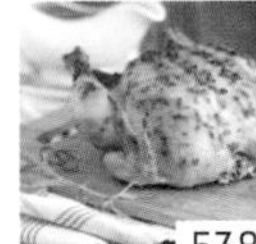 538 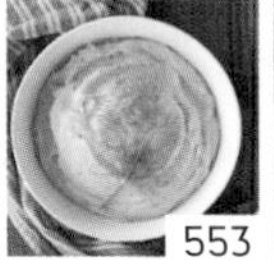 553 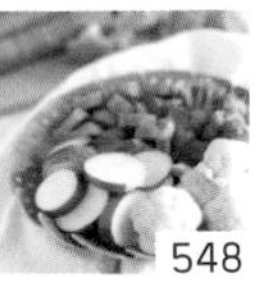 548 Mustard & Rosemary Roasted Chicken with Pan Sauce, Parsnip & Fennel Puree, and DIY Steamed Veggies
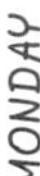 MONDAY	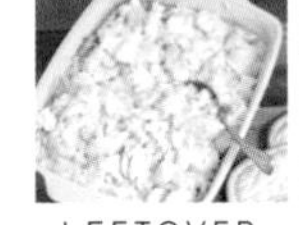 LEFTOVER 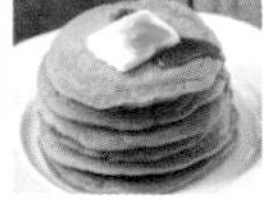 LEFTOVER 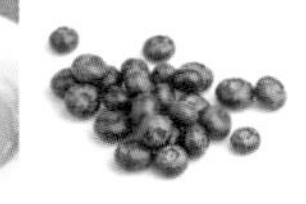 Leftover Oven Scrambled Eggs and DIY Pancakes and berries	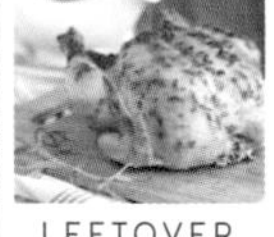 519 LEFTOVER DIY Salad and leftover Mustard & Rosemary Roasted Chicken with Pan Sauce *Wrap in coconut wraps, if desired.*	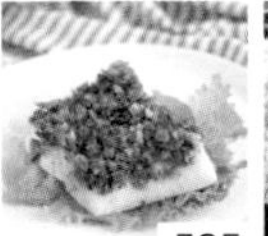 525 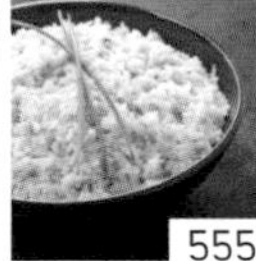 555 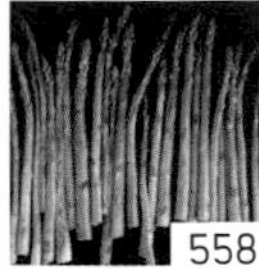 558 Gremolata-Topped Fish Fillets, Lemon Parsley Cauli-rice, and Broiled Asparagus
TUESDAY	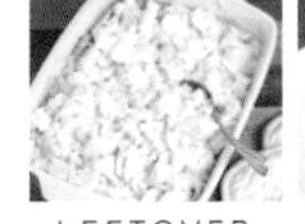 LEFTOVER 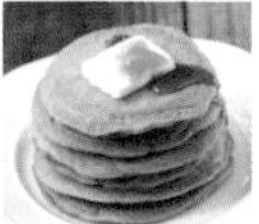 LEFTOVER 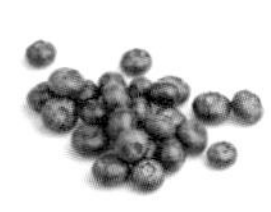 Leftover Oven Scrambled Eggs and DIY Pancakes and berries	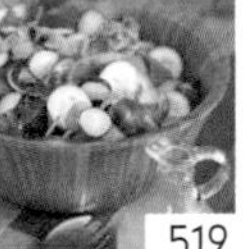 519 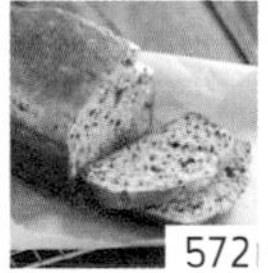 572 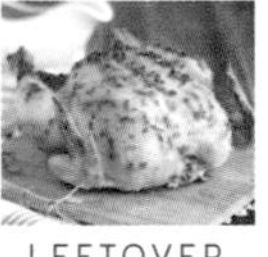 LEFTOVER DIY Salad, "Multigrain" Quick Bread, and leftover Roasted Chicken *Make chicken sandwiches!*	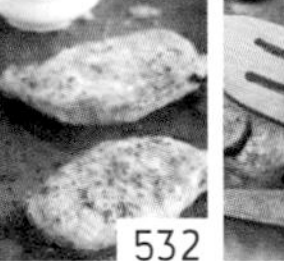 532 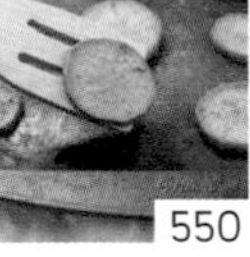 550 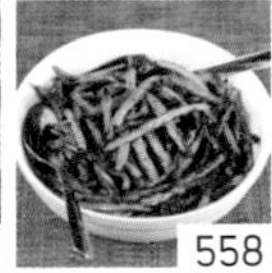 558 Broiled Pork Chops, DIY Roasted Roots, and Roasted Green Beans
WEDNESDAY	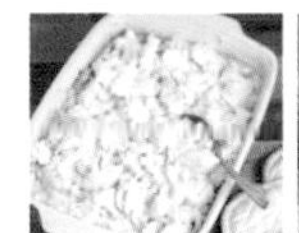 LEFTOVER 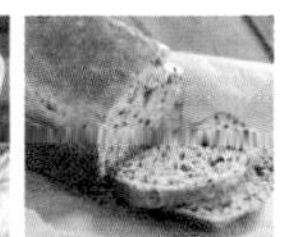 LEFTOVER 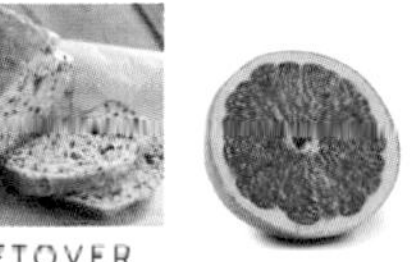 Leftover Oven Scrambled Eggs, toast made with leftover "Multigrain" Quick Bread, and half a grapefruit	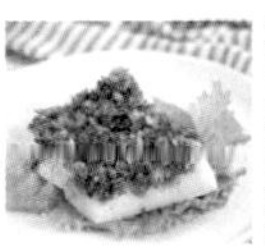 LEFTOVER 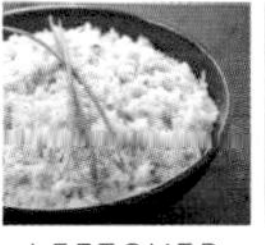 LEFTOVER 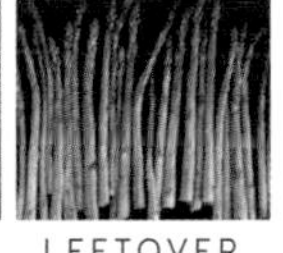 LEFTOVER Leftover Gremolata-Topped Fish Fillets, Lemon Parsley Cauli-rice, and Broiled Asparagus	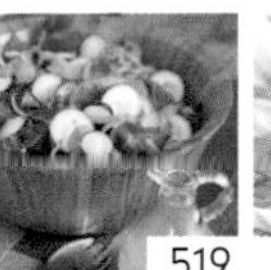 519 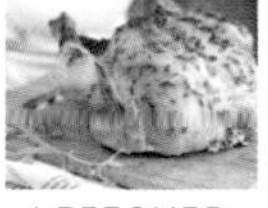 LEFTOVER 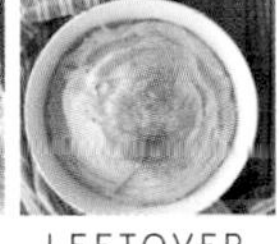 LEFTOVER DIY Salad and leftover Mustard & Rosemary Roasted Chicken with Pan Sauce and Parsnip & Fennel Puree
THURSDAY	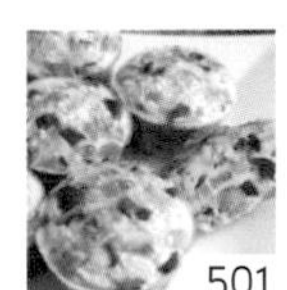 501 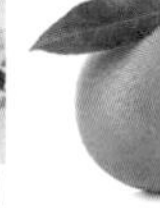 Ham & Sweet Potato Egg Muffins and an orange	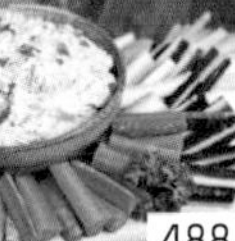 488 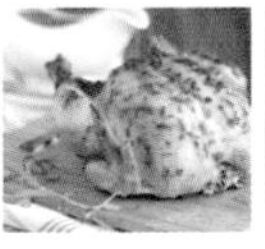 LEFTOVER 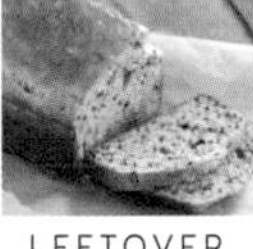 LEFTOVER Cauliflower Hummus with veggies and chicken sandwiches made with leftover Roasted Chicken and "Multigrain" Quick Bread	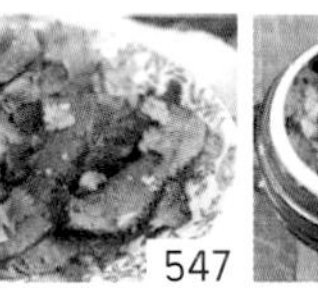 547 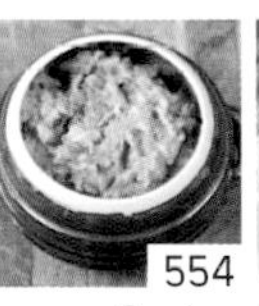 554 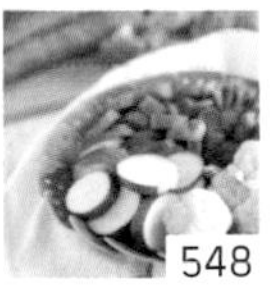 548 Balsamic Pressure Cooker Roast Beef, Mashed Plantains, and DIY Steamed Veggies
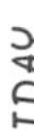 FRIDAY	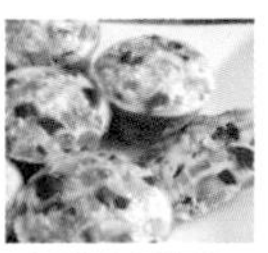 LEFTOVER 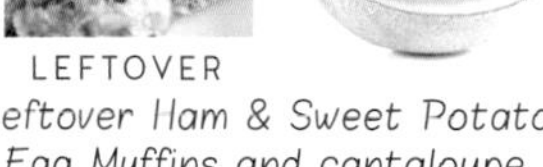 Leftover Ham & Sweet Potato Egg Muffins and cantaloupe	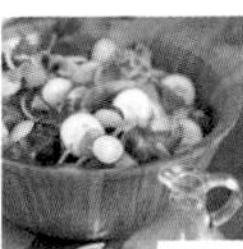 519 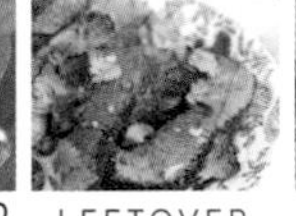 LEFTOVER LEFTOVER DIY Salad and leftover Balsamic Pressure Cooker Roast Beef and Mashed Plantains	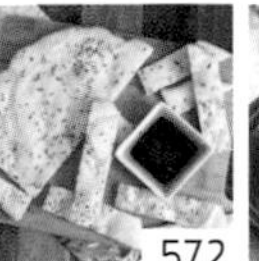 572 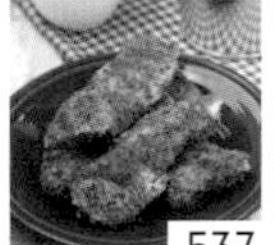 537 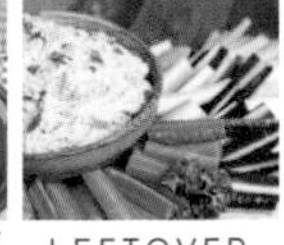 LEFTOVER Flatbread, Chicken Fingers, and leftover Cauliflower Hummus with veggies
SATURDAY 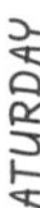	 502 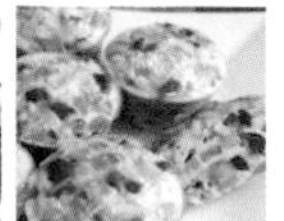 LEFTOVER 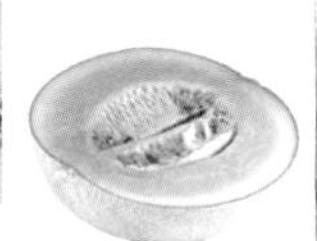 Crispy Bacon, leftover Ham & Sweet Potato Egg Muffins, and cantaloupe	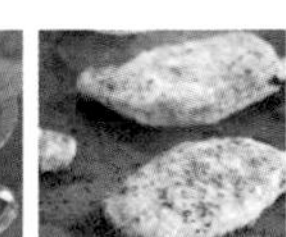 519 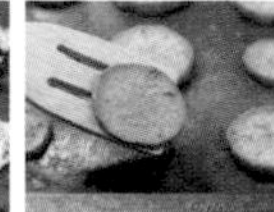 LEFTOVER LEFTOVER DIY Salad and leftover Broiled Pork Chops and DIY Roasted Roots	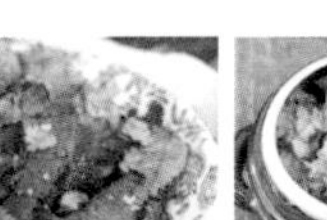 LEFTOVER 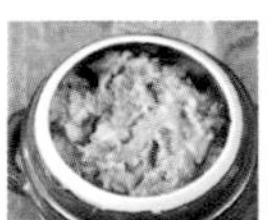 LEFTOVER 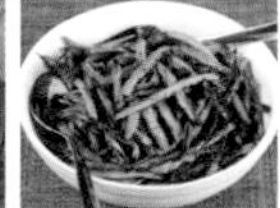 LEFTOVER Leftover Balsamic Pressure Cooker Roast Beef, Mashed Plantains, and Roasted Green Beans

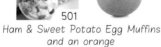

WEIGHT-LOSS MEAL PLAN

With a focus on low-caloric-density veggies and seafood, plus nutrients needed for fat metabolism, this meal plan has portion control built right in! Of course, caloric needs vary from person to person, so you may find that you need to serve yourself smaller portions and freeze some leftovers. Pair this plan with plenty of sleep, tons of low-intensity movement (in addition to hitting your weekly targets for moderately intense activity), and stress management. When in doubt, talk to your doctor about potential underlying causes of weight-loss resistance, like insulin resistance and hypothyroidism.

SHOPPING LIST

PRODUCE

arugula - 4 cups
asparagus - 1 pound
basil - 3 tablespoons
berries of choice - 2 pounds
broccoli slaw - 1 package
carrots - 3
cauliflower - 1½ heads
celery - 2 stalks
celery root - 2
chives - 2 tablespoons
cilantro - 1 bunch
English cucumbers - 1½
ginger root - 1 inch
garlic - 3 heads
grapefruit - 2
green beans - 1½ pounds
green onions - 9
kabocha squash (or other winter squash) - 3 cups
kale - 2 cups
lemons - 5
limes - 6
mint - 1 bunch plus 2 tablespoons
mushrooms - 1½ cups
oranges - 2
oregano - 3 tablespoons
parsley - ½ cup
red bell peppers - 2
romaine lettuce - 1 head
sage - 1 tablespoon
spinach - 6 cups
thyme - 2 sprigs plus 1 tablespoon
turnips - 1 pound
yellow onions - 2
zucchini - 2
salad veggies of choice for DIY Salad (page 519) - 4 meals
veggies of choice for DIY Steamed Veggies (page 548) - 1 meal

VINEGARS & OILS

apple cider vinegar
avocado oil
coconut oil
coconut water vinegar
olive oil
ingredients for salad dressing of choice (pages 484 to 485)

DELI & PREPARED FOODS

beef bone stock - 2 cups (or ingredients to make homemade, page 486)
bone stock - 2 cups (or ingredients to make homemade, page 486)

BULK

roasted unsalted cashews - ⅓ cup

SWEETENERS & BAKING SUPPLIES

blackstrap molasses - 1 tablespoon

CANNED & JARRED GOODS

beef broth - 2 cups
black olives - 1 cup
coconut aminos - 3 tablespoons
coconut milk yogurt - ½ cup (or ingredients to make homemade, page 481)
prepared yellow mustard - 1 tablespoon

ASIAN FOODS

fish sauce - 7 tablespoons

OTHER

plantain chips - ¼ cup

MEAT & SEAFOOD

bacon - 10 ounces
chicken thighs - 10
chicken (whole or pieces) - 3 pounds
duck fat - ¼ cup
fish fillets (such as sea bass, mahi mahi, halibut, or swordfish) - 1 to 1½ pounds
ground beef - 3 pounds
ground pork - 2 pounds
liver - 1 pound
salad shrimp, precooked - 1 pound

EGGS & DAIRY

butter - 1 tablespoon
eggs - 28
ghee - 2 tablespoons

DRIED HERBS & SPICES

black pepper
cayenne pepper
coarse sea salt
fennel seeds
fenugreek
garam masala
garlic powder
ginger powder
ground coriander
ground cumin
ground mace
onion powder
paprika
sea salt
truffle salt
turmeric powder
ingredients for salad dressing of choice (pages 484 to 485)

MAKE AHEAD OR PURCHASE QUALITY OPTIONS

salad dressing, bone stock

	BREAKFAST	LUNCH	DINNER
SUNDAY	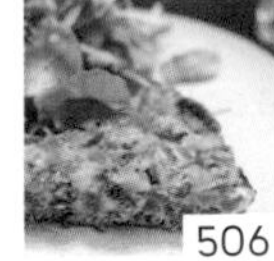 506 Pork & Winter Squash Frittata and berries	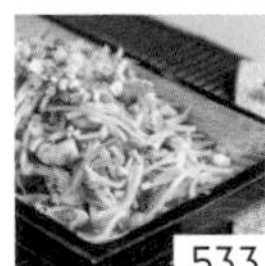 533 Shrimp Pad Thai	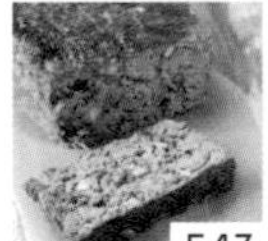 543 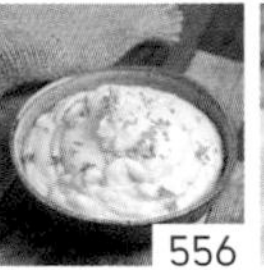 556 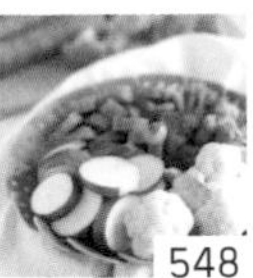 548 Meatloaf, Celery Root Puree, and DIY Steamed Veggies
MONDAY	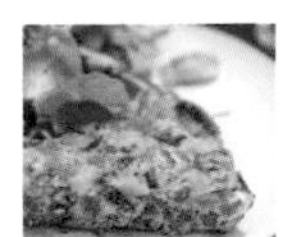 LEFTOVER Leftover Pork & Winter Squash Frittata and berries	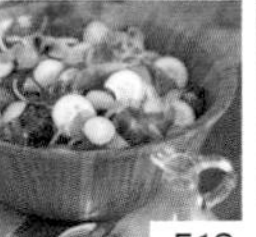 519 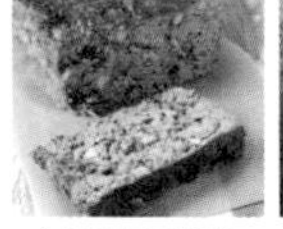 LEFTOVER 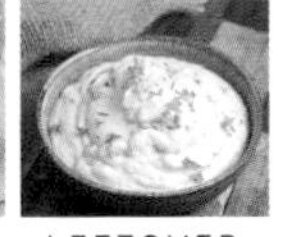 LEFTOVER DIY Salad and leftover Meatloaf and Celery Root Puree	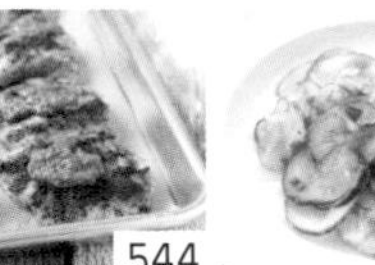 544 521 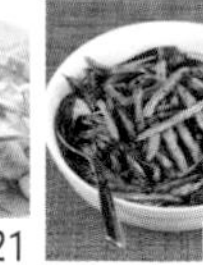 558 Barbecue Chicken with Arugula Pesto, Simple Cucumber Salad, and Roasted Green Beans
TUESDAY	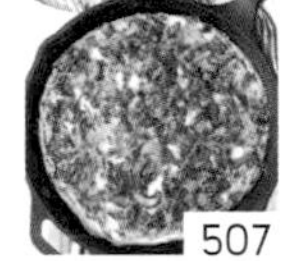 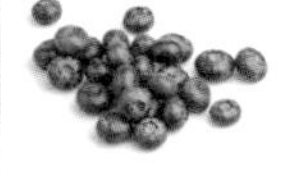 507 Veggie Frittata and berries	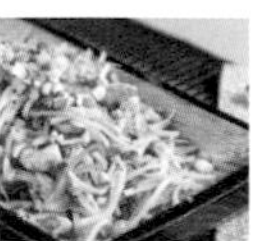 LEFTOVER Leftover Shrimp Pad Thai	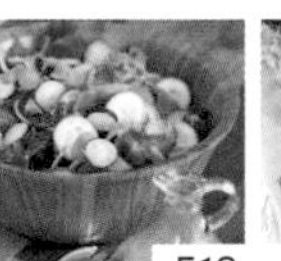 519 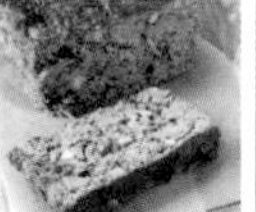 LEFTOVER 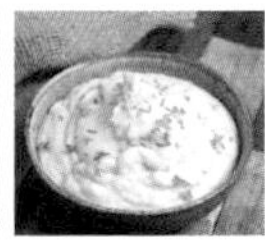 LEFTOVER DIY Salad and leftover Meatloaf and Celery Root Puree
WEDNESDAY	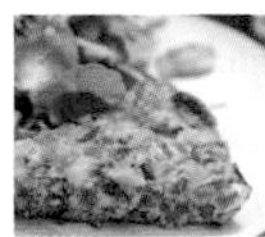 LEFTOVER 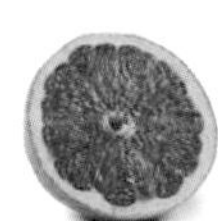 Leftover Pork & Winter Squash Frittata and half a grapefruit	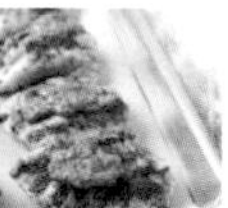 LEFTOVER 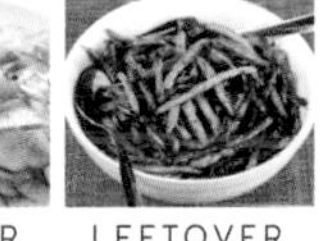 LEFTOVER LEFTOVER Leftover Barbecue Chicken with Arugula Pesto, Simple Cucumber Salad, and Roasted Green Beans	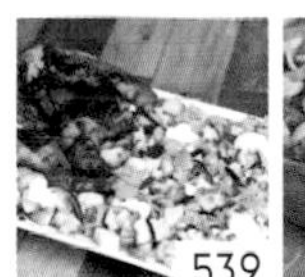 539 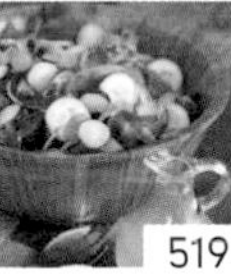 519 Bengali Tandoori Chicken with Aloo Gobi and DIY Salad
THURSDAY	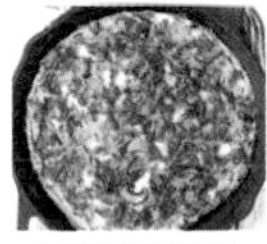 LEFTOVER Leftover Veggie Frittata and half a grapefruit	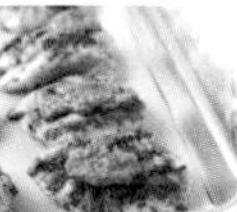 LEFTOVER 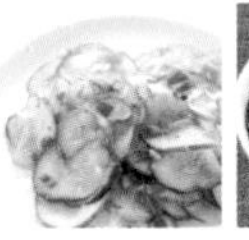 LEFTOVER 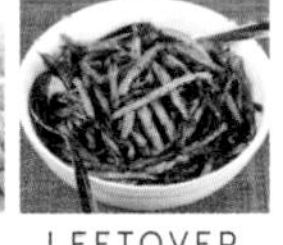 LEFTOVER Leftover Barbecue Chicken with Arugula Pesto, Simple Cucumber Salad, and Roasted Green Beans	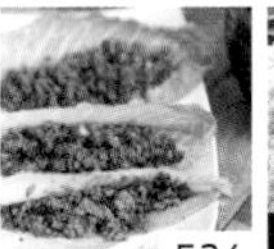 526 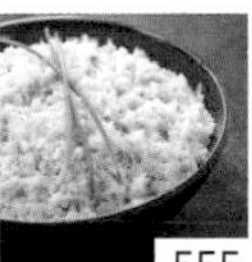 555 Thai Beef Lettuce Wraps and Asian Cauli-rice
FRIDAY	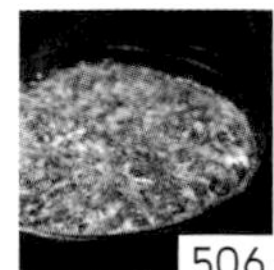 506 Bacon, Spinach & Olive Frittata and an orange	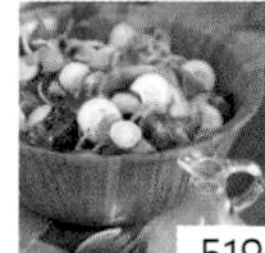 519 LEFTOVER DIY Salad and leftover Bengali Tandoori Chicken with Aloo Gobi	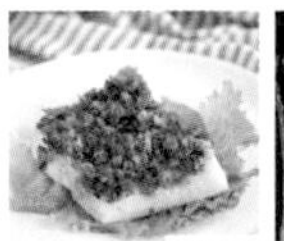 525 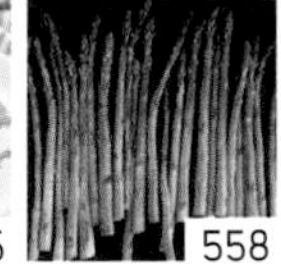 558 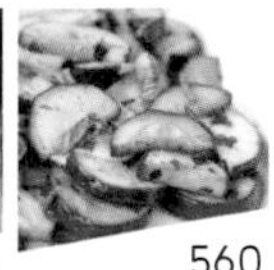 560 Gremolata-Topped Fish Fillets, Broiled Asparagus, and Minted Zucchini
SATURDAY 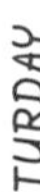	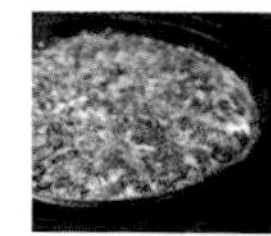 LEFTOVER 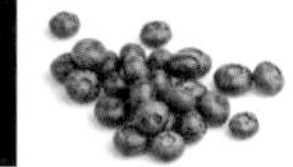 Leftover Bacon, Spinach & Olive Frittata and berries	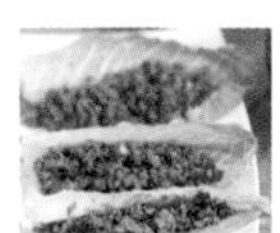 LEFTOVER LEFTOVER Leftover Thai Beef Lettuce Wraps and Asian Cauli-rice	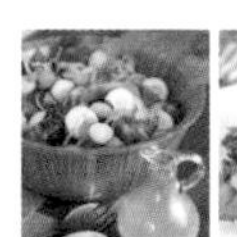 519 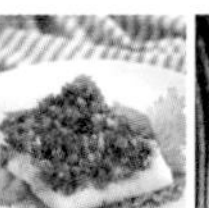 LEFTOVER 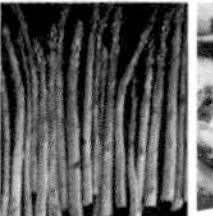 LEFTOVER 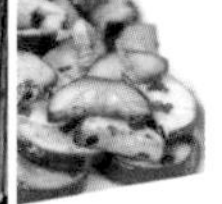 LEFTOVER DIY Salad and leftover Gremolata-Topped Fish Fillets, Broiled Asparagus, and Minted Zucchini

AIP MEAL PLAN

If you're looking to mitigate a suspected or diagnosed autoimmune disease with diet and lifestyle, this meal plan is for you! This plan combines nutrient-dense recipes with AIP re-creations of American comfort foods as a basic introduction to the Paleo Autoimmune Protocol. Remember to pair this meal plan with plenty of sleep, exposure to sunlight, moderate activity, and stress management. Also, check out *The Paleo Approach Cookbook* and *The Healing Kitchen* for more AIP recipes and meal plans.

SHOPPING LIST

PRODUCE

asparagus - 1 pound
avocados - 3
basil - ¾ teaspoon
berries of choice - 2 pounds
broccoli - 8 cups
cabbage - 3 pounds (or use store-bought raw sauerkraut)
carrots - 1 pound
cauliflower - 1 head
celery - 6 stalks
celery root - 2
cilantro - 1 large bunch
fennel bulb - 1¼ pounds
garlic - 3 heads
grapefruit - 1
lemons - 7
limes - 5
mango - 1
onions - 2
oranges - 2
oregano - 2 tablespoons
parsley - 2 cups
plantains, green - 3
red onions - 1½
romaine lettuce - 1 head
rosemary - ½ teaspoon
sage - 1 tablespoon
spinach - 6 cups
thyme - 4 sprigs plus 1 teaspoon
turnip - 1
winter squash - 2 pounds
greens of choice for DIY Braised Greens (page 549) - 3 meals
salad veggies of choice for DIY Salad (page 519) - 4 meals

MEAT & SEAFOOD

bacon - 4 slices
beef shoulder or brisket - 5 to 7 pounds
chicken - 1 whole (4 to 5 pounds)
clams - 3 (5- to 6-ounce) cans
duck fat - ¾ cup
fish fillets (such as sea bass, mahi mahi, halibut, or swordfish) - 1 to 1½ pounds
ground pork - 3 pounds
pork chops - 2 pounds
shrimp, precooked - 1 pound

DRIED HERBS & SPICES

bay leaf
cinnamon sticks
coarse sea salt
garlic powder
ginger powder
marjoram leaves
onion powder
oregano
rosemary
rubbed sage
savory
sea salt
tarragon
thyme
truffle salt
turmeric powder
ingredients for salad dressing of choice (pages 484 to 485)

VINEGARS & OILS

apple cider vinegar
avocado oil
coconut oil
olive oil
ingredients for salad dressing of choice (pages 484 to 485)

DELI & PREPARED FOODS

beef bone stock - 1 quart (or ingredients to make homemade, page 486)
bone stock - 2½ quarts (or ingredients to make homemade, page 486)

SWEETENERS & BAKING SUPPLIES

baking soda - ⅛ teaspoon
blackstrap molasses - 1 tablespoon
cassava flour - 1½ cups
cream of tartar - ¼ teaspoon
maple sugar - 2 tablespoons

CANNED & JARRED GOODS

coconut cream - 2 cups (or ingredients to make homemade, page 480)

ASIAN FOODS

fish sauce - 5 tablespoons

OTHER

plantain chips - ¼ cup

NOTE: Make sure to follow AIP modifications for recipes, if required.

MAKE AHEAD OR PURCHASE QUALITY OPTIONS

salad dressing, bone stock, sauerkraut

	BREAKFAST	LUNCH	DINNER
SUNDAY	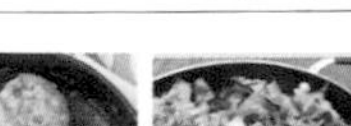 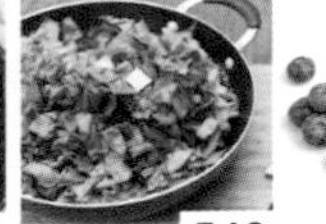 502 549 Replace ½ to 1 pound of ground pork in the sausage with liver, following instructions in "Sneaky Liver" Ground Beef on page 498. *Sweet Italian Sausage, DIY Braised Greens, and berries* *Make half of the sausage mix into small meatballs for soup. Make enough braised greens for 3 breakfasts.*	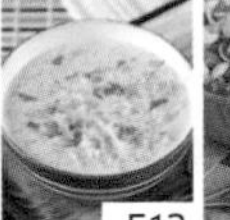 512 519 *Clam Chowder and DIY Salad* *Freeze half of the chowder for later in the week.*	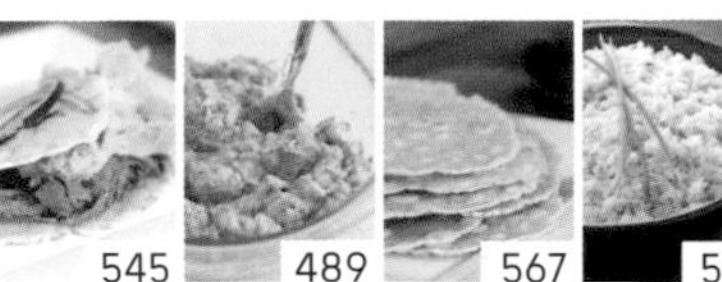 545 489 567 555 *Mild Barbacoa, Guacamole, Tortillas, and Lemon Parsley Cauli-rice* *Serve with shredded romaine lettuce, chopped cilantro, and lime wedges.*
MONDAY	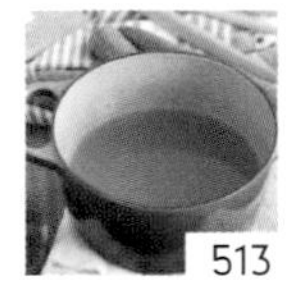 513 *Use Sweet Italian Sausage meatballs, carrots, celery, onion, spinach, and fresh parsley. Make enough soup for 3 breakfasts.* *DIY Soup*	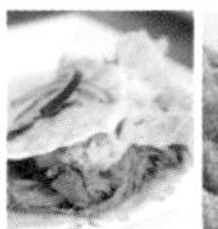 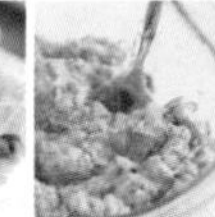 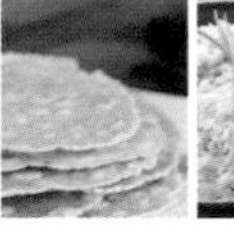 LEFTOVER LEFTOVER LEFTOVER LEFTOVER *Leftover Mild Barbacoa, Guacamole, Tortillas, and Lemon Parsley Cauli-rice*	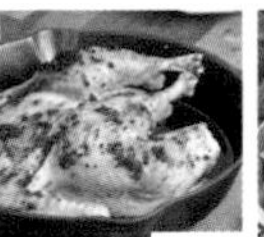 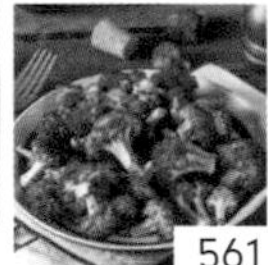 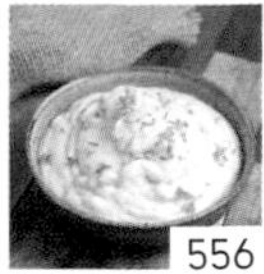 531 561 556 *Spatchcocked Chicken, Roasted Broccoli, and Celery Root Puree*
TUESDAY	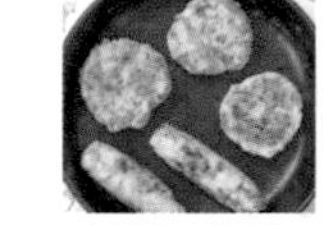 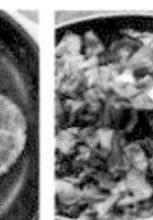 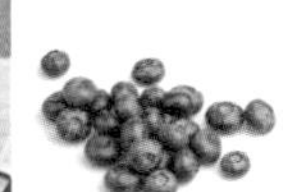 LEFTOVER LEFTOVER *Leftover Sweet Italian Sausage and DIY Braised Greens and berries*	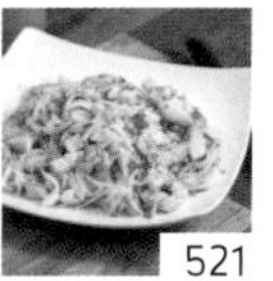 521 *Shrimp Salad*	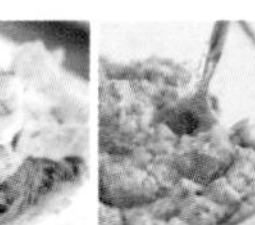 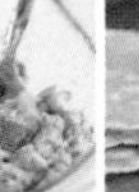 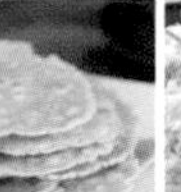 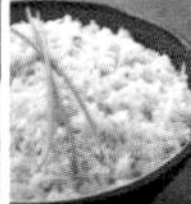 LEFTOVER LEFTOVER LEFTOVER LEFTOVER *Leftover Mild Barbacoa, Guacamole, Tortillas, and Lemon Parsley Cauli-rice*
WEDNESDAY	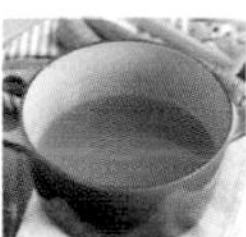 LEFTOVER *Leftover DIY Soup*	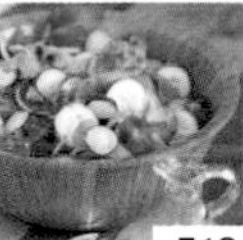 519 LEFTOVER *DIY Salad and leftover Clam Chowder*	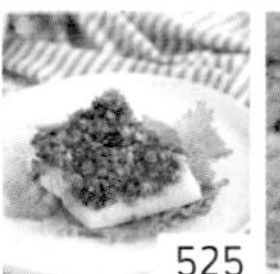 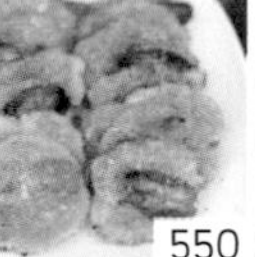 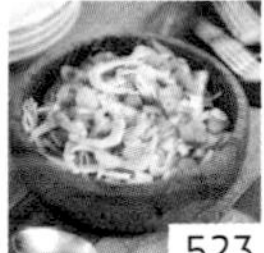 525 550 523 *Gremolata-Topped Fish Fillets, Tostones, and Simple Fennel Salad*
THURSDAY	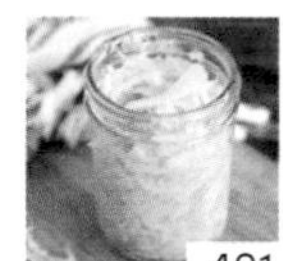 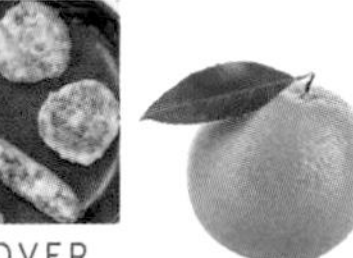 491 LEFTOVER *Sauerkraut, leftover Sweet Italian Sausage, and an orange*	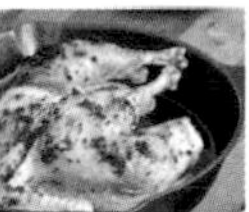 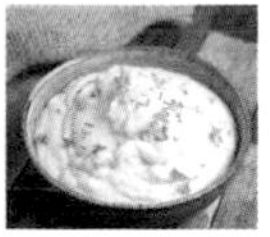 LEFTOVER LEFTOVER LEFTOVER *Leftover Spatchcocked Chicken, Roasted Broccoli, and Celery Root Puree*	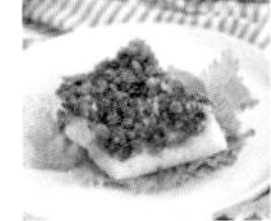 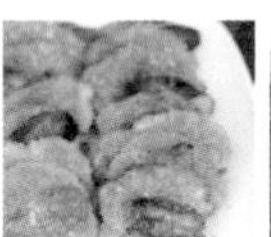 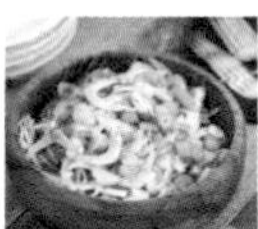 LEFTOVER LEFTOVER LEFTOVER *Leftover Gremolata-Topped Fish Fillets, Tostones, and Simple Fennel Salad*
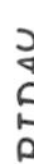 FRIDAY	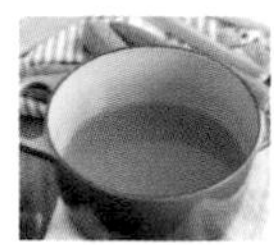 LEFTOVER *Leftover DIY Soup*	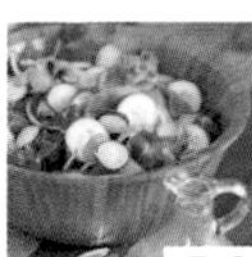 519 LEFTOVER *DIY Salad and leftover Clam Chowder*	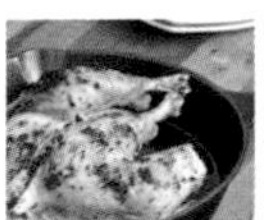 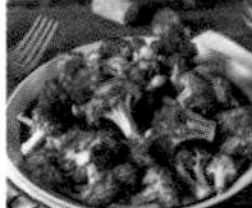 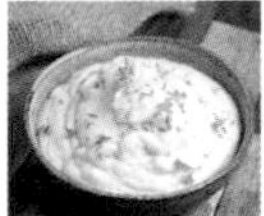 LEFTOVER LEFTOVER LEFTOVER *Leftover Spatchcocked Chicken, Roasted Broccoli, and Celery Root Puree*
SATURDAY	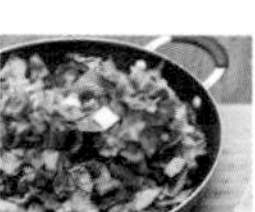 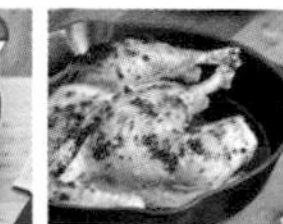 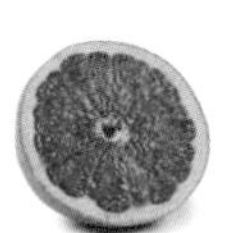 LEFTOVER LEFTOVER *Leftover DIY Braised Greens and Spatchcocked Chicken, Sweet Italian Sausage, or Mild Barbacoa, and half a grapefruit*	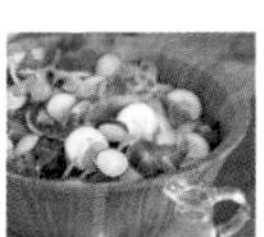 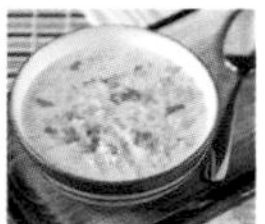 519 LEFTOVER *DIY Salad and leftover Clam Chowder*	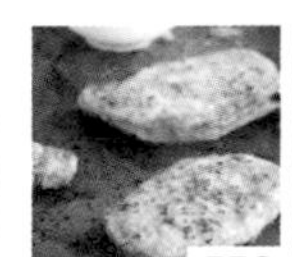 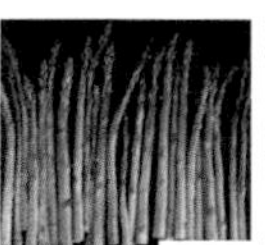 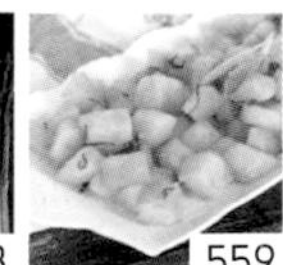 532 558 559 *Broiled Pork Chops, Broiled Asparagus, and Maple & Sage Roasted Winter Squash*

LOW-FODMAP MEAL PLAN

Need to try a low-FODMAP diet to reduce digestive symptoms? This meal plan is all about emphasizing just how many tasty foods you can eat even while following a low-FODMAP Paleo plan. Aim for as much variety in leafy greens as you can for DIY Salads and DIY Braised Greens (think every variety of lettuce, chard, collards, kale, arugula, beet tops, mustard greens, mâche, spinach, chervil, and fresh herbs). Other great low-FODMAP salad ingredients include cucumbers, radishes, carrots, celery, sunflower sprouts, chives, olives, nuts (except almonds, cashews, and pistachios), and seeds. Pair this low-FODMAP plan with an evaluation for potential causes of your digestive symptoms, such as small intestinal bacterial overgrowth (SIBO), by a qualified health-care professional.

SHOPPING LIST

PRODUCE

- arugula - 2½ ounces
- baby spinach - 3 cups
- bananas, green-tipped - 2
- berries of choice - 1 pound
- bok choy - 1 large bunch
- carrots - 1½ pounds
- cilantro - 2 tablespoons
- dill - 3 tablespoons
- English cucumbers - 2
- ginger root - 1½ teaspoons
- green beans - 1½ pounds
- green onions - 4
- kale - 2 large bunches
- lemons - 5
- pie pumpkin - 1
- parsnips - 2 pounds
- plantains, green - 6
- raspberries - 1 pound
- rosemary - 3 tablespoons
- rutabaga - 1 pound
- sage - 1 tablespoon
- strawberries - 1 pound
- tarragon - 3 tablespoons
- thyme - 1½ teaspoons
- turnips - 1 pound
- greens of choice for DIY Braised Greens (page 549) - 3 meals
- salad veggies of choice for DIY Salad (page 519) - 2 meals

MEAT & SEAFOOD

- bacon - 1 package
- beef roast - 5 pounds
- Canadian bacon - 4 slices
- chicken breasts - 4 pounds
- duck fat - ¾ cup
- fish steaks or fillets - 2 (6 to 8 ounces each)
- ground pork - 3 pounds
- pork chops - 2 pounds
- salmon fillets - 4 (6 to 8 ounces each)
- steaks - 4 (6 to 8 ounces each)

EGGS & DAIRY

- eggs - 29

DRIED HERBS & SPICES

- anise seed
- black pepper
- fennel seeds
- ginger powder
- ground allspice
- ground cardamom
- ground cinnamon
- ground mace
- ground nutmeg
- marjoram leaves
- oregano leaves
- rosemary
- rubbed sage
- savory
- sea salt
- tarragon
- thyme
- truffle salt
- ingredients for salad dressing of choice (pages 484 to 485)

VINEGARS & OILS

- avocado oil
- coconut oil
- coconut water vinegar
- lard
- olive oil
- ingredients for salad dressing of choice (pages 484 to 485)

DELI & PREPARED FOODS

- beef stock - 2 cups (or ingredients to make homemade, page 486)
- chicken stock - 2 quarts (or ingredients to make homemade, page 486)

BULK

- pecan halves - 1 cup

SWEETENERS & BAKING SUPPLIES

- active dry yeast - 1 teaspoon
- arrowroot powder - ¼ cup
- baking soda - 1½ teaspoons
- maple syrup - 2 teaspoons
- palm shortening - ½ cup
- vanilla extract - 2 teaspoons

CANNED & JARRED GOODS

- capers - 3 tablespoons
- mayonnaise - ½ cup (or ingredients to make homemade, page 487)

ASIAN FOODS

- bamboo shoots - 1 (5-ounce) can
- kelp noodles - 1 bag

NOTE: Make sure to follow low-FODMAP modifications for recipes, if required.

MAKE AHEAD OR PURCHASE QUALITY OPTIONS

salad dressing, bone stock, mayonnaise, pork seasoning

	BREAKFAST	LUNCH	DINNER
SUNDAY	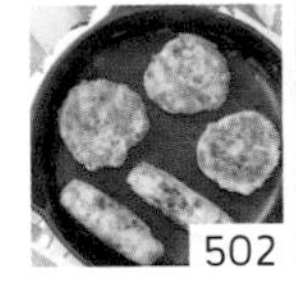 502 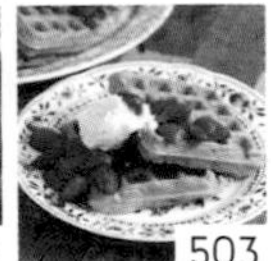 503 Breakfast Sausage and Waffles with strawberries and raspberries	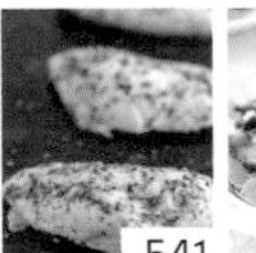 541 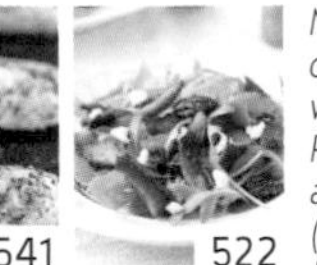 522 DIY Baked Chicken Breast and Strawberry & Arugula Salad with Candied Pecans *Make 4 pounds of chicken. Season half with AIP Herbes de Provence (page 482) and half with just salt (for DIY Stir-Fry later in the week). Omit goat cheese from salad and substitute maple syrup for honey in Candied Pecans.*	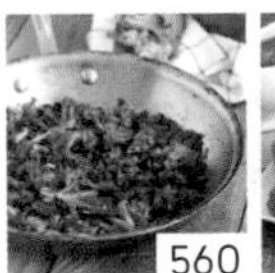 560 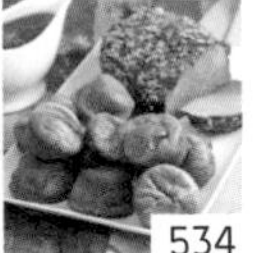 534 Bacon-Braised Kale and Herb-Crusted Roast Beef with Paleo Yorkshire Puddings & Pan Gravy *Omit garlic from Bacon-Braised Kale and Roast Beef herb rub.*
MONDAY	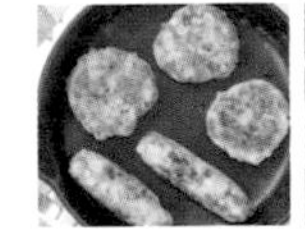 LEFTOVER 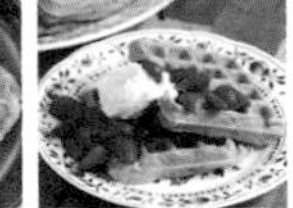 LEFTOVER Leftover Breakfast Sausage and Waffles with strawberries and raspberries	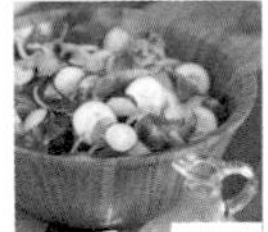 519 LEFTOVER DIY Salad and leftover Herb-Crusted Roast Beef with Paleo Yorkshire Puddings & Pan Gravy	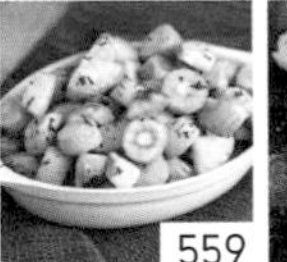 559 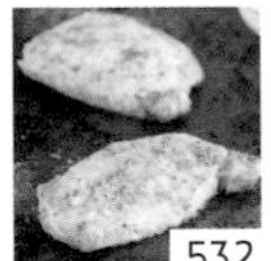 532 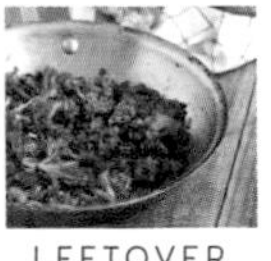 LEFTOVER Rosemary & Sage Roasted Parsnips, Broiled Pork Chops, and leftover Bacon-Braised Kale
TUESDAY	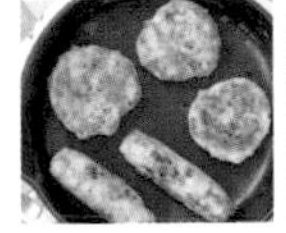 LEFTOVER 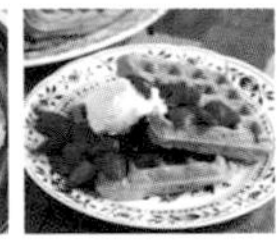 LEFTOVER 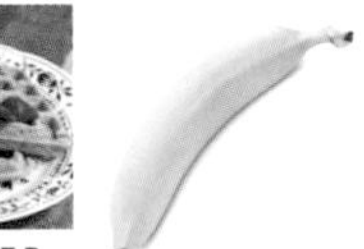 Leftover Breakfast Sausage and Waffles with sliced green-tipped banana	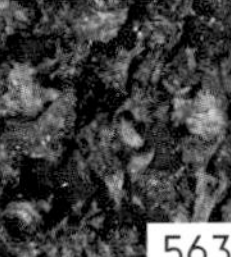 563 LEFTOVER 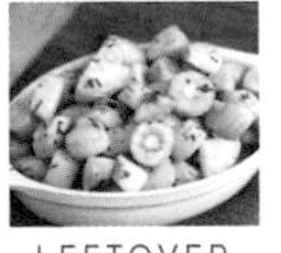 LEFTOVER Kale Chips and leftover DIY Baked Chicken Breast and Rosemary & Sage Roasted Parsnips	550 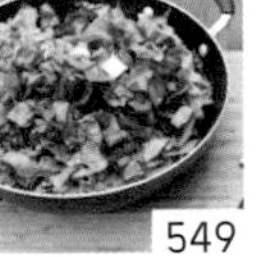 549 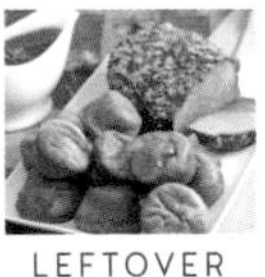 LEFTOVER DIY Roasted Roots, DIY Braised Greens, and leftover Herb-Crusted Roast Beef with Paleo Yorkshire Puddings & Pan Gravy *Use carrots, pumpkin, and turnips for Roasted Roots.*
WEDNESDAY	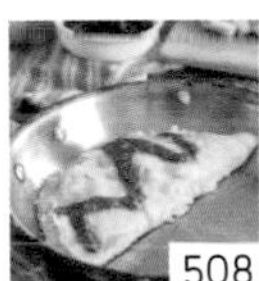 508 DIY Omelet *Use bacon, chopped plantain, and spinach for the filling.*	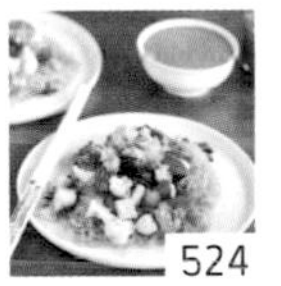 524 DIY Stir-Fry *Make enough for 2 lunches. Use leftover DIY Baked Chicken Breast, carrots, bamboo shoots, bok choy, and kelp noodles.*	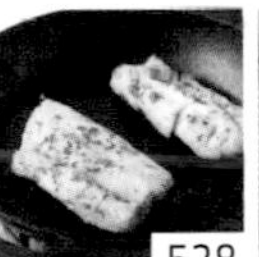 528 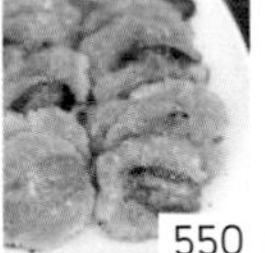 550 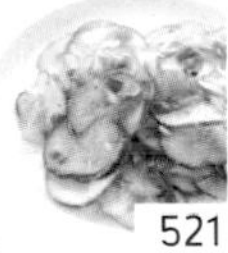 521 Tarragon-Seared Fish Fillets, Tostones, and Simple Cucumber Salad
THURSDAY	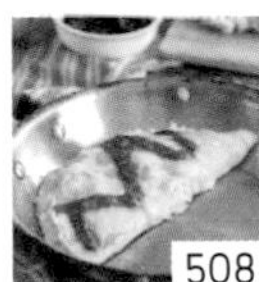 508 DIY Omelet *Use bacon, chopped plantain, and spinach for the filling.*	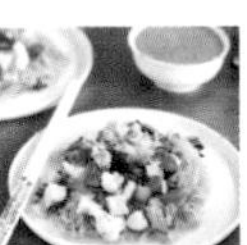 LEFTOVER Leftover DIY Stir-Fry	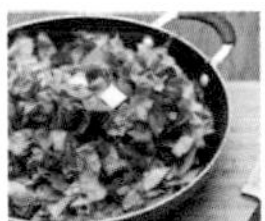 549 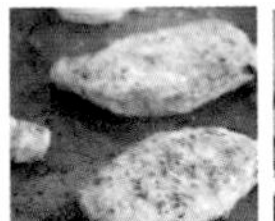 LEFTOVER 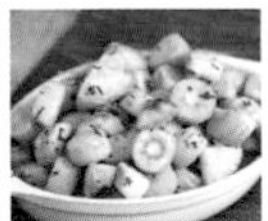 LEFTOVER DIY Braised Greens and leftover Broiled Pork Chops and Rosemary & Sage Roasted Parsnips
FRIDAY	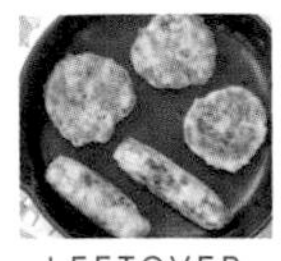 LEFTOVER LEFTOVER Leftover Breakfast Sausage and Waffles with strawberries and raspberries	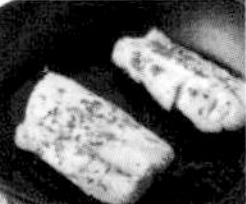 LEFTOVER LEFTOVER 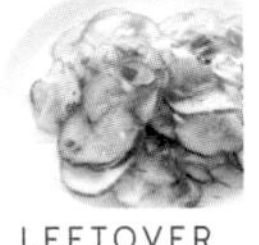 LEFTOVER Leftover Tarragon-Seared Fish Fillets, Tostones, and Simple Cucumber Salad	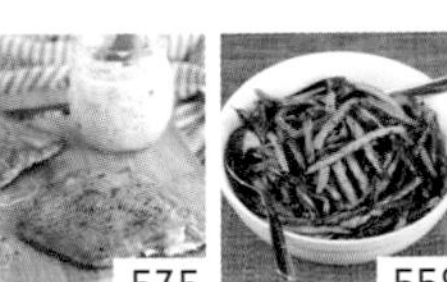 535 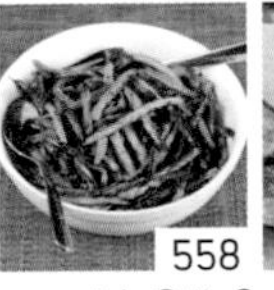 558 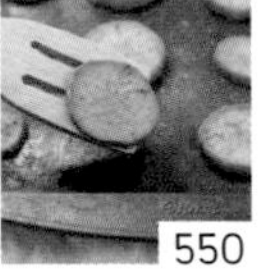 550 Broiled Salmon with Dill-Caper Sauce, Roasted Green Beans, and DIY Roasted Roots *Use turnips and rutabaga for DIY Roasted Roots.*
SATURDAY	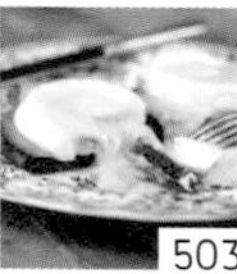 503 Eggs Benedict	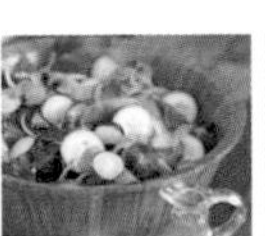 519 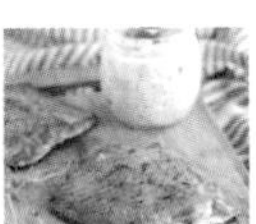 LEFTOVER 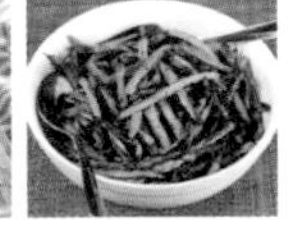 LEFTOVER DIY Salad and leftover Broiled Salmon with Dill-Caper Sauce and Roasted Green Beans	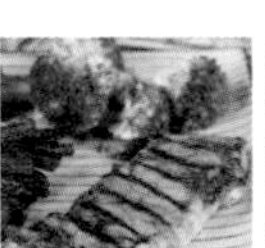 547 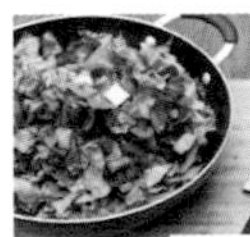 549 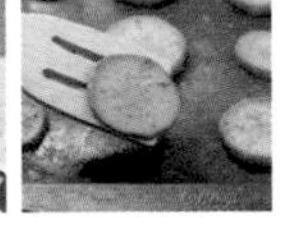 LEFTOVER Simple Steak, DIY Braised Greens, and leftover DIY Roasted Roots *Season steak with salt and pepper or truffle salt.*

NIGHTSHADE-FREE MEAL PLAN

Think going nightshade-free means missing out on your favorite comfort foods? This meal plan features dishes classically teeming with tomatoes, potatoes, and peppers, all reinvented to do away with these potentially inflammatory ingredients while still retaining those wonderfully familiar flavors. Make sure to follow the nightshade-free variations of the recipes and choose nightshade-free options for DIY recipes.

SHOPPING LIST

PRODUCE

- apple - 1
- avocados - 1½
- basil - 1 large bunch
- berries - 1½ pounds
- bok choy - 1 pound
- carrots - 1½ pounds
- cauliflower - 2½ heads
- celery - 3 stalks
- cherries - 3 cups
- chives - 1 tablespoon
- cilantro - 1½ cups
- English cucumbers - 2
- ginger root - 4 inches plus 1 tablespoon
- garlic - 3 heads
- green onions - 4
- plantains, green - 1 very large or 2 medium
- kabocha squash (or other winter squash) - 3 cups
- kaffir limes - 2 (or use regular limes)
- lemons - 5
- lemongrass - 1 stalk
- lime - 1
- mushrooms - 10 ounces
- radishes - 1 bunch
- romaine lettuce - 1 head
- sage - 1 tablespoon
- shallots - 3
- spaghetti squash - 4 pounds
- spinach - 6 ounces
- sweet potatoes - 4 small
- Thai basil - ½ cup
- thyme - 2 sprigs
- turnips - 2½ pounds
- white onion - 1
- yellow onions - 3
- greens of choice for DIY Braised Greens (page 549) - 1 meal
- salad veggies of choice for DIY Salad (page 519) - 4 meals
- veggies of choice for DIY Steamed Veggies (page 548) - 1 meal

MEAT & SEAFOOD

- bacon - 8 ounces
- chicken (whole or pieces) - 3 pounds
- chicken thighs - 2 pounds
- ground beef - 5 pounds (optional: swap in 1 pound ground liver and make "Sneaky Liver" Ground Beef, page 498)
- ground pork - 4 pounds
- ham - 4 ounces
- lamb stew meat - 3 pounds
- pork chops - 2 pounds
- steaks - 4 (6 to 8 ounces each)

EGGS & DAIRY

- eggs - 14
- ghee - ½ cup
- unsalted butter - ½ cup

VINEGARS & OILS

- apple cider vinegar
- avocado oil
- coconut oil
- coconut water vinegar
- olive oil
- red palm oil
- ingredients for salad dressing of choice (pages 484 to 485)

DRIED HERBS & SPICES

- anise powder
- bay leaf
- black pepper
- caraway seeds
- cinnamon stick
- curry powder (or ingredients to make homemade, page 483)
- fennel seeds
- fenugreek
- galangal
- garam masala
- garlic powder
- ginger powder
- granulated onion
- ground cardamom
- ground cinnamon
- ground coriander
- ground cumin
- ground mace
- ground mustard
- marjoram
- onion powder
- oregano
- sage
- sea salt
- thyme
- truffle salt
- turmeric powder
- ingredients for salad dressing of choice (pages 484 to 485)

DELI & PREPARED FOODS

- bone stock - 4 quarts (or ingredients to make homemade, page 486)

BULK

- dried apricots - ½ cup

SWEETENERS & BAKING SUPPLIES

- baking soda - ¾ teaspoon
- cassava flour - 1½ cups
- cream of tartar - ¼ teaspoon
- gelatin - 1 tablespoon
- honey - 3 tablespoons
- molasses - ¼ cup
- vanilla extract - 1 tablespoon

CANNED & JARRED GOODS

- coconut cream concentrate - 2 tablespoons
- coconut milk - 1 (13½-ounce) can (or ingredients to make homemade, page 480)
- coconut milk yogurt - ¼ cup (or ingredients to make homemade, page 481)
- Kalamata olives - ⅓ cup
- olives, sliced - 3 (5-ounce) cans
- prepared yellow mustard - 1 tablespoon
- pumpkin puree - 1 (16-ounce) can

ASIAN FOODS

- fish sauce - 3½ tablespoons
- shrimp paste - 1 teaspoon
- wasabi powder - ¼ teaspoon

MAKE AHEAD OR PURCHASE QUALITY OPTIONS

salad dressing, Thai green curry paste, bone stock, coconut milk yogurt

	BREAKFAST	LUNCH	DINNER
SUNDAY	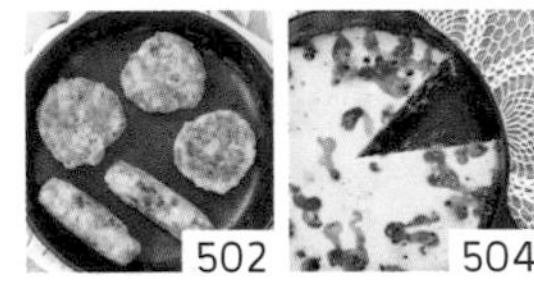 502 504 Breakfast Sausage and Clafoutis	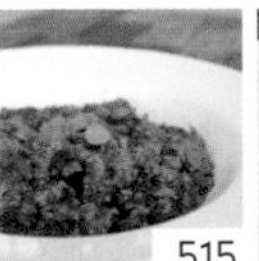 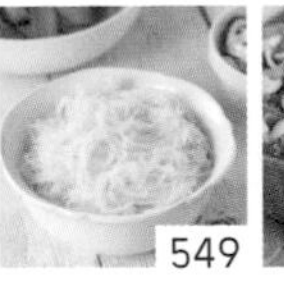 515 549 519 Spanish Picadillo over Spaghetti Squash Noodles and DIY Salad	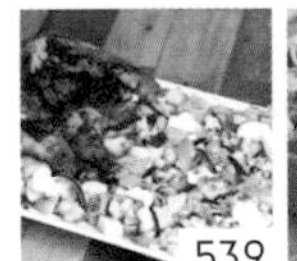 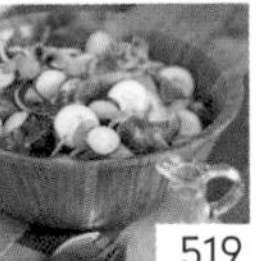 539 519 Bengali Tandoori Chicken with Aloo Gobi and DIY Salad
MONDAY 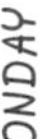	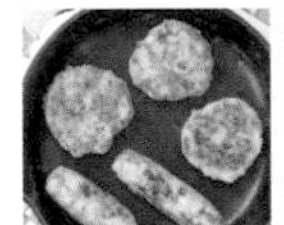 LEFTOVER LEFTOVER Leftover Breakfast Sausage and Clafoutis	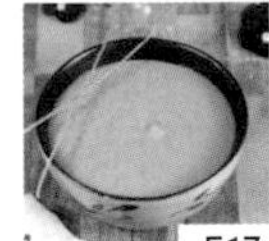 513 LEFTOVER Curry Carrot Soup with Nightshade-Free Curry Powder and leftover Bengali Tandoori Chicken with Aloo Gobi	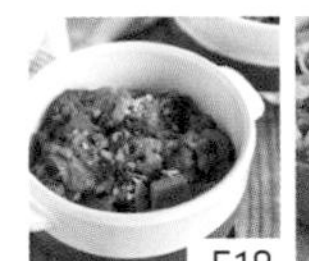 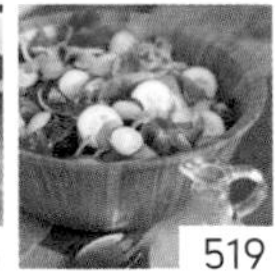 518 519 Moroccan Lamb Stew and DIY Salad
TUESDAY	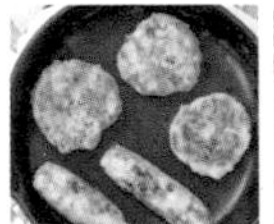 LEFTOVER LEFTOVER Leftover Breakfast Sausage and Clafoutis	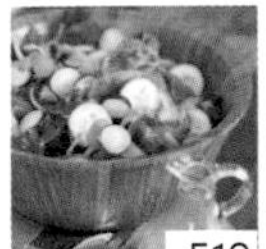 519 LEFTOVER DIY Salad and leftover Moroccan Lamb Stew	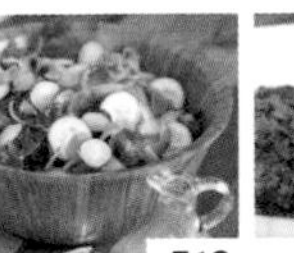 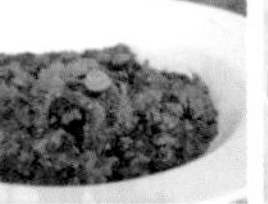 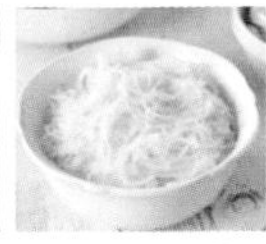 519 LEFTOVER LEFTOVER DIY Salad and leftover Spanish Picadillo over Spaghetti Squash Noodles
WEDNESDAY	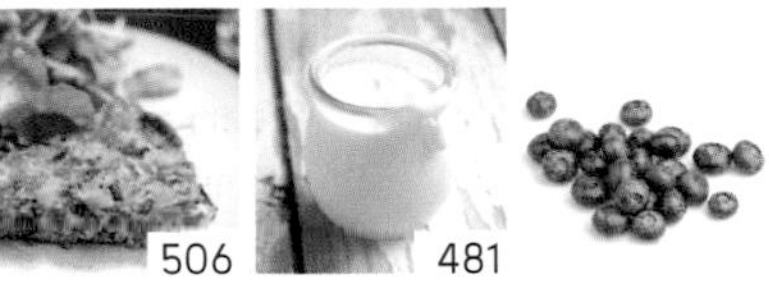 506 481 Pork & Winter Squash Frittata and Coconut Milk Yogurt with berries	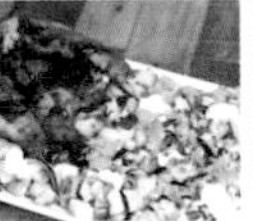 LEFTOVER LEFTOVER Leftover Bengali Tandoori Chicken with Aloo Gobi and Curry Carrot Soup	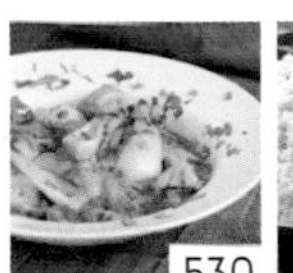 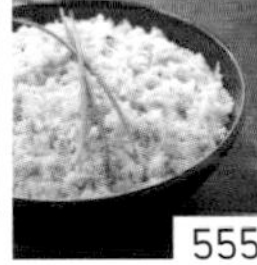 530 555 Thai Green Curry and Asian Cauli-rice
THURSDAY	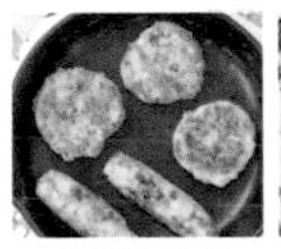 LEFTOVER LEFTOVER Leftover Breakfast Sausage and Clafoutis	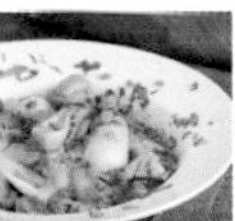 LEFTOVER LEFTOVER Leftover Thai Green Curry and Asian Cauli-rice	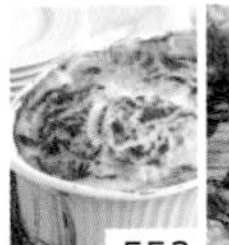 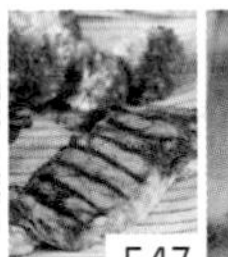 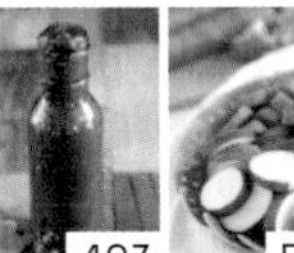 552 547 493 548 Scalloped Notatoes, Simple Steak, AIP Barbecue Sauce, and DIY Steamed Veggies
FRIDAY	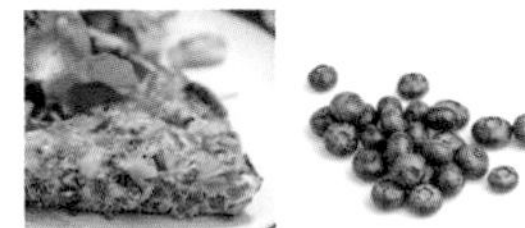 LEFTOVER Leftover Pork & Winter Squash Frittata and berries	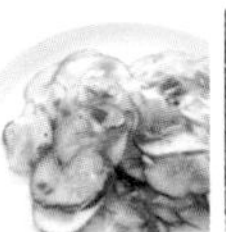 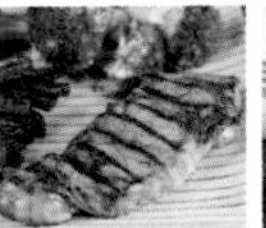 521 LEFTOVER LEFTOVER Simple Cucumber Salad and leftover Simple Steak and Scalloped Notatoes	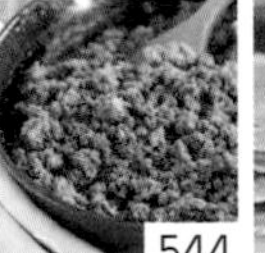 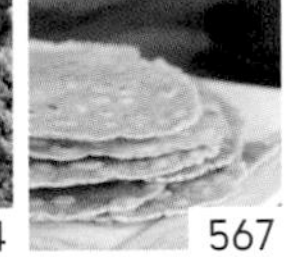 489 544 567 Guacamole, AIP Taco Meat, and Tortillas *Serve with shredded romaine lettuce and chopped cucumber.*
SATURDAY	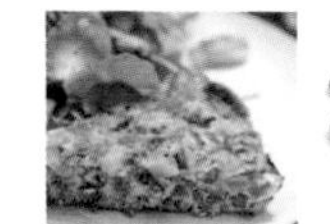 LEFTOVER Leftover Pork & Winter Squash Frittata and berries	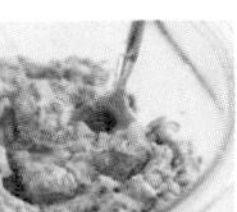 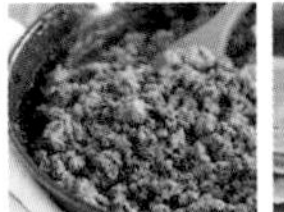 LEFTOVER LEFTOVER LEFTOVER Leftover Guacamole, AIP Taco Meat, and Tortillas	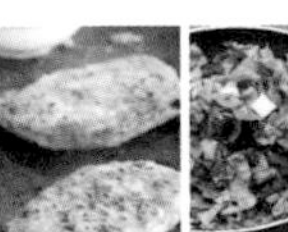 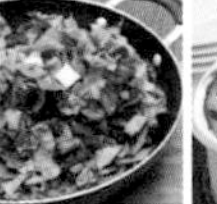 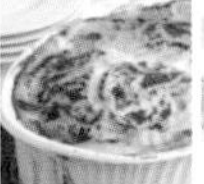 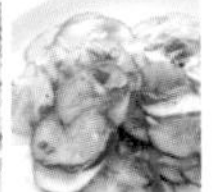 532 549 LEFTOVER LEFTOVER Broiled Pork Chops, DIY Braised Greens, and leftover Scalloped Notatoes and Simple Cucumber Salad

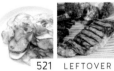

NUT-FREE MEAL PLAN

This meal plan features some fun recipes of which typical Paleo versions often rely on nut flours, butters, or milks. These recipes are all 100 percent tree nut-free. (Note for those who are also sensitive to coconut: use alternate cooking fat options in recipes where coconut oil is called for, and use apple cider vinegar or white wine vinegar in place of coconut water vinegar.) Enjoy!

SHOPPING LIST

PRODUCE

asparagus - 1 pound
bananas - 2
berries of choice - 1 pound
broccoli slaw - 1 package
carrots - 4
cauliflower - 2 heads
cilantro - 5 tablespoons
dill - ¼ cup
garlic - 3 heads
grapefruit - 2
green bell peppers - ½ cup
green cabbage - ½ head
green onions - 5
green plantain - 1
kale - 2 cups
kiwi - 2
lemons - 4
limes - 2
mushrooms - 1½ cups
parsley - ½ cup
plantains, ripe (nearly black) - 6
red bell peppers - 3
romaine lettuce - 1 head
rosemary - 2 tablespoons
spinach - 6 cups
sweet potatoes - 1½ pounds
thyme - 2 tablespoons
yellow onions - 3
yellow summer squash - 1 pound
root vegetables of choice for Root Vegetable Casserole (page 551) - 4 pounds
salad veggies of choice for DIY Salad (page 519) - 5 meals
veggies of choice for DIY Steamed Veggies (page 548) - 1 meal

MEAT & SEAFOOD

bacon - 10 ounces
Canadian bacon - 4 slices
chicken breast - 1 pound
fish steaks or fillets (such as sea bass, mahi mahi, halibut, or swordfish) - 1 to 1½ pounds
ground beef - 2 pounds
pork center loin - 4 pounds
salad shrimp, precooked - 1 pound
white fish fillets (such as cod or halibut) - 1½ pounds

EGGS & DAIRY

butter - 1 tablespoon
eggs - 47

DRIED HERBS & SPICES

bay leaf
black pepper
ginger powder
ground allspice
ground cinnamon
ground cloves
ground cumin
ground nutmeg
paprika
sea salt
truffle salt
turmeric powder
ingredients for salad dressing of choice (pages 484 to 485)
ingredients for seasoning of choice for DIY Baked Chicken Breast (pages 482 to 483)

VINEGARS & OILS

apple cider vinegar
avocado oil
coconut oil
coconut water vinegar
lard
olive oil
high-smoke-point fat for deep-frying (see page 467)
ingredients for salad dressing of choice (pages 484 to 485)

DELI & PREPARED FOODS

bone stock - 2½ cups (or ingredients to make homemade, page 486)

SWEETENERS & BAKING SUPPLIES

active dry yeast - 1 teaspoon
arrowroot powder - 3 tablespoons
baking soda - 1 teaspoon
cream of tartar - 1 teaspoon
honey - 2 tablespoons
pumpkin powder - ½ cup (may need to order online)
tapioca flour - 1 cup

CANNED & JARRED GOODS

anchovy paste - 1 teaspoon
black olives - 1 cup
coconut aminos - 1 tablespoon
Dijon mustard - 1 tablespoon
mayonnaise - 1 cup (or ingredients to make homemade, page 487)
tahini - ⅓ cup
tomato paste - 1 can

ASIAN FOODS

fish sauce - 3 tablespoons

DRINKS

white wine - 1½ cups

OTHER

plantain chips - ¼ cup

MAKE AHEAD OR PURCHASE QUALITY OPTIONS

mayonnaise, bone stock, salad dressing of choice

	BREAKFAST	LUNCH	DINNER
SUNDAY	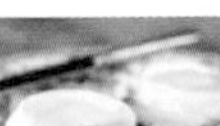 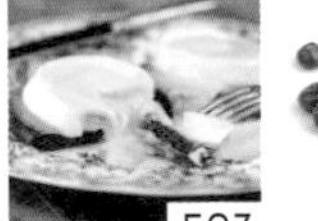 503 Eggs Benedict and berries	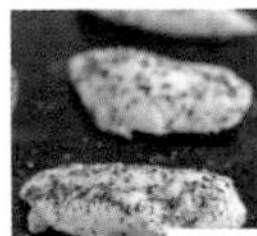 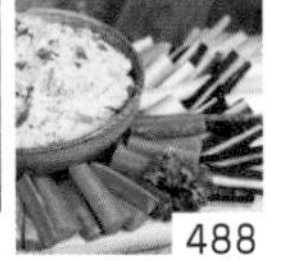 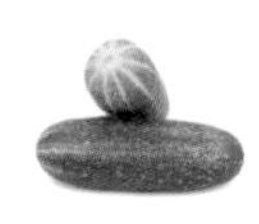 541 488 DIY Baked Chicken Breast, Cauliflower Hummus, and raw veggies for dipping	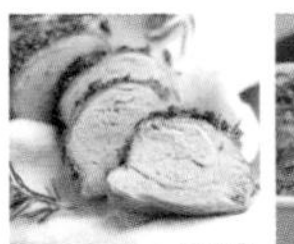 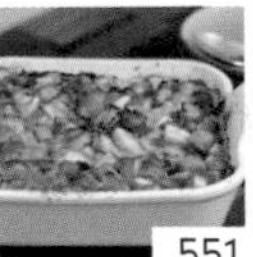 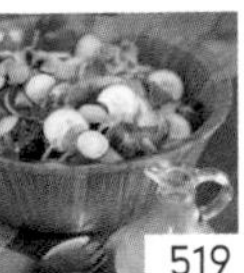 540 551 519 Herb-Crusted Pork Loin, Root Vegetable Casserole, and DIY Salad
MONDAY	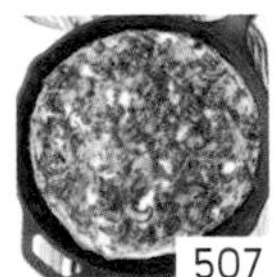 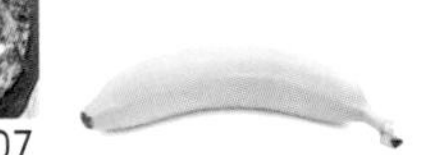 507 Veggie Frittata and a banana	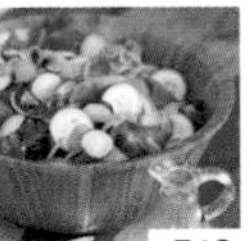 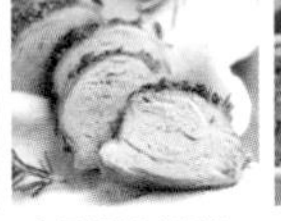 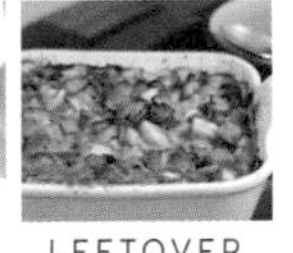 519 LEFTOVER LEFTOVER DIY Salad and leftover Herb-Crusted Pork Loin and Root Vegetable Casserole	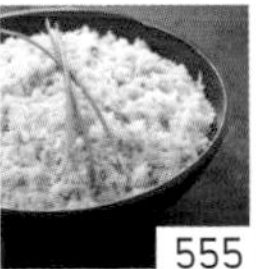 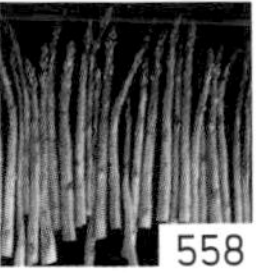 525 555 558 Gremolata-Topped Fish Fillets, Lemon Parsley Cauli-rice, and Broiled Asparagus *Serve with Hollandaise (page 497).*
TUESDAY	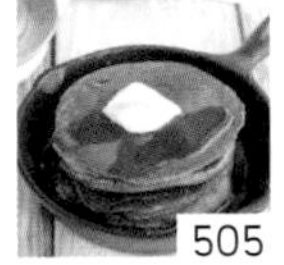 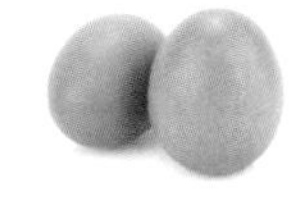 505 Pumpkin Pancakes and 2 eggs, any style	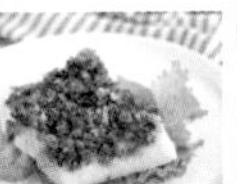 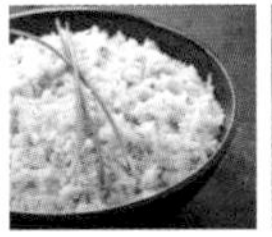 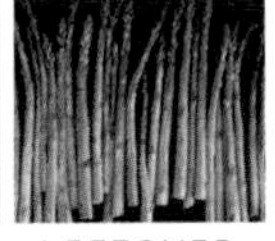 LEFTOVER LEFTOVER LEFTOVER Leftover Gremolata-Topped Fish Fillets, Lemon Parsley Cauli-rice, and Broiled Asparagus	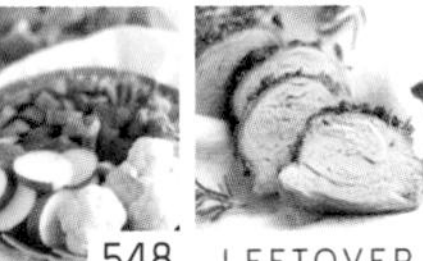 548 LEFTOVER LEFTOVER DIY Steamed Veggies and leftover Herb-Crusted Pork Loin and Root Vegetable Casserole
WEDNESDAY	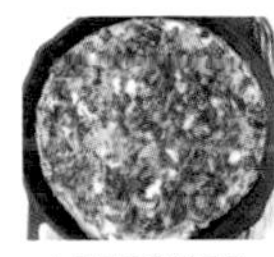 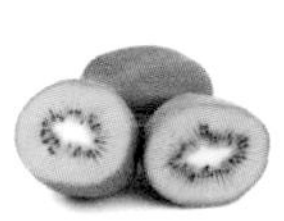 LEFTOVER Leftover Veggie Frittata and a kiwi	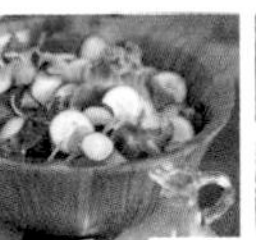 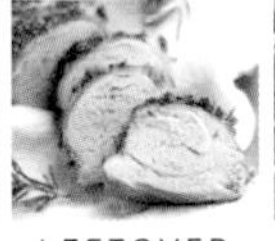 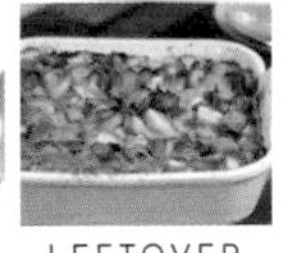 519 LEFTOVER LEFTOVER DIY Salad and leftover Herb-Crusted Pork Loin and Root Vegetable Casserole	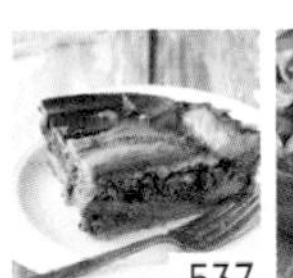 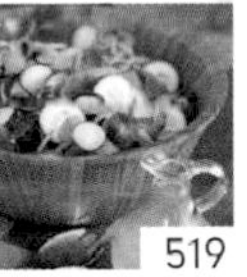 537 519 Puerto Rican Lasagna and DIY Salad
THURSDAY	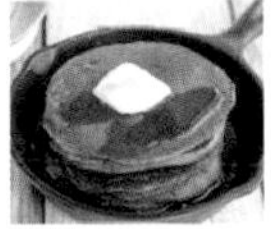 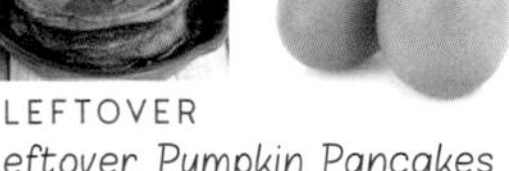 LEFTOVER Leftover Pumpkin Pancakes and 2 eggs, any style	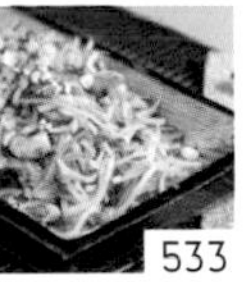 533 Shrimp Pad Thai *Omit cashews.*	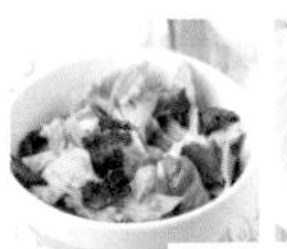 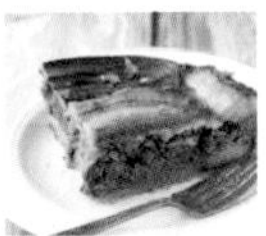 520 LEFTOVER Paleo Caesar Salad and leftover Puerto Rican Lasagna
FRIDAY	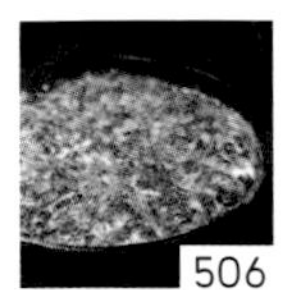 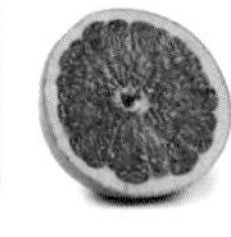 506 Bacon, Spinach & Olive Frittata and half a grapefruit	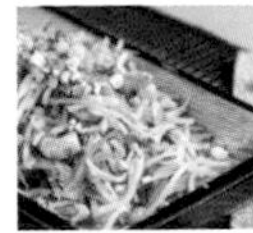 LEFTOVER Leftover Shrimp Pad Thai	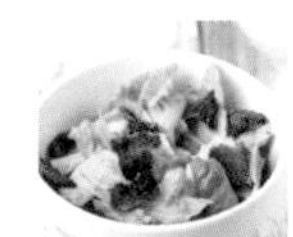 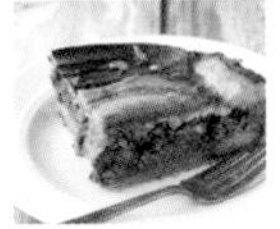 LEFTOVER LEFTOVER Leftover Paleo Caesar Salad and Puerto Rican Lasagna
SATURDAY	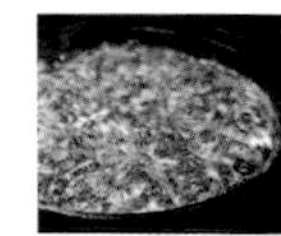 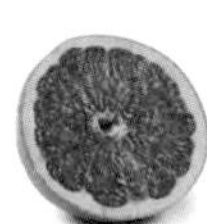 LEFTOVER Leftover Bacon, Spinach & Olive Frittata and half a grapefruit	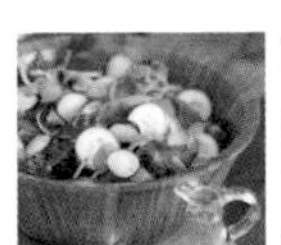 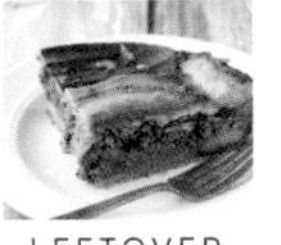 519 LEFTOVER DIY Salad and leftover Puerto Rican Lasagna	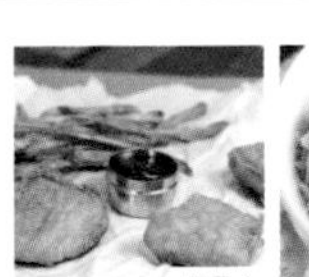 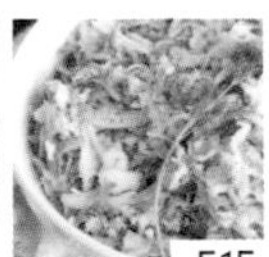 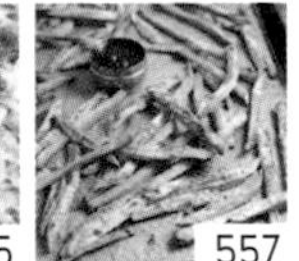 536 515 557 Fish n' Chips, Creamy Coleslaw, and Oven-Baked Sweet Potato Fries

FAMILY FAVORITES MEAL PLAN

With many re-creations of American favorites and classic kids' favorites, this meal plan is designed to cater to picky eaters and ease the whole family into a healthier way of eating!

NOTE: This plan is designed to feed four people.

SHOPPING LIST

PRODUCE

avocados - 1½
berries of choice - 3 pounds
cantaloupe - 1
carrots - 7
cassava - 2½ pounds
celery - 8 stalks
cilantro - 1 cup
garlic - 1 head
green and red bell peppers - 1½ cups
green beans - 1½ pounds
jalapeño pepper - 1
kabocha squash (or other winter squash) - 3 cups
kale - 8 cups
lemons - 3
lime - 1
oranges - 4
oregano - 3 tablespoons
parsley - 1 tablespoon
plantains, green - 7
red onion - ½
rosemary - ½ teaspoon
sage - 1 tablespoon
spaghetti squash - 4 pounds
sweet potatoes - 2½ pounds
thyme - 2 sprigs plus 1 teaspoon
tomatoes - 1½ pounds
white onions - 2
raw veggies of choice for dipping - 3 meals
root vegetables of choice for DIY Roasted Roots (page 550) - 2 pounds
salad veggies of choice for DIY Salad (page 519) - 3 meals
toppings of choice and sauce ingredients for DIY Pizza - 1 meal
veggies of choice for DIY Steamed Veggies (page 548) - 2 meals

MEAT & SEAFOOD

bacon - 1¼ pounds
chicken - 1 whole (4 to 5 pounds)
chicken tenders - 1 pound
chicken wings - 3 pounds
duck fat - ½ cup
flank steak or chicken - 2 pounds
ground beef - 5 pounds
ground pork - 1 pound
ham - 10 ounces
liver - 1 pound
pancetta - 4 ounces
tallow - 2 tablespoons
meat of choice for sandwiches - 2 meals
meat of choice for DIY Pizza (page 529)

EGGS & DAIRY

eggs - 88
mozzarella cheese (optional)

CANNED & JARRED GOODS

coconut aminos - 2 tablespoons
coconut cream - 1 cup (or ingredients to make homemade, page 480) (optional, for crepes)
coconut milk - 2⅔ cups (or ingredients to make homemade, page 480)
crushed tomatoes - 1 (15-ounce) can
mayonnaise - ½ cup (or ingredients to make homemade, page 487)
toppings of choice for DIY Pizza (page 529)

DRIED HERBS & SPICES

bay leaf
black pepper
cayenne pepper
chili powder
ginger powder
granulated garlic
granulated onion
ground coriander
ground cumin
ground mace
oregano
paprika
sea salt
truffle salt
ingredients for salad dressing of choice (pages 484 to 485)

DELI & PREPARED FOODS

bone stock - 7 cups (or ingredients to make homemade, page 486)

VINEGARS & OILS

apple cider vinegar
avocado oil
coconut oil
lard
olive oil
ingredients for salad dressing of choice (pages 484 to 485)

BULK

almonds - ½ cup
black sesame seeds - 2 tablespoons
raw pepitas - 1 cup
raw walnuts - ½ cup
sesame seeds - ¾ cup
sunflower seeds - ½ cup

SWEETENERS & BAKING SUPPLIES

almond flour - 3½ cups
arrowroot powder - 1¾ cups
baking soda - 3¼ teaspoons
cassava flour - 1¾ cups
coconut flour - 1 cup
cream of tartar - 1¼ teaspoons
evaporated cane juice - ¼ cup
gelatin - 1 tablespoon
honey - ½ cup plus 3 tablespoons
palm shortening - ½ cup
tapioca starch - 2½ cups
unsweetened shredded coconut - ½ cup
vanilla extract - 2 tablespoons
ingredients for pie crust of choice (page 499)

FROZEN FOODS

frozen peas - 1 cup

DRINKS

dry white wine - 1 cup

MAKE AHEAD OR PURCHASE QUALITY OPTIONS

salad dressing, mayonnaise, bone stock, pizza sauce, "multigrain" quick bread, marinade for Honey Garlic Chicken Wings

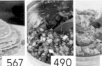

	BREAKFAST	LUNCH	DINNER
SUNDAY	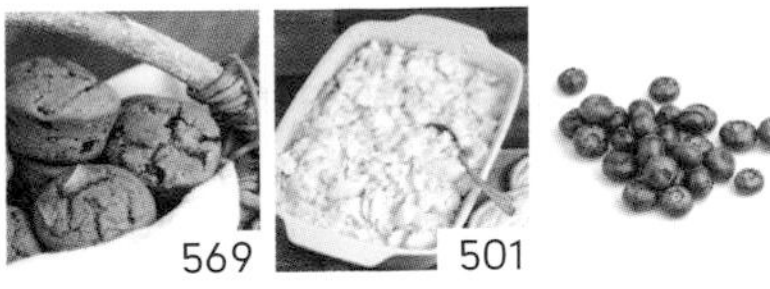 569 501 DIY Muffins, Oven Scrambled Eggs, and berries	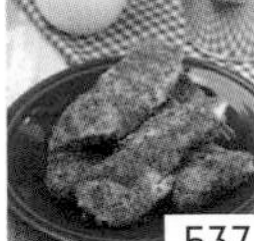 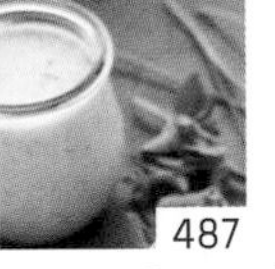 537 487 Chicken Fingers, Ranch Dip, and raw veggies for dipping	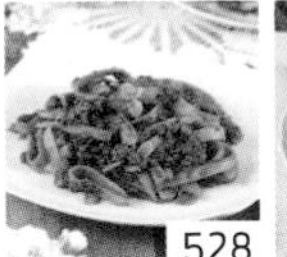 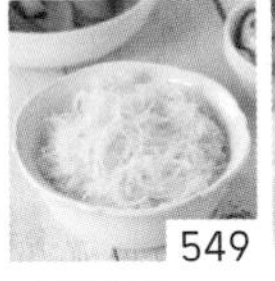 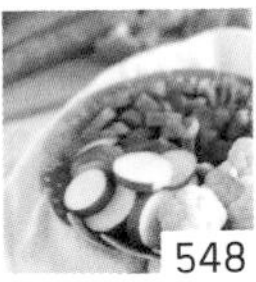 528 549 548 "Spaghetti" Bolognese over Spaghetti Squash Noodles and DIY Steamed Veggies
MONDAY	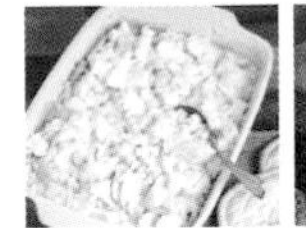 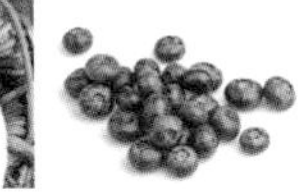 LEFTOVER LEFTOVER Leftover Oven Scrambled Eggs and DIY Muffins and berries	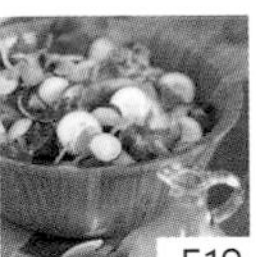 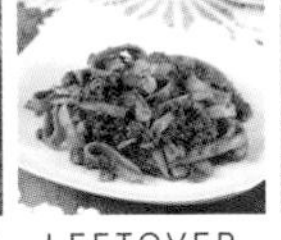 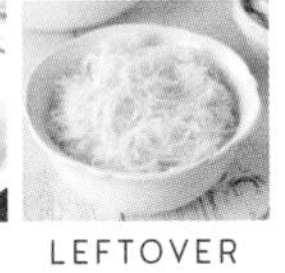 519 LEFTOVER LEFTOVER DIY Salad and leftover "Spaghetti" Bolognese over Spaghetti Squash Noodles	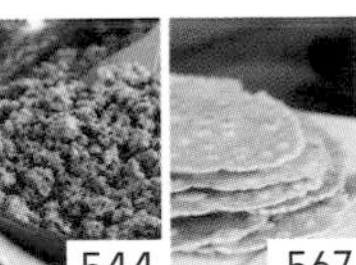 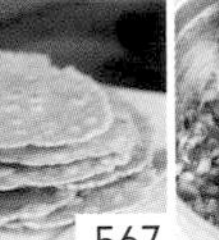 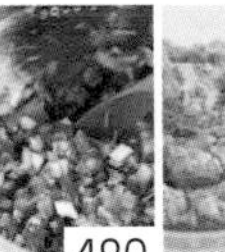 544 567 490 489 Taco Meat, Tortillas, Pico de Gallo, and Guacamole
TUESDAY	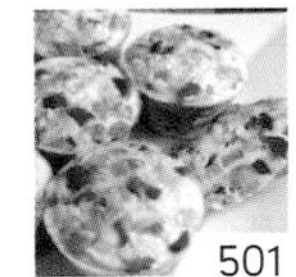 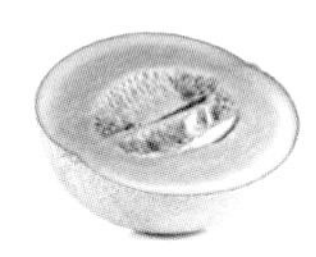 501 Ham & Sweet Potato Egg Muffins and cantaloupe	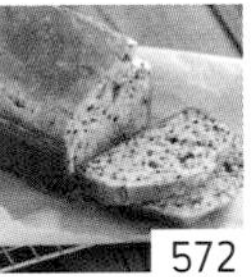 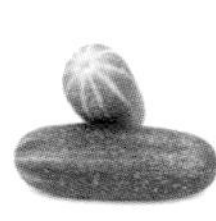 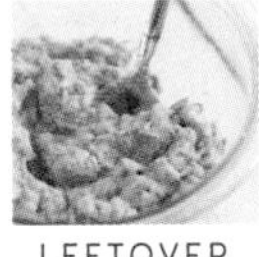 572 LEFTOVER "Multigrain" Quick Bread and raw veggies and leftover Guacamole or Ranch Dip *Use bread to make sandwiches with your filling of choice.*	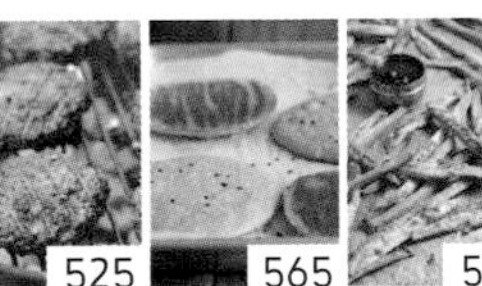 525 565 557 519 50/50/50 Burgers, Sesame Seed Buns, Oven-Baked Sweet Potato Fries, and DIY Salad *Make double batch of Sesame Seed Buns.*
WEDNESDAY	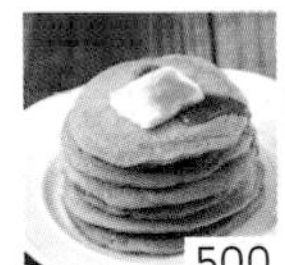 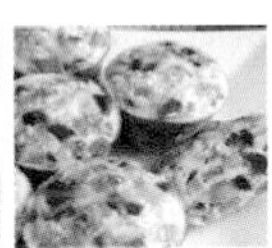 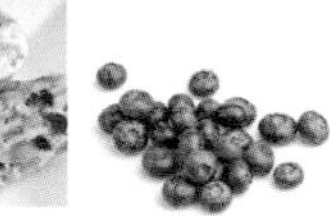 500 LEFTOVER DIY Pancakes, leftover Ham & Sweet Potato Egg Muffins, and berries	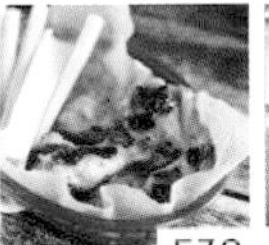 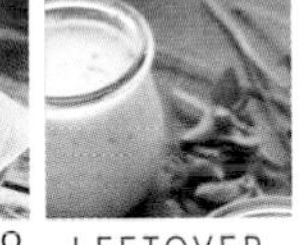 539 LEFTOVER Honey Garlic Chicken Wings, leftover Ranch Dip, and raw veggies	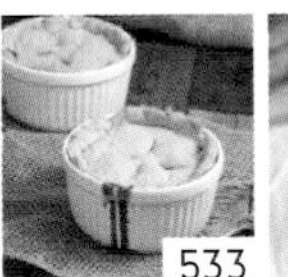 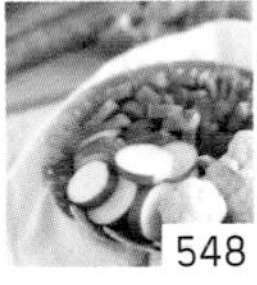 533 548 Chicken or Beef Pot Pie and DIY Steamed Veggies
THURSDAY	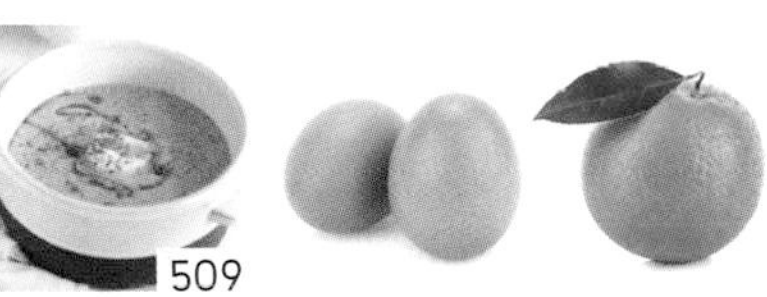 509 DIY Paleo Porridge, 2 eggs, any style, and an orange *Make double batch of porridge.*	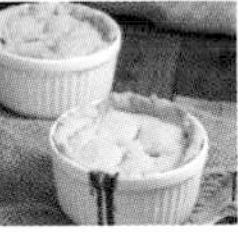 LEFTOVER Leftover Chicken or Beef Pot Pie	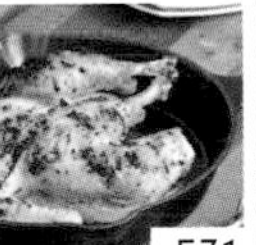 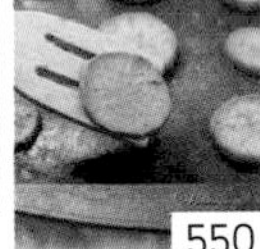 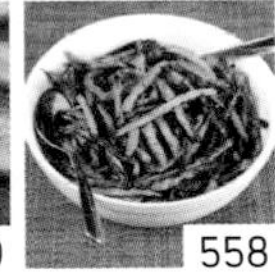 531 550 558 Spatchcocked Chicken, DIY Roasted Roots, and Roasted Green Beans
FRIDAY	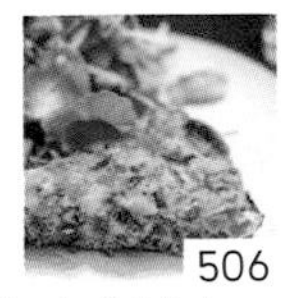 506 Pork & Winter Squash Frittata and cantaloupe	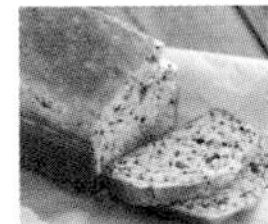 LEFTOVER 563 Leftover "Multigrain" Quick Bread and Kale Chips *Use bread to make sandwiches with your filling of choice.*	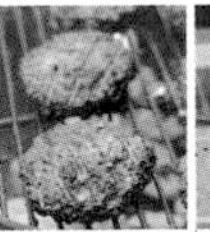 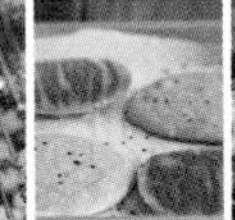 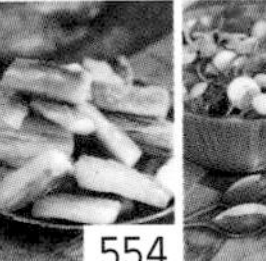 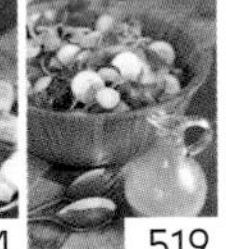 LEFTOVER LEFTOVER 554 519 Leftover 50/50/50 Burgers and Sesame Seed Buns with Cassava Oven Fries and DIY Salad *Make double batch of Sesame Seed Buns.*
SATURDAY	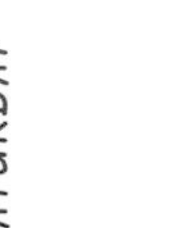 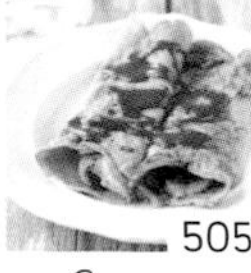 505 Crepes *Serve with berries and coconut cream, if desired. Add any leftovers from the week.*	Leftovers! You probably have quite a few bits and pieces left over from meals during the week. Let everyone pick their favorite!	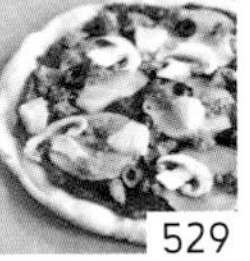 529 DIY Pizza *Top with leftover Spatchcocked Chicken, if desired.*

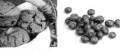

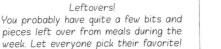

NUTRIENT NUT MEAL PLAN

Looking to address nutrient deficiencies or put healing on the fast track? This meal plan is chock-full of organ meat, seafood, and tons of vegetables to pack a nutrient punch! Even breakfast is an opportunity for nutrient-dense options! Up the ante by drinking kombucha with one meal per day, using raw sauerkraut as a salad ingredient, adding some nuts or seeds to salads, and challenging yourself to make different steamed veggies and salads during the week.

SHOPPING LIST

PRODUCE

asparagus - 1 pound
avocados - 2
basil - 3 tablespoons
beets - 8
berries of choice - 1 pound
Brussels sprouts - 2 pounds
carrots - 10
cauliflower - 1 head
celery - 10 stalks
chives - ¼ cup
cilantro - ½ cup
cucumbers - 2 cups
daikon - 2 cups
dried seaweed - 2 ounces
fennel bulb - 1¼ pounds
garlic - 3 heads
ginger root - 3 inches
Granny Smith apple - 1
green onions - 2
honeydew melon - 1
kiwis - 2
lemons - 2
lime basil - 2 cups (or use regular basil)
limes - 2
mango - 1
mint - ⅓ cup
mushrooms - 1¼ pounds
onions - 3
oregano - 3 tablespoons
parsley - ½ cup
parsnips - 1½ pounds
plantains, green - 3
portobello mushrooms - 6 ounces
red bell pepper - ½
red onions - ½ cup
rosemary - 2 sprigs plus 1 teaspoon
tarragon - 3 tablespoons
thyme - 14 sprigs plus 2 tablespoons
turnip - 1
white onion - 1
yellow onions - 3
yuca - 1 pound
zucchini - 6
greens of choice for DIY Braised Greens (page 549) - 1 meal
salad veggies of choice for DIY Salad (page 519) - 5 meals
veggies of choice for DIY Steamed Veggies (page 548) - 2 meals

MEAT & SEAFOOD

bacon - 4 slices
beef tongue - 3 pounds
clams - 3 (5- to 6-ounce) cans
duck fat - 2 tablespoons
fish steaks or fillets - 2 (6 to 8 ounces each)
ground beef - 4 pounds
ground pork - 1 pound
lamb kidneys - 1½ pounds
liver - 2 pounds
pancetta - 4 ounces
pork sausage - 8 ounces
shrimp, precooked - 1 pound
steak - 3 pounds

EGGS & DAIRY

eggs - 21
unsalted butter - ¼ cup

DELI & PREPARED FOODS

beef bone stock - 5 cups (or ingredients to make homemade, page 486)
bone stock - 2 quarts (or ingredients to make homemade, page 486)

DRIED HERBS & SPICES

bay leaf
black pepper
cayenne pepper
coarse sea salt
fennel seeds
garlic powder
ground cinnamon
ground cloves
paprika
sage
sea salt
truffle salt
ingredients for salad dressing of choice (pages 484 to 485)

VINEGARS & OILS

apple cider vinegar
avocado oil
balsamic vinegar
coconut oil
coconut water vinegar
lard
olive oil
sesame oil
ingredients for salad dressing of choice (pages 484 to 485) - 2 varieties

BULK

pine nuts - ¼ cup
raw hazelnuts - 1 cup
sunflower seeds - ½ cup

SWEETENERS & BAKING SUPPLIES

arrowroot powder - 1 cup
baking soda - ¼ teaspoon
blackstrap molasses - 1 tablespoon
coconut flour - ½ cup
cream of tartar - ½ teaspoon
gelatin - 1¼ teaspoons
honey - 3 tablespoons
palm shortening - ½ cup
tapioca starch - ⅓ cup

CANNED & JARRED GOODS

coconut aminos - 6 tablespoons
coconut cream - 2 cups (or ingredients to make homemade, page 480)
coconut milk - 2¾ cups (or ingredients to make homemade, page 480)
mayonnaise - 1 cup (or ingredients to make homemade, page 487)
whole-grain mustard - 2 tablespoons

ASIAN FOODS

fish sauce - 5 tablespoons

SUPPLEMENTS

Lactobacillus-based probiotic supplement capsules or nondairy yogurt starter

MAKE AHEAD OR PURCHASE QUALITY OPTIONS

salad dressing (2 varieties to mix it up), bone stock, mayonnaise, coconut milk yogurt

	BREAKFAST	LUNCH	DINNER
SUNDAY	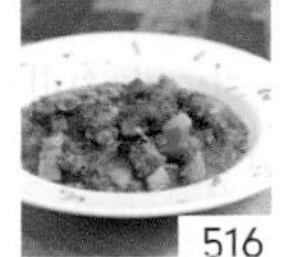 516 Hamburger Stew and a kiwi Use "Sneaky Liver" Ground Beef to make Hamburger Stew.	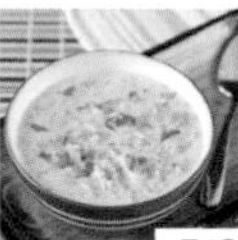 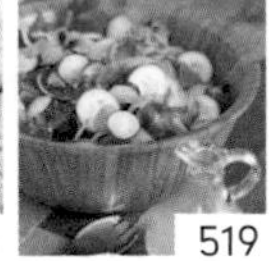 512 566 519 Clam Chowder, Yuca Biscuits, and DIY Salad	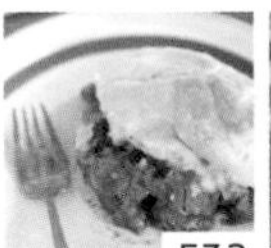 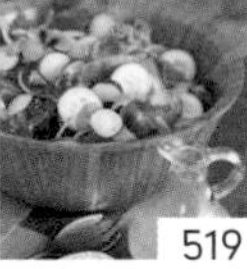 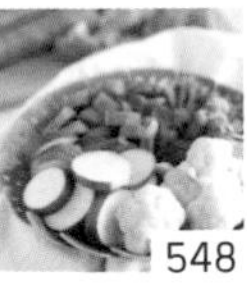 532 519 548 Steak & Kidney Pot Pie, DIY Salad, and DIY Steamed Veggies
MONDAY	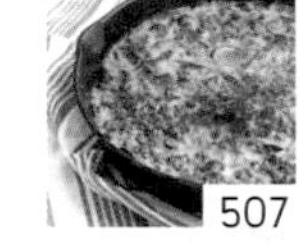 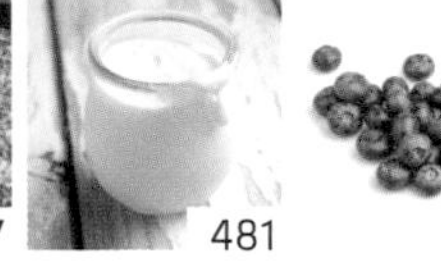 507 481 Sausage & Mushroom Frittata and Coconut Milk Yogurt with berries	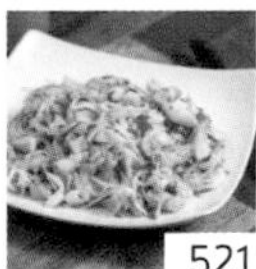 521 Shrimp Salad	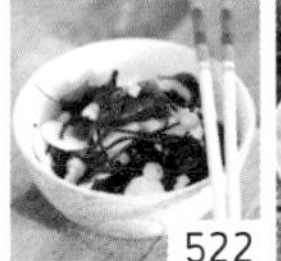 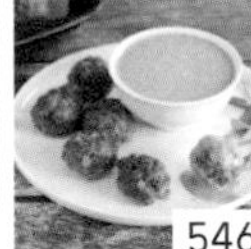 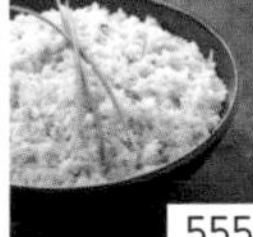 522 546 555 Seaweed Salad, Meatballs with Asian Dipping Sauce, and Asian Cauli-rice Use "Sneaky Liver" Ground Beef to make meatballs.
TUESDAY	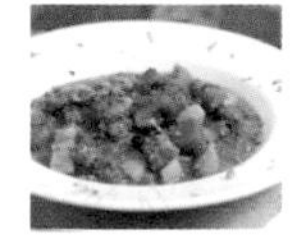 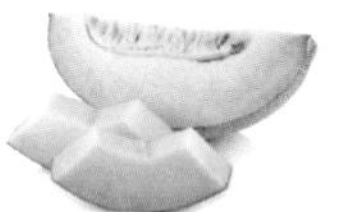 LEFTOVER Leftover Hamburger Stew and honeydew melon	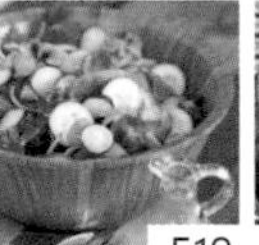 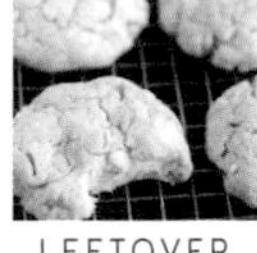 519 LEFTOVER LEFTOVER DIY Salad and leftover Clam Chowder and Yuca Biscuits	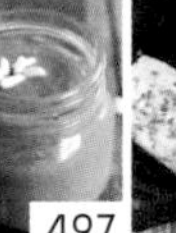 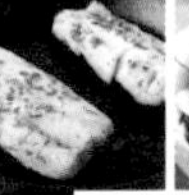 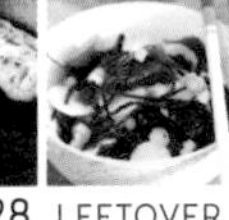 553 497 528 LEFTOVER Zoodles, Lemon Basil Pesto, Tarragon-Seared Fish Fillets, and leftover Seaweed Salad
WEDNESDAY	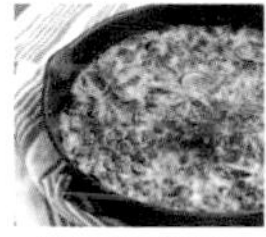 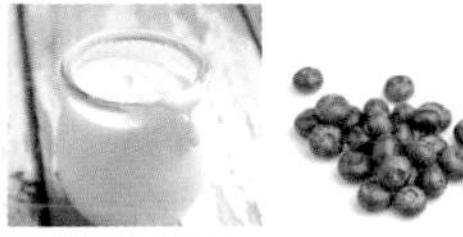 LEFTOVER LEFTOVER Leftover Sausage & Mushroom Frittata and Coconut Milk Yogurt with berries	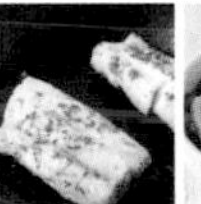 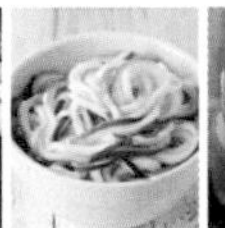 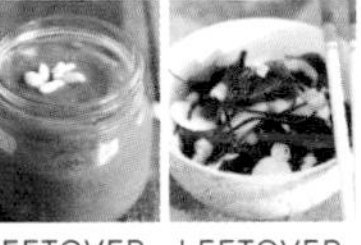 LEFTOVER LEFTOVER LEFTOVER LEFTOVER Leftover Tarragon-Seared Fish Fillets, Zoodles, Lemon Basil Pesto, and Seaweed Salad	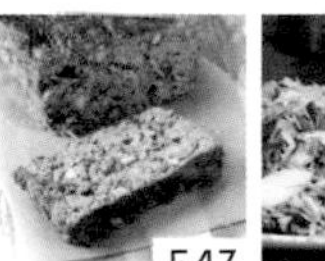 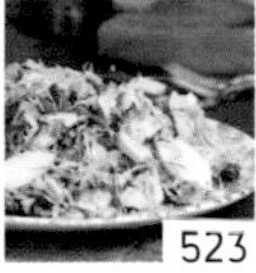 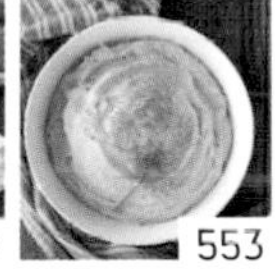 543 523 553 Meatloaf, Shaved Brussels Slaw with Hazelnuts, Apple & Mint, and Parsnip & Fennel Puree
THURSDAY	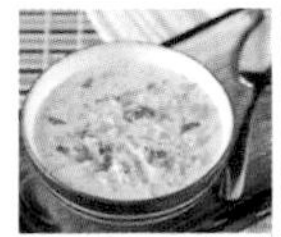 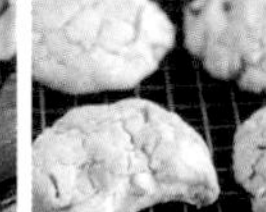 LEFTOVER LEFTOVER Leftover Clam Chowder and Yuca Biscuits	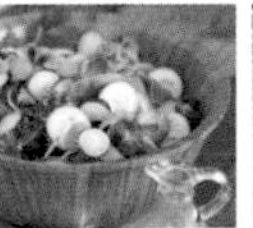 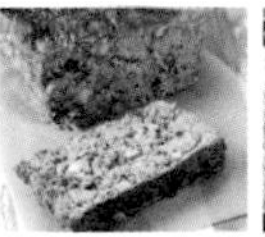 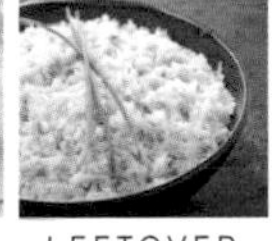 519 LEFTOVER LEFTOVER DIY Salad and leftover Meatloaf and Asian Cauli-rice	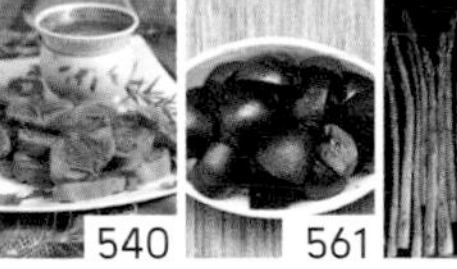 540 561 558 548 Beef Tongue with Rosemary-Mustard Reduction, Balsamic-Roasted Beets, Broiled Asparagus, and DIY Steamed Veggies
FRIDAY	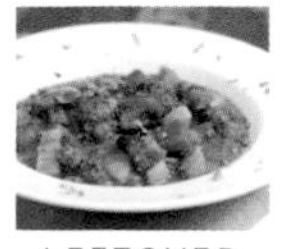 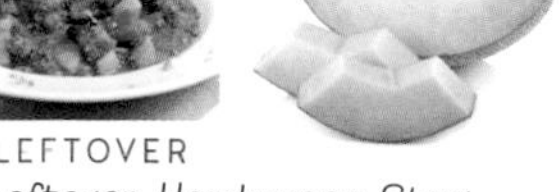 LEFTOVER Leftover Hamburger Stew and honeydew melon	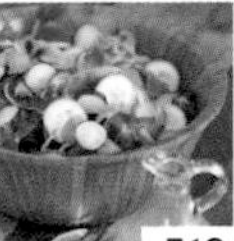 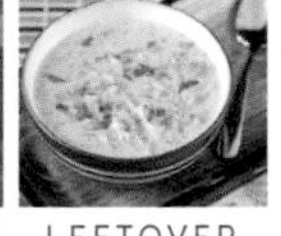 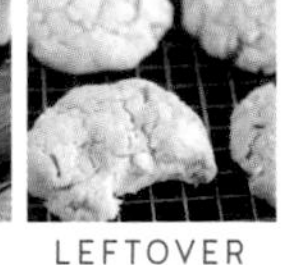 519 LEFTOVER LEFTOVER DIY Salad, leftover Clam Chowder, and Yuca Biscuits	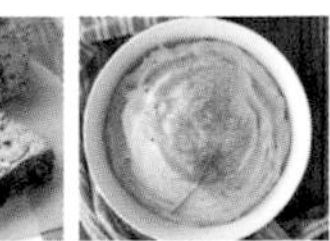 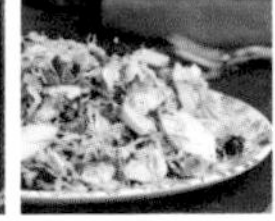 LEFTOVER LEFTOVER LEFTOVER Leftover Meatloaf, Parsnip & Fennel Puree, and Shaved Brussels Slaw with Hazelnuts, Apple & Mint
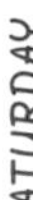 SATURDAY	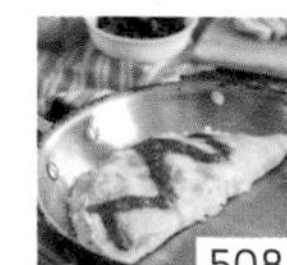 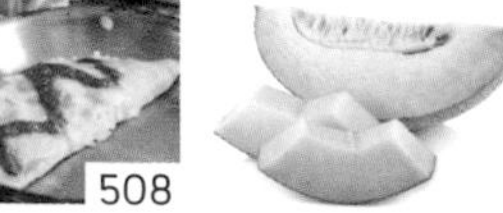 508 DIY Omelet and honeydew melon	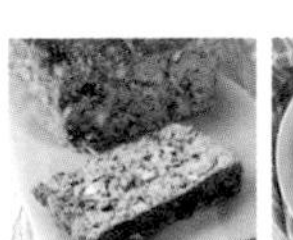 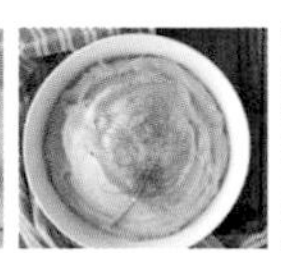 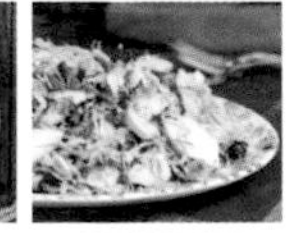 LEFTOVER LEFTOVER LEFTOVER Leftover Meatloaf, Parsnip & Fennel Puree, and Shaved Brussels Slaw with Hazelnuts, Apple & Mint	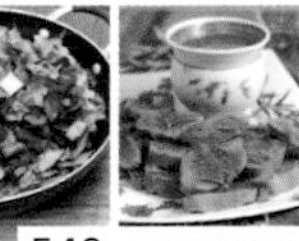 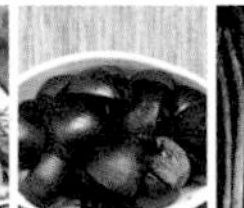 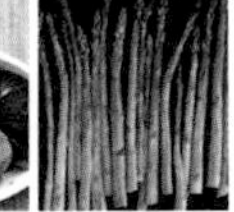 549 LEFTOVER LEFTOVER LEFTOVER DIY Braised Greens and leftover Beef Tongue with Rosemary-Mustard Reduction, Balsamic-Roasted Beets, and Broiled Asparagus

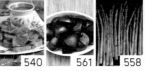

PERFORMANCE MEAL PLAN

Packed with protein and slow-burning starchy carbs, this meal plan is about providing fuel for movement and nutrients for muscle repair. Pair this plan with adequate recovery time between workouts, plenty of mobility work (stretching, foam rolling, and so on), sleep, and stress-reducing practices like mindful meditation and nature walks. Consider drinking coconut water as a sports drink during long and vigorous training sessions.

SHOPPING LIST

PRODUCE

- bananas - 2
- beets - 8
- berries of choice - 2 pounds
- butternut squash - 2 large
- carrots - 4
- cassava - 2½ pounds
- celery - 4 stalks
- cilantro - 1 cup
- English cucumbers - 1½
- garlic - 2 heads
- grapefruit - 2
- green beans - 1½ pounds
- green onions - 8
- jalapeño pepper - 1 (optional)
- kabocha squash - 3 cups (or any winter squash)
- lemons - 5
- lime - 1
- onion - 1
- oregano - 3 tablespoons
- plantains, green - 4
- red onions - ½
- romaine lettuce - 1 head
- rosemary - ½ teaspoon
- sage - 1 tablespoon
- sweet potatoes - 3
- tarragon - 3 tablespoons
- thyme - 2 sprigs plus ½ teaspoon
- tomatoes - 1½ pounds
- salad veggies of choice for DIY Salad (page 519) - 7 meals
- veggies of choice for DIY Steamed Veggies (page 548) - 2 meals

MEAT & SEAFOOD

- bacon - 33 slices
- chicken - 1 whole (4 to 5 pounds)
- duck fat - 1 cup
- fish steaks or fillets (such as mahi mahi, amberjack, grouper, or halibut) - 2 (6 to 8 ounces each)
- ground beef - 5 pounds
- ground pork - 1 pound
- pancetta - 4 ounces
- steaks - 2 to 4 (6 to 8 ounces each)
- tallow - 2 tablespoons

EGGS & DAIRY

- eggs - 38

DRIED HERBS & SPICES

- black pepper
- coarse sea salt
- curry powder (or ingredients to make homemade, page 483)
- ground mace
- sea salt
- truffle salt
- ingredients for steak seasoning of choice (page 482)
- ingredients for salad dressing of choice (pages 484 to 485) - 2 varieties

VINEGARS & OILS

- avocado oil
- balsamic vinegar
- coconut oil
- olive oil
- ingredients for salad dressing of choice (pages 484 to 485)

DELI & PREPARED FOODS

- bone stock - 2 cups (or ingredients to make homemade, page 486)

SWEETENERS & BAKING SUPPLIES

- baking soda - ½ teaspoon
- vanilla extract - 2 teaspoons

CANNED & JARRED GOODS

- anchovy paste - 1 teaspoon
- coconut milk - 1 (13½-ounce) can (or ingredients to make homemade, page 480)
- crushed tomatoes - 1 (15-ounce) can
- mayonnaise - ½ cup (or ingredients to make homemade, page 487)

DRINKS

- dry white wine - 1 cup

OTHER

- coconut wraps or ingredients to make Tortillas (page 567) (optional)

MAKE AHEAD OR PURCHASE QUALITY OPTIONS

salad dressing (2 varieties to mix it up), bone stock, mayonnaise, curry powder

	BREAKFAST	LUNCH	DINNER
SUNDAY	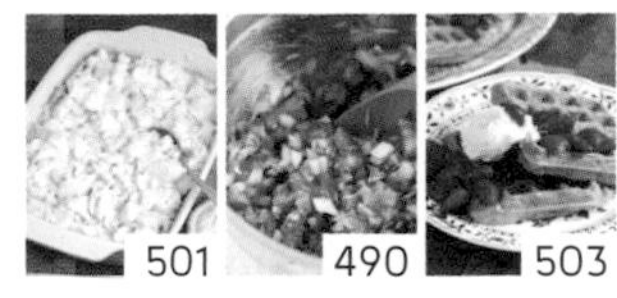 501 490 503 Oven Scrambled Eggs with Pico de Gallo and Waffles with berries	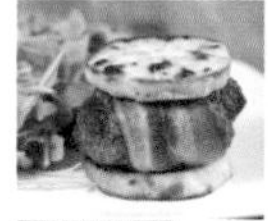 531 519 Bacon-Wrapped Curry Burgers with Sweet Potato "Buns" and DIY Salad	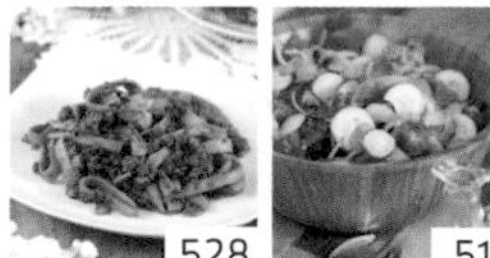 528 519 "Spaghetti" Bolognese over Butternut Squash "Linguine" and DIY Salad *Freeze half of the Bolognese for later in the week.*
MONDAY	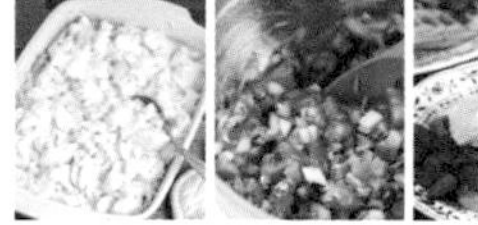 LEFTOVER LEFTOVER LEFTOVER Leftover Oven Scrambled Eggs with Pico de Gallo and Waffles with berries	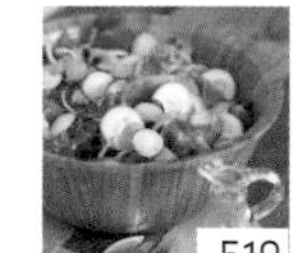 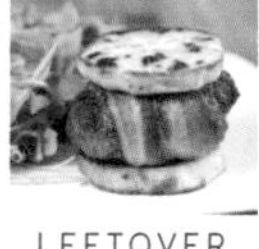 519 LEFTOVER DIY Salad and leftover Bacon-Wrapped Curry Burgers with Sweet Potato "Buns"	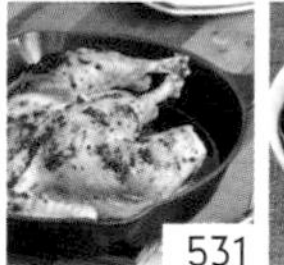 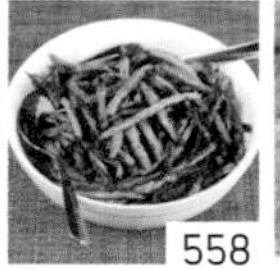 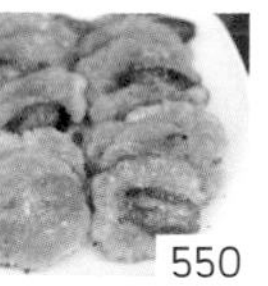 531 558 550 Spatchcocked Chicken, Roasted Green Beans, and Tostones
TUESDAY	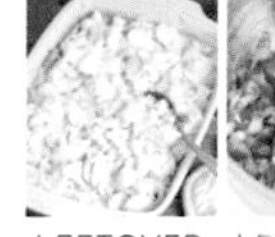 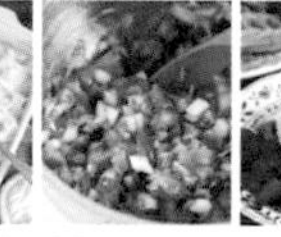 LEFTOVER LEFTOVER LEFTOVER Leftover Oven Scrambled Eggs with Pico de Gallo and Waffles with sliced banana	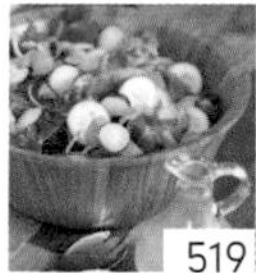 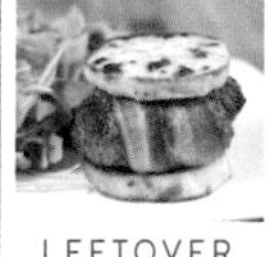 519 LEFTOVER DIY Salad and leftover Bacon-Wrapped Curry Burgers with Sweet Potato "Buns"	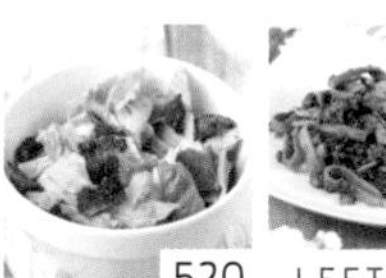 520 LEFTOVER Paleo Caesar Salad and leftover "Spaghetti" Bolognese over Butternut Squash "Linguine"
WEDNESDAY	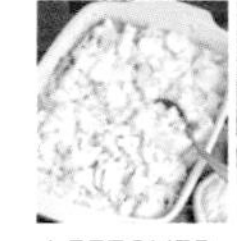 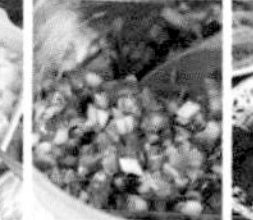 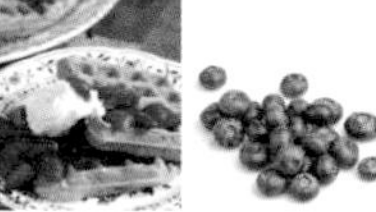 LEFTOVER LEFTOVER LEFTOVER Leftover Oven Scrambled Eggs with Pico de Gallo and Waffles with berries	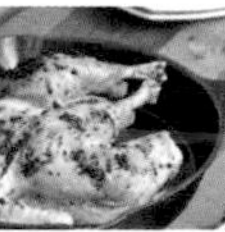 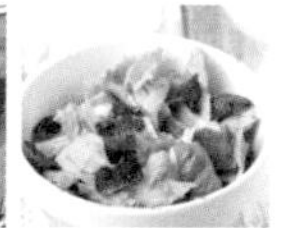 LEFTOVER LEFTOVER Leftover Spatchcocked Chicken and Paleo Caesar Salad *Wrap in coconut wraps or Tortillas, if desired.*	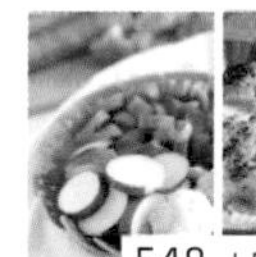 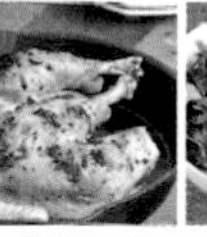 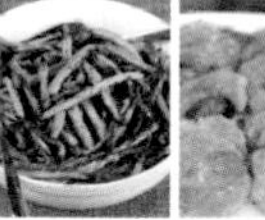 548 LEFTOVER LEFTOVER LEFTOVER DIY Steamed Veggies and leftover Spatchcocked Chicken, Roasted Green Beans, and Tostones
THURSDAY	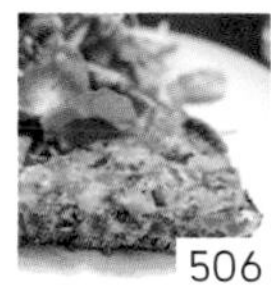 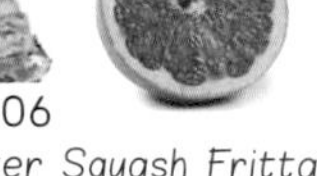 506 Pork & Winter Squash Frittata and half a grapefruit	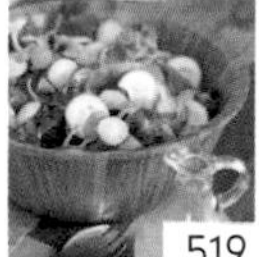 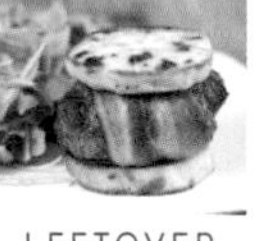 519 LEFTOVER DIY Salad and leftover Bacon-Wrapped Curry Burgers with Sweet Potato "Buns"	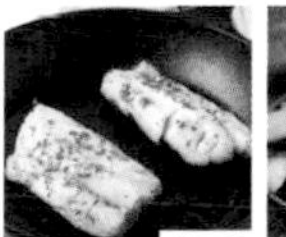 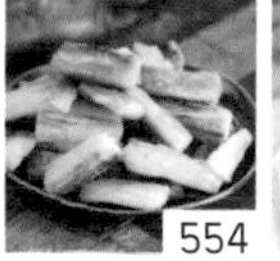 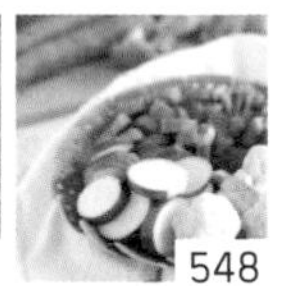 528 554 548 Tarragon-Seared Fish Fillets, Cassava Oven Fries, and DIY Steamed Veggies
FRIDAY	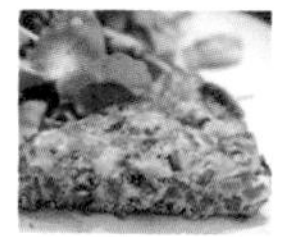 LEFTOVER Leftover Pork & Winter Squash Frittata and half a grapefruit	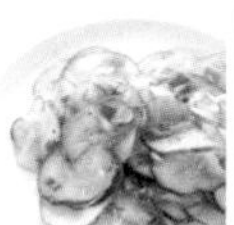 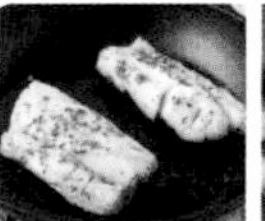 521 LEFTOVER LEFTOVER Simple Cucumber Salad and leftover Tarragon-Seared Fish Fillets and Cassava Oven Fries	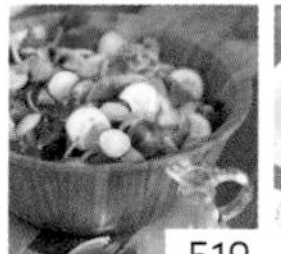 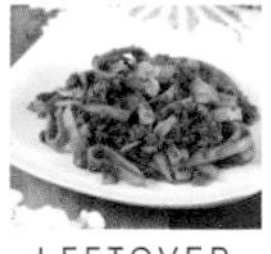 519 LEFTOVER DIY Salad and leftover "Spaghetti" Bolognese over Butternut Squash "Linguine"
SATURDAY	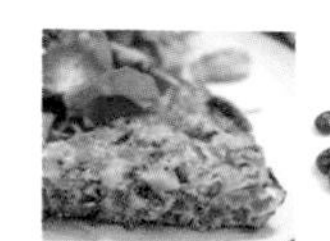 LEFTOVER Leftover Pork & Winter Squash Frittata and berries	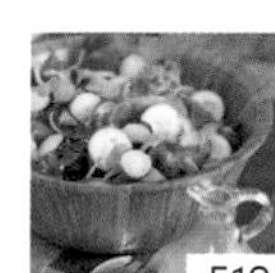 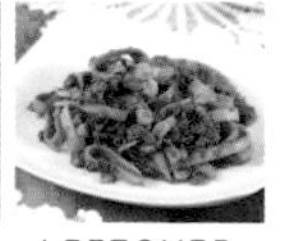 519 LEFTOVER DIY Salad and leftover "Spaghetti" Bolognese over Butternut Squash "Linguine"	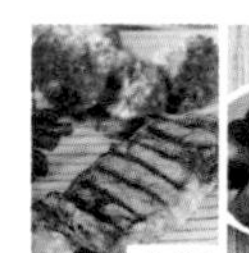 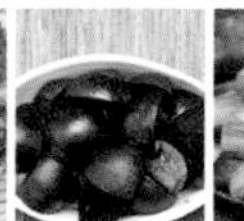 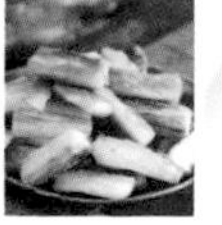 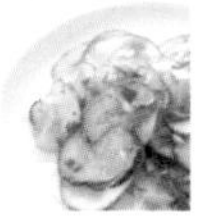 547 561 LEFTOVER LEFTOVER Simple Steak, Balsamic-Roasted Beets, and leftover Cassava Fries and Simple Cucumber Salad *Optional: Make half batch of Simple Steak.*

MENTAL HEALTH MEAL PLAN

This meal plan features foods rich in omega-3 fatty acids, zinc, B vitamins, and essential amino acids. While there are some great food sources of vitamin D included in this plan, it's important to get your levels tested and supplement accordingly. Pair this meal plan with exercise, plenty of sleep, and stress-reducing practices like mindfulness meditation.

SHOPPING LIST

PRODUCE

- arugula - 2½ ounces
- avocados - 2
- basil - 3 tablespoons
- berries of choice - 1 pound
- broccoli crowns - 3
- broccoli slaw - 1 package
- carrots - 5
- cauliflower - 1 head
- celery - 4 stalks
- chives - 1 tablespoon
- cilantro - 1½ cups
- cremini mushrooms - 8 ounces
- English cucumber - 1
- fennel bulbs - 2½
- garlic - 3 heads
- green onions - 5
- lemons - 2
- limes - 8
- mango - 1
- onion - 1
- oregano - 3 tablespoons
- parsley - 1 cup
- parsnips - 2 pounds
- plantain, green - 1
- plantains, green or ripe - 3
- red bell peppers - 1½ cups
- red onion - 1
- spinach - 4 cups
- strawberries - ½ pound
- tarragon - 1 tablespoon
- thyme - 4 sprigs plus 1 tablespoon
- turnip - 1
- white onion - ½
- yellow onions - 2½
- greens of choice for DIY Braised Greens (page 549) - 1 meal
- salad veggies of choice for DIY Salad (page 519) - 1 meal
- veggies of choice for DIY Steamed Veggies (page 548) - 1 meal
- veggies of choice for DIY Omelet (page 508) - 2 meals

MEAT & SEAFOOD

- ahi tuna, sushi-quality - 12 ounces
- bacon - 1 pound
- clams - 3 (5- to 6-ounce) cans
- fish fillets (such as sea bass, mahi mahi, halibut, or swordfish) - 1½ pounds
- ground beef - 2 pounds
- ground pork - 1¾ pounds
- lamb chops - 4 pounds
- liver - 1 pound
- salad shrimp, precooked - 2 pounds

EGGS & DAIRY

- butter - 1 tablespoon
- eggs - 23
- goat cheese - ¼ cup (optional)

VINEGARS & OILS

- apple cider vinegar
- avocado oil
- coconut oil
- coconut water vinegar
- olive oil
- red palm oil
- ingredients for salad dressing of choice (pages 484 to 485)

DRIED HERBS & SPICES

- bay leaf
- black pepper
- cardamom
- cayenne pepper
- coarse sea salt
- fennel seeds
- ginger powder
- ground allspice
- ground cinnamon
- ground cloves
- ground coriander
- ground cumin
- ground mace
- ground nutmeg
- paprika
- sage
- sea salt
- thyme
- truffle salt
- ingredients for salad dressing of choice (pages 484 to 485)

DELI & PREPARED FOODS

- bone stock - 7 cups (or ingredients to make homemade, page 486)

BULK

- pepitas - ½ cup
- raw pecan halves - 1 cup
- roasted unsalted cashews - ⅓ cup
- sesame seeds - 2½ tablespoons

SWEETENERS & BAKING SUPPLIES

- baking soda - ¾ teaspoon
- blackstrap molasses - 1 tablespoon
- cream of tartar - 1 teaspoon
- honey - ¼ cup
- pumpkin powder - ½ cup (may need to order online)

CANNED & JARRED GOODS

- black olives, sliced - 1 cup
- coconut aminos - 3 tablespoons
- coconut cream - 2 cups (or ingredients to make homemade, page 480)
- coconut milk - ½ cup (or ingredients to make homemade, page 480)
- pomegranate molasses - 1 tablespoon

ASIAN FOODS

- fish sauce - 6 tablespoons

OTHER

- plantain chips - 1 bag

MAKE AHEAD OR PURCHASE QUALITY OPTIONS

salad dressing, bone stock

	BREAKFAST	LUNCH	DINNER
SUNDAY	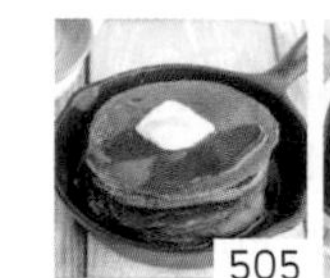 505 502 Pumpkin Pancakes and Breakfast Sausage	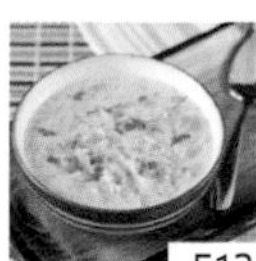 512 Clam Chowder	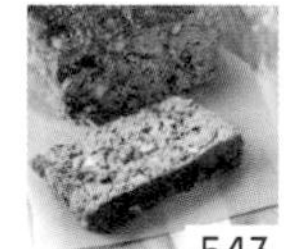 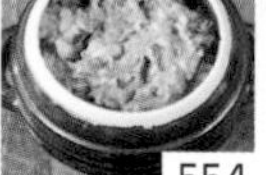 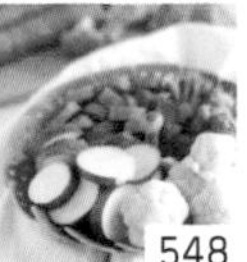 543 554 548 Meatloaf, Mashed Plantains, and DIY Steamed Veggies
MONDAY	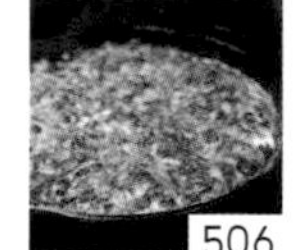 506 Bacon, Spinach & Olive Frittata and berries	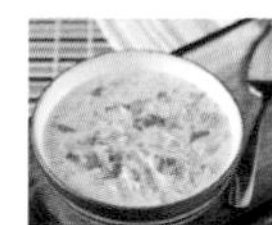 LEFTOVER Leftover Clam Chowder	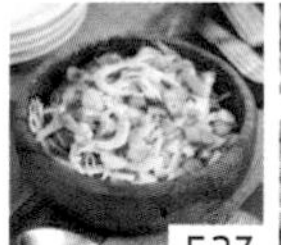 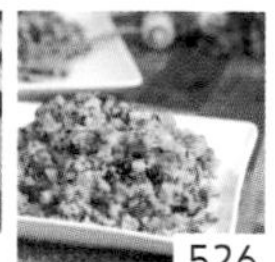 523 526 Simple Fennel Salad and Beef & Mushroom Risotto
TUESDAY	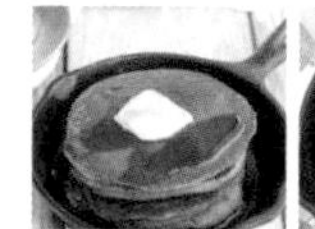 LEFTOVER LEFTOVER Leftover Pumpkin Pancakes and Breakfast Sausage	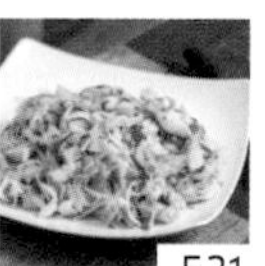 521 Shrimp Salad	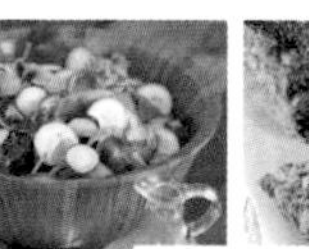 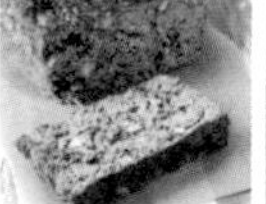 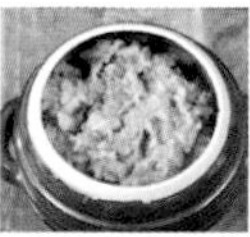 519 LEFTOVER LEFTOVER DIY Salad and leftover Meatloaf and Mashed Plantains
WEDNESDAY	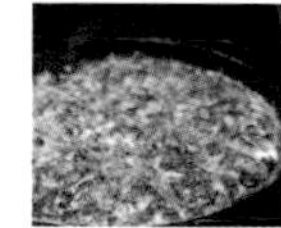 LEFTOVER Leftover Bacon, Spinach & Olive Frittata and berries	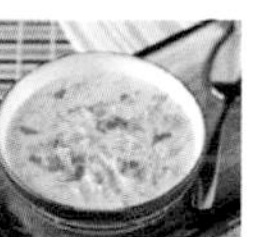 LEFTOVER Leftover Clam Chowder	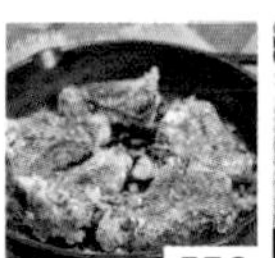 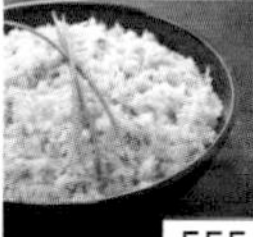 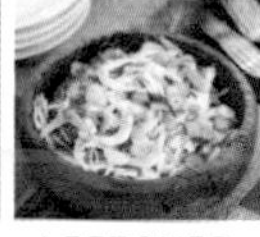 538 555 LEFTOVER Middle Eastern Dukkah-Crusted Lamb Chops, Cumin Cauli-rice, and leftover Simple Fennel Salad
THURSDAY	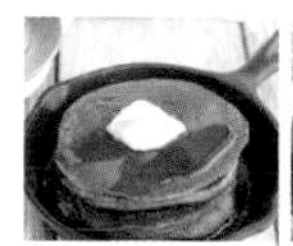 LEFTOVER LEFTOVER Leftover Pumpkin Pancakes and Breakfast Sausage	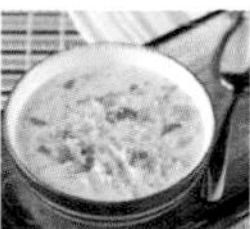 LEFTOVER Leftover Clam Chowder	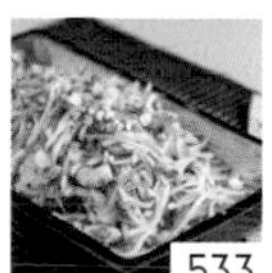 533 Shrimp Pad Thai
FRIDAY	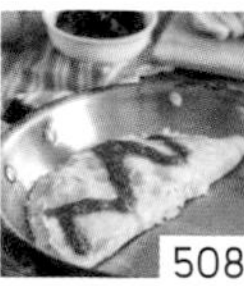 508 DIY Omelet	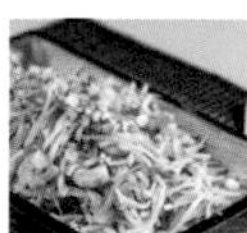 LEFTOVER Leftover Shrimp Pad Thai	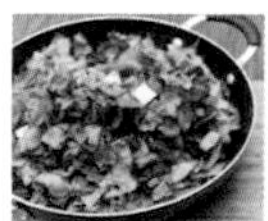 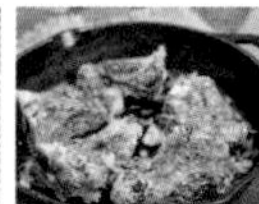 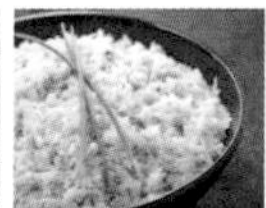 549 LEFTOVER LEFTOVER DIY Braised Greens and leftover Middle Eastern Dukkah-Crusted Lamb Chops and Cumin Cauli-rice
SATURDAY	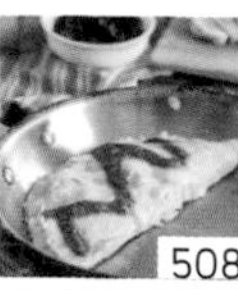 508 DIY Omelet	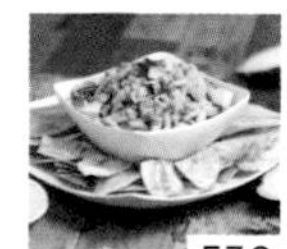 530 Ceviche with plantain chips and sliced English cucumber	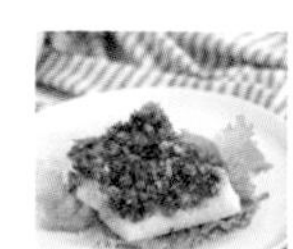 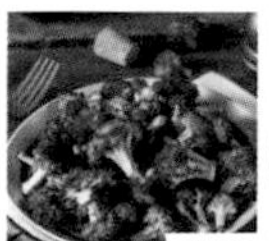 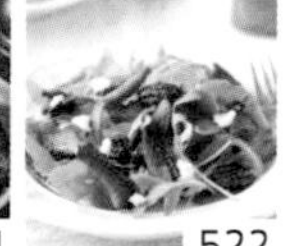 525 561 522 Gremolata-Topped Fish Fillets, Roasted Broccoli, and Strawberry & Arugula Salad with Candied Pecans

DIABETES MANAGEMENT MEAL PLAN

With measured carbohydrates, balanced meals, and plenty of vegetables, seafood, and satiating healthy fats, this meal plan can both help regulate blood sugar levels and provide nutrients that can reduce the risk of developing diabetes. Make sure to check your blood sugar levels and adjust carbohydrate servings and/or medication doses accordingly. Also, pair this plan with plenty of sleep, activity, and stress management!

SHOPPING LIST

PRODUCE

arugula - 4 cups
avocado - 1
bananas - 2
berries of choice - 2 pounds
broccoli crown - 1
Brussels sprouts - 4 pounds
carrot - 1
cauliflower - 1 head
celery - 2 stalks
cilantro - ½ cup
dill - 3 tablespoons
English cucumbers - 2
fennel bulb - 1 pound
garlic - 2 heads
grapefruit - 2
green bell pepper - 1
green onions - 4
jicama - ½ cup
kale - 8 cups
kumquats - 8
lavender - ½ teaspoon (or use rosemary)
lemons - 2
lettuce (romaine, butter, or Bibb) - 2 heads
mint - 3 tablespoons
mushrooms - 1½ cups
oranges - 2
parsley - ¼ cup
parsnips - 1½ pounds
peaches - 2
plantain, green - 1
red bell peppers - 2
red onions - 1 cup
shallots - 3
spinach - 9 cups
sweet potatoes - 3 cups
thyme - 1½ teaspoons
watermelon - 5 cups
white onions - 2
yellow onion - 1
zucchini - 2
salad veggies of choice for DIY Salad (page 519) - 3 meals

MEAT & SEAFOOD

bacon - 6 ounces
beef shoulder roast - 4 pounds
chicken thighs - 10
duck fat - 2 tablespoons
ham - 10 ounces
lox - 12 ounces
salmon fillets - 4 (6 to 8 ounces each)
steaks - 4 (6 to 8 ounces each)

EGGS & DAIRY

eggs - 28

DRIED HERBS & SPICES

black pepper
coarse sea salt
garlic powder
ground cardamom
ground coriander
ground cumin
paprika
sea salt
truffle salt
ingredients for salad dressing of choice (pages 484 to 485)

VINEGARS & OILS

avocado oil
balsamic vinegar
coconut oil
olive oil
white wine vinegar
ingredients for salad dressing of choice (pages 484 to 485)

DELI & PREPARED FOODS

bone stock - 3 quarts (or ingredients to make homemade, page 486)

BULK

almonds, sliced - 2 tablespoons
dried cranberries - ¼ cup
dried figs - 6
raw walnuts - 1 cup

SWEETENERS & BAKING SUPPLIES

gelatin - 1¼ teaspoons
honey - 1⅔ tablespoons

CANNED & JARRED GOODS

black olives, sliced - 1 cup
capers - 3 tablespoons
coconut aminos - 1 tablespoon
coconut milk - 1 (13½-ounce) can (or ingredients to make homemade, page 480)
mayonnaise - ½ cup (or ingredients to make homemade, page 487)

ASIAN FOODS

fish sauce - 1 tablespoon

SUPPLEMENTS

Lactobacillus-based probiotic supplement capsules or nondairy yogurt starter

MAKE AHEAD OR PURCHASE QUALITY OPTIONS

mayonnaise, salad dressing, coconut milk yogurt, bone stock

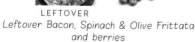

	BREAKFAST	LUNCH	DINNER
SUNDAY	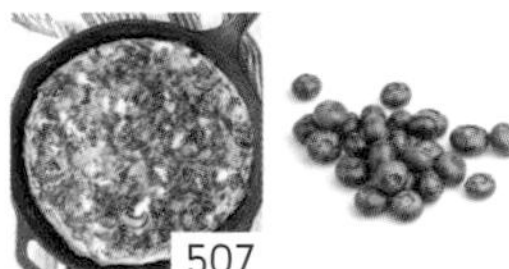 507 *Veggie Frittata and berries*	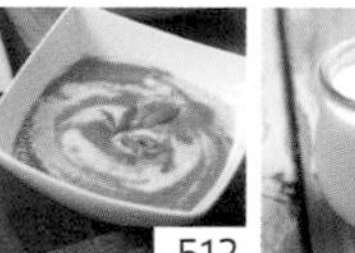 512 481 *Lettuce Soup, Coconut Milk Yogurt, and lox*	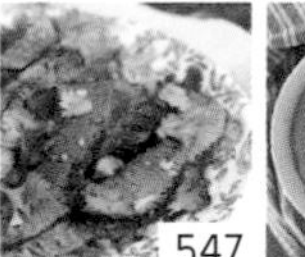 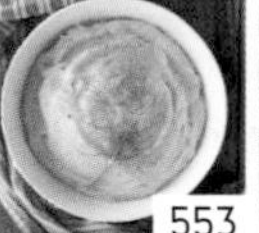 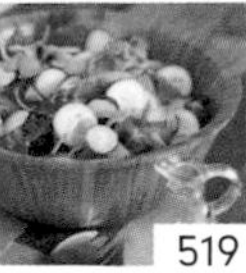 547 553 519 *Balsamic Pressure Cooker Roast Beef, Parsnip & Fennel Puree, and DIY Salad*
MONDAY	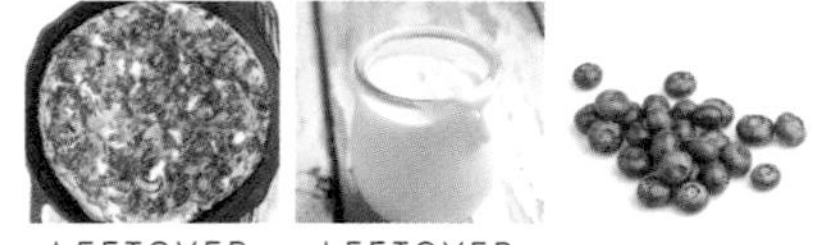 LEFTOVER LEFTOVER *Leftover Veggie Frittata and Coconut Milk Yogurt with berries*	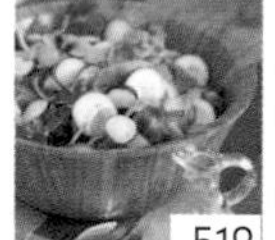 519 LEFTOVER *DIY Salad and leftover Balsamic Pressure Cooker Roast Beef*	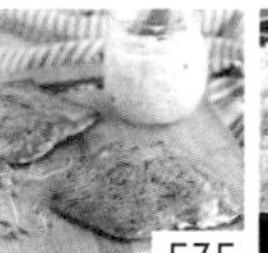 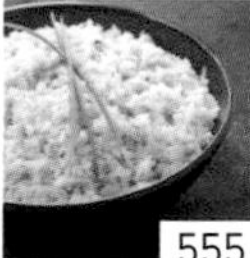 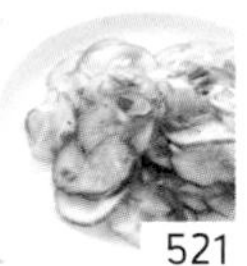 535 555 521 *Broiled Salmon with Dill-Caper Sauce, Lemon Parsley Cauli-rice, and Simple Cucumber Salad*
TUESDAY	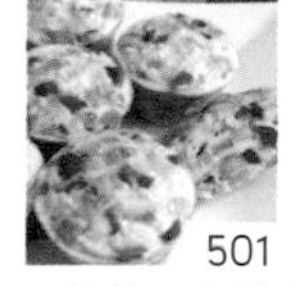 501 *Ham & Sweet Potato Egg Muffins and half a grapefruit*	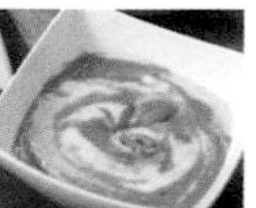 LEFTOVER LEFTOVER *Leftover Lettuce Soup, Coconut Milk Yogurt, and lox*	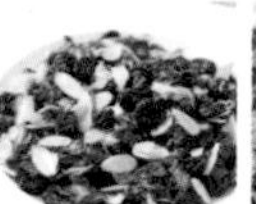 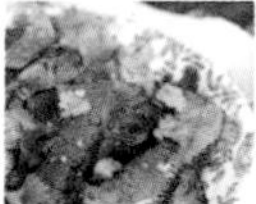 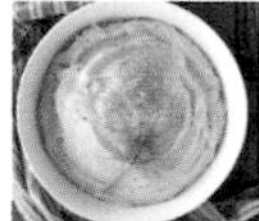 520 LEFTOVER LEFTOVER *Wilted Spinach Salad with Almonds & Cranberries and leftover Balsamic Pressure Cooker Roast Beef and Parsnip & Fennel Puree*
WEDNESDAY	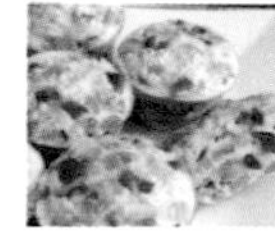 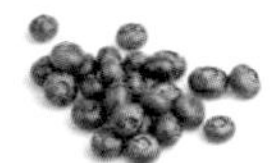 LEFTOVER *Leftover Ham & Sweet Potato Egg Muffins and berries*	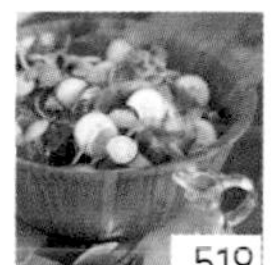 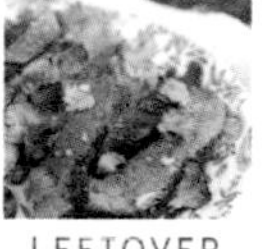 519 LEFTOVER *DIY Salad and leftover Balsamic Pressure Cooker Roast Beef*	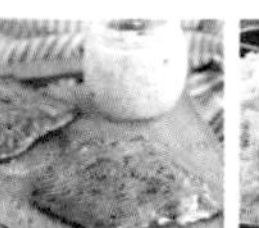 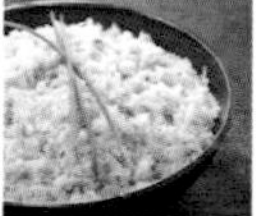 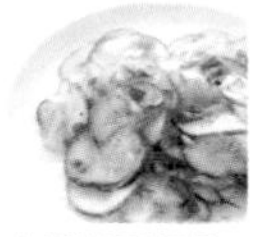 LEFTOVER LEFTOVER LEFTOVER *Leftover Broiled Salmon with Dill-Caper Sauce, Lemon Parsley Cauli-rice, and Simple Cucumber Salad*
THURSDAY	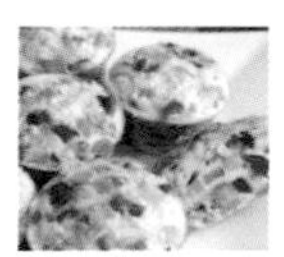 LEFTOVER *Leftover Ham & Sweet Potato Egg Muffins and half a grapefruit*	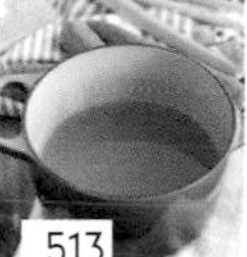 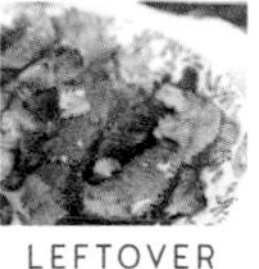 513 LEFTOVER *DIY Soup* Use leftover Balsamic Pressure Cooker Roast Beef with carrots, celery, onions, broccoli, and sweet potatoes. Make enough for 2 lunches.	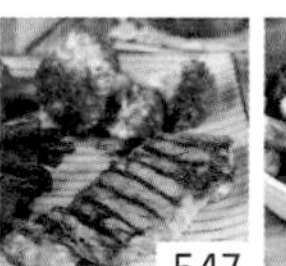 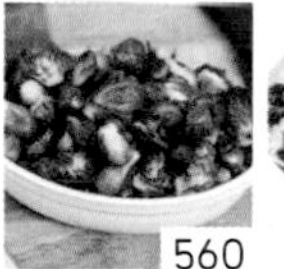 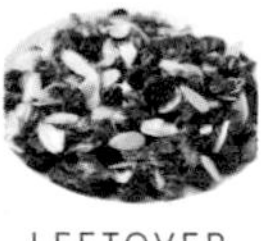 547 560 LEFTOVER *Simple Steak, Roasted Brussels Sprouts, and leftover Wilted Spinach Salad with Almonds & Cranberries*
FRIDAY	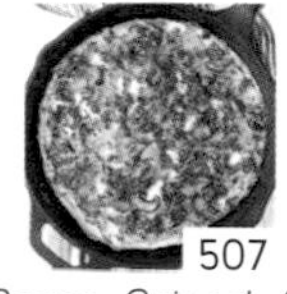 507 *Bacon, Spinach & Olive Frittata and sliced peaches*	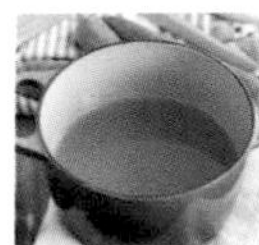 LEFTOVER *Leftover DIY Soup*	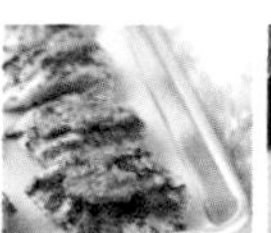 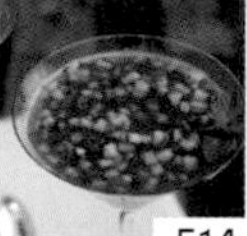 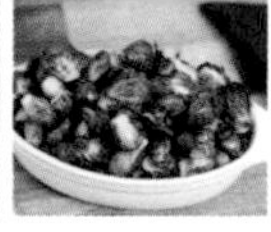 544 514 LEFTOVER *Barbecue Chicken with Arugula Pesto, Watermelon Gazpacho, and leftover Roasted Brussels Sprouts*
SATURDAY	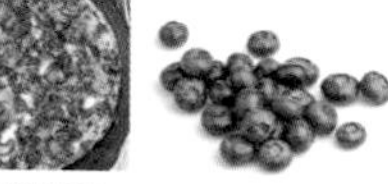 LEFTOVER *Leftover Bacon, Spinach & Olive Frittata and berries*	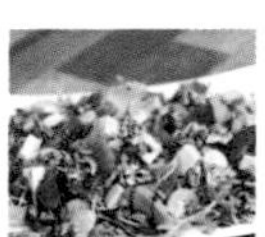 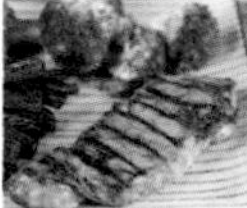 520 LEFTOVER *Citrus, Fig & Walnut Salad and leftover Simple Steak*	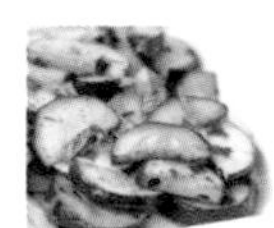 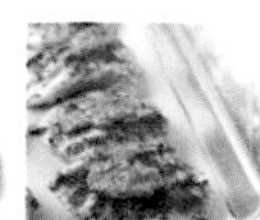 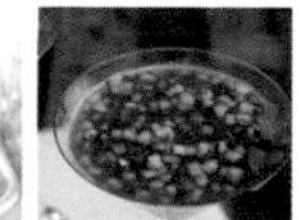 560 LEFTOVER LEFTOVER *Minted Zucchini and leftover Barbecue Chicken with Arugula Pesto and Watermelon Gazpacho*

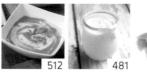

CARDIOVASCULAR DISEASE PREVENTION MEAL PLAN

Featuring plenty of veggies, fruit, and fresh herbs plus lots of seafood, potassium-rich foods, and monounsaturated fat-rich olives and olive oil, this meal plan is packed with phytochemicals, fiber, vitamins, minerals, and both monounsaturated and omega-3 fats to reduce cardiovascular disease risk. Pair this plan with lots of sleep, activity, and stress management. Also, make sure to get your vitamin D levels checked and supplement accordingly!

SHOPPING LIST

PRODUCE

asparagus - 1 pound
avocados - 2
bananas - 2
berries of choice - 2 pounds
broccoli - 2 large heads
Brussels sprouts - 2 pounds
cauliflower - 2 heads
cilantro - ½ cup
dill - ½ cup
fennel bulb - ½ large
garlic - 2 heads
Granny Smith apple - 1
grapefruit - 2
kabocha squash (or other winter squash) - 3 cups
lemons - 3
lime basil - 2 cups (or use regular basil)
limes - 2
mango - 1
mint - ⅓ cup
orange - 1
parsley - 1 large bunch
plantains, green - 2
red bell peppers - 1½ cups
red onions - ½ cup
romaine lettuce - 1 head
sage - 1 tablespoon
spinach - 4 cups
tarragon - 3 tablespoons
thyme - 2 sprigs
yellow onion - ½
zucchini - 4
root vegetables of choice for DIY Roasted Roots (page 550) - 2 pounds
veggies of choice for DIY Salad (page 519) - 2 meals
veggies of choice for DIY Steamed Veggies (page 548) - 2 meals

MEAT & SEAFOOD

bacon - 1 pound
chicken breast - 3 pounds
fish steaks or fillets (such as mahi mahi, amberjack, grouper, or halibut) - 2 (6 to 8 ounces each)
ground pork - 1 pound
lamb chops - 4 pounds
pancetta - 4 ounces
salad shrimp, precooked - 1½ pounds
salmon fillets - 4 (6 to 8 ounces each)
steaks - 4 (6 to 8 ounces each)

EGGS & DAIRY

butter - 1 cup
eggs - 34

DRIED HERBS & SPICES

black pepper
ground cinnamon
ground coriander
ground cumin
ground mace
ground nutmeg
sea salt
truffle salt
turmeric powder
ingredients for salad dressing of choice (pages 484 to 485)
ingredients for seasoning of choice for DIY Baked Chicken Breast (pages 482 to 483)
ingredients for steak seasoning of choice (page 482)

VINEGARS & OILS

apple cider vinegar
avocado oil
coconut oil
olive oil
red palm oil
ingredients for salad dressing of choice (pages 484 to 485)

DELI & PREPARED FOODS

bone stock - 2 cups (or ingredients to make homemade, page 486)
Medjool dates - ⅓ cup

BULK

almonds, sliced - 3 tablespoons
crystallized ginger - 2 tablespoons
pepitas - ½ cup
pine nuts - ¼ cup
raisins - ½ cup
raw cashews - ¾ cup
raw hazelnuts - 1 cup
sesame seeds - 2½ tablespoons

SWEETENERS & BAKING SUPPLIES

baking soda - ½ teaspoon
honey - 1 tablespoon
vanilla extract - 2 teaspoons

CANNED & JARRED GOODS

anchovy paste - 1 teaspoon
black olives, sliced - 2 cans
mayonnaise - ½ cup (or ingredients to make homemade, page 487)
pomegranate molasses - 1 tablespoon

ASIAN FOODS

fish sauce - 2 tablespoons

OTHER

coconut wraps (optional)

MAKE AHEAD OR PURCHASE QUALITY OPTIONS

salad dressing, mayonnaise, pesto, bone stock

	BREAKFAST	LUNCH	DINNER
SUNDAY	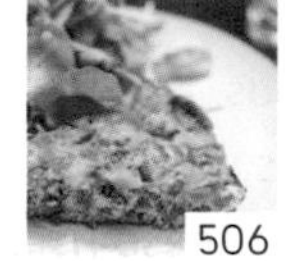 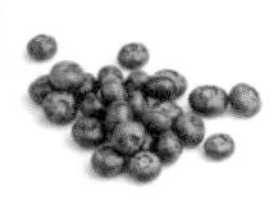 506 Pork & Winter Squash Frittata and berries	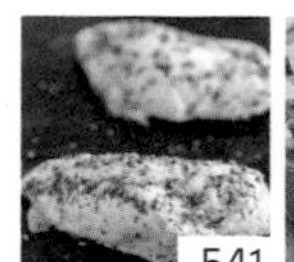 541 519 DIY Baked Chicken Breast and DIY Salad Make enough chicken for 4 lunches.	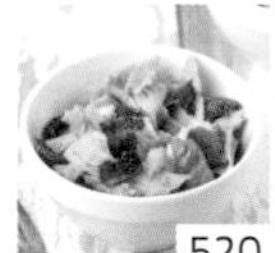 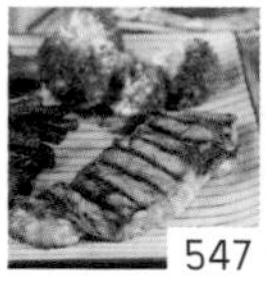 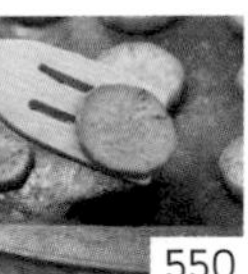 520 547 550 Paleo Caesar Salad, Simple Steak, and DIY Roasted Roots
MONDAY	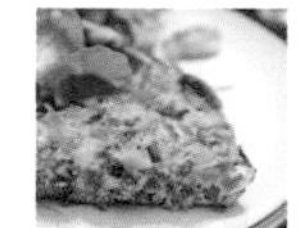 LEFTOVER Leftover Pork & Winter Squash Frittata and berries	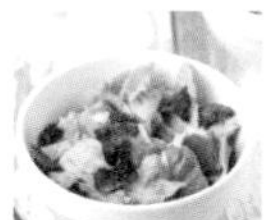 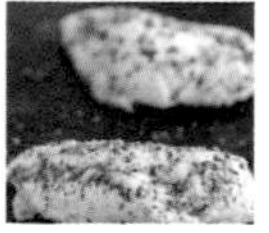 LEFTOVER LEFTOVER Leftover Paleo Caesar Salad with DIY Baked Chicken Breast Wrap in coconut wraps, if desired.	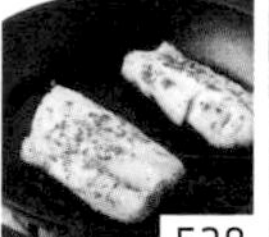 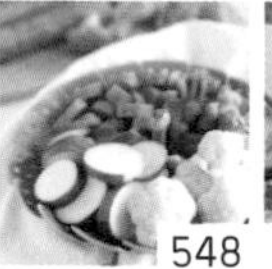 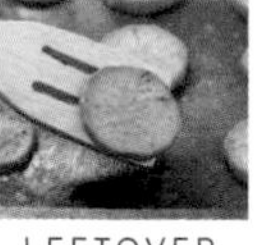 528 548 LEFTOVER Tarragon-Seared Fish Fillets, DIY Steamed Veggies, and leftover DIY Roasted Roots
TUESDAY	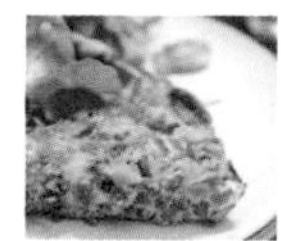 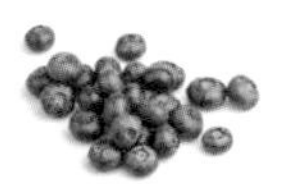 LEFTOVER Leftover Pork & Winter Squash Frittata and berries	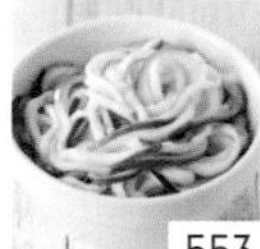 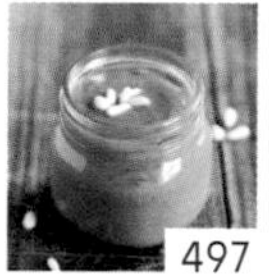 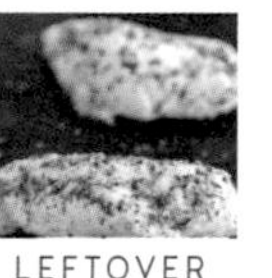 553 497 LEFTOVER Zoodles and Lemon Basil Pesto with sliced black olives and leftover DIY Baked Chicken Breast	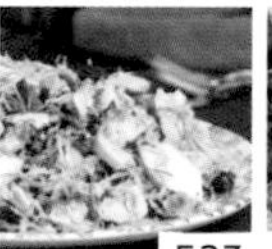 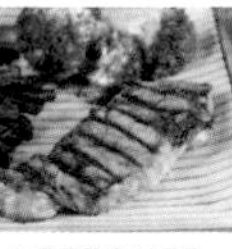 523 LEFTOVER Shaved Brussels Slaw with Hazelnuts, Apple & Mint and leftover Simple Steak
WEDNESDAY	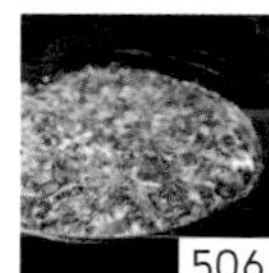 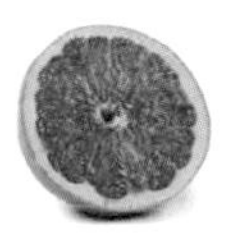 506 Bacon, Spinach & Olive Frittata and half a grapefruit	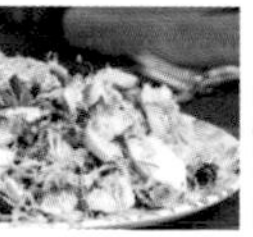 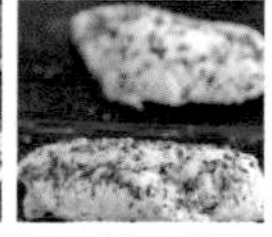 LEFTOVER LEFTOVER Leftover Shaved Brussels Slaw with Hazelnuts, Apple & Mint and DIY Baked Chicken Breast	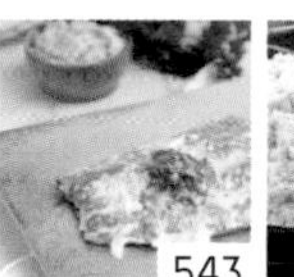 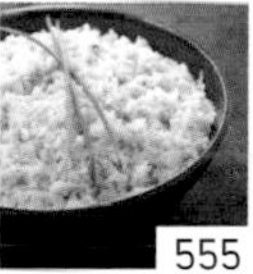 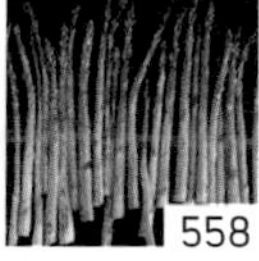 543 555 558 Salmon en Papillote with Maître d' Butter, Lemon Parsley Cauli-rice, and Broiled Asparagus
THURSDAY	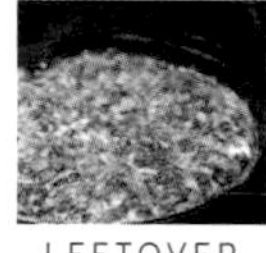 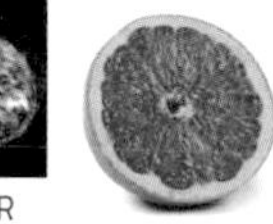 LEFTOVER Leftover Bacon, Spinach & Olive Frittata and half a grapefruit	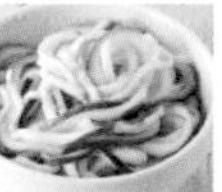 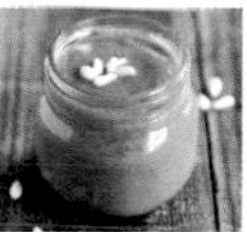 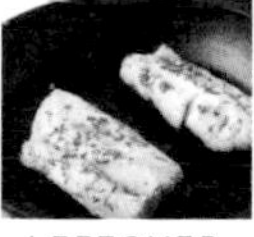 LEFTOVER LEFTOVER LEFTOVER Leftover Zoodles, Lemon Basil Pesto, and Tarragon-Seared Fish Fillets	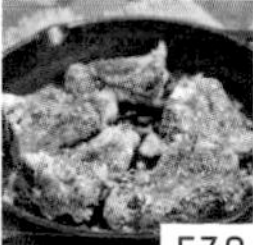 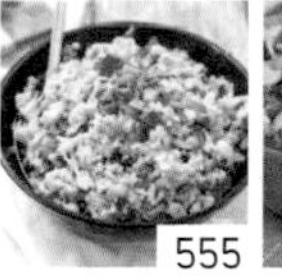 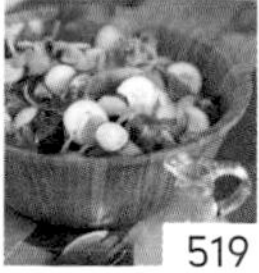 538 555 519 Middle Eastern Dukkah-Crusted Lamb Chops, Moroccan "Couscous," and DIY Salad
FRIDAY	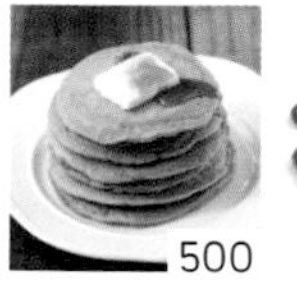 500 DIY Pancakes with berries and 2 eggs, any style	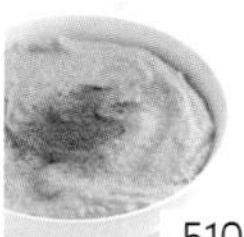 510 "Cream" of Broccoli Soup with salad shrimp and sliced almonds	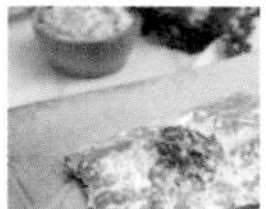 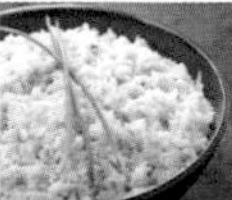 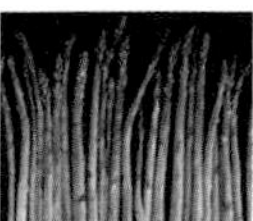 LEFTOVER LEFTOVER LEFTOVER Leftover Salmon en Papillote with Maître d' Butter, Lemon-Parsley Cauli-rice, and Broiled Asparagus
SATURDAY 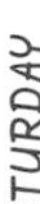	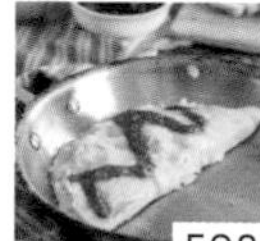 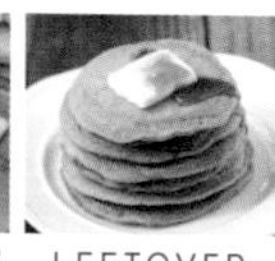 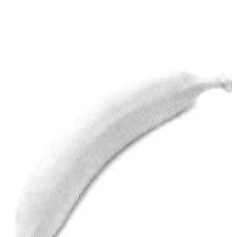 508 LEFTOVER DIY Omelet and leftover pancakes with sliced banana	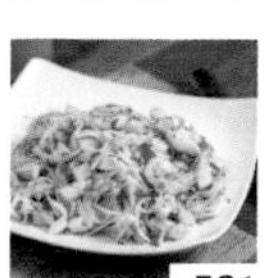 521 Shrimp Salad	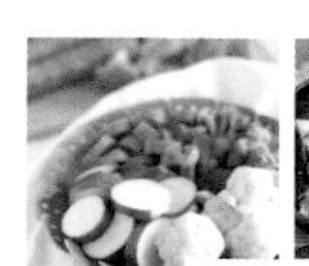 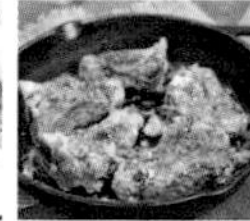 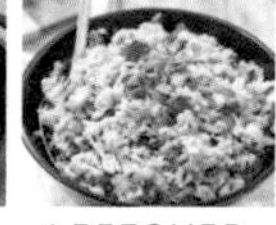 548 LEFTOVER LEFTOVER DIY Steamed Veggies and leftover Middle Eastern Dukkah-Crusted Lamb Chops and Moroccan "Couscous"

CANCER PREVENTION MEAL PLAN

Featuring plenty of veggies, fruit, and fresh herbs plus lots of seafood, this meal plan is packed with phytochemicals, fiber, vitamins, minerals, and omega-3 fats to reduce cancer risk. Pair this plan with lots of sleep, activity, and stress management. Also, make sure to get your vitamin D levels checked and supplement accordingly!

SHOPPING LIST

PRODUCE

- arugula - 2 cups
- asparagus - 1 pound
- avocados - 2
- baby kale - 2 cups
- berries - 2 pounds
- broccoli slaw - 1 package
- cabbage - 3 pounds (or use store-bought sauerkraut)
- carrots - 1 pound plus 2 medium
- cauliflower - 1 head
- celery root - 2
- chives - 1 tablespoon
- cilantro - 1½ cups
- daikon - 2 cups
- English cucumbers - 2½
- fennel bulb - ½
- garlic - 2 heads
- ginger root - 4 inches
- grapefruit - 1
- green bell pepper - 1 large
- green onions - 14
- kale - 2 cups
- kumquats - 4
- lemons - 2
- limes - 5
- lime basil - 2 cups (or use regular basil)
- mango - 1
- mushrooms - 1½ cups
- oranges - 2
- parsley - ¼ cup
- pear - 1
- red bell pepper - 1 large
- red onions - ¾ cup
- spaghetti squash - 4 pounds
- spinach - 2 cups
- sweet potatoes - 2 cups
- white onions - ½ cup
- yellow onion - 1
- salad veggies of choice for DIY Salad (page 519) - 3 meals
- veggies of choice for DIY Steamed Veggies (page 548) - 1 meal

MEAT & SEAFOOD

- chicken breasts - 3½ pounds
- duck fat - ¼ cup
- fish fillets (such as sea bass, mahi mahi, halibut, or swordfish) - 1½ pounds
- ground pork - 3 pounds
- ham - 10 ounces
- pork chops - 2 pounds
- salad shrimp, precooked - 2 pounds
- short ribs - 6 pounds

EGGS & DAIRY

- butter or ghee - 1 tablespoon
- eggs - 20

DRIED HERBS & SPICES

- black pepper
- curry powder (or ingredients to make homemade, page 483)
- ginger powder
- ground mace
- sage
- sea salt
- thyme
- truffle salt
- ingredients for salad dressing of choice (pages 484 to 485)
- ingredients for seasoning of choice for DIY Baked Chicken Breast (pages 482 to 483)

VINEGARS & OILS

- apple cider vinegar
- avocado oil
- balsamic vinegar
- coconut oil
- coconut water vinegar
- olive oil
- sesame oil
- ingredients for salad dressing of choice (pages 484 to 485)

DELI & PREPARED FOODS

- bone stock - 2 cups (or ingredients to make homemade, page 486)

BULK

- dried figs - 3
- pine nuts - ¼ cup
- raw walnut halves - ½ cup
- roasted unsalted cashews - ⅓ cup

SWEETENERS & BAKING SUPPLIES

- baking soda - ½ teaspoon
- honey - 3 tablespoons

CANNED & JARRED GOODS

- coconut aminos - 2 tablespoons
- coconut cream concentrate - 2 tablespoons

ASIAN FOODS

- fish sauce - 7 tablespoons
- dried seaweed - 2 ounces

OTHER

- plantain chips - ¼ cup

MAKE AHEAD OR PURCHASE QUALITY OPTIONS

salad dressing, bone stock, sauerkraut

	BREAKFAST	LUNCH	DINNER
SUNDAY	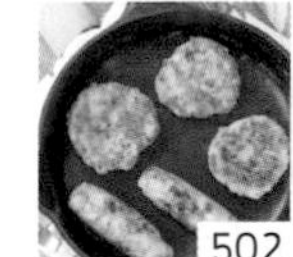 502 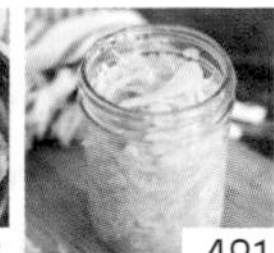 491 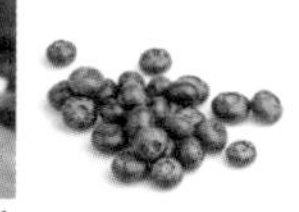 Breakfast Sausage, Sauerkraut, and berries Freeze sausage patties for later in the week.	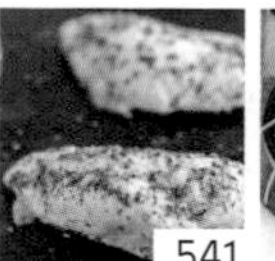 541 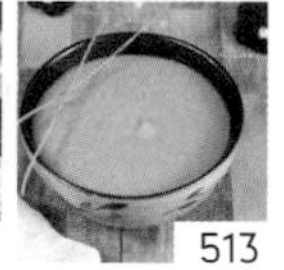 513 DIY Baked Chicken Breast and Curry Carrot Soup Make enough chicken for 1 dinner and 3 lunches.	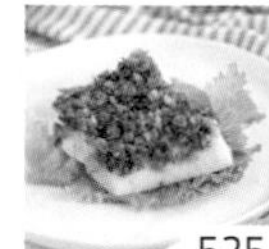 525 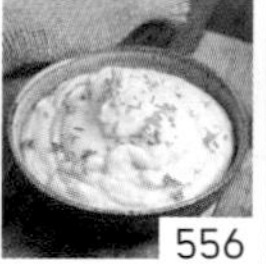 556 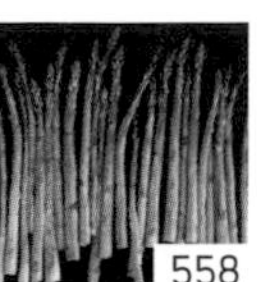 558 Gremolata-Topped Fish Fillets, Celery Root Puree, and Broiled Asparagus
MONDAY	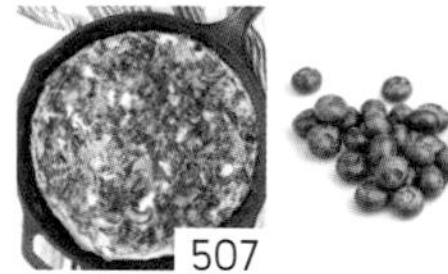 507 Veggie Frittata and berries	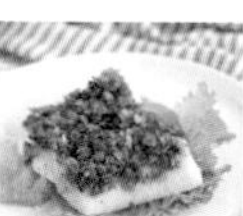 LEFTOVER 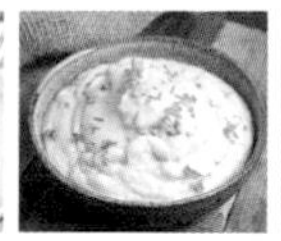 LEFTOVER 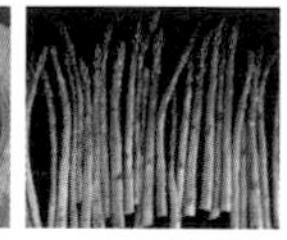 LEFTOVER Leftover Gremolata-Topped Fish Fillets, Celery Root Puree, and Broiled Asparagus	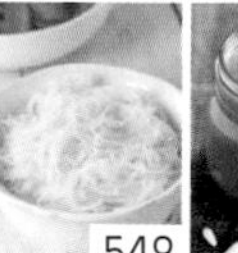 549 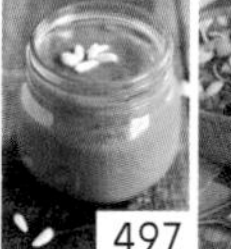 497 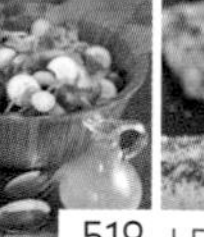 519 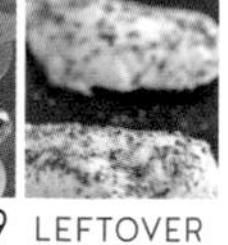 LEFTOVER Spaghetti Squash Noodles, Lemon Basil Pesto, DIY Salad, and leftover DIY Baked Chicken Breast
TUESDAY	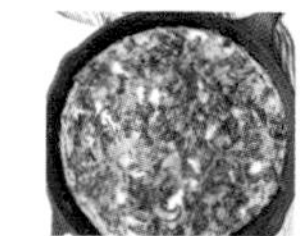 LEFTOVER 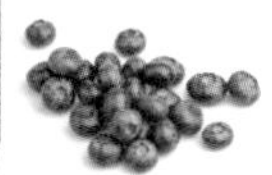 Leftover Veggie Frittata and berries	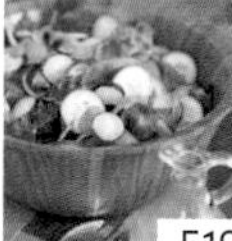 519 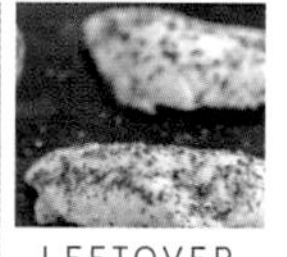 LEFTOVER DIY Salad with leftover DIY Baked Chicken Breast	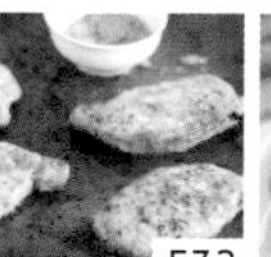 532 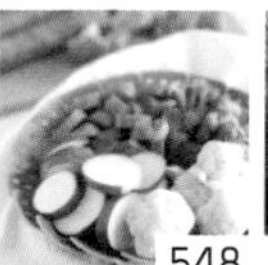 548 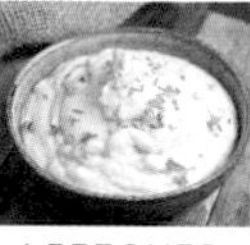 LEFTOVER Broiled Pork Chops, DIY Steamed Veggies, and leftover Celery Root Puree
WEDNESDAY	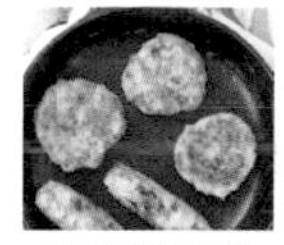 LEFTOVER 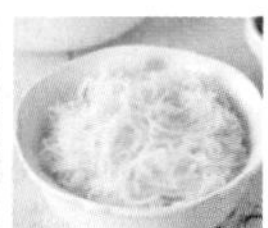 LEFTOVER 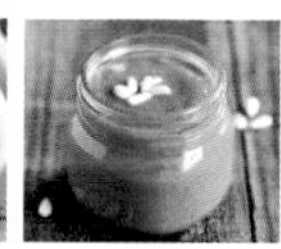 LEFTOVER Leftover Breakfast Sausage, Spaghetti Squash Noodles, and Lemon Basil Pesto	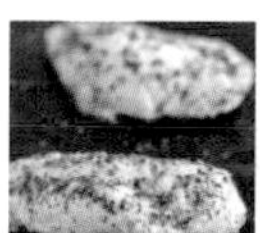 LEFTOVER LEFTOVER Leftover DIY Baked Chicken Breast and Curry Carrot Soup	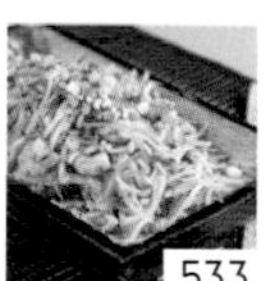 533 Shrimp Pad Thai
THURSDAY	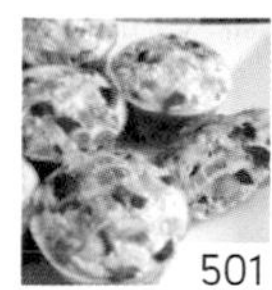 501 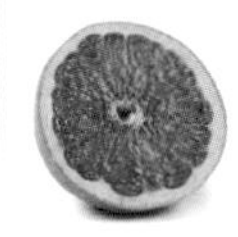 Ham & Sweet Potato Egg Muffins and half a grapefruit	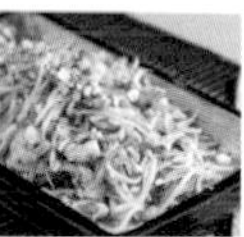 LEFTOVER Leftover Shrimp Pad Thai	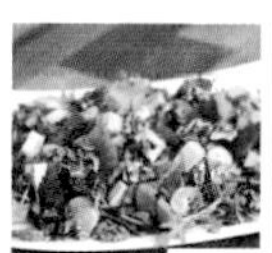 520 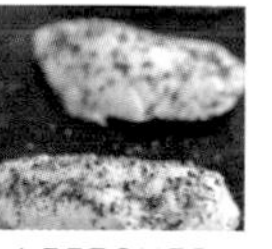 LEFTOVER Citrus, Fig & Walnut Salad and leftover DIY Baked Chicken Breast
FRIDAY	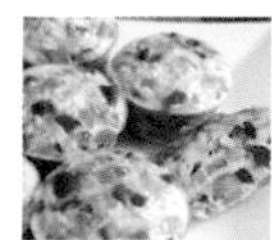 LEFTOVER 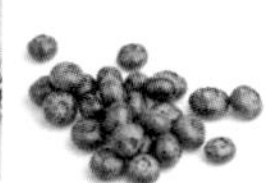 Leftover Ham & Sweet Potato Egg Muffins and berries	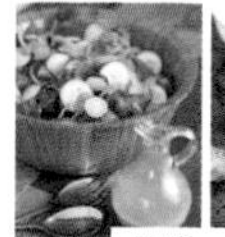 519 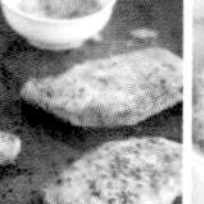 LEFTOVER 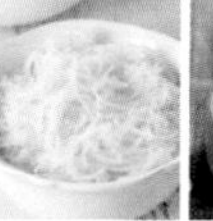 LEFTOVER 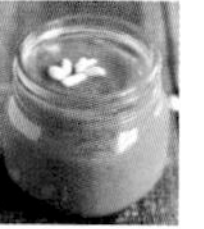 LEFTOVER DIY Salad and leftover Broiled Pork Chops, Spaghetti Squash Noodles, and Lemon Basil Pesto	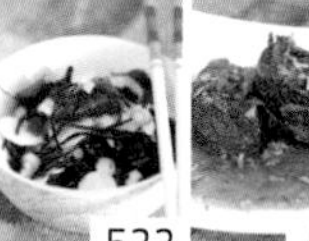 522 541 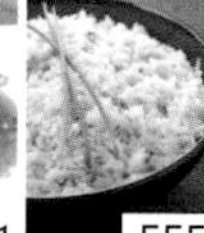 555 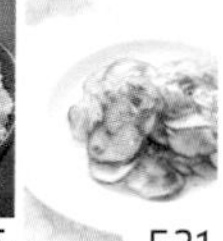 521 Seaweed Salad, Korean Short Ribs, Asian Cauli-rice, and Simple Cucumber Salad
SATURDAY	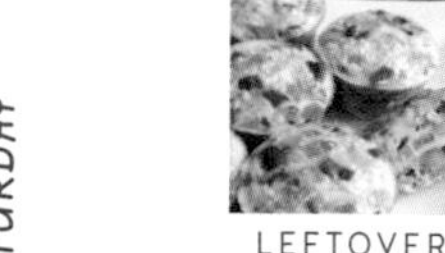 LEFTOVER 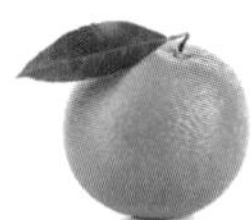 Leftover Ham & Sweet Potato Egg Muffins and an orange	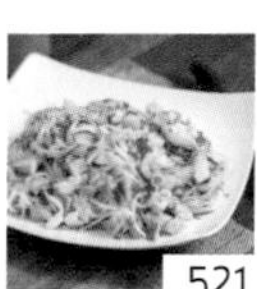 521 Shrimp Salad	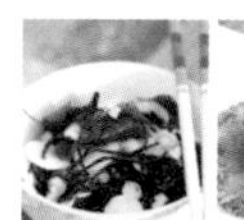 LEFTOVER 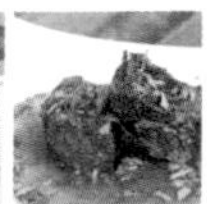 LEFTOVER 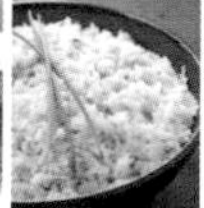 LEFTOVER 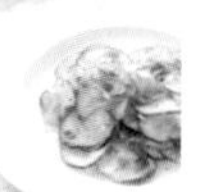 LEFTOVER Leftover Seaweed Salad, Korean Short Ribs, Asian Cauli-rice, and Simple Cucumber Salad

GUT HEALTH MEAL PLAN

Featuring plenty of soups and stews for their bone broth, easily digested protein, and veggies, as well as coconut oil, seafood, and fermented foods, this meal plan is both easy on a sensitive digestive tract and full of important nutrients and fiber to support gut barrier health and a healthy gut microbiota. Pair this plan with plenty of sleep, light activity, and stress management.

SHOPPING LIST

PRODUCE

- arugula - 2 cups
- Asian pear - 1
- asparagus - 2 bunches
- basil - ¼ cup
- berries of choice - 1½ pounds
- cabbage - 3 pounds (or use store-bought raw sauerkraut)
- carrots - 1 pound
- cauliflower - 1½ heads
- celery - 14 stalks
- chives - ¼ cup
- fennel bulb - 1 pound
- garlic - 2 heads
- ginger root - 1 inch
- lemon - 1
- lettuce (romaine, butter, or Bibb) - 2 heads
- onions - 2
- oregano - 3 tablespoons
- parsley - 1½ cups
- parsnips - 2¼ pounds
- pie pumpkins - 2 (3 to 4 pounds each) (or use winter squash)
- plantains, green - 3
- rosemary - 1 sprig
- shallots - 3
- spinach - 4 cups
- thyme - 4 sprigs plus 3 tablespoons
- turnip - 1
- yellow onions - 6
- yuca - 1 pound
- greens of choice for DIY Braised Greens (page 549) - 1 meal
- veggies of choice for DIY Salad (page 519) - 1 meal

MEAT & SEAFOOD

- bacon - 1¼ pounds
- beef stew meat - 3 pounds
- clams - 3 (5- to 6-ounce) cans
- crabmeat or salad shrimp (for Lettuce Soup) - 1 pound
- duck fat - 2 tablespoons
- ground beef - 1 pound
- ground pork - 4 pounds
- liver - 1 pound
- lox - 12 ounces
- tilapia fillets - 4 (6 to 7 ounces each)

EGGS & DAIRY

- eggs - 3

DRIED HERBS & SPICES

- bay leaf
- black pepper
- cayenne pepper
- coarse sea salt
- fennel seeds
- ground cardamom
- ground coriander
- ground nutmeg
- oregano
- paprika
- rosemary
- sea salt
- tarragon

VINEGARS & OILS

- apple cider vinegar
- avocado oil
- coconut oil
- coconut water vinegar
- lard
- olive oil
- sesame oil

DELI & PREPARED FOODS

- bone stock - 6½ to 7 quarts (or ingredients to make 3 batches of homemade, page 486)

BULK

- sesame seeds - 1 tablespoon

SWEETENERS & BAKING SUPPLIES

- arrowroot powder - ½ cup
- baking soda - ¼ teaspoon
- blackstrap molasses - 1 tablespoon
- coconut flour - 2 tablespoons
- cream of tartar - ½ teaspoon
- gelatin - 2½ teaspoons
- honey - 4 teaspoons

CANNED & JARRED GOODS

- coconut aminos - 2 tablespoons
- coconut cream - 2 cups
- coconut milk - 2 (13½-ounce) cans (or ingredients to make homemade, page 480)
- tomato paste - ½ can

ASIAN FOODS

- fish sauce - 1 tablespoon

SUPPLEMENTS

- *Lactobacillus*-based probiotic supplement capsules or nondairy yogurt starter

DRINKS

- dry red wine - 2 cups
- kombucha (or ingredients to make homemade, page 492)

MAKE AHEAD OR PURCHASE QUALITY OPTIONS

kombucha (to drink with 1 meal per day), sauerkraut, coconut milk yogurt, lard, bone stock

	BREAKFAST	LUNCH	DINNER
SUNDAY	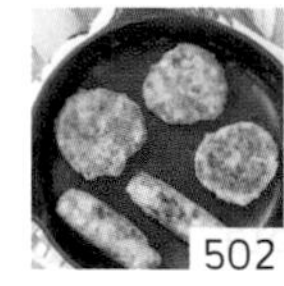 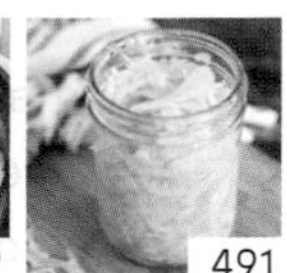 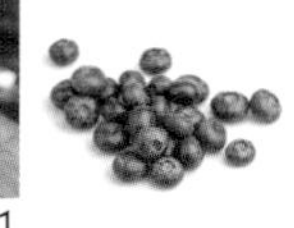 502 491 Sweet Italian Sausage, Sauerkraut, and berries *Make a third of the sausage mix into small meatballs for soup. Freeze leftover patties and meatballs for later in the week.*	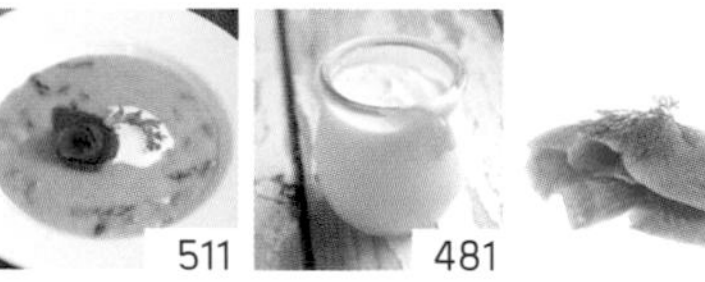 511 481 Asparagus Soup, Coconut Milk Yogurt, and lox *Make double batch of yogurt.*	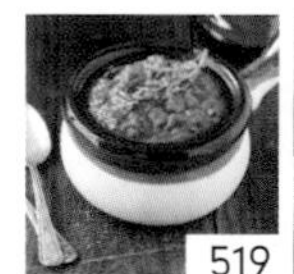 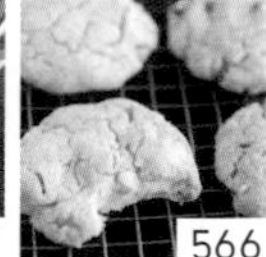 519 566 Hearty Beef Stew and Yuca Biscuits *Freeze half of the biscuits for later in the week.*
MONDAY	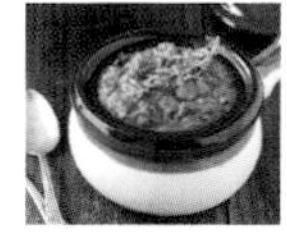 LEFTOVER Leftover Hearty Beef Stew	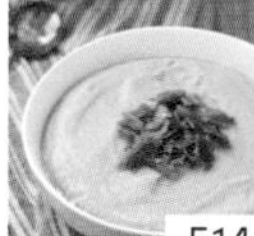 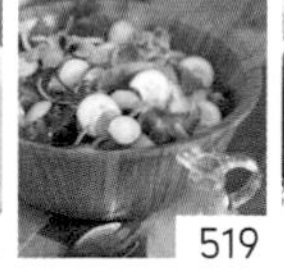 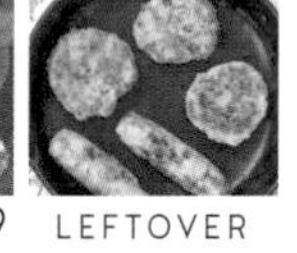 514 519 LEFTOVER Rustic Bacon & Pumpkin Soup, DIY Salad, and leftover Sweet Italian Sausage	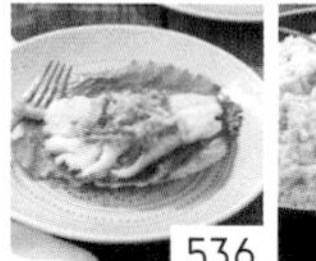 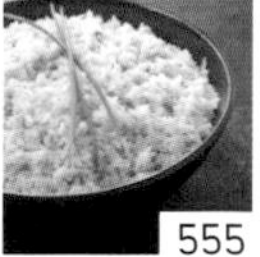 536 555 Coconut Oil-Poached Tilapia with Asian Pear Slaw and Asian Cauli-rice
TUESDAY	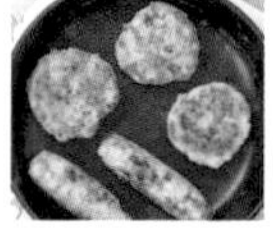 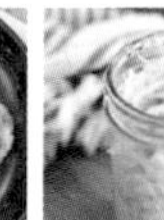 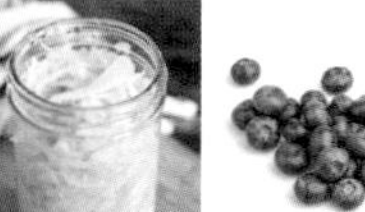 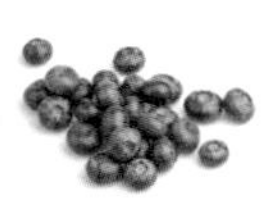 LEFTOVER LEFTOVER Leftover Sweet Italian Sausage, Sauerkraut, and berries (serve berries with Coconut Milk Yogurt, if desired)	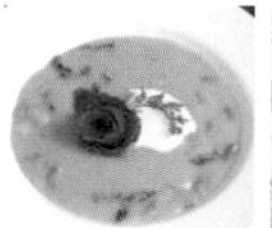 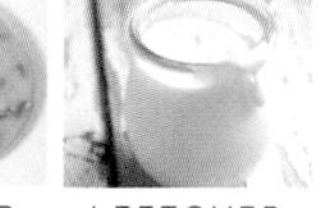 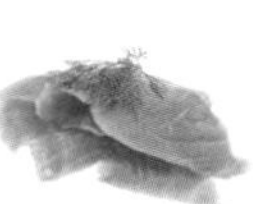 LEFTOVER LEFTOVER Leftover Asparagus Soup, Coconut Milk Yogurt, and lox	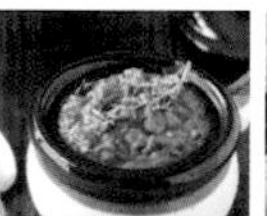 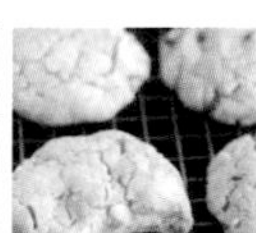 LEFTOVER LEFTOVER Leftover Hearty Beef Stew and Yuca Biscuits
WEDNESDAY	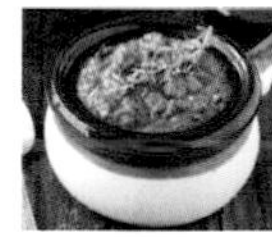 LEFTOVER Leftover Hearty Beef Stew	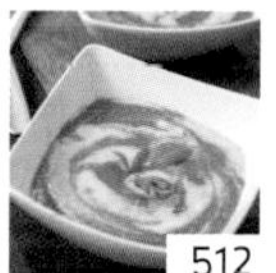 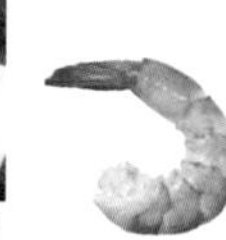 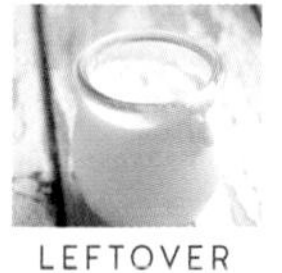 512 LEFTOVER Lettuce Soup with crabmeat or salad shrimp and leftover Coconut Milk Yogurt	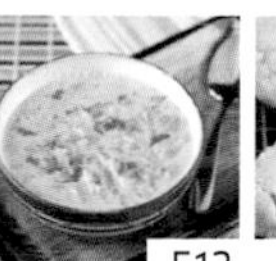 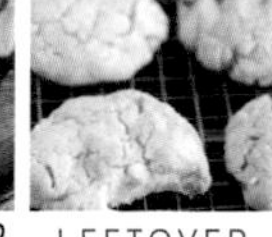 512 LEFTOVER Clam Chowder and leftover Yuca Biscuits
THURSDAY	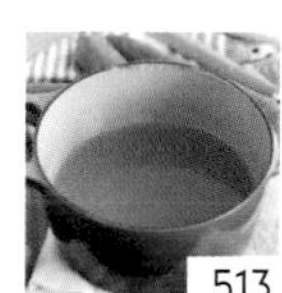 513 DIY Soup *Use sausage meatballs, carrots, celery, onions, spinach, and fresh parsley.*	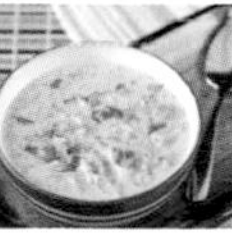 LEFTOVER Leftover Clam Chowder	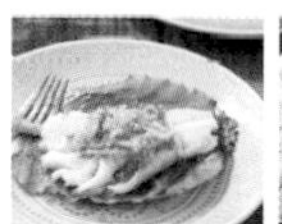 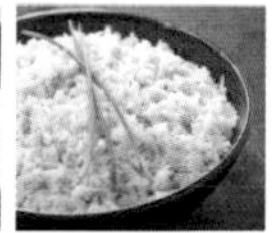 LEFTOVER LEFTOVER Leftover Coconut Oil-Poached Tilapia with Asian Pear Slaw and Asian Cauli-rice
FRIDAY	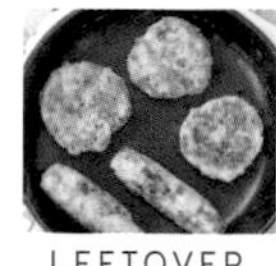 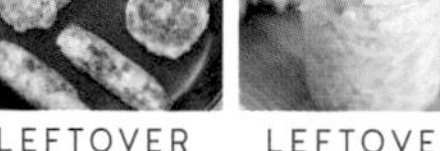 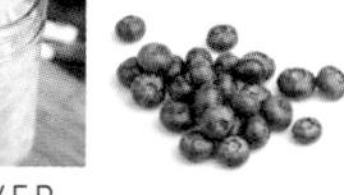 LEFTOVER LEFTOVER Leftover Sweet Italian Sausage, Sauerkraut, and berries (serve berries with Coconut Milk Yogurt, if desired)	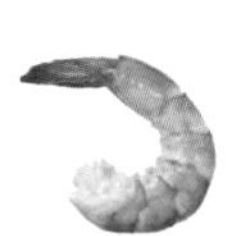 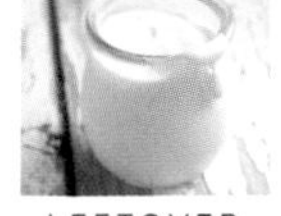 LEFTOVER LEFTOVER Leftover Lettuce Soup with crabmeat or salad shrimp and Coconut Milk Yogurt	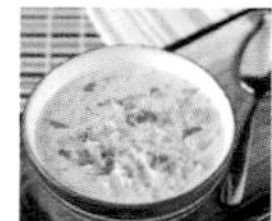 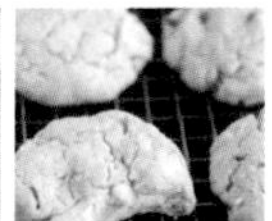 LEFTOVER LEFTOVER Leftover Clam Chowder and Yuca Biscuits
SATURDAY	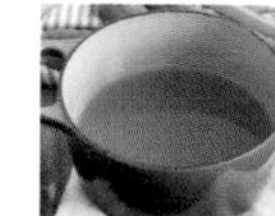 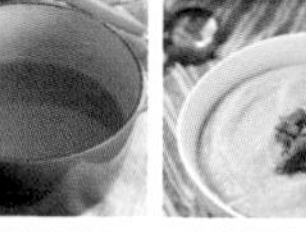 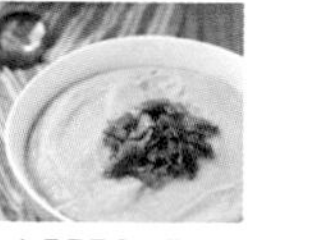 LEFTOVER LEFTOVER Leftover DIY Soup or Rustic Bacon & Pumpkin Soup	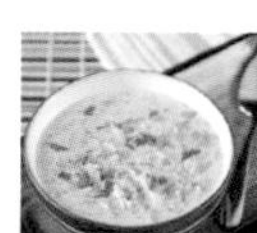 LEFTOVER Leftover Clam Chowder	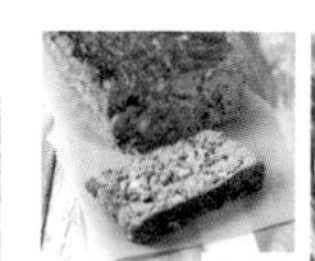 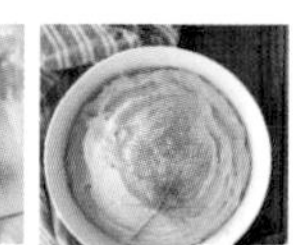 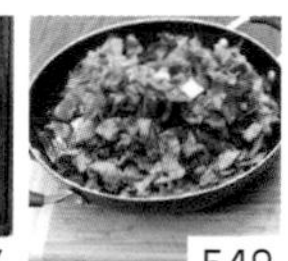 543 553 549 Meatloaf, Parsnip & Fennel Puree, and DIY Braised Greens

APPENDIXES

ONLINE SHOPPING GUIDE

The following are my recommendations for vendors and companies selling and producing quality products catering to the Paleo community.

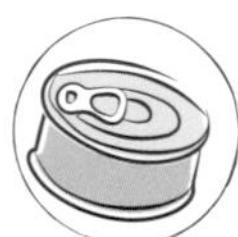

PANTRY STAPLES

Amazon
www.amazon.com

Barefoot Provisions
www.barefootprovisions.com

One Stop Paleo Shop
www.onestoppaleoshop.com

Thrive Market
www.thrivemarket.com

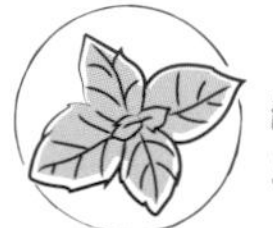

HERBS & SPICES

Changing Habits
www.changinghabits.com.au/product-category/healthy-whole-foods

Paleo Powder
www.paleopowderseasoning.com

Primal Palate
www.primalpalate.com/organic-spices

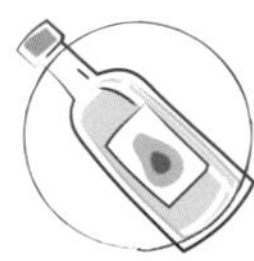

QUALITY FATS

Epic animal oils
www.epicbar.com/animal-oils-overview

Fatworks Foods
www.fatworksfoods.com

Kasandrinos International olive oil
www.kasandrinos.com

Primal Kitchen avocado oil
www.primalblueprint.com/primal-kitchen

Pure Indian Foods
www.pureindianfoods.com

Tropical Traditions
www.healthytraditions.com/tropicaltraditions

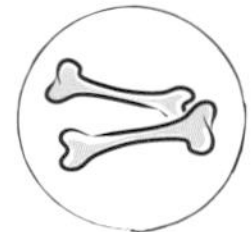

BONE BROTH

Epic
www.epicbar.com/bone-broth-overview

Kettle & Fire
www.kettleandfire.com

HERBAL TEA

Klio Tea
www.kliotea.com

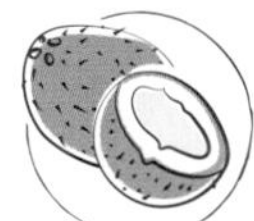

COCONUT & PALM PRODUCTS

Tropical Traditions
www.healthytraditions.com/tropicaltraditions

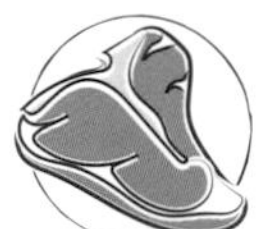

GRASS-FED & PASTURE-RAISED MEATS

ButcherBox
www.butcherbox.com

GrassFed Traditions
www.healthytraditions.com/grassfedtraditions

Pasturebird
www.pasturebird.com

US Wellness Meats
www.grasslandbeef.com

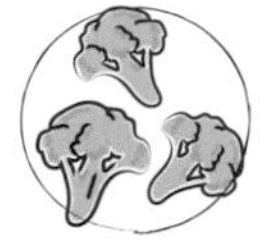

ORGANIC VEGETABLES

Farmbox Direct
www.farmboxdirect.com

PREMADE PALEO MEALS

Paleo on the Go
www.paleoonthego.com

Pete's Paleo
www.petespaleo.com

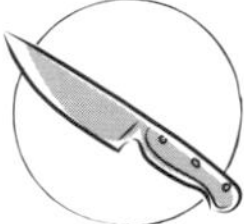

KITCHEN TOOLS

Misen knives
www.misen.co

Instant Pot
www.instantpot.com

High-speed blender
www.vitamix.com

Ice cream maker
www.cuisinart.com/products/ice_cream

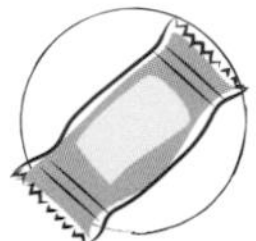

PORTABLE PROTEIN-RICH SNACKS

Epic bars, bites, and sticks
www.epicbar.com

Exo Bars
www.exoprotein.com

Mountain Strips
www.wildmountainpaleo.com

Paleo Angel Power Balls
www.paleoangel.com

Rx Bars
www.rxbar.com

Wild Zora
www.wildzora.com

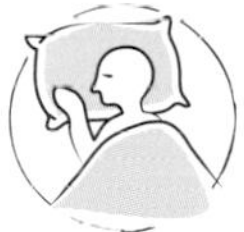

BIOHACKS & TRACKERS

Oura Ring
www.ouraring.com

Swannies blue-blocking glasses
www.swanwicksleep.com

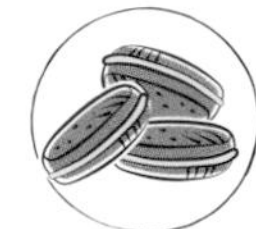

PALEO TREATS

Cappello's cookie dough
www.cappellos.com

Paleo Angel Power Balls
www.paleoangel.com

Paleo Treats
www.paleotreats.com

Rickaroons
www.rickaroons.com

Sweet Apricity caramels
www.sweetapricity.com

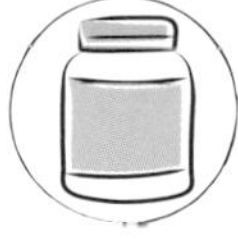

FOOD-BASED SUPPLEMENTS

Dr. Ron's Ultrapure
www.drrons.com

Vital Proteins
www.vitalproteins.com

Vital Proteins Collagen Veggie Blend
www.thepaleomom.com/go/ppveggieblend

See pages 473 to 477 for a complete list of recommended cooking tools and gadgets.

USEFUL COOKING GUIDES

Need to know what temperature to set the oven to when you're cooking a leg of lamb? Need help converting imperial units to metric? Want to look up the smoke point of a fat to figure out what temperature to set your deep-fryer to? I've got you covered.

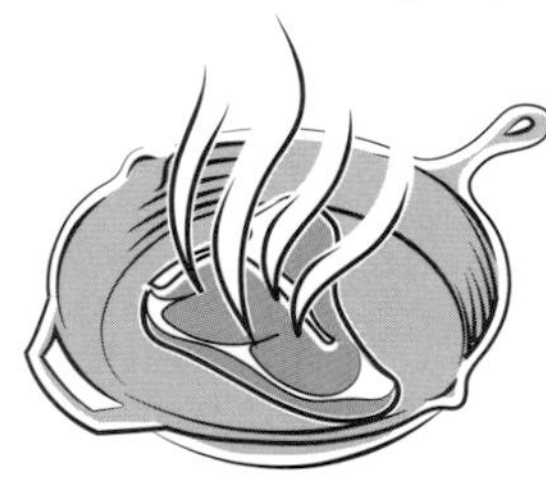

Meat Cooking Times and Temperatures

The single most important tool when it comes to cooking meat is an oven-safe meat thermometer. Grass-fed and pasture-raised meats often cook much faster than conventionally produced meats, and many factors can influence just how much faster. For example, the pasture-raised turkey I bought for Thanksgiving dinner 2 years ago cooked in 3¼ hours. Last year, it cooked in 2¾ hours. Both years, the turkey weighed 15 pounds and, stuffed, should have taken at least 4 hours to cook. If I hadn't had a meat thermometer in place, my family would have been eating very dry, overcooked turkey!

The following list is based on USDA recommendations and should be considered a general guide and starting place for cooking fresh or fully thawed (not frozen) meat. It is often recommended to reduce the oven temperature by 25°F when cooking grass-fed and pasture-raised meats.

Grilling is direct heat unless otherwise noted.

BEEF CUT	SIZE/WEIGHT	COOKING METHOD	COOKING TIME	INTERNAL TEMPERATURE AND REST TIME
Chuck roast, brisket	3–4 pounds	Braise at 325°F	2–3 hours	145°F for medium-rare; 160°F for medium. Let rest for at least 3 minutes.
Hamburger patties	4 ounces	Grill, broil, or fry, turning halfway through	6–10 minutes	160°F
Rib roast, bone-in	4–6 pounds	Roast at 325°F	23–25 minutes per pound	145°F for medium-rare; 160°F for medium. Let rest for at least 3 minutes.
Rib roast, boneless, rolled	4–6 pounds	Roast at 325°F	Add 5–8 minutes per pound to above	
Round or rump roast	2½–4 pounds	Roast at 325°F	30–35 minutes per pound	
Steaks	¾ inch thick	Broil or grill, turning halfway through	8–10 minutes	
Stew or shank cross-cuts	1–1½ inches thick	Cover with liquid and simmer	2–3 hours	
Short ribs	4 inches long and 2 inches thick	Braise at 325°F	1½–2½ hours	
Tenderloin, whole	4–6 pounds	Roast at 425°F	45–60 minutes	

LAMB CUT	SIZE/WEIGHT	COOKING METHOD	COOKING TIME	INTERNAL TEMPERATURE AND REST TIME
Breast, rolled	1½–2 pounds	Braise at 325°F	1½–2 hours	145°F for medium-rare; 160°F for medium. Let rest for at least 3 minutes
Chops, rib, or loin	1–1½ inches thick	Broil or grill	7–11 minutes	
Kabobs	1–1½ inches	Broil or grill	8–12 minutes	
Ground lamb patties	2 inches thick	Broil or grill, turning halfway through	5–8 minutes	160°F
Leg, bone-in	5–7 pounds	Roast at 325°F	20–25 minutes per pound	145°F for medium-rare; 160°F for medium. Let rest for at least 3 minutes.
	7–9 pounds	Roast at 325°F	15–20 minutes per pound	
Leg, boneless, rolled	4–7 pounds	Roast at 325°F	25–30 minutes per pound	
Leg steaks	¾ inch thick	Broil or grill	14–18 minutes	
Shoulder roast or shank leg half	3–4 pounds	Roast at 325°F	30–35 minutes per pound	
Stew meat	1–1½-inch pieces	Cover with liquid and simmer	1½–2 hours	
Shanks	¾–1 pound	Cover with liquid and simmer	1½–2 hours	

TURKEY TYPE	SIZE/WEIGHT	COOKING METHOD	COOKING TIME	INTERNAL TEMPERATURE AND REST TIME
Turkey breast	4–6 pounds	Roast at 325°F	1½–2¼ hours	165°F
	6–8 pounds		2¼–3¼ hours	
Whole turkey, unstuffed	8–12 pounds		2¾–3 hours	
	12–14 pounds		3–3¾ hours	
	14–18 pounds		3¾–4¼ hours	
	18–20 pounds		4¼–4½ hours	
	20–24 pounds		4½–5 hours	
Whole turkey, stuffed	8–12 pounds		3–3½ hours	
	12–14 pounds		3½–4 hours	
	14–18 pounds		4–4¼ hours	
	18–20 pounds		4¼–4¾ hours	
	20–24 pounds		4¾–5¼ hours	

PORK CUT	SIZE/WEIGHT	COOKING METHOD	COOKING TIME	INTERNAL TEMPERATURE AND REST TIME
Boston butt	3–6 pounds	Roast at 350°F in a shallow pan, uncovered	45 minutes per pound	145°F for medium; 160°F for well-done. Let rest for at least 3 minutes.
Crown roast	10 pounds	Roast at 350°F in a shallow pan, uncovered	12 minutes per pound	
Ground pork patties	1/2 inch thick	Fry in a skillet, turning halfway through	8–10 minutes	160°F
		Broil or grill, turning halfway through	8–10 minutes	
Leg, (fresh ham) half, bone-in	5–8 pounds	Roast at 350°F in a shallow pan, uncovered	22–25 minutes per pound	
Leg, (fresh ham) whole, bone-in	18–20 pounds	Roast at 350°F in a shallow pan, uncovered	15 minutes per pound	145°F for medium; 160°F for well-done. Let rest for at least 3 minutes.
Loin chops or cutlets	1/4 inch thick	Fry in a skillet, turning halfway through	3–4 minutes	
	3/4 inch thick	Fry in a skillet, turning halfway through	7–8 minutes	
Loin chops, bone-in or boneless	1/4–3/4 inch thick	Braise	6–8 minutes	
	1 1/2 inches thick	Broil or grill, turning halfway through	12–16 minutes	
Loin cubes or tenderloin medallions	1/2–1 inch thick	Braise	8–10 minutes	
Loin kabobs	1-inch cubes	Broil or grill, turning halfway through	10–15 minutes	
Loin or shoulder cubes	1-inch cubes	Stew	45–60 minutes	
Loin roast, bone-in or boneless	2–5 pounds	Roast at 350°F in a shallow pan, uncovered	20 minutes per pound	
Ribs (baby-back, country-style, or spareribs)	2–4 pounds	Roast at 350°F in a shallow pan, uncovered	1 1/2–2 hours	
Ribs, all types	2–4 pounds	Broil or grill (indirect heat), turning halfway through	1 1/2–2 hours	
		Braise	1 1/2–2 hours	
Shoulder, boneless	3–6 pounds	Braise	2–2 1/2 hours	
Tenderloin	1/2–1 1/2 pounds	Broil or grill, turning halfway through	20 minutes	
		Roast at 425°F–450°F	20–27 minutes	
Tenderloin medallions	1/4–1/2 inch thick	Fry in a skillet	4–8 minutes	

CHICKEN TYPE	SIZE/WEIGHT	COOKING METHOD	COOKING TIME	INTERNAL TEMPERATURE AND REST TIME
Breast halves, bone-in	6–8 ounces	Roast at 350°F	30–40 minutes	165°F
		Cover with liquid and simmer	35–45 minutes	
		Broil or grill, turning halfway through	20–30 minutes	
Breast halves, boneless	4 ounces	Roast at 350°F	20–30 minutes	
		Cover with liquid and simmer	25–30 minutes	
		Broil or grill, turning halfway through	12–16 minutes	
Drumsticks	4 ounces	Roast at 350°F	35–45 minutes	
		Cover with liquid and simmer	40–50 minutes	
		Broil or grill, turning halfway through	16–24 minutes	
Legs or thighs	4–8 ounces	Roast at 350°F or cover with liquid and simmer	40–50 minutes	
		Broil or grill, turning halfway through	20–30 minutes	
Whole broiler-fryer*	3–4 pounds	Roast at 350°F	1 1/4–1 1/2 hours	
		Broil, grill, or cover with liquid and simmer	60–75 minutes**	
Whole roasting hen*	5–7 pounds	Roast at 350°F	2–2 1/4 hours	
		Cover with liquid and simmer	1 3/4–2 hours	
		Broil or grill	18–25 minutes per pound**	
Whole capon*	4–8 pounds	Roast at 350°F	2–3 hours	
		Broil or grill	15–20 minutes per pound**	
Whole Cornish hens*	18–24 ounces	Roast at 350°F	50–60 minutes	
		Cover with liquid and simmer	35–40 minutes	
		Broil or grill	45–55 minutes**	
Wings or wingettes	2–3 ounces	Roast at 350°F	30–40 minutes	
		Cover with liquid and simmer	35–45 minutes	
		Broil or grill, turning halfway through	16–24 minutes	

* Unstuffed. If stuffed, add 15–30 minutes. **Indirect method using drip pan.

Cooking Fish

In general, fish is cooked when it just begins to flake easily when tested with a fork and loses its translucent or raw appearance. To be thoroughly cooked, fish should reach a minimum internal temperature of 145°F.

One helpful guideline for cooking fish is the 10-minute rule. Apply it when baking, broiling, grilling, steaming, and poaching fillets, steaks, or whole fish. (Do not apply the 10-minute rule to microwave cooking or deep-frying.)

Here's how to use the 10-minute rule:

1. Measure the fish at its thickest point. If it is to be stuffed or rolled, measure it after stuffing or rolling.
2. Cook the fish at 450°F for 10 minutes per inch of thickness, turning the fish halfway through the cooking time. For example, a 1-inch-thick fish steak should be cooked for 5 minutes per side for a total cooking time of 10 minutes. Pieces of fish that are less than ½ inch thick do not have to be turned.
3. Add 5 minutes to the total cooking time if you are cooking the fish in aluminum foil or in a sauce.

Other Guides Scattered Throughout This Book

Measurement Conversions

LIQUID OR VOLUME MEASUREMENTS (APPROXIMATE)

1 teaspoon		1/3 tablespoon	5 ml
1 tablespoon	1/2 fl. oz.	3 teaspoons	15 ml or 15 cc
2 tablespoons	1 fl. oz.	1/8 cup or 6 teaspoons	30 ml or 30 cc
1/4 cup	2 fl. oz.	4 tablespoons	59 ml
1/3 cup	2 2/3 fl. oz.	5 tablespoons plus 1 teaspoon	79 ml
1/2 cup	4 fl. oz.	8 tablespoons	118 ml
2/3 cup	5 1/3 fl. oz.	10 tablespoons plus 2 teaspoons	158 ml
3/4 cup	6 fl. oz.	12 tablespoons	177 ml
7/8 cup	7 fl. oz.	14 tablespoons	207 ml
1 cup	8 fl. oz. or 1/2 pint	16 tablespoons	237 ml
2 cups	16 fl. oz. or 1 pint	32 tablespoons	473 ml
4 cups	32 fl. oz.	1 quart	946 ml
1 pint	16 fl. oz. or 2 cups	32 tablespoons	473 ml
2 pints	32 fl. oz.	1 quart	946 ml or 0.946 liter
8 pints	1 gallon or 128 fl. oz.	4 quarts	3,785 ml or 3.78 liters
4 quarts	1 gallon or 128 fl. oz.	1 gallon	3,785 ml or 3.78 liters
1 liter	1.057 quarts		1,000 ml
1 gallon	4 quarts	128 fl. oz.	3,785 ml or 3.785 liters

DRY OR WEIGHT MEASUREMENTS (APPROXIMATE)

1 ounce		30 g
2 ounces		55 g
3 ounces		85 g
4 ounces	1/4 pound	125 g
8 ounces	1/2 pound	240 g
12 ounces	3/4 pound	375 g
16 ounces	1 pound	454 g
32 ounces	2 pounds	907 g
1/4 pound	4 ounces	125 g
1/2 pound	8 ounces	240 g
3/4 pound	12 ounces	375 g
1 pound	16 ounces	454 g
2 pounds	32 ounces	907 g
1 kg	2.2 pounds or 35.2 ounces	1,000 g

GLOSSARY OF TERMS

AA: Arachidonic acid, an omega-6 fatty acid.

Adaptive immune system: The part of the immune system that is specifically for a particular foreign invader.

Adenosine triphosphate (ATP): A high-energy molecule that stores and supplies every cell with needed energy; the energy currency of all cells.

Adjuvant: A substance that stimulates the adaptive immune system. In vaccines, adjuvants are added to stimulate the immune system because the antigen, typically a dead or inert virus or bacteria, is non-infectious—the adjuvant is needed for immunity to develop because the dead virus can't replicate and stimulate the immune system effectively on its own.

Aerobic: Refers to something that requires oxygen.

Agglutinin: A protein capable of making red blood cells clump together.

All-cause mortality: All the deaths that occur in a population, regardless of the cause. It is measured in clinical trials as an indicator of the overall health and longevity of a population, which can be used to determine the safety or hazard of an intervention.

Allergy: A damaging immune response to a normally harmless substance, such as pollen, dander, dust, or food, to which the body has become hypersensitive. See also IgE antibodies.

Alpha-amylase: See amylase.

Amino acids: The basic building blocks of all proteins.

AMY1 copy number: The number of repeated sections of the genome that contain the AMY1 gene, which encodes salivary α-amylase, a starch-digesting enzyme found in saliva. The more copies of AMY1 we have, the more α-amylase we produce.

Amylase: A digestive enzyme that breaks down starch. One example is α-amylase, which is found in saliva.

Anaerobic: Refers to something that does not require oxygen.

Antibody: A specialized protein, produced by cells of the immune system, that recognizes and binds to small sequences of amino acids in other (typically foreign) proteins.

Antigen: A small fragment of a protein on a pathogen to which antibodies bind.

Anti-inflammatory: Anything that counteracts or helps resolve inflammation.

Antinutrient: A substance that prevents the absorption or utilization of nutrients.

Apoptosis: A controlled form a cell death, akin to cell suicide. Uncontrolled cell death is called necrosis. The difference is that apoptosis does not cause cell fragments or proteins to be released into the body, but necrosis does.

ATP: See adenosine triphosphate.

Autocrine: A fat-based molecule that acts as a signal for communication within a cell (from one part of a cell to another).

Autoimmune disease: A disease caused by the immune system attacking cells, tissues, or organs in the body.

Autoimmunity: Immunity targeted against oneself. Autoimmunity does not become an autoimmune disease until damage accumulates and symptoms appear.

B cells: Lymphocytes produced in the bone marrow that circulate through blood and lymphatic vessels, patrolling the body for antigens. When they find an antigen, they become antibody factories, releasing thousands of antibodies into the blood or connective tissues. B cells are the main cell type of the humoral adaptive immune system.

Basophil: A type of white blood cell that can phagocytose, produce histamine, and produce heparin, which prevents blood clotting.

Bioavailable: The amount of a substance that becomes available for biological activity by being modified, if necessary, to a form that is usable by the body and by reaching its target organ or systemic circulation.

Blood-brain barrier: A filtering mechanism of the capillaries in the brain and spinal cord tissue, blocking the passage of certain substances to protect the brain.

Blue Zones: Areas that boast a high concentration of centenarians that are studied for longevity clues.

Calcitriol: The hormonally active metabolite of vitamin D, also called 1,25-dihydroxycholecalciferol or 1,25-dihydroxyvitamin D3.

Carbohydrate: A molecule composed of a chain of sugar molecules. Carbohydrates are both important fuel for the body and important molecular components of many chemicals (glycoproteins, glycolipids, and membrane carbohydrates) used or produced by the cells of the body.

Carcinogenic: Having the potential to cause cancer.

Cardiovascular: Relating to the heart and blood vessels.

Cardiovascular disease: Any chronic health condition that involves the heart and/or blood vessels.

Catalyst: A substance that speeds up the rate of a chemical reaction. In biology, this usually means a substance (such as a mineral) that speeds up the activity of an enzyme (which facilitates the chemical reaction).

Cellular respiration: A series of chemical reactions in cells in which energy molecules from food (carbohydrates, fats, and protein) are converted to adenosine triphosphate.

Cholesterol: A type of fat (technically a type of lipid called a sterol) that is an essential structural component of cell membranes, steroid hormones, vitamin D, and bile acids. See also low-density lipoprotein and high-density lipoprotein.

Chyme: The thick acidic fluid, consisting of gastric juices and partly digested food, that passes from the stomach to the small intestine.

Circadian rhythm: The cycling of biological functions with the 24-hour clock. It is controlled by specific cells in the brain, but all cells have an internal clock that is synchronized with the brain's clock through the rhythm of hormones that circulate through the body.

Circulation: The system of vessels through which blood flows. When something is "in circulation," it is traveling throughout the body in the blood.

Cofactor: A substance that is necessary for an enzyme to perform its activity (and is not what the enzyme acts on).

Colorectal adenoma: A type of colonic polyp that is a precursor of colorectal cancer.

Correlate: A statistical term meaning that two things being measured follow the same pattern. While correlation does not prove causation (just because two things correlate, that does not necessarily mean that one thing causes the other), it generally implies a link between the two things being measured, even if that link is indirect.

Cortisol: The main stress hormone. Cortisol plays diverse roles in the body, including controlling metabolism and the immune system. It is also an important circadian rhythm hormone.

Cross-reactive antibody: An antibody that binds to an antigen that is not specific to one protein, but instead can be found on two or more proteins.

Cross-reactor: When an antibody binds to more than one protein, any protein that is not the primary protein the antibody formed against is called a cross-reactor. For example, if an antibody formed against gluten can also bind to proteins in milk, milk is a cross-reactor.

Cytokines: Chemical messengers of inflammation. Some act as pro-inflammatory signals to turn on inflammation, and some act as anti-inflammatory signals to turn off inflammation.

Cytotoxic T cells: White blood cells (T lymphocytes) that are members of the adaptive immune system and specialize in attacking cells of the body infected by viruses and some bacteria. They release chemicals called cytotoxins, which cause their target cell to die by a process called apoptosis.

Dendritic cells: Immune cells that reside in barrier tissues of the body (such as the gut and skin) and act as sentinels. They are also phagocytes.

DHA: Docosahexaenoic acid, a very long-chain omega-3 polyunsaturated fatty acid with important functions in the body, especially in regulating inflammation and neural health.

Disaccharide: A simple carbohydrate composed of two sugar molecules; for example, sucrose, which is composed of one glucose and one fructose molecule.

Duodenum: The first segment of the small intestine.

Electron transport chain: The site of oxidative phosphorylation, the last step in ATP production, in the mitochondrion of the cell. See also oxidative phosphorylation.

Endocrine: Pertaining to hormones, especially organs or glands that secrete hormones. The endocrine system encompasses everything in the body related to hormones.

Endocytosis: The process by which a cell transports something from outside the cell to inside the cell by wrapping its surface membrane around the target to form a bubblelike structure (the surface membrane then closes around the bubble and the target is then inside the cell). When this "bubble" is internalized, it may be called an endosome, vesicle, or vacuole (depending on the size of the bubble, the exact makeup of the membrane, and what's inside the bubble).

Endogenous: Produced in or otherwise originating from the body. The opposite of exogenous.

Enterocyte: The main cell type that forms the gut barrier. Also called intestinal absorptive cells, enterocytes are a type of epithelial cell and are responsible for transporting nutrients from inside the gut to the inside of the body.

Enzyme: A protein whose function is to coordinate, stimulate, or otherwise control a specific chemical reaction.

EPA: Eicosapentaenoic acid, a long-chain omega-3 polyunsaturated fatty acid with important functions in the body, especially in regulating inflammation.

Epidemiology: The branch of medicine that deals with the incidence, distribution, and control of diseases, based largely on statistics. Epidemiologists look for correlations between populations and disease.

Epithelial barrier: A barrier composed predominantly of epithelial cells. The gut barrier is a type of epithelial barrier.

Epithelial cell: A special type of cell found in all barrier tissues. Epithelial cells are characterized by having a top (also called the apical side of the cell, where the membrane is organized into fingerlike projections called microvilli), sides, and a bottom (also called the basolateral side of the cell, and the cell differentiates apical from basolateral via the tight junctions).

Epithelium: Tissue composed predominantly of epithelial cells. Gut epithelium is another way to say gut barrier or gut epithelial barrier.

Ethnography: The scientific description of the customs of individual peoples and cultures.

Etiology: The cause(s) of a disease or condition.

Eukaryote (aka eukaryotic cell): An organism whose cells contain complex structures enclosed within membranes. All animals and plants are eukaryotes.

Exocytosis: The opposite of endocytosis. In exocytosis, a bubblelike structure enclosed by a membrane (an endosome, vesicle, or vacuole) merges with the cell's surface membrane, expelling its contents outside of the cell in the process. See also endocytosis.

Exogenous: Originating outside the body. The opposite of endogenous.

Expression: Gene expression means that the gene is used to form a functional product, typically a protein. Protein expression means the protein is made, modified appropriately, and has been transported to the area where it can do its job.

Fatty acid: The basic building block of all fats, composed of a hydrocarbon chain with a carboxyl group at one end of the chain. A fatty acid may be saturated, monounsaturated, or polyunsaturated.

Ferritin: An iron storage protein.

Flare: A sudden appearance or worsening of symptoms of an autoimmune disease.

Food intolerance: A negative reaction to a food that involves production of antibodies other than IgE antibodies.

Food sensitivity: A negative reaction to a food that does not involve the production of antibodies.

Free radical: A highly chemically reactive molecule, typically containing oxygen. (If it contains oxygen, it may also be called an oxidant.)

GALT (gut associated lymphoid tissue): All the immune tissues surrounding the gut.

Genera: The plural of genus.

Genus: The second to lowest level of taxonomy grouping (the science of grouping organisms based on common characteristics). The lowest level is species.

Ghrelin: The main hunger-stimulating hormone. Also an important regulator of the immune system.

Gliadin: A class of proteins found in wheat and several other cereal grains. The protein fraction of gluten.

Gluten: A type of prolamin found in wheat, rye, and barley.

Glycemic Index: A measure of how quickly the carbohydrates from a specific food impact blood sugar levels. The higher the glycemic index, the higher and faster blood sugar will rise after that food is eaten.

Glycemic load: A measure of how quickly the carbohydrates from a specific food impact blood sugar levels, adjusting for how many carbohydrates are likely to be consumed in a serving.

Glycoalkaloid: A type of saponin (a molecule with detergent-like properties) found in nightshade plants that has adjuvant properties.

Glycocalyx layer: A layer formed by sticky molecules (glycoproteins, glycolipids, proteoglycans, and polysaccharides). Glycocalyx layers, which function as semipermeable barriers and structural support, are produced by a variety of cell types, including the gut epithelial cells.

Glycolipid: A molecule composed of a type of fat called a lipid and a carbohydrate.

Glycoprotein: A molecule composed of a protein and a carbohydrate.

Gram-negative bacteria: A type of bacteria that does not retain the color of the crystal violet stain in the Gram staining technique. Gram-negative bacteria have more complex cell membranes than Gram-positive bacteria and tend to be pathogenic. *E. coli* is one example.

Gram-positive bacteria: A type of bacteria that retains the color of the crystal violet stain in the Gram staining technique. Gram-positive bacteria have less complex cell membranes than Gram-negative bacteria and tend to be harmless or probiotic. *Lactobacillus* is one example.

Gut barrier: See intestinal barrier.

Gut dysbiosis: A microbial imbalance in the gastrointestinal tract. This may include microorganisms that are the wrong kinds, wrong diversity, or wrong numbers and/or are in the wrong part of the gastrointestinal tract. An example of gut dysbiosis is small intestinal bacterial overgrowth (SIBO).

Gut microbiota: The microbe population living in the intestine. The gut is inhabited by bacteria, archaea (similar to bacteria), viruses, and single-cell eukaryotes (like yeast), which collectively play an important role in human health.

Gut motility: The movements of the digestive system and the transit of the contents within it.

Gut-brain axis: The biochemical signaling that takes place between the gastrointestinal tract and the central nervous system.

HbA1c: See hemoglobin A1c.

Hedonic hyperphagia: The drive to eat to obtain pleasure in the absence of an energy deficit.

Helper T cells: A group of T cells that are important for directing other components of the innate and adaptive immune system. There are several subtypes of helper T cells, including Th1, Th2, Th3 Th9, Th17, Th22, Tr1, and Tfh.

Hemoglobin A1c (HbA1c): A fraction of the red blood cell protein hemoglobin to which glucose is bound, sometimes called glycated hemoglobin, that acts as an indicator of average blood glucose concentration over the previous 3 months.

High-density lipoprotein (HDL): A blood constituent involved in cholesterol transport. HDL delivers excess cholesterol from cells back to the liver for excretion in bile. This lipoprotein is composed of a high proportion of protein with little triglyceride and cholesterol. It is correlated with a reduced risk of atherosclerosis—called also "good" cholesterol.

Histamine: A chemical released from mast cells and basophils that causes the symptoms normally associated with allergies, including hives, rashes, swelling (lips, eyes, ears, face, tongue, throat), flushing or burning sensation in skin, abdominal pain, bloating, vomiting, diarrhea, ear pain, sneezing, coughing, bronchoconstriction, wheezing, feeling breathless, red or itchy eyes, swelling of nasal tissues, runny nose, and increased heart rate.

HLA gene (human leukocyte antigen gene): The name of the major histocompatibility complex in humans, often used interchangeably with major histocompatibility complex, which is a set of proteins on every cell's surface that displays fragments of proteins from the inside of the cell, including fragments of normal proteins and fragments from invading microorganisms. A way for the cell to raise a red flag if it gets infected. The HLA-DQ2 or the HLA-DQ8 gene variants are associated with celiac disease and increased zonulin secretion in response to gluten consumption.

Hormesis: Any generally favorable biological response to low-level exposures to toxins and other stressors.

Hormetic effect: See hormesis.

Hormone: A fat-based molecule produced by many different organs in the body (endocrine organs, collectively referred to as the endocrine system) that acts as a signal throughout the body, controlling a vast variety of functions. A long-distance communication system in the body.

HPA axis: The hypothalamic-pituitary-adrenal axis, sometimes called the limbic-hypothalamic-pituitary-adrenal axis, which describes the cross-talk between the hypothalamus (a region of the brain), the pituitary gland (in the brain), and the adrenal glands (located on top of the kidneys).

Humoral immune system: The components of the immune system that are not cells, but rather secreted proteins, such as antibodies, cytokines, and complement proteins.

Hyponatremia: A condition of having too little sodium in the blood.

IgA antibody: A type of antibody found in barrier tissues such as the gut, respiratory tract, and genitourinary tract, as well as in saliva, tears, and breast milk. Their main function is to prevent pathogens from entering the circulatory system.

IgD antibody: A type of antibody that functions mainly as antigen receptors on the cell membranes of B cells that have not yet been exposed to antigens. They are also known to activate other immune cells (basophils and mast cells) to produce cytokines.

IgE antibody: A type of antibody that binds to allergens and triggers histamine release from specialized cells (mast cells and basophils), thereby causing the symptoms of allergy. They also have an important role in protection from parasites.

IgG antibody: A type of antibody secreted by B cells and providing the majority of antibody-based immunity from pathogens. Approximately 75 percent of the antibodies circulating in the blood at any given time are IgGs. They are also the only antibodies capable of crossing the placenta to provide passive immunity to the fetus.

IgM antibody: A type of antibody found on the surface of B cells that are secreted in the early stages of humoral immunity before there is sufficient IgG.

Immune system: A complex system that encompasses everything the body does to protect itself from pathogens.

Immune tolerance: The process by which the immune system does not attack an antigen. Immune tolerance is important during pregnancy (so that the immune system doesn't attack the fetus), organ transplantation, and to prevent hypersensitivity to food antigens. Used interchangeably with immunologic tolerance.

Immunity: The ability to resist infection by a specific pathogen. The body acquires immunity when the adaptive immune system "remembers" which pathogens have infected the body before (via memory B and T cells); also called immunological memory. Vaccines confer immunity by stimulating the adaptive immune system to produce antibodies against a specific antigen (the inert or dead virus or bacteria in the vaccine).

Immunogenic: Relating to or denoting substances able to produce an immune response.

Immunological memory: See immunity.

Immunomodulator: A substance that adjusts the immune response to a desired level. An immunomodulator can stimulate or suppress all or a subset of the immune system (it can stimulate one subset while suppressing another), or cause the loss or acquisition of immune tolerance.

Immunoregulator: A substance that adjusts the immune system so that it functions normally.

Immunosuppressant: Something that suppresses the immune system, hindering or lowering its normal activity; typically a drug or treatment, such as radiation.

Immunosuppression: The activity of an immunosuppressant. The suppression of the immune system, typically by a drug or radiation.

Immunotoxic: A substance that is toxic to the immune system, altering (typically suppressing) immune function.

Innate immune system: The part of the immune system that is fastest to respond, but is not specific to the invading pathogen. The part of the immune system responsible for inflammation.

Insoluble fiber: A type of fiber that does not dissolve in water and that tends to speed up the movement of material through the digestive system.

Insulin resistance: A pathological condition in which cells fail to respond normally to insulin; someone who is insulin resistant has low insulin sensitivity and needs more insulin to normalize blood glucose levels than someone who is not insulin resistant. Insulin resistance can lead to type 2 diabetes.

Insulin sensitivity: Refers to how sensitive the body is to the effects of insulin; if you have normal insulin sensitivity, your body needs less insulin to normalize blood glucose levels compared to someone who has impaired insulin sensitivity.

Intestinal barrier: The lining of the intestines, which provides a physical barrier between the inside of the gut and the inside of the body. Used interchangeably with gut barrier, gut epithelial barrier, and mucosal barrier of the gut.

Intestinal permeability: The quantification of how permeable the intestinal barrier is. When intestinal permeability increases, substances that normally can't cross the intestinal barrier do. This is also called leaky gut.

Jejunum: The middle section of the small intestine, between the duodenum and the ileum.

Krebs cycle: The sequence of chemical reactions by which cells generate energy in the form of ATP during the process of cellular respiration. Also called the citric acid cycle.

Leaky gut: See intestinal permeability.

Lectin: A large class of glycoproteins that are also carbohydrate-binding proteins, meaning that they bind to specific carbohydrates (such as membrane carbohydrates).

Leptin: A hunger hormone and adiposity hormone, important for appetite suppression and regulation of the immune system.

Leukocyte: The technical term for a white blood cell.

Leukotriene: A group of hormonelike molecules that act as autocrines and paracrines. Leukotrienes figure prominently in the development of inflammation through their action as pro-inflammatory signaling molecules.

Lipid metabolism: The degradation of lipids to produce energy in the form of ATP or the synthesis of lipids for the storage of energy in the cells.

Low-density lipoprotein (LDL): A blood constituent involved in transporting cholesterol. LDL delivers cholesterol to cells in the body. This lipoprotein is composed of a low proportion of protein with a high amount of triglyceride and cholesterol. Also called "bad" cholesterol, it is correlated with increased risk of atherosclerosis.

Lymph: A fluid that is essentially recycled blood plasma and lymphocytes. When blood circulates in the smallest blood vessels in the body, called capillaries, plasma is filtered out of the blood vessels and bathes all the cells of the body; this is called interstitial fluid. Interstitial fluid is then collected back into the lymphatic system (the fluid component of lymph) to be returned to the blood.

Lymphatic system: A network of organs, lymph nodes, lymph ducts, and lymph vessels that make and move lymph from tissues to the bloodstream. The lymphatic system is also a major part of the immune system and important for the transport of fatty acids and fats from the digestive system.

Lymphocyte: A type of white blood cell found predominantly in the lymphatic system, but also in the blood and infected tissues. Lymphocytes are produced in the bone marrow.

Lysosome: An organelle that contains degradative enzymes. Lysosomes are important for breaking down waste products and digesting substances internalized via phagocytosis or endocytosis. Akin to the stomach of a cell.

Lysozyme: An enzyme that breaks down components of bacterial cell walls (called peptidoglycans).

M cell: A special cell type in the gut barrier responsible for testing the environment inside the gut and reporting any pathogens or other problematic substances to the immune system.

Macronutrients: The chemical constituents of food required in large amounts to sustain life: carbohydrates, fats, and proteins.

Macrophages: Immune cells that reside in connective tissues and organs and act as sentinels. They are also phagocytes.

Markers of inflammation: Inflammation cannot actually be directly measured, so in studies, inflammation is inferred by measuring markers such as C-reactive protein and certain pro-inflammatory cytokines.

Mast cell: A type of immune cell that resides in most tissues surrounding blood vessels and nerves. When activated, mast cells release histamine and the anticoagulant heparin as well as cytokines.

Mediator: A compound that stimulates or activates functions in other cells, acting like a signal or directive.

Melatonin: A hormone that is produced by the pineal gland and that regulates the sleep-wake cycles, among other processes. An important circadian rhythm hormone.

Membrane receptor: A specialized type of protein embedded in the cell membrane that enables communication between the cell and the outside world. Molecules that serve as signals (for example, hormones, neurotransmitters, cytokines, paracrines) attach to the receptor, triggering changes in the function of the cell. The terms *membrane receptor, cell surface receptor,* and *transmembrane receptor* are all used interchangeably.

Memory cell: A subtype of B or T cells produced when the body is defending itself from a pathogen that is responsible for "remembering" that specific pathogen. Memory cells protect against future infections by making an accelerated response to that antigen if they encounter it again.

Metabolic syndrome: A cluster of conditions—hypertension, insulin resistance, being overweight (especially excess weight in the abdominal area), and having abnormal cholesterol or triglyceride levels—that occur together, increasing risk of heart disease, stroke, and diabetes.

Metabolism: The collection of life-sustaining chemical reactions within cells. Metabolism includes the conversion of food to energy and the conversion of food to building blocks for cellular structures

Methyl cycle: A complex system in which methyl groups are transported throughout and recycled by the body. The terms methyl cycle and methylation cycle are used interchangeably.

Methyl group: A molecule, derived from methane, composed of one carbon atom and three hydrogen atoms (CH3), used to methylate proteins.

Methylation: A type of post-translational modification in which a methyl group is added to certain amino acids (lysine or arginine). Adding this methyl group may activate or deactivate a protein (depending on the protein) and affect its ability to bind to a receptor or substrate (like an on-off switch).

Microbiome: The collective genome of our microbiota.

Microbiota: The microbe population living on and in our bodies. Also called microflora.

Micronutrient: A chemical element or substance required in trace amounts but necessary to sustain life. Among micronutrients are minerals, vitamins, and other organic compounds, such as phytochemicals and antioxidants.

Mitochondria: The organelles (typically found in large numbers in most cells) responsible for energy production in the cell. Mitochondria use glucose and oxygen to produce energy (in the form of the molecule adenine triphosphate, ATP) and release carbon dioxide and water in the process.

Monocyte: A type of white blood cell that is part of the innate immune system.

Monosaccharide: A simple carbohydrate composed of a single sugar molecule.

Monounsaturated fatty acid: A fatty acid with only one double bond between carbon atoms.

Mucosa: A membrane that consists of one or more layers of epithelial cells overlying a layer of loose connective tissue that surrounds body organs and body orifices. It protects the body from infection and prevents tissues from becoming dehydrated. Some mucous membranes secrete mucus, a thick protective fluid. The terms mucous membrane and mucosa are used interchangeably.

Mucosal barrier: See intestinal barrier.

Natural killer cell: A type of white blood cell—part of the innate immune system—recruited to the site of infection specifically to destroy virally infected cells of the body. Similar to cytotoxic T cells, but natural killer cells respond quicker.

Neurotransmitter: A chemical released by nerve cells to send signals to other nerve cells.

Neutrophil: A type of white blood cell that is a phagocyte. Neutrophils are rapidly recruited to a site of infection, where they engulf cells coated with antibodies and secrete cytokines that can kill pathogens and stimulate more macrophages and dendritic cells.

Nutrient density: The concentration of micronutrients (mainly vitamins and minerals, but also phytochemicals, essential fatty acids, and essential amino acids) per calorie of food.

Omega-3 fatty acid: A type of polyunsaturated fatty acid in which the first double bond occurs between the third and fourth carbons in the hydrocarbon chain. DHA and EPA are omega-3 fatty acids.

Omega-6 fatty acid: A type of polyunsaturated fatty acid in which the first double bond occurs between the sixth and seventh carbons in the hydrocarbon chain.

Organelle: A membrane-bound, specialized structure within a cell. There are many different types of organelles, each with a specific function within the cell, akin to little organs.

Oxidant: A highly chemically reactive molecule that contains oxygen. The terms oxidant, oxygen radicals, and reactive oxygen species are used interchangeably. Oxidants are a type of free radical but not all free radicals are oxidants.

Oxidative phosphorylation: The last step of cellular respiration. A series of redox chemical reactions, in which electrons are transferred from one molecule to another, releasing energy that is used to produce ATP.

Oxidative stress: Stress on cells and tissues caused by an imbalance between the damage caused by oxidants and the body's ability to readily detoxify the chemicals produced by reactions with oxidants and to repair the resulting damage.

Oxygen radicals: See oxidant.

Paracrine: A fat-based molecule that acts as a signal for communication between adjacent cells (from cell to neighboring cell).

Pathogen: A foreign organism that can make you sick; for example, a virus, bacterium, or parasite.

Pathogenesis: The genesis or origin of a disease; that is, how the disease starts and develops.

Pathology: Something abnormal or affected by disease. Also refers to the study of the causes and effects of disease and the branch of medicine responsible for analyzing samples to evaluate the presence of disease.

Peptide: A short sequence of amino acids, like a mini protein. Some proteins are composed of several peptides, or polypeptides, bound together. A peptide typically has 30 or fewer amino acids, but there is no firm cutoff point to differentiate between a peptide and a polypeptide or a small protein (peptide and polypeptide are often used interchangeably). Some chains of 500 amino acids are considered peptides, based on the fact that they combine with other peptides to create a protein (such as an antibody).

Peristalsis: The wavelike contraction and relaxation of the muscles of the intestine that push food through the digestive tract. Also refers to this motion in connection with any other muscular tube in the body.

Permeability: The quantification of how permeable a substance is; that is, how easily it lets liquids or gases pass through it.

Permeable: A material that allows liquids or gases to pass through it.

Peyer's patches: Areas of the small intestine that are designed to allow more direct interaction between the immune system and the environment inside the gut. The reason for Peyer's patches is one of vigilance: the immune cells within the patch are able to evaluate whether there are pathogens inside the gut that the body should prepare to defend itself from.

Phagocytes: Cells that engulf and destroy pathogens, akin to eating pathogens.

Phagocytose: See phagocytosis.

Phagocytosis: The ingestion of a pathogen (like a bacterium) by phagocytes (amoebas do this, too). When a phagocyte phagocytoses a pathogen, the process is called phagocytosis.

Phytochemicals: An umbrella term for a huge array of helpful plant-derived compounds that support health in a number of ways. Many phytochemicals possess antioxidant, anti-inflammatory, and anticancer properties.

Plasma: The fluid portion of blood in which red and white blood cells are suspended.

Polypeptide: A longer sequence of amino acids than a peptide (typically 30 to 50 amino acids long). Sometimes used interchangeably with peptide, since there is no firm cutoff point to differentiate between a peptide, a polypeptide, and a short protein. For example, heavy chain, a polypeptide component of antibodies, is between 450 and 550 amino acids long.

Polysaccharide: A carbohydrate chain made of many sugar molecules; for example, starch or fiber.

Polyunsaturated fatty acid: A fatty acid with two or more double bonds between carbon atoms. Omega-3 and omega-6 fats are polyunsaturated fatty acids.

Postprandial: Occurring after a meal.

Post-translational modifications: A variety of modifications that can be made to proteins after they are synthesized (that is, built by the protein factories in your cells), which affect the protein's function.

Prebiotic: A nondigestible food ingredient (such as fiber) that promotes the growth of beneficial microorganisms in the intestines.

Probiotics: Beneficial microorganisms that live in the body (primarily within the gastrointestinal tract).

Pro-inflammatory: Refers to something that promotes or stimulates inflammation.

Prolamin: A type of lectin. Prolamins are plant storage proteins found in the seeds of cereal grains that are high in the amino acid proline.

Proliferation: The reproduction or multiplication of cells via cell division.

Prostaglandin: A group of hormonelike molecules that act as autocrines and paracrines. Prostaglandins figure prominently in blood clotting, pain signaling, cell growth, kidney function, stomach acid secretion, and inflammation through their actions as signaling molecules.

Proteases: Enzymes that break apart, or lyse, proteins. The terms protease and proteolytic enzyme are used interchangeably.

Proteoglycan: Glycoproteins that have a negative electric charge. An important component of the gut glycocalyx layer.

Proteolysis: The process of breaking apart, or lysing, a protein.

Proteolytic enzymes: See proteases.

Pseudograins: The starchy seeds or fruits of broadleaf plants—the most common of which are amaranth, buckwheat, chia, and quinoa.

Pyruvate oxidation: The step in cellular respiration that follows glycolysis in which pyruvate molecules are converted to carbon dioxide, acetyl coenzyme A, and NADH.

Reactive oxygen species: See oxidant.

Receptor: A specialized type of protein that takes part in communication between the cell and the outside world or within the cell. Molecules that serve as signals (such as hormones, neurotransmitters, cytokines, autocrines, and paracrines) attach to the receptor, triggering changes in the function of the cell. Membrane receptors are a type of receptor.

Recruitment: The process by which white blood cells leave blood vessels and enter the tissue. This is a complex, multistep process that involves the interactions of many proteins, including proteins on the surface of the white blood cells and the cells that line the blood vessels, as well as cytokines.

Regulatory T cell: A type of T cell that suppresses the activity of immune and inflammatory cells to shut down immune response toward the end of an immune reaction (once the pathogen has been eradicated). Regulatory T cells also suppress activation of dendritic cells and suppress the activity of any T cells that recognize self and therefore have the ability to attack healthy cells within the body. Some helper T cells, including Th3 cells, perform a similar function.

Renal: Pertaining to the kidneys.

Retrotranscytosis: A type of transcytosis, or transport of small molecules from one side of a cell to the other. In the case of retrotranscytosis, the transport is in the opposite direction of normal transport for that specific molecule. For example, IgA antibodies are normally transcytosed from inside the body across the gut epithelial cells into the gut as part of normal immune defenses. When antibodies are recycled back into the body, this is transport across the cell in the opposite direction, or retrotranscytosis. See also transcytosis.

Saponin: A substance found in many plants that has detergent-like properties.

Saturated fatty acid: A fatty acid with all single bonds between all carbon atoms, therefore containing the most hydrogen atoms possible; that is, it is saturated with hydrogen.

Semipermeable: Refers to any material that allows some liquids or gases to pass through it but not others.

Serum: Similar to blood plasma, but with all the substances involved in blood clotting removed.

Small intestinal bacterial overgrowth (SIBO): A pathological condition characterized by higher-than-normal levels of bacteria and other microorganisms growing in the small intestine.

Soluble fiber: A type of fiber that dissolves in water to form a gel-like material in the gut that tends to slow the movement of material through the digestive system.

Stem cell: An important type of cell that has the ability to differentiate (mature) into many different cell types. Stem cells are necessary for normal cell turnover (where cells die and are replaced with new cells), growth, and repair. A progenitor cell is a type of stem cell that can differentiate into fewer different types of cells.

Steroid hormone: A class of hormones with a specific molecular structure (called a steroid structure) that includes cortisol, estrogen, and testosterone.

Substrate: A molecule that is acted upon by an enzyme.

Systemic: Relating to or affecting the entire body. For example, systemic inflammation is bodywide inflammation.

T cells: Lymphocytes produced in the bone marrow and matured in the thymus gland that circulate through the blood and lymphatic vessels, patrolling the body for antigens. Their functions include activating B cells, activating inflammatory cells, killing infected cells, and directly killing pathogens. T cells are one of two main cell types involved in the cellular adaptive immune system.

T lymphocyte: See T cell.

Thermogenesis: The production of heat, which burns calories.

Thromboxanes: A group of hormonelike molecules that act as autocrines and paracrines; important regulators of blood clotting.

Thymocyte: A type of progenitor cell that lives in the thymus gland. Thymocytes can differentiate into the many types of T cells.

Thymus gland: A specialized organ of the immune system responsible for controlling the differentiation and survival of T cells and B cells.

Tight junction: A specialized connection between two cells formed by the knitting together of special proteins. The tight junction holds cells tightly together but also helps cells divide their cell membranes into regions, which is important for the function of barrier cells such as enterocytes.

Toll-like receptor: A special type of membrane receptor in cells of the innate immune system (especially macrophages and dendritic cells) that binds to proteins unique to microbes. Important for initial recognition of a pathogen.

Transcytosis: A type of transport of small molecules across a cell, required for innumerable and diverse functions of the cell, including absorption of nutrients across the intestinal barrier. Molecules (such as proteins) are captured by the cell via endocytosis and expelled on the other side of the cell via exocytosis.

Triglyceride: A molecule made up of three fatty acids combined with a molecule of the alcohol glycerol. Triglycerides are the main fat constituent of animals and vegetables. Having high serum triglycerides increases the risk for cardiovascular disease.

Trypsin: A specific protease.

Villi: An important aspect of the structure of the small intestine. Intestinal villus refers to any of the small, finger-shaped outgrowths of the epithelial lining of the wall of the intestine, formed by columns of cells, collectively called the intestinal villi.

Zonulin: A protein that modulates the permeability of tight junctions between cells of the wall of the digestive tract.

ACKNOWLEDGMENTS

Denise Minger, your contribution to this book cannot be overstated. I love having a research assistant who values science the same way that I do, caring about the big picture, digging deep into mechanisms, and never dismissing any evidence, even when it doesn't conform to our understanding. *Paleo Principles* quite literally would not exist without all your help, support, and dedication to this project. Thank you.

Kiersten Peterson, your photographs are just so, so beautiful. Thank you for making this project manageable for me by taking on so much of the food photography and recipe testing, as well as helping with the editing and formatting. This book is so much prettier thanks to you!

Charissa Talbot, not only are you the person who holds the entire Paleo Mom team together, but you are a dear friend. Thank you for running such a tight ship, keeping me on task, listening to my gripes, sharing my excitement, protecting my time and health, and generally just being awesome.

Katie Pickworth, much of your detailed research into topics for my website ended up supporting chapters in this book! Your perspective and scientific thoroughness are invaluable to my writing and my mission to improve public health by increasing scientific literacy.

Nicole Pittman, your graphic design genius shines through on my website and is even reflected in much of this book! Thank you for your amazing ability to translate the essence of me and my message to a cohesive visual palette and style.

Claire Wiseman, thank you for filling in the gaps and taking on such a diversity of roles within the Paleo Mom team that it's impossible to figure out a job title that appropriately reflects how vital you are to everything I do.

David Schmeltzle and the BizBudding Inc. team, thank you not just for your technical expertise in all things website, but also for being a true partner in this amazing adventure of affecting positive change in the world.

My husband, David, your support, love, and dedication are the reason I am able to do everything that I do. Thank you for supporting me through the creation of yet another beast of a book, for being a wonderful father and husband, and for sharing this adventurous and wonderful life with me. I love you.

My daughters, Adele and Mira, you two are my true motivation for wanting to make the world a better place. You fill my life with meaning, love, laughter, pride, joy, music, curiosity, and *raison d'etre*.

My mom, Patsy, I am who I am because of you. Without the passion, strength, work ethic, and dedication that I learned from you, I would be unable to complete a project of this magnitude! Thank you for being my greatest cheerleader, shoulder to cry on, sounding board for new ideas, and rock to lean on.

The Awkward Selfies, every girl needs a safe place to be a dork. Thank you for making me laugh, challenging my creativity, and always having my back.

CrossFit Dwala and Anne Marie, there's something tremendously therapeutic about a hard workout, and many days I owe my sanity in addition to my physical strength, agility, and endurance to you.

Heritage Sandy Springs Farmers Market, my passion for supporting the local food movement came from connecting with the wonderful farmers and vendors at your market. Thank you for your continued commitment to this community!

Flowers Medical Group, your care and support, both emotional and medical, are the reason why I was able to stay healthy through such a demanding and ambitious project.

The Paleo community, your enduring support, enthusiasm, and connection are the best encouragement! Thank you for all your likes, shares, comments, personal stories, and hugs at events. And thank you for helping prove that people do care about science through your continued patronage and engagement.

Victory Belt Publishing Inc., it never ceases to amaze me how awesome the entire team at VB is to work with. Thank you for supporting me in yet another ridiculously huge project, for your flexibility in letting me work at the pace I needed to in order to protect my health, and for contributing all your amazing talents to this project. Thank you, Erich, Pam, Holly, Donna, Lance, Susan, Matt, the design team, the sales team, and everyone who had a hand, big or small, in making this book a reality.

DR. SARAH'S STORY

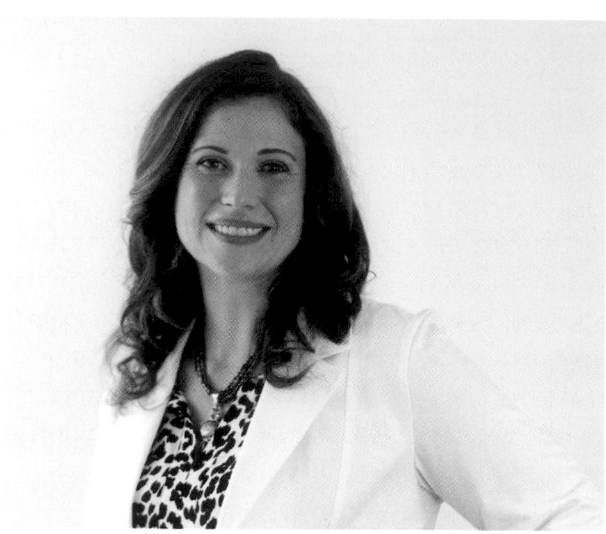

Passionate is a word that most people would use to describe me (along with some other choice words, like *geek*, *nerd*, and *nerdy geek*). Two of my biggest passions are improving scientific literacy and improving public health, which I believe go hand in hand. I see the biggest barrier to changing the epidemic of chronic illness in our society as the fact that most of us don't have the foundation of scientific knowledge needed to truly understand what the best choices are and to be motivated to implement them. And it's become my *raison d'être* to help people regain their health by providing health education rooted in science.

This passion originates from my personal history of health struggles and my own scientific education—which I didn't even think to apply to my health until it got bad enough to compel me to give up my career in science.

I was the kid who fell asleep in the car every time we drove more than a few miles. I always liked waking up to discover that we were already at our destination, and both my family and I didn't think it was anything more than my "just being a sleeper." But sleeping a lot wasn't my only symptom. I started getting teased for being the "fat kid" at 7 years old; I hit puberty extremely early, just after my tenth birthday, when I also stopped growing; I battled constipation for most of my life and dealt with mild depression and anxiety throughout my teens and twenties; and I was morbidly obese by my twentieth birthday, my heaviest weight being close to 300 pounds in my late twenties. And from age 7 on, I was always getting sick with whatever was going around, or strep throat if nothing was going around. From puberty on, I always had dry skin, acne, crazy dandruff, thin hair, eyebrows that would cyclically thin out and then grow back in, and random rashes and allergic reactions to things I touched. I don't remember when my joints and muscles started aching and feeling stiff, but by my late twenties, I had repetitive strain injuries, carpal tunnel syndrome, and early arthritis. I developed infrequent but debilitating migraines at the age of 18 and severe adult-onset asthma at the age of 25. I had diagnoses of irritable bowel syndrome, gastroesophageal reflux disease, eczema, psoriasis, and an additional skin condition called lichen planus. Yet none of these symptoms or conditions was severe. It was a collection of annoyances, some things my doctors would dismiss (or just treat with painkillers, steroids, bronchodilators, or laxatives) and many things I didn't even think to mention to my doctors. My blood pressure was borderline high, my blood sugar levels were borderline diabetic, and my LDL cholesterol was just above the normal range. Nothing was off the charts, but I wasn't healthy by any metric.

Being tired and prone to illness throughout my formative years kept me out of trouble like no threat of grounding could. I willingly went to bed at 8 p.m. on school nights and slept on the bus on the way to school instead of playing poker with the other kids my age. Instead of running around or hanging out with the smokers at recess, I preferred to find a quiet place to do my homework. Being too tired for mischief combined with some innate geekiness and ambition meant that my energy was focused on schoolwork and on playing the violin. Because I didn't know any different, I worked hard despite not feeling energetic or physically comfortable most of the time. In fact, not feeling great somehow translated to a stubborn drive to work harder, a determination to do whatever I needed to do to succeed at everything I set my mind to, and a habit of breaking molds along the way.

I started my academic career in physics, earning an honors bachelor of science degree with distinction from the University of Victoria, Canada, in 1999. I went on to earn a doctorate degree in medical biophysics at Western University, Canada, in 2003, at the age of 26, and spent the next 4 years doing medical research as a postdoctoral fellow, first in the cardiology department at St. Michael's Hospital in Toronto and then in the Department of Cell Biology at the University of Arizona.

During my training and research career, I switched fields repeatedly, moving from physics to medical biophysics to physiology to cell biology, with focuses ranging from immunology to vascular health to gene therapy to cancer biology. The specific goals of my research also ran the gamut from simply increasing basic scientific understanding of a particular system to more medically based research that included preclinical and clinical trial work. Yes, I like to make unconventional and fairly dramatic career shifts. Normally, each step in an academic career builds on the knowledge and experience learned in the previous steps. The way I did it, each time I moved on to a new degree or position, I had experience to draw on but had to teach myself an entire bachelor's degree worth of knowledge, plus learn new lab and experimental techniques in order to continue to do high-quality research at the level I expected of myself.

Despite that added hurdle, I earned a variety of awards throughout my academic career, including awards for research excellence, many scholarships and fellowships, and even my own research grant. I was prolific during these years, too, publishing fourteen papers in peer-reviewed scientific journals (including seven first-author papers, several of which continue to be widely cited today) and presenting twenty-five abstracts at international conferences.

But my academic career was cut short. Although I didn't know it yet, I suffered from Hashimoto's thyroiditis and fibromyalgia in addition to the two secondary autoimmune diseases that affect my skin (psoriasis and lichen planus). By the time my first daughter was born when I was 30 years old, at the end of my second postdoctoral research fellowship, my body couldn't keep up with the demands of my burgeoning academic career. I was sick and incapable of finding balance between my ambitions as a scientist and my goals as a mother. I made the decision to stay home with my baby and put my academic career on hold. Yes, another unconventional choice.

Staying home with my daughters (I had a second one 3 years later) gave me the space I needed to focus on my health. I lost 100 pounds, got fit, and lived happily ever after—er, or not. I did lose 100 pounds and became physically active, but while my blood sugar levels and blood pressure improved, nothing else did. In fact, my energy levels tanked, my headaches grew more frequent, my joints felt stiff and sore every morning, and the condition of my skin continued to deteriorate. The frustration of getting thinner and thinner while feeling worse and worse motivated me to start digging deeper. I finally began to apply my scientific background and broad knowledge base to the problem of my health—and that brought me to the Paleo diet and the Autoimmune Protocol.

Within 2 weeks of adopting a Paleo diet, I was able to discontinue 6 prescription medications, one of which I had been taking for 12 years. Further refining my diet by adopting the Autoimmune Protocol allowed me to put my autoimmune diseases into remission. My weight stabilized, my skin improved, my energy levels soared, my body stopped hurting all the time, and symptoms that I had endured for nearly 3 decades melted away. Needless to say, my rapid health turnaround convinced me of the healing power of the right foods.

Finding a solution to my health problems—a solution as simple as changing the foods I was eating—lit a fire under me. I couldn't sit back and simply enjoy better health myself; I had to tell the world and help others who were going through the same thing I had. I found my voice through my blog, *The Paleo Mom*, where I could combine all my interests: science, health, cooking, and art. It became my mission to effectively communicate that some foods can support health by providing a wealth and diversity of essential and nonessential nutrients while others undermine health by disrupting the gut, dysregulating hormones, or instigating inflammation. I needed to help people understand how sleep, stress, and activity affect the health equation. And perhaps more important, I needed to create resources so that people could actually implement the choices they made to improve their health.

And so enters *Paleo Principles*, my fourth book. The goal of this book is to provide readers with a scientific foundation from which to draw on when making day-to-day choices that affect health. I want to educate the public about what truly are the best foods and lifestyle practices, admitting the limits of current scientific knowledge and where individual variability comes into play. I want to establish the scientific validity of the Paleo diet while positioning this framework to transcend labels and enter the mainstream simply as the definition of making healthy choices. I guess that's a pretty ambitious set of goals, but that's what the Western world needs.

INDEX

A

D

Q

R

T

U

V

W

X

Y

Z

MORE PRAISE FOR *PALEO PRINCIPLES*

"*There is no one diet that is right for everyone. How do you know if one is better than the other for you? Dr. Ballantyne has outdone herself once again. Like a fine wine that just gets better over time, Sarah Ballantyne continues to lead the field on showing us why the Paleo diet is valid and how to implement it successfully for you and your family.* Paleo Principles *is the cutting-edge encyclopedia of the why's and the most user-friendly guide I've ever seen of the 'how-to's'. This book is the complete one-stop-shop resource. This is the type of book that will be dog-eared again and again. You'll be grateful it's on your shelf.*"

Tom O'Bryan, DC, CCN, DACBN, adjunct faculty, Institute for Functional Medicine, and author of *The Autoimmune Fix*

"*For many years, Sarah Ballantyne, PhD, has been one of the leading lights of the ancestral health movement, synthesizing her scientific expertise with personal experiences—her own and those of her many fans—to become one of our most reliable guides to natural healing. In* Paleo Principles, *Sarah presents her magnum opus. Years in the making,* Paleo Principles *is not to be missed!*"

Paul Jaminet, PhD, author of *Perfect Health Diet*

"*If you want to restore your digestive health, balance hormones, and support your immune system, then* Paleo Principles *is the book for you. Dr. Ballantyne offers the latest medical research, nutrition advice, and Paleo recipes to transform your health. She has created a comprehensive and well-researched guide to better health through nutrition and lifestyle. Not only will* Paleo Principles *help you reach your health goals, but it will most likely have you feeling better than ever before.*"

Josh Axe, DNM, CNS, DC, founder of DrAxe.com, bestselling author of *Eat Dirt* and co-founder of Ancient Nutrition

"*Sarah's latest heartfelt offering is a superbly guided journey into vibrant health and an easy-to-follow and truly inspirational source of pure goodness, or, shall we just say, THE TRUTH!*"

Chef Pete Evans

"*Reading* Paleo Principles *is like chatting with a dear friend who happens to have deep knowledge and the compassion to help you fine-tune your individual nutrition and lifestyle.*"

Amy Myers, MD, *New York Times* bestselling author of *The Autoimmune Solution* and *The Thyroid Connection*

"*Twenty years ago the Paleo diet had a few review papers or references in anthropology books and papers. Many detractors cited a "lack of research" to support the Paleo diet/Ancestral health template. That story has changed. We now have well-conducted human trails on a host of different topics, with a consistent theme which paints the Paleo diet as safe, effective, and beneficial over the long haul. There are still detractors who cite a paucity of research, but we now have Dr. Sarah Ballantyne's Magnum Opus,* Paleo Principles, *which compiles and puts into context the vast body of research which now encompasses the Paleo diet.*"

Robb Wolf, *New York Times* bestselling author of *The Paleo Solution* and *Wired to Eat*

"Paleo Principles *is the book we've all been waiting for. Being sick, tired, and unhealthy may be common, but it's NOT normal. I love that it focuses beyond just Paleo foods; finally, an in-depth resource on the overall lifestyle to nourish and heal you to live your best life. It will be your end-all-be-all resource for everything healthy, an in-depth science textbook and cookbook in one, presented like never before!*"

Stacy Toth, author of *Real Life Paleo* and *Beyond Bacon*

"*Reading* Paleo Principles *is like having a heart-to-heart with one of the world's foremost experts on health in your kitchen—not only does Dr. Ballantyne take the time to thoroughly explain the science behind the Paleo template, but her understanding and compassion shine through in her writing. With this book, not only will you find answers to your health challenges, but an ally for your health journey.*"

Izabella Wentz, PharmD, FASCP, pharmacist and *New York Times* bestselling author of *Hashimoto's Protocol*

"*In* Paleo Principles, *Dr. Ballantyne lays the complete scientific foundation for the Paleo lifestyle while providing a huge collection of practical tips, visual guides, delicious recipes, and meal plans. Her book is a complete guide to achieving your best health.*"

Chris Kresser MS, LAc, *New York Times* bestselling author of *The Paleo Cure*

"Paleo Principles *methodically reviews the rich scientific foundation for the Paleo diet and lifestyle while providing the tips, tools, and recipes you need to achieve your best health. This is a must-have book for every home!*"

Dr. Terry Wahls, MD, author of *The Wahls Protocol*